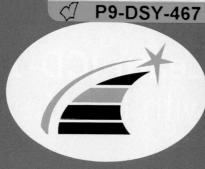
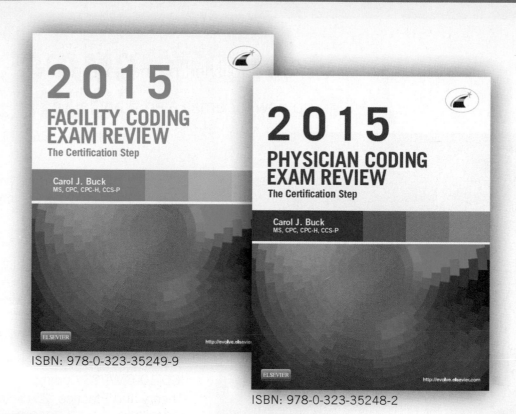

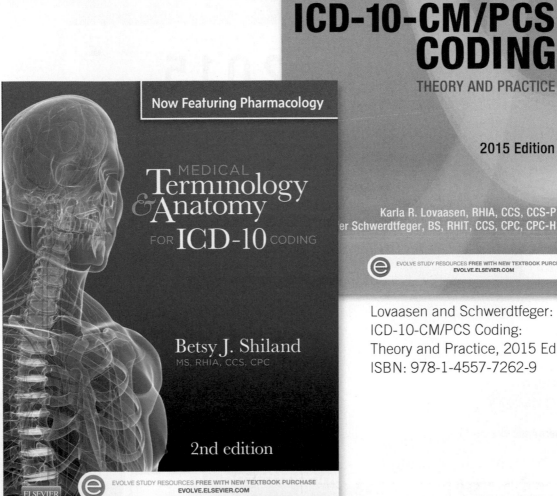
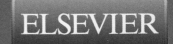

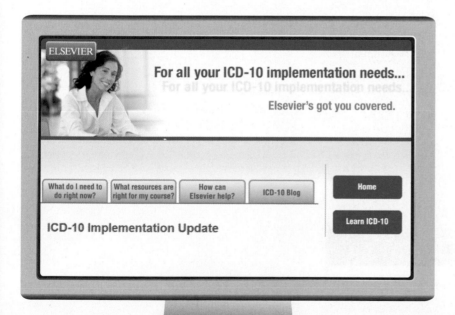

2015

ICD-10-PCS

DRAFT

INCLUDES NETTER'S ANATOMY ART

Carol J. Buck
MS, CPC, CPC-H, CCS-P

Former Program Director
Medical Secretary Programs
Northwest Technical College
East Grand Forks, Minnesota

ELSEVIER

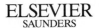

3251 Riverport Lane
St. Louis, Missouri 63043

2015 ICD-10-PCS DRAFT

ISBN: 978-0-323-35255-0

Notice

Knowledge and best practice in this field are constantly changing. As new research and experience broaden our understanding, changes in research methods, professional practices, or medical treatment may become necessary.

Practitioners and researchers must always rely on their own experience and knowledge in evaluating and using any information, methods, compounds, or experiments described herein. In using such information or methods they should be mindful of their own safety and the safety of others, including parties for whom they have a professional responsibility.

With respect to any drug or pharmaceutical products identified, readers are advised to check the most current information provided (i) on procedures featured or (ii) by the manufacturer of each product to be administered, to verify the recommended dose or formula, the method and duration of administration, and contraindications. It is the responsibility of practitioners, relying on their own experience and knowledge of their patients, to make diagnoses, to determine dosages and the best treatment for each individual patient, and to take all appropriate safety precautions.

To the fullest extent of the law, neither the Publisher nor the authors, contributors, or editors, assume any liability for any injury and/or damage to persons or property as a matter of products liability, negligence or otherwise, or from any use or operation of any methods, products, instructions, or ideas contained in the material herein.

Library of Congress Cataloging-in-Publication Data

Buck, Carol J., author.
[ICD-10-PCS draft]
2015 ICD-10-PCS draft / Carol J. Buck.
    p. ; cm.
ICD-10-PCS draft
Preceded by: 2014 ICD-10-PCS draft / Carol J. Buck. 2013.
ISBN 978-0-323-35255-0 (pbk. : alk. paper)
I. Title. II. Title: ICD-10-PCS draft.
    [DNLM: 1. International statistical classification of diseases and related health problems. 10th revision.
Procedure coding system. 2. Disease--classification. 3. Forms and Records Control--methods.
4. International Classification of Diseases. 5. Medical Records. WB 15]
    R728.8
    616.001'2--dc23

2014023369

Director, Private Sector Education & Professional/References: Jeanne R. Olson
Senior Content Development Specialist: Jenna Price
Publishing Services Manager: Pat Joiner
Project Manager: Lisa A. P. Bushey
Senior Designer: Amy Buxton

Printed in Canada

Last digit is the print number: 9 8 7 6 5 4 3 2 1

CONTENTS

SYMBOLS AND CONVENTIONS

Annotated

Throughout the manual, revisions, additions, and deleted codes or words are indicated by the following symbols:

- ⬅ **Revised:** Revisions within the line or code from the previous edition are indicated by the arrow.
- ◄ **New:** Additions to the previous edition are indicated by the triangle.
- ~~deleted~~ **Deleted:** Deletions from the previous edition are struck through.

ICD-10-PCS Table Symbols

Throughout the manual information is indicated by the following symbols:

♀♂ **Sex conflict:** *Definitions of Medicare Code Edits*, Version 31 (MCE) detects inconsistencies between a patient's sex and any diagnosis or procedure on the patient's record. For example, a male patient with cervical cancer (diagnosis) or a female patient with a prostatectomy (procedure). In both instances, the indicated diagnosis or the procedure conflicts with the stated sex of the patient. Therefore, either the patient's diagnosis, procedure, or sex is presumed to be incorrect.

🚫 **Noncovered:** There are some procedures for which Medicare does not provide reimbursement. There are also procedures that would normally not be reimbursed by Medicare but due to the presence of certain diagnoses are reimbursed.

🚫 **Limited Coverage:** For certain procedures whose medical complexity and serious nature incur extraordinary associated costs, Medicare limits coverage to a portion of the cost.

🚫 **Hospital-Acquired Condition:** Some procedures are always associated with Hospital Acquired Conditions (HAC) according to the MS-DRG.

Coding Clinic: American Hospital Association's *Coding Clinic®* citations provide reference information to official ICD-10-PCS coding advice.

If a symbol does not apply to all possible code combinations within the table, a list of the applicable codes will appear below the table. For example, on table 00F, applicable Noncovered codes are listed after the Noncovered symbol.

SECTION: 0 MEDICAL AND SURGICAL
BODY SYSTEM: 0 CENTRAL NERVOUS SYSTEM
OPERATION: F FRAGMENTATION: Breaking solid matter in a body part into pieces

Body Part	Approach	Device	Qualifier
3 Epidural Space 🚫 4 Subdural Space 🚫 5 Subarachnoid Space 🚫 6 Cerebral Ventricle U Spinal Canal	0 Open 3 Percutaneous 4 Percutaneous Endoscopic X External	Z No Device	Z No Qualifier

🚫 00F3XZZ, 00F4XZZ, 00F5XZZ, 00F6XZZ

Introduction

ICD-10-PCS Official Guidelines for Coding and Reporting

2015

The Centers for Medicare and Medicaid Services (CMS) and the National Center for Health Statistics (NCHS), two departments within the U.S. Federal Government's Department of Health and Human Services (DHHS) provide the following guidelines for coding and reporting using the International Classification of Diseases, 10th Revision, Procedure Coding System (ICD-10-PCS). These guidelines should be used as a companion document to the official version of the ICD-10-PCS as published on the CMS website. The ICD-10-PCS is a procedure classification published by the United States for classifying procedures performed in hospital inpatient health care settings.

These guidelines have been approved by the four organizations that make up the Cooperating Parties for the ICD-10-PCS: the American Hospital Association (AHA), the American Health Information Management Association (AHIMA), CMS, and NCHS.

These guidelines are a set of rules that have been developed to accompany and complement the official conventions and instructions provided within the ICD-10-PCS itself. The instructions and conventions of the classification take precedence over guidelines. These guidelines are based on the coding and sequencing instructions in the Tables, Index and Definitions of ICD-10-PCS, but provide additional instruction. Adherence to these guidelines when assigning ICD-10-PCS procedure codes is required under the Health Insurance Portability and Accountability Act (HIPAA). The procedure codes have been adopted under HIPAA for hospital inpatient healthcare settings. A joint effort between the healthcare provider and the coder is essential to achieve complete and accurate documentation, code assignment, and reporting of diagnoses and procedures. These guidelines have been developed to assist both the healthcare provider and the coder in identifying those procedures that are to be reported. The importance of consistent, complete documentation in the medical record cannot be overemphasized. Without such documentation accurate coding cannot be achieved.

Table of Contents

Conventions

A1
ICD-10-PCS codes are composed of seven characters. Each character is an axis of classification that specifies information about the procedure performed. Within a defined code range, a character specifies the same type of information in that axis of classification.
Example: The fifth axis of classification specifies the approach in sections 0 through 4 and 7 through 9 of the system.

A2
One of 34 possible values can be assigned to each axis of classification in the seven-character code: they are the numbers 0 through 9 and the alphabet (except I and O because they are easily confused with the numbers 1 and 0). The number of unique values used in an axis of classification differs as needed.
Example: Where the fifth axis of classification specifies the approach, seven different approach values are currently used to specify the approach.

A3
The valid values for an axis of classification can be added to as needed.
Example: If a significantly distinct type of device is used in a new procedure, a new device value can be added to the system.

A4

As with words in their context, the meaning of any single value is a combination of its axis of classification and any preceding values on which it may be dependent.

Example: The meaning of a body part value in the Medical and Surgical section is always dependent on the body system value. The body part value 0 in the Central Nervous body system specifies Brain and the body part value 0 in the Peripheral Nervous body system specifies Cervical Plexus.

A5

As the system is expanded to become increasingly detailed, over time more values will depend on preceding values for their meaning.

Example: In the Lower Joints body system, the device value 3 in the root operation Insertion specifies Infusion Device and the device value 3 in the root operation Replacement specifies Ceramic Synthetic Substitute.

A6

The purpose of the alphabetic index is to locate the appropriate table that contains all information necessary to construct a procedure code. The PCS Tables should always be consulted to find the most appropriate valid code.

A7

It is not required to consult the index first before proceeding to the tables to complete the code. A valid code may be chosen directly from the tables.

A8

All seven characters must be specified to be a valid code. If the documentation is incomplete for coding purposes, the physician should be queried for the necessary information.

A9

Within a PCS table, valid codes include all combinations of choices in characters 4 through 7 contained in the same row of the table. In the example below, 0JHT3VZ is a valid code, and 0JHW3VZ is *not* a valid code.

A10

"And," when used in a code description, means "and/or."

Example: Lower Arm and Wrist Muscle means lower arm and/or wrist muscle.

A11

Many of the terms used to construct PCS codes are defined within the system. It is the coder's responsibility to determine what the documentation in the medical record equates to in the PCS definitions. The physician is not expected to use the terms used in PCS code descriptions, nor is the coder required to query the physician when the correlation between the documentation and the defined PCS terms is clear.

Example: When the physician documents "partial resection" the coder can independently correlate "partial resection" to the root operation Excision without querying the physician for clarification.

Medical and Surgical Section Guidelines (section 0)

B2. Body System

General guidelines

B2.1a

The procedure codes in the general anatomical regions body systems should only be used when the procedure is performed on an anatomical region rather than a specific body part (e.g., root operations Control and Detachment, Drainage of a body cavity) or on the rare occasion when no information is available to support assignment of a code to a specific body part.

Example: Control of postoperative hemorrhage is coded to the root operation Control found in the general anatomical regions body systems.

B2.1b

Where the general body part values "upper" and "lower" are provided as an option in the Upper Arteries, Lower Arteries, Upper Veins, Lower Veins, Muscles and Tendons body systems, "upper" or "lower" specifies body parts located above or below the diaphragm respectively.

Example: Vein body parts above the diaphragm are found in the Upper Veins body system; vein body parts below the diaphragm are found in the Lower Veins body system.

B3. Root Operation

General guidelines

B3.1a

In order to determine the appropriate root operation, the full definition of the root operation as contained in the PCS Tables must be applied.

B3.1b

Components of a procedure specified in the root operation definition and explanation are not coded separately. Procedural steps necessary to reach the operative site and close the operative site, including anastomosis of a tubular body part, are also not coded separately.

Example: Resection of a joint as part of a joint replacement procedure is included in the root operation definition of Replacement and is not coded separately. Laparotomy performed to reach the site of an open liver biopsy is not coded separately. In a resection of sigmoid colon with anastomosis of descending colon to rectum, the anastomosis is not coded separately.

SECTION: 0 MEDICAL AND SURGICAL

BODY SYSTEM: J SUBCUTANEOUS TISSUE AND FASCIA

OPERATION: H INSERTION: Putting in a nonbiological appliance that monitors, assists, performs, or prevents a physiological function but does not physically take the place of a body part

Body Part	Approach	Device	Qualifier
S Subcutaneous Tissue and Fascia, Head and Neck V Subcutaneous Tissue and Fascia, Upper Extremity W Subcutaneous Tissue and Fascia, Lower Extremity	0 Open 3 Percutaneous	1 Radioactive Element 3 Infusion Device	Z No Qualifier
T Subcutaneous Tissue and Fascia, Trunk	0 Open 3 Percutaneous	1 Radioactive Element 3 Infusion Device V Infusion Pump	Z No Qualifier

Multiple procedures
B3.2
During the same operative episode, multiple procedures are coded if:
  a. The same root operation is performed on different body parts as defined by distinct values of the body part character.
     Example: Diagnostic excision of liver and pancreas are coded separately.
  b. The same root operation is repeated at different body sites that are included in the same body part value.
     Example: Excision of the sartorius muscle and excision of the gracilis muscle are both included in the upper leg muscle body part value, and multiple procedures are coded.
  c. Multiple root operations with distinct objectives are performed on the same body part.
     Example: Destruction of sigmoid lesion and bypass of sigmoid colon are coded separately.
  d. The intended root operation is attempted using one approach, but is converted to a different approach.
     Example: Laparoscopic cholecystectomy converted to an open cholecystectomy is coded as percutaneous endoscopic Inspection and open Resection.

Discontinued procedures
B3.3
If the intended procedure is discontinued, code the procedure to the root operation performed. If a procedure is discontinued before any other root operation is performed, code the root operation Inspection of the body part or anatomical region inspected.
Example: A planned aortic valve replacement procedure is discontinued after the initial thoracotomy and before any incision is made in the heart muscle, when the patient becomes hemodynamically unstable. This procedure is coded as an open Inspection of the mediastinum.

Biopsy procedures
B3.4a
Biopsy procedures are coded using the root operations Excision, Extraction, or Drainage and the qualifier Diagnostic. The qualifier Diagnostic is used only for biopsies.
Examples: Fine needle aspiration biopsy of lung is coded to the root operation Drainage with the qualifier Diagnostic. Biopsy of bone marrow is coded to the root operation Extraction with the qualifier Diagnostic. Lymph node sampling for biopsy is coded to the root operation Excision with the qualifier Diagnostic.

Biopsy followed by more definitive treatment
B3.4b
If a diagnostic Excision, Extraction, or Drainage procedure (biopsy) is followed by a more definitive procedure, such as Destruction, Excision or Resection at the same procedure site, both the biopsy and the more definitive treatment are coded.
Example: Biopsy of breast followed by partial mastectomy at the same procedure site, both the biopsy and the partial mastectomy procedure are coded.

Overlapping body layers
B3.5
If the root operations Excision, Repair or Inspection are performed on overlapping layers of the musculoskeletal system, the body part specifying the deepest layer is coded.
Example: Excisional debridement that includes skin and subcutaneous tissue and muscle is coded to the muscle body part.

Bypass procedures
B3.6a
Bypass procedures are coded by identifying the body part bypassed "from" and the body part bypassed "to." The fourth character body part specifies the body part bypassed from, and the qualifier specifies the body part bypassed to.
Example: Bypass from stomach to jejunum, stomach is the body part and jejunum is the qualifier.
B3.6b
Coronary arteries are classified by number of distinct sites treated, rather than number of coronary arteries or anatomic name of a coronary artery (e.g., left anterior descending). Coronary artery bypass procedures are coded differently than other bypass procedures as described in the previous guideline. Rather than identifying the body part bypassed from, the body part identifies the number of coronary artery sites bypassed to, and the qualifier specifies the vessel bypassed from.
Example: Aortocoronary artery bypass of one site on the left anterior descending coronary artery and one site on the obtuse marginal coronary artery is classified in the body part axis of classification as two coronary artery sites and the qualifier specifies the aorta as the body part bypassed from.
B3.6c
If multiple coronary artery sites are bypassed, a separate procedure is coded for each coronary artery site that uses a different device and/or qualifier.
Example: Aortocoronary artery bypass and internal mammary coronary artery bypass are coded separately.

Control vs. more definitive root operations
B3.7
The root operation Control is defined as, "Stopping, or attempting to stop, postprocedural bleeding." If an attempt to stop postprocedural bleeding is initially unsuccessful, and to stop the bleeding requires performing any of the definitive root operations Bypass, Detachment, Excision, Extraction, Reposition, Replacement, or Resection, then that root operation is coded instead of Control.
Example: Resection of spleen to stop postprocedural bleeding is coded to Resection instead of Control.

Excision vs. Resection
B3.8
PCS contains specific body parts for anatomical subdivisions of a body part, such as lobes of the lungs or liver and regions of the intestine. Resection of the specific body part is coded whenever all of the body part is cut out or off, rather than coding Excision of a less specific body part.
Example: Left upper lung lobectomy is coded to Resection of Upper Lung Lobe, Left rather than Excision of Lung, Left.

Excision for graft
B3.9
If an autograft is obtained from a different body part in order to complete the objective of the procedure, a separate procedure is coded.
Example: Coronary bypass with excision of saphenous vein graft, excision of saphenous vein is coded separately.

Fusion procedures of the spine
B3.10a
The body part coded for a spinal vertebral joint(s) rendered immobile by a spinal fusion procedure is classified by the level of the spine (e.g. thoracic). There are distinct body part values for a single vertebral joint and for multiple vertebral joints at each spinal level.
Example: Body part values specify Lumbar Vertebral Joint, Lumbar Vertebral Joints, 2 or More and Lumbosacral Vertebral Joint.

B3.10b

If multiple vertebral joints are fused, a separate procedure is coded for each vertebral joint that uses a different device and/ or qualifier.

Example: Fusion of lumbar vertebral joint, posterior approach, anterior column and fusion of lumbar vertebral joint, posterior approach, posterior column are coded separately.

B3.10c

Combinations of devices and materials are often used on a vertebral joint to render the joint immobile. When combinations of devices are used on the same vertebral joint, the device value coded for the procedure is as follows:

- If an interbody fusion device is used to render the joint immobile (alone or containing other material like bone graft), the procedure is coded with the device value Interbody Fusion Device
- If bone graft is the *only* device used to render the joint immobile, the procedure is coded with the device value Nonautologous Tissue Substitute or Autologous Tissue Substitute
- If a mixture of autologous and nonautologous bone graft (with or without biological or synthetic extenders or binders) is used to render the joint immobile, code the procedure with the device value Autologous Tissue Substitute

Examples: Fusion of a vertebral joint using a cage style interbody fusion device containing morsellized bone graft is coded to the device Interbody Fusion Device. Fusion of a vertebral joint using a bone dowel interbody fusion device made of cadaver bone and packed with a mixture of local morsellized bone and demineralized bone matrix is coded to the device Interbody Fusion Device.
Fusion of a vertebral joint using both autologous bone graft and bone bank bone graft is coded to the device Autologous Tissue Substitute.

Inspection procedures
B3.11a

Inspection of a body part(s) performed in order to achieve the objective of a procedure is not coded separately.

Example: Fiberoptic bronchoscopy performed for irrigation of bronchus, only the irrigation procedure is coded.

B3.11b

If multiple tubular body parts are inspected, the most distal body part inspected is coded. If multiple non-tubular body parts in a region are inspected, the body part that specifies the entire area inspected is coded.

Examples: Cystoureteroscopy with inspection of bladder and ureters is coded to the ureter body part value. Exploratory laparotomy with general inspection of abdominal contents is coded to the peritoneal cavity body part value.

B3.11c

When both an Inspection procedure and another procedure are performed on the same body part during the same episode, if the Inspection procedure is performed using a different approach than the other procedure, the Inspection procedure is coded separately.

Example: Endoscopic Inspection of the duodenum is coded separately when open
Excision of the duodenum is performed during the same procedural episode.

Occlusion vs. Restriction for vessel embolization procedures
B3.12

If the objective of an embolization procedure is to completely close a vessel, the root operation Occlusion is coded. If the objective of an embolization procedure is to narrow the lumen of a vessel, the root operation Restriction is coded.

Examples: Tumor embolization is coded to the root operation Occlusion, because the objective of the procedure is to cut off the blood supply to the vessel.
Embolization of a cerebral aneurysm is coded to the root operation Restriction, because the objective of the procedure is not to close off the vessel entirely, but to narrow the lumen of the vessel at the site of the aneurysm where it is abnormally wide.

Release procedures
B3.13

In the root operation Release, the body part value coded is the body part being freed and not the tissue being manipulated or cut to free the body part.

Example: Lysis of intestinal adhesions is coded to the specific intestine body part value.

Release vs. Division
B3.14

If the sole objective of the procedure is freeing a body part without cutting the body part, the root operation is Release. If the sole objective of the procedure is separating or transecting a body part, the root operation is Division.

Examples: Freeing a nerve root from surrounding scar tissue to relieve pain is coded to the root operation Release. Severing a nerve root to relieve pain is coded to the root operation Division.

Reposition for fracture treatment
B3.15

Reduction of a displaced fracture is coded to the root operation Reposition and the application of a cast or splint in conjunction with the Reposition procedure is not coded separately. Treatment of a nondisplaced fracture is coded to the procedure performed.

Examples: Casting of a nondisplaced fracture is coded to the root operation Immobilization in the Placement section.
Putting a pin in a nondisplaced fracture is coded to the root operation Insertion.

Transplantation vs. Administration
B3.16

Putting in a mature and functioning living body part taken from another individual or animal is coded to the root operation Transplantation. Putting in autologous or nonautologous cells is coded to the Administration section.

Example: Putting in autologous or nonautologous bone marrow, pancreatic islet cells or stem cells is coded to the Administration section.

B4. Body Part

General guidelines
B4.1a

If a procedure is performed on a portion of a body part that does not have a separate body part value, code the body part value corresponding to the whole body part.

Example: A procedure performed on the alveolar process of the mandible is coded to the mandible body part.

B4.1b

If the prefix "peri" is combined with a body part to identify the site of the procedure, the procedure is coded to the body part named.

Example: A procedure site identified as perirenal is coded to the kidney body part.

Branches of body parts
B4.2

Where a specific branch of a body part does not have its own body part value in PCS, the body part is coded to the closest proximal branch that has a specific body part value.

Example: A procedure performed on the mandibular branch of the trigeminal nerve is coded to the trigeminal nerve body part value.

Bilateral body part values
B4.3
Bilateral body part values are available for a limited number of body parts. If the identical procedure is performed on contralateral body parts, and a bilateral body part value exists for that body part, a single procedure is coded using the bilateral body part value. If no bilateral body part value exists, each procedure is coded separately using the appropriate body part value.
Example: The identical procedure performed on both fallopian tubes is coded once using the body part value Fallopian Tube, Bilateral. The identical procedure performed on both knee joints is coded twice using the body part values Knee Joint, Right and Knee Joint, Left.

Coronary arteries
B4.4
The coronary arteries are classified as a single body part that is further specified by number of sites treated and not by name or number of arteries. Separate body part values are used to specify the number of sites treated when the same procedure is performed on multiple sites in the coronary arteries.
Examples: Angioplasty of two distinct sites in the left anterior descending coronary artery with placement of two stents is coded as Dilation of Coronary Arteries, Two Sites, with Intraluminal Device.
Angioplasty of two distinct sites in the left anterior descending coronary artery, one with stent placed and one without, is coded separately as Dilation of Coronary Artery, One Site with Intraluminal Device, and Dilation of Coronary Artery, One Site with no device.

Tendons, ligaments, bursae and fascia near a joint
B4.5
Procedures performed on tendons, ligaments, bursae and fascia supporting a joint are coded to the body part in the respective body system that is the focus of the procedure. Procedures performed on joint structures themselves are coded to the body part in the joint body systems.
Example: Repair of the anterior cruciate ligament of the knee is coded to the knee bursae and ligament body part in the bursae and ligaments body system. Knee arthroscopy with shaving of articular cartilage is coded to the knee joint body part in the Lower Joints body system.

Skin, subcutaneous tissue and fascia overlying a joint
B4.6
If a procedure is performed on the skin, subcutaneous tissue or fascia overlying a joint, the procedure is coded to the following body part:
- Shoulder is coded to Upper Arm
- Elbow is coded to Lower Arm
- Wrist is coded to Lower Arm
- Hip is coded to Upper Leg
- Knee is coded to Lower Leg
- Ankle is coded to Foot

Fingers and toes
B4.7
If a body system does not contain a separate body part value for fingers, procedures performed on the fingers are coded to the body part value for the hand. If a body system does not contain a separate body part value for toes, procedures performed on the toes are coded to the body part value for the foot.
Example: Excision of finger muscle is coded to one of the hand muscle body part values in the Muscles body system.

Upper and lower intestinal tract
B4.8
In the Gastrointestinal body system, the general body part values Upper Intestinal Tract and Lower Intestinal Tract are provided as an option for the root operations Change, Inspection, Removal and Revision. Upper Intestinal Tract includes the portion of the gastrointestinal tract from the esophagus down to and including the duodenum, and Lower Intestinal Tract includes the portion of the gastrointestinal tract from the jejunum down to and including the rectum and anus.
Example: In the root operation Change table, change of a device in the jejunum is coded using the body part Lower Intestinal Tract.

B5. Approach
Open approach with percutaneous endoscopic assistance
B5.2
Procedures performed using the open approach with percutaneous endoscopic assistance are coded to the approach Open.
Example: Laparoscopic-assisted sigmoidectomy is coded to the approach Open.

External approach
B5.3a
Procedures performed within an orifice on structures that are visible without the aid of any instrumentation are coded to the approach External.
Example: Resection of tonsils is coded to the approach External.
B5.3b
Procedures performed indirectly by the application of external force through the intervening body layers are coded to the approach External.
Example: Closed reduction of fracture is coded to the approach External.

Percutaneous procedure via device
B5.4
Procedures performed percutaneously via a device placed for the procedure are coded to the approach Percutaneous.
Example: Fragmentation of kidney stone performed via percutaneous nephrostomy is coded to the approach Percutaneous.

B6. Device
General guidelines
B6.1a
A device is coded only if a device remains after the procedure is completed. If no device remains, the device value No Device is coded.

B6.1b
Materials such as sutures, ligatures, radiological markers and temporary post-operative wound drains are considered integral to the performance of a procedure and are not coded as devices.

B6.1c
Procedures performed on a device only and not on a body part are specified in the root operations Change, Irrigation, Removal and Revision, and are coded to the procedure performed.
Example: Irrigation of percutaneous nephrostomy tube is coded to the root operation Irrigation of indwelling device in the Administration section.

Drainage device
B6.2
A separate procedure to put in a drainage device is coded to the root operation Drainage with the device value Drainage Device.

Obstetric Section Guidelines (section 1)

C. Obstetrics Section
Products of conception
C1
Procedures performed on the products of conception are coded to the Obstetrics section. Procedures performed on the pregnant female other than the products of conception are coded to the appropriate root operation in the Medical and Surgical section.
Example: Amniocentesis is coded to the products of conception body part in the Obstetrics section. Repair of obstetric urethral laceration is coded to the urethra body part in the Medical and Surgical section.

Procedures following delivery or abortion
C2
Procedures performed following a delivery or abortion for curettage of the endometrium or evacuation of retained products of conception are all coded in the Obstetrics section, to the root operation Extraction and the body part Products of Conception, Retained. Diagnostic or therapeutic dilation and curettage performed during times other than the postpartum or post-abortion period are all coded in the Medical and Surgical section, to the root operation Extraction and the body part Endometrium.

Selection of Principal Procedure
The following instructions should be applied in the selection of principal procedure and clarification on the importance of the relation to the principal diagnosis when more than one procedure is performed:

1. Procedure performed for definitive treatment of both principal diagnosis and secondary diagnosis
   a. Sequence procedure performed for definitive treatment most related to principal diagnosis as principal procedure.
2. Procedure performed for definitive treatment and diagnostic procedures performed for both principal diagnosis and secondary diagnosis
   a. Sequence procedure performed for definitive treatment most related to principal diagnosis as principal procedure
3. A diagnostic procedure was performed for the principal diagnosis and a procedure is performed for definitive treatment of a secondary diagnosis.
   a. Sequence diagnostic procedure as principal procedure, since the procedure most related to the principal diagnosis takes precedence.
4. No procedures performed that are related to principal diagnosis; procedures performed for definitive treatment and diagnostic procedures were performed for secondary diagnosis
   a. Sequence procedure performed for definitive treatment of secondary diagnosis as principal procedure, since there are no procedures (definitive or nondefinitive treatment) related to principal diagnosis.

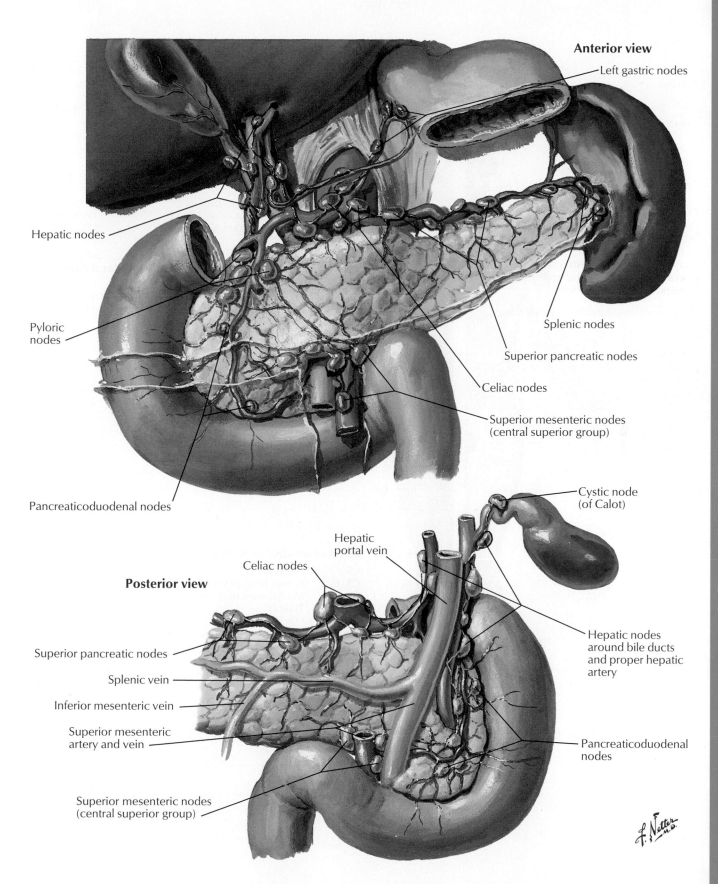

Anterior view

Left gastric nodes

Hepatic nodes

Pyloric nodes

Splenic nodes

Superior pancreatic nodes

Celiac nodes

Superior mesenteric nodes
(central superior group)

Pancreaticoduodenal nodes

Cystic node
(of Calot)

Hepatic portal vein

Celiac nodes

Posterior view

Hepatic nodes around bile ducts and proper hepatic artery

Superior pancreatic nodes

Splenic vein

Inferior mesenteric vein

Superior mesenteric artery and vein

Pancreaticoduodenal nodes

Superior mesenteric nodes (central superior group)

Plate 315 Lymph Vessels and Nodes of Pancreas. (Netter: Atlas of Human Anatomy, 4 ed, 2006, Saunders.)

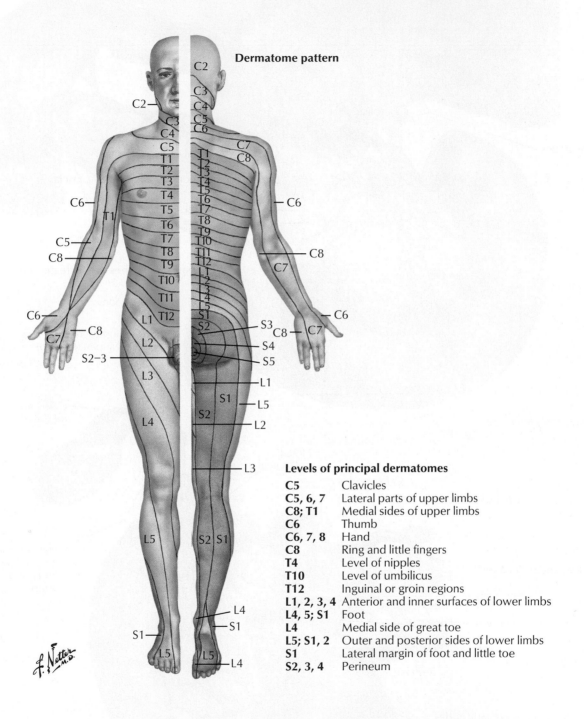

Dermatome pattern

Levels of principal dermatomes

C5	Clavicles
C5, 6, 7	Lateral parts of upper limbs
C8; T1	Medial sides of upper limbs
C6	Thumb
C6, 7, 8	Hand
C8	Ring and little fingers
T4	Level of nipples
T10	Level of umbilicus
T12	Inguinal or groin regions
L1, 2, 3, 4	Anterior and inner surfaces of lower limbs
L4, 5; S1	Foot
L4	Medial side of great toe
L5; S1, 2	Outer and posterior sides of lower limbs
S1	Lateral margin of foot and little toe
S2, 3, 4	Perineum

Plate 164   Dermatomes. (Netter: Atlas of Human Anatomy, 4 ed, 2006, Saunders.)

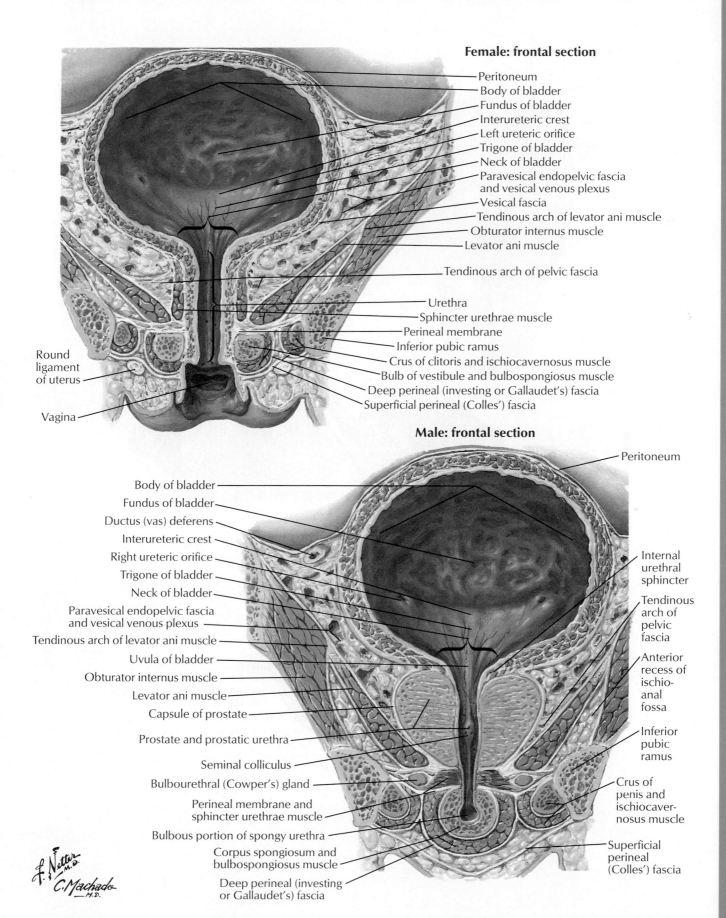

Female: frontal section

- Peritoneum
- Body of bladder
- Fundus of bladder
- Interureteric crest
- Left ureteric orifice
- Trigone of bladder
- Neck of bladder
- Paravesical endopelvic fascia and vesical venous plexus
- Vesical fascia
- Tendinous arch of levator ani muscle
- Obturator internus muscle
- Levator ani muscle
- Tendinous arch of pelvic fascia
- Urethra
- Sphincter urethrae muscle
- Perineal membrane
- Inferior pubic ramus
- Crus of clitoris and ischiocavernosus muscle
- Bulb of vestibule and bulbospongiosus muscle
- Deep perineal (investing or Gallaudet's) fascia
- Superficial perineal (Colles') fascia

- Round ligament of uterus
- Vagina

Male: frontal section

- Peritoneum
- Body of bladder
- Fundus of bladder
- Ductus (vas) deferens
- Interureteric crest
- Right ureteric orifice
- Trigone of bladder
- Neck of bladder
- Paravesical endopelvic fascia and vesical venous plexus
- Tendinous arch of levator ani muscle
- Uvula of bladder
- Obturator internus muscle
- Levator ani muscle
- Capsule of prostate
- Prostate and prostatic urethra
- Seminal colliculus
- Bulbourethral (Cowper's) gland
- Perineal membrane and sphincter urethrae muscle
- Bulbous portion of spongy urethra
- Corpus spongiosum and bulbospongiosus muscle
- Deep perineal (investing or Gallaudet's) fascia

- Internal urethral sphincter
- Tendinous arch of pelvic fascia
- Anterior recess of ischio-anal fossa
- Inferior pubic ramus
- Crus of penis and ischiocavernosus muscle
- Superficial perineal (Colles') fascia

Plate 366 Urinary Bladder: Female and Male. (Netter: Atlas of Human Anatomy, 4 ed, 2006, Saunders.)

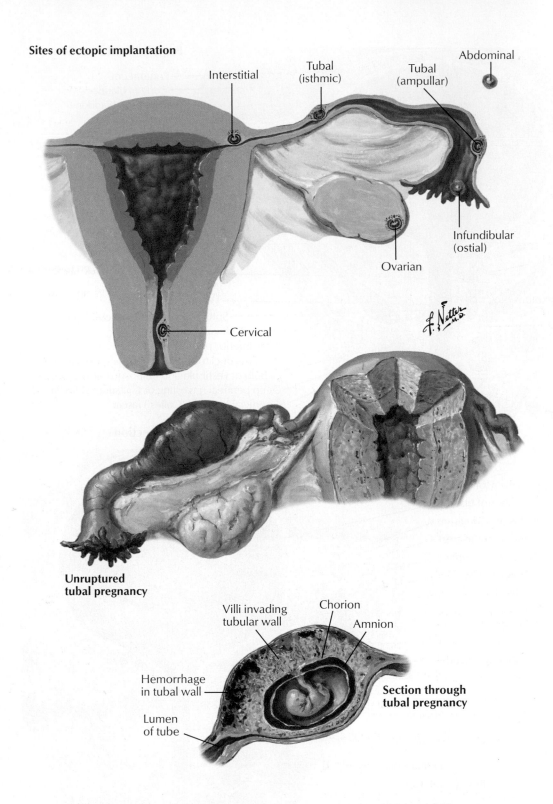

Sites of ectopic implantation

Interstitial

Tubal (isthmic)

Tubal (ampullar)

Abdominal

Infundibular (ostial)

Ovarian

Cervical

Unruptured tubal pregnancy

Villi invading tubular wall

Chorion

Amnion

Hemorrhage in tubal wall

Lumen of tube

Section through tubal pregnancy

Plate 375 Ectopic Pregnancy. (Netter: Atlas of Human Anatomy, 4 ed, 2006, Saunders.)

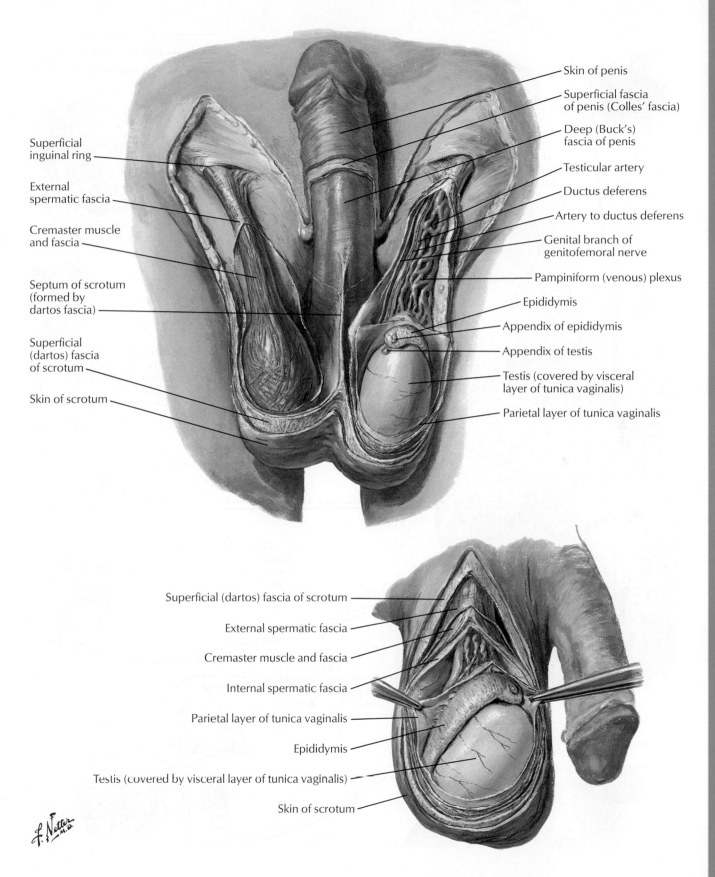

Skin of penis

Superficial fascia
of penis (Colles' fascia)

Deep (Buck's)
fascia of penis

Testicular artery

Ductus deferens

Artery to ductus deferens

Genital branch of
genitofemoral nerve

Pampiniform (venous) plexus

Epididymis

Appendix of epididymis

Appendix of testis

Testis (covered by visceral
layer of tunica vaginalis)

Parietal layer of tunica vaginalis

Superficial
inguinal ring

External
spermatic fascia

Cremaster muscle
and fascia

Septum of scrotum
(formed by
dartos fascia)

Superficial
(dartos) fascia
of scrotum

Skin of scrotum

Superficial (dartos) fascia of scrotum

External spermatic fascia

Cremaster muscle and fascia

Internal spermatic fascia

Parietal layer of tunica vaginalis

Epididymis

Testis (covered by visceral layer of tunica vaginalis)

Skin of scrotum

Plate 387   Scrotum and Contents. (Netter: Atlas of Human Anatomy, 4 ed, 2006, Saunders.)

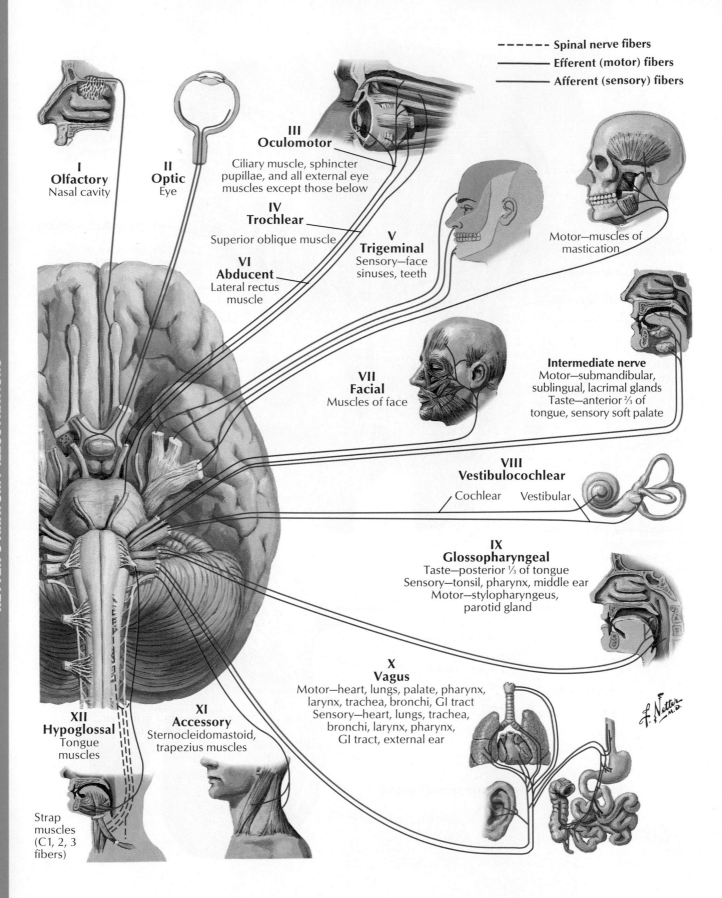

- - - - - Spinal nerve fibers
———— Efferent (motor) fibers
———— Afferent (sensory) fibers

I
Olfactory
Nasal cavity

II
Optic
Eye

III
Oculomotor
Ciliary muscle, sphincter
pupillae, and all external eye
muscles except those below

IV
Trochlear
Superior oblique muscle

V
Trigeminal
Sensory—face
sinuses, teeth

VI
Abducent
Lateral rectus
muscle

Motor—muscles of
mastication

VII
Facial
Muscles of face

Intermediate nerve
Motor—submandibular,
sublingual, lacrimal glands
Taste—anterior ⅔ of
tongue, sensory soft palate

VIII
Vestibulocochlear

Cochlear   Vestibular

IX
Glossopharyngeal
Taste—posterior ⅓ of tongue
Sensory—tonsil, pharynx, middle ear
Motor—stylopharyngeus,
parotid gland

X
Vagus
Motor—heart, lungs, palate, pharynx,
larynx, trachea, bronchi, GI tract
Sensory—heart, lungs, trachea,
bronchi, larynx, pharynx,
GI tract, external ear

XII
Hypoglossal
Tongue
muscles

XI
Accessory
Sternocleidomastoid,
trapezius muscles

Strap
muscles
(C1, 2, 3
fibers)

Plate 118 Cranial Nerves (Motor and Sensory Distribution): Schema. (Netter: Atlas of Human Anatomy, 4 ed, 2006, Saunders.)

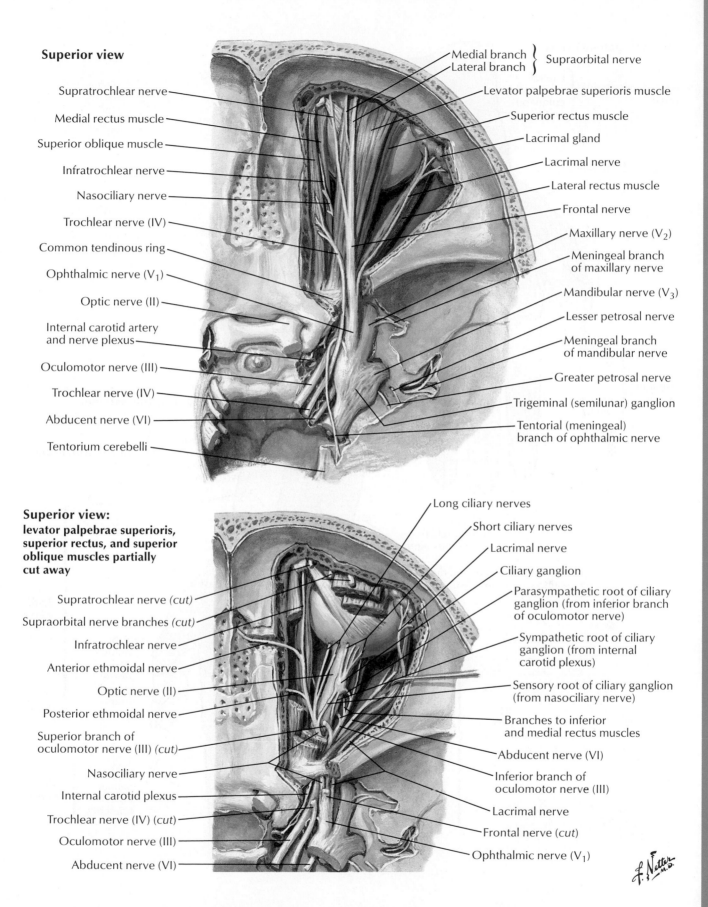

Superior view

Supratrochlear nerve
Medial rectus muscle
Superior oblique muscle
Infratrochlear nerve
Nasociliary nerve
Trochlear nerve (IV)
Common tendinous ring
Ophthalmic nerve (V₁)
Optic nerve (II)
Internal carotid artery and nerve plexus
Oculomotor nerve (III)
Trochlear nerve (IV)
Abducent nerve (VI)
Tentorium cerebelli

Medial branch ⎱ Supraorbital nerve
Lateral branch ⎰
Levator palpebrae superioris muscle
Superior rectus muscle
Lacrimal gland
Lacrimal nerve
Lateral rectus muscle
Frontal nerve
Maxillary nerve (V₂)
Meningeal branch of maxillary nerve
Mandibular nerve (V₃)
Lesser petrosal nerve
Meningeal branch of mandibular nerve
Greater petrosal nerve
Trigeminal (semilunar) ganglion
Tentorial (meningeal) branch of ophthalmic nerve

Superior view:
levator palpebrae superioris, superior rectus, and superior oblique muscles partially cut away

Supratrochlear nerve (cut)
Supraorbital nerve branches (cut)
Infratrochlear nerve
Anterior ethmoidal nerve
Optic nerve (II)
Posterior ethmoidal nerve
Superior branch of oculomotor nerve (III) (cut)
Nasociliary nerve
Internal carotid plexus
Trochlear nerve (IV) (cut)
Oculomotor nerve (III)
Abducent nerve (VI)

Long ciliary nerves
Short ciliary nerves
Lacrimal nerve
Ciliary ganglion
Parasympathetic root of ciliary ganglion (from inferior branch of oculomotor nerve)
Sympathetic root of ciliary ganglion (from internal carotid plexus)
Sensory root of ciliary ganglion (from nasociliary nerve)
Branches to inferior and medial rectus muscles
Abducent nerve (VI)
Inferior branch of oculomotor nerve (III)
Lacrimal nerve
Frontal nerve (cut)
Ophthalmic nerve (V₁)

Plate 86 Nerves of Orbit. (Netter: Atlas of Human Anatomy, 4 ed, 2006, Saunders.)

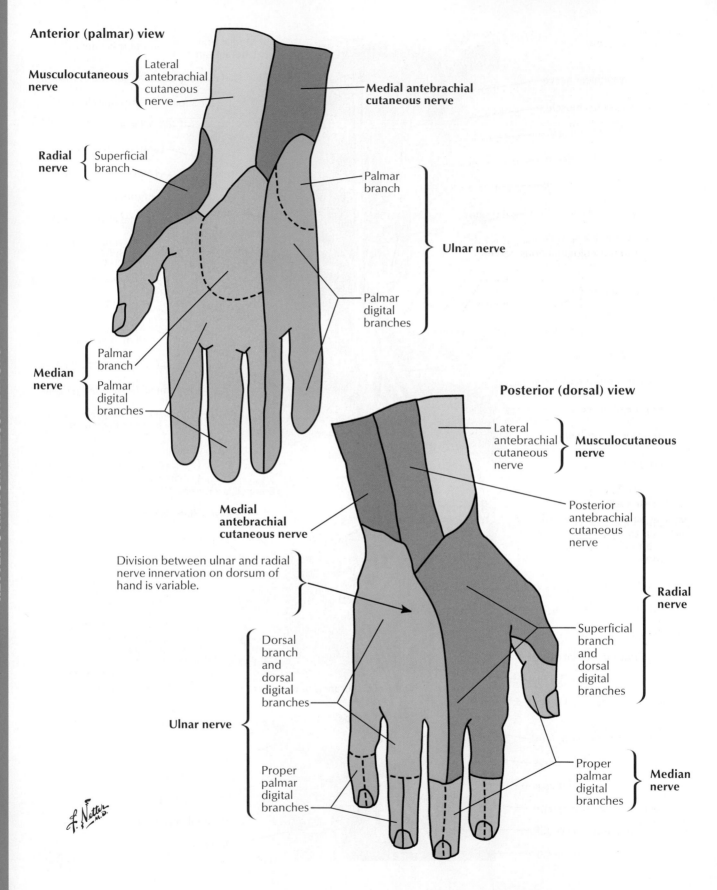

Anterior (palmar) view

Musculocutaneous nerve { Lateral antebrachial cutaneous nerve

Medial antebrachial cutaneous nerve

Radial nerve { Superficial branch

Palmar branch

Ulnar nerve

Palmar digital branches

Palmar branch
Median nerve { Palmar digital branches

Posterior (dorsal) view

Lateral antebrachial cutaneous nerve **Musculocutaneous nerve**

Medial antebrachial cutaneous nerve

Posterior antebrachial cutaneous nerve

Division between ulnar and radial nerve innervation on dorsum of hand is variable.

Radial nerve

Dorsal branch and dorsal digital branches

Superficial branch and dorsal digital branches

Ulnar nerve

Proper palmar digital branches

Proper palmar digital branches **Median nerve**

f. Netter m.d.

Plate 472 Cutaneous Innervation of Wrist and Hand. (Netter: Atlas of Human Anatomy, 4 ed, 2006, Saunders.)

Anterior view

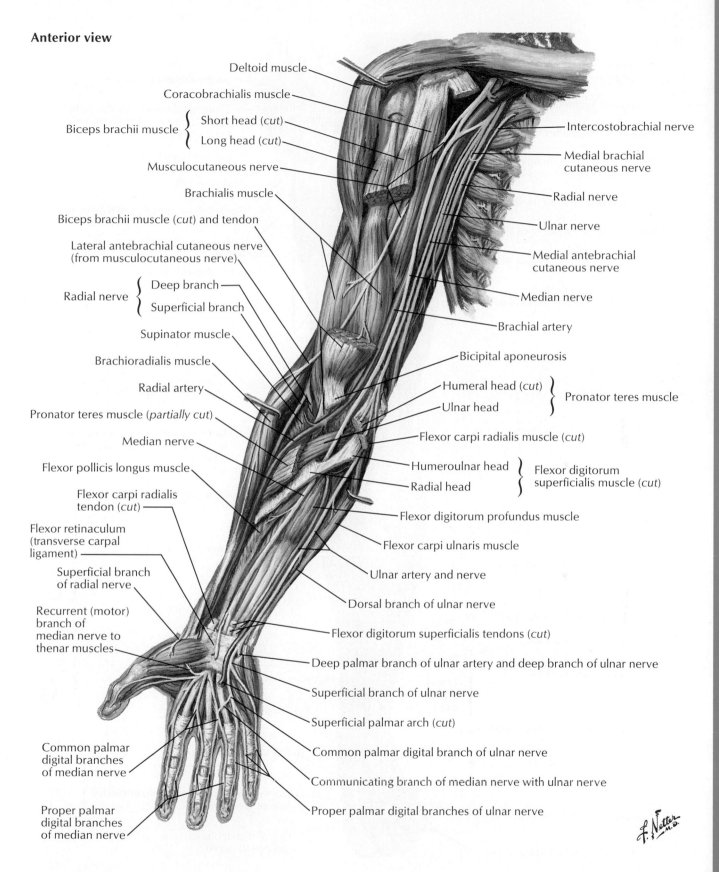

Deltoid muscle

Coracobrachialis muscle

Biceps brachii muscle { Short head (*cut*)
Long head (*cut*)

Musculocutaneous nerve

Brachialis muscle

Biceps brachii muscle (*cut*) and tendon

Lateral antebrachial cutaneous nerve (from musculocutaneous nerve)

Radial nerve { Deep branch
Superficial branch

Supinator muscle

Brachioradialis muscle

Radial artery

Pronator teres muscle (*partially cut*)

Median nerve

Flexor pollicis longus muscle

Flexor carpi radialis tendon (*cut*)

Flexor retinaculum (transverse carpal ligament)

Superficial branch of radial nerve

Recurrent (motor) branch of median nerve to thenar muscles

Common palmar digital branches of median nerve

Proper palmar digital branches of median nerve

Intercostobrachial nerve

Medial brachial cutaneous nerve

Radial nerve

Ulnar nerve

Medial antebrachial cutaneous nerve

Median nerve

Brachial artery

Bicipital aponeurosis

Humeral head (*cut*) } Pronator teres muscle
Ulnar head

Flexor carpi radialis muscle (*cut*)

Humeroulnar head } Flexor digitorum superficialis muscle (*cut*)
Radial head

Flexor digitorum profundus muscle

Flexor carpi ulnaris muscle

Ulnar artery and nerve

Dorsal branch of ulnar nerve

Flexor digitorum superficialis tendons (*cut*)

Deep palmar branch of ulnar artery and deep branch of ulnar nerve

Superficial branch of ulnar nerve

Superficial palmar arch (*cut*)

Common palmar digital branch of ulnar nerve

Communicating branch of median nerve with ulnar nerve

Proper palmar digital branches of ulnar nerve

Plate 473 Arteries and Nerves of Upper Limb. (Netter: Atlas of Human Anatomy, 4 ed, 2006, Saunders.)

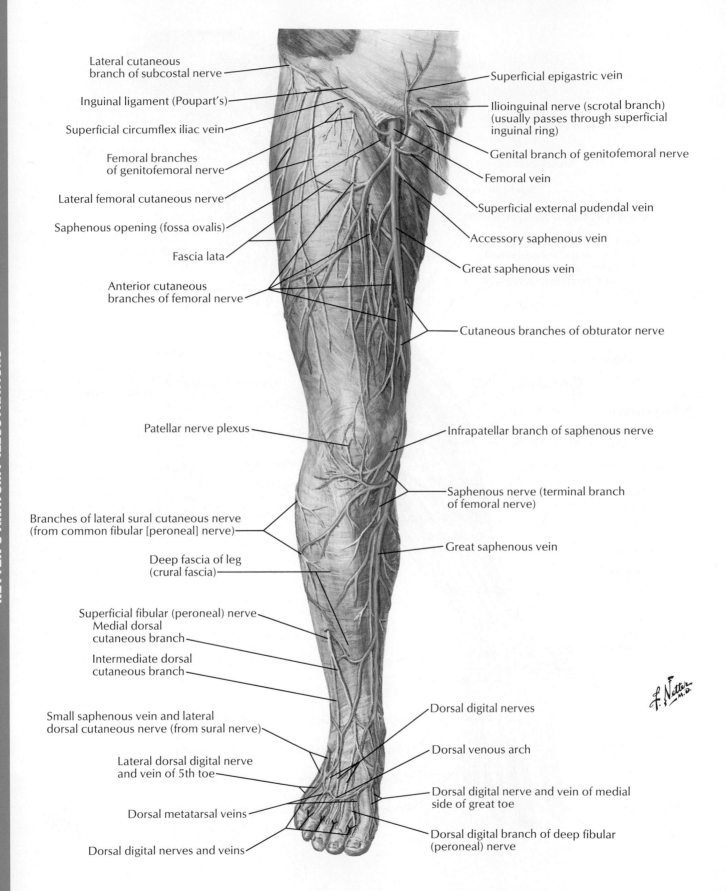

Lateral cutaneous branch of subcostal nerve

Inguinal ligament (Poupart's)

Superficial circumflex iliac vein

Femoral branches of genitofemoral nerve

Lateral femoral cutaneous nerve

Saphenous opening (fossa ovalis)

Fascia lata

Anterior cutaneous branches of femoral nerve

Patellar nerve plexus

Branches of lateral sural cutaneous nerve (from common fibular [peroneal] nerve)

Deep fascia of leg (crural fascia)

Superficial fibular (peroneal) nerve
Medial dorsal cutaneous branch

Intermediate dorsal cutaneous branch

Small saphenous vein and lateral dorsal cutaneous nerve (from sural nerve)

Lateral dorsal digital nerve and vein of 5th toe

Dorsal metatarsal veins

Dorsal digital nerves and veins

Superficial epigastric vein

Ilioinguinal nerve (scrotal branch) (usually passes through superficial inguinal ring)

Genital branch of genitofemoral nerve

Femoral vein

Superficial external pudendal vein

Accessory saphenous vein

Great saphenous vein

Cutaneous branches of obturator nerve

Infrapatellar branch of saphenous nerve

Saphenous nerve (terminal branch of femoral nerve)

Great saphenous vein

Dorsal digital nerves

Dorsal venous arch

Dorsal digital nerve and vein of medial side of great toe

Dorsal digital branch of deep fibular (peroneal) nerve

Plate 544 Superficial Nerves and Veins of Lower Limb: Anterior View. (Netter: Atlas of Human Anatomy, 4 ed, 2006, Saunders.)

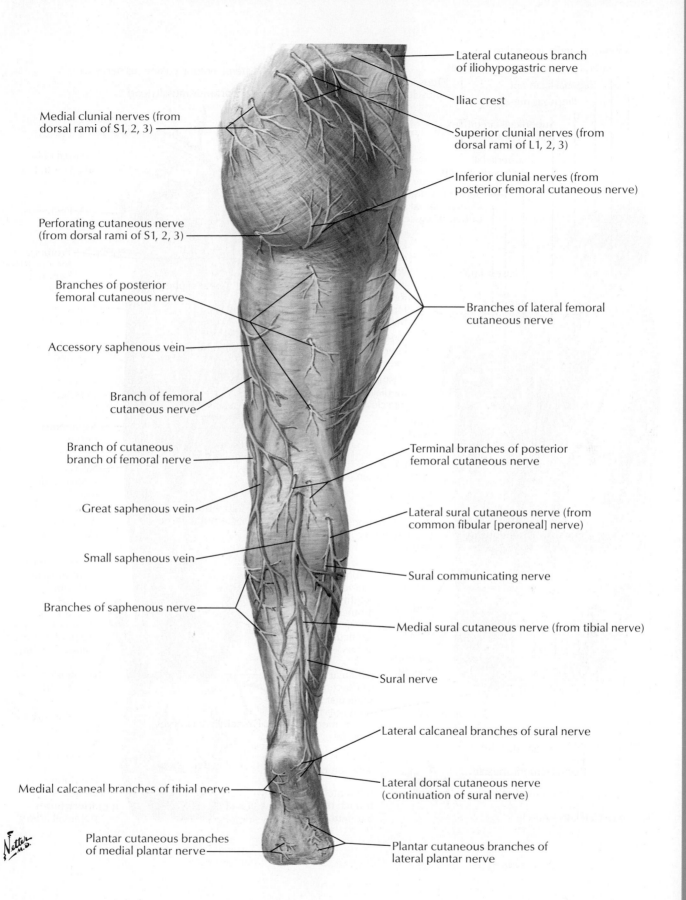

Lateral cutaneous branch of iliohypogastric nerve

Iliac crest

Medial clunial nerves (from dorsal rami of S1, 2, 3)

Superior clunial nerves (from dorsal rami of L1, 2, 3)

Inferior clunial nerves (from posterior femoral cutaneous nerve)

Perforating cutaneous nerve (from dorsal rami of S1, 2, 3)

Branches of posterior femoral cutaneous nerve

Branches of lateral femoral cutaneous nerve

Accessory saphenous vein

Branch of femoral cutaneous nerve

Branch of cutaneous branch of femoral nerve

Terminal branches of posterior femoral cutaneous nerve

Great saphenous vein

Lateral sural cutaneous nerve (from common fibular [peroneal] nerve)

Small saphenous vein

Sural communicating nerve

Branches of saphenous nerve

Medial sural cutaneous nerve (from tibial nerve)

Sural nerve

Lateral calcaneal branches of sural nerve

Medial calcaneal branches of tibial nerve

Lateral dorsal cutaneous nerve (continuation of sural nerve)

Plantar cutaneous branches of medial plantar nerve

Plantar cutaneous branches of lateral plantar nerve

Plate 545 Superficial Nerves and Veins of Lower Limb: Posterior View. (Netter: Atlas of Human Anatomy, 4 ed, 2006, Saunders.)

Superficial dissections

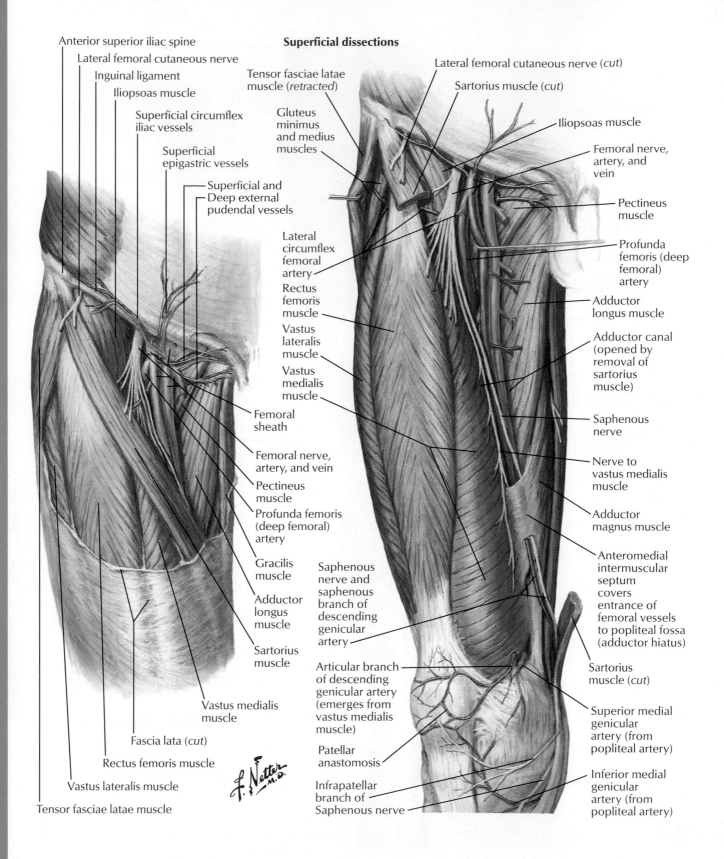

Anterior superior iliac spine
Lateral femoral cutaneous nerve
Inguinal ligament
Iliopsoas muscle
Superficial circumflex iliac vessels
Superficial epigastric vessels
Superficial and Deep external pudendal vessels
Tensor fasciae latae muscle (retracted)
Gluteus minimus and medius muscles
Lateral circumflex femoral artery
Rectus femoris muscle
Vastus lateralis muscle
Vastus medialis muscle
Femoral sheath
Femoral nerve, artery, and vein
Pectineus muscle
Profunda femoris (deep femoral) artery
Gracilis muscle
Adductor longus muscle
Sartorius muscle
Vastus medialis muscle
Fascia lata (cut)
Rectus femoris muscle
Vastus lateralis muscle
Tensor fasciae latae muscle

Lateral femoral cutaneous nerve (cut)
Sartorius muscle (cut)
Iliopsoas muscle
Femoral nerve, artery, and vein
Pectineus muscle
Profunda femoris (deep femoral) artery
Adductor longus muscle
Adductor canal (opened by removal of sartorius muscle)
Saphenous nerve
Nerve to vastus medialis muscle
Adductor magnus muscle
Anteromedial intermuscular septum covers entrance of femoral vessels to popliteal fossa (adductor hiatus)
Sartorius muscle (cut)
Superior medial genicular artery (from popliteal artery)
Inferior medial genicular artery (from popliteal artery)

Saphenous nerve and saphenous branch of descending genicular artery
Articular branch of descending genicular artery (emerges from vastus medialis muscle)
Patellar anastomosis
Infrapatellar branch of Saphenous nerve

F. Netter M.D.

Plate 500   Arteries and Nerves of Thigh: Anterior Views. (Netter: Atlas of Human Anatomy, 4 ed, 2006, Saunders.)

Deep dissection

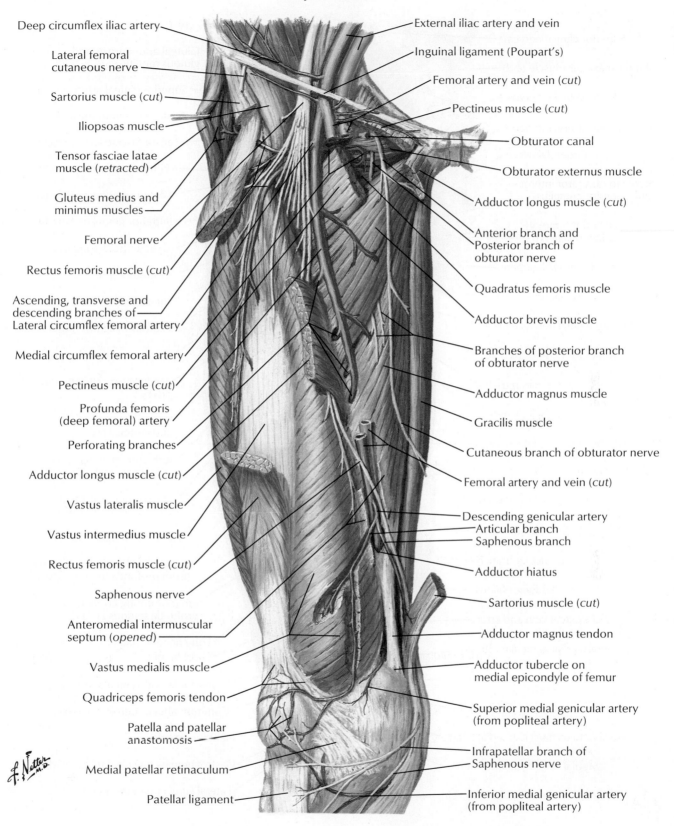

Deep circumflex iliac artery

Lateral femoral cutaneous nerve

Sartorius muscle (*cut*)

Iliopsoas muscle

Tensor fasciae latae muscle (*retracted*)

Gluteus medius and minimus muscles

Femoral nerve

Rectus femoris muscle (*cut*)

Ascending, transverse and descending branches of Lateral circumflex femoral artery

Medial circumflex femoral artery

Pectineus muscle (*cut*)

Profunda femoris (deep femoral) artery

Perforating branches

Adductor longus muscle (*cut*)

Vastus lateralis muscle

Vastus intermedius muscle

Rectus femoris muscle (*cut*)

Saphenous nerve

Anteromedial intermuscular septum (*opened*)

Vastus medialis muscle

Quadriceps femoris tendon

Patella and patellar anastomosis

Medial patellar retinaculum

Patellar ligament

External iliac artery and vein

Inguinal ligament (Poupart's)

Femoral artery and vein (*cut*)

Pectineus muscle (*cut*)

Obturator canal

Obturator externus muscle

Adductor longus muscle (*cut*)

Anterior branch and Posterior branch of obturator nerve

Quadratus femoris muscle

Adductor brevis muscle

Branches of posterior branch of obturator nerve

Adductor magnus muscle

Gracilis muscle

Cutaneous branch of obturator nerve

Femoral artery and vein (*cut*)

Descending genicular artery
Articular branch
Saphenous branch

Adductor hiatus

Sartorius muscle (*cut*)

Adductor magnus tendon

Adductor tubercle on medial epicondyle of femur

Superior medial genicular artery (from popliteal artery)

Infrapatellar branch of Saphenous nerve

Inferior medial genicular artery (from popliteal artery)

Plate 501   Arteries and Nerves of Thigh: Posterior View. (Netter: Atlas of Human Anatomy, 4 ed, 2006, Saunders.)

Deep dissection

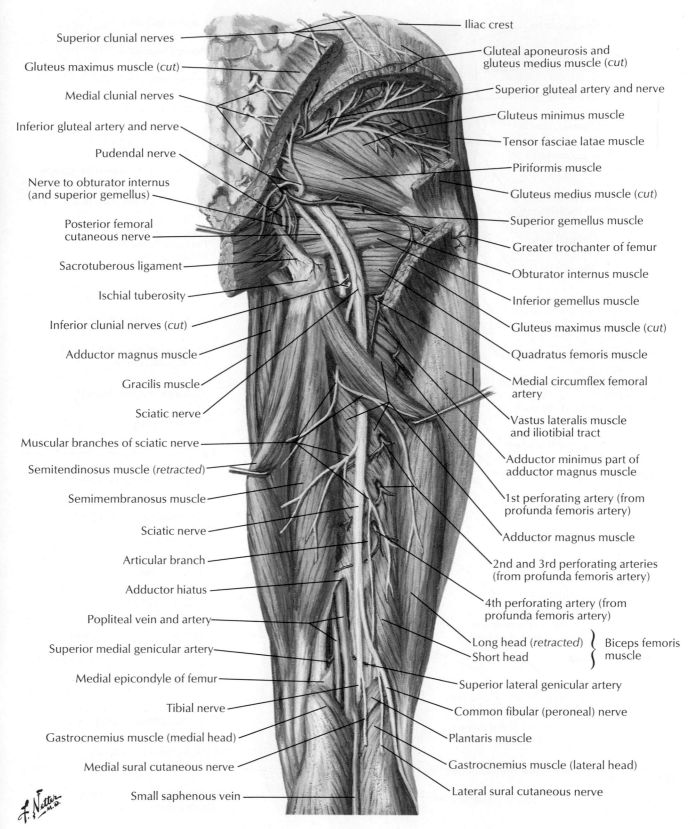

Superior clunial nerves

Gluteus maximus muscle (*cut*)

Medial clunial nerves

Inferior gluteal artery and nerve

Pudendal nerve

Nerve to obturator internus (and superior gemellus)

Posterior femoral cutaneous nerve

Sacrotuberous ligament

Ischial tuberosity

Inferior clunial nerves (*cut*)

Adductor magnus muscle

Gracilis muscle

Sciatic nerve

Muscular branches of sciatic nerve

Semitendinosus muscle (*retracted*)

Semimembranosus muscle

Sciatic nerve

Articular branch

Adductor hiatus

Popliteal vein and artery

Superior medial genicular artery

Medial epicondyle of femur

Tibial nerve

Gastrocnemius muscle (medial head)

Medial sural cutaneous nerve

Small saphenous vein

Iliac crest

Gluteal aponeurosis and gluteus medius muscle (*cut*)

Superior gluteal artery and nerve

Gluteus minimus muscle

Tensor fasciae latae muscle

Piriformis muscle

Gluteus medius muscle (*cut*)

Superior gemellus muscle

Greater trochanter of femur

Obturator internus muscle

Inferior gemellus muscle

Gluteus maximus muscle (*cut*)

Quadratus femoris muscle

Medial circumflex femoral artery

Vastus lateralis muscle and iliotibial tract

Adductor minimus part of adductor magnus muscle

1st perforating artery (from profunda femoris artery)

Adductor magnus muscle

2nd and 3rd perforating arteries (from profunda femoris artery)

4th perforating artery (from profunda femoris artery)

Long head (*retracted*) ⎫ Biceps femoris
Short head   ⎭ muscle

Superior lateral genicular artery

Common fibular (peroneal) nerve

Plantaris muscle

Gastrocnemius muscle (lateral head)

Lateral sural cutaneous nerve

Plate 502 Arteries and Nerves of Thigh: Posterior View. (Netter: Atlas of Human Anatomy, 4 ed, 2006, Saunders.)

Horizontal section

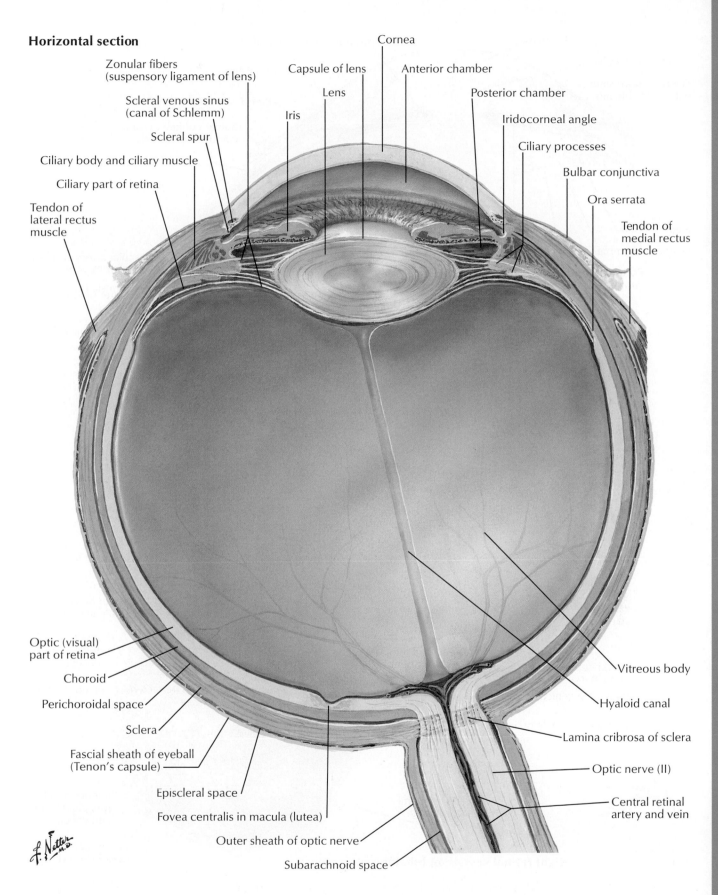

Zonular fibers
(suspensory ligament of lens)

Scleral venous sinus
(canal of Schlemm)

Scleral spur

Ciliary body and ciliary muscle

Ciliary part of retina

Tendon of
lateral rectus
muscle

Iris

Capsule of lens

Lens

Cornea

Anterior chamber

Posterior chamber

Iridocorneal angle

Ciliary processes

Bulbar conjunctiva

Ora serrata

Tendon of
medial rectus
muscle

Optic (visual)
part of retina

Choroid

Perichoroidal space

Sclera

Fascial sheath of eyeball
(Tenon's capsule)

Episcleral space

Fovea centralis in macula (lutea)

Outer sheath of optic nerve

Subarachnoid space

Vitreous body

Hyaloid canal

Lamina cribrosa of sclera

Optic nerve (II)

Central retinal
artery and vein

Plate 87   Eyeball. (Netter: Atlas of Human Anatomy, 4 ed, 2006, Saunders.)

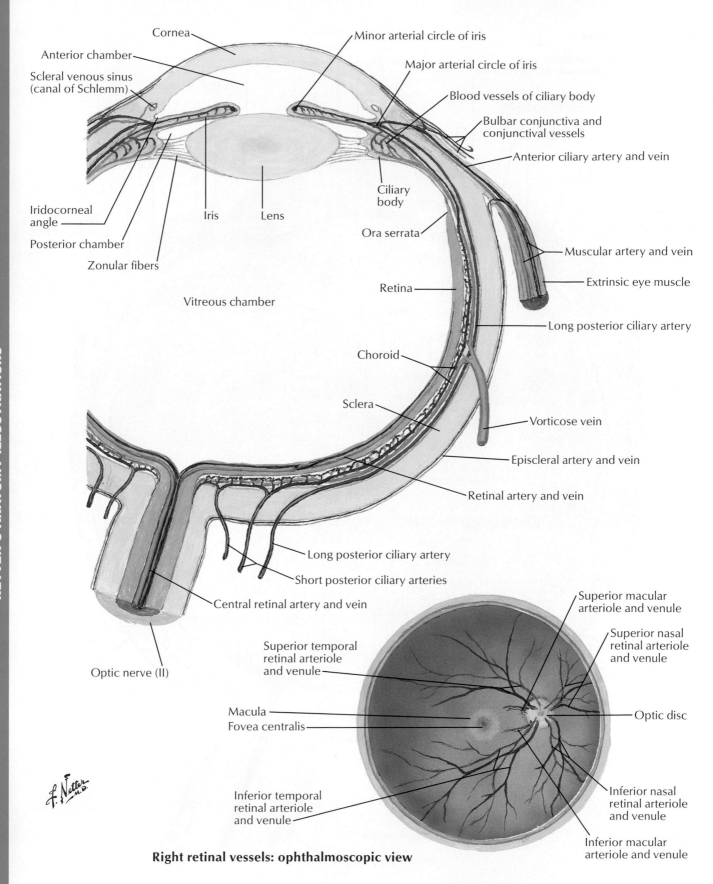

Cornea

Anterior chamber

Scleral venous sinus
(canal of Schlemm)

Minor arterial circle of iris

Major arterial circle of iris

Blood vessels of ciliary body

Bulbar conjunctiva and
conjunctival vessels

Anterior ciliary artery and vein

Iridocorneal
angle

Iris

Lens

Ciliary
body

Posterior chamber

Zonular fibers

Ora serrata

Muscular artery and vein

Extrinsic eye muscle

Retina

Long posterior ciliary artery

Vitreous chamber

Choroid

Sclera

Vorticose vein

Episcleral artery and vein

Retinal artery and vein

Long posterior ciliary artery

Short posterior ciliary arteries

Central retinal artery and vein

Optic nerve (II)

Superior temporal
retinal arteriole
and venule

Macula

Fovea centralis

Inferior temporal
retinal arteriole
and venule

Superior macular
arteriole and venule

Superior nasal
retinal arteriole
and venule

Optic disc

Inferior nasal
retinal arteriole
and venule

Inferior macular
arteriole and venule

Right retinal vessels: ophthalmoscopic view

Plate 90   Intrinsic Arteries and Veins of Eye. (Netter: Atlas of Human Anatomy, 4 ed, 2006, Saunders.)

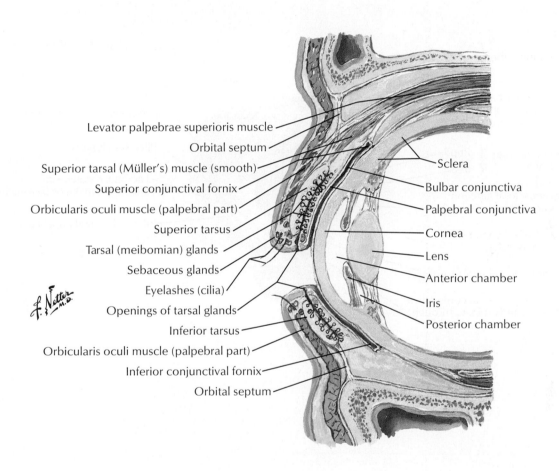

Levator palpebrae superioris muscle
Orbital septum
Superior tarsal (Müller's) muscle (smooth)
Superior conjunctival fornix
Orbicularis oculi muscle (palpebral part)
Superior tarsus
Tarsal (meibomian) glands
Sebaceous glands
Eyelashes (cilia)
Openings of tarsal glands
Inferior tarsus
Orbicularis oculi muscle (palpebral part)
Inferior conjunctival fornix
Orbital septum

Sclera
Bulbar conjunctiva
Palpebral conjunctiva
Cornea
Lens
Anterior chamber
Iris
Posterior chamber

Plate 81, Middle Eyelids. (Netter: Atlas of Human Anatomy, 4 ed, 2006, Saunders.)

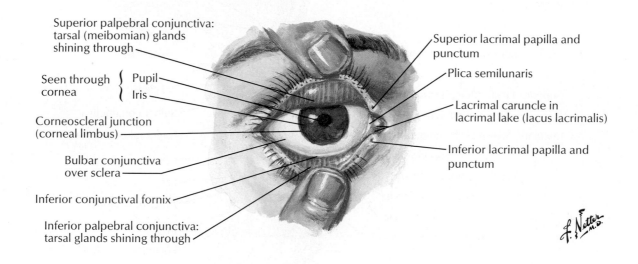

Superior palpebral conjunctiva: tarsal (meibomian) glands shining through

Seen through cornea { Pupil / Iris }

Corneoscleral junction (corneal limbus)

Bulbar conjunctiva over sclera

Inferior conjunctival fornix

Inferior palpebral conjunctiva: tarsal glands shining through

Superior lacrimal papilla and punctum

Plica semilunaris

Lacrimal caruncle in lacrimal lake (lacus lacrimalis)

Inferior lacrimal papilla and punctum

Plate 81, Upper Eyelid. (Netter: Atlas of Human Anatomy, 4 ed, 2006, Saunders.)

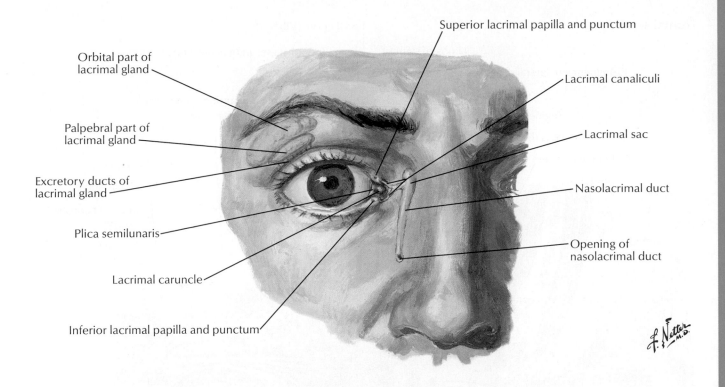

Superior lacrimal papilla and punctum

Orbital part of lacrimal gland

Palpebral part of lacrimal gland

Excretory ducts of lacrimal gland

Plica semilunaris

Lacrimal caruncle

Inferior lacrimal papilla and punctum

Lacrimal canaliculi

Lacrimal sac

Nasolacrimal duct

Opening of nasolacrimal duct

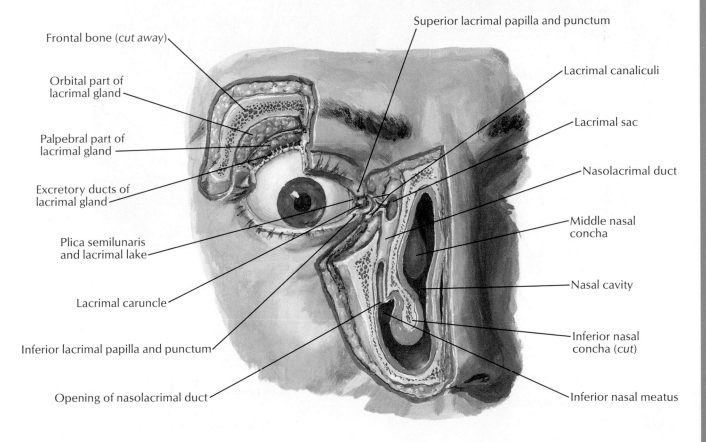

Frontal bone (cut away)

Orbital part of lacrimal gland

Palpebral part of lacrimal gland

Excretory ducts of lacrimal gland

Plica semilunaris and lacrimal lake

Lacrimal caruncle

Inferior lacrimal papilla and punctum

Opening of nasolacrimal duct

Superior lacrimal papilla and punctum

Lacrimal canaliculi

Lacrimal sac

Nasolacrimal duct

Middle nasal concha

Nasal cavity

Inferior nasal concha (cut)

Inferior nasal meatus

Plate 82 Lacrimal Apparatus. (Netter: Atlas of Human Anatomy, 4 ed, 2006, Saunders.)

Frontal section

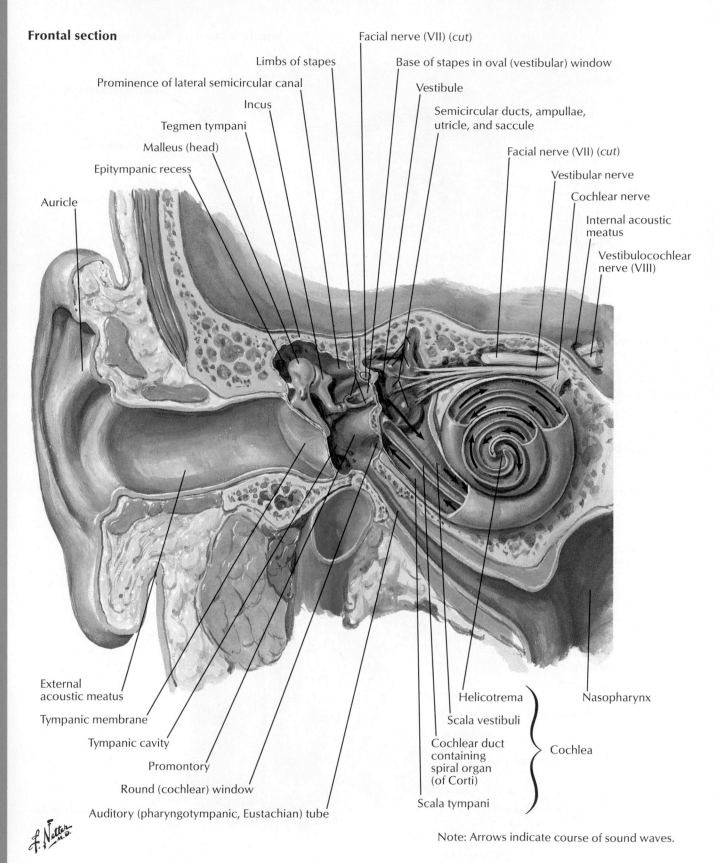

Limbs of stapes

Prominence of lateral semicircular canal

Incus

Tegmen tympani

Malleus (head)

Epitympanic recess

Auricle

Facial nerve (VII) (*cut*)

Base of stapes in oval (vestibular) window

Vestibule

Semicircular ducts, ampullae, utricle, and saccule

Facial nerve (VII) (*cut*)

Vestibular nerve

Cochlear nerve

Internal acoustic meatus

Vestibulocochlear nerve (VIII)

External acoustic meatus

Tympanic membrane

Tympanic cavity

Promontory

Round (cochlear) window

Auditory (pharyngotympanic, Eustachian) tube

Helicotrema

Scala vestibuli

Cochlear duct containing spiral organ (of Corti)

Scala tympani

Nasopharynx

Cochlea

Note: Arrows indicate course of sound waves.

Plate 92 Pathway of Sound Reception. (Netter: Atlas of Human Anatomy, 4 ed, 2006, Saunders.)

Medial wall of tympanic cavity: lateral view

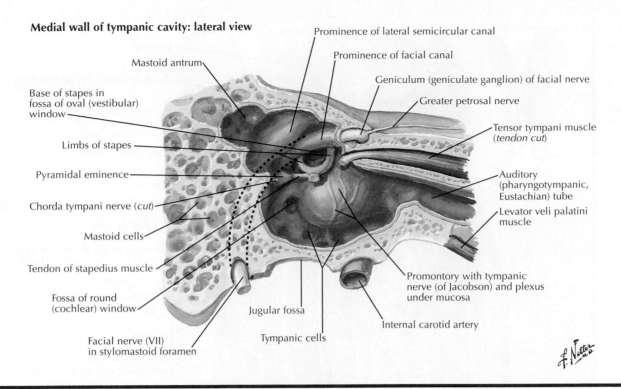

Prominence of lateral semicircular canal

Prominence of facial canal

Geniculum (geniculate ganglion) of facial nerve

Greater petrosal nerve

Mastoid antrum

Base of stapes in fossa of oval (vestibular) window

Limbs of stapes

Pyramidal eminence

Chorda tympani nerve (cut)

Mastoid cells

Tendon of stapedius muscle

Fossa of round (cochlear) window

Facial nerve (VII) in stylomastoid foramen

Jugular fossa

Tympanic cells

Tensor tympani muscle (tendon cut)

Auditory (pharyngotympanic, Eustachian) tube

Levator veli palatini muscle

Promontory with tympanic nerve (of Jacobson) and plexus under mucosa

Internal carotid artery

Plate 94   Tympanic Cavity. (Netter: Atlas of Human Anatomy, 4 ed, 2006, Saunders.)

Otoscopic view of right tympanic membrane

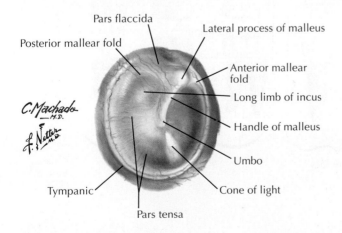

Pars flaccida

Posterior mallear fold

Lateral process of malleus

Anterior mallear fold

Long limb of incus

Handle of malleus

Umbo

Cone of light

Tympanic

Pars tensa

Plate 93   Tympanic Cavity. (Netter: Atlas of Human Anatomy, 4 ed, 2006, Saunders.)

Dissected right bony labyrinth (otic capsule): membranous labyrinth removed

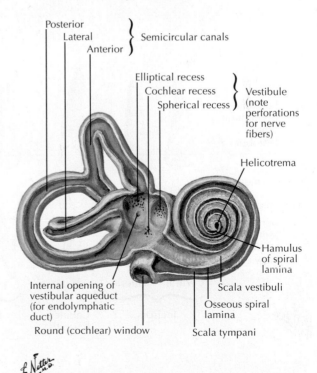

Posterior

Lateral

Anterior

Semicircular canals

Elliptical recess

Cochlear recess

Spherical recess

Vestibule (note perforations for nerve fibers)

Helicotrema

Hamulus of spiral lamina

Scala vestibuli

Osseous spiral lamina

Scala tympani

Internal opening of vestibular aqueduct (for endolymphatic duct)

Round (cochlear) window

Plate 95   Bony Membranous Labyrinth. (Netter: Atlas of Human Anatomy, 4 ed, 2006, Saunders.)

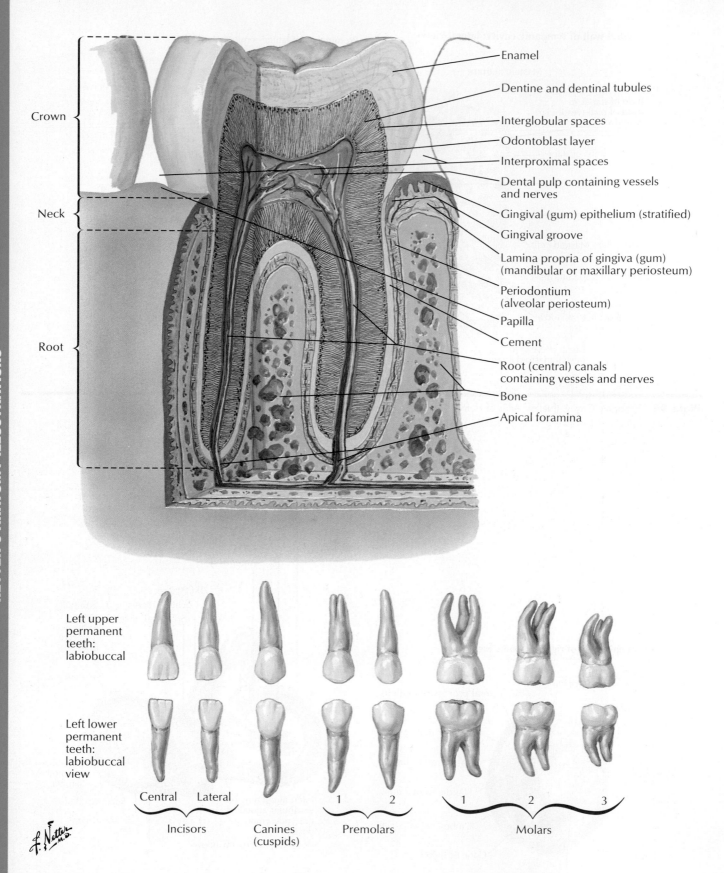

Crown

Enamel

Dentine and dentinal tubules

Interglobular spaces

Odontoblast layer

Interproximal spaces

Dental pulp containing vessels and nerves

Neck

Gingival (gum) epithelium (stratified)

Gingival groove

Lamina propria of gingiva (gum) (mandibular or maxillary periosteum)

Periodontium (alveolar periosteum)

Papilla

Cement

Root

Root (central) canals containing vessels and nerves

Bone

Apical foramina

Left upper permanent teeth: labiobuccal

Left lower permanent teeth: labiobuccal view

Central   Lateral

Incisors

Canines (cuspids)

1   2

Premolars

1   2   3

Molars

Plate 57   Teeth. (Netter: Atlas of Human Anatomy, 4 ed, 2006, Saunders.)

Tongue

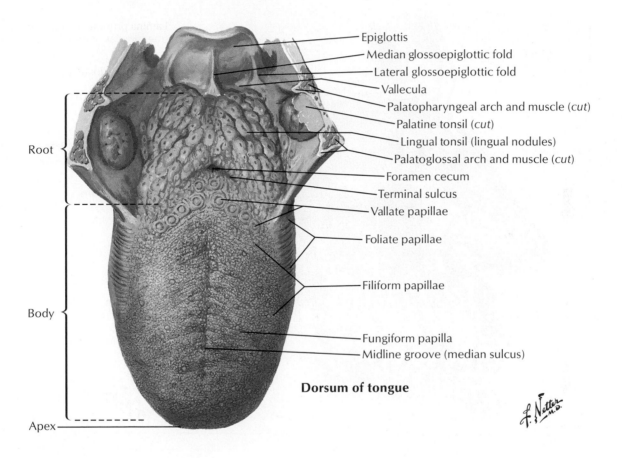

Epiglottis

Median glossoepiglottic fold

Lateral glossoepiglottic fold

Vallecula

Palatopharyngeal arch and muscle (*cut*)

Palatine tonsil (*cut*)

Lingual tonsil (lingual nodules)

Palatoglossal arch and muscle (*cut*)

Foramen cecum

Terminal sulcus

Vallate papillae

Foliate papillae

Filiform papillae

Fungiform papilla

Midline groove (median sulcus)

Root

Body

Apex

Dorsum of tongue

Plate 58   Tongue. (Netter: Atlas of Human Anatomy, 4 ed, 2006, Saunders.)

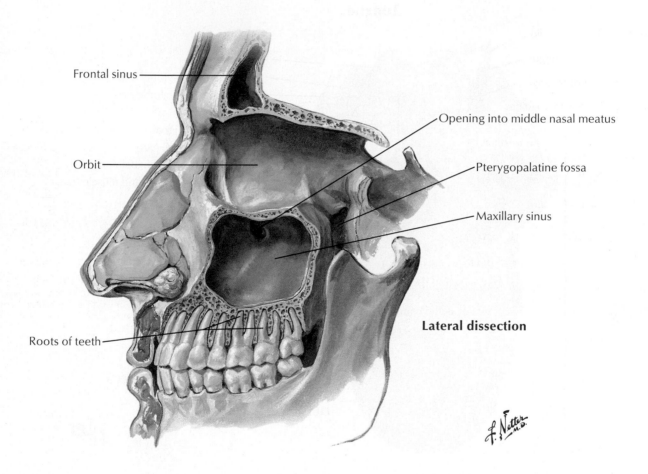

Frontal sinus

Orbit

Roots of teeth

Opening into middle nasal meatus

Pterygopalatine fossa

Maxillary sinus

Lateral dissection

Plate 49 Paranasal Sinuses. (Netter: Atlas of Human Anatomy, 4 ed, 2006, Saunders.)

30

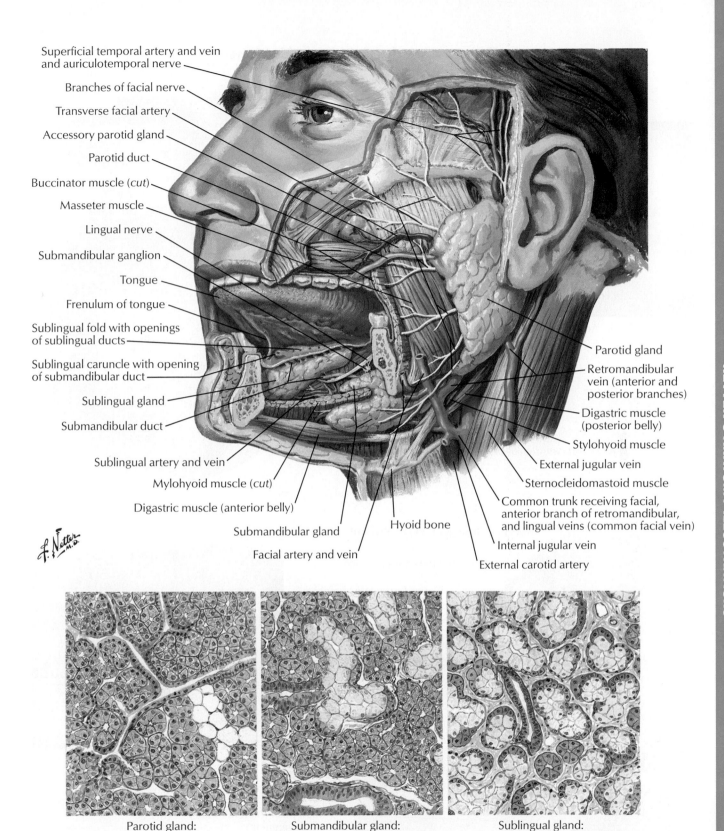

Superficial temporal artery and vein and auriculotemporal nerve

Branches of facial nerve

Transverse facial artery

Accessory parotid gland

Parotid duct

Buccinator muscle (*cut*)

Masseter muscle

Lingual nerve

Submandibular ganglion

Tongue

Frenulum of tongue

Sublingual fold with openings of sublingual ducts

Sublingual caruncle with opening of submandibular duct

Sublingual gland

Submandibular duct

Sublingual artery and vein

Mylohyoid muscle (*cut*)

Digastric muscle (anterior belly)

Submandibular gland

Facial artery and vein

Parotid gland

Retromandibular vein (anterior and posterior branches)

Digastric muscle (posterior belly)

Stylohyoid muscle

External jugular vein

Sternocleidomastoid muscle

Common trunk receiving facial, anterior branch of retromandibular, and lingual veins (common facial vein)

Internal jugular vein

External carotid artery

Hyoid bone

Parotid gland: totally serous

Submandibular gland: mostly serous, partially mucous

Sublingual gland: almost completely mucous

NETTER'S ANATOMY ILLUSTRATIONS

Plate 61   Salivary Glands. (Netter: Atlas of Human Anatomy, 4 ed, 2006, Saunders.)

Coronary Arteries: Arteriographic Views

Right coronary artery: left anterior oblique view

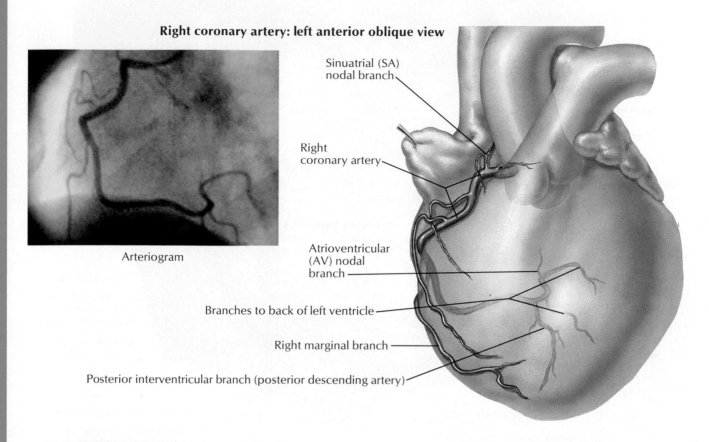

Arteriogram

Sinuatrial (SA) nodal branch

Right coronary artery

Atrioventricular (AV) nodal branch

Branches to back of left ventricle

Right marginal branch

Posterior interventricular branch (posterior descending artery)

Right coronary artery: right anterior oblique view

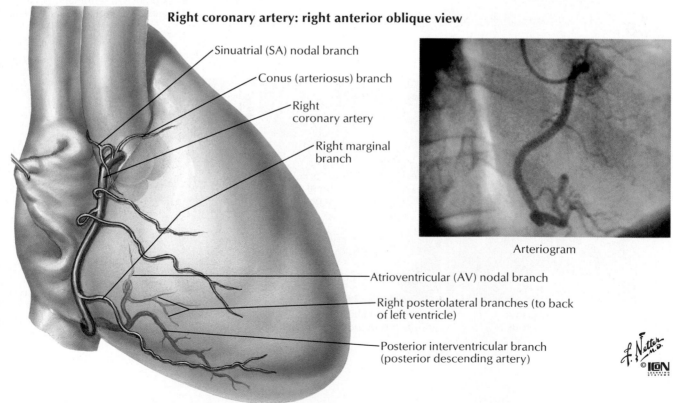

Sinuatrial (SA) nodal branch

Conus (arteriosus) branch

Right coronary artery

Right marginal branch

Arteriogram

Atrioventricular (AV) nodal branch

Right posterolateral branches (to back of left ventricle)

Posterior interventricular branch (posterior descending artery)

Plate 218   Coronary Arteries: Arteriographic Views. (Netter: Atlas of Human Anatomy, 4 ed, 2006, Saunders.)

32

Left coronary artery: left anterior oblique view

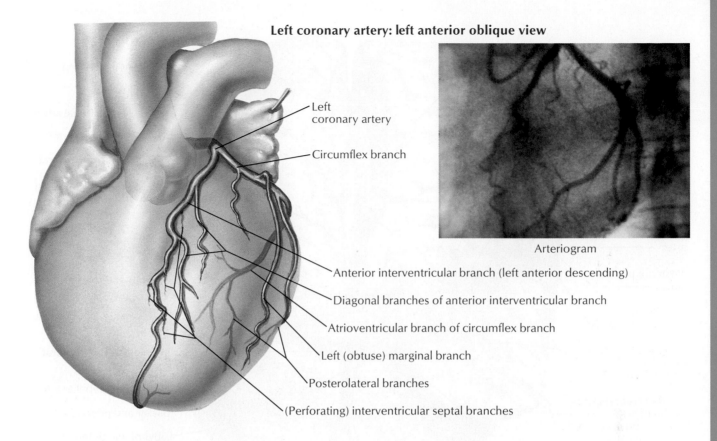

Left coronary artery

Circumflex branch

Arteriogram

Anterior interventricular branch (left anterior descending)

Diagonal branches of anterior interventricular branch

Atrioventricular branch of circumflex branch

Left (obtuse) marginal branch

Posterolateral branches

(Perforating) interventricular septal branches

Left coronary artery: right anterior oblique view

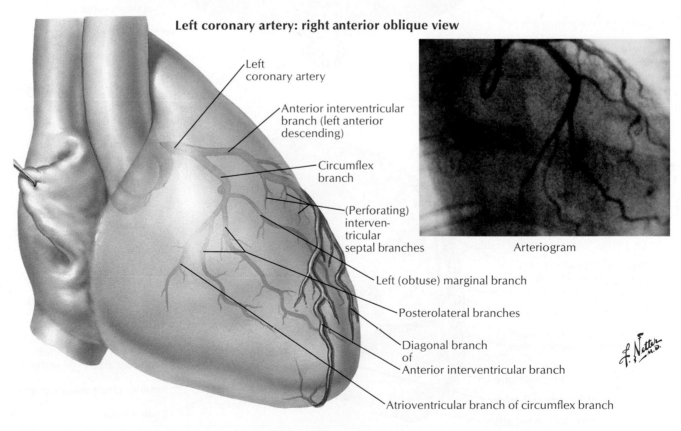

Left coronary artery

Anterior interventricular branch (left anterior descending)

Circumflex branch

(Perforating) interventricular septal branches

Arteriogram

Left (obtuse) marginal branch

Posterolateral branches

Diagonal branch of Anterior interventricular branch

Atrioventricular branch of circumflex branch

Plate 219   Coronary Arteries: Arteriographic Views. (Netter: Atlas of Human Anatomy, 4 ed, 2006, Saunders.)

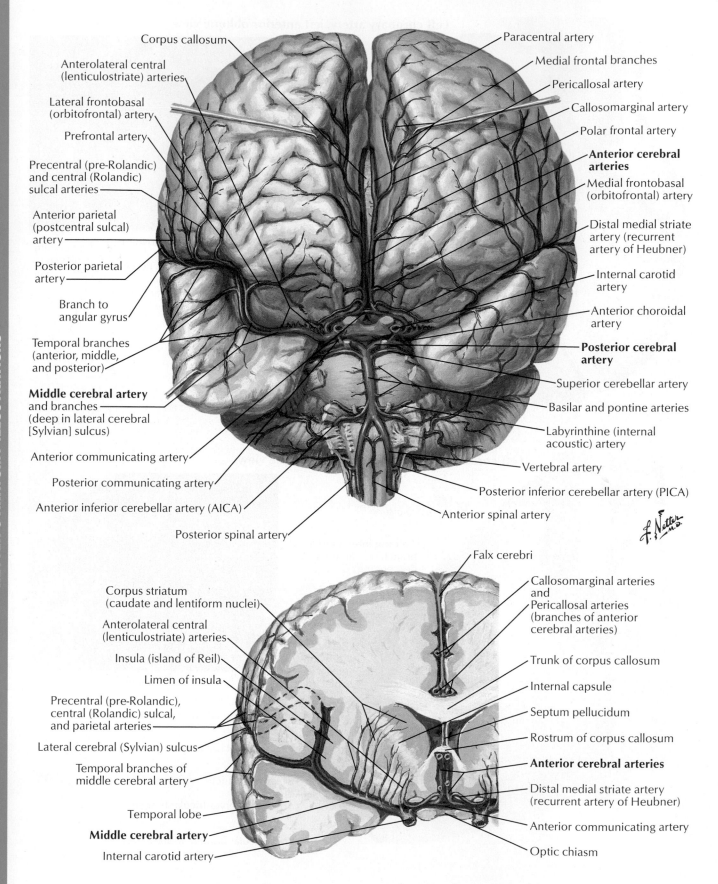

Corpus callosum

Anterolateral central (lenticulostriate) arteries

Lateral frontobasal (orbitofrontal) artery

Prefrontal artery

Precentral (pre-Rolandic) and central (Rolandic) sulcal arteries

Anterior parietal (postcentral sulcal) artery

Posterior parietal artery

Branch to angular gyrus

Temporal branches (anterior, middle, and posterior)

Middle cerebral artery and branches (deep in lateral cerebral [Sylvian] sulcus)

Anterior communicating artery

Posterior communicating artery

Anterior inferior cerebellar artery (AICA)

Posterior spinal artery

Paracentral artery

Medial frontal branches

Pericallosal artery

Callosomarginal artery

Polar frontal artery

Anterior cerebral arteries

Medial frontobasal (orbitofrontal) artery

Distal medial striate artery (recurrent artery of Heubner)

Internal carotid artery

Anterior choroidal artery

Posterior cerebral artery

Superior cerebellar artery

Basilar and pontine arteries

Labyrinthine (internal acoustic) artery

Vertebral artery

Posterior inferior cerebellar artery (PICA)

Anterior spinal artery

Falx cerebri

Corpus striatum (caudate and lentiform nuclei)

Anterolateral central (lenticulostriate) arteries

Insula (island of Reil)

Limen of insula

Precentral (pre-Rolandic), central (Rolandic) sulcal, and parietal arteries

Lateral cerebral (Sylvian) sulcus

Temporal branches of middle cerebral artery

Temporal lobe

Middle cerebral artery

Internal carotid artery

Callosomarginal arteries and Pericallosal arteries (branches of anterior cerebral arteries)

Trunk of corpus callosum

Internal capsule

Septum pellucidum

Rostrum of corpus callosum

Anterior cerebral arteries

Distal medial striate artery (recurrent artery of Heubner)

Anterior communicating artery

Optic chiasm

NETTER'S ANATOMY ILLUSTRATIONS

Plate 141 Arteries of Brain: Frontal View and Section. (Netter: Atlas of Human Anatomy, 4 ed, 2006, Saunders.)

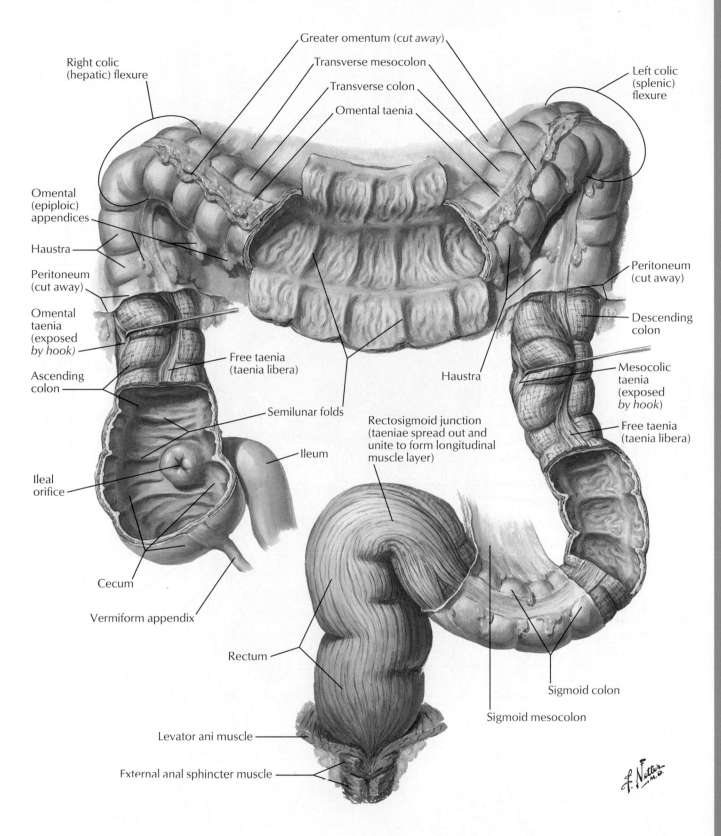

Right colic (hepatic) flexure

Greater omentum (cut away)

Transverse mesocolon

Transverse colon

Omental taenia

Left colic (splenic) flexure

Omental (epiploic) appendices

Haustra

Peritoneum (cut away)

Omental taenia (exposed by hook)

Ascending colon

Free taenia (taenia libera)

Semilunar folds

Ileal orifice

Ileum

Cecum

Vermiform appendix

Rectosigmoid junction (taeniae spread out and unite to form longitudinal muscle layer)

Haustra

Peritoneum (cut away)

Descending colon

Mesocolic taenia (exposed by hook)

Free taenia (taenia libera)

Rectum

Sigmoid colon

Sigmoid mesocolon

Levator ani muscle

External anal sphincter muscle

Plate 284 Mucosa and Musculature of Large Intestine. (Netter: Atlas of Human Anatomy, 4 ed, 2006, Saunders.)

Transverse Section: T3–4 Intervertebral Disc, Manubrium

Plate 244   T3–4

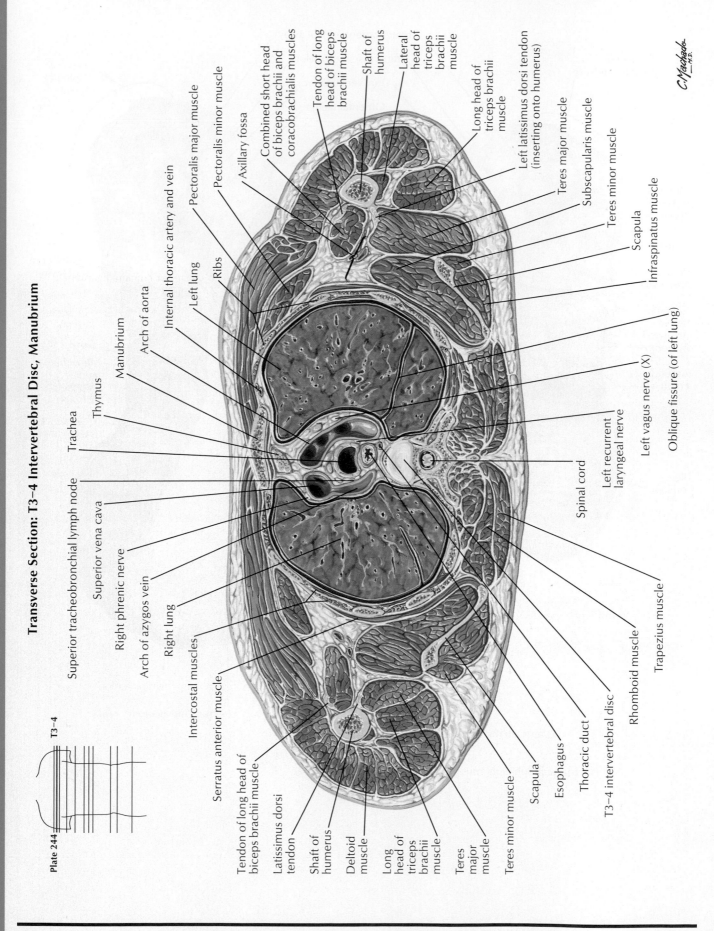

Superior tracheobronchial lymph node

Trachea

Thymus

Manubrium

Arch of aorta

Internal thoracic artery and vein

Left lung

Ribs

Axillary fossa

Pectoralis minor muscle

Pectoralis major muscle

Combined short head of biceps brachii and coracobrachialis muscles

Tendon of long head of biceps brachii muscle

Shaft of humerus

Lateral head of triceps brachii muscle

Long head of triceps brachii muscle

Left latissimus dorsi tendon (inserting onto humerus)

Teres major muscle

Subscapularis muscle

Teres minor muscle

Scapula

Infraspinatus muscle

Oblique fissure (of left lung)

Left vagus nerve (X)

Left recurrent laryngeal nerve

Spinal cord

Trapezius muscle

Rhomboid muscle

T3–4 intervertebral disc

Thoracic duct

Esophagus

Scapula

Teres minor muscle

Teres major muscle

Long head of triceps brachii muscle

Deltoid muscle

Shaft of humerus

Latissimus dorsi tendon

Tendon of long head of biceps brachii muscle

Serratus anterior muscle

Intercostal muscles

Right lung

Arch of azygos vein

Right phrenic nerve

Superior vena cava

Plate 244   Cross Section of Thorax at T3-4 Disc Level. (Netter: Atlas of Human Anatomy, 4 ed, 2006, Saunders.)

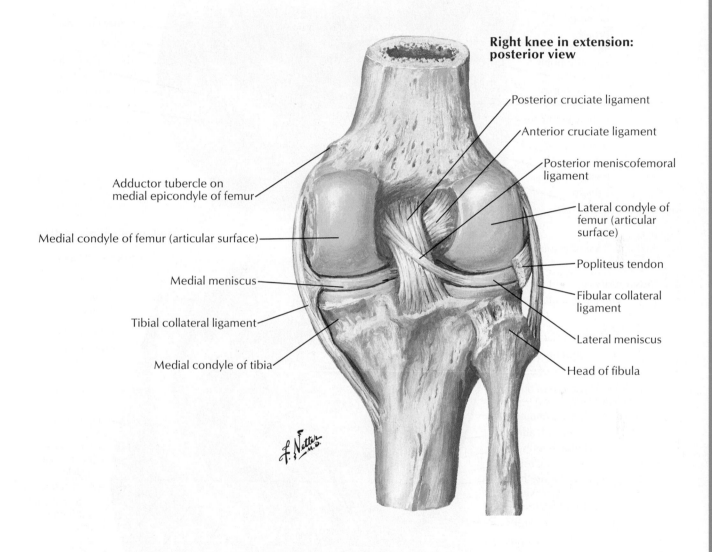

Right knee in extension: posterior view

Posterior cruciate ligament

Anterior cruciate ligament

Posterior meniscofemoral ligament

Lateral condyle of femur (articular surface)

Popliteus tendon

Fibular collateral ligament

Lateral meniscus

Head of fibula

Adductor tubercle on medial epicondyle of femur

Medial condyle of femur (articular surface)

Medial meniscus

Tibial collateral ligament

Medial condyle of tibia

Plate 509 Knee: Cruciate and Collateral Ligaments. (Netter: Atlas of Human Anatomy, 4 ed, 2006, Saunders.)

Paramedian (sagittal) dissection

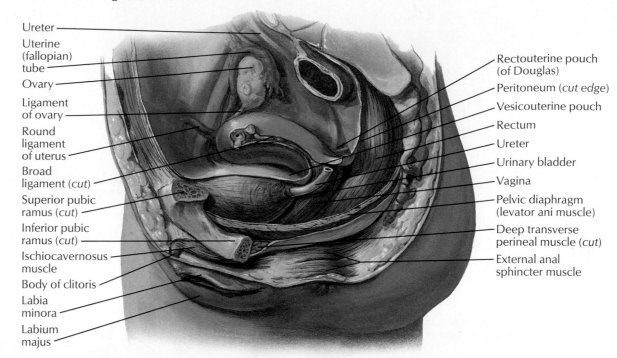

Ureter

Uterine (fallopian) tube

Ovary

Ligament of ovary

Round ligament of uterus

Broad ligament (*cut*)

Superior pubic ramus (*cut*)

Inferior pubic ramus (*cut*)

Ischiocavernosus muscle

Body of clitoris

Labia minora

Labium majus

Rectouterine pouch (of Douglas)

Peritoneum (*cut edge*)

Vesicouterine pouch

Rectum

Ureter

Urinary bladder

Vagina

Pelvic diaphragm (levator ani muscle)

Deep transverse perineal muscle (*cut*)

External anal sphincter muscle

Median (sagittal) section

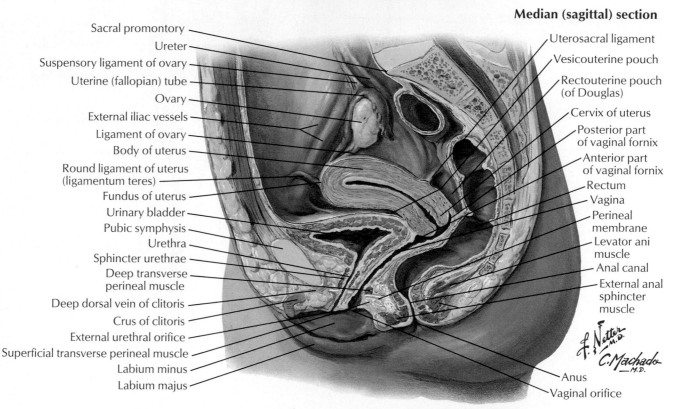

Sacral promontory

Ureter

Suspensory ligament of ovary

Uterine (fallopian) tube

Ovary

External iliac vessels

Ligament of ovary

Body of uterus

Round ligament of uterus (ligamentum teres)

Fundus of uterus

Urinary bladder

Pubic symphysis

Urethra

Sphincter urethrae

Deep transverse perineal muscle

Deep dorsal vein of clitoris

Crus of clitoris

External urethral orifice

Superficial transverse perineal muscle

Labium minus

Labium majus

Uterosacral ligament

Vesicouterine pouch

Rectouterine pouch (of Douglas)

Cervix of uterus

Posterior part of vaginal fornix

Anterior part of vaginal fornix

Rectum

Vagina

Perineal membrane

Levator ani muscle

Anal canal

External anal sphincter muscle

Anus

Vaginal orifice

Plate 360 Pelvic Viscera and Perineum: Female. (Netter: Atlas of Human Anatomy, 4 ed, 2006, Saunders.)

Medical and Surgical

◀ New   ◀〰 Revised   deleted Deleted   ♀ Females Only   ♂ Males Only
Noncovered   Limited Coverage   Hospital-Acquired Condition   **Coding Clinic**

SECTION: 0 MEDICAL AND SURGICAL

BODY SYSTEM: 0 CENTRAL NERVOUS SYSTEM

OPERATION: 1 **BYPASS:** Altering the route of passage of the contents of a tubular body part

Body Part	Approach	Device	Qualifier
6 Cerebral Ventricle	0 Open 3 Percutaneous	7 Autologous Tissue Substitute J Synthetic Substitute K Nonautologous Tissue Substitute	0 Nasopharynx 1 Mastoid Sinus 2 Atrium 3 Blood Vessel 4 Pleural Cavity 5 Intestine 6 Peritoneal Cavity 7 Urinary Tract 8 Bone Marrow B Cerebral Cisterns
U Spinal Canal	0 Open 3 Percutaneous	7 Autologous Tissue Substitute J Synthetic Substitute K Nonautologous Tissue Substitute	4 Pleural Cavity 6 Peritoneal Cavity 7 Urinary Tract 9 Fallopian Tube

Coding Clinic: 2013, Q2, P37 – 00163J6

SECTION: 0 MEDICAL AND SURGICAL

BODY SYSTEM: 0 CENTRAL NERVOUS SYSTEM

OPERATION: 2 **CHANGE:** Taking out or off a device from a body part and putting back an identical or similar device in or on the same body part without cutting or puncturing the skin or a mucous membrane

Body Part	Approach	Device	Qualifier
0 Brain E Cranial Nerve U Spinal Canal	X External	0 Drainage Device Y Other Device	Z No Qualifier

◀ New   ◀ Revised   ~~deleted~~ Deleted   ♀ Females Only   ♂ Males Only
Noncovered   Limited Coverage   Hospital-Acquired Condition   **Coding Clinic**   41

0: M/S 0: CENTRAL NERVOUS SYSTEM 1: BYPASS 2: CHANGE

SECTION: 0 MEDICAL AND SURGICAL
BODY SYSTEM: 0 CENTRAL NERVOUS SYSTEM
OPERATION: 5 DESTRUCTION: Physical eradication of all or a portion of a body part by the direct use of energy, force, or a destructive agent

Body Part	Approach	Device	Qualifier
0 Brain	0 Open	Z No Device	Z No Qualifier
1 Cerebral Meninges	3 Percutaneous		
2 Dura Mater	4 Percutaneous Endoscopic		
6 Cerebral Ventricle			
7 Cerebral Hemisphere			
8 Basal Ganglia			
9 Thalamus			
A Hypothalamus			
B Pons			
C Cerebellum			
D Medulla Oblongata			
F Olfactory Nerve			
G Optic Nerve			
H Oculomotor Nerve			
J Trochlear Nerve			
K Trigeminal Nerve			
L Abducens Nerve			
M Facial Nerve			
N Acoustic Nerve			
P Glossopharyngeal Nerve			
Q Vagus Nerve			
R Accessory Nerve			
S Hypoglossal Nerve			
T Spinal Meninges			
W Cervical Spinal Cord			
X Thoracic Spinal Cord			
Y Lumbar Spinal Cord			

5: DESTRUCTION

0: CENTRAL NERVOUS SYSTEM

0: M/S

◄ New ◄ Revised ~~deleted~~ Deleted ♀ Females Only ♂ Males Only
Noncovered Limited Coverage Hospital-Acquired Condition **Coding Clinic**

SECTION: 0 MEDICAL AND SURGICAL

BODY SYSTEM: 0 CENTRAL NERVOUS SYSTEM

OPERATION: 8 **DIVISION:** Cutting into a body part, without draining fluids and/or gases from the body part, in order to separate or transect a body part

Body Part	Approach	Device	Qualifier
0 Brain 7 Cerebral Hemisphere 8 Basal Ganglia F Olfactory Nerve G Optic Nerve H Oculomotor Nerve J Trochlear Nerve K Trigeminal Nerve L Abducens Nerve M Facial Nerve N Acoustic Nerve P Glossopharyngeal Nerve Q Vagus Nerve R Accessory Nerve S Hypoglossal Nerve W Cervical Spinal Cord X Thoracic Spinal Cord Y Lumbar Spinal Cord	0 Open 3 Percutaneous 4 Percutaneous Endoscopic	Z No Device	Z No Qualifier

◀ New   ◀ⅢⅢ Revised   ~~deleted~~ Deleted   ♀ Females Only   ♂ Males Only

⊘ Noncovered   ⊘ Limited Coverage   ⊘ Hospital-Acquired Condition   **Coding Clinic**

SECTION: 0 MEDICAL AND SURGICAL

BODY SYSTEM: 0 CENTRAL NERVOUS SYSTEM

OPERATION: 9 DRAINAGE: *(on multiple pages)*
Taking or letting out fluids and/or gases from a body part

Body Part	Approach	Device	Qualifier
0 Brain	0 Open	0 Drainage Device	Z No Qualifier
1 Cerebral Meninges	3 Percutaneous		
2 Dura Mater	4 Percutaneous Endoscopic		
3 Epidural Space			
4 Subdural Space			
5 Subarachnoid Space			
6 Cerebral Ventricle			
7 Cerebral Hemisphere			
8 Basal Ganglia			
9 Thalamus			
A Hypothalamus			
B Pons			
C Cerebellum			
D Medulla Oblongata			
F Olfactory Nerve			
G Optic Nerve			
H Oculomotor Nerve			
J Trochlear Nerve			
K Trigeminal Nerve			
L Abducens Nerve			
M Facial Nerve			
N Acoustic Nerve			
P Glossopharyngeal Nerve			
Q Vagus Nerve			
R Accessory Nerve			
S Hypoglossal Nerve			
T Spinal Meninges			
U Spinal Canal			
W Cervical Spinal Cord			
X Thoracic Spinal Cord			
Y Lumbar Spinal Cord			

9: DRAINAGE

0: CENTRAL NERVOUS SYSTEM

0: M/S

◀ New ◀▥ Revised ~~deleted~~ Deleted ♀ Females Only ♂ Males Only
Ⓝ Noncovered Ⓛ Limited Coverage Ⓗ Hospital-Acquired Condition **Coding Clinic**

SECTION: 0 MEDICAL AND SURGICAL
BODY SYSTEM: 0 CENTRAL NERVOUS SYSTEM
OPERATION: 9 DRAINAGE: *(continued)*
Taking or letting out fluids and/or gases from a body part

Body Part	Approach	Device	Qualifier
0 Brain	0 Open	Z No Device	X Diagnostic
1 Cerebral Meninges	3 Percutaneous		Z No Qualifier
2 Dura Mater	4 Percutaneous Endoscopic		
3 Epidural Space			
4 Subdural Space			
5 Subarachnoid Space			
6 Cerebral Ventricle			
7 Cerebral Hemisphere			
8 Basal Ganglia			
9 Thalamus			
A Hypothalamus			
B Pons			
C Cerebellum			
D Medulla Oblongata			
F Olfactory Nerve			
G Optic Nerve			
H Oculomotor Nerve			
J Trochlear Nerve			
K Trigeminal Nerve			
L Abducens Nerve			
M Facial Nerve			
N Acoustic Nerve			
P Glossopharyngeal Nerve			
Q Vagus Nerve			
R Accessory Nerve			
S Hypoglossal Nerve			
T Spinal Meninges			
U Spinal Canal			
W Cervical Spinal Cord			
X Thoracic Spinal Cord			
Y Lumbar Spinal Cord			

0: M/S

0: CENTRAL NERVOUS SYSTEM

9: DRAINAGE

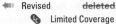

◀ New   ◀▬ Revised   ~~deleted~~ Deleted   ♀ Females Only   ♂ Males Only
Ⓝ Noncovered   Ⓛ Limited Coverage   Ⓗ Hospital-Acquired Condition   **Coding Clinic**

SECTION: 0 MEDICAL AND SURGICAL
BODY SYSTEM: 0 CENTRAL NERVOUS SYSTEM
OPERATION: B EXCISION: Cutting out or off, without replacement, a portion of a body part

Body Part	Approach	Device	Qualifier
0 Brain	0 Open	Z No Device	X Diagnostic
1 Cerebral Meninges	3 Percutaneous		Z No Qualifier
2 Dura Mater	4 Percutaneous Endoscopic		
6 Cerebral Ventricle			
7 Cerebral Hemisphere			
8 Basal Ganglia			
9 Thalamus			
A Hypothalamus			
B Pons			
C Cerebellum			
D Medulla Oblongata			
F Olfactory Nerve			
G Optic Nerve			
H Oculomotor Nerve			
J Trochlear Nerve			
K Trigeminal Nerve			
L Abducens Nerve			
M Facial Nerve			
N Acoustic Nerve			
P Glossopharyngeal Nerve			
Q Vagus Nerve			
R Accessory Nerve			
S Hypoglossal Nerve			
T Spinal Meninges			
W Cervical Spinal Cord			
X Thoracic Spinal Cord			
Y Lumbar Spinal Cord			

B: EXCISION

0: CENTRAL NERVOUS SYSTEM

0: M/S

◀ New ◀◁ Revised ~~deleted~~ Deleted ♀ Females Only ♂ Males Only
Ⓝⓒ Noncovered Ⓛⓒ Limited Coverage Ⓗⓐⓒ Hospital-Acquired Condition **Coding Clinic**

SECTION: 0 MEDICAL AND SURGICAL
BODY SYSTEM: 0 CENTRAL NERVOUS SYSTEM
OPERATION: C EXTIRPATION: Taking or cutting out solid matter from a body part

Body Part	Approach	Device	Qualifier
0 Brain	0 Open	Z No Device	Z No Qualifier
1 Cerebral Meninges	3 Percutaneous		
2 Dura Mater	4 Percutaneous Endoscopic		
3 Epidural Space			
4 Subdural Space			
5 Subarachnoid Space			
6 Cerebral Ventricle			
7 Cerebral Hemisphere			
8 Basal Ganglia			
9 Thalamus			
A Hypothalamus			
B Pons			
C Cerebellum			
D Medulla Oblongata			
F Olfactory Nerve			
G Optic Nerve			
H Oculomotor Nerve			
J Trochlear Nerve			
K Trigeminal Nerve			
L Abducens Nerve			
M Facial Nerve			
N Acoustic Nerve			
P Glossopharyngeal Nerve			
Q Vagus Nerve			
R Accessory Nerve			
S Hypoglossal Nerve			
T Spinal Meninges			
W Cervical Spinal Cord			
X Thoracic Spinal Cord			
Y Lumbar Spinal Cord			

SECTION: 0 MEDICAL AND SURGICAL
BODY SYSTEM: 0 CENTRAL NERVOUS SYSTEM
OPERATION: D EXTRACTION: Pulling or stripping out or off all or a portion of a body part by the use of force

Body Part	Approach	Device	Qualifier
1 Cerebral Meninges	0 Open	Z No Device	Z No Qualifier
2 Dura Mater	3 Percutaneous		
F Olfactory Nerve	4 Percutaneous Endoscopic		
G Optic Nerve			
H Oculomotor Nerve			
J Trochlear Nerve			
K Trigeminal Nerve			
L Abducens Nerve			
M Facial Nerve			
N Acoustic Nerve			
P Glossopharyngeal Nerve			
Q Vagus Nerve			
R Accessory Nerve			
S Hypoglossal Nerve			
T Spinal Meninges			

◀ New ◀▬ Revised ~~deleted~~ Deleted ♀ Females Only ♂ Males Only
⬤ Noncovered ⬤ Limited Coverage ⬤ Hospital-Acquired Condition **Coding Clinic**

SECTION: 0 MEDICAL AND SURGICAL
BODY SYSTEM: 0 CENTRAL NERVOUS SYSTEM
OPERATION: F FRAGMENTATION: Breaking solid matter in a body part into pieces

Body Part	Approach	Device	Qualifier
3 Epidural Space ⊗ 4 Subdural Space ⊗ 5 Subarachnoid Space ⊗ 6 Cerebral Ventricle U Spinal Canal	0 Open 3 Percutaneous 4 Percutaneous Endoscopic X External	Z No Device	Z No Qualifier

⊗ 00F3XZZ, 00F4XZZ, 00F5XZZ, 00F6XZZ

SECTION: 0 MEDICAL AND SURGICAL
BODY SYSTEM: 0 CENTRAL NERVOUS SYSTEM
OPERATION: H INSERTION: Putting in a nonbiological appliance that monitors, assists, performs, or prevents a physiological function but does not physically take the place of a body part

Body Part	Approach	Device	Qualifier
0 Brain 6 Cerebral Ventricle E Cranial Nerve U Spinal Canal V Spinal Cord	0 Open 3 Percutaneous 4 Percutaneous Endoscopic	2 Monitoring Device 3 Infusion Device M Neurostimulator Lead	Z No Qualifier

SECTION: 0 MEDICAL AND SURGICAL
BODY SYSTEM: 0 CENTRAL NERVOUS SYSTEM
OPERATION: J INSPECTION: Visually and/or manually exploring a body part

Body Part	Approach	Device	Qualifier
0 Brain E Cranial Nerve U Spinal Canal V Spinal Cord	0 Open 3 Percutaneous 4 Percutaneous Endoscopic	Z No Device	Z No Qualifier

SECTION: 0 MEDICAL AND SURGICAL
BODY SYSTEM: 0 CENTRAL NERVOUS SYSTEM
OPERATION: **K MAP:** Locating the route of passage of electrical impulses and/or locating functional areas in a body part

Body Part	Approach	Device	Qualifier
0 Brain	0 Open	Z No Device	Z No Qualifier
7 Cerebral Hemisphere	3 Percutaneous		
8 Basal Ganglia	4 Percutaneous Endoscopic		
9 Thalamus			
A Hypothalamus			
B Pons			
C Cerebellum			
D Medulla Oblongata			

SECTION: 0 MEDICAL AND SURGICAL
BODY SYSTEM: 0 CENTRAL NERVOUS SYSTEM
OPERATION: **N RELEASE:** Freeing a body part from an abnormal physical constraint by cutting or by the use of force

Body Part	Approach	Device	Qualifier
0 Brain	0 Open	Z No Device	Z No Qualifier
1 Cerebral Meninges	3 Percutaneous		
2 Dura Mater	4 Percutaneous Endoscopic		
6 Cerebral Ventricle			
7 Cerebral Hemisphere			
8 Basal Ganglia			
9 Thalamus			
A Hypothalamus			
B Pons			
C Cerebellum			
D Medulla Oblongata			
F Olfactory Nerve			
G Optic Nerve			
H Oculomotor Nerve			
J Trochlear Nerve			
K Trigeminal Nerve			
L Abducens Nerve			
M Facial Nerve			
N Acoustic Nerve			
P Glossopharyngeal Nerve			
Q Vagus Nerve			
R Accessory Nerve			
S Hypoglossal Nerve			
T Spinal Meninges			
W Cervical Spinal Cord			
X Thoracic Spinal Cord			
Y Lumbar Spinal Cord			

◀ New ◀ Revised ~~deleted~~ Deleted ♀ Females Only ♂ Males Only
Noncovered Limited Coverage Hospital-Acquired Condition **Coding Clinic**

49

0: M/S 0: CENTRAL NERVOUS SYSTEM K: MAP N: RELEASE

SECTION: 0 MEDICAL AND SURGICAL
BODY SYSTEM: 0 CENTRAL NERVOUS SYSTEM
OPERATION: P REMOVAL: Taking out or off a device from a body part

Body Part	Approach	Device	Qualifier
0 Brain V Spinal Cord	0 Open 3 Percutaneous 4 Percutaneous Endoscopic	0 Drainage Device 2 Monitoring Device 3 Infusion Device 7 Autologous Tissue Substitute J Synthetic Substitute K Nonautologous Tissue Substitute M Neurostimulator Lead	Z No Qualifier
0 Brain V Spinal Cord	X External	0 Drainage Device 2 Monitoring Device 3 Infusion Device M Neurostimulator Lead	Z No Qualifier
6 Cerebral Ventricle U Spinal Canal	0 Open 3 Percutaneous 4 Percutaneous Endoscopic	0 Drainage Device 2 Monitoring Device 3 Infusion Device J Synthetic Substitute M Neurostimulator Lead	Z No Qualifier
6 Cerebral Ventricle U Spinal Canal	X External	0 Drainage Device 2 Monitoring Device 3 Infusion Device M Neurostimulator Lead	Z No Qualifier
E Cranial Nerve	0 Open 3 Percutaneous 4 Percutaneous Endoscopic	0 Drainage Device 2 Monitoring Device 3 Infusion Device 7 Autologous Tissue Substitute M Neurostimulator Lead	Z No Qualifier
E Cranial Nerve	X External	0 Drainage Device 2 Monitoring Device 3 Infusion Device M Neurostimulator Lead	Z No Qualifier

P: REMOVAL

0: CENTRAL NERVOUS SYSTEM

0: M/S

◀ New ◀ Revised ~~deleted~~ Deleted ♀ Females Only ♂ Males Only
Noncovered Limited Coverage Hospital-Acquired Condition **Coding Clinic**

SECTION: 0 MEDICAL AND SURGICAL
BODY SYSTEM: 0 CENTRAL NERVOUS SYSTEM
OPERATION: Q REPAIR: Restoring, to the extent possible, a body part to its normal anatomic structure and function

Body Part	Approach	Device	Qualifier
0 Brain	0 Open	Z No Device	Z No Qualifier
1 Cerebral Meninges	3 Percutaneous		
2 Dura Mater	4 Percutaneous Endoscopic		
6 Cerebral Ventricle			
7 Cerebral Hemisphere			
8 Basal Ganglia			
9 Thalamus			
A Hypothalamus			
B Pons			
C Cerebellum			
D Medulla Oblongata			
F Olfactory Nerve			
G Optic Nerve			
H Oculomotor Nerve			
J Trochlear Nerve			
K Trigeminal Nerve			
L Abducens Nerve			
M Facial Nerve			
N Acoustic Nerve			
P Glossopharyngeal Nerve			
Q Vagus Nerve			
R Accessory Nerve			
S Hypoglossal Nerve			
T Spinal Meninges			
W Cervical Spinal Cord			
X Thoracic Spinal Cord			
Y Lumbar Spinal Cord			

Coding Clinic: 2013, Q3, P25 – 00Q20ZZ

SECTION: 0 MEDICAL AND SURGICAL
BODY SYSTEM: 0 CENTRAL NERVOUS SYSTEM
OPERATION: S REPOSITION: Moving to its normal location, or other suitable location, all or a portion of a body part

Body Part	Approach	Device	Qualifier
F Olfactory Nerve	0 Open	Z No Device	Z No Qualifier
G Optic Nerve	3 Percutaneous		
H Oculomotor Nerve	4 Percutaneous Endoscopic		
J Trochlear Nerve			
K Trigeminal Nerve			
L Abducens Nerve			
M Facial Nerve			
N Acoustic Nerve			
P Glossopharyngeal Nerve			
Q Vagus Nerve			
R Accessory Nerve			
S Hypoglossal Nerve			
W Cervical Spinal Cord			
X Thoracic Spinal Cord			
Y Lumbar Spinal Cord			

◀ New   ◀ Revised   deleted Deleted   ♀ Females Only   ♂ Males Only
Noncovered   Limited Coverage   Hospital-Acquired Condition   **Coding Clinic**

51

SECTION: 0 MEDICAL AND SURGICAL
BODY SYSTEM: 0 CENTRAL NERVOUS SYSTEM
OPERATION: **T** **RESECTION:** Cutting out or off, without replacement, all of a body part

Body Part	Approach	Device	Qualifier
7 Cerebral Hemisphere	0 Open 3 Percutaneous 4 Percutaneous Endoscopic	Z No Device	Z No Qualifier

SECTION: 0 MEDICAL AND SURGICAL
BODY SYSTEM: 0 CENTRAL NERVOUS SYSTEM
OPERATION: **U** **SUPPLEMENT:** Putting in or on biological or synthetic material that physically reinforces and/or augments the function of a portion of a body part

Body Part	Approach	Device	Qualifier
1 Cerebral Meninges 2 Dura Mater T Spinal Meninges	0 Open 3 Percutaneous 4 Percutaneous Endoscopic	7 Autologous Tissue Substitute J Synthetic Substitute K Nonautologous Tissue Substitute	Z No Qualifier
F Olfactory Nerve G Optic Nerve H Oculomotor Nerve J Trochlear Nerve K Trigeminal Nerve L Abducens Nerve M Facial Nerve N Acoustic Nerve P Glossopharyngeal Nerve Q Vagus Nerve R Accessory Nerve S Hypoglossal Nerve	0 Open 3 Percutaneous 4 Percutaneous Endoscopic	7 Autologous Tissue Substitute	Z No Qualifier

T: RESECTION   U: SUPPLEMENT

0: CENTRAL NERVOUS SYSTEM

0: M/S

SECTION: 0 MEDICAL AND SURGICAL
BODY SYSTEM: 0 CENTRAL NERVOUS SYSTEM
OPERATION: W REVISION: Correcting, to the extent possible, a portion of a malfunctioning device or the position of a displaced device

Body Part	Approach	Device	Qualifier
0 Brain V Spinal Cord	0 Open 3 Percutaneous 4 Percutaneous Endoscopic X External	0 Drainage Device 2 Monitoring Device 3 Infusion Device 7 Autologous Tissue Substitute J Synthetic Substitute K Nonautologous Tissue Substitute M Neurostimulator Lead	Z No Qualifier
6 Cerebral Ventricle U Spinal Canal	0 Open 3 Percutaneous 4 Percutaneous Endoscopic X External	0 Drainage Device 2 Monitoring Device 3 Infusion Device J Synthetic Substitute M Neurostimulator Lead	Z No Qualifier
E Cranial Nerve	0 Open 3 Percutaneous 4 Percutaneous Endoscopic X External	0 Drainage Device 2 Monitoring Device 3 Infusion Device 7 Autologous Tissue Substitute M Neurostimulator Lead	Z No Qualifier

SECTION: 0 MEDICAL AND SURGICAL
BODY SYSTEM: 0 CENTRAL NERVOUS SYSTEM
OPERATION: X TRANSFER: Moving, without taking out, all or a portion of a body part to another location to take over the function of all or a portion of a body part

Body Part	Approach	Device	Qualifier
F Olfactory Nerve G Optic Nerve H Oculomotor Nerve J Trochlear Nerve K Trigeminal Nerve L Abducens Nerve M Facial Nerve N Acoustic Nerve P Glossopharyngeal Nerve Q Vagus Nerve R Accessory Nerve S Hypoglossal Nerve	0 Open 4 Percutaneous Endoscopic	Z No Device	F Olfactory Nerve G Optic Nerve H Oculomotor Nerve J Trochlear Nerve K Trigeminal Nerve L Abducens Nerve M Facial Nerve N Acoustic Nerve P Glossopharyngeal Nerve Q Vagus Nerve R Accessory Nerve S Hypoglossal Nerve

0: M/S

0: CENTRAL NERVOUS SYSTEM

W: REVISION X: TRANSFER

◀ New ◀▦ Revised ~~deleted~~ Deleted ♀ Females Only ♂ Males Only
Ⓝ Noncovered Ⓛ Limited Coverage Ⓗ Hospital-Acquired Condition **Coding Clinic**

SECTION: 0 MEDICAL AND SURGICAL
BODY SYSTEM: 1 PERIPHERAL NERVOUS SYSTEM
OPERATION: 2 CHANGE: Taking out or off a device from a body part and putting back an identical or similar device in or on the same body part without cutting or puncturing the skin or a mucous membrane

Body Part	Approach	Device	Qualifier
Y Peripheral Nerve	X External	0 Drainage Device Y Other Device	Z No Qualifier

SECTION: 0 MEDICAL AND SURGICAL
BODY SYSTEM: 1 PERIPHERAL NERVOUS SYSTEM
OPERATION: 5 DESTRUCTION: Physical eradication of all or a portion of a body part by the direct use of energy, force, or a destructive agent

Body Part	Approach	Device	Qualifier
0 Cervical Plexus 1 Cervical Nerve 2 Phrenic Nerve 3 Brachial Plexus 4 Ulnar Nerve 5 Median Nerve 6 Radial Nerve 8 Thoracic Nerve 9 Lumbar Plexus A Lumbosacral Plexus B Lumbar Nerve C Pudendal Nerve D Femoral Nerve F Sciatic Nerve G Tibial Nerve H Peroneal Nerve K Head and Neck Sympathetic Nerve L Thoracic Sympathetic Nerve M Abdominal Sympathetic Nerve N Lumbar Sympathetic Nerve P Sacral Sympathetic Nerve Q Sacral Plexus R Sacral Nerve	0 Open 3 Percutaneous 4 Percutaneous Endoscopic	Z No Device	Z No Qualifier

SECTION: 0 MEDICAL AND SURGICAL
BODY SYSTEM: 1 PERIPHERAL NERVOUS SYSTEM
OPERATION: 8 **DIVISION:** Cutting into a body part, without draining fluids and/or gases from the body part, in order to separate or transect a body part

Body Part	Approach	Device	Qualifier
0 Cervical Plexus	0 Open	Z No Device	Z No Qualifier
1 Cervical Nerve	3 Percutaneous		
2 Phrenic Nerve	4 Percutaneous Endoscopic		
3 Brachial Plexus			
4 Ulnar Nerve			
5 Median Nerve			
6 Radial Nerve			
8 Thoracic Nerve			
9 Lumbar Plexus			
A Lumbosacral Plexus			
B Lumbar Nerve			
C Pudendal Nerve			
D Femoral Nerve			
F Sciatic Nerve			
G Tibial Nerve			
H Peroneal Nerve			
K Head and Neck Sympathetic Nerve			
L Thoracic Sympathetic Nerve			
M Abdominal Sympathetic Nerve			
N Lumbar Sympathetic Nerve			
P Sacral Sympathetic Nerve			
Q Sacral Plexus			
R Sacral Nerve			

8: DIVISION

1: PERIPHERAL NERVOUS SYSTEM

0: M/S

◀ New ◀▥ Revised deleted Deleted ♀ Females Only ♂ Males Only
🅠 Noncovered 🅠 Limited Coverage 🅠 Hospital-Acquired Condition **Coding Clinic**

SECTION: 0 MEDICAL AND SURGICAL
BODY SYSTEM: 1 PERIPHERAL NERVOUS SYSTEM
OPERATION: 9 DRAINAGE: Taking or letting out fluids and/or gases from a body part

Body Part	Approach	Device	Qualifier
0 Cervical Plexus 1 Cervical Nerve 2 Phrenic Nerve 3 Brachial Plexus 4 Ulnar Nerve 5 Median Nerve 6 Radial Nerve 8 Thoracic Nerve 9 Lumbar Plexus A Lumbosacral Plexus B Lumbar Nerve C Pudendal Nerve D Femoral Nerve F Sciatic Nerve G Tibial Nerve H Peroneal Nerve K Head and Neck Sympathetic Nerve L Thoracic Sympathetic Nerve M Abdominal Sympathetic Nerve N Lumbar Sympathetic Nerve P Sacral Sympathetic Nerve Q Sacral Plexus R Sacral Nerve	0 Open 3 Percutaneous 4 Percutaneous Endoscopic	0 Drainage Device	Z No Qualifier
0 Cervical Plexus 1 Cervical Nerve 2 Phrenic Nerve 3 Brachial Plexus 4 Ulnar Nerve 5 Median Nerve 6 Radial Nerve 8 Thoracic Nerve 9 Lumbar Plexus A Lumbosacral Plexus B Lumbar Nerve C Pudendal Nerve D Femoral Nerve F Sciatic Nerve G Tibial Nerve H Peroneal Nerve K Head and Neck Sympathetic Nerve L Thoracic Sympathetic Nerve M Abdominal Sympathetic Nerve N Lumbar Sympathetic Nerve P Sacral Sympathetic Nerve Q Sacral Plexus R Sacral Nerve	0 Open 3 Percutaneous 4 Percutaneous Endoscopic	Z No Device	X Diagnostic Z No Qualifier

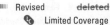

◀ New　◀■ Revised　deleted Deleted　♀ Females Only　♂ Males Only
Ⓝ Noncovered　Ⓛ Limited Coverage　Ⓗ Hospital-Acquired Condition　**Coding Clinic**

SECTION: 0 MEDICAL AND SURGICAL
BODY SYSTEM: 1 PERIPHERAL NERVOUS SYSTEM
OPERATION: B EXCISION: Cutting out or off, without replacement, a portion of a body part

Body Part	Approach	Device	Qualifier
0 Cervical Plexus	0 Open	Z No Device	X Diagnostic
1 Cervical Nerve	3 Percutaneous		Z No Qualifier
2 Phrenic Nerve	4 Percutaneous Endoscopic		
3 Brachial Plexus			
4 Ulnar Nerve			
5 Median Nerve			
6 Radial Nerve			
8 Thoracic Nerve			
9 Lumbar Plexus			
A Lumbosacral Plexus			
B Lumbar Nerve			
C Pudendal Nerve			
D Femoral Nerve			
F Sciatic Nerve			
G Tibial Nerve			
H Peroneal Nerve			
K Head and Neck Sympathetic Nerve			
L Thoracic Sympathetic Nerve			
M Abdominal Sympathetic Nerve			
N Lumbar Sympathetic Nerve			
P Sacral Sympathetic Nerve			
Q Sacral Plexus			
R Sacral Nerve			

SECTION: 0 MEDICAL AND SURGICAL
BODY SYSTEM: 1 PERIPHERAL NERVOUS SYSTEM
OPERATION: C EXTIRPATION: Taking or cutting out solid matter from a body part

Body Part	Approach	Device	Qualifier
0 Cervical Plexus	0 Open	Z No Device	Z No Qualifier
1 Cervical Nerve	3 Percutaneous		
2 Phrenic Nerve	4 Percutaneous Endoscopic		
3 Brachial Plexus			
4 Ulnar Nerve			
5 Median Nerve			
6 Radial Nerve			
8 Thoracic Nerve			
9 Lumbar Plexus			
A Lumbosacral Plexus			
B Lumbar Nerve			
C Pudendal Nerve			
D Femoral Nerve			
F Sciatic Nerve			
G Tibial Nerve			
H Peroneal Nerve			
K Head and Neck Sympathetic Nerve			
L Thoracic Sympathetic Nerve			
M Abdominal Sympathetic Nerve			
N Lumbar Sympathetic Nerve			
P Sacral Sympathetic Nerve			
Q Sacral Plexus			
R Sacral Nerve			

◀ New   ◀▥ Revised   deleted Deleted   ♀ Females Only   ♂ Males Only
Noncovered   Limited Coverage   Hospital-Acquired Condition   **Coding Clinic**

SECTION: 0 MEDICAL AND SURGICAL
BODY SYSTEM: 1 PERIPHERAL NERVOUS SYSTEM
OPERATION: D EXTRACTION: Pulling or stripping out or off all or a portion of a body part by the use of force

Body Part	Approach	Device	Qualifier
0 Cervical Plexus 1 Cervical Nerve 2 Phrenic Nerve 3 Brachial Plexus 4 Ulnar Nerve 5 Median Nerve 6 Radial Nerve 8 Thoracic Nerve 9 Lumbar Plexus A Lumbosacral Plexus B Lumbar Nerve C Pudendal Nerve D Femoral Nerve F Sciatic Nerve G Tibial Nerve H Peroneal Nerve K Head and Neck Sympathetic Nerve L Thoracic Sympathetic Nerve M Abdominal Sympathetic Nerve N Lumbar Sympathetic Nerve P Sacral Sympathetic Nerve Q Sacral Plexus R Sacral Nerve	0 Open 3 Percutaneous 4 Percutaneous Endoscopic	Z No Device	Z No Qualifier

SECTION: 0 MEDICAL AND SURGICAL
BODY SYSTEM: 1 PERIPHERAL NERVOUS SYSTEM
OPERATION: H INSERTION: Putting in a nonbiological appliance that monitors, assists, performs, or prevents a physiological function but does not physically take the place of a body part

Body Part	Approach	Device	Qualifier
Y Peripheral Nerve	0 Open 3 Percutaneous 4 Percutaneous Endoscopic	2 Monitoring Device M Neurostimulator Lead	Z No Qualifier

SECTION: 0 MEDICAL AND SURGICAL
BODY SYSTEM: 1 PERIPHERAL NERVOUS SYSTEM
OPERATION: J INSPECTION: Visually and/or manually exploring a body part

Body Part	Approach	Device	Qualifier
Y Peripheral Nerve	0 Open 3 Percutaneous 4 Percutaneous Endoscopic	Z No Device	Z No Qualifier

◀ New ◀ Revised ~~deleted~~ Deleted ♀ Females Only ♂ Males Only
Noncovered Limited Coverage Hospital-Acquired Condition **Coding Clinic**

59

SECTION: 0 MEDICAL AND SURGICAL
BODY SYSTEM: 1 PERIPHERAL NERVOUS SYSTEM
OPERATION: N RELEASE: Freeing a body part from an abnormal physical constraint by cutting or by the use of force

Body Part	Approach	Device	Qualifier
0 Cervical Plexus 1 Cervical Nerve 2 Phrenic Nerve 3 Brachial Plexus 4 Ulnar Nerve 5 Median Nerve 6 Radial Nerve 8 Thoracic Nerve 9 Lumbar Plexus A Lumbosacral Plexus B Lumbar Nerve C Pudendal Nerve D Femoral Nerve F Sciatic Nerve G Tibial Nerve H Peroneal Nerve K Head and Neck Sympathetic Nerve L Thoracic Sympathetic Nerve M Abdominal Sympathetic Nerve N Lumbar Sympathetic Nerve P Sacral Sympathetic Nerve Q Sacral Plexus R Sacral Nerve	0 Open 3 Percutaneous 4 Percutaneous Endoscopic	Z No Device	Z No Qualifier

SECTION: 0 MEDICAL AND SURGICAL
BODY SYSTEM: 1 PERIPHERAL NERVOUS SYSTEM
OPERATION: P REMOVAL: Taking out or off a device from a body part

Body Part	Approach	Device	Qualifier
Y Peripheral Nerve	0 Open 3 Percutaneous 4 Percutaneous Endoscopic	0 Drainage Device 2 Monitoring Device 7 Autologous Tissue Substitute M Neurostimulator Lead	Z No Qualifier
Y Peripheral Nerve	X External	0 Drainage Device 2 Monitoring Device M Neurostimulator Lead	Z No Qualifier

◀ New   ◀▥ Revised   ~~deleted~~ Deleted   ♀ Females Only   ♂ Males Only
🅝 Noncovered   🅛 Limited Coverage   🅗 Hospital-Acquired Condition   **Coding Clinic**

SECTION: 0 MEDICAL AND SURGICAL
BODY SYSTEM: 1 PERIPHERAL NERVOUS SYSTEM
OPERATION: Q **REPAIR:** Restoring, to the extent possible, a body part to its normal anatomic structure and function

Body Part	Approach	Device	Qualifier
0 Cervical Plexus	0 Open	Z No Device	Z No Qualifier
1 Cervical Nerve	3 Percutaneous		
2 Phrenic Nerve	4 Percutaneous Endoscopic		
3 Brachial Plexus			
4 Ulnar Nerve			
5 Median Nerve			
6 Radial Nerve			
8 Thoracic Nerve			
9 Lumbar Plexus			
A Lumbosacral Plexus			
B Lumbar Nerve			
C Pudendal Nerve			
D Femoral Nerve			
F Sciatic Nerve			
G Tibial Nerve			
H Peroneal Nerve			
K Head and Neck Sympathetic Nerve			
L Thoracic Sympathetic Nerve			
M Abdominal Sympathetic Nerve			
N Lumbar Sympathetic Nerve			
P Sacral Sympathetic Nerve			
Q Sacral Plexus			
R Sacral Nerve			

SECTION: 0 MEDICAL AND SURGICAL
BODY SYSTEM: 1 PERIPHERAL NERVOUS SYSTEM
OPERATION: S **REPOSITION:** Moving to its normal location, or other suitable location, all or a portion of a body part

Body Part	Approach	Device	Qualifier
0 Cervical Plexus	0 Open	Z No Device	Z No Qualifier
1 Cervical Nerve	3 Percutaneous		
2 Phrenic Nerve	4 Percutaneous Endoscopic		
3 Brachial Plexus			
4 Ulnar Nerve			
5 Median Nerve			
6 Radial Nerve			
8 Thoracic Nerve			
9 Lumbar Plexus			
A Lumbosacral Plexus			
B Lumbar Nerve			
C Pudendal Nerve			
D Femoral Nerve			
F Sciatic Nerve			
G Tibial Nerve			
H Peroneal Nerve			
Q Sacral Plexus			
R Sacral Nerve			

SECTION: 0 MEDICAL AND SURGICAL
BODY SYSTEM: 1 PERIPHERAL NERVOUS SYSTEM
OPERATION: U SUPPLEMENT: Putting in or on biological or synthetic material that physically reinforces and/or augments the function of a portion of a body part

Body Part	Approach	Device	Qualifier
1 Cervical Nerve 2 Phrenic Nerve 4 Ulnar Nerve 5 Median Nerve 6 Radial Nerve 8 Thoracic Nerve B Lumbar Nerve C Pudendal Nerve D Femoral Nerve F Sciatic Nerve G Tibial Nerve H Peroneal Nerve R Sacral Nerve	0 Open 3 Percutaneous 4 Percutaneous Endoscopic	7 Autologous Tissue Substitute	Z No Qualifier

SECTION: 0 MEDICAL AND SURGICAL
BODY SYSTEM: 1 PERIPHERAL NERVOUS SYSTEM
OPERATION: W REVISION: Correcting, to the extent possible, a portion of a malfunctioning device or the position of a displaced device

Body Part	Approach	Device	Qualifier
Y Peripheral Nerve	0 Open 3 Percutaneous 4 Percutaneous Endoscopic X External	0 Drainage Device 2 Monitoring Device 7 Autologous Tissue Substitute M Neurostimulator Lead	Z No Qualifier

◀ New ◀ Revised ~~deleted~~ Deleted ♀ Females Only ♂ Males Only
🅝 Noncovered 🅛 Limited Coverage 🅗 Hospital-Acquired Condition **Coding Clinic**

SECTION: 0 MEDICAL AND SURGICAL
BODY SYSTEM: 1 PERIPHERAL NERVOUS SYSTEM
OPERATION: X TRANSFER: Moving, without taking out, all or a portion of a body part to another location to take over the function of all or a portion of a body part

Body Part	Approach	Device	Qualifier
1 Cervical Nerve 2 Phrenic Nerve	0 Open 4 Percutaneous Endoscopic	Z No Device	1 Cervical Nerve 2 Phrenic Nerve
4 Ulnar Nerve 5 Median Nerve 6 Radial Nerve	0 Open 4 Percutaneous Endoscopic	Z No Device	4 Ulnar Nerve 5 Median Nerve 6 Radial Nerve
8 Thoracic Nerve	0 Open 4 Percutaneous Endoscopic	Z No Device	8 Thoracic Nerve
B Lumbar Nerve C Pudendal Nerve	0 Open 4 Percutaneous Endoscopic	Z No Device	B Lumbar Nerve C Pudendal Nerve
D Femoral Nerve F Sciatic Nerve G Tibial Nerve H Peroneal Nerve	0 Open 4 Percutaneous Endoscopic	Z No Device	D Femoral Nerve F Sciatic Nerve G Tibial Nerve H Peroneal Nerve

◀ New ◀▥ Revised deleted Deleted ♀ Females Only ♂ Males Only
🚫 Noncovered 🚫 Limited Coverage 🚫 Hospital-Acquired Condition **Coding Clinic**

63

◀ New　◀▥ Revised　deleted Deleted　♀ Females Only　♂ Males Only
🅝 Noncovered　🅛 Limited Coverage　🅗 Hospital-Acquired Condition　**Coding Clinic**

SECTION: 0 MEDICAL AND SURGICAL

BODY SYSTEM: 2 HEART AND GREAT VESSELS

OPERATION: **1** **BYPASS:** *(on multiple pages)*

Altering the route of passage of the contents of a tubular body part

Body Part	Approach	Device	Qualifier
0 Coronary Artery, One Site 🔲 1 Coronary Artery, Two Sites 🔲 2 Coronary Artery, Three Sites 🔲 3 Coronary Artery, Four or More Sites 🔲	0 Open	9 Autologous Venous Tissue A Autologous Arterial Tissue J Synthetic Substitute K Nonautologous Tissue Substitute	3 Coronary Artery 8 Internal Mammary, Right 9 Internal Mammary, Left C Thoracic Artery F Abdominal Artery W Aorta
0 Coronary Artery, One Site 🔲 1 Coronary Artery, Two Sites 🔲 2 Coronary Artery, Three Sites 🔲 3 Coronary Artery, Four or More Sites 🔲	0 Open	Z No Device	3 Coronary Artery 8 Internal Mammary, Right 9 Internal Mammary, Left C Thoracic Artery F Abdominal Artery
0 Coronary Artery, One Site 1 Coronary Artery, Two Sites 2 Coronary Artery, Three Sites 3 Coronary Artery, Four or More Sites	3 Percutaneous	4 Drug-eluting Intraluminal Device D Intraluminal Device	4 Coronary Vein
0 Coronary Artery, One Site 1 Coronary Artery, Two Sites 2 Coronary Artery, Three Sites 3 Coronary Artery, Four or More Sites	4 Percutaneous Endoscopic	4 Drug-eluting Intraluminal Device D Intraluminal Device	4 Coronary Vein
0 Coronary Artery, One Site 🔲 1 Coronary Artery, Two Sites 🔲 2 Coronary Artery, Three Sites 🔲 3 Coronary Artery, Four or More Sites 🔲	4 Percutaneous Endoscopic	9 Autologous Venous Tissue A Autologous Arterial Tissue J Synthetic Substitute K Nonautologous Tissue Substitute	3 Coronary Artery 8 Internal Mammary, Right 9 Internal Mammary, Left C Thoracic Artery F Abdominal Artery W Aorta
0 Coronary Artery, One Site 🔲 1 Coronary Artery, Two Sites 🔲 2 Coronary Artery, Three Sites 🔲 3 Coronary Artery, Four or More Sites 🔲	4 Percutaneous Endoscopic	Z No Device	3 Coronary Artery 8 Internal Mammary, Right 9 Internal Mammary, Left C Thoracic Artery F Abdominal Artery
6 Atrium, Right	0 Open 4 Percutaneous Endoscopic	9 Autologous Venous Tissue A Autologous Arterial Tissue J Synthetic Substitute K Nonautologous Tissue Substitute	P Pulmonary Trunk Q Pulmonary Artery, Right R Pulmonary Artery, Left
6 Atrium, Right	0 Open 4 Percutaneous Endoscopic	Z No Device	7 Atrium, Left P Pulmonary Trunk Q Pulmonary Artery, Right R Pulmonary Artery, Left
7 Atrium, Left V Superior Vena Cava	0 Open 4 Percutaneous Endoscopic	9 Autologous Venous Tissue A Autologous Arterial Tissue J Synthetic Substitute K Nonautologous Tissue Substitute Z No Device	P Pulmonary Trunk Q Pulmonary Artery, Right R Pulmonary Artery, Left
K Ventricle, Right L Ventricle, Left	0 Open 4 Percutaneous Endoscopic	9 Autologous Venous Tissue A Autologous Arterial Tissue J Synthetic Substitute K Nonautologous Tissue Substitute	P Pulmonary Trunk Q Pulmonary Artery, Right R Pulmonary Artery, Left

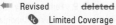

◀ New ⬅ Revised ~~deleted~~ Deleted ♀ Females Only ♂ Males Only
🔲 Noncovered 🔲 Limited Coverage 🔲 Hospital-Acquired Condition **Coding Clinic**

2: HEART AND GREAT VESSELS   **1: BYPASS**   **5: DESTRUCTION**   **0: M/S**

SECTION: 0 MEDICAL AND SURGICAL

BODY SYSTEM: 2 HEART AND GREAT VESSELS

OPERATION: 1 BYPASS: *(continued)*

Altering the route of passage of the contents of a tubular body part

Body Part	Approach	Device	Qualifier
K Ventricle, Right L Ventricle, Left	0 Open 4 Percutaneous Endoscopic	Z No Device	5 Coronary Circulation 8 Internal Mammary, Right 9 Internal Mammary, Left C Thoracic Artery F Abdominal Artery P Pulmonary Trunk Q Pulmonary Artery, Right R Pulmonary Artery, Left W Aorta
W Thoracic Aorta	0 Open 4 Percutaneous Endoscopic	9 Autologous Venous Tissue A Autologous Arterial Tissue J Synthetic Substitute K Nonautologous Tissue Substitute Z No Device	B Subclavian D Carotid P Pulmonary Trunk Q Pulmonary Artery, Right R Pulmonary Artery, Left

SECTION: 0 MEDICAL AND SURGICAL

BODY SYSTEM: 2 HEART AND GREAT VESSELS

OPERATION: 5 DESTRUCTION: Physical eradication of all or a portion of a body part by the direct use of energy, force, or a destructive agent

Body Part	Approach	Device	Qualifier
4 Coronary Vein 5 Atrial Septum 6 Atrium, Right 7 Atrium, Left 8 Conduction Mechanism 9 Chordae Tendineae D Papillary Muscle F Aortic Valve G Mitral Valve H Pulmonary Valve J Tricuspid Valve K Ventricle, Right L Ventricle, Left M Ventricular Septum N Pericardium P Pulmonary Trunk Q Pulmonary Artery, Right R Pulmonary Artery, Left S Pulmonary Vein, Right T Pulmonary Vein, Left V Superior Vena Cava W Thoracic Aorta	0 Open 3 Percutaneous 4 Percutaneous Endoscopic	Z No Device	Z No Qualifier
7 Atrium, Left	0 Open 3 Percutaneous 4 Percutaneous Endoscopic	Z No Device	K Left Atrial Appendage Z No Qualifier

Coding Clinic: 2013, Q2, P39 – 025S3ZZ, 025T3ZZ

◀ New   ◀▥ Revised   ~~deleted~~ Deleted   ♀ Females Only   ♂ Males Only
🔖 Noncovered   🔖 Limited Coverage   🔖 Hospital-Acquired Condition   **Coding Clinic**

SECTION: 0 MEDICAL AND SURGICAL
BODY SYSTEM: 2 HEART AND GREAT VESSELS
OPERATION: 7 DILATION: Expanding an orifice or the lumen of a tubular body part

Body Part	Approach	Device	Qualifier
0 Coronary Artery, One Site 1 Coronary Artery, Two Sites 2 Coronary Artery, Three Sites 3 Coronary Artery, Four or More Sites	0 Open 3 Percutaneous 4 Percutaneous Endoscopic	4 Drug-eluting Intraluminal Device D Intraluminal Device T Radioactive Intraluminal Device Z No Device	6 Bifurcation Z No Qualifier
F Aortic Valve G Mitral Valve H Pulmonary Valve J Tricuspid Valve K Ventricle, Right P Pulmonary Trunk Q Pulmonary Artery, Right S Pulmonary Vein, Right T Pulmonary Vein, Left V Superior Vena Cava W Thoracic Aorta	0 Open 3 Percutaneous 4 Percutaneous Endoscopic	4 Drug-eluting Intraluminal Device D Intraluminal Device Z No Device	Z No Qualifier
R Pulmonary Artery, Left	0 Open 3 Percutaneous 4 Percutaneous Endoscopic	4 Drug-eluting Intraluminal Device D Intraluminal Device Z No Device	T Ductus Arteriosus Z No Qualifier

SECTION: 0 MEDICAL AND SURGICAL
BODY SYSTEM: 2 HEART AND GREAT VESSELS
OPERATION: 8 DIVISION: Cutting into a body part, without draining fluids and/or gases from the body part, in order to separate or transect a body part

Body Part	Approach	Device	Qualifier
8 Conduction Mechanism 9 Chordae Tendineae D Papillary Muscle	0 Open 3 Percutaneous 4 Percutaneous Endoscopic	Z No Device	Z No Qualifier

0: M/S 2: HEART AND GREAT VESSELS 7: DILATION 8: DIVISION

SECTION: 0 MEDICAL AND SURGICAL
BODY SYSTEM: 2 HEART AND GREAT VESSELS
OPERATION: B EXCISION: Cutting out or off, without replacement, a portion of a body part

Body Part	Approach	Device	Qualifier
4 Coronary Vein 5 Atrial Septum 6 Atrium, Right 8 Conduction Mechanism 9 Chordae Tendineae D Papillary Muscle F Aortic Valve G Mitral Valve H Pulmonary Valve J Tricuspid Valve K Ventricle, Right 🚱 L Ventricle, Left 🚱 M Ventricular Septum N Pericardium P Pulmonary Trunk Q Pulmonary Artery, Right R Pulmonary Artery, Left S Pulmonary Vein, Right T Pulmonary Vein, Left V Superior Vena Cava W Thoracic Aorta	0 Open 3 Percutaneous 4 Percutaneous Endoscopic	Z No Device	X Diagnostic Z No Qualifier
7 Atrium, Left	0 Open 3 Percutaneous 4 Percutaneous Endoscopic	Z No Device	K Left Atrial Appendage X Diagnostic Z No Qualifier

🚱 02BK0ZZ, 02BK3ZZ, 02BK4ZZ
🚱 02BL0ZZ, 02BL3ZZ, 02BL4ZZ

◀ New   ◀▥ Revised   ~~deleted~~ Deleted   ♀ Females Only   ♂ Males Only
🚱 Noncovered   🚱 Limited Coverage   🚱 Hospital-Acquired Condition   **Coding Clinic**

SECTION: 0 MEDICAL AND SURGICAL
BODY SYSTEM: 2 HEART AND GREAT VESSELS
OPERATION: C EXTIRPATION: Taking or cutting out solid matter from a body part

Body Part	Approach	Device	Qualifier
0 Coronary Artery, One Site 1 Coronary Artery, Two Sites 2 Coronary Artery, Three Sites 3 Coronary Artery, Four or More Sites 4 Coronary Vein 5 Atrial Septum 6 Atrium, Right 7 Atrium, Left 8 Conduction Mechanism 9 Chordae Tendineae D Papillary Muscle F Aortic Valve G Mitral Valve H Pulmonary Valve J Tricuspid Valve K Ventricle, Right L Ventricle, Left M Ventricular Septum N Pericardium P Pulmonary Trunk Q Pulmonary Artery, Right R Pulmonary Artery, Left S Pulmonary Vein, Right T Pulmonary Vein, Left V Superior Vena Cava W Thoracic Aorta	0 Open 3 Percutaneous 4 Percutaneous Endoscopic	Z No Device	Z No Qualifier

SECTION: 0 MEDICAL AND SURGICAL
BODY SYSTEM: 2 HEART AND GREAT VESSELS
OPERATION: F FRAGMENTATION: Breaking solid matter in a body part into pieces

Body Part	Approach	Device	Qualifier
N Pericardium	0 Open 3 Percutaneous 4 Percutaneous Endoscopic X External	Z No Device	Z No Qualifier

SECTION: 0 MEDICAL AND SURGICAL
BODY SYSTEM: 2 HEART AND GREAT VESSELS
OPERATION: H INSERTION: Putting in a nonbiological appliance that monitors, assists, performs, or prevents a physiological function but does not physically take the place of a body part

Body Part	Approach	Device	Qualifier
4 Coronary Vein ✅ 6 Atrium, Right ✅ 7 Atrium, Left ✅ K Ventricle, Right ✅ L Ventricle, Left ✅	0 Open 3 Percutaneous 4 Percutaneous Endoscopic	0 Monitoring Device, Pressure Sensor 2 Monitoring Device 3 Infusion Device D Intraluminal Device J Cardiac Lead, Pacemaker K Cardiac Lead, Defibrillator M Cardiac Lead	Z No Qualifier
A Heart	0 Open 3 Percutaneous 4 Percutaneous Endoscopic	Q Implantable Heart Assist System ✅	Z No Qualifier
A Heart	0 Open 3 Percutaneous 4 Percutaneous Endoscopic	R External Heart Assist System	S Biventricular Z No Qualifier
N Pericardium	0 Open 3 Percutaneous 4 Percutaneous Endoscopic	0 Monitoring Device, Pressure Sensor 2 Monitoring Device J Cardiac Lead, Pacemaker ✅ K Cardiac Lead, Defibrillator M Cardiac Lead ✅	Z No Qualifier
P Pulmonary Trunk Q Pulmonary Artery, Right R Pulmonary Artery, Left S Pulmonary Vein, Right T Pulmonary Vein, Left V Superior Vena Cava W Thoracic Aorta	0 Open 3 Percutaneous 4 Percutaneous Endoscopic	0 Monitoring Device, Pressure Sensor 2 Monitoring Device 3 Infusion Device D Intraluminal Device	Z No Qualifier

✅ 02H43JZ, 02H43KZ, 02H43MZ
✅ 02H63JZ, 02H63MZ
✅ 02H73JZ, 02H73MZ
✅ 02HK3JZ
✅ 02HL3JZ

Coding Clinic: 2013, Q3, P18 – 02HV33Z

New ◄ Revised ◄ ~~deleted~~ Deleted ♀ Females Only ♂ Males Only
✅ Noncovered ✅ Limited Coverage ✅ Hospital-Acquired Condition **Coding Clinic**

SECTION: 0 MEDICAL AND SURGICAL
BODY SYSTEM: 2 HEART AND GREAT VESSELS
OPERATION: J INSPECTION: Visually and/or manually exploring a body part

Body Part	Approach	Device	Qualifier
A Heart Y Great Vessel	0 Open 3 Percutaneous 4 Percutaneous Endoscopic	Z No Device	Z No Qualifier

SECTION: 0 MEDICAL AND SURGICAL
BODY SYSTEM: 2 HEART AND GREAT VESSELS
OPERATION: K MAP: Locating the route of passage of electrical impulses and/or locating functional areas in a body part

Body Part	Approach	Device	Qualifier
8 Conduction Mechanism	0 Open 3 Percutaneous 4 Percutaneous Endoscopic	Z No Device	Z No Qualifier

SECTION: 0 MEDICAL AND SURGICAL
BODY SYSTEM: 2 HEART AND GREAT VESSELS
OPERATION: L OCCLUSION: Completely closing an orifice or the lumen of a tubular body part

Body Part	Approach	Device	Qualifier
7 Atrium, Left	0 Open 3 Percutaneous 4 Percutaneous Endoscopic	C Extraluminal Device D Intraluminal Device Z No Device	K Left Atrial Appendage
R Pulmonary Artery, Left	0 Open 3 Percutaneous 4 Percutaneous Endoscopic	C Extraluminal Device D Intraluminal Device Z No Device	T Ductus Arteriosus
S Pulmonary Vein, Right T Pulmonary Vein, Left V Superior Vena Cava	0 Open 3 Percutaneous 4 Percutaneous Endoscopic	C Extraluminal Device D Intraluminal Device Z No Device	Z No Qualifier

0: M/S   2: HEART AND GREAT VESSELS   J: INSPECTION   K: MAP   L: OCCLUSION

SECTION: 0 MEDICAL AND SURGICAL
BODY SYSTEM: 2 HEART AND GREAT VESSELS
OPERATION: N RELEASE: Freeing a body part from an abnormal physical constraint by cutting or by the use of force

Body Part	Approach	Device	Qualifier
4 Coronary Vein	0 Open	Z No Device	Z No Qualifier
5 Atrial Septum	3 Percutaneous		
6 Atrium, Right	4 Percutaneous Endoscopic		
7 Atrium, Left			
8 Conduction Mechanism			
9 Chordae Tendineae			
D Papillary Muscle			
F Aortic Valve			
G Mitral Valve			
H Pulmonary Valve			
J Tricuspid Valve			
K Ventricle, Right			
L Ventricle, Left			
M Ventricular Septum			
N Pericardium			
P Pulmonary Trunk			
Q Pulmonary Artery, Right			
R Pulmonary Artery, Left			
S Pulmonary Vein, Right			
T Pulmonary Vein, Left			
V Superior Vena Cava			
W Thoracic Aorta			

N: RELEASE

2: HEART AND GREAT VESSELS

0: M/S

◀ New ◀ Revised ~~deleted~~ Deleted ♀ Females Only ♂ Males Only
Noncovered Limited Coverage Hospital-Acquired Condition **Coding Clinic**

SECTION: 0 MEDICAL AND SURGICAL

BODY SYSTEM: 2 HEART AND GREAT VESSELS

OPERATION: **P** **REMOVAL:** Taking out or off a device from a body part

Body Part	Approach	Device	Qualifier
A Heart	0 Open 3 Percutaneous 4 Percutaneous Endoscopic	2 Monitoring Device 3 Infusion Device 7 Autologous Tissue Substitute 8 Zooplastic Tissue C Extraluminal Device D Intraluminal Device J Synthetic Substitute K Nonautologous Tissue Substitute M Cardiac Lead 🔊 Q Implantable Heart Assist System R External Heart Assist System	Z No Qualifier
A Heart	X External	2 Monitoring Device 3 Infusion Device D Intraluminal Device M Cardiac Lead	Z No Qualifier
Y Great Vessel	0 Open 3 Percutaneous 4 Percutaneous Endoscopic	2 Monitoring Device 3 Infusion Device 7 Autologous Tissue Substitute 8 Zooplastic Tissue C Extraluminal Device D Intraluminal Device J Synthetic Substitute K Nonautologous Tissue Substitute	Z No Qualifier
Y Great Vessel	X External	2 Monitoring Device 3 Infusion Device D Intraluminal Device	Z No Qualifier

0: M/S

2: HEART AND GREAT VESSELS

P: REMOVAL

◀ New　◀▥ Revised　deleted Deleted　♀ Females Only　♂ Males Only

🔊 Noncovered　🔊 Limited Coverage　🔊 Hospital-Acquired Condition　**Coding Clinic**

SECTION: 0 MEDICAL AND SURGICAL
BODY SYSTEM: 2 HEART AND GREAT VESSELS

OPERATION: **Q REPAIR:** Restoring, to the extent possible, a body part to its normal anatomic structure and function

Body Part	Approach	Device	Qualifier
0 Coronary Artery, One Site	0 Open	Z No Device	Z No Qualifier
1 Coronary Artery, Two Sites	3 Percutaneous		
2 Coronary Artery, Three Sites	4 Percutaneous Endoscopic		
3 Coronary Artery, Four or More Sites			
4 Coronary Vein			
5 Atrial Septum			
6 Atrium, Right			
7 Atrium, Left			
8 Conduction Mechanism			
9 Chordae Tendineae			
A Heart			
B Heart, Right			
C Heart, Left			
D Papillary Muscle			
F Aortic Valve			
G Mitral Valve			
H Pulmonary Valve			
J Tricuspid Valve			
K Ventricle, Right			
L Ventricle, Left			
M Ventricular Septum			
N Pericardium			
P Pulmonary Trunk			
Q Pulmonary Artery, Right			
R Pulmonary Artery, Left			
S Pulmonary Vein, Right			
T Pulmonary Vein, Left			
V Superior Vena Cava			
W Thoracic Aorta			

◀ New   ◀▥ Revised   ~~deleted~~ Deleted   ♀ Females Only   ♂ Males Only
❀ Noncovered   ❀ Limited Coverage   ❀ Hospital-Acquired Condition   **Coding Clinic**

SECTION: 0 MEDICAL AND SURGICAL
BODY SYSTEM: 2 HEART AND GREAT VESSELS
OPERATION: R REPLACEMENT: Putting in or on biological or synthetic material that physically takes the place and/or function of all or a portion of a body part

Body Part	Approach	Device	Qualifier
5 Atrial Septum 6 Atrium, Right 7 Atrium, Left 9 Chordae Tendineae D Papillary Muscle J Tricuspid Valve K Ventricle, Right 🦠 🦠 L Ventricle, Left 🦠 🦠 M Ventricular Septum N Pericardium P Pulmonary Trunk Q Pulmonary Artery, Right R Pulmonary Artery, Left S Pulmonary Vein, Right T Pulmonary Vein, Left V Superior Vena Cava W Thoracic Aorta	0 Open 4 Percutaneous Endoscopic	7 Autologous Tissue Substitute 8 Zooplastic Tissue J Synthetic Substitute K Nonautologous Tissue Substitute	Z No Qualifier
F Aortic Valve G Mitral Valve H Pulmonary Valve	0 Open 4 Percutaneous Endoscopic	7 Autologous Tissue Substitute 8 Zooplastic Tissue J Synthetic Substitute K Nonautologous Tissue Substitute	Z No Qualifier
F Aortic Valve G Mitral Valve H Pulmonary Valve	3 Percutaneous	7 Autologous Tissue Substitute 8 Zooplastic Tissue J Synthetic Substitute K Nonautologous Tissue Substitute	H Transapical Z No Qualifier

🦠 02RK0JZ, 02RL0JZ: except when combined with diagnosis code Z00.6.
🦠 02RK0JZ, 02RL0JZ: when combined with Z00.6

SECTION: 0 MEDICAL AND SURGICAL
BODY SYSTEM: 2 HEART AND GREAT VESSELS
OPERATION: S REPOSITION: Moving to its normal location, or other suitable location, all or a portion of a body part

Body Part	Approach	Device	Qualifier
P Pulmonary Trunk Q Pulmonary Artery, Right R Pulmonary Artery, Left S Pulmonary Vein, Right T Pulmonary Vein, Left V Superior Vena Cava W Thoracic Aorta	0 Open	Z No Device	Z No Qualifier

◀ New   ◀▥ Revised   ~~deleted~~ Deleted   ♀ Females Only   ♂ Males Only
🦠 Noncovered   🦠 Limited Coverage   🦠 Hospital-Acquired Condition   **Coding Clinic**

75

0: M/S   2: HEART AND GREAT VESSELS   R: REPLACEMENT   S: REPOSITION

T: RESECTION   U: SUPPLEMENT

2: HEART AND GREAT VESSELS

0: M/S

SECTION: 0 MEDICAL AND SURGICAL
BODY SYSTEM: 2 HEART AND GREAT VESSELS
OPERATION: T RESECTION: Cutting out or off, without replacement, all of a body part

Body Part	Approach	Device	Qualifier
5 Atrial Septum 8 Conduction Mechanism 9 Chordae Tendineae D Papillary Muscle H Pulmonary Valve M Ventricular Septum N Pericardium	0 Open 3 Percutaneous 4 Percutaneous Endoscopic	Z No Device	Z No Qualifier

SECTION: 0 MEDICAL AND SURGICAL
BODY SYSTEM: 2 HEART AND GREAT VESSELS
OPERATION: U SUPPLEMENT: Putting in or on biological or synthetic material that physically reinforces and/or augments the function of a portion of a body part

Body Part	Approach	Device	Qualifier
5 Atrial Septum 6 Atrium, Right 7 Atrium, Left 9 Chordae Tendineae A Heart D Papillary Muscle F Aortic Valve G Mitral Valve H Pulmonary Valve J Tricuspid Valve K Ventricle, Right L Ventricle, Left M Ventricular Septum N Pericardium P Pulmonary Trunk Q Pulmonary Artery, Right R Pulmonary Artery, Left S Pulmonary Vein, Right T Pulmonary Vein, Left V Superior Vena Cava W Thoracic Aorta	0 Open 3 Percutaneous 4 Percutaneous Endoscopic	7 Autologous Tissue Substitute 8 Zooplastic Tissue J Synthetic Substitute K Nonautologous Tissue Substitute	Z No Qualifier

◀ New   ◀▥ Revised   ~~deleted~~ Deleted   ♀ Females Only   ♂ Males Only
Ⓝ Noncovered   Ⓛ Limited Coverage   Ⓗ Hospital-Acquired Condition   **Coding Clinic**

SECTION: 0 MEDICAL AND SURGICAL
BODY SYSTEM: 2 HEART AND GREAT VESSELS
OPERATION: V **RESTRICTION:** Partially closing an orifice or the lumen of a tubular body part

Body Part	Approach	Device	Qualifier
A Heart	0 Open 3 Percutaneous 4 Percutaneous Endoscopic	C Extraluminal Device Z No Device	Z No Qualifier
P Pulmonary Trunk Q Pulmonary Artery, Right S Pulmonary Vein, Right T Pulmonary Vein, Left V Superior Vena Cava W Thoracic Aorta	0 Open 3 Percutaneous 4 Percutaneous Endoscopic	C Extraluminal Device D Intraluminal Device Z No Device	Z No Qualifier
R Pulmonary Artery, Left	0 Open 3 Percutaneous 4 Percutaneous Endoscopic	C Extraluminal Device D Intraluminal Device Z No Device	T Ductus Arteriosus Z No Qualifier

SECTION: **0 MEDICAL AND SURGICAL**
BODY SYSTEM: **2 HEART AND GREAT VESSELS**
OPERATION: **W REVISION:** Correcting, to the extent possible, a portion of a malfunctioning device or the position of a displaced device

Body Part	Approach	Device	Qualifier
5 Atrial Septum M Ventricular Septum	0 Open 4 Percutaneous Endoscopic	J Synthetic Substitute	Z No Qualifier
A Heart	0 Open 🜩 🜩 3 Percutaneous 🜩 🜩 4 Percutaneous Endoscopic 🜩 🜩 X External	2 Monitoring Device 3 Infusion Device 7 Autologous Tissue Substitute 8 Zooplastic Tissue C Extraluminal Device D Intraluminal Device J Synthetic Substitute K Nonautologous Tissue Substitute M Cardiac Lead Q Implantable Heart Assist System R External Heart Assist System	Z No Qualifier
F Aortic Valve G Mitral Valve H Pulmonary Valve J Tricuspid Valve	0 Open 4 Percutaneous Endoscopic	7 Autologous Tissue Substitute 8 Zooplastic Tissue J Synthetic Substitute K Nonautologous Tissue Substitute	Z No Qualifier
Y Great Vessel	0 Open 3 Percutaneous 4 Percutaneous Endoscopic X External	2 Monitoring Device 3 Infusion Device 7 Autologous Tissue Substitute 8 Zooplastic Tissue C Extraluminal Device D Intraluminal Device J Synthetic Substitute K Nonautologous Tissue Substitute	Z No Qualifier

🜩 02WA0JZ, 02WA0QZ
🜩 02WA3QZ, 02WA4QZ
🜩 02WA0MZ, 02WA3MZ, 02WA4MZ

◀ New ◀▥ Revised ~~deleted~~ Deleted ♀ Females Only ♂ Males Only
🜩 Noncovered 🜩 Limited Coverage 🜩 Hospital-Acquired Condition **Coding Clinic**

SECTION: 0 MEDICAL AND SURGICAL
BODY SYSTEM: 2 HEART AND GREAT VESSELS
OPERATION: Y TRANSPLANTATION: Putting in or on all or a portion of a living body part taken from another individual or animal to physically take the place and/or function of all or a portion of a similar body part

Body Part	Approach	Device	Qualifier
A Heart 🔖	0 Open	Z No Device	0 Allogeneic 1 Syngeneic 2 Zooplastic

Coding Clinic: 2013, Q3, P19 – 02YA0Z0

◄ New   ◄ Revised   deleted Deleted   ♀ Females Only   ♂ Males Only
Noncovered   Limited Coverage   Hospital-Acquired Condition   **Coding Clinic**

SECTION: 0 MEDICAL AND SURGICAL
BODY SYSTEM: 3 UPPER ARTERIES
OPERATION: 1 BYPASS: *(on multiple pages)*

Altering the route of passage of the contents of a tubular body part

Body Part	Approach	Device	Qualifier
2 Innominate Artery 5 Axillary Artery, Right 6 Axillary Artery, Left	0 Open	9 Autologous Venous Tissue A Autologous Arterial Tissue J Synthetic Substitute K Nonautologous Tissue Substitute Z No Device	0 Upper Arm Artery, Right 1 Upper Arm Artery, Left 2 Upper Arm Artery, Bilateral 3 Lower Arm Artery, Right 4 Lower Arm Artery, Left 5 Lower Arm Artery, Bilateral 6 Upper Leg Artery, Right 7 Upper Leg Artery, Left 8 Upper Leg Artery, Bilateral 9 Lower Leg Artery, Right B Lower Leg Artery, Left C Lower Leg Artery, Bilateral D Upper Arm Vein F Lower Arm Vein J Extracranial Artery, Right K Extracranial Artery, Left
3 Subclavian Artery, Right 4 Subclavian Artery, Left	0 Open	9 Autologous Venous Tissue A Autologous Arterial Tissue J Synthetic Substitute K Nonautologous Tissue Substitute Z No Device	0 Upper Arm Artery, Right 1 Upper Arm Artery, Left 2 Upper Arm Artery, Bilateral 3 Lower Arm Artery, Right 4 Lower Arm Artery, Left 5 Lower Arm Artery, Bilateral 6 Upper Leg Artery, Right 7 Upper Leg Artery, Left 8 Upper Leg Artery, Bilateral 9 Lower Leg Artery, Right B Lower Leg Artery, Left C Lower Leg Artery, Bilateral D Upper Arm Vein F Lower Arm Vein J Extracranial Artery, Right K Extracranial Artery, Left M Pulmonary Artery, Right N Pulmonary Artery, Left
7 Brachial Artery, Right	0 Open	9 Autologous Venous Tissue A Autologous Arterial Tissue J Synthetic Substitute K Nonautologous Tissue Substitute Z No Device	0 Upper Arm Artery, Right 3 Lower Arm Artery, Right D Upper Arm Vein F Lower Arm Vein
8 Brachial Artery, Left	0 Open	9 Autologous Venous Tissue A Autologous Arterial Tissue J Synthetic Substitute K Nonautologous Tissue Substitute Z No Device	1 Upper Arm Artery, Left 4 Lower Arm Artery, Left D Upper Arm Vein F Lower Arm Vein
9 Ulnar Artery, Right B Radial Artery, Right	0 Open	9 Autologous Venous Tissue A Autologous Arterial Tissue J Synthetic Substitute K Nonautologous Tissue Substitute Z No Device	3 Lower Arm Artery, Right F Lower Arm Vein

◀ New ◀ Revised deleted Deleted ♀ Females Only ♂ Males Only
Noncovered Limited Coverage Hospital-Acquired Condition **Coding Clinic**

0: M/S 3: UPPER ARTERIES 1: BYPASS

SECTION: 0 MEDICAL AND SURGICAL
BODY SYSTEM: 3   UPPER ARTERIES
OPERATION: 1   BYPASS: *(continued)*
Altering the route of passage of the contents of a tubular body part

Body Part	Approach	Device	Qualifier
A Ulnar Artery, Left C Radial Artery, Left	0 Open	9 Autologous Venous Tissue A Autologous Arterial Tissue J Synthetic Substitute K Nonautologous Tissue Substitute Z No Device	4 Lower Arm Artery, Left F Lower Arm Vein
G Intracranial Artery S Temporal Artery, Right 🕲 T Temporal Artery, Left 🕲	0 Open	9 Autologous Venous Tissue A Autologous Arterial Tissue J Synthetic Substitute K Nonautologous Tissue Substitute Z No Device	G Intracranial Artery
H Common Carotid Artery, Right	0 Open	9 Autologous Venous Tissue A Autologous Arterial Tissue J Synthetic Substitute K Nonautologous Tissue Substitute Z No Device	G Intracranial Artery J Extracranial Artery, Right 🕲
J Common Carotid Artery, Left	0 Open	9 Autologous Venous Tissue A Autologous Arterial Tissue J Synthetic Substitute K Nonautologous Tissue Substitute Z No Device	G Intracranial Artery K Extracranial Artery, Left 🕲
K Internal Carotid Artery, Right 🕲 M External Carotid Artery, Right 🕲	0 Open	9 Autologous Venous Tissue A Autologous Arterial Tissue J Synthetic Substitute K Nonautologous Tissue Substitute Z No Device	J Extracranial Artery, Right
L Internal Carotid Artery, Left 🕲 N External Carotid Artery, Left 🕲	0 Open	9 Autologous Venous Tissue A Autologous Arterial Tissue J Synthetic Substitute K Nonautologous Tissue Substitute Z No Device	K Extracranial Artery, Left

Coding Clinic: 2013, Q1, P228 – 031C0ZF

1: BYPASS

3: UPPER ARTERIES

0: M/S

◀ New   ◀ Revised   ~~deleted~~ Deleted   ♀ Females Only   ♂ Males Only
🕲 Noncovered   🕲 Limited Coverage   🕲 Hospital-Acquired Condition   **Coding Clinic**

SECTION: 0 MEDICAL AND SURGICAL
BODY SYSTEM: 3 UPPER ARTERIES
OPERATION: 5 DESTRUCTION: Physical eradication of all or a portion of a body part by the direct use of energy, force, or a destructive agent

Body Part	Approach	Device	Qualifier
0 Internal Mammary Artery, Right	0 Open	Z No Device	Z No Qualifier
1 Internal Mammary Artery, Left	3 Percutaneous		
2 Innominate Artery	4 Percutaneous Endoscopic		
3 Subclavian Artery, Right			
4 Subclavian Artery, Left			
5 Axillary Artery, Right			
6 Axillary Artery, Left			
7 Brachial Artery, Right			
8 Brachial Artery, Left			
9 Ulnar Artery, Right			
A Ulnar Artery, Left			
B Radial Artery, Right			
C Radial Artery, Left			
D Hand Artery, Right			
F Hand Artery, Left			
G Intracranial Artery			
H Common Carotid Artery, Right			
J Common Carotid Artery, Left			
K Internal Carotid Artery, Right			
L Internal Carotid Artery, Left			
M External Carotid Artery, Right			
N External Carotid Artery, Left			
P Vertebral Artery, Right			
Q Vertebral Artery, Left			
R Face Artery			
S Temporal Artery, Right			
T Temporal Artery, Left			
U Thyroid Artery, Right			
V Thyroid Artery, Left			
Y Upper Artery			

0: M/S

3: UPPER ARTERIES

5: DESTRUCTION

SECTION: 0 MEDICAL AND SURGICAL
BODY SYSTEM: 3 UPPER ARTERIES
OPERATION: 7 DILATION: Expanding an orifice or the lumen of a tubular body part

Body Part	Approach	Device	Qualifier
0 Internal Mammary Artery, Right	0 Open	4 Drug-eluting Intraluminal Device	Z No Qualifier
1 Internal Mammary Artery, Left	3 Percutaneous	D Intraluminal Device	
2 Innominate Artery	4 Percutaneous Endoscopic	Z No Device	
3 Subclavian Artery, Right			
4 Subclavian Artery, Left			
5 Axillary Artery, Right			
6 Axillary Artery, Left			
7 Brachial Artery, Right			
8 Brachial Artery, Left			
9 Ulnar Artery, Right			
A Ulnar Artery, Left			
B Radial Artery, Right			
C Radial Artery, Left			
D Hand Artery, Right			
F Hand Artery, Left			
G Intracranial Artery ⬙			
H Common Carotid Artery, Right			
J Common Carotid Artery, Left			
K Internal Carotid Artery, Right			
L Internal Carotid Artery, Left			
M External Carotid Artery, Right			
N External Carotid Artery, Left			
P Vertebral Artery, Right			
Q Vertebral Artery, Left			
R Face Artery			
S Temporal Artery, Right			
T Temporal Artery, Left			
U Thyroid Artery, Right			
V Thyroid Artery, Left			
Y Upper Artery			

⬙ 037G3ZZ, 037G4ZZ

7: DILATION

3: UPPER ARTERIES

0: M/S

SECTION: 0 MEDICAL AND SURGICAL
BODY SYSTEM: 3 UPPER ARTERIES
OPERATION: 9 DRAINAGE: *(on multiple pages)*

Taking or letting out fluids and/or gases from a body part

Body Part	Approach	Device	Qualifier
0 Internal Mammary Artery, Right	0 Open	0 Drainage Device	Z No Qualifier
1 Internal Mammary Artery, Left	3 Percutaneous		
2 Innominate Artery	4 Percutaneous Endoscopic		
3 Subclavian Artery, Right			
4 Subclavian Artery, Left			
5 Axillary Artery, Right			
6 Axillary Artery, Left			
7 Brachial Artery, Right			
8 Brachial Artery, Left			
9 Ulnar Artery, Right			
A Ulnar Artery, Left			
B Radial Artery, Right			
C Radial Artery, Left			
D Hand Artery, Right			
F Hand Artery, Left			
G Intracranial Artery			
H Common Carotid Artery, Right			
J Common Carotid Artery, Left			
K Internal Carotid Artery, Right			
L Internal Carotid Artery, Left			
M External Carotid Artery, Right			
N External Carotid Artery, Left			
P Vertebral Artery, Right			
Q Vertebral Artery, Left			
R Face Artery			
S Temporal Artery, Right			
T Temporal Artery, Left			
U Thyroid Artery, Right			
V Thyroid Artery, Left			
Y Upper Artery			

0: M/S

3: UPPER ARTERIES

9: DRAINAGE

◀ New   ◀≡ Revised   ~~deleted~~ Deleted   ♀ Females Only   ♂ Males Only
Ⓝ Noncovered   Ⓛ Limited Coverage   Ⓗ Hospital-Acquired Condition   **Coding Clinic**

SECTION: 0 MEDICAL AND SURGICAL
BODY SYSTEM: 3 UPPER ARTERIES
OPERATION: 9 DRAINAGE: *(continued)*

Taking or letting out fluids and/or gases from a body part

Body Part	Approach	Device	Qualifier
0 Internal Mammary Artery, Right	0 Open	Z No Device	X Diagnostic
1 Internal Mammary Artery, Left	3 Percutaneous		Z No Qualifier
2 Innominate Artery	4 Percutaneous Endoscopic		
3 Subclavian Artery, Right			
4 Subclavian Artery, Left			
5 Axillary Artery, Right			
6 Axillary Artery, Left			
7 Brachial Artery, Right			
8 Brachial Artery, Left			
9 Ulnar Artery, Right			
A Ulnar Artery, Left			
B Radial Artery, Right			
C Radial Artery, Left			
D Hand Artery, Right			
F Hand Artery, Left			
G Intracranial Artery			
H Common Carotid Artery, Right			
J Common Carotid Artery, Left			
K Internal Carotid Artery, Right			
L Internal Carotid Artery, Left			
M External Carotid Artery, Right			
N External Carotid Artery, Left			
P Vertebral Artery, Right			
Q Vertebral Artery, Left			
R Face Artery			
S Temporal Artery, Right			
T Temporal Artery, Left			
U Thyroid Artery, Right			
V Thyroid Artery, Left			
Y Upper Artery			

9: DRAINAGE

3: UPPER ARTERIES

0: M/S

◀ New ◀▥ Revised ~~deleted~~ Deleted ♀ Females Only ♂ Males Only
🔖 Noncovered 🔖 Limited Coverage 🔖 Hospital-Acquired Condition **Coding Clinic**

SECTION: 0 MEDICAL AND SURGICAL
BODY SYSTEM: 3 UPPER ARTERIES
OPERATION: B **EXCISION:** Cutting out or off, without replacement, a portion of a body part

Body Part	Approach	Device	Qualifier
0 Internal Mammary Artery, Right 1 Internal Mammary Artery, Left 2 Innominate Artery 3 Subclavian Artery, Right 4 Subclavian Artery, Left 5 Axillary Artery, Right 6 Axillary Artery, Left 7 Brachial Artery, Right 8 Brachial Artery, Left 9 Ulnar Artery, Right A Ulnar Artery, Left B Radial Artery, Right C Radial Artery, Left D Hand Artery, Right F Hand Artery, Left G Intracranial Artery H Common Carotid Artery, Right J Common Carotid Artery, Left K Internal Carotid Artery, Right L Internal Carotid Artery, Left M External Carotid Artery, Right N External Carotid Artery, Left P Vertebral Artery, Right Q Vertebral Artery, Left R Face Artery S Temporal Artery, Right T Temporal Artery, Left U Thyroid Artery, Right V Thyroid Artery, Left Y Upper Artery	0 Open 3 Percutaneous 4 Percutaneous Endoscopic	Z No Device	X Diagnostic Z No Qualifier

SECTION: 0 MEDICAL AND SURGICAL
BODY SYSTEM: 3 UPPER ARTERIES
OPERATION: C EXTIRPATION: Taking or cutting out solid matter from a body part

Body Part	Approach	Device	Qualifier
0 Internal Mammary Artery, Right 1 Internal Mammary Artery, Left 2 Innominate Artery 3 Subclavian Artery, Right 4 Subclavian Artery, Left 5 Axillary Artery, Right 6 Axillary Artery, Left 7 Brachial Artery, Right 8 Brachial Artery, Left 9 Ulnar Artery, Right A Ulnar Artery, Left B Radial Artery, Right C Radial Artery, Left D Hand Artery, Right F Hand Artery, Left G Intracranial Artery % H Common Carotid Artery, Right J Common Carotid Artery, Left K Internal Carotid Artery, Right L Internal Carotid Artery, Left M External Carotid Artery, Right N External Carotid Artery, Left P Vertebral Artery, Right Q Vertebral Artery, Left R Face Artery S Temporal Artery, Right T Temporal Artery, Left U Thyroid Artery, Right V Thyroid Artery, Left Y Upper Artery	0 Open 3 Percutaneous 4 Percutaneous Endoscopic	Z No Device	Z No Qualifier

% 03CG3ZZ, 03CG4ZZ

C: EXTIRPATION

3: UPPER ARTERIES

0: M/S

◄ New ◄ Revised ~~deleted~~ Deleted ♀ Females Only ♂ Males Only
% Noncovered % Limited Coverage % Hospital-Acquired Condition **Coding Clinic**

SECTION: 0 MEDICAL AND SURGICAL

BODY SYSTEM: 3 UPPER ARTERIES
OPERATION: H INSERTION: Putting in a nonbiological appliance that monitors, assists, performs, or prevents a physiological function but does not physically take the place of a body part

Body Part	Approach	Device	Qualifier
0 Internal Mammary Artery, Right 1 Internal Mammary Artery, Left 2 Innominate Artery 3 Subclavian Artery, Right 4 Subclavian Artery, Left 5 Axillary Artery, Right 6 Axillary Artery, Left 7 Brachial Artery, Right 8 Brachial Artery, Left 9 Ulnar Artery, Right A Ulnar Artery, Left B Radial Artery, Right C Radial Artery, Left D Hand Artery, Right F Hand Artery, Left G Intracranial Artery H Common Carotid Artery, Right J Common Carotid Artery, Left M External Carotid Artery, Right N External Carotid Artery, Left P Vertebral Artery, Right Q Vertebral Artery, Left R Face Artery S Temporal Artery, Right T Temporal Artery, Left U Thyroid Artery, Right V Thyroid Artery, Left	0 Open 3 Percutaneous 4 Percutaneous Endoscopic	3 Infusion Device D Intraluminal Device	Z No Qualifier
K Internal Carotid Artery, Right L Internal Carotid Artery, Left	0 Open 3 Percutaneous 4 Percutaneous Endoscopic	3 Infusion Device D Intraluminal Device M Stimulator Lead	Z No Qualifier
Y Upper Artery	0 Open 3 Percutaneous 4 Percutaneous Endoscopic	2 Monitoring Device 3 Infusion Device D Intraluminal Device	Z No Qualifier

SECTION: 0 MEDICAL AND SURGICAL

BODY SYSTEM: 3 UPPER ARTERIES
OPERATION: J INSPECTION: Visually and/or manually exploring a body part

Body Part	Approach	Device	Qualifier
Y Upper Artery	0 Open 3 Percutaneous 4 Percutaneous Endoscopic X External	Z No Device	Z No Qualifier

◀ New   ◀▬ Revised   deleted Deleted   ♀ Females Only   ♂ Males Only
🚫 Noncovered   🚫 Limited Coverage   🚫 Hospital-Acquired Condition   **Coding Clinic**

89

SECTION: 0 MEDICAL AND SURGICAL
BODY SYSTEM: 3 UPPER ARTERIES
OPERATION: **L OCCLUSION:** Completely closing an orifice or the lumen of a tubular body part

Body Part	Approach	Device	Qualifier
0 Internal Mammary Artery, Right 1 Internal Mammary Artery, Left 2 Innominate Artery 3 Subclavian Artery, Right 4 Subclavian Artery, Left 5 Axillary Artery, Right 6 Axillary Artery, Left 7 Brachial Artery, Right 8 Brachial Artery, Left 9 Ulnar Artery, Right A Ulnar Artery, Left B Radial Artery, Right C Radial Artery, Left D Hand Artery, Right F Hand Artery, Left R Face Artery S Temporal Artery, Right T Temporal Artery, Left U Thyroid Artery, Right V Thyroid Artery, Left Y Upper Artery	0 Open 3 Percutaneous 4 Percutaneous Endoscopic	C Extraluminal Device D Intraluminal Device Z No Device	Z No Qualifier
G Intracranial Artery H Common Carotid Artery, Right J Common Carotid Artery, Left K Internal Carotid Artery, Right L Internal Carotid Artery, Left M External Carotid Artery, Right N External Carotid Artery, Left P Vertebral Artery, Right Q Vertebral Artery, Left	0 Open 3 Percutaneous 4 Percutaneous Endoscopic	B Intraluminal Device, Bioactive C Extraluminal Device D Intraluminal Device Z No Device	Z No Qualifier

◀ New   ◀▥ Revised   ~~deleted~~ Deleted   ♀ Females Only   ♂ Males Only
🏵 Noncovered   🏵 Limited Coverage   🏵 Hospital-Acquired Condition   **Coding Clinic**

SECTION: 0 MEDICAL AND SURGICAL
BODY SYSTEM: 3 UPPER ARTERIES
OPERATION: N RELEASE: Freeing a body part from an abnormal physical constraint by cutting or by the use of force

Body Part	Approach	Device	Qualifier
0 Internal Mammary Artery, Right	0 Open	Z No Device	Z No Qualifier
1 Internal Mammary Artery, Left	3 Percutaneous		
2 Innominate Artery	4 Percutaneous Endoscopic		
3 Subclavian Artery, Right			
4 Subclavian Artery, Left			
5 Axillary Artery, Right			
6 Axillary Artery, Left			
7 Brachial Artery, Right			
8 Brachial Artery, Left			
9 Ulnar Artery, Right			
A Ulnar Artery, Left			
B Radial Artery, Right			
C Radial Artery, Left			
D Hand Artery, Right			
F Hand Artery, Left			
G Intracranial Artery			
H Common Carotid Artery, Right			
J Common Carotid Artery, Left			
K Internal Carotid Artery, Right			
L Internal Carotid Artery, Left			
M External Carotid Artery, Right			
N External Carotid Artery, Left			
P Vertebral Artery, Right			
Q Vertebral Artery, Left			
R Face Artery			
S Temporal Artery, Right			
T Temporal Artery, Left			
U Thyroid Artery, Right			
V Thyroid Artery, Left			
Y Upper Artery			

◀ New   ◀━ Revised   deleted Deleted   ♀ Females Only   ♂ Males Only
Noncovered   Limited Coverage   Hospital-Acquired Condition   **Coding Clinic**

91

SECTION: 0 MEDICAL AND SURGICAL
BODY SYSTEM: 3 UPPER ARTERIES
OPERATION: P REMOVAL: Taking out or off a device from a body part

Body Part	Approach	Device	Qualifier
Y Upper Artery	0 Open 3 Percutaneous 4 Percutaneous Endoscopic	0 Drainage Device 2 Monitoring Device 3 Infusion Device 7 Autologous Tissue Substitute C Extraluminal Device D Intraluminal Device J Synthetic Substitute K Nonautologous Tissue Substitute M Stimulator Lead	Z No Qualifier
Y Upper Artery	X External	0 Drainage Device 2 Monitoring Device 3 Infusion Device D Intraluminal Device M Stimulator Lead	Z No Qualifier

P: REMOVAL

3: UPPER ARTERIES

0: M/S

◀ New ◀ Revised ~~deleted~~ Deleted ♀ Females Only ♂ Males Only
🐾 Noncovered 🐾 Limited Coverage 🐾 Hospital-Acquired Condition **Coding Clinic**

SECTION: 0 MEDICAL AND SURGICAL
BODY SYSTEM: 3 UPPER ARTERIES
OPERATION: Q REPAIR: Restoring, to the extent possible, a body part to its normal anatomic structure and function

Body Part	Approach	Device	Qualifier
0 Internal Mammary Artery, Right	0 Open	Z No Device	Z No Qualifier
1 Internal Mammary Artery, Left	3 Percutaneous		
2 Innominate Artery	4 Percutaneous Endoscopic		
3 Subclavian Artery, Right			
4 Subclavian Artery, Left			
5 Axillary Artery, Right			
6 Axillary Artery, Left			
7 Brachial Artery, Right			
8 Brachial Artery, Left			
9 Ulnar Artery, Right			
A Ulnar Artery, Left			
B Radial Artery, Right			
C Radial Artery, Left			
D Hand Artery, Right			
F Hand Artery, Left			
G Intracranial Artery			
H Common Carotid Artery, Right			
J Common Carotid Artery, Left			
K Internal Carotid Artery, Right			
L Internal Carotid Artery, Left			
M External Carotid Artery, Right			
N External Carotid Artery, Left			
P Vertebral Artery, Right			
Q Vertebral Artery, Left			
R Face Artery			
S Temporal Artery, Right			
T Temporal Artery, Left			
U Thyroid Artery, Right			
V Thyroid Artery, Left			
Y Upper Artery			

0: M/S

3: UPPER ARTERIES

Q: REPAIR

SECTION: 0 MEDICAL AND SURGICAL
BODY SYSTEM: 3 UPPER ARTERIES
OPERATION: R REPLACEMENT: Putting in or on biological or synthetic material that physically takes the place and/or function of all or a portion of a body part

Body Part	Approach	Device	Qualifier
0 Internal Mammary Artery, Right 1 Internal Mammary Artery, Left 2 Innominate Artery 3 Subclavian Artery, Right 4 Subclavian Artery, Left 5 Axillary Artery, Right 6 Axillary Artery, Left 7 Brachial Artery, Right 8 Brachial Artery, Left 9 Ulnar Artery, Right A Ulnar Artery, Left B Radial Artery, Right C Radial Artery, Left D Hand Artery, Right F Hand Artery, Left G Intracranial Artery H Common Carotid Artery, Right J Common Carotid Artery, Left K Internal Carotid Artery, Right L Internal Carotid Artery, Left M External Carotid Artery, Right N External Carotid Artery, Left P Vertebral Artery, Right Q Vertebral Artery, Left R Face Artery S Temporal Artery, Right T Temporal Artery, Left U Thyroid Artery, Right V Thyroid Artery, Left Y Upper Artery	0 Open 4 Percutaneous Endoscopic	7 Autologous Tissue Substitute J Synthetic Substitute K Nonautologous Tissue Substitute	Z No Qualifier

◀ New   ◀▥ Revised   ~~deleted~~ Deleted   ♀ Females Only   ♂ Males Only
🚫 Noncovered   🚫 Limited Coverage   🚫 Hospital-Acquired Condition   **Coding Clinic**

SECTION: 0 MEDICAL AND SURGICAL
BODY SYSTEM: 3 UPPER ARTERIES
OPERATION: S REPOSITION: Moving to its normal location, or other suitable location, all or a portion of a body part

Body Part	Approach	Device	Qualifier
0 Internal Mammary Artery, Right	0 Open	Z No Device	Z No Qualifier
1 Internal Mammary Artery, Left	3 Percutaneous		
2 Innominate Artery	4 Percutaneous Endoscopic		
3 Subclavian Artery, Right			
4 Subclavian Artery, Left			
5 Axillary Artery, Right			
6 Axillary Artery, Left			
7 Brachial Artery, Right			
8 Brachial Artery, Left			
9 Ulnar Artery, Right			
A Ulnar Artery, Left			
B Radial Artery, Right			
C Radial Artery, Left			
D Hand Artery, Right			
F Hand Artery, Left			
G Intracranial Artery			
H Common Carotid Artery, Right			
J Common Carotid Artery, Left			
K Internal Carotid Artery, Right			
L Internal Carotid Artery, Left			
M External Carotid Artery, Right			
N External Carotid Artery, Left			
P Vertebral Artery, Right			
Q Vertebral Artery, Left			
R Face Artery			
S Temporal Artery, Right			
T Temporal Artery, Left			
U Thyroid Artery, Right			
V Thyroid Artery, Left			
Y Upper Artery			

0: M/S 3: UPPER ARTERIES S: REPOSITION

SECTION: 0 MEDICAL AND SURGICAL
BODY SYSTEM: 3 UPPER ARTERIES
OPERATION: U **SUPPLEMENT:** Putting in or on biological or synthetic material that physically reinforces and/or augments the function of a portion of a body part

Body Part	Approach	Device	Qualifier
0 Internal Mammary Artery, Right 1 Internal Mammary Artery, Left 2 Innominate Artery 3 Subclavian Artery, Right 4 Subclavian Artery, Left 5 Axillary Artery, Right 6 Axillary Artery, Left 7 Brachial Artery, Right 8 Brachial Artery, Left 9 Ulnar Artery, Right A Ulnar Artery, Left B Radial Artery, Right C Radial Artery, Left D Hand Artery, Right F Hand Artery, Left G Intracranial Artery H Common Carotid Artery, Right J Common Carotid Artery, Left K Internal Carotid Artery, Right L Internal Carotid Artery, Left M External Carotid Artery, Right N External Carotid Artery, Left P Vertebral Artery, Right Q Vertebral Artery, Left R Face Artery S Temporal Artery, Right T Temporal Artery, Left U Thyroid Artery, Right V Thyroid Artery, Left Y Upper Artery	0 Open 3 Percutaneous 4 Percutaneous Endoscopic	7 Autologous Tissue Substitute J Synthetic Substitute K Nonautologous Tissue Substitute	Z No Qualifier

SECTION: 0 MEDICAL AND SURGICAL
BODY SYSTEM: 3 UPPER ARTERIES
OPERATION: V RESTRICTION: Partially closing an orifice or the lumen of a tubular body part

Body Part	Approach	Device	Qualifier
0 Internal Mammary Artery, Right 1 Internal Mammary Artery, Left 2 Innominate Artery 3 Subclavian Artery, Right 4 Subclavian Artery, Left 5 Axillary Artery, Right 6 Axillary Artery, Left 7 Brachial Artery, Right 8 Brachial Artery, Left 9 Ulnar Artery, Right A Ulnar Artery, Left B Radial Artery, Right C Radial Artery, Left D Hand Artery, Right F Hand Artery, Left R Face Artery S Temporal Artery, Right T Temporal Artery, Left U Thyroid Artery, Right V Thyroid Artery, Left Y Upper Artery	0 Open 3 Percutaneous 4 Percutaneous Endoscopic	C Extraluminal Device D Intraluminal Device Z No Device	Z No Qualifier
G Intracranial Artery H Common Carotid Artery, Right J Common Carotid Artery, Left K Internal Carotid Artery, Right L Internal Carotid Artery, Left M External Carotid Artery, Right N External Carotid Artery, Left P Vertebral Artery, Right Q Vertebral Artery, Left	0 Open 3 Percutaneous 4 Percutaneous Endoscopic	B Intraluminal Device, Bioactive C Extraluminal Device D Intraluminal Device Z No Device	Z No Qualifier

SECTION: 0 MEDICAL AND SURGICAL
BODY SYSTEM: 3 UPPER ARTERIES
OPERATION: W REVISION: Correcting, to the extent possible, a portion of a malfunctioning device or the position of a displaced device

Body Part	Approach	Device	Qualifier
Y Upper Artery	0 Open 3 Percutaneous 4 Percutaneous Endoscopic X External	0 Drainage Device 2 Monitoring Device 3 Infusion Device 7 Autologous Tissue Substitute C Extraluminal Device D Intraluminal Device J Synthetic Substitute K Nonautologous Tissue Substitute M Stimulator Lead	Z No Qualifier

◀ New   ◀ Revised   deleted Deleted   ♀ Females Only   ♂ Males Only
🄽 Noncovered   🄻 Limited Coverage   🄷 Hospital-Acquired Condition   **Coding Clinic**

97

◀ New   ◀▥ Revised   ~~deleted~~ Deleted   ♀ Females Only   ♂ Males Only
Ⓝⓒ Noncovered   Ⓛⓒ Limited Coverage   Ⓗⓐⓒ Hospital-Acquired Condition   **Coding Clinic**

SECTION: 0 MEDICAL AND SURGICAL
BODY SYSTEM: 4 LOWER ARTERIES
OPERATION: 1 BYPASS: Altering the route of passage of the contents of a tubular body part

Body Part	Approach	Device	Qualifier
0 Abdominal Aorta C Common Iliac Artery, Right D Common Iliac Artery, Left	0 Open 4 Percutaneous Endoscopic	9 Autologous Venous Tissue A Autologous Arterial Tissue J Synthetic Substitute K Nonautologous Tissue Substitute Z No Device	0 Abdominal Aorta 1 Celiac Artery 2 Mesenteric Artery 3 Renal Artery, Right 4 Renal Artery, Left 5 Renal Artery, Bilateral 6 Common Iliac Artery, Right 7 Common Iliac Artery, Left 8 Common Iliac Arteries, Bilateral 9 Internal Iliac Artery, Right B Internal Iliac Artery, Left C Internal Iliac Arteries, Bilateral D External Iliac Artery, Right F External Iliac Artery, Left G External Iliac Arteries, Bilateral H Femoral Artery, Right J Femoral Artery, Left K Femoral Arteries, Bilateral Q Lower Extremity Artery R Lower Artery
4 Splenic Artery	0 Open 4 Percutaneous Endoscopic	9 Autologous Venous Tissue A Autologous Arterial Tissue J Synthetic Substitute K Nonautologous Tissue Substitute Z No Device	3 Renal Artery, Right 4 Renal Artery, Left 5 Renal Artery, Bilateral
E Internal Iliac Artery, Right F Internal Iliac Artery, Left H External Iliac Artery, Right J External Iliac Artery, Left	0 Open 4 Percutaneous Endoscopic	9 Autologous Venous Tissue A Autologous Arterial Tissue J Synthetic Substitute K Nonautologous Tissue Substitute Z No Device	9 Internal Iliac Artery, Right B Internal Iliac Artery, Left C Internal Iliac Arteries, Bilateral D External Iliac Artery, Right F External Iliac Artery, Left G External Iliac Arteries, Bilateral H Femoral Artery, Right J Femoral Artery, Left K Femoral Arteries, Bilateral P Foot Artery Q Lower Extremity Artery
K Femoral Artery, Right L Femoral Artery, Left	0 Open 4 Percutaneous Endoscopic	9 Autologous Venous Tissue A Autologous Arterial Tissue J Synthetic Substitute K Nonautologous Tissue Substitute Z No Device	H Femoral Artery, Right J Femoral Artery, Left K Femoral Arteries, Bilateral L Popliteal Artery M Peroneal Artery N Posterior Tibial Artery P Foot Artery Q Lower Extremity Artery S Lower Extremity Vein
M Popliteal Artery, Right N Popliteal Artery, Left	0 Open 4 Percutaneous Endoscopic	9 Autologous Venous Tissue A Autologous Arterial Tissue J Synthetic Substitute K Nonautologous Tissue Substitute Z No Device	L Popliteal Artery M Peroneal Artery P Foot Artery Q Lower Extremity Artery S Lower Extremity Vein

0: M/S   4: LOWER ARTERIES   1: BYPASS

◄ New   ◄▥ Revised   ~~deleted~~ Deleted   ♀ Females Only   ♂ Males Only
🅡 Noncovered   🅡 Limited Coverage   🅡 Hospital-Acquired Condition   **Coding Clinic**

99

SECTION: 0 MEDICAL AND SURGICAL

BODY SYSTEM: 4 LOWER ARTERIES

OPERATION: 5 DESTRUCTION: Physical eradication of all or a portion of a body part by the direct use of energy, force, or a destructive agent

Body Part	Approach	Device	Qualifier
0 Abdominal Aorta 1 Celiac Artery 2 Gastric Artery 3 Hepatic Artery 4 Splenic Artery 5 Superior Mesenteric Artery 6 Colic Artery, Right 7 Colic Artery, Left 8 Colic Artery, Middle 9 Renal Artery, Right A Renal Artery, Left B Inferior Mesenteric Artery C Common Iliac Artery, Right D Common Iliac Artery, Left E Internal Iliac Artery, Right F Internal Iliac Artery, Left H External Iliac Artery, Right J External Iliac Artery, Left K Femoral Artery, Right L Femoral Artery, Left M Popliteal Artery, Right N Popliteal Artery, Left P Anterior Tibial Artery, Right Q Anterior Tibial Artery, Left R Posterior Tibial Artery, Right S Posterior Tibial Artery, Left T Peroneal Artery, Right U Peroneal Artery, Left V Foot Artery, Right W Foot Artery, Left Y Lower Artery	0 Open 3 Percutaneous 4 Percutaneous Endoscopic	Z No Device	Z No Qualifier

5: DESTRUCTION

4: LOWER ARTERIES

0: M/S

◀ New ◀ Revised ~~deleted~~ Deleted ♀ Females Only ♂ Males Only
Noncovered Limited Coverage Hospital-Acquired Condition **Coding Clinic**

SECTION: 0 MEDICAL AND SURGICAL
BODY SYSTEM: 4 LOWER ARTERIES
OPERATION: 7 DILATION: Expanding an orifice or the lumen of a tubular body part

Body Part	Approach	Device	Qualifier
0 Abdominal Aorta	0 Open	4 Intraluminal Device, Drug-eluting	Z No Qualifier
1 Celiac Artery	3 Percutaneous	D Intraluminal Device	
2 Gastric Artery	4 Percutaneous Endoscopic	Z No Device	
3 Hepatic Artery			
4 Splenic Artery			
5 Superior Mesenteric Artery			
6 Colic Artery, Right			
7 Colic Artery, Left			
8 Colic Artery, Middle			
9 Renal Artery, Right			
A Renal Artery, Left			
B Inferior Mesenteric Artery			
C Common Iliac Artery, Right			
D Common Iliac Artery, Left			
E Internal Iliac Artery, Right			
F Internal Iliac Artery, Left			
H External Iliac Artery, Right			
J External Iliac Artery, Left			
K Femoral Artery, Right			
L Femoral Artery, Left			
M Popliteal Artery, Right			
N Popliteal Artery, Left			
P Anterior Tibial Artery, Right			
Q Anterior Tibial Artery, Left			
R Posterior Tibial Artery, Right			
S Posterior Tibial Artery, Left			
T Peroneal Artery, Right			
U Peroneal Artery, Left			
V Foot Artery, Right			
W Foot Artery, Left			
Y Lower Artery			

0: M/S

4: LOWER ARTERIES

7: DILATION

SECTION: 0 MEDICAL AND SURGICAL
BODY SYSTEM: 4 LOWER ARTERIES
OPERATION: 9 DRAINAGE: *(on multiple pages)*
Taking or letting out fluids and/or gases from a body part

Body Part	Approach	Device	Qualifier
0 Abdominal Aorta	0 Open	0 Drainage Device	Z No Qualifier
1 Celiac Artery	3 Percutaneous		
2 Gastric Artery	4 Percutaneous Endoscopic		
3 Hepatic Artery			
4 Splenic Artery			
5 Superior Mesenteric Artery			
6 Colic Artery, Right			
7 Colic Artery, Left			
8 Colic Artery, Middle			
9 Renal Artery, Right			
A Renal Artery, Left			
B Inferior Mesenteric Artery			
C Common Iliac Artery, Right			
D Common Iliac Artery, Left			
E Internal Iliac Artery, Right			
F Internal Iliac Artery, Left			
H External Iliac Artery, Right			
J External Iliac Artery, Left			
K Femoral Artery, Right			
L Femoral Artery, Left			
M Popliteal Artery, Right			
N Popliteal Artery, Left			
P Anterior Tibial Artery, Right			
Q Anterior Tibial Artery, Left			
R Posterior Tibial Artery, Right			
S Posterior Tibial Artery, Left			
T Peroneal Artery, Right			
U Peroneal Artery, Left			
V Foot Artery, Right			
W Foot Artery, Left			
Y Lower Artery			

9: DRAINAGE

4: LOWER ARTERIES

0: M/S

◀ New   ◀▥ Revised   ~~deleted~~ Deleted   ♀ Females Only   ♂ Males Only
℞ Noncovered   ℞ Limited Coverage   ℞ Hospital-Acquired Condition   **Coding Clinic**

SECTION: 0 MEDICAL AND SURGICAL
BODY SYSTEM: 4 LOWER ARTERIES
OPERATION: 9 DRAINAGE: *(continued)*
Taking or letting out fluids and/or gases from a body part

Body Part	Approach	Device	Qualifier
0 Abdominal Aorta	0 Open	Z No Device	X Diagnostic
1 Celiac Artery	3 Percutaneous		Z No Qualifier
2 Gastric Artery	4 Percutaneous Endoscopic		
3 Hepatic Artery			
4 Splenic Artery			
5 Superior Mesenteric Artery			
6 Colic Artery, Right			
7 Colic Artery, Left			
8 Colic Artery, Middle			
9 Renal Artery, Right			
A Renal Artery, Left			
B Inferior Mesenteric Artery			
C Common Iliac Artery, Right			
D Common Iliac Artery, Left			
E Internal Iliac Artery, Right			
F Internal Iliac Artery, Left			
H External Iliac Artery, Right			
J External Iliac Artery, Left			
K Femoral Artery, Right			
L Femoral Artery, Left			
M Popliteal Artery, Right			
N Popliteal Artery, Left			
P Anterior Tibial Artery, Right			
Q Anterior Tibial Artery, Left			
R Posterior Tibial Artery, Right			
S Posterior Tibial Artery, Left			
T Peroneal Artery, Right			
U Peroneal Artery, Left			
V Foot Artery, Right			
W Foot Artery, Left			
Y Lower Artery			

0: M/S

4: LOWER ARTERIES

9: DRAINAGE

◀ New ◀ Revised ~~deleted~~ Deleted ♀ Females Only ♂ Males Only
Noncovered Limited Coverage Hospital-Acquired Condition **Coding Clinic**

103

SECTION: 0 MEDICAL AND SURGICAL
BODY SYSTEM: 4 LOWER ARTERIES
OPERATION: B **EXCISION:** Cutting out or off, without replacement, a portion of a body part

Body Part	Approach	Device	Qualifier
0 Abdominal Aorta	0 Open	Z No Device	X Diagnostic
1 Celiac Artery	3 Percutaneous		Z No Qualifier
2 Gastric Artery	4 Percutaneous Endoscopic		
3 Hepatic Artery			
4 Splenic Artery			
5 Superior Mesenteric Artery			
6 Colic Artery, Right			
7 Colic Artery, Left			
8 Colic Artery, Middle			
9 Renal Artery, Right			
A Renal Artery, Left			
B Inferior Mesenteric Artery			
C Common Iliac Artery, Right			
D Common Iliac Artery, Left			
E Internal Iliac Artery, Right			
F Internal Iliac Artery, Left			
H External Iliac Artery, Right			
J External Iliac Artery, Left			
K Femoral Artery, Right			
L Femoral Artery, Left			
M Popliteal Artery, Right			
N Popliteal Artery, Left			
P Anterior Tibial Artery, Right			
Q Anterior Tibial Artery, Left			
R Posterior Tibial Artery, Right			
S Posterior Tibial Artery, Left			
T Peroneal Artery, Right			
U Peroneal Artery, Left			
V Foot Artery, Right			
W Foot Artery, Left			
Y Lower Artery			

◀ New   ◀▬ Revised   ~~deleted~~ Deleted   ♀ Females Only   ♂ Males Only
🚫 Noncovered   🚫 Limited Coverage   🚫 Hospital-Acquired Condition   **Coding Clinic**

SECTION: 0 MEDICAL AND SURGICAL
BODY SYSTEM: 4 LOWER ARTERIES
OPERATION: C EXTIRPATION: Taking or cutting out solid matter from a body part

Body Part	Approach	Device	Qualifier
0 Abdominal Aorta	0 Open	Z No Device	Z No Qualifier
1 Celiac Artery	3 Percutaneous		
2 Gastric Artery	4 Percutaneous Endoscopic		
3 Hepatic Artery			
4 Splenic Artery			
5 Superior Mesenteric Artery			
6 Colic Artery, Right			
7 Colic Artery, Left			
8 Colic Artery, Middle			
9 Renal Artery, Right			
A Renal Artery, Left			
B Inferior Mesenteric Artery			
C Common Iliac Artery, Right			
D Common Iliac Artery, Left			
E Internal Iliac Artery, Right			
F Internal Iliac Artery, Left			
H External Iliac Artery, Right			
J External Iliac Artery, Left			
K Femoral Artery, Right			
L Femoral Artery, Left			
M Popliteal Artery, Right			
N Popliteal Artery, Left			
P Anterior Tibial Artery, Right			
Q Anterior Tibial Artery, Left			
R Posterior Tibial Artery, Right			
S Posterior Tibial Artery, Left			
T Peroneal Artery, Right			
U Peroneal Artery, Left			
V Foot Artery, Right			
W Foot Artery, Left			
Y Lower Artery			

◀ New ◀▥ Revised ~~deleted~~ Deleted ♀ Females Only ♂ Males Only
Noncovered Limited Coverage Hospital-Acquired Condition **Coding Clinic**

105

SECTION: 0 **MEDICAL AND SURGICAL**
BODY SYSTEM: 4 **LOWER ARTERIES**
OPERATION: H **INSERTION:** Putting in a nonbiological appliance that monitors, assists, performs, or prevents a physiological function but does not physically take the place of a body part

Body Part	Approach	Device	Qualifier
0 Abdominal Aorta Y Lower Artery	0 Open 3 Percutaneous 4 Percutaneous Endoscopic	2 Monitoring Device 3 Infusion Device D Intraluminal Device	Z No Qualifier
1 Celiac Artery 2 Gastric Artery 3 Hepatic Artery 4 Splenic Artery 5 Superior Mesenteric Artery 6 Colic Artery, Right 7 Colic Artery, Left 8 Colic Artery, Middle 9 Renal Artery, Right A Renal Artery, Left B Inferior Mesenteric Artery C Common Iliac Artery, Right D Common Iliac Artery, Left E Internal Iliac Artery, Right F Internal Iliac Artery, Left H External Iliac Artery, Right J External Iliac Artery, Left K Femoral Artery, Right L Femoral Artery, Left M Popliteal Artery, Right N Popliteal Artery, Left P Anterior Tibial Artery, Right Q Anterior Tibial Artery, Left R Posterior Tibial Artery, Right S Posterior Tibial Artery, Left T Peroneal Artery, Right U Peroneal Artery, Left V Foot Artery, Right W Foot Artery, Left	0 Open 3 Percutaneous 4 Percutaneous Endoscopic	3 Infusion Device D Intraluminal Device	Z No Qualifier

SECTION: 0 **MEDICAL AND SURGICAL**
BODY SYSTEM: 4 **LOWER ARTERIES**
OPERATION: J **INSPECTION:** Visually and/or manually exploring a body part

Body Part	Approach	Device	Qualifier
Y Lower Artery	0 Open 3 Percutaneous 4 Percutaneous Endoscopic X External	Z No Device	Z No Qualifier

H: INSERTION   J: INSPECTION

4: LOWER ARTERIES

0: M/S

◀ New   ◀▥ Revised   ~~deleted~~ Deleted   ♀ Females Only   ♂ Males Only
Noncovered   Limited Coverage   Hospital-Acquired Condition   **Coding Clinic**

SECTION: 0 MEDICAL AND SURGICAL
BODY SYSTEM: 4 LOWER ARTERIES
OPERATION: L OCCLUSION: Completely closing an orifice or the lumen of a tubular body part

Body Part	Approach	Device	Qualifier
0 Abdominal Aorta 1 Celiac Artery 2 Gastric Artery 3 Hepatic Artery 4 Splenic Artery 5 Superior Mesenteric Artery 6 Colic Artery, Right 7 Colic Artery, Left 8 Colic Artery, Middle 9 Renal Artery, Right A Renal Artery, Left B Inferior Mesenteric Artery C Common Iliac Artery, Right D Common Iliac Artery, Left H External Iliac Artery, Right J External Iliac Artery, Left K Femoral Artery, Right L Femoral Artery, Left M Popliteal Artery, Right N Popliteal Artery, Left P Anterior Tibial Artery, Right Q Anterior Tibial Artery, Left R Posterior Tibial Artery, Right S Posterior Tibial Artery, Left T Peroneal Artery, Right U Peroneal Artery, Left V Foot Artery, Right W Foot Artery, Left Y Lower Artery	0 Open 3 Percutaneous 4 Percutaneous Endoscopic	C Extraluminal Device D Intraluminal Device Z No Device	Z No Qualifier
E Internal Iliac Artery, Right	0 Open 3 Percutaneous 4 Percutaneous Endoscopic	C Extraluminal Device D Intraluminal Device Z No Device	T Uterine Artery, Right ♀ Z No Qualifier
F Internal Iliac Artery, Left	0 Open 3 Percutaneous 4 Percutaneous Endoscopic	C Extraluminal Device D Intraluminal Device Z No Device	U Uterine Artery, Left ♀ Z No Qualifier

◀ New   ◀▥ Revised   ~~deleted~~ Deleted   ♀ Females Only   ♂ Males Only
 Noncovered   Limited Coverage   Hospital-Acquired Condition   **Coding Clinic**

SECTION: 0 MEDICAL AND SURGICAL
BODY SYSTEM: 4 LOWER ARTERIES
OPERATION: N RELEASE: Freeing a body part from an abnormal physical constraint by cutting or by the use of force

Body Part	Approach	Device	Qualifier
0 Abdominal Aorta	0 Open	Z No Device	Z No Qualifier
1 Celiac Artery	3 Percutaneous		
2 Gastric Artery	4 Percutaneous Endoscopic		
3 Hepatic Artery			
4 Splenic Artery			
5 Superior Mesenteric Artery			
6 Colic Artery, Right			
7 Colic Artery, Left			
8 Colic Artery, Middle			
9 Renal Artery, Right			
A Renal Artery, Left			
B Inferior Mesenteric Artery			
C Common Iliac Artery, Right			
D Common Iliac Artery, Left			
E Internal Iliac Artery, Right			
F Internal Iliac Artery, Left			
H External Iliac Artery, Right			
J External Iliac Artery, Left			
K Femoral Artery, Right			
L Femoral Artery, Left			
M Popliteal Artery, Right			
N Popliteal Artery, Left			
P Anterior Tibial Artery, Right			
Q Anterior Tibial Artery, Left			
R Posterior Tibial Artery, Right			
S Posterior Tibial Artery, Left			
T Peroneal Artery, Right			
U Peroneal Artery, Left			
V Foot Artery, Right			
W Foot Artery, Left			
Y Lower Artery			

N: RELEASE

4: LOWER ARTERIES

0: M/S

◀ New ◀ Revised deleted Deleted ♀ Females Only ♂ Males Only
Noncovered Limited Coverage Hospital-Acquired Condition **Coding Clinic**

SECTION: 0 MEDICAL AND SURGICAL
BODY SYSTEM: 4 LOWER ARTERIES
OPERATION: **P REMOVAL:** Taking out or off a device from a body part

Body Part	Approach	Device	Qualifier
Y Lower Artery	0 Open 3 Percutaneous 4 Percutaneous Endoscopic	0 Drainage Device 2 Monitoring Device 3 Infusion Device 7 Autologous Tissue Substitute C Extraluminal Device D Intraluminal Device J Synthetic Substitute K Nonautologous Tissue Substitute	Z No Qualifier
Y Lower Artery	X External	0 Drainage Device 1 Radioactive Element 2 Monitoring Device 3 Infusion Device D Intraluminal Device	Z No Qualifier

SECTION: 0 MEDICAL AND SURGICAL
BODY SYSTEM: 4 LOWER ARTERIES
OPERATION: Q REPAIR: Restoring, to the extent possible, a body part to its normal anatomic structure and function

Body Part	Approach	Device	Qualifier
0 Abdominal Aorta	0 Open	Z No Device	Z No Qualifier
1 Celiac Artery	3 Percutaneous		
2 Gastric Artery	4 Percutaneous Endoscopic		
3 Hepatic Artery			
4 Splenic Artery			
5 Superior Mesenteric Artery			
6 Colic Artery, Right			
7 Colic Artery, Left			
8 Colic Artery, Middle			
9 Renal Artery, Right			
A Renal Artery, Left			
B Inferior Mesenteric Artery			
C Common Iliac Artery, Right			
D Common Iliac Artery, Left			
E Internal Iliac Artery, Right			
F Internal Iliac Artery, Left			
H External Iliac Artery, Right			
J External Iliac Artery, Left			
K Femoral Artery, Right			
L Femoral Artery, Left			
M Popliteal Artery, Right			
N Popliteal Artery, Left			
P Anterior Tibial Artery, Right			
Q Anterior Tibial Artery, Left			
R Posterior Tibial Artery, Right			
S Posterior Tibial Artery, Left			
T Peroneal Artery, Right			
U Peroneal Artery, Left			
V Foot Artery, Right			
W Foot Artery, Left			
Y Lower Artery			

Q: REPAIR

4: LOWER ARTERIES

0: M/S

◀ New   ◀ Revised   ~~deleted~~ Deleted   ♀ Females Only   ♂ Males Only
Noncovered   Limited Coverage   Hospital-Acquired Condition   **Coding Clinic**

SECTION: 0 MEDICAL AND SURGICAL
BODY SYSTEM: 4 LOWER ARTERIES
OPERATION: R **REPLACEMENT:** Putting in or on biological or synthetic material that physically takes the place and/or function of all or a portion of a body part

Body Part	Approach	Device	Qualifier
0 Abdominal Aorta 1 Celiac Artery 2 Gastric Artery 3 Hepatic Artery 4 Splenic Artery 5 Superior Mesenteric Artery 6 Colic Artery, Right 7 Colic Artery, Left 8 Colic Artery, Middle 9 Renal Artery, Right A Renal Artery, Left B Inferior Mesenteric Artery C Common Iliac Artery, Right D Common Iliac Artery, Left E Internal Iliac Artery, Right F Internal Iliac Artery, Left H External Iliac Artery, Right J External Iliac Artery, Left K Femoral Artery, Right L Femoral Artery, Left M Popliteal Artery, Right N Popliteal Artery, Left P Anterior Tibial Artery, Right Q Anterior Tibial Artery, Left R Posterior Tibial Artery, Right S Posterior Tibial Artery, Left T Peroneal Artery, Right U Peroneal Artery, Left V Foot Artery, Right W Foot Artery, Left Y Lower Artery	0 Open 4 Percutaneous Endoscopic	7 Autologous Tissue Substitute J Synthetic Substitute K Nonautologous Tissue Substitute	Z No Qualifier

0: M/S   4: LOWER ARTERIES   R: REPLACEMENT

SECTION: 0 MEDICAL AND SURGICAL
BODY SYSTEM: 4 LOWER ARTERIES
OPERATION: S REPOSITION: Moving to its normal location, or other suitable location, all or a portion of a body part

Body Part	Approach	Device	Qualifier
0 Abdominal Aorta 1 Celiac Artery 2 Gastric Artery 3 Hepatic Artery 4 Splenic Artery 5 Superior Mesenteric Artery 6 Colic Artery, Right 7 Colic Artery, Left 8 Colic Artery, Middle 9 Renal Artery, Right A Renal Artery, Left B Inferior Mesenteric Artery C Common Iliac Artery, Right D Common Iliac Artery, Left E Internal Iliac Artery, Right F Internal Iliac Artery, Left H External Iliac Artery, Right J External Iliac Artery, Left K Femoral Artery, Right L Femoral Artery, Left M Popliteal Artery, Right N Popliteal Artery, Left P Anterior Tibial Artery, Right Q Anterior Tibial Artery, Left R Posterior Tibial Artery, Right S Posterior Tibial Artery, Left T Peroneal Artery, Right U Peroneal Artery, Left V Foot Artery, Right W Foot Artery, Left Y Lower Artery	0 Open 3 Percutaneous 4 Percutaneous Endoscopic	Z No Device	Z No Qualifier

S: REPOSITION

4: LOWER ARTERIES

0: M/S

◀ New ◀▥ Revised ~~deleted~~ Deleted ♀ Females Only ♂ Males Only
Noncovered Limited Coverage Hospital-Acquired Condition **Coding Clinic**

SECTION: 0 MEDICAL AND SURGICAL
BODY SYSTEM: 4 LOWER ARTERIES
OPERATION: U SUPPLEMENT: Putting in or on biological or synthetic material that physically reinforces and/or augments the function of a portion of a body part

Body Part	Approach	Device	Qualifier
0 Abdominal Aorta	0 Open	7 Autologous Tissue Substitute	Z No Qualifier
1 Celiac Artery	3 Percutaneous	J Synthetic Substitute	
2 Gastric Artery	4 Percutaneous Endoscopic	K Nonautologous Tissue	
3 Hepatic Artery		Substitute	
4 Splenic Artery			
5 Superior Mesenteric Artery			
6 Colic Artery, Right			
7 Colic Artery, Left			
8 Colic Artery, Middle			
9 Renal Artery, Right			
A Renal Artery, Left			
B Inferior Mesenteric Artery			
C Common Iliac Artery, Right			
D Common Iliac Artery, Left			
E Internal Iliac Artery, Right			
F Internal Iliac Artery, Left			
H External Iliac Artery, Right			
J External Iliac Artery, Left			
K Femoral Artery, Right			
L Femoral Artery, Left			
M Popliteal Artery, Right			
N Popliteal Artery, Left			
P Anterior Tibial Artery, Right			
Q Anterior Tibial Artery, Left			
R Posterior Tibial Artery, Right			
S Posterior Tibial Artery, Left			
T Peroneal Artery, Right			
U Peroneal Artery, Left			
V Foot Artery, Right			
W Foot Artery, Left			
Y Lower Artery			

◀ New   ◀▥ Revised   ~~deleted~~ Deleted   ♀ Females Only   ♂ Males Only
℞ Noncovered   ℞ Limited Coverage   ℞ Hospital-Acquired Condition   **Coding Clinic**

113

SECTION: 0   MEDICAL AND SURGICAL
BODY SYSTEM: 4   LOWER ARTERIES
OPERATION: V   RESTRICTION: Partially closing an orifice or the lumen of a tubular body part

Body Part	Approach	Device	Qualifier
0 Abdominal Aorta	0 Open 3 Percutaneous 4 Percutaneous Endoscopic	C Extraluminal Device Z No Device	Z No Qualifier
0 Abdominal Aorta	0 Open 3 Percutaneous 4 Percutaneous Endoscopic	D Intraluminal Device	J Temporary Z No Qualifier
1 Celiac Artery 2 Gastric Artery 3 Hepatic Artery 4 Splenic Artery 5 Superior Mesenteric Artery 6 Colic Artery, Right 7 Colic Artery, Left 8 Colic Artery, Middle 9 Renal Artery, Right A Renal Artery, Left B Inferior Mesenteric Artery C Common Iliac Artery, Right D Common Iliac Artery, Left E Internal Iliac Artery, Right F Internal Iliac Artery, Left H External Iliac Artery, Right J External Iliac Artery, Left K Femoral Artery, Right L Femoral Artery, Left M Popliteal Artery, Right N Popliteal Artery, Left P Anterior Tibial Artery, Right Q Anterior Tibial Artery, Left R Posterior Tibial Artery, Right S Posterior Tibial Artery, Left T Peroneal Artery, Right U Peroneal Artery, Left V Foot Artery, Right W Foot Artery, Left Y Lower Artery	0 Open 3 Percutaneous 4 Percutaneous Endoscopic	C Extraluminal Device D Intraluminal Device Z No Device	Z No Qualifier

SECTION: 0   MEDICAL AND SURGICAL
BODY SYSTEM: 4   LOWER ARTERIES
OPERATION: W   REVISION: Correcting, to the extent possible, a portion of a malfunctioning device or the position of a displaced device

Body Part	Approach	Device	Qualifier
Y Lower Artery	0 Open 3 Percutaneous 4 Percutaneous Endoscopic X External	0 Drainage Device 2 Monitoring Device 3 Infusion Device 7 Autologous Tissue Substitute C Extraluminal Device D Intraluminal Device J Synthetic Substitute K Nonautologous Tissue Substitute	Z No Qualifier

114

◀ New   ◀▥ Revised   deleted Deleted   ♀ Females Only   ♂ Males Only
🅽 Noncovered   🅛 Limited Coverage   🅗 Hospital-Acquired Condition   **Coding Clinic**

◀ New   ◀◀◀ Revised   ~~deleted~~ Deleted   ♀ Females Only   ♂ Males Only
🚫 Noncovered   🚫 Limited Coverage   🚫 Hospital-Acquired Condition   **Coding Clinic**

SECTION: 0 MEDICAL AND SURGICAL

BODY SYSTEM: 5 UPPER VEINS

OPERATION: 1 **BYPASS:** Altering the route of passage of the contents of a tubular body part

Body Part	Approach	Device	Qualifier
0 Azygos Vein	0 Open	7 Autologous Tissue Substitute	Y Upper Vein
1 Hemiazygos Vein	4 Percutaneous Endoscopic	9 Autologous Venous Tissue	
3 Innominate Vein, Right		A Autologous Arterial Tissue	
4 Innominate Vein, Left		J Synthetic Substitute	
5 Subclavian Vein, Right		K Nonautologous Tissue	
6 Subclavian Vein, Left		Substitute	
7 Axillary Vein, Right		Z No Device	
8 Axillary Vein, Left			
9 Brachial Vein, Right			
A Brachial Vein, Left			
B Basilic Vein, Right			
C Basilic Vein, Left			
D Cephalic Vein, Right			
F Cephalic Vein, Left			
G Hand Vein, Right			
H Hand Vein, Left			
L Intracranial Vein			
M Internal Jugular Vein, Right			
N Internal Jugular Vein, Left			
P External Jugular Vein, Right			
Q External Jugular Vein, Left			
R Vertebral Vein, Right			
S Vertebral Vein, Left			
T Face Vein, Right			
V Face Vein, Left			

1: BYPASS

5: UPPER VEINS

0: M/S

◄ New   ◄ Revised   deleted Deleted   ♀ Females Only   ♂ Males Only
Noncovered   Limited Coverage   Hospital-Acquired Condition   **Coding Clinic**

SECTION: 0 MEDICAL AND SURGICAL
BODY SYSTEM: 5 UPPER VEINS
OPERATION: 5 **DESTRUCTION:** Physical eradication of all or a portion of a body part by the direct use of energy, force, or a destructive agent

Body Part	Approach	Device	Qualifier
0 Azygos Vein	0 Open	Z No Device	Z No Qualifier
1 Hemiazygos Vein	3 Percutaneous		
3 Innominate Vein, Right	4 Percutaneous Endoscopic		
4 Innominate Vein, Left			
5 Subclavian Vein, Right			
6 Subclavian Vein, Left			
7 Axillary Vein, Right			
8 Axillary Vein, Left			
9 Brachial Vein, Right			
A Brachial Vein, Left			
B Basilic Vein, Right			
C Basilic Vein, Left			
D Cephalic Vein, Right			
F Cephalic Vein, Left			
G Hand Vein, Right			
H Hand Vein, Left			
L Intracranial Vein			
M Internal Jugular Vein, Right			
N Internal Jugular Vein, Left			
P External Jugular Vein, Right			
Q External Jugular Vein, Left			
R Vertebral Vein, Right			
S Vertebral Vein, Left			
T Face Vein, Right			
V Face Vein, Left			
Y Upper Vein			

0: M/S

5: UPPER VEINS

5: DESTRUCTION

SECTION: 0 MEDICAL AND SURGICAL

BODY SYSTEM: 5 UPPER VEINS

OPERATION: 7 DILATION: Expanding an orifice or the lumen of a tubular body part

Body Part	Approach	Device	Qualifier
0 Azygos Vein	0 Open	D Intraluminal Device	Z No Qualifier
1 Hemiazygos Vein	3 Percutaneous	Z No Device	
3 Innominate Vein, Right	4 Percutaneous Endoscopic		
4 Innominate Vein, Left			
5 Subclavian Vein, Right			
6 Subclavian Vein, Left			
7 Axillary Vein, Right			
8 Axillary Vein, Left			
9 Brachial Vein, Right			
A Brachial Vein, Left			
B Basilic Vein, Right			
C Basilic Vein, Left 🜂			
D Cephalic Vein, Right			
F Cephalic Vein, Left			
G Hand Vein, Right			
H Hand Vein, Left			
L Intracranial Vein 🜂			
M Internal Jugular Vein, Right			
N Internal Jugular Vein, Left			
P External Jugular Vein, Right			
Q External Jugular Vein, Left			
R Vertebral Vein, Right			
S Vertebral Vein, Left			
T Face Vein, Right			
V Face Vein, Left			
Y Upper Vein			

🜂 057L3ZZ, 057L4ZZ
🜂 05CL3ZZ, 05CL4ZZ

◀ New   ◀▥ Revised   deleted Deleted   ♀ Females Only   ♂ Males Only
🜂 Noncovered   🜂 Limited Coverage   🜂 Hospital-Acquired Condition   **Coding Clinic**

SECTION: 0 MEDICAL AND SURGICAL

BODY SYSTEM: 5 UPPER VEINS

OPERATION: 9 DRAINAGE: Taking or letting out fluids and/or gases from a body part

Body Part	Approach	Device	Qualifier
0 Azygos Vein 1 Hemiazygos Vein 3 Innominate Vein, Right 4 Innominate Vein, Left 5 Subclavian Vein, Right 6 Subclavian Vein, Left 7 Axillary Vein, Right 8 Axillary Vein, Left 9 Brachial Vein, Right A Brachial Vein, Left B Basilic Vein, Right C Basilic Vein, Left D Cephalic Vein, Right F Cephalic Vein, Left G Hand Vein, Right H Hand Vein, Left L Intracranial Vein M Internal Jugular Vein, Right N Internal Jugular Vein, Left P External Jugular Vein, Right Q External Jugular Vein, Left R Vertebral Vein, Right S Vertebral Vein, Left T Face Vein, Right V Face Vein, Left Y Upper Vein	0 Open 3 Percutaneous 4 Percutaneous Endoscopic	0 Drainage Device	Z No Qualifier
0 Azygos Vein 1 Hemiazygos Vein 3 Innominate Vein, Right 4 Innominate Vein, Left 5 Subclavian Vein, Right 6 Subclavian Vein, Left 7 Axillary Vein, Right 8 Axillary Vein, Left 9 Brachial Vein, Right A Brachial Vein, Left B Basilic Vein, Right C Basilic Vein, Left D Cephalic Vein, Right F Cephalic Vein, Left G Hand Vein, Right H Hand Vein, Left L Intracranial Vein M Internal Jugular Vcin, Right N Internal Jugular Vein, Left P External Jugular Vein, Right Q External Jugular Vein, Left R Vertebral Vein, Right S Vertebral Vein, Left T Face Vein, Right V Face Vein, Left Y Upper Vein	0 Open 3 Percutaneous 4 Percutaneous Endoscopic	Z No Device	X Diagnostic Z No Qualifier

0: M/S 5: UPPER VEINS 9: DRAINAGE

 New ◀ Revised ~~deleted~~ Deleted ♀ Females Only ♂ Males Only
Noncovered Limited Coverage Hospital-Acquired Condition **Coding Clinic**

119

SECTION: 0 MEDICAL AND SURGICAL
BODY SYSTEM: 5 UPPER VEINS
OPERATION: B **EXCISION:** Cutting out or off, without replacement, a portion of a body part

Body Part	Approach	Device	Qualifier
0 Azygos Vein	0 Open	Z No Device	X Diagnostic
1 Hemiazygos Vein	3 Percutaneous		Z No Qualifier
3 Innominate Vein, Right	4 Percutaneous Endoscopic		
4 Innominate Vein, Left			
5 Subclavian Vein, Right			
6 Subclavian Vein, Left			
7 Axillary Vein, Right			
8 Axillary Vein, Left			
9 Brachial Vein, Right			
A Brachial Vein, Left			
B Basilic Vein, Right			
C Basilic Vein, Left			
D Cephalic Vein, Right			
F Cephalic Vein, Left			
G Hand Vein, Right			
H Hand Vein, Left			
L Intracranial Vein			
M Internal Jugular Vein, Right			
N Internal Jugular Vein, Left			
P External Jugular Vein, Right			
Q External Jugular Vein, Left			
R Vertebral Vein, Right			
S Vertebral Vein, Left			
T Face Vein, Right			
V Face Vein, Left			
Y Upper Vein			

◀ New ◀▥ Revised ~~deleted~~ Deleted ♀ Females Only ♂ Males Only
🅝 Noncovered 🅛 Limited Coverage 🅗 Hospital-Acquired Condition **Coding Clinic**

SECTION: 0 MEDICAL AND SURGICAL

BODY SYSTEM: 5 UPPER VEINS

OPERATION: C EXTIRPATION: Taking or cutting out solid matter from a body part

Body Part	Approach	Device	Qualifier
0 Azygos Vein	0 Open	Z No Device	Z No Qualifier
1 Hemiazygos Vein	3 Percutaneous		
3 Innominate Vein, Right	4 Percutaneous Endoscopic		
4 Innominate Vein, Left			
5 Subclavian Vein, Right			
6 Subclavian Vein, Left			
7 Axillary Vein, Right			
8 Axillary Vein, Left			
9 Brachial Vein, Right			
A Brachial Vein, Left			
B Basilic Vein, Right			
C Basilic Vein, Left			
D Cephalic Vein, Right			
F Cephalic Vein, Left			
G Hand Vein, Right			
H Hand Vein, Left			
L Intracranial Vein			
M Internal Jugular Vein, Right			
N Internal Jugular Vein, Left			
P External Jugular Vein, Right			
Q External Jugular Vein, Left			
R Vertebral Vein, Right			
S Vertebral Vein, Left			
T Face Vein, Right			
V Face Vein, Left			
Y Upper Vein			

MCE: Always non-covered procedures:
05CL3ZZ
05CL4ZZ

SECTION: 0 MEDICAL AND SURGICAL

BODY SYSTEM: 5 UPPER VEINS

OPERATION: D EXTRACTION: Pulling or stripping out or off all or a portion of a body part by the use of force

Body Part	Approach	Device	Qualifier
9 Brachial Vein, Right	0 Open	Z No Device	Z No Qualifier
A Brachial Vein, Left	3 Percutaneous		
B Basilic Vein, Right			
C Basilic Vein, Left			
D Cephalic Vein, Right			
F Cephalic Vein, Left			
G Hand Vein, Right			
H Hand Vein, Left			
Y Upper Vein			

◀ New ◀ Revised ~~deleted~~ Deleted ♀ Females Only ♂ Males Only
🚫 Noncovered 🚫 Limited Coverage 🚫 Hospital-Acquired Condition **Coding Clinic**

121

SECTION: 0 MEDICAL AND SURGICAL

BODY SYSTEM: 5 UPPER VEINS

OPERATION: H INSERTION: Putting in a nonbiological appliance that monitors, assists, performs, or prevents a physiological function but does not physically take the place of a body part

Body Part	Approach	Device	Qualifier
0 Azygos Vein 1 Hemiazygos Vein 3 Innominate Vein, Right 4 Innominate Vein, Left 5 Subclavian Vein, Right 6 Subclavian Vein, Left 7 Axillary Vein, Right 8 Axillary Vein, Left 9 Brachial Vein, Right A Brachial Vein, Left B Basilic Vein, Right C Basilic Vein, Left D Cephalic Vein, Right F Cephalic Vein, Left G Hand Vein, Right H Hand Vein, Left L Intracranial Vein M Internal Jugular Vein, Right ⚕ N Internal Jugular Vein, Left ⚕ P External Jugular Vein, Right ⚕ Q External Jugular Vein, Left ⚕ R Vertebral Vein, Right S Vertebral Vein, Left T Face Vein, Right V Face Vein, Left	0 Open 3 Percutaneous 4 Percutaneous Endoscopic	3 Infusion Device D Intraluminal Device	Z No Qualifier
Y Upper Vein	0 Open 3 Percutaneous 4 Percutaneous Endoscopic	2 Monitoring Device 3 Infusion Device D Intraluminal Device	Z No Qualifier

⚕ 05HM33Z, 05HN33Z, 05HP33Z, 05HQ33Z

SECTION: 0 MEDICAL AND SURGICAL

BODY SYSTEM: 5 UPPER VEINS

OPERATION: J INSPECTION: Visually and/or manually exploring a body part

Body Part	Approach	Device	Qualifier
Y Upper Vein	0 Open 3 Percutaneous 4 Percutaneous Endoscopic X External	Z No Device	Z No Qualifier

◀ New ◀ Revised ~~deleted~~ Deleted ♀ Females Only ♂ Males Only
⚕ Noncovered ⚕ Limited Coverage ⚕ Hospital-Acquired Condition **Coding Clinic**

Sidebar: H: INSERTION J: INSPECTION 5: UPPER VEINS 0: M/S

SECTION: 0 MEDICAL AND SURGICAL

BODY SYSTEM: 5 UPPER VEINS

OPERATION: L OCCLUSION: Completely closing an orifice or the lumen of a tubular body part

Body Part	Approach	Device	Qualifier
0 Azygos Vein	0 Open	C Extraluminal Device	Z No Qualifier
1 Hemiazygos Vein	3 Percutaneous	D Intraluminal Device	
3 Innominate Vein, Right	4 Percutaneous Endoscopic	Z No Device	
4 Innominate Vein, Left			
5 Subclavian Vein, Right			
6 Subclavian Vein, Left			
7 Axillary Vein, Right			
8 Axillary Vein, Left			
9 Brachial Vein, Right			
A Brachial Vein, Left			
B Basilic Vein, Right			
C Basilic Vein, Left			
D Cephalic Vein, Right			
F Cephalic Vein, Left			
G Hand Vein, Right			
H Hand Vein, Left			
L Intracranial Vein			
M Internal Jugular Vein, Right			
N Internal Jugular Vein, Left			
P External Jugular Vein, Right			
Q External Jugular Vein, Left			
R Vertebral Vein, Right			
S Vertebral Vein, Left			
T Face Vein, Right			
V Face Vein, Left			
Y Upper Vein			

0: M/S

5: UPPER VEINS

L: OCCLUSION

◀ New ◀▥ Revised deleted Deleted ♀ Females Only ♂ Males Only
Noncovered Limited Coverage Hospital-Acquired Condition Coding Clinic

123

N: RELEASE   P: REMOVAL

5: UPPER VEINS

0: M/S

SECTION: 0 MEDICAL AND SURGICAL
BODY SYSTEM: 5 UPPER VEINS
OPERATION: N RELEASE: Freeing a body part from an abnormal physical constraint

Body Part	Approach	Device	Qualifier
0 Azygos Vein 1 Hemiazygos Vein 3 Innominate Vein, Right 4 Innominate Vein, Left 5 Subclavian Vein, Right 6 Subclavian Vein, Left 7 Axillary Vein, Right 8 Axillary Vein, Left 9 Brachial Vein, Right A Brachial Vein, Left B Basilic Vein, Right C Basilic Vein, Left D Cephalic Vein, Right F Cephalic Vein, Left G Hand Vein, Right H Hand Vein, Left L Intracranial Vein M Internal Jugular Vein, Right N Internal Jugular Vein, Left P External Jugular Vein, Right Q External Jugular Vein, Left R Vertebral Vein, Right S Vertebral Vein, Left T Face Vein, Right V Face Vein, Left Y Upper Vein	0 Open 3 Percutaneous 4 Percutaneous Endoscopic	Z No Device	Z No Qualifier

SECTION: 0 MEDICAL AND SURGICAL
BODY SYSTEM: 5 UPPER VEINS
OPERATION: P REMOVAL: Taking out or off a device from a body part

Body Part	Approach	Device	Qualifier
Y Upper Vein	0 Open 3 Percutaneous 4 Percutaneous Endoscopic	0 Drainage Device 2 Monitoring Device 3 Infusion Device 7 Autologous Tissue Substitute C Extraluminal Device D Intraluminal Device J Synthetic Substitute K Nonautologous Tissue Substitute	Z No Qualifier
Y Upper Vein	X External	0 Drainage Device 2 Monitoring Device 3 Infusion Device D Intraluminal Device	Z No Qualifier

◀ New   ◀▥ Revised   ~~deleted~~ Deleted   ♀ Females Only   ♂ Males Only
▥ Noncovered   ▥ Limited Coverage   ▥ Hospital-Acquired Condition   **Coding Clinic**

SECTION: 0 MEDICAL AND SURGICAL

BODY SYSTEM: 5 UPPER VEINS

OPERATION: **Q REPAIR:** Restoring, to the extent possible, a body part to its normal anatomic structure and function

Body Part	Approach	Device	Qualifier
0 Azygos Vein	0 Open	Z No Device	Z No Qualifier
1 Hemiazygos Vein	3 Percutaneous		
3 Innominate Vein, Right	4 Percutaneous Endoscopic		
4 Innominate Vein, Left			
5 Subclavian Vein, Right			
6 Subclavian Vein, Left			
7 Axillary Vein, Right			
8 Axillary Vein, Left			
9 Brachial Vein, Right			
A Brachial Vein, Left			
B Basilic Vein, Right			
C Basilic Vein, Left			
D Cephalic Vein, Right			
F Cephalic Vein, Left			
G Hand Vein, Right			
H Hand Vein, Left			
L Intracranial Vein			
M Internal Jugular Vein, Right			
N Internal Jugular Vein, Left			
P External Jugular Vein, Right			
Q External Jugular Vein, Left			
R Vertebral Vein, Right			
S Vertebral Vein, Left			
T Face Vein, Right			
V Face Vein, Left			
Y Upper Vein			

◀ New ◀▦ Revised ~~deleted~~ Deleted ♀ Females Only ♂ Males Only
🅝 Noncovered 🅛 Limited Coverage 🅗 Hospital-Acquired Condition **Coding Clinic**

125

SECTION: 0 MEDICAL AND SURGICAL
BODY SYSTEM: 5 UPPER VEINS
OPERATION: R REPLACEMENT: Putting in or on biological or synthetic material that physically takes the place and/or function of all or a portion of a body part

Body Part	Approach	Device	Qualifier
0 Azygos Vein	0 Open	7 Autologous Tissue Substitute	Z No Qualifier
1 Hemiazygos Vein	4 Percutaneous Endoscopic	J Synthetic Substitute	
3 Innominate Vein, Right		K Nonautologous Tissue Substitute	
4 Innominate Vein, Left			
5 Subclavian Vein, Right			
6 Subclavian Vein, Left			
7 Axillary Vein, Right			
8 Axillary Vein, Left			
9 Brachial Vein, Right			
A Brachial Vein, Left			
B Basilic Vein, Right			
C Basilic Vein, Left			
D Cephalic Vein, Right			
F Cephalic Vein, Left			
G Hand Vein, Right			
H Hand Vein, Left			
L Intracranial Vein			
M Internal Jugular Vein, Right			
N Internal Jugular Vein, Left			
P External Jugular Vein, Right			
Q External Jugular Vein, Left			
R Vertebral Vein, Right			
S Vertebral Vein, Left			
T Face Vein, Right			
V Face Vein, Left			
Y Upper Vein			

R: REPLACEMENT

5: UPPER VEINS

0: M/S

◀ New ◀▥ Revised ~~deleted~~ Deleted ♀ Females Only ♂ Males Only
℞ Noncovered ℞ Limited Coverage ℞ Hospital-Acquired Condition **Coding Clinic**

SECTION: 0 MEDICAL AND SURGICAL
BODY SYSTEM: 5 UPPER VEINS
OPERATION: S REPOSITION: Moving to its normal location, or other suitable location, all or a portion of a body part

Body Part	Approach	Device	Qualifier
0 Azygos Vein	0 Open	Z No Device	Z No Qualifier
1 Hemiazygos Vein	3 Percutaneous		
3 Innominate Vein, Right	4 Percutaneous Endoscopic		
4 Innominate Vein, Left			
5 Subclavian Vein, Right			
6 Subclavian Vein, Left			
7 Axillary Vein, Right			
8 Axillary Vein, Left			
9 Brachial Vein, Right			
A Brachial Vein, Left			
B Basilic Vein, Right			
C Basilic Vein, Left			
D Cephalic Vein, Right			
F Cephalic Vein, Left			
G Hand Vein, Right			
H Hand Vein, Left			
L Intracranial Vein			
M Internal Jugular Vein, Right			
N Internal Jugular Vein, Left			
P External Jugular Vein, Right			
Q External Jugular Vein, Left			
R Vertebral Vein, Right			
S Vertebral Vein, Left			
T Face Vein, Right			
V Face Vein, Left			
Y Upper Vein			

SECTION: 0 MEDICAL AND SURGICAL
BODY SYSTEM: 5 UPPER VEINS
OPERATION: U SUPPLEMENT: Putting in or on biological or synthetic material that physically reinforces and/or augments the function of a portion of a body part

Body Part	Approach	Device	Qualifier
0 Azygos Vein	0 Open	7 Autologous Tissue Substitute	Z No Qualifier
1 Hemiazygos Vein	3 Percutaneous	J Synthetic Substitute	
3 Innominate Vein, Right	4 Percutaneous Endoscopic	K Nonautologous Tissue Substitute	
4 Innominate Vein, Left			
5 Subclavian Vein, Right			
6 Subclavian Vein, Left			
7 Axillary Vein, Right			
8 Axillary Vein, Left			
9 Brachial Vein, Right			
A Brachial Vein, Left			
B Basilic Vein, Right			
C Basilic Vein, Left			
D Cephalic Vein, Right			
F Cephalic Vein, Left			
G Hand Vein, Right			
H Hand Vein, Left			
L Intracranial Vein			
M Internal Jugular Vein, Right			
N Internal Jugular Vein, Left			
P External Jugular Vein, Right			
Q External Jugular Vein, Left			
R Vertebral Vein, Right			
S Vertebral Vein, Left			
T Face Vein, Right			
V Face Vein, Left			
Y Upper Vein			

U: SUPPLEMENT

5: UPPER VEINS

0: M/S

◀ New   ◀▦ Revised   deleted Deleted   ♀ Females Only   ♂ Males Only
℞ Noncovered   ℞ Limited Coverage   ℞ Hospital-Acquired Condition   **Coding Clinic**

SECTION: 0 MEDICAL AND SURGICAL
BODY SYSTEM: 5 UPPER VEINS
OPERATION: V RESTRICTION: Partially closing an orifice or the lumen of a tubular body part

Body Part	Approach	Device	Qualifier
0 Azygos Vein 1 Hemiazygos Vein 3 Innominate Vein, Right 4 Innominate Vein, Left 5 Subclavian Vein, Right 6 Subclavian Vein, Left 7 Axillary Vein, Right 8 Axillary Vein, Left 9 Brachial Vein, Right A Brachial Vein, Left B Basilic Vein, Right C Basilic Vein, Left D Cephalic Vein, Right F Cephalic Vein, Left G Hand Vein, Right H Hand Vein, Left L Intracranial Vein M Internal Jugular Vein, Right N Internal Jugular Vein, Left P External Jugular Vein, Right Q External Jugular Vein, Left R Vertebral Vein, Right S Vertebral Vein, Left T Face Vein, Right V Face Vein, Left Y Upper Vein	0 Open 3 Percutaneous 4 Percutaneous Endoscopic	C Extraluminal Device D Intraluminal Device Z No Device	Z No Qualifier

SECTION: 0 MEDICAL AND SURGICAL
BODY SYSTEM: 5 UPPER VEINS
OPERATION: W REVISION: Correcting, to the extent possible, a portion of a malfunctioning device or the position of a displaced device

Body Part	Approach	Device	Qualifier
Y Upper Vein	0 Open 3 Percutaneous 4 Percutaneous Endoscopic X External	0 Drainage Device 2 Monitoring Device 3 Infusion Device 7 Autologous Tissue Substitute C Extraluminal Device D Intraluminal Device J Synthetic Substitute K Nonautologous Tissue Substitute	Z No Qualifier

0: M/S   5: UPPER VEINS   V: RESTRICTION   W: REVISION

◀ New   ◀▥ Revised   ~~deleted~~ Deleted   ♀ Females Only   ♂ Males Only

Ⓝ Noncovered   Ⓛ Limited Coverage   Ⓗ Hospital-Acquired Condition   **Coding Clinic**

SECTION: 0 MEDICAL AND SURGICAL

BODY SYSTEM: 6 LOWER VEINS
OPERATION: 1 BYPASS: Altering the route of passage of the contents of a tubular body part

Body Part	Approach	Device	Qualifier
0 Inferior Vena Cava	0 Open 4 Percutaneous Endoscopic	7 Autologous Tissue Substitute 9 Autologous Venous Tissue A Autologous Arterial Tissue J Synthetic Substitute K Nonautologous Tissue Substitute Z No Device	5 Superior Mesenteric Vein 6 Inferior Mesenteric Vein Y Lower Vein
1 Splenic Vein	0 Open 4 Percutaneous Endoscopic	7 Autologous Tissue Substitute 9 Autologous Venous Tissue A Autologous Arterial Tissue J Synthetic Substitute K Nonautologous Tissue Substitute Z No Device	9 Renal Vein, Right B Renal Vein, Left Y Lower Vein
2 Gastric Vein 3 Esophageal Vein 4 Hepatic Vein 5 Superior Mesenteric Vein 6 Inferior Mesenteric Vein 7 Colic Vein 9 Renal Vein, Right B Renal Vein, Left C Common Iliac Vein, Right D Common Iliac Vein, Left F External Iliac Vein, Right G External Iliac Vein, Left H Hypogastric Vein, Right J Hypogastric Vein, Left M Femoral Vein, Right N Femoral Vein, Left P Greater Saphenous Vein, Right Q Greater Saphenous Vein, Left R Lesser Saphenous Vein, Right S Lesser Saphenous Vein, Left T Foot Vein, Right V Foot Vein, Left	0 Open 4 Percutaneous Endoscopic	7 Autologous Tissue Substitute 9 Autologous Venous Tissue A Autologous Arterial Tissue J Synthetic Substitute K Nonautologous Tissue Substitute Z No Device	Y Lower Vein
8 Portal Vein	0 Open	7 Autologous Tissue Substitute 9 Autologous Venous Tissue A Autologous Arterial Tissue J Synthetic Substitute K Nonautologous Tissue Substitute Z No Device	9 Renal Vein, Right B Renal Vein, Left Y Lower Vein
8 Portal Vein	3 Percutaneous	D Intraluminal Device	Y Lower Vein
8 Portal Vein	4 Percutaneous Endoscopic	7 Autologous Tissue Substitute 9 Autologous Venous Tissue A Autologous Arterial Tissue J Synthetic Substitute K Nonautologous Tissue Substitute Z No Device	9 Renal Vein, Right B Renal Vein, Left Y Lower Vein
8 Portal Vein	4 Percutaneous Endoscopic	D Intraluminal Device	Y Lower Vein

SECTION: 0 MEDICAL AND SURGICAL
BODY SYSTEM: 6 LOWER VEINS
OPERATION: 5 DESTRUCTION: Physical eradication of all or a portion of a body part by the direct use of energy, force, or a destructive agent

Body Part	Approach	Device	Qualifier
0 Inferior Vena Cava 1 Splenic Vein 2 Gastric Vein 3 Esophageal Vein 4 Hepatic Vein 5 Superior Mesenteric Vein 6 Inferior Mesenteric Vein 7 Colic Vein 8 Portal Vein 9 Renal Vein, Right B Renal Vein, Left C Common Iliac Vein, Right D Common Iliac Vein, Left F External Iliac Vein, Right G External Iliac Vein, Left H Hypogastric Vein, Right J Hypogastric Vein, Left M Femoral Vein, Right N Femoral Vein, Left P Greater Saphenous Vein, Right Q Greater Saphenous Vein, Left R Lesser Saphenous Vein, Right S Lesser Saphenous Vein, Left T Foot Vein, Right V Foot Vein, Left	0 Open 3 Percutaneous 4 Percutaneous Endoscopic	Z No Device	Z No Qualifier
Y Lower Vein	0 Open 3 Percutaneous 4 Percutaneous Endoscopic	Z No Device	C Hemorrhoidal Plexus Z No Qualifier

5: DESTRUCTION

6: LOWER VEINS

0: M/S

◄ New ◄▦ Revised ~~deleted~~ Deleted ♀ Females Only ♂ Males Only
Noncovered Limited Coverage Hospital-Acquired Condition **Coding Clinic**

SECTION: 0 MEDICAL AND SURGICAL
BODY SYSTEM: 6 LOWER VEINS
OPERATION: 7 DILATION: Expanding an orifice or the lumen of a tubular body part

Body Part	Approach	Device	Qualifier
0 Inferior Vena Cava	0 Open	D Intraluminal Device	Z No Qualifier
1 Splenic Vein	3 Percutaneous	Z No Device	
2 Gastric Vein	4 Percutaneous Endoscopic		
3 Esophageal Vein			
4 Hepatic Vein			
5 Superior Mesenteric Vein			
6 Inferior Mesenteric Vein			
7 Colic Vein			
8 Portal Vein			
9 Renal Vein, Right			
B Renal Vein, Left			
C Common Iliac Vein, Right			
D Common Iliac Vein, Left			
F External Iliac Vein, Right			
G External Iliac Vein, Left			
H Hypogastric Vein, Right			
J Hypogastric Vein, Left			
M Femoral Vein, Right			
N Femoral Vein, Left			
P Greater Saphenous Vein, Right			
Q Greater Saphenous Vein, Left			
R Lesser Saphenous Vein, Right			
S Lesser Saphenous Vein, Left			
T Foot Vein, Right			
V Foot Vein, Left			
Y Lower Vein			

0: M/S

6: LOWER VEINS

7: DILATION

SECTION: 0 MEDICAL AND SURGICAL
BODY SYSTEM: 6 LOWER VEINS
OPERATION: 9 DRAINAGE: Taking or letting out fluids and/or gases from a body part

9: DRAINAGE

6: LOWER VEINS

0: M/S

Body Part	Approach	Device	Qualifier
0 Inferior Vena Cava 1 Splenic Vein 2 Gastric Vein 3 Esophageal Vein 4 Hepatic Vein 5 Superior Mesenteric Vein 6 Inferior Mesenteric Vein 7 Colic Vein 8 Portal Vein 9 Renal Vein, Right B Renal Vein, Left C Common Iliac Vein, Right D Common Iliac Vein, Left F External Iliac Vein, Right G External Iliac Vein, Left H Hypogastric Vein, Right J Hypogastric Vein, Left M Femoral Vein, Right N Femoral Vein, Left P Greater Saphenous Vein, Right Q Greater Saphenous Vein, Left R Lesser Saphenous Vein, Right S Lesser Saphenous Vein, Left T Foot Vein, Right V Foot Vein, Left Y Lower Vein	0 Open 3 Percutaneous 4 Percutaneous Endoscopic	0 Drainage Device	Z No Qualifier
0 Inferior Vena Cava 1 Splenic Vein 2 Gastric Vein 3 Esophageal Vein 4 Hepatic Vein 5 Superior Mesenteric Vein 6 Inferior Mesenteric Vein 7 Colic Vein 8 Portal Vein 9 Renal Vein, Right B Renal Vein, Left C Common Iliac Vein, Right D Common Iliac Vein, Left F External Iliac Vein, Right G External Iliac Vein, Left H Hypogastric Vein, Right J Hypogastric Vein, Left M Femoral Vein, Right N Femoral Vein, Left P Greater Saphenous Vein, Right Q Greater Saphenous Vein, Left R Lesser Saphenous Vein, Right S Lesser Saphenous Vein, Left T Foot Vein, Right V Foot Vein, Left Y Lower Vein	0 Open 3 Percutaneous 4 Percutaneous Endoscopic	Z No Device	X Diagnostic Z No Qualifier

 New   Revised   deleted Deleted   ♀ Females Only   ♂ Males Only
Noncovered   Limited Coverage   Hospital-Acquired Condition   **Coding Clinic**

SECTION: 0 MEDICAL AND SURGICAL
BODY SYSTEM: 6 LOWER VEINS
OPERATION: B EXCISION: Cutting out or off, without replacement, a portion of a body part

Body Part	Approach	Device	Qualifier
0 Inferior Vena Cava 1 Splenic Vein 2 Gastric Vein 3 Esophageal Vein 4 Hepatic Vein 5 Superior Mesenteric Vein 6 Inferior Mesenteric Vein 7 Colic Vein 8 Portal Vein 9 Renal Vein, Right B Renal Vein, Left C Common Iliac Vein, Right D Common Iliac Vein, Left F External Iliac Vein, Right G External Iliac Vein, Left H Hypogastric Vein, Right J Hypogastric Vein, Left M Femoral Vein, Right N Femoral Vein, Left P Greater Saphenous Vein, Right Q Greater Saphenous Vein, Left R Lesser Saphenous Vein, Right S Lesser Saphenous Vein, Left T Foot Vein, Right V Foot Vein, Left	0 Open 3 Percutaneous 4 Percutaneous Endoscopic	Z No Device	X Diagnostic Z No Qualifier
Y Lower Vein	0 Open 3 Percutaneous 4 Percutaneous Endoscopic	Z No Device	C Hemorrhoidal Plexus X Diagnostic Z No Qualifier

SECTION: 0 MEDICAL AND SURGICAL
BODY SYSTEM: 6 LOWER VEINS
OPERATION: C EXTIRPATION: Taking or cutting out solid matter from a body part

Body Part	Approach	Device	Qualifier
0 Inferior Vena Cava 1 Splenic Vein 2 Gastric Vein 3 Esophageal Vein 4 Hepatic Vein 5 Superior Mesenteric Vein 6 Inferior Mesenteric Vein 7 Colic Vein 8 Portal Vein 9 Renal Vein, Right B Renal Vein, Left C Common Iliac Vein, Right D Common Iliac Vein, Left F External Iliac Vein, Right G External Iliac Vein, Left H Hypogastric Vein, Right J Hypogastric Vein, Left M Femoral Vein, Right N Femoral Vein, Left P Greater Saphenous Vein, Right Q Greater Saphenous Vein, Left R Lesser Saphenous Vein, Right S Lesser Saphenous Vein, Left T Foot Vein, Right V Foot Vein, Left Y Lower Vein	0 Open 3 Percutaneous 4 Percutaneous Endoscopic	Z No Device	Z No Qualifier

SECTION: 0 MEDICAL AND SURGICAL
BODY SYSTEM: 6 LOWER VEINS
OPERATION: D EXTRACTION: Pulling or stripping out or off all or a portion of a body part by the use of force

Body Part	Approach	Device	Qualifier
M Femoral Vein, Right N Femoral Vein, Left P Greater Saphenous Vein, Right Q Greater Saphenous Vein, Left R Lesser Saphenous Vein, Right S Lesser Saphenous Vein, Left T Foot Vein, Right V Foot Vein, Left Y Lower Vein	0 Open 3 Percutaneous 4 Percutaneous Endoscopic	Z No Device	Z No Qualifier

C: EXTIRPATION   D: EXTRACTION

6: LOWER VEINS   0: M/S

◀ New   ◀▥ Revised   ~~deleted~~ Deleted   ♀ Females Only   ♂ Males Only
Ⓝ Noncovered   Ⓛ Limited Coverage   Ⓗ Hospital-Acquired Condition   **Coding Clinic**

SECTION: 0 MEDICAL AND SURGICAL

BODY SYSTEM: 6 LOWER VEINS

OPERATION: H INSERTION: Putting in a nonbiological appliance that monitors, assists, performs, or prevents a physiological function but does not physically take the place of a body part

Body Part	Approach	Device	Qualifier
0 Inferior Vena Cava	0 Open 3 Percutaneous	3 Infusion Device	T Via Unbilical Vein Z No Qualifier
0 Inferior Vena Cava	0 Open 3 Percutaneous	D Intraluminal Device	Z No Qualifier
0 Inferior Vena Cava	4 Percutaneous Endoscopic	3 Infusion Device D Intraluminal Device	Z No Qualifier
1 Splenic Vein 2 Gastric Vein 3 Esophageal Vein 4 Hepatic Vein 5 Superior Mesenteric Vein 6 Inferior Mesenteric Vein 7 Colic Vein 8 Portal Vein 9 Renal Vein, Right B Renal Vein, Left C Common Iliac Vein, Right D Common Iliac Vein, Left F External Iliac Vein, Right G External Iliac Vein, Left H Hypogastric Vein, Right J Hypogastric Vein, Left M Femoral Vein, Right N Femoral Vein, Left P Greater Saphenous Vein, Right Q Greater Saphenous Vein, Left R Lesser Saphenous Vein, Right S Lesser Saphenous Vein, Left T Foot Vein, Right V Foot Vein, Left	0 Open 3 Percutaneous 4 Percutaneous Endoscopic	3 Infusion Device D Intraluminal Device	Z No Qualifier
Y Lower Vein	0 Open 3 Percutaneous 4 Percutaneous Endoscopic	2 Monitoring Device 3 Infusion Device D Intraluminal Device	Z No Qualifier

Coding Clinic: 2013, Q3, P19 – 06H033Z

SECTION: 0 MEDICAL AND SURGICAL

BODY SYSTEM: 6 LOWER VEINS

OPERATION: J INSPECTION: Visually and/or manually exploring a body part

Body Part	Approach	Device	Qualifier
Y Lower Vein	0 Open 3 Percutaneous 4 Percutaneous Endoscopic X External	Z No Device	Z No Qualifier

SECTION: 0 MEDICAL AND SURGICAL
BODY SYSTEM: 6 LOWER VEINS
OPERATION: L OCCLUSION: Completely closing an orifice or the lumen of a tubular body part

Body Part	Approach	Device	Qualifier
0 Inferior Vena Cava 1 Splenic Vein 2 Gastric Vein 3 Esophageal Vein 4 Hepatic Vein 5 Superior Mesenteric Vein 6 Inferior Mesenteric Vein 7 Colic Vein 8 Portal Vein 9 Renal Vein, Right B Renal Vein, Left C Common Iliac Vein, Right D Common Iliac Vein, Left F External Iliac Vein, Right G External Iliac Vein, Left H Hypogastric Vein, Right J Hypogastric Vein, Left M Femoral Vein, Right N Femoral Vein, Left P Greater Saphenous Vein, Right Q Greater Saphenous Vein, Left R Lesser Saphenous Vein, Right S Lesser Saphenous Vein, Left T Foot Vein, Right V Foot Vein, Left	0 Open 3 Percutaneous 4 Percutaneous Endoscopic	C Extraluminal Device D Intraluminal Device Z No Device	Z No Qualifier
Y Lower Vein	0 Open 3 Percutaneous 4 Percutaneous Endoscopic	C Extraluminal Device D Intraluminal Device Z No Device	C Hemorrhoidal Plexus Z No Qualifier

L: OCCLUSION 6: LOWER VEINS 0: M/S

◀ New ◀ Revised deleted Deleted ♀ Females Only ♂ Males Only Noncovered Limited Coverage Hospital-Acquired Condition Coding Clinic

SECTION: 0 MEDICAL AND SURGICAL
BODY SYSTEM: 6 LOWER VEINS
OPERATION: N RELEASE: Freeing a body part from an abnormal physical constraint by cutting or by the use of force

Body Part	Approach	Device	Qualifier
0 Inferior Vena Cava 1 Splenic Vein 2 Gastric Vein 3 Esophageal Vein 4 Hepatic Vein 5 Superior Mesenteric Vein 6 Inferior Mesenteric Vein 7 Colic Vein 8 Portal Vein 9 Renal Vein, Right B Renal Vein, Left C Common Iliac Vein, Right D Common Iliac Vein, Left F External Iliac Vein, Right G External Iliac Vein, Left H Hypogastric Vein, Right J Hypogastric Vein, Left M Femoral Vein, Right N Femoral Vein, Left P Greater Saphenous Vein, Right Q Greater Saphenous Vein, Left R Lesser Saphenous Vein, Right S Lesser Saphenous Vein, Left T Foot Vein, Right V Foot Vein, Left Y Lower Vein	0 Open 3 Percutaneous 4 Percutaneous Endoscopic	Z No Device	Z No Qualifier

SECTION: 0 MEDICAL AND SURGICAL
BODY SYSTEM: 6 LOWER VEINS
OPERATION: P REMOVAL: Taking out or off a device from a body part

Body Part	Approach	Device	Qualifier
Y Lower Vein	0 Open 3 Percutaneous 4 Percutaneous Endoscopic	0 Drainage Device 2 Monitoring Device 3 Infusion Device 7 Autologous Tissue Substitute C Extraluminal Device D Intraluminal Device J Synthetic Substitute K Nonautologous Tissue Substitute	Z No Qualifier
Y Lower Vein	X External	0 Drainage Device 2 Monitoring Device 3 Infusion Device D Intraluminal Device	Z No Qualifier

◀ New ◀ Revised ~~deleted~~ Deleted ♀ Females Only ♂ Males Only
Ⓝ Noncovered Ⓛ Limited Coverage Ⓗ Hospital-Acquired Condition **Coding Clinic**

SECTION: 0 MEDICAL AND SURGICAL
BODY SYSTEM: 6 LOWER VEINS
OPERATION: Q REPAIR: Restoring, to the extent possible, a body part to its normal anatomic structure and function

Body Part	Approach	Device	Qualifier
0 Inferior Vena Cava 1 Splenic Vein 2 Gastric Vein 3 Esophageal Vein 4 Hepatic Vein 5 Superior Mesenteric Vein 6 Inferior Mesenteric Vein 7 Colic Vein 8 Portal Vein 9 Renal Vein, Right B Renal Vein, Left C Common Iliac Vein, Right D Common Iliac Vein, Left F External Iliac Vein, Right G External Iliac Vein, Left H Hypogastric Vein, Right J Hypogastric Vein, Left M Femoral Vein, Right N Femoral Vein, Left P Greater Saphenous Vein, Right Q Greater Saphenous Vein, Left R Lesser Saphenous Vein, Right S Lesser Saphenous Vein, Left T Foot Vein, Right V Foot Vein, Left Y Lower Vein	0 Open 3 Percutaneous 4 Percutaneous Endoscopic	Z No Device	Z No Qualifier

Q: REPAIR

6: LOWER VEINS

0: M/S

◄ New ◄▦ Revised ~~deleted~~ Deleted ♀ Females Only ♂ Males Only
Ⓝ🅒 Noncovered Ⓛ🅒 Limited Coverage 🅗🅐🅒 Hospital-Acquired Condition **Coding Clinic**

SECTION: 0 MEDICAL AND SURGICAL

BODY SYSTEM: 6 LOWER VEINS

OPERATION: R REPLACEMENT: Putting in or on biological or synthetic material that physically takes the place and/or function of all or a portion of a body part

Body Part	Approach	Device	Qualifier
0 Inferior Vena Cava 1 Splenic Vein 2 Gastric Vein 3 Esophageal Vein 4 Hepatic Vein 5 Superior Mesenteric Vein 6 Inferior Mesenteric Vein 7 Colic Vein 8 Portal Vein 9 Renal Vein, Right B Renal Vein, Left C Common Iliac Vein, Right D Common Iliac Vein, Left F External Iliac Vein, Right G External Iliac Vein, Left H Hypogastric Vein, Right J Hypogastric Vein, Left M Femoral Vein, Right N Femoral Vein, Left P Greater Saphenous Vein, Right Q Greater Saphenous Vein, Left R Lesser Saphenous Vein, Right S Lesser Saphenous Vein, Left T Foot Vein, Right V Foot Vein, Left Y Lower Vein	0 Open 4 Percutaneous Endoscopic	7 Autologous Tissue Substitute J Synthetic Substitute K Nonautologous Tissue Substitute	Z No Qualifier

SECTION: 0 MEDICAL AND SURGICAL
BODY SYSTEM: 6 LOWER VEINS
OPERATION: S REPOSITION: Moving to its normal location, or other suitable location, all or a portion of a body part

Body Part	Approach	Device	Qualifier
0 Inferior Vena Cava	0 Open	Z No Device	Z No Qualifier
1 Splenic Vein	3 Percutaneous		
2 Gastric Vein	4 Percutaneous Endoscopic		
3 Esophageal Vein			
4 Hepatic Vein			
5 Superior Mesenteric Vein			
6 Inferior Mesenteric Vein			
7 Colic Vein			
8 Portal Vein			
9 Renal Vein, Right			
B Renal Vein, Left			
C Common Iliac Vein, Right			
D Common Iliac Vein, Left			
F External Iliac Vein, Right			
G External Iliac Vein, Left			
H Hypogastric Vein, Right			
J Hypogastric Vein, Left			
M Femoral Vein, Right			
N Femoral Vein, Left			
P Greater Saphenous Vein, Right			
Q Greater Saphenous Vein, Left			
R Lesser Saphenous Vein, Right			
S Lesser Saphenous Vein, Left			
T Foot Vein, Right			
V Foot Vein, Left			
Y Lower Vein			

S: REPOSITION

6: LOWER VEINS

0: M/S

◀ New   ◀▥ Revised   deleted Deleted   ♀ Females Only   ♂ Males Only
℞ Noncovered   ℞ Limited Coverage   ℞ Hospital-Acquired Condition   **Coding Clinic**

SECTION: 0 MEDICAL AND SURGICAL
BODY SYSTEM: 6 LOWER VEINS
OPERATION: **U SUPPLEMENT:** Putting in or on biological or synthetic material that physically reinforces and/or augments the function of a portion of a body part

Body Part	Approach	Device	Qualifier
0 Inferior Vena Cava 1 Splenic Vein 2 Gastric Vein 3 Esophageal Vein 4 Hepatic Vein 5 Superior Mesenteric Vein 6 Inferior Mesenteric Vein 7 Colic Vein 8 Portal Vein 9 Renal Vein, Right B Renal Vein, Left C Common Iliac Vein, Right D Common Iliac Vein, Left F External Iliac Vein, Right G External Iliac Vein, Left H Hypogastric Vein, Right J Hypogastric Vein, Left M Femoral Vein, Right N Femoral Vein, Left P Greater Saphenous Vein, Right Q Greater Saphenous Vein, Left R Lesser Saphenous Vein, Right S Lesser Saphenous Vein, Left T Foot Vein, Right V Foot Vein, Left Y Lower Vein	0 Open 3 Percutaneous 4 Percutaneous Endoscopic	7 Autologous Tissue Substitute J Synthetic Substitute K Nonautologous Tissue Substitute	Z No Qualifier

◀ New   ◀▥ Revised   ~~deleted~~ Deleted   ♀ Females Only   ♂ Males Only
◐ Noncovered   ◐ Limited Coverage   ◐ Hospital-Acquired Condition   **Coding Clinic**

143

SECTION: 0 MEDICAL AND SURGICAL
BODY SYSTEM: 6 LOWER VEINS
OPERATION: V RESTRICTION: Partially closing an orifice or the lumen of a tubular body part

Body Part	Approach	Device	Qualifier
0 Inferior Vena Cava 1 Splenic Vein 2 Gastric Vein 3 Esophageal Vein 4 Hepatic Vein 5 Superior Mesenteric Vein 6 Inferior Mesenteric Vein 7 Colic Vein 8 Portal Vein 9 Renal Vein, Right B Renal Vein, Left C Common Iliac Vein, Right D Common Iliac Vein, Left F External Iliac Vein, Right G External Iliac Vein, Left H Hypogastric Vein, Right J Hypogastric Vein, Left M Femoral Vein, Right N Femoral Vein, Left P Greater Saphenous Vein, Right Q Greater Saphenous Vein, Left R Lesser Saphenous Vein, Right S Lesser Saphenous Vein, Left T Foot Vein, Right V Foot Vein, Left Y Lower Vein	0 Open 3 Percutaneous 4 Percutaneous Endoscopic	C Extraluminal Device D Intraluminal Device Z No Device	Z No Qualifier

SECTION: 0 MEDICAL AND SURGICAL
BODY SYSTEM: 6 LOWER VEINS
OPERATION: W REVISION: Correcting, to the extent possible, a portion of a malfunctioning device or the position of a displaced device

Body Part	Approach	Device	Qualifier
Y Lower Vein	0 Open 3 Percutaneous 4 Percutaneous Endoscopic X External	0 Drainage Device 2 Monitoring Device 3 Infusion Device 7 Autologous Tissue Substitute C Extraluminal Device D Intraluminal Device J Synthetic Substitute K Nonautologous Tissue Substitute	Z No Qualifier

◄ New ◄ Revised ~~deleted~~ Deleted ♀ Females Only ♂ Males Only
Noncovered Limited Coverage Hospital-Acquired Condition **Coding Clinic**

SECTION: 0 MEDICAL AND SURGICAL
BODY SYSTEM: 7 LYMPHATIC AND HEMIC SYSTEMS
OPERATION: 2 CHANGE: Taking out or off a device from a body part and putting back an identical or similar device in or on the same body part without cutting or puncturing the skin or a mucous membrane

Body Part	Approach	Device	Qualifier
K Thoracic Duct L Cisterna Chyli M Thymus N Lymphatic P Spleen T Bone Marrow	X External	0 Drainage Device Y Other Device	Z No Qualifier

SECTION: 0 MEDICAL AND SURGICAL
BODY SYSTEM: 7 LYMPHATIC AND HEMIC SYSTEMS
OPERATION: 5 DESTRUCTION: Physical eradication of all or a portion of a body part by the direct use of energy, force, or a destructive agent

Body Part	Approach	Device	Qualifier
0 Lymphatic, Head 1 Lymphatic, Right Neck 2 Lymphatic, Left Neck 3 Lymphatic, Right Upper Extremity 4 Lymphatic, Left Upper Extremity 5 Lymphatic, Right Axillary 6 Lymphatic, Left Axillary 7 Lymphatic, Thorax 8 Lymphatic, Internal Mammary, Right 9 Lymphatic, Internal Mammary, Left B Lymphatic, Mesenteric C Lymphatic, Pelvis D Lymphatic, Aortic F Lymphatic, Right Lower Extremity G Lymphatic, Left Lower Extremity H Lymphatic, Right Inguinal J Lymphatic, Left Inguinal K Thoracic Duct L Cisterna Chyli M Thymus P Spleen	0 Open 3 Percutaneous 4 Percutaneous Endoscopic	Z No Device	Z No Qualifier

Side tabs: 2: CHANGE 5: DESTRUCTION | 7: LYMPHATIC AND HEMIC SYSTEMS | 0: M/S

◀ New ◀ Revised ~~deleted~~ Deleted ♀ Females Only ♂ Males Only
Noncovered Limited Coverage Hospital-Acquired Condition **Coding Clinic**

SECTION: 0 MEDICAL AND SURGICAL
BODY SYSTEM: 7 **LYMPHATIC AND HEMIC SYSTEMS**
OPERATION: 9 **DRAINAGE:** Taking or letting out fluids and/or gases from a body part

Body Part	Approach	Device	Qualifier
0 Lymphatic, Head 1 Lymphatic, Right Neck 2 Lymphatic, Left Neck 3 Lymphatic, Right Upper Extremity 4 Lymphatic, Left Upper Extremity 5 Lymphatic, Right Axillary 6 Lymphatic, Left Axillary 7 Lymphatic, Thorax 8 Lymphatic, Internal Mammary, Right 9 Lymphatic, Internal Mammary, Left B Lymphatic, Mesenteric C Lymphatic, Pelvis D Lymphatic, Aortic F Lymphatic, Right Lower Extremity G Lymphatic, Left Lower Extremity H Lymphatic, Right Inguinal J Lymphatic, Left Inguinal K Thoracic Duct L Cisterna Chyli M Thymus P Spleen T Bone Marrow	0 Open 3 Percutaneous 4 Percutaneous Endoscopic	0 Drainage Device	Z No Qualifier
0 Lymphatic, Head 1 Lymphatic, Right Neck 2 Lymphatic, Left Neck 3 Lymphatic, Right Upper Extremity 4 Lymphatic, Left Upper Extremity 5 Lymphatic, Right Axillary 6 Lymphatic, Left Axillary 7 Lymphatic, Thorax 8 Lymphatic, Internal Mammary, Right 9 Lymphatic, Internal Mammary, Left B Lymphatic, Mesenteric C Lymphatic, Pelvis D Lymphatic, Aortic F Lymphatic, Right Lower Extremity G Lymphatic, Left Lower Extremity H Lymphatic, Right Inguinal J Lymphatic, Left Inguinal K Thoracic Duct L Cisterna Chyli M Thymus P Spleen T Bone Marrow	0 Open 3 Percutaneous 4 Percutaneous Endoscopic	Z No Device	X Diagnostic Z No Qualifier

B: EXCISION C: EXTIRPATION

7: LYMPHATIC AND HEMIC SYSTEMS

0: M/S

SECTION: 0 MEDICAL AND SURGICAL
BODY SYSTEM: 7 **LYMPHATIC AND HEMIC SYSTEMS**
OPERATION: B **EXCISION:** Cutting out or off, without replacement, a portion of a body part

Body Part	Approach	Device	Qualifier
0 Lymphatic, Head 1 Lymphatic, Right Neck 2 Lymphatic, Left Neck 3 Lymphatic, Right Upper Extremity 4 Lymphatic, Left Upper Extremity 5 Lymphatic, Right Axillary 6 Lymphatic, Left Axillary 7 Lymphatic, Thorax 8 Lymphatic, Internal Mammary, Right 9 Lymphatic, Internal Mammary, Left B Lymphatic, Mesenteric C Lymphatic, Pelvis D Lymphatic, Aortic F Lymphatic, Right Lower Extremity G Lymphatic, Left Lower Extremity H Lymphatic, Right Inguinal J Lymphatic, Left Inguinal K Thoracic Duct L Cisterna Chyli M Thymus P Spleen	0 Open 3 Percutaneous 4 Percutaneous Endoscopic	Z No Device	X Diagnostic Z No Qualifier

SECTION: 0 MEDICAL AND SURGICAL
BODY SYSTEM: 7 **LYMPHATIC AND HEMIC SYSTEMS**
OPERATION: C **EXTIRPATION:** Taking or cutting out solid matter from a body part

Body Part	Approach	Device	Qualifier
0 Lymphatic, Head 1 Lymphatic, Right Neck 2 Lymphatic, Left Neck 3 Lymphatic, Right Upper Extremity 4 Lymphatic, Left Upper Extremity 5 Lymphatic, Right Axillary 6 Lymphatic, Left Axillary 7 Lymphatic, Thorax 8 Lymphatic, Internal Mammary, Right 9 Lymphatic, Internal Mammary, Left B Lymphatic, Mesenteric C Lymphatic, Pelvis D Lymphatic, Aortic F Lymphatic, Right Lower Extremity G Lymphatic, Left Lower Extremity H Lymphatic, Right Inguinal J Lymphatic, Left Inguinal K Thoracic Duct L Cisterna Chyli M Thymus P Spleen	0 Open 3 Percutaneous 4 Percutaneous Endoscopic	Z No Device	Z No Qualifier

◄ New   ◄ Revised   ~~deleted~~ Deleted   ♀ Females Only   ♂ Males Only
No Noncovered   Limited Coverage   Hospital-Acquired Condition   **Coding Clinic**

SECTION: **0 MEDICAL AND SURGICAL**
BODY SYSTEM: **7 LYMPHATIC AND HEMIC SYSTEMS**
OPERATION: **D EXTRACTION:** Pulling or stripping out or off all or a portion of a body part by the use of force

Body Part	Approach	Device	Qualifier
Q Bone Marrow, Sternum R Bone Marrow, Iliac S Bone Marrow, Vertebral	0 Open 3 Percutaneous	Z No Device	X Diagnostic Z No Qualifier

SECTION: **0 MEDICAL AND SURGICAL**
BODY SYSTEM: **7 LYMPHATIC AND HEMIC SYSTEMS**
OPERATION: **H INSERTION:** Putting in a nonbiological appliance that monitors, assists, performs, or prevents a physiological function but does not physically take the place of a body part

Body Part	Approach	Device	Qualifier
K Thoracic Duct L Cisterna Chyli M Thymus N Lymphatic P Spleen	0 Open 3 Percutaneous 4 Percutaneous Endoscopic	3 Infusion Device	Z No Qualifier

SECTION: **0 MEDICAL AND SURGICAL**
BODY SYSTEM: **7 LYMPHATIC AND HEMIC SYSTEMS**
OPERATION: **J INSPECTION:** Visually and/or manually exploring a body part

Body Part	Approach	Device	Qualifier
K Thoracic Duct L Cisterna Chyli M Thymus T Bone Marrow	0 Open 3 Percutaneous 4 Percutaneous Endoscopic	Z No Device	Z No Qualifier
N Lymphatic P Spleen	0 Open 3 Percutaneous 4 Percutaneous Endoscopic X External	Z No Device	Z No Qualifier

◀ New　◀▥ Revised　~~deleted~~ Deleted　♀ Females Only　♂ Males Only
⊘ Noncovered　⊘ Limited Coverage　⊘ Hospital-Acquired Condition　**Coding Clinic**

149

SECTION: **0** **MEDICAL AND SURGICAL**
BODY SYSTEM: 7 **LYMPHATIC AND HEMIC SYSTEMS**
OPERATION: **L** **OCCLUSION:** Completely closing an orifice or the lumen of a tubular body part

Body Part	Approach	Device	Qualifier
0 Lymphatic, Head 1 Lymphatic, Right Neck 2 Lymphatic, Left Neck 3 Lymphatic, Right Upper Extremity 4 Lymphatic, Left Upper Extremity 5 Lymphatic, Right Axillary 6 Lymphatic, Left Axillary 7 Lymphatic, Thorax 8 Lymphatic, Internal Mammary, Right 9 Lymphatic, Internal Mammary, Left B Lymphatic, Mesenteric C Lymphatic, Pelvis D Lymphatic, Aortic F Lymphatic, Right Lower Extremity G Lymphatic, Left Lower Extremity H Lymphatic, Right Inguinal J Lymphatic, Left Inguinal K Thoracic Duct L Cisterna Chyli	0 Open 3 Percutaneous 4 Percutaneous Endoscopic	C Extraluminal Device D Intraluminal Device Z No Device	Z No Qualifier

SECTION: **0** **MEDICAL AND SURGICAL**
BODY SYSTEM: 7 **LYMPHATIC AND HEMIC SYSTEMS**
OPERATION: **N** **RELEASE:** Freeing a body part from an abnormal physical constraint by cutting or by the use of force

Body Part	Approach	Device	Qualifier
0 Lymphatic, Head 1 Lymphatic, Right Neck 2 Lymphatic, Left Neck 3 Lymphatic, Right Upper Extremity 4 Lymphatic, Left Upper Extremity 5 Lymphatic, Right Axillary 6 Lymphatic, Left Axillary 7 Lymphatic, Thorax 8 Lymphatic, Internal Mammary, Right 9 Lymphatic, Internal Mammary, Left B Lymphatic, Mesenteric C Lymphatic, Pelvis D Lymphatic, Aortic F Lymphatic, Right Lower Extremity G Lymphatic, Left Lower Extremity H Lymphatic, Right Inguinal J Lymphatic, Left Inguinal K Thoracic Duct L Cisterna Chyli M Thymus P Spleen	0 Open 3 Percutaneous 4 Percutaneous Endoscopic	Z No Device	Z No Qualifier

◀ New   ◀ Revised   ~~deleted~~ Deleted   ♀ Females Only   ♂ Males Only
◈ Noncovered   ◈ Limited Coverage   ◈ Hospital-Acquired Condition   **Coding Clinic**

SECTION: 0 MEDICAL AND SURGICAL

BODY SYSTEM: 7 LYMPHATIC AND HEMIC SYSTEMS

OPERATION: P REMOVAL: Taking out or off a device from a body part

Body Part	Approach	Device	Qualifier
K Thoracic Duct L Cisterna Chyli N Lymphatic	0 Open 3 Percutaneous 4 Percutaneous Endoscopic	0 Drainage Device 3 Infusion Device 7 Autologous Tissue Substitute C Extraluminal Device D Intraluminal Device J Synthetic Substitute K Nonautologous Tissue 　 Substitute	Z No Qualifier
K Thoracic Duct L Cisterna Chyli N Lymphatic	X External	0 Drainage Device 3 Infusion Device D Intraluminal Device	Z No Qualifier
M Thymus P Spleen	0 Open 3 Percutaneous 4 Percutaneous Endoscopic X External	0 Drainage Device 3 Infusion Device	Z No Qualifier
T Bone Marrow	0 Open 3 Percutaneous 4 Percutaneous Endoscopic X External	0 Drainage Device	Z No Qualifier

SECTION: 0 MEDICAL AND SURGICAL

BODY SYSTEM: 7 LYMPHATIC AND HEMIC SYSTEMS

OPERATION: Q REPAIR: Restoring, to the extent possible, a body part to its normal anatomic structure and function

Body Part	Approach	Device	Qualifier
0 Lymphatic, Head 1 Lymphatic, Right Neck 2 Lymphatic, Left Neck 3 Lymphatic, Right Upper Extremity 4 Lymphatic, Left Upper Extremity 5 Lymphatic, Right Axillary 6 Lymphatic, Left Axillary 7 Lymphatic, Thorax 8 Lymphatic, Internal Mammary, Right 9 Lymphatic, Internal Mammary, Left B Lymphatic, Mesenteric C Lymphatic, Pelvis D Lymphatic, Aortic F Lymphatic, Right Lower Extremity G Lymphatic, Left Lower Extremity H Lymphatic, Right Inguinal J Lymphatic, Left Inguinal K Thoracic Duct L Cisterna Chyli M Thymus P Spleen	0 Open 3 Percutaneous 4 Percutaneous Endoscopic	Z No Device	Z No Qualifier

◀ New　　◀ Revised　　~~deleted~~ Deleted　　♀ Females Only　　♂ Males Only

🔾 Noncovered　　🔾 Limited Coverage　　🔾 Hospital-Acquired Condition　　**Coding Clinic**

SECTION: 0 MEDICAL AND SURGICAL
BODY SYSTEM: 7 LYMPHATIC AND HEMIC SYSTEMS
OPERATION: S REPOSITION: Moving to its normal location, or other suitable location, all or a portion of a body part

Body Part	Approach	Device	Qualifier
M Thymus P Spleen	0 Open	Z No Device	Z No Qualifier

SECTION: 0 MEDICAL AND SURGICAL
BODY SYSTEM: 7 LYMPHATIC AND HEMIC SYSTEMS
OPERATION: T RESECTION: Cutting out or off, without replacement, all of a body part

Body Part	Approach	Device	Qualifier
0 Lymphatic, Head 1 Lymphatic, Right Neck 2 Lymphatic, Left Neck 3 Lymphatic, Right Upper Extremity 4 Lymphatic, Left Upper Extremity 5 Lymphatic, Right Axillary 6 Lymphatic, Left Axillary 7 Lymphatic, Thorax 8 Lymphatic, Internal Mammary, Right 9 Lymphatic, Internal Mammary, Left B Lymphatic, Mesenteric C Lymphatic, Pelvis D Lymphatic, Aortic F Lymphatic, Right Lower Extremity G Lymphatic, Left Lower Extremity H Lymphatic, Right Inguinal J Lymphatic, Left Inguinal K Thoracic Duct L Cisterna Chyli M Thymus P Spleen	0 Open 4 Percutaneous Endoscopic	Z No Device	Z No Qualifier

◀ New   ◀▦ Revised   ~~deleted~~ Deleted   ♀ Females Only   ♂ Males Only
🅝 Noncovered   🅛 Limited Coverage   🅗 Hospital-Acquired Condition   **Coding Clinic**

SECTION: 0 MEDICAL AND SURGICAL
BODY SYSTEM: 7 LYMPHATIC AND HEMIC SYSTEMS
OPERATION: U SUPPLEMENT: Putting in or on biological or synthetic material that physically reinforces and/or augments the function of a portion of a body part

Body Part	Approach	Device	Qualifier
0 Lymphatic, Head	0 Open	7 Autologous Tissue Substitute	Z No Qualifier
1 Lymphatic, Right Neck	4 Percutaneous Endoscopic	J Synthetic Substitute	
2 Lymphatic, Left Neck		K Nonautologous Tissue Substitute	
3 Lymphatic, Right Upper Extremity			
4 Lymphatic, Left Upper Extremity			
5 Lymphatic, Right Axillary			
6 Lymphatic, Left Axillary			
7 Lymphatic, Thorax			
8 Lymphatic, Internal Mammary, Right			
9 Lymphatic, Internal Mammary, Left			
B Lymphatic, Mesenteric			
C Lymphatic, Pelvis			
D Lymphatic, Aortic			
F Lymphatic, Right Lower Extremity			
G Lymphatic, Left Lower Extremity			
H Lymphatic, Right Inguinal			
J Lymphatic, Left Inguinal			
K Thoracic Duct			
L Cisterna Chyli			

SECTION: 0 MEDICAL AND SURGICAL
BODY SYSTEM: 7 LYMPHATIC AND HEMIC SYSTEMS
OPERATION: V RESTRICTION: Partially closing an orifice or the lumen of a tubular body part

Body Part	Approach	Device	Qualifier
0 Lymphatic, Head	0 Open	C Extraluminal Device	Z No Qualifier
1 Lymphatic, Right Neck	3 Percutaneous	D Intraluminal Device	
2 Lymphatic, Left Neck	4 Percutaneous Endoscopic	Z No Device	
3 Lymphatic, Right Upper Extremity			
4 Lymphatic, Left Upper Extremity			
5 Lymphatic, Right Axillary			
6 Lymphatic, Left Axillary			
7 Lymphatic, Thorax			
8 Lymphatic, Internal Mammary, Right			
9 Lymphatic, Internal Mammary, Left			
B Lymphatic, Mesenteric			
C Lymphatic, Pelvis			
D Lymphatic, Aortic			
F Lymphatic, Right Lower Extremity			
G Lymphatic, Left Lower Extremity			
H Lymphatic, Right Inguinal			
J Lymphatic, Left Inguinal			
K Thoracic Duct			
L Cisterna Chyli			

◀ New   ◀█ Revised   deleted Deleted   ♀ Females Only   ♂ Males Only
🚫 Noncovered   🚫 Limited Coverage   🚫 Hospital-Acquired Condition   **Coding Clinic**

SECTION: 0 MEDICAL AND SURGICAL
BODY SYSTEM: 7 LYMPHATIC AND HEMIC SYSTEMS
OPERATION: W REVISION: Correcting, to the extent possible, a portion of a malfunctioning device or the position of a displaced device

Body Part	Approach	Device	Qualifier
K Thoracic Duct L Cisterna Chyli N Lymphatic	0 Open 3 Percutaneous 4 Percutaneous Endoscopic X External	0 Drainage Device 3 Infusion Device 7 Autologous Tissue Substitute C Extraluminal Device D Intraluminal Device J Synthetic Substitute K Nonautologous Tissue Substitute	Z No Qualifier
M Thymus P Spleen	0 Open 3 Percutaneous 4 Percutaneous Endoscopic X External	0 Drainage Device 3 Infusion Device	Z No Qualifier
T Bone Marrow	0 Open 3 Percutaneous 4 Percutaneous Endoscopic X External	0 Drainage Device	Z No Qualifier

SECTION: 0 MEDICAL AND SURGICAL
BODY SYSTEM: 7 LYMPHATIC AND HEMIC SYSTEMS
OPERATION: Y TRANSPLANTATION: Putting in or on all or a portion of a living body part taken from another individual or animal to physically take the place and/or function of all or a portion of a similar body part

Body Part	Approach	Device	Qualifier
M Thymus P Spleen	0 Open	Z No Device	0 Allogeneic 1 Syngeneic 2 Zooplastic

◀ New   ◀▥ Revised   ~~deleted~~ Deleted   ♀ Females Only   ♂ Males Only
🚫 Noncovered   🚫 Limited Coverage   🚫 Hospital-Acquired Condition   **Coding Clinic**

Vertical side text: W: REVISION   Y: TRANSPLANTATION   7: LYMPHATIC AND HEMIC SYSTEMS   0: M/S

SECTION: 0 MEDICAL AND SURGICAL
BODY SYSTEM: 8 EYE
OPERATION: 0 ALTERATION: Modifying the anatomic structure of a body part without affecting the function of the body part

Body Part	Approach	Device	Qualifier
N Upper Eyelid, Right P Upper Eyelid, Left Q Lower Eyelid, Right R Lower Eyelid, Left	0 Open 3 Percutaneous X External	7 Autologous Tissue Substitute J Synthetic Substitute K Nonautologous Tissue Substitute Z No Device	Z No Qualifier

SECTION: 0 MEDICAL AND SURGICAL
BODY SYSTEM: 8 EYE
OPERATION: 1 BYPASS: Altering the route of passage of the contents of a tubular body part

Body Part	Approach	Device	Qualifier
2 Anterior Chamber, Right 3 Anterior Chamber, Left	3 Percutaneous	J Synthetic Substitute K Nonautologous Tissue Substitute Z No Device	4 Sclera
X Lacrimal Duct, Right Y Lacrimal Duct, Left	0 Open 3 Percutaneous	J Synthetic Substitute K Nonautologous Tissue Substitute Z No Device	3 Nasal Cavity

SECTION: 0 MEDICAL AND SURGICAL
BODY SYSTEM: 8 EYE
OPERATION: 2 CHANGE: Taking out or off a device from a body part and putting back an identical or similar device in or on the same body part without cutting or puncturing the skin or a mucous membrane

Body Part	Approach	Device	Qualifier
0 Eye, Right 1 Eye, Left	X External	0 Drainage Device Y Other Device	Z No Qualifier

Sidebar: 0: ALTERATION 1: BYPASS 2: CHANGE / 8: EYE / 0: M/S

◄ New ◄ Revised ~~deleted~~ Deleted ♀ Females Only ♂ Males Only
Ⓝ Noncovered Ⓛ Limited Coverage Ⓗ Hospital-Acquired Condition **Coding Clinic**

SECTION: 0 MEDICAL AND SURGICAL

BODY SYSTEM: 8 EYE
OPERATION: 5 **DESTRUCTION:** Physical eradication of all or a portion of a body part by the direct use of energy, force, or a destructive agent

Body Part	Approach	Device	Qualifier
0 Eye, Right 1 Eye, Left 6 Sclera, Right 7 Sclera, Left 8 Cornea, Right 9 Cornea, Left S Conjunctiva, Right T Conjunctiva, Left	X External	Z No Device	Z No Qualifier
2 Anterior Chamber, Right 3 Anterior Chamber, Left 4 Vitreous, Right 5 Vitreous, Left C Iris, Right D Iris, Left E Retina, Right F Retina, Left G Retinal Vessel, Right H Retinal Vessel, Left J Lens, Right K Lens, Left	3 Percutaneous	Z No Device	Z No Qualifier
A Choroid, Right B Choroid, Left L Extraocular Muscle, Right M Extraocular Muscle, Left V Lacrimal Gland, Right W Lacrimal Gland, Left	0 Open 3 Percutaneous	Z No Device	Z No Qualifier
N Upper Eyelid, Right P Upper Eyelid, Left Q Lower Eyelid, Right R Lower Eyelid, Left	0 Open 3 Percutaneous X External	Z No Device	Z No Qualifier
X Lacrimal Duct, Right Y Lacrimal Duct, Left	0 Open 3 Percutaneous 7 Via Natural or Artificial Opening 8 Via Natural or Artificial Opening Endoscopic	Z No Device	Z No Qualifier

SECTION: 0 MEDICAL AND SURGICAL

BODY SYSTEM: 8 EYE
OPERATION: 7 **DILATION:** Expanding an orifice or the lumen of a tubular body part

Body Part	Approach	Device	Qualifier
X Lacrimal Duct, Right Y Lacrimal Duct, Left	0 Open 3 Percutaneous 7 Via Natural or Artificial Opening 8 Via Natural or Artificial Opening Endoscopic	D Intraluminal Device Z No Device	Z No Qualifier

◀ New ◀ Revised deleted Deleted ♀ Females Only ♂ Males Only
⬡ Noncovered ⬡ Limited Coverage ⬡ Hospital-Acquired Condition **Coding Clinic**

SECTION: 0 MEDICAL AND SURGICAL
BODY SYSTEM: 8 EYE
OPERATION: 9 DRAINAGE: *(on multiple pages)*
Taking or letting out fluids and/or gases from a body part

Body Part	Approach	Device	Qualifier
0 Eye, Right 1 Eye, Left 6 Sclera, Right 7 Sclera, Left 8 Cornea, Right 9 Cornea, Left S Conjunctiva, Right T Conjunctiva, Left	X External	0 Drainage Device	Z No Qualifier
0 Eye, Right 1 Eye, Left 6 Sclera, Right 7 Sclera, Left 8 Cornea, Right 9 Cornea, Left S Conjunctiva, Right T Conjunctiva, Left	X External	Z No Device	X Diagnostic Z No Qualifier
2 Anterior Chamber, Right 3 Anterior Chamber, Left 4 Vitreous, Right 5 Vitreous, Left C Iris, Right D Iris, Left E Retina, Right F Retina, Left G Retinal Vessel, Right H Retinal Vessel, Left J Lens, Right K Lens, Left	3 Percutaneous	0 Drainage Device	Z No Qualifier
2 Anterior Chamber, Right 3 Anterior Chamber, Left 4 Vitreous, Right 5 Vitreous, Left C Iris, Right D Iris, Left E Retina, Right F Retina, Left G Retinal Vessel, Right H Retinal Vessel, Left J Lens, Right K Lens, Left	3 Percutaneous	Z No Device	X Diagnostic Z No Qualifier
A Choroid, Right B Choroid, Left L Extraocular Muscle, Right M Extraocular Muscle, Left V Lacrimal Gland, Right W Lacrimal Gland, Left	0 Open 3 Percutaneous	0 Drainage Device	Z No Qualifier

9: DRAINAGE **8: EYE** **0: M/S**

◀ New   ◀▥ Revised   ~~deleted~~ Deleted   ♀ Females Only   ♂ Males Only
🟤 Noncovered   🟤 Limited Coverage   🟤 Hospital-Acquired Condition   **Coding Clinic**

SECTION: 0 MEDICAL AND SURGICAL
BODY SYSTEM: 8 EYE
OPERATION: 9 DRAINAGE: *(continued)*
Taking or letting out fluids and/or gases from a body part

Body Part	Approach	Device	Qualifier
A Choroid, Right B Choroid, Left L Extraocular Muscle, Right M Extraocular Muscle, Left V Lacrimal Gland, Right W Lacrimal Gland, Left	0 Open 3 Percutaneous	Z No Device	X Diagnostic Z No Qualifier
N Upper Eyelid, Right P Upper Eyelid, Left Q Lower Eyelid, Right R Lower Eyelid, Left	0 Open 3 Percutaneous X External	0 Drainage Device	Z No Qualifier
N Upper Eyelid, Right P Upper Eyelid, Left Q Lower Eyelid, Right R Lower Eyelid, Left	0 Open 3 Percutaneous X External	Z No Device	X Diagnostic Z No Qualifier
X Lacrimal Duct, Right Y Lacrimal Duct, Left	0 Open 3 Percutaneous 7 Via Natural or Artificial Opening 8 Via Natural or Artificial Opening Endoscopic	0 Drainage Device	Z No Qualifier
X Lacrimal Duct, Right Y Lacrimal Duct, Left	0 Open 3 Percutaneous 7 Via Natural or Artificial Opening 8 Via Natural or Artificial Opening Endoscopic	Z No Device	X Diagnostic Z No Qualifier

0: M/S

8: EYE

9: DRAINAGE

◀ New   ◀▥ Revised   ~~deleted~~ Deleted   ♀ Females Only   ♂ Males Only
⊗ Noncovered   ⊗ Limited Coverage   ⊗ Hospital-Acquired Condition   **Coding Clinic**
159

SECTION: 0 MEDICAL AND SURGICAL
BODY SYSTEM: 8 EYE
OPERATION: B EXCISION: Cutting out or off, without replacement, a portion of a body part

Body Part	Approach	Device	Qualifier
0 Eye, Right 1 Eye, Left N Upper Eyelid, Right P Upper Eyelid, Left Q Lower Eyelid, Right R Lower Eyelid, Left	0 Open 3 Percutaneous X External	Z No Device	X Diagnostic Z No Qualifier
4 Vitreous, Right 5 Vitreous, Left C Iris, Right D Iris, Left E Retina, Right F Retina, Left J Lens, Right K Lens, Left	3 Percutaneous	Z No Device	X Diagnostic Z No Qualifier
6 Sclera, Right 7 Sclera, Left 8 Cornea, Right 9 Cornea, Left S Conjunctiva, Right T Conjunctiva, Left	X External	Z No Device	X Diagnostic Z No Qualifier
A Choroid, Right B Choroid, Left L Extraocular Muscle, Right M Extraocular Muscle, Left V Lacrimal Gland, Right W Lacrimal Gland, Left	0 Open 3 Percutaneous	Z No Device	X Diagnostic Z No Qualifier
X Lacrimal Duct, Right Y Lacrimal Duct, Left	0 Open 3 Percutaneous 7 Via Natural or Artificial Opening 8 Via Natural or Artificial Opening Endoscopic	Z No Device	X Diagnostic Z No Qualifier

B: EXCISION

8: EYE

0: M/S

◀ New   ◀ Revised   deleted Deleted   ♀ Females Only   ♂ Males Only
Noncovered   Limited Coverage   Hospital-Acquired Condition   **Coding Clinic**

SECTION: 0 MEDICAL AND SURGICAL

BODY SYSTEM: 8 EYE

OPERATION: C EXTIRPATION: Taking or cutting out solid matter from a body part

Body Part	Approach	Device	Qualifier
0 Eye, Right 1 Eye, Left 6 Sclera, Right 7 Sclera, Left 8 Cornea, Right 9 Cornea, Left S Conjunctiva, Right T Conjunctiva, Left	X External	Z No Device	Z No Qualifier
2 Anterior Chamber, Right 3 Anterior Chamber, Left 4 Vitreous, Right 5 Vitreous, Left C Iris, Right D Iris, Left E Retina, Right F Retina, Left G Retinal Vessel, Right H Retinal Vessel, Left J Lens, Right K Lens, Left	3 Percutaneous X External	Z No Device	Z No Qualifier
A Choroid, Right B Choroid, Left L Extraocular Muscle, Right M Extraocular Muscle, Left N Upper Eyelid, Right P Upper Eyelid, Left Q Lower Eyelid, Right R Lower Eyelid, Left V Lacrimal Gland, Right W Lacrimal Gland, Left	0 Open 3 Percutaneous X External	Z No Device	Z No Qualifier
X Lacrimal Duct, Right Y Lacrimal Duct, Left	0 Open 3 Percutaneous 7 Via Natural or Artificial Opening 8 Via Natural or Artificial Opening Endoscopic	Z No Device	Z No Qualifier

SECTION: 0 MEDICAL AND SURGICAL

BODY SYSTEM: 8 EYE

OPERATION: D EXTRACTION: Pulling or stripping out or off all or a portion of a body part by the use of force

Body Part	Approach	Device	Qualifier
8 Cornea, Right 9 Cornea, Left	X External	Z No Device	X Diagnostic Z No Qualifier
J Lens, Right K Lens, Left	3 Percutaneous	Z No Device	Z No Qualifier

◀ New ◀ Revised ~~deleted~~ Deleted ♀ Females Only ♂ Males Only
Noncovered Limited Coverage Hospital-Acquired Condition **Coding Clinic**

161

0: M/S   8: EYE   C: EXTIRPATION   D: EXTRACTION

SECTION: 0 MEDICAL AND SURGICAL
BODY SYSTEM: 8 EYE
OPERATION: F FRAGMENTATION: Breaking solid matter in a body part into pieces

Body Part	Approach	Device	Qualifier
4 Vitreous, Right 5 Vitreous, Left	3 Percutaneous X External ⊗	Z No Device	Z No Qualifier

SECTION: 0 MEDICAL AND SURGICAL
BODY SYSTEM: 8 EYE
OPERATION: H INSERTION: Putting in a nonbiological appliance that monitors, assists, performs, or prevents a physiological function but does not physically take the place of a body part

Body Part	Approach	Device	Qualifier
0 Eye, Right 1 Eye, Left	0 Open	5 Epiretinal Visual Prosthesis	Z No Qualifier
0 Eye, Right 1 Eye, Left	3 Percutaneous X External	1 Radioactive Element 3 Infusion Device	Z No Qualifier

SECTION: 0 MEDICAL AND SURGICAL
BODY SYSTEM: 8 EYE
OPERATION: J INSPECTION: Visually and/or manually exploring a body part

Body Part	Approach	Device	Qualifier
0 Eye, Right 1 Eye, Left J Lens, Right K Lens, Left	X External	Z No Device	Z No Qualifier
L Extraocular Muscle, Right M Extraocular Muscle, Left	0 Open X External	Z No Device	Z No Qualifier

SECTION: 0 MEDICAL AND SURGICAL
BODY SYSTEM: 8 EYE
OPERATION: L OCCLUSION: Completely closing an orifice or the lumen of a tubular body part

Body Part	Approach	Device	Qualifier
X Lacrimal Duct, Right Y Lacrimal Duct, Left	0 Open 3 Percutaneous	C Extraluminal Device D Intraluminal Device Z No Device	Z No Qualifier
X Lacrimal Duct, Right Y Lacrimal Duct, Left	7 Via Natural or Artificial Opening 8 Via Natural or Artificial Opening Endoscopic	D Intraluminal Device Z No Device	Z No Qualifier

◀ New   ◀ Revised   ~~deleted~~ Deleted   ♀ Females Only   ♂ Males Only
⊗ Noncovered   ⊗ Limited Coverage   ⊗ Hospital-Acquired Condition   **Coding Clinic**

Side tab: F: FRAGMENTATION   H: INSERTION   J: INSPECTION   L: OCCLUSION   8: EYE   0: M/S

SECTION: 0 MEDICAL AND SURGICAL
BODY SYSTEM: 8 EYE

OPERATION: M REATTACHMENT: Putting back in or on all or a portion of a separated body part to its normal location or other suitable location

Body Part	Approach	Device	Qualifier
N Upper Eyelid, Right P Upper Eyelid, Left Q Lower Eyelid, Right R Lower Eyelid, Left	X External	Z No Device	Z No Qualifier

SECTION: 0 MEDICAL AND SURGICAL
BODY SYSTEM: 8 EYE

OPERATION: N RELEASE: Freeing a body part from an abnormal physical constraint by cutting or by the use of force

Body Part	Approach	Device	Qualifier
0 Eye, Right 1 Eye, Left 6 Sclera, Right 7 Sclera, Left 8 Cornea, Right 9 Cornea, Left S Conjunctiva, Right T Conjunctiva, Left	X External	Z No Device	Z No Qualifier
2 Anterior Chamber, Right 3 Anterior Chamber, Left 4 Vitreous, Right 5 Vitreous, Left C Iris, Right D Iris, Left E Retina, Right F Retina, Left G Retinal Vessel, Right H Retinal Vessel, Left J Lens, Right K Lens, Left	3 Percutaneous	Z No Device	Z No Qualifier
A Choroid, Right B Choroid, Left L Extraocular Muscle, Right M Extraocular Muscle, Left V Lacrimal Gland, Right W Lacrimal Gland, Left	0 Open 3 Percutaneous	Z No Device	Z No Qualifier
N Upper Eyelid, Right P Upper Eyelid, Left Q Lower Eyelid, Right R Lower Eyelid, Left	0 Open 3 Percutaneous X External	Z No Device	Z No Qualifier
X Lacrimal Duct, Right Y Lacrimal Duct, Left	0 Open 3 Percutaneous 7 Via Natural or Artificial Opening 8 Via Natural or Artificial Opening Endoscopic	Z No Device	Z No Qualifier

0: M/S

8: EYE

M: REATTACHMENT N: RELEASE

◀ New　◀◀ Revised　deleted Deleted　♀ Females Only　♂ Males Only
Noncovered　Limited Coverage　Hospital-Acquired Condition　**Coding Clinic**

SECTION: 0 MEDICAL AND SURGICAL
BODY SYSTEM: 8 EYE
OPERATION: P REMOVAL: Taking out or off a device from a body part

Body Part	Approach	Device	Qualifier
0 Eye, Right 1 Eye, Left	0 Open 3 Percutaneous 7 Via Natural or Artificial Opening 8 Via Natural or Artificial Opening Endoscopic X External	0 Drainage Device 1 Radioactive Element 3 Infusion Device 7 Autologous Tissue Substitute C Extraluminal Device D Intraluminal Device J Synthetic Substitute K Nonautologous Tissue Substitute	Z No Qualifier
J Lens, Right K Lens, Left	3 Percutaneous	J Synthetic Substitute	Z No Qualifier
L Extraocular Muscle, Right M Extraocular Muscle, Left	0 Open 3 Percutaneous	0 Drainage Device 7 Autologous Tissue Substitute J Synthetic Substitute K Nonautologous Tissue Substitute	Z No Qualifier

P: REMOVAL 8: EYE 0: M/S

◀ New   ⬅ Revised   ~~deleted~~ Deleted   ♀ Females Only   ♂ Males Only
Noncovered   Limited Coverage   Hospital-Acquired Condition   **Coding Clinic**

SECTION: 0 MEDICAL AND SURGICAL
BODY SYSTEM: 8 EYE
OPERATION: Q REPAIR: Restoring, to the extent possible, a body part to its normal anatomic structure and function

Body Part	Approach	Device	Qualifier
0 Eye, Right 1 Eye, Left 6 Sclera, Right 7 Sclera, Left 8 Cornea, Right ⓠ 9 Cornea, Left ⓠ S Conjunctiva, Right T Conjunctiva, Left	X External	Z No Device	Z No Qualifier
2 Anterior Chamber, Right 3 Anterior Chamber, Left 4 Vitreous, Right 5 Vitreous, Left C Iris, Right D Iris, Left E Retina, Right F Retina, Left G Retinal Vessel, Right H Retinal Vessel, Left J Lens, Right K Lens, Left	3 Percutaneous	Z No Device	Z No Qualifier
A Choroid, Right B Choroid, Left L Extraocular Muscle, Right M Extraocular Muscle, Left V Lacrimal Gland, Right W Lacrimal Gland, Left	0 Open 3 Percutaneous	Z No Device	Z No Qualifier
N Upper Eyelid, Right P Upper Eyelid, Left Q Lower Eyelid, Right R Lower Eyelid, Left	0 Open 3 Percutaneous X External	Z No Device	Z No Qualifier
X Lacrimal Duct, Right Y Lacrimal Duct, Left	0 Open 3 Percutaneous 7 Via Natural or Artificial Opening 8 Via Natural or Artificial Opening Endoscopic	Z No Device	Z No Qualifier

SECTION: 0 MEDICAL AND SURGICAL
BODY SYSTEM: 8 EYE
OPERATION: R **REPLACEMENT:** Putting in or on biological or synthetic material that physically takes the place and/or function of all or a portion of a body part

Body Part	Approach	Device	Qualifier
0 Eye, Right 1 Eye, Left A Choroid, Right B Choroid, Left	0 Open 3 Percutaneous	7 Autologous Tissue Substitute J Synthetic Substitute K Nonautologous Tissue Substitute	Z No Qualifier
4 Vitreous, Right 5 Vitreous, Left C Iris, Right D Iris, Left G Retinal Vessel, Right H Retinal Vessel, Left	3 Percutaneous	7 Autologous Tissue Substitute J Synthetic Substitute K Nonautologous Tissue Substitute	Z No Qualifier
6 Sclera, Right 7 Sclera, Left S Conjunctiva, Right T Conjunctiva, Left	X External	7 Autologous Tissue Substitute J Synthetic Substitute K Nonautologous Tissue Substitute	Z No Qualifier
8 Cornea, Right 9 Cornea, Left	3 Percutaneous X External	7 Autologous Tissue Substitute J Synthetic Substitute K Nonautologous Tissue Substitute	Z No Qualifier
J Lens, Right K Lens, Left	3 Percutaneous	0 Synthetic Substitute, Intraocular Telescope 7 Autologous Tissue Substitute J Synthetic Substitute K Nonautologous Tissue Substitute	Z No Qualifier
N Upper Eyelid, Right P Upper Eyelid, Left Q Lower Eyelid, Right R Lower Eyelid, Left	0 Open 3 Percutaneous X External	7 Autologous Tissue Substitute J Synthetic Substitute K Nonautologous Tissue Substitute	Z No Qualifier
X Lacrimal Duct, Right Y Lacrimal Duct, Left	0 Open 3 Percutaneous 7 Via Natural or Artificial Opening 8 Via Natural or Artificial Opening Endoscopic	7 Autologous Tissue Substitute J Synthetic Substitute K Nonautologous Tissue Substitute	Z No Qualifier

R: REPLACEMENT

8: EYE

0: M/S

◀ New   ◀ Revised   ~~deleted~~ Deleted   ♀ Females Only   ♂ Males Only
Noncovered   Limited Coverage   Hospital-Acquired Condition   **Coding Clinic**

SECTION: 0 MEDICAL AND SURGICAL
BODY SYSTEM: 8 EYE
OPERATION: S REPOSITION: Moving to its normal location, or other suitable location, all or a portion of a body part

Body Part	Approach	Device	Qualifier
C Iris, Right D Iris, Left G Retinal Vessel, Right H Retinal Vessel, Left J Lens, Right K Lens, Left	3 Percutaneous	Z No Device	Z No Qualifier
L Extraocular Muscle, Right M Extraocular Muscle, Left V Lacrimal Gland, Right W Lacrimal Gland, Left	0 Open 3 Percutaneous	Z No Device	Z No Qualifier
N Upper Eyelid, Right P Upper Eyelid, Left Q Lower Eyelid, Right R Lower Eyelid, Left	0 Open 3 Percutaneous X External	Z No Device	Z No Qualifier
X Lacrimal Duct, Right Y Lacrimal Duct, Left	0 Open 3 Percutaneous 7 Via Natural or Artificial Opening 8 Via Natural or Artificial Opening Endoscopic	Z No Device	Z No Qualifier

◀ New   ◀▥ Revised   deleted Deleted   ♀ Females Only   ♂ Males Only
Noncovered   Limited Coverage   Hospital-Acquired Condition   **Coding Clinic**

167

SECTION: 0 MEDICAL AND SURGICAL
BODY SYSTEM: 8 EYE
OPERATION: T RESECTION: Cutting out or off, without replacement, all of a body part

Body Part	Approach	Device	Qualifier
0 Eye, Right 1 Eye, Left 8 Cornea, Right 9 Cornea, Left	X External	Z No Device	Z No Qualifier
4 Vitreous, Right 5 Vitreous, Left C Iris, Right D Iris, Left J Lens, Right K Lens, Left	3 Percutaneous	Z No Device	Z No Qualifier
L Extraocular Muscle, Right M Extraocular Muscle, Left V Lacrimal Gland, Right W Lacrimal Gland, Left	0 Open 3 Percutaneous	Z No Device	Z No Qualifier
N Upper Eyelid, Right P Upper Eyelid, Left Q Lower Eyelid, Right R Lower Eyelid, Left	0 Open X External	Z No Device	Z No Qualifier
X Lacrimal Duct, Right Y Lacrimal Duct, Left	0 Open 3 Percutaneous 7 Via Natural or Artificial Opening 8 Via Natural or Artificial Opening Endoscopic	Z No Device	Z No Qualifier

T: RESECTION   8: EYE   0: M/S

◀ New ◀▥ Revised ~~deleted~~ Deleted ♀ Females Only ♂ Males Only
🔒 Noncovered 🔒 Limited Coverage 🔒 Hospital-Acquired Condition **Coding Clinic**

SECTION: 0 MEDICAL AND SURGICAL

BODY SYSTEM: 8 EYE

OPERATION: U SUPPLEMENT: Putting in or on biological or synthetic material that physically reinforces and/or augments the function of a portion of a body part

Body Part	Approach	Device	Qualifier
0 Eye, Right 1 Eye, Left C Iris, Right D Iris, Left E Retina, Right F Retina, Left G Retinal Vessel, Right H Retinal Vessel, Left L Extraocular Muscle, Right M Extraocular Muscle, Left	0 Open 3 Percutaneous	7 Autologous Tissue Substitute J Synthetic Substitute K Nonautologous Tissue Substitute	Z No Qualifier
8 Cornea, Right ⚭ 9 Cornea, Left ⚭ N Upper Eyelid, Right P Upper Eyelid, Left Q Lower Eyelid, Right R Lower Eyelid, Left	0 Open 3 Percutaneous X External	7 Autologous Tissue Substitute J Synthetic Substitute K Nonautologous Tissue Substitute	Z No Qualifier

X Lacrimal Duct, Right
Y Lacrimal Duct, Left
	0 Open
	3 Percutaneous
	7 Via Natural or Artificial
	   Opening
	8 Via Natural or Artificial
	   Opening Endoscopic
		7 Autologous Tissue Substitute
		J Synthetic Substitute
		K Nonautologous Tissue
		   Substitute
			Z No Qualifier

⚭ 08U80KZ, 08U83KZ, 08U8XKZ
⚭ 08U90KZ, 08U93KZ, 08U9XKZ

SECTION: 0 MEDICAL AND SURGICAL

BODY SYSTEM: 8 EYE

OPERATION: V RESTRICTION: Partially closing an orifice or the lumen of a tubular body part

Body Part	Approach	Device	Qualifier
X Lacrimal Duct, Right Y Lacrimal Duct, Left	0 Open 3 Percutaneous	C Extraluminal Device D Intraluminal Device Z No Device	Z No Qualifier

X Lacrimal Duct, Right
Y Lacrimal Duct, Left
	7 Via Natural or Artificial
	   Opening
	8 Via Natural or Artificial
	   Opening Endoscopic
		D Intraluminal Device
		Z No Device
			Z No Qualifier

◀ New ◀▬ Revised ~~deleted~~ Deleted ♀ Females Only ♂ Males Only
⚭ Noncovered ⚭ Limited Coverage ⚭ Hospital-Acquired Condition **Coding Clinic**

SECTION: 0 MEDICAL AND SURGICAL
BODY SYSTEM: 8 EYE
OPERATION: W REVISION: Correcting, to the extent possible, a portion of a malfunctioning device or the positon of a displaced device

Body Part	Approach	Device	Qualifier
0 Eye, Right 1 Eye, Left	0 Open 3 Percutaneous 7 Via Natural or Artificial Opening 8 Via Natural or Artificial Opening Endoscopic X External	0 Drainage Device 3 Infusion Device 7 Autologous Tissue Substitute C Extraluminal Device D Intraluminal Device J Synthetic Substitute K Nonautologous Tissue Substitute	Z No Qualifier
J Lens, Right K Lens, Left	3 Percutaneous X External	J Synthetic Substitute	Z No Qualifier
L Extraocular Muscle, Right M Extraocular Muscle, Left	0 Open 3 Percutaneous	0 Drainage Device 7 Autologous Tissue Substitute J Synthetic Substitute K Nonautologous Tissue Substitute	Z No Qualifier

SECTION: 0 MEDICAL AND SURGICAL
BODY SYSTEM: 8 EYE
OPERATION: X TRANSFER: Moving, without taking out, all or a portion of a body part to another location to take over the function of all or a portion of a body part

Body Part	Approach	Device	Qualifier
L Extraocular Muscle, Right M Extraocular Muscle, Left	0 Open 3 Percutaneous	Z No Device	Z No Qualifier

W: REVISION X: TRANSFER

8: EYE

0: M/S

◀ New   ◀▥ Revised   ~~deleted~~ Deleted   ♀ Females Only   ♂ Males Only
⊘ Noncovered   ⊘ Limited Coverage   ⊘ Hospital-Acquired Condition   **Coding Clinic**

SECTION: 0 MEDICAL AND SURGICAL
BODY SYSTEM: 9 EAR, NOSE, SINUS
OPERATION: 0 ALTERATION: Modifying the anatomic structure of a body part without affecting the function of the body part

Body Part	Approach	Device	Qualifier
0 External Ear, Right 1 External Ear, Left 2 External Ear, Bilateral K Nose	0 Open 3 Percutaneous 4 Percutaneous Endoscopic X External	7 Autologous Tissue Substitute J Synthetic Substitute K Nonautologous Tissue Substitute Z No Device	Z No Qualifier

SECTION: 0 MEDICAL AND SURGICAL
BODY SYSTEM: 9 EAR, NOSE, SINUS
OPERATION: 1 BYPASS: Altering the route of passage of the contents of a tubular body part

Body Part	Approach	Device	Qualifier
D Inner Ear, Right E Inner Ear, Left	0 Open	7 Autologous Tissue Substitute J Synthetic Substitute K Nonautologous Tissue Substitute Z No Device	0 Endolymphatic

SECTION: 0 MEDICAL AND SURGICAL
BODY SYSTEM: 9 EAR, NOSE, SINUS
OPERATION: 2 CHANGE: Taking out or off a device from a body part and putting back an identical or similar device in or on the same body part without cutting or puncturing the skin or a mucous membrane

Body Part	Approach	Device	Qualifier
H Ear, Right J Ear, Left K Nose Y Sinus	X External	0 Drainage Device Y Other Device	Z No Qualifier

0: ALTERATION   1: BYPASS   2: CHANGE

9: EAR, NOSE, SINUS

0: M/S

◀ New   ◀▯▯▯ Revised   ~~deleted~~ Deleted   ♀ Females Only   ♂ Males Only
🚫 Noncovered   🚫 Limited Coverage   🚫 Hospital-Acquired Condition   **Coding Clinic**

SECTION: 0 MEDICAL AND SURGICAL
BODY SYSTEM: 9 EAR, NOSE, SINUS
OPERATION: 5 DESTRUCTION: Physical eradication of all or a portion of a body part by the direct use of energy, force, or a destructive agent

Body Part	Approach	Device	Qualifier
0 External Ear, Right 1 External Ear, Left K Nose	0 Open 3 Percutaneous 4 Percutaneous Endoscopic X External	Z No Device	Z No Qualifier
3 External Auditory Canal, Right 4 External Auditory Canal, Left	0 Open 3 Percutaneous 4 Percutaneous Endoscopic 7 Via Natural or Artificial Opening 8 Via Natural or Artificial Opening Endoscopic X External	Z No Device	Z No Qualifier
5 Middle Ear, Right 6 Middle Ear, Left 9 Auditory Ossicle, Right A Auditory Ossicle, Left D Inner Ear, Right E Inner Ear, Left	0 Open	Z No Device	Z No Qualifier
7 Tympanic Membrane, Right 8 Tympanic Membrane, Left F Eustachian Tube, Right G Eustachian Tube, Left L Nasal Turbinate N Nasopharynx	0 Open 3 Percutaneous 4 Percutaneous Endoscopic 7 Via Natural or Artificial Opening 8 Via Natural or Artificial Opening Endoscopic	Z No Device	Z No Qualifier
B Mastoid Sinus, Right C Mastoid Sinus, Left M Nasal Septum P Accessory Sinus Q Maxillary Sinus, Right R Maxillary Sinus, Left S Frontal Sinus, Right T Frontal Sinus, Left U Ethmoid Sinus, Right V Ethmoid Sinus, Left W Sphenoid Sinus, Right X Sphenoid Sinus, Left	0 Open 3 Percutaneous 4 Percutaneous Endoscopic	Z No Device	Z No Qualifier

0: M/S

9: EAR, NOSE, SINUS

5: DESTRUCTION

◀ New   ◀▦ Revised   ~~deleted~~ Deleted   ♀ Females Only   ♂ Males Only
🚫 Noncovered   🅢 Limited Coverage   🅗 Hospital-Acquired Condition   **Coding Clinic**

SECTION: 0 MEDICAL AND SURGICAL
BODY SYSTEM: 9 EAR, NOSE, SINUS
OPERATION: 7 DILATION: Expanding an orifice or the lumen of a tubular body part

Body Part	Approach	Device	Qualifier
F Eustachian Tube, Right G Eustachian Tube, Left	0 Open 7 Via Natural or Artificial Opening 8 Via Natural or Artificial Opening Endoscopic	D Intraluminal Device Z No Device	Z No Qualifier
F Eustachian Tube, Right G Eustachian Tube, Left	3 Percutaneous 4 Percutaneous Endoscopic	Z No Device	Z No Qualifier

SECTION: 0 MEDICAL AND SURGICAL
BODY SYSTEM: 9 EAR, NOSE, SINUS
OPERATION: 8 DIVISION: Cutting into a body part, without draining fluids and/or gases from the body part, in order to separate or transect a body part

Body Part	Approach	Device	Qualifier
L Nasal Turbinate	0 Open 3 Percutaneous 4 Percutaneous Endoscopic 7 Via Natural or Artificial Opening 8 Via Natural or Artificial Opening Endoscopic	Z No Device	Z No Qualifier

◀ New ◀ Revised ~~deleted~~ Deleted ♀ Females Only ♂ Males Only
Noncovered Limited Coverage Hospital-Acquired Condition **Coding Clinic**

SECTION: 0 MEDICAL AND SURGICAL
BODY SYSTEM: 9 EAR, NOSE, SINUS
OPERATION: 9 DRAINAGE: *(on multiple pages)*
Taking or letting out fluids and/or gases from a body part

Body Part	Approach	Device	Qualifier
0 External Ear, Right 1 External Ear, Left K Nose	0 Open 3 Percutaneous 4 Percutaneous Endoscopic X External	0 Drainage Device	Z No Qualifier
0 External Ear, Right 1 External Ear, Left K Nose	0 Open 3 Percutaneous 4 Percutaneous Endoscopic X External	Z No Device	X Diagnostic Z No Qualifier
3 External Auditory Canal, Right 4 External Auditory Canal, Left	0 Open 3 Percutaneous 4 Percutaneous Endoscopic 7 Via Natural or Artificial Opening 8 Via Natural or Artificial Opening Endoscopic X External	0 Drainage Device	Z No Qualifier
3 External Auditory Canal, Right 4 External Auditory Canal, Left	0 Open 3 Percutaneous 4 Percutaneous Endoscopic 7 Via Natural or Artificial Opening 8 Via Natural or Artificial Opening Endoscopic X External	Z No Device	X Diagnostic Z No Qualifier
5 Middle Ear, Right 6 Middle Ear, Left 9 Auditory Ossicle, Right A Auditory Ossicle, Left D Inner Ear, Right E Inner Ear, Left	0 Open	0 Drainage Device	Z No Qualifier
5 Middle Ear, Right 6 Middle Ear, Left 9 Auditory Ossicle, Right A Auditory Ossicle, Left D Inner Ear, Right E Inner Ear, Left	0 Open	Z No Device	X Diagnostic Z No Qualifier
7 Tympanic Membrane, Right 8 Tympanic Membrane, Left F Eustachian Tube, Right G Eustachian Tube, Left L Nasal Turbinate N Nasopharynx	0 Open 3 Percutaneous 4 Percutaneous Endoscopic 7 Via Natural or Artificial Opening 8 Via Natural or Artificial Opening Endoscopic	0 Drainage Device	Z No Qualifier

0: M/S

9: EAR, NOSE, SINUS

9: DRAINAGE

◄ New ◄ Revised ~~deleted~~ Deleted ♀ Females Only ♂ Males Only
Noncovered Limited Coverage Hospital-Acquired Condition **Coding Clinic**

175

SECTION: 0 MEDICAL AND SURGICAL
BODY SYSTEM: 9 EAR, NOSE, SINUS
OPERATION: 9 DRAINAGE: *(continued)*
Taking or letting out fluids and/or gases from a body part

Body Part	Approach	Device	Qualifier
7 Tympanic Membrane, Right 8 Tympanic Membrane, Left F Eustachian Tube, Right G Eustachian Tube, Left L Nasal Turbinate N Nasopharynx	0 Open 3 Percutaneous 4 Percutaneous Endoscopic 7 Via Natural or Artificial Opening 8 Via Natural or Artificial Opening Endoscopic	Z No Device	X Diagnostic Z No Qualifier
B Mastoid Sinus, Right C Mastoid Sinus, Left M Nasal Septum P Accessory Sinus Q Maxillary Sinus, Right R Maxillary Sinus, Left S Frontal Sinus, Right T Frontal Sinus, Left U Ethmoid Sinus, Right V Ethmoid Sinus, Left W Sphenoid Sinus, Right X Sphenoid Sinus, Left	0 Open 3 Percutaneous 4 Percutaneous Endoscopic	0 Drainage Device	Z No Qualifier
B Mastoid Sinus, Right C Mastoid Sinus, Left M Nasal Septum P Accessory Sinus Q Maxillary Sinus, Right R Maxillary Sinus, Left S Frontal Sinus, Right T Frontal Sinus, Left U Ethmoid Sinus, Right V Ethmoid Sinus, Left W Sphenoid Sinus, Right X Sphenoid Sinus, Left	0 Open 3 Percutaneous 4 Percutaneous Endoscopic	Z No Device	X Diagnostic Z No Qualifier

9: DRAINAGE

9: EAR, NOSE, SINUS

0: M/S

◀ New ◀ Revised ~~deleted~~ Deleted ♀ Females Only ♂ Males Only
Noncovered Limited Coverage Hospital-Acquired Condition **Coding Clinic**

SECTION: 0 MEDICAL AND SURGICAL
BODY SYSTEM: 9 EAR, NOSE, SINUS
OPERATION: B EXCISION: Cutting out or off, without replacement, a portion of a body part

Body Part	Approach	Device	Qualifier
0 External Ear, Right 1 External Ear, Left K Nose	0 Open 3 Percutaneous 4 Percutaneous Endoscopic X External	Z No Device	X Diagnostic Z No Qualifier
3 External Auditory Canal, Right 4 External Auditory Canal, Left	0 Open 3 Percutaneous 4 Percutaneous Endoscopic 7 Via Natural or Artificial Opening 8 Via Natural or Artificial Opening Endoscopic X External	Z No Device	X Diagnostic Z No Qualifier
5 Middle Ear, Right 6 Middle Ear, Left 9 Auditory Ossicle, Right A Auditory Ossicle, Left D Inner Ear, Right E Inner Ear, Left	0 Open	Z No Device	X Diagnostic Z No Qualifier
7 Tympanic Membrane, Right 8 Tympanic Membrane, Left F Eustachian Tube, Right G Eustachian Tube, Left L Nasal Turbinate N Nasopharynx	0 Open 3 Percutaneous 4 Percutaneous Endoscopic 7 Via Natural or Artificial Opening 8 Via Natural or Artificial Opening Endoscopic	Z No Device	X Diagnostic Z No Qualifier
B Mastoid Sinus, Right C Mastoid Sinus, Left M Nasal Septum P Accessory Sinus Q Maxillary Sinus, Right R Maxillary Sinus, Left S Frontal Sinus, Right T Frontal Sinus, Left U Ethmoid Sinus, Right V Ethmoid Sinus, Left W Sphenoid Sinus, Right X Sphenoid Sinus, Left	0 Open 3 Percutaneous 4 Percutaneous Endoscopic	Z No Device	X Diagnostic Z No Qualifier

0: M/S

9: EAR, NOSE, SINUS

B: EXCISION

◀ New ◀▥ Revised ~~deleted~~ Deleted ♀ Females Only ♂ Males Only
⬭ Noncovered ⬭ Limited Coverage ⬭ Hospital-Acquired Condition **Coding Clinic**

SECTION: 0 MEDICAL AND SURGICAL
BODY SYSTEM: 9 EAR, NOSE, SINUS
OPERATION: C EXTIRPATION: Taking or cutting out solid matter from a body part

Body Part	Approach	Device	Qualifier
0 External Ear, Right 1 External Ear, Left K Nose	0 Open 3 Percutaneous 4 Percutaneous Endoscopic X External	Z No Device	Z No Qualifier
3 External Auditory Canal, Right 4 External Auditory Canal, Left	0 Open 3 Percutaneous 4 Percutaneous Endoscopic 7 Via Natural or Artificial Opening 8 Via Natural or Artificial Opening Endoscopic X External	Z No Device	Z No Qualifier
5 Middle Ear, Right 6 Middle Ear, Left 9 Auditory Ossicle, Right A Auditory Ossicle, Left D Inner Ear, Right E Inner Ear, Left	0 Open	Z No Device	Z No Qualifier
7 Tympanic Membrane, Right 8 Tympanic Membrane, Left F Eustachian Tube, Right G Eustachian Tube, Left L Nasal Turbinate N Nasopharynx	0 Open 3 Percutaneous 4 Percutaneous Endoscopic 7 Via Natural or Artificial Opening 8 Via Natural or Artificial Opening Endoscopic	Z No Device	Z No Qualifier
B Mastoid Sinus, Right C Mastoid Sinus, Left M Nasal Septum P Accessory Sinus Q Maxillary Sinus, Right R Maxillary Sinus, Left S Frontal Sinus, Right T Frontal Sinus, Left U Ethmoid Sinus, Right V Ethmoid Sinus, Left W Sphenoid Sinus, Right X Sphenoid Sinus, Left	0 Open 3 Percutaneous 4 Percutaneous Endoscopic	Z No Device	Z No Qualifier

C: EXTIRPATION

9: EAR, NOSE, SINUS

0: M/S

◀ New   ◀▥ Revised   ~~deleted~~ Deleted   ♀ Females Only   ♂ Males Only
🅝🅒 Noncovered   🅛🅒 Limited Coverage   🅗🅐🅒 Hospital-Acquired Condition   **Coding Clinic**

SECTION: 0 MEDICAL AND SURGICAL
BODY SYSTEM: 9 EAR, NOSE, SINUS
OPERATION: D EXTRACTION: Pulling or stripping out or off all or a portion of a body part by the use of force

Body Part	Approach	Device	Qualifier
7 Tympanic Membrane, Right 8 Tympanic Membrane, Left L Nasal Turbinate	0 Open 3 Percutaneous 4 Percutaneous Endoscopic 7 Via Natural or Artificial Opening 8 Via Natural or Artificial Opening Endoscopic	Z No Device	Z No Qualifier
9 Auditory Ossicle, Right A Auditory Ossicle, Left	0 Open	Z No Device	Z No Qualifier
B Mastoid Sinus, Right C Mastoid Sinus, Left M Nasal Septum P Accessory Sinus Q Maxillary Sinus, Right R Maxillary Sinus, Left S Frontal Sinus, Right T Frontal Sinus, Left U Ethmoid Sinus, Right V Ethmoid Sinus, Left W Sphenoid Sinus, Right X Sphenoid Sinus, Left	0 Open 3 Percutaneous 4 Percutaneous Endoscopic	Z No Device	Z No Qualifier

SECTION: 0 MEDICAL AND SURGICAL
BODY SYSTEM: 9 EAR, NOSE, SINUS
OPERATION: H INSERTION: Putting in a nonbiological appliance that monitors, assists, performs, or prevents a physiological function but does not physically take the place of a body part

Body Part	Approach	Device	Qualifier
D Inner Ear, Right E Inner Ear, Left	0 Open 3 Percutaneous 4 Percutaneous Endoscopic	4 Hearing Device, Bone Conduction 5 Hearing Device, Single Channel Cochlear Prosthesis 6 Hearing Device, Multiple Channel Cochlear Prosthesis S Hearing Device	Z No Qualifier
N Nasopharynx	7 Via Natural or Artificial Opening 8 Via Natural or Artificial Opening Endoscopic	B Intraluminal Device, Airway	Z No Qualifier

◀ New ◀ Revised ~~deleted~~ Deleted ♀ Females Only ♂ Males Only
Noncovered Limited Coverage Hospital-Acquired Condition **Coding Clinic**

179

SECTION: 0 MEDICAL AND SURGICAL

BODY SYSTEM: 9 EAR, NOSE, SINUS
OPERATION: J INSPECTION: Visually and/or manually exploring a body part

Body Part	Approach	Device	Qualifier
7 Tympanic Membrane, Right 8 Tympanic Membrane, Left H Ear, Right J Ear, Left	0 Open 3 Percutaneous 4 Percutaneous Endoscopic 7 Via Natural or Artificial Opening 8 Via Natural or Artificial Opening Endoscopic X External	Z No Device	Z No Qualifier
D Inner Ear, Right E Inner Ear, Left K Nose Y Sinus	0 Open 3 Percutaneous 4 Percutaneous Endoscopic X External	Z No Device	Z No Qualifier

SECTION: 0 MEDICAL AND SURGICAL

BODY SYSTEM: 9 EAR, NOSE, SINUS
OPERATION: M REATTACHMENT: Putting back in or on all or a portion of a separated body part to its normal location or other suitable location

Body Part	Approach	Device	Qualifier
0 External Ear, Right 1 External Ear, Left K Nose	X External	Z No Device	Z No Qualifier

SECTION: 0 MEDICAL AND SURGICAL
BODY SYSTEM: 9 EAR, NOSE, SINUS
OPERATION: N RELEASE: Freeing a body part from an abnormal physical constraint

Body Part	Approach	Device	Qualifier
0 External Ear, Right 1 External Ear, Left K Nose	0 Open 3 Percutaneous 4 Percutaneous Endoscopic X External	Z No Device	Z No Qualifier
3 External Auditory Canal, Right 4 External Auditory Canal, Left	0 Open 3 Percutaneous 4 Percutaneous Endoscopic 7 Via Natural or Artificial Opening 8 Via Natural or Artificial Opening Endoscopic X External	Z No Device	Z No Qualifier
5 Middle Ear, Right 6 Middle Ear, Left 9 Auditory Ossicle, Right A Auditory Ossicle, Left D Inner Ear, Right E Inner Ear, Left	0 Open	Z No Device	Z No Qualifier
7 Tympanic Membrane, Right 8 Tympanic Membrane, Left F Eustachian Tube, Right G Eustachian Tube, Left L Nasal Turbinate N Nasopharynx	0 Open 3 Percutaneous 4 Percutaneous Endoscopic 7 Via Natural or Artificial Opening 8 Via Natural or Artificial Opening Endoscopic	Z No Device	Z No Qualifier
B Mastoid Sinus, Right C Mastoid Sinus, Left M Nasal Septum P Accessory Sinus Q Maxillary Sinus, Right R Maxillary Sinus, Left S Frontal Sinus, Right T Frontal Sinus, Left U Ethmoid Sinus, Right V Ethmoid Sinus, Left W Sphenoid Sinus, Right X Sphenoid Sinus, Left	0 Open 3 Percutaneous 4 Percutaneous Endoscopic	Z No Device	Z No Qualifier

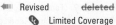

◀ New ◀ Revised ~~deleted~~ Deleted ♀ Females Only ♂ Males Only
ⓃⒸ Noncovered ⓁⒸ Limited Coverage ⒽⒶⒸ Hospital-Acquired Condition **Coding Clinic**

SECTION: 0 MEDICAL AND SURGICAL

BODY SYSTEM: 9 EAR, NOSE, SINUS
OPERATION: P REMOVAL: Taking out or off a device from a body part

Body Part	Approach	Device	Qualifier
7 Tympanic Membrane, Right 8 Tympanic Membrane, Left	0 Open 7 Via Natural or Artificial Opening 8 Via Natural or Artificial Opening Endoscopic X External	0 Drainage Device	Z No Qualifier
D Inner Ear, Right E Inner Ear, Left	0 Open 7 Via Natural or Artificial Opening 8 Via Natural or Artificial Opening Endoscopic	S Hearing Device	Z No Qualifier
H Ear, Right J Ear, Left K Nose	0 Open 3 Percutaneous 4 Percutaneous Endoscopic 7 Via Natural or Artificial Opening 8 Via Natural or Artificial Opening Endoscopic X External	0 Drainage Device 7 Autologous Tissue Substitute D Intraluminal Device J Synthetic Substitute K Nonautologous Tissue Substitute	Z No Qualifier
Y Sinus	0 Open 3 Percutaneous 4 Percutaneous Endoscopic X External	0 Drainage Device	Z No Qualifier

◄ New ◄▬▬ Revised ~~deleted~~ Deleted ♀ Females Only ♂ Males Only
℞ Noncovered ℞ Limited Coverage ℞ Hospital-Acquired Condition **Coding Clinic**

SECTION: 0 MEDICAL AND SURGICAL
BODY SYSTEM: 9 EAR, NOSE, SINUS
OPERATION: Q REPAIR: Restoring, to the extent possible, a body part to its normal anatomic structure and function

Body Part	Approach	Device	Qualifier
0 External Ear, Right 1 External Ear, Left 2 External Ear, Bilateral K Nose	0 Open 3 Percutaneous 4 Percutaneous Endoscopic X External	Z No Device	Z No Qualifier
3 External Auditory Canal, Right 4 External Auditory Canal, Left F Eustachian Tube, Right G Eustachian Tube, Left	0 Open 3 Percutaneous 4 Percutaneous Endoscopic 7 Via Natural or Artificial Opening 8 Via Natural or Artificial Opening Endoscopic X External	Z No Device	Z No Qualifier
5 Middle Ear, Right 6 Middle Ear, Left 9 Auditory Ossicle, Right A Auditory Ossicle, Left D Inner Ear, Right E Inner Ear, Left	0 Open	Z No Device	Z No Qualifier
7 Tympanic Membrane, Right 8 Tympanic Membrane, Left L Nasal Turbinate N Nasopharynx	0 Open 3 Percutaneous 4 Percutaneous Endoscopic 7 Via Natural or Artificial Opening 8 Via Natural or Artificial Opening Endoscopic	Z No Device	Z No Qualifier
B Mastoid Sinus, Right C Mastoid Sinus, Left M Nasal Septum P Accessory Sinus Q Maxillary Sinus, Right R Maxillary Sinus, Left S Frontal Sinus, Right T Frontal Sinus, Left U Ethmoid Sinus, Right V Ethmoid Sinus, Left W Sphenoid Sinus, Right X Sphenoid Sinus, Left	0 Open 3 Percutaneous 4 Percutaneous Endoscopic	Z No Device	Z No Qualifier

SECTION: 0 MEDICAL AND SURGICAL
BODY SYSTEM: 9 EAR, NOSE, SINUS
OPERATION: R REPLACEMENT: Putting in or on biological or synthetic material that physically takes the place and/or function of all or a portion of a body part

Body Part	Approach	Device	Qualifier
0 External Ear, Right 1 External Ear, Left 2 External Ear, Bilateral K Nose	0 Open X External	7 Autologous Tissue Substitute J Synthetic Substitute K Nonautologous Tissue Substitute	Z No Qualifier
5 Middle Ear, Right 6 Middle Ear, Left 9 Auditory Ossicle, Right A Auditory Ossicle, Left D Inner Ear, Right E Inner Ear, Left	0 Open	7 Autologous Tissue Substitute J Synthetic Substitute K Nonautologous Tissue Substitute	Z No Qualifier
7 Tympanic Membrane, Right 8 Tympanic Membrane, Left N Nasopharynx	0 Open 7 Via Natural or Artificial Opening 8 Via Natural or Artificial Opening Endoscopic	7 Autologous Tissue Substitute J Synthetic Substitute K Nonautologous Tissue Substitute	Z No Qualifier
L Nasal Turbinate	0 Open 3 Percutaneous 4 Percutaneous Endoscopic 7 Via Natural or Artificial Opening 8 Via Natural or Artificial Opening Endoscopic	7 Autologous Tissue Substitute J Synthetic Substitute K Nonautologous Tissue Substitute	Z No Qualifier
M Nasal Septum	0 Open 3 Percutaneous 4 Percutaneous Endoscopic	7 Autologous Tissue Substitute J Synthetic Substitute K Nonautologous Tissue Substitute	Z No Qualifier

SECTION: 0 MEDICAL AND SURGICAL
BODY SYSTEM: 9 EAR, NOSE, SINUS
OPERATION: S REPOSITION: Moving to its normal location, or other suitable location, all or a portion of a body part

Body Part	Approach	Device	Qualifier
0 External Ear, Right 1 External Ear, Left 2 External Ear, Bilateral K Nose	0 Open 4 Percutaneous Endoscopic X External	Z No Device	Z No Qualifier
7 Tympanic Membrane, Right 8 Tympanic Membrane, Left F Eustachian Tube, Right G Eustachian Tube, Left L Nasal Turbinate	0 Open 4 Percutaneous Endoscopic 7 Via Natural or Artificial Opening 8 Via Natural or Artificial Opening Endoscopic	Z No Device	Z No Qualifier
9 Auditory Ossicle, Right A Auditory Ossicle, Left M Nasal Septum	0 Open 4 Percutaneous Endoscopic	Z No Device	Z No Qualifier

◀ New   ◀▥ Revised   ~~deleted~~ Deleted   ♀ Females Only   ♂ Males Only
🅝 Noncovered   🅛 Limited Coverage   🅗 Hospital-Acquired Condition   **Coding Clinic**

SECTION: 0 MEDICAL AND SURGICAL
BODY SYSTEM: 9 EAR, NOSE, SINUS
OPERATION: **T RESECTION:** Cutting out or off, without replacement, all of a body part

Body Part	Approach	Device	Qualifier
0 External Ear, Right 1 External Ear, Left K Nose	0 Open 4 Percutaneous Endoscopic X External	Z No Device	Z No Qualifier
5 Middle Ear, Right 6 Middle Ear, Left 9 Auditory Ossicle, Right A Auditory Ossicle, Left D Inner Ear, Right E Inner Ear, Left	0 Open	Z No Device	Z No Qualifier

7 Tympanic Membrane, Right
8 Tympanic Membrane, Left
F Eustachian Tube, Right
G Eustachian Tube, Left
L Nasal Turbinate
N Nasopharynx
	0 Open
	4 Percutaneous Endoscopic
	7 Via Natural or Artificial
	    Opening
	8 Via Natural or Artificial
	    Opening Endoscopic
		Z No Device	Z No Qualifier

B Mastoid Sinus, Right C Mastoid Sinus, Left M Nasal Septum P Accessory Sinus Q Maxillary Sinus, Right R Maxillary Sinus, Left S Frontal Sinus, Right T Frontal Sinus, Left U Ethmoid Sinus, Right V Ethmoid Sinus, Left W Sphenoid Sinus, Right X Sphenoid Sinus, Left	0 Open 4 Percutaneous Endoscopic	Z No Device	Z No Qualifier

0: M/S

9: EAR, NOSE, SINUS

T: RESECTION

SECTION: 0 MEDICAL AND SURGICAL
BODY SYSTEM: 9 EAR, NOSE, SINUS
OPERATION: U SUPPLEMENT: Putting in or on biological or synthetic material that physically reinforces and/or augments the function of a portion of a body part

Body Part	Approach	Device	Qualifier
0 External Ear, Right 1 External Ear, Left 2 External Ear, Bilateral K Nose	0 Open X External	7 Autologous Tissue Substitute J Synthetic Substitute K Nonautologous Tissue Substitute	Z No Qualifier
5 Middle Ear, Right 6 Middle Ear, Left 9 Auditory Ossicle, Right A Auditory Ossicle, Left D Inner Ear, Right E Inner Ear, Left	0 Open	7 Autologous Tissue Substitute J Synthetic Substitute K Nonautologous Tissue Substitute	Z No Qualifier
7 Tympanic Membrane, Right 8 Tympanic Membrane, Left N Nasopharynx	0 Open 7 Via Natural or Artificial Opening 8 Via Natural or Artificial Opening Endoscopic	7 Autologous Tissue Substitute J Synthetic Substitute K Nonautologous Tissue Substitute	Z No Qualifier
L Nasal Turbinate	0 Open 3 Percutaneous 4 Percutaneous Endoscopic 7 Via Natural or Artificial Opening 8 Via Natural or Artificial Opening Endoscopic	7 Autologous Tissue Substitute J Synthetic Substitute K Nonautologous Tissue Substitute	Z No Qualifier
M Nasal Septum	0 Open 3 Percutaneous 4 Percutaneous Endoscopic	7 Autologous Tissue Substitute J Synthetic Substitute K Nonautologous Tissue Substitute	Z No Qualifier

U: SUPPLEMENT

9: EAR, NOSE, SINUS

0: M/S

◀ New   ◀▥ Revised   ~~deleted~~ Deleted   ♀ Females Only   ♂ Males Only
🅝 Noncovered   🅛 Limited Coverage   🅗 Hospital-Acquired Condition   **Coding Clinic**

SECTION: 0 MEDICAL AND SURGICAL
BODY SYSTEM: 9 EAR, NOSE, SINUS
OPERATION: W REVISION: Correcting, to the extent possible, a portion of a malfunctioning device or the position of a displaced device

Body Part	Approach	Device	Qualifier
7 Tympanic Membrane, Right 8 Tympanic Membrane, Left 9 Auditory Ossicle, Right A Auditory Ossicle, Left	0 Open 7 Via Natural or Artificial Opening 8 Via Natural or Artificial Opening Endoscopic	7 Autologous Tissue Substitute J Synthetic Substitute K Nonautologous Tissue Substitute	Z No Qualifier
D Inner Ear, Right E Inner Ear, Left	0 Open 7 Via Natural or Artificial Opening 8 Via Natural or Artificial Opening Endoscopic	S Hearing Device	Z No Qualifier
H Ear, Right J Ear, Left K Nose	0 Open 3 Percutaneous 4 Percutaneous Endoscopic 7 Via Natural or Artificial Opening 8 Via Natural or Artificial Opening Endoscopic X External	0 Drainage Device 7 Autologous Tissue Substitute D Intraluminal Device J Synthetic Substitute K Nonautologous Tissue Substitute	Z No Qualifier
Y Sinus	0 Open 3 Percutaneous 4 Percutaneous Endoscopic X External	0 Drainage Device	Z No Qualifier

◀ New   ◀ Revised   deleted Deleted   ♀ Females Only   ♂ Males Only
Noncovered   Limited Coverage   Hospital-Acquired Condition   **Coding Clinic**

187

◀ New   ◀▥ Revised   deleted Deleted   ♀ Females Only   ♂ Males Only
🅝 Noncovered   🅛 Limited Coverage   🅗 Hospital-Acquired Condition   **Coding Clinic**

SECTION: 0 MEDICAL AND SURGICAL

BODY SYSTEM: B RESPIRATORY SYSTEM

OPERATION: 1 BYPASS: Altering the route of passage of the contents of a tubular body part

Body Part	Approach	Device	Qualifier
1 Trachea	0 Open	D Intraluminal Device	6 Esophagus
1 Trachea	0 Open	F Tracheostomy Device Z No Device	4 Cutaneous
1 Trachea	3 Percutaneous 4 Percutaneous Endoscopic	F Tracheostomy Device Z No Device	4 Cutaneous

SECTION: 0 MEDICAL AND SURGICAL

BODY SYSTEM: B RESPIRATORY SYSTEM

OPERATION: 2 CHANGE: Taking out or off a device from a body part and putting back an identical or similar device in or on the same body part without cutting or puncturing the skin or a mucous membrane

Body Part	Approach	Device	Qualifier
0 Tracheobronchial Tree K Lung, Right L Lung, Left Q Pleura T Diaphragm	X External	0 Drainage Device Y Other Device	Z No Qualifier
1 Trachea	X External	0 Drainage Device E Intraluminal Device, Endotracheal Airway F Tracheostomy Device Y Other Device	Z No Qualifier

SECTION: 0 MEDICAL AND SURGICAL
BODY SYSTEM: B RESPIRATORY SYSTEM
OPERATION: 5 DESTRUCTION: Physical eradication of all or a portion of a body part by the direct use of energy, force, or a destructive agent

Body Part	Approach	Device	Qualifier
1 Trachea 2 Carina 3 Main Bronchus, Right 4 Upper Lobe Bronchus, Right 5 Middle Lobe Bronchus, Right 6 Lower Lobe Bronchus, Right 7 Main Bronchus, Left 8 Upper Lobe Bronchus, Left 9 Lingula Bronchus B Lower Lobe Bronchus, Left C Upper Lung Lobe, Right D Middle Lung Lobe, Right F Lower Lung Lobe, Right G Upper Lung Lobe, Left H Lung Lingula J Lower Lung Lobe, Left K Lung, Right L Lung, Left M Lungs, Bilateral	0 Open 3 Percutaneous 4 Percutaneous Endoscopic 7 Via Natural or Artificial Opening 8 Via Natural or Artificial Opening Endoscopic	Z No Device	Z No Qualifier
N Pleura, Right P Pleura, Left R Diaphragm, Right S Diaphragm, Left	0 Open 3 Percutaneous 4 Percutaneous Endoscopic	Z No Device	Z No Qualifier

SECTION: 0 MEDICAL AND SURGICAL
BODY SYSTEM: B RESPIRATORY SYSTEM
OPERATION: 7 DILATION: Expanding an orifice or the lumen of a tubular body part

Body Part	Approach	Device	Qualifier
1 Trachea 2 Carina 3 Main Bronchus, Right 4 Upper Lobe Bronchus, Right 5 Middle Lobe Bronchus, Right 6 Lower Lobe Bronchus, Right 7 Main Bronchus, Left 8 Upper Lobe Bronchus, Left 9 Lingula Bronchus B Lower Lobe Bronchus, Left	0 Open 3 Percutaneous 4 Percutaneous Endoscopic 7 Via Natural or Artificial Opening 8 Via Natural or Artificial Opening Endoscopic	D Intraluminal Device Z No Device	Z No Qualifier

SECTION: 0 MEDICAL AND SURGICAL
BODY SYSTEM: B RESPIRATORY SYSTEM
OPERATION: 9 DRAINAGE: Taking or letting out fluids and/or gases from a body part

Body Part	Approach	Device	Qualifier
1 Trachea 2 Carina 3 Main Bronchus, Right 4 Upper Lobe Bronchus, Right 5 Middle Lobe Bronchus, Right 6 Lower Lobe Bronchus, Right 7 Main Bronchus, Left 8 Upper Lobe Bronchus, Left 9 Lingula Bronchus B Lower Lobe Bronchus, Left C Upper Lung Lobe, Right D Middle Lung Lobe, Right F Lower Lung Lobe, Right G Upper Lung Lobe, Left H Lung Lingula J Lower Lung Lobe, Left K Lung, Right L Lung, Left M Lungs, Bilateral	0 Open 3 Percutaneous 4 Percutaneous Endoscopic 7 Via Natural or Artificial Opening 8 Via Natural or Artificial Opening Endoscopic	0 Drainage Device	Z No Qualifier
1 Trachea 2 Carina 3 Main Bronchus, Right 4 Upper Lobe Bronchus, Right 5 Middle Lobe Bronchus, Right 6 Lower Lobe Bronchus, Right 7 Main Bronchus, Left 8 Upper Lobe Bronchus, Left 9 Lingula Bronchus B Lower Lobe Bronchus, Left C Upper Lung Lobe, Right D Middle Lung Lobe, Right F Lower Lung Lobe, Right G Upper Lung Lobe, Left H Lung Lingula J Lower Lung Lobe, Left K Lung, Right L Lung, Left M Lungs, Bilateral	0 Open 3 Percutaneous 4 Percutaneous Endoscopic 7 Via Natural or Artificial Opening 8 Via Natural or Artificial Opening Endoscopic	Z No Device	X Diagnostic Z No Qualifier
N Pleura, Right P Pleura, Left R Diaphragm, Right S Diaphragm, Left	0 Open 3 Percutaneous 4 Percutaneous Endoscopic	0 Drainage Device	Z No Qualifier
N Pleura, Right P Pleura, Left R Diaphragm, Right S Diaphragm, Left	0 Open 3 Percutaneous 4 Percutaneous Endoscopic	Z No Device	X Diagnostic Z No Qualifier

◀ New   ◀ Revised   ~~deleted~~ Deleted   ♀ Females Only   ♂ Males Only

 Noncovered   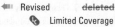 Limited Coverage   Hospital-Acquired Condition   **Coding Clinic**

SECTION: **0** **MEDICAL AND SURGICAL**
BODY SYSTEM: **B** RESPIRATORY SYSTEM
OPERATION: **B** **EXCISION:** Cutting out or off, without replacement, a portion of a body part

Body Part	Approach	Device	Qualifier
1 Trachea 2 Carina 3 Main Bronchus, Right 4 Upper Lobe Bronchus, Right 5 Middle Lobe Bronchus, Right 6 Lower Lobe Bronchus, Right 7 Main Bronchus, Left 8 Upper Lobe Bronchus, Left 9 Lingula Bronchus B Lower Lobe Bronchus, Left C Upper Lung Lobe, Right D Middle Lung Lobe, Right F Lower Lung Lobe, Right G Upper Lung Lobe, Left H Lung Lingula J Lower Lung Lobe, Left K Lung, Right L Lung, Left M Lungs, Bilateral	0 Open 3 Percutaneous 4 Percutaneous Endoscopic 7 Via Natural or Artificial Opening 8 Via Natural or Artificial Opening Endoscopic	Z No Device	X Diagnostic Z No Qualifier
N Pleura, Right P Pleura, Left R Diaphragm, Right S Diaphragm, Left	0 Open 3 Percutaneous 4 Percutaneous Endoscopic	Z No Device	X Diagnostic Z No Qualifier

SECTION: **0** **MEDICAL AND SURGICAL**
BODY SYSTEM: **B** RESPIRATORY SYSTEM
OPERATION: **C** **EXTIRPATION:** Taking or cutting out solid matter from a body part

Body Part	Approach	Device	Qualifier
1 Trachea 2 Carina 3 Main Bronchus, Right 4 Upper Lobe Bronchus, Right 5 Middle Lobe Bronchus, Right 6 Lower Lobe Bronchus, Right 7 Main Bronchus, Left 8 Upper Lobe Bronchus, Left 9 Lingula Bronchus B Lower Lobe Bronchus, Left C Upper Lung Lobe, Right D Middle Lung Lobe, Right F Lower Lung Lobe, Right G Upper Lung Lobe, Left H Lung Lingula J Lower Lung Lobe, Left K Lung, Right L Lung, Left M Lungs, Bilateral	0 Open 3 Percutaneous 4 Percutaneous Endoscopic 7 Via Natural or Artificial Opening 8 Via Natural or Artificial Opening Endoscopic	Z No Device	Z No Qualifier
N Pleura, Right P Pleura, Left R Diaphragm, Right S Diaphragm, Left	0 Open 3 Percutaneous 4 Percutaneous Endoscopic	Z No Device	Z No Qualifier

B: RESPIRATORY SYSTEM   B: EXCISION   C: EXTIRPATION   0: M/S

◄ New   ◄◼ Revised   ~~deleted~~ Deleted   ♀ Females Only   ♂ Males Only
Ⓝ Noncovered   Ⓛ Limited Coverage   Ⓗ Hospital-Acquired Condition   **Coding Clinic**

SECTION: 0 MEDICAL AND SURGICAL
BODY SYSTEM: B RESPIRATORY SYSTEM
OPERATION: D EXTRACTION: Pulling or stripping out or off all or a portion of a body part by the use of force

Body Part	Approach	Device	Qualifier
N Pleura, Right P Pleura, Left	0 Open 3 Percutaneous 4 Percutaneous Endoscopic	Z No Device	X Diagnostic Z No Qualifier

SECTION: 0 MEDICAL AND SURGICAL
BODY SYSTEM: B RESPIRATORY SYSTEM
OPERATION: F FRAGMENTATION: Breaking solid matter in a body part into pieces

Body Part	Approach	Device	Qualifier
1 Trachea 2 Carina 3 Main Bronchus, Right 4 Upper Lobe Bronchus, Right 5 Middle Lobe Bronchus, Right 6 Lower Lobe Bronchus, Right 7 Main Bronchus, Left 8 Upper Lobe Bronchus, Left 9 Lingula Bronchus B Lower Lobe Bronchus, Left	0 Open 3 Percutaneous 4 Percutaneous Endoscopic 7 Via Natural or Artificial Opening 8 Via Natural or Artificial Opening Endoscopic X External ⚕	Z No Device	Z No Qualifier

◀ New   ◀ Revised   ~~deleted~~ Deleted   ♀ Females Only   ♂ Males Only
⚕ Noncovered   ⚕ Limited Coverage   ⚕ Hospital-Acquired Condition   **Coding Clinic**

193

SECTION: 0 MEDICAL AND SURGICAL

BODY SYSTEM: **B RESPIRATORY SYSTEM**

OPERATION: **H INSERTION:** Putting in a nonbiological appliance that monitors, assists, performs, or prevents a physiological function but does not physically take the place of a body part

Body Part	Approach	Device	Qualifier
0 Tracheobronchial Tree	0 Open 3 Percutaneous 4 Percutaneous Endoscopic 7 Via Natural or Artificial Opening 8 Via Natural or Artificial Opening Endoscopic	1 Radioactive Element 2 Monitoring Device 3 Infusion Device D Intraluminal Device	Z No Qualifier
1 Trachea	0 Open	2 Monitoring Device D Intraluminal Device	Z No Qualifier
1 Trachea	3 Percutaneous	D Intraluminal Device E Intraluminal Device, Endotracheal Airway	Z No Qualifier
1 Trachea	4 Percutaneous Endoscopic	D Intraluminal Device	Z No Qualifier
1 Trachea	7 Via Natural or Artificial Opening 8 Via Natural or Artificial Opening Endoscopic	2 Monitoring Device D Intraluminal Device E Intraluminal Device, Endotracheal Airway	Z No Qualifier
3 Main Bronchus, Right 4 Upper Lobe Bronchus, Right 5 Middle Lobe Bronchus, Right 6 Lower Lobe Bronchus, Right 7 Main Bronchus, Left 8 Upper Lobe Bronchus, Left 9 Lingula Bronchus B Lower Lobe Bronchus, Left	0 Open 3 Percutaneous 4 Percutaneous Endoscopic 7 Via Natural or Artificial Opening 8 Via Natural or Artificial Opening Endoscopic	G Endobronchial Device	Z No Qualifier
K Lung, Right L Lung, Left	0 Open 3 Percutaneous 4 Percutaneous Endoscopic 7 Via Natural or Artificial Opening 8 Via Natural or Artificial Opening Endoscopic	1 Radioactive Element 2 Monitoring Device 3 Infusion Device	Z No Qualifier
R Diaphragm, Right S Diaphragm, Left	0 Open 3 Percutaneous 4 Percutaneous Endoscopic	2 Monitoring Device M Diaphragmatic Pacemaker Lead	Z No Qualifier

◀ New ◀ Revised ~~deleted~~ Deleted ♀ Females Only ♂ Males Only
Noncovered Limited Coverage Hospital-Acquired Condition **Coding Clinic**

SECTION: 0 MEDICAL AND SURGICAL
BODY SYSTEM: B RESPIRATORY SYSTEM
OPERATION: J INSPECTION: Visually and/or manually exploring a body part

Body Part	Approach	Device	Qualifier
0 Tracheobronchial Tree 1 Trachea K Lung, Right L Lung, Left Q Pleura T Diaphragm	0 Open 3 Percutaneous 4 Percutaneous Endoscopic 7 Via Natural or Artificial Opening 8 Via Natural or Artificial Opening Endoscopic X External	Z No Device	Z No Qualifier

SECTION: 0 MEDICAL AND SURGICAL
BODY SYSTEM: B RESPIRATORY SYSTEM
OPERATION: L OCCLUSION: Completely closing an orifice or the lumen of a tubular body part

Body Part	Approach	Device	Qualifier
1 Trachea 2 Carina 3 Main Bronchus, Right 4 Upper Lobe Bronchus, Right 5 Middle Lobe Bronchus, Right 6 Lower Lobe Bronchus, Right 7 Main Bronchus, Left 8 Upper Lobe Bronchus, Left 9 Lingula Bronchus B Lower Lobe Bronchus, Left	0 Open 3 Percutaneous 4 Percutaneous Endoscopic	C Extraluminal Device D Intraluminal Device Z No Device	Z No Qualifier
1 Trachea 2 Carina 3 Main Bronchus, Right 4 Upper Lobe Bronchus, Right 5 Middle Lobe Bronchus, Right 6 Lower Lobe Bronchus, Right 7 Main Bronchus, Left 8 Upper Lobe Bronchus, Left 9 Lingula Bronchus B Lower Lobe Bronchus, Left	7 Via Natural or Artificial Opening 8 Via Natural or Artificial Opening Endoscopic	D Intraluminal Device Z No Device	Z No Qualifier

◀ New   ◀▥ Revised   ~~deleted~~ Deleted   ♀ Females Only   ♂ Males Only
🜚 Noncovered   🜚 Limited Coverage   🜚 Hospital-Acquired Condition   **Coding Clinic**

195

SECTION: **0 MEDICAL AND SURGICAL**
BODY SYSTEM: **B RESPIRATORY SYSTEM**
OPERATION: **M REATTACHMENT:** Putting back in or on all or a portion of a separated body part to its normal location or other suitable location

Body Part	Approach	Device	Qualifier
1 Trachea 2 Carina 3 Main Bronchus, Right 4 Upper Lobe Bronchus, Right 5 Middle Lobe Bronchus, Right 6 Lower Lobe Bronchus, Right 7 Main Bronchus, Left 8 Upper Lobe Bronchus, Left 9 Lingula Bronchus B Lower Lobe Bronchus, Left C Upper Lung Lobe, Right D Middle Lung Lobe, Right F Lower Lung Lobe, Right G Upper Lung Lobe, Left H Lung Lingula J Lower Lung Lobe, Left K Lung, Right L Lung, Left R Diaphragm, Right S Diaphragm, Left	0 Open	Z No Device	Z No Qualifier

SECTION: **0 MEDICAL AND SURGICAL**
BODY SYSTEM: **B RESPIRATORY SYSTEM**
OPERATION: **N RELEASE:** Freeing a body part from an abnormal physical constraint

Body Part	Approach	Device	Qualifier
1 Trachea 2 Carina 3 Main Bronchus, Right 4 Upper Lobe Bronchus, Right 5 Middle Lobe Bronchus, Right 6 Lower Lobe Bronchus, Right 7 Main Bronchus, Left 8 Upper Lobe Bronchus, Left 9 Lingula Bronchus B Lower Lobe Bronchus, Left C Upper Lung Lobe, Right D Middle Lung Lobe, Right F Lower Lung Lobe, Right G Upper Lung Lobe, Left H Lung Lingula J Lower Lung Lobe, Left K Lung, Right L Lung, Left M Lungs, Bilateral	0 Open 3 Percutaneous 4 Percutaneous Endoscopic 7 Via Natural or Artificial Opening 8 Via Natural or Artificial Opening Endoscopic	Z No Device	Z No Qualifier
N Pleura, Right P Pleura, Left R Diaphragm, Right S Diaphragm, Left	0 Open 3 Percutaneous 4 Percutaneous Endoscopic	Z No Device	Z No Qualifier

M: REATTACHMENT   N: RELEASE

B: RESPIRATORY SYSTEM

0: M/S

◀ New ◀ Revised ~~deleted~~ Deleted ♀ Females Only ♂ Males Only
Noncovered Limited Coverage Hospital-Acquired Condition **Coding Clinic**

SECTION: 0 MEDICAL AND SURGICAL
BODY SYSTEM: B RESPIRATORY SYSTEM
OPERATION: P REMOVAL: *(on multiple pages)*
Taking out or off a device from a body part

Body Part	Approach	Device	Qualifier
0 Tracheobronchial Tree	0 Open 3 Percutaneous 4 Percutaneous Endoscopic 7 Via Natural or Artificial Opening 8 Via Natural or Artificial Opening Endoscopic	0 Drainage Device 1 Radioactive Element 2 Monitoring Device 3 Infusion Device 7 Autologous Tissue Substitute C Extraluminal Device D Intraluminal Device J Synthetic Substitute K Nonautologous Tissue Substitute	Z No Qualifier
0 Tracheobronchial Tree	X External	0 Drainage Device 1 Radioactive Element 2 Monitoring Device 3 Infusion Device D Intraluminal Device	Z No Qualifier
1 Trachea	0 Open 3 Percutaneous 4 Percutaneous Endoscopic 7 Via Natural or Artificial Opening 8 Via Natural or Artificial Opening Endoscopic	0 Drainage Device 2 Monitoring Device 7 Autologous Tissue Substitute C Extraluminal Device D Intraluminal Device F Tracheostomy Device J Synthetic Substitute K Nonautologous Tissue Substitute	Z No Qualifier
1 Trachea	X External	0 Drainage Device 2 Monitoring Device D Intraluminal Device F Tracheostomy Device	Z No Qualifier
K Lung, Right L Lung, Left	0 Open 3 Percutaneous 4 Percutaneous Endoscopic 7 Via Natural or Artificial Opening 8 Via Natural or Artificial Opening Endoscopic X External	0 Drainage Device 1 Radioactive Element 2 Monitoring Device 3 Infusion Device	Z No Qualifier
Q Pleura	0 Open 3 Percutaneous 4 Percutaneous Endoscopic 7 Via Natural or Artificial Opening 8 Via Natural or Artificial Opening Endoscopic X External	0 Drainage Device 1 Radioactive Element 2 Monitoring Device	Z No Qualifier

SECTION: 0 MEDICAL AND SURGICAL
BODY SYSTEM: B RESPIRATORY SYSTEM
OPERATION: P REMOVAL: *(continued)*
Taking out or off a device from a body part

Body Part	Approach	Device	Qualifier
T Diaphragm	0 Open 3 Percutaneous 4 Percutaneous Endoscopic 7 Via Natural or Artificial Opening 8 Via Natural or Artificial Opening Endoscopic	0 Drainage Device 2 Monitoring Device 7 Autologous Tissue Substitute J Synthetic Substitute K Nonautologous Tissue Substitute M Electrode	Z No Qualifier
T Diaphragm	X External	0 Drainage Device 2 Monitoring Device M Electrode	Z No Qualifier

SECTION: 0 MEDICAL AND SURGICAL
BODY SYSTEM: B RESPIRATORY SYSTEM
OPERATION: Q REPAIR: Restoring, to the extent possible, a body part to its normal anatomic structure and function

Body Part	Approach	Device	Qualifier
1 Trachea 2 Carina 3 Main Bronchus, Right 4 Upper Lobe Bronchus, Right 5 Middle Lobe Bronchus, Right 6 Lower Lobe Bronchus, Right 7 Main Bronchus, Left 8 Upper Lobe Bronchus, Left 9 Lingula Bronchus B Lower Lobe Bronchus, Left C Upper Lung Lobe, Right D Middle Lung Lobe, Right F Lower Lung Lobe, Right G Upper Lung Lobe, Left H Lung Lingula J Lower Lung Lobe, Left K Lung, Right L Lung, Left M Lungs, Bilateral	0 Open 3 Percutaneous 4 Percutaneous Endoscopic 7 Via Natural or Artificial Opening 8 Via Natural or Artificial Opening Endoscopic	Z No Device	Z No Qualifier
N Pleura, Right P Pleura, Left R Diaphragm, Right S Diaphragm, Left	0 Open 3 Percutaneous 4 Percutaneous Endoscopic	Z No Device	Z No Qualifier

◀ New   ◀ Revised   ~~deleted~~ Deleted   ♀ Females Only   ♂ Males Only
Noncovered   Limited Coverage   Hospital-Acquired Condition   **Coding Clinic**

P: REMOVAL   Q: REPAIR

B: RESPIRATORY SYSTEM

0: M/S

SECTION: 0 MEDICAL AND SURGICAL

BODY SYSTEM: B RESPIRATORY SYSTEM

OPERATION: S REPOSITION: Moving to its normal location, or other suitable location, all or a portion of a body part

Body Part	Approach	Device	Qualifier
1 Trachea	0 Open	Z No Device	Z No Qualifier
2 Carina			
3 Main Bronchus, Right			
4 Upper Lobe Bronchus, Right			
5 Middle Lobe Bronchus, Right			
6 Lower Lobe Bronchus, Right			
7 Main Bronchus, Left			
8 Upper Lobe Bronchus, Left			
9 Lingula Bronchus			
B Lower Lobe Bronchus, Left			
C Upper Lung Lobe, Right			
D Middle Lung Lobe, Right			
F Lower Lung Lobe, Right			
G Upper Lung Lobe, Left			
H Lung Lingula			
J Lower Lung Lobe, Left			
K Lung, Right			
L Lung, Left			
R Diaphragm, Right			
S Diaphragm, Left			

SECTION: 0 MEDICAL AND SURGICAL

BODY SYSTEM: B RESPIRATORY SYSTEM

OPERATION: T RESECTION: Cutting out or off, without replacement, all of a body part

Body Part	Approach	Device	Qualifier
1 Trachea	0 Open	Z No Device	Z No Qualifier
2 Carina	4 Percutaneous Endoscopic		
3 Main Bronchus, Right			
4 Upper Lobe Bronchus, Right			
5 Middle Lobe Bronchus, Right			
6 Lower Lobe Bronchus, Right			
7 Main Bronchus, Left			
8 Upper Lobe Bronchus, Left			
9 Lingula Bronchus			
B Lower Lobe Bronchus, Left			
C Upper Lung Lobe, Right			
D Middle Lung Lobe, Right			
F Lower Lung Lobe, Right			
G Upper Lung Lobe, Left			
H Lung Lingula			
J Lower Lung Lobe, Left			
K Lung, Right			
L Lung, Left			
M Lungs, Bilateral			
R Diaphragm, Right			
S Diaphragm, Left			

◀ New   ◀▥ Revised   ~~deleted~~ Deleted   ♀ Females Only   ♂ Males Only
🜲 Noncovered   🜲 Limited Coverage   🜲 Hospital-Acquired Condition   **Coding Clinic**

199

0: M/S   B: RESPIRATORY SYSTEM   S: REPOSITION   T: RESECTION

SECTION: 0 MEDICAL AND SURGICAL
BODY SYSTEM: B RESPIRATORY SYSTEM
OPERATION: U SUPPLEMENT: Putting in or on biological or synthetic material that physically reinforces and/or augments the function of a portion of a body part

Body Part	Approach	Device	Qualifier
1 Trachea 2 Carina 3 Main Bronchus, Right 4 Upper Lobe Bronchus, Right 5 Middle Lobe Bronchus, Right 6 Lower Lobe Bronchus, Right 7 Main Bronchus, Left 8 Upper Lobe Bronchus, Left 9 Lingula Bronchus B Lower Lobe Bronchus, Left R Diaphragm, Right S Diaphragm, Left	0 Open 4 Percutaneous Endoscopic	7 Autologous Tissue Substitute J Synthetic Substitute K Nonautologous Tissue Substitute	Z No Qualifier

SECTION: 0 MEDICAL AND SURGICAL
BODY SYSTEM: B RESPIRATORY SYSTEM
OPERATION: V RESTRICTION: Partially closing an orifice or the lumen of a tubular body part

Body Part	Approach	Device	Qualifier
1 Trachea 2 Carina 3 Main Bronchus, Right 4 Upper Lobe Bronchus, Right 5 Middle Lobe Bronchus, Right 6 Lower Lobe Bronchus, Right 7 Main Bronchus, Left 8 Upper Lobe Bronchus, Left 9 Lingula Bronchus B Lower Lobe Bronchus, Left	0 Open 3 Percutaneous 4 Percutaneous Endoscopic	C Extraluminal Device D Intraluminal Device Z No Device	Z No Qualifier
1 Trachea 2 Carina 3 Main Bronchus, Right 4 Upper Lobe Bronchus, Right 5 Middle Lobe Bronchus, Right 6 Lower Lobe Bronchus, Right 7 Main Bronchus, Left 8 Upper Lobe Bronchus, Left 9 Lingula Bronchus B Lower Lobe Bronchus, Left	7 Via Natural or Artificial Opening 8 Via Natural or Artificial Opening Endoscopic	D Intraluminal Device Z No Device	Z No Qualifier

◀ New   ◀ Revised   ~~deleted~~ Deleted   ♀ Females Only   ♂ Males Only
Noncovered   Limited Coverage   Hospital-Acquired Condition   **Coding Clinic**

(left margin) U: SUPPLEMENT   V: RESTRICTION   B: RESPIRATORY SYSTEM   0: M/S

SECTION: 0 MEDICAL AND SURGICAL
BODY SYSTEM: B RESPIRATORY SYSTEM
OPERATION: W REVISION: Correcting, to the extent possible, a portion of a malfunctioning device or the position of a displaced device

Body Part	Approach	Device	Qualifier
0 Tracheobronchial Tree	0 Open 3 Percutaneous 4 Percutaneous Endoscopic 7 Via Natural or Artificial Opening 8 Via Natural or Artificial Opening Endoscopic X External	0 Drainage Device 2 Monitoring Device 3 Infusion Device 7 Autologous Tissue Substitute C Extraluminal Device D Intraluminal Device J Synthetic Substitute K Nonautologous Tissue Substitute	Z No Qualifier
1 Trachea	0 Open 3 Percutaneous 4 Percutaneous Endoscopic 7 Via Natural or Artificial Opening 8 Via Natural or Artificial Opening Endoscopic X External	0 Drainage Device 2 Monitoring Device 7 Autologous Tissue Substitute C Extraluminal Device D Intraluminal Device F Tracheostomy Device J Synthetic Substitute K Nonautologous Tissue Substitute	Z No Qualifier
K Lung, Right L Lung, Left	0 Open 3 Percutaneous 4 Percutaneous Endoscopic 7 Via Natural or Artificial Opening 8 Via Natural or Artificial Opening Endoscopic X External	0 Drainage Device 2 Monitoring Device 3 Infusion Device	Z No Qualifier
Q Pleura	0 Open 3 Percutaneous 4 Percutaneous Endoscopic 7 Via Natural or Artificial Opening 8 Via Natural or Artificial Opening Endoscopic X External	0 Drainage Device 2 Monitoring Device	Z No Qualifier
T Diaphragm	0 Open 3 Percutaneous 4 Percutaneous Endoscopic 7 Via Natural or Artificial Opening 8 Via Natural or Artificial Opening Endoscopic X External	0 Drainage Device 2 Monitoring Device 7 Autologous Tissue Substitute J Synthetic Substitute K Nonautologous Tissue Substitute M Electrode	Z No Qualifier

◀ New   ◀▥ Revised   ~~deleted~~ Deleted   ♀ Females Only   ♂ Males Only
🚫 Noncovered   🚫 Limited Coverage   🚫 Hospital-Acquired Condition   **Coding Clinic**

Y: TRANSPLANTATION

B: RESPIRATORY SYSTEM

0: M/S

SECTION: 0 MEDICAL AND SURGICAL

BODY SYSTEM: B RESPIRATORY SYSTEM

OPERATION: Y TRANSPLANTATION: Putting in or on all or a portion of a living body part taken from another individual or animal to physically take the place and/or function of all or a portion of a similar body part

Body Part	Approach	Device	Qualifier
C Upper Lung Lobe, Right ⚕	0 Open	Z No Device	0 Allogeneic
D Middle Lung Lobe, Right ⚕			1 Syngeneic
F Lower Lung Lobe, Right ⚕			2 Zooplastic
G Upper Lung Lobe, Left ⚕			
H Lung Lingula ⚕			
J Lower Lung Lobe, Left ⚕			
K Lung, Right ⚕			
L Lung, Left ⚕			
M Lungs, Bilateral ⚕			

◀ New ◀▦ Revised ~~deleted~~ Deleted ♀ Females Only ♂ Males Only
⚕ Noncovered ⚕ Limited Coverage ⚕ Hospital-Acquired Condition **Coding Clinic**

SECTION: 0 MEDICAL AND SURGICAL

BODY SYSTEM: C MOUTH AND THROAT

OPERATION: 0 **ALTERATION:** Modifying the anatomic structure of a body part without affecting the function of the body part

Body Part	Approach	Device	Qualifier
0 Upper Lip 1 Lower Lip	X External	7 Autologous Tissue Substitute J Synthetic Substitute K Nonautologous Tissue Substitute Z No Device	Z No Qualifier

SECTION: 0 MEDICAL AND SURGICAL

BODY SYSTEM: C MOUTH AND THROAT

OPERATION: 2 **CHANGE:** Taking out or off a device from a body part and putting back an identical or similar device in or on the same body part without cutting or puncturing the skin or a mucous membrane

Body Part	Approach	Device	Qualifier
A Salivary Gland S Larynx Y Mouth and Throat	X External	0 Drainage Device Y Other Device	Z No Qualifier

0: ALTERATION   2: CHANGE

C: MOUTH AND THROAT

0: M/S

◀ New   ◀▥ Revised   ~~deleted~~ Deleted   ♀ Females Only   ♂ Males Only
🔖 Noncovered   🔖 Limited Coverage   🔖 Hospital-Acquired Condition   **Coding Clinic**

SECTION: 0 MEDICAL AND SURGICAL

BODY SYSTEM: C MOUTH AND THROAT

OPERATION: 5 DESTRUCTION: Physical eradication of all or a portion of a body part by the use of direct energy, force, or a destructive agent

Body Part	Approach	Device	Qualifier
0 Upper Lip 1 Lower Lip 2 Hard Palate 3 Soft Palate 4 Buccal Mucosa 5 Upper Gingiva 6 Lower Gingiva 7 Tongue N Uvula P Tonsils Q Adenoids	0 Open 3 Percutaneous X External	Z No Device	Z No Qualifier
8 Parotid Gland, Right 9 Parotid Gland, Left B Parotid Duct, Right C Parotid Duct, Left D Sublingual Gland, Right F Sublingual Gland, Left G Submaxillary Gland, Right H Submaxillary Gland, Left J Minor Salivary Gland	0 Open 3 Percutaneous	Z No Device	Z No Qualifier
M Pharynx R Epiglottis S Larynx T Vocal Cord, Right V Vocal Cord, Left	0 Open 3 Percutaneous 4 Percutaneous Endoscopic 7 Via Natural or Artificial Opening 8 Via Natural or Artificial Opening Endoscopic	Z No Device	Z No Qualifier
W Upper Tooth X Lower Tooth	0 Open X External	Z No Device	0 Single 1 Multiple 2 All

SECTION: 0 MEDICAL AND SURGICAL

BODY SYSTEM: C MOUTH AND THROAT

OPERATION: 7 DILATION: Expanding an orifice or the lumen of a tubular body part

Body Part	Approach	Device	Qualifier
B Parotid Duct, Right C Parotid Duct, Left	0 Open 3 Percutaneous 7 Via Natural or Artificial Opening	D Intraluminal Device Z No Device	Z No Qualifier
M Pharynx	7 Via Natural or Artificial Opening 8 Via Natural or Artificial Opening Endoscopic	D Intraluminal Device Z No Device	Z No Qualifier
S Larynx	0 Open 3 Percutaneous 4 Percutaneous Endoscopic 7 Via Natural or Artificial Opening 8 Via Natural or Artificial Opening Endoscopic	D Intraluminal Device Z No Device	Z No Qualifier

◀ New   ◀ Revised   ~~deleted~~ Deleted   ♀ Females Only   ♂ Males Only

🚫 Noncovered   🚫 Limited Coverage   🚫 Hospital-Acquired Condition   **Coding Clinic**

SECTION: 0 MEDICAL AND SURGICAL
BODY SYSTEM: C MOUTH AND THROAT
OPERATION: 9 DRAINAGE: *(on multiple pages)*
Taking or letting out fluids and/or gases from a body part

Body Part	Approach	Device	Qualifier
0 Upper Lip 1 Lower Lip 2 Hard Palate 3 Soft Palate 4 Buccal Mucosa 5 Upper Gingiva 6 Lower Gingiva 7 Tongue N Uvula P Tonsils Q Adenoids	0 Open 3 Percutaneous X External	0 Drainage Device	Z No Qualifier
0 Upper Lip 1 Lower Lip 2 Hard Palate 3 Soft Palate 4 Buccal Mucosa 5 Upper Gingiva 6 Lower Gingiva 7 Tongue N Uvula P Tonsils Q Adenoids	0 Open 3 Percutaneous X External	Z No Device	X Diagnostic Z No Qualifier
8 Parotid Gland, Right 9 Parotid Gland, Left B Parotid Duct, Right C Parotid Duct, Left D Sublingual Gland, Right F Sublingual Gland, Left G Submaxillary Gland, Right H Submaxillary Gland, Left J Minor Salivary Gland	0 Open 3 Percutaneous	0 Drainage Device	Z No Qualifier
8 Parotid Gland, Right 9 Parotid Gland, Left B Parotid Duct, Right C Parotid Duct, Left D Sublingual Gland, Right F Sublingual Gland, Left G Submaxillary Gland, Right H Submaxillary Gland, Left J Minor Salivary Gland	0 Open 3 Percutaneous	Z No Device	X Diagnostic Z No Qualifier
M Pharynx R Epiglottis S Larynx T Vocal Cord, Right V Vocal Cord, Left	0 Open 3 Percutaneous 4 Percutaneous Endoscopic 7 Via Natural or Artificial Opening 8 Via Natural or Artificial Opening Endoscopic	0 Drainage Device	Z No Qualifier

Left margin: 9: DRAINAGE   C: MOUTH AND THROAT   0: M/S

 New 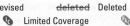 Revised ~~deleted~~ Deleted ♀ Females Only ♂ Males Only
Noncovered Limited Coverage Hospital-Acquired Condition **Coding Clinic**

SECTION: 0 MEDICAL AND SURGICAL
BODY SYSTEM: C MOUTH AND THROAT
OPERATION: 9 DRAINAGE: *(continued)*
Taking or letting out fluids and/or gases from a body part

Body Part	Approach	Device	Qualifier
M Pharynx R Epiglottis S Larynx T Vocal Cord, Right V Vocal Cord, Left	0 Open 3 Percutaneous 4 Percutaneous Endoscopic 7 Via Natural or Artificial Opening 8 Via Natural or Artificial Opening Endoscopic	Z No Device	X Diagnostic Z No Qualifier
W Upper Tooth X Lower Tooth	0 Open X External	0 Drainage Device Z No Device	0 Single 1 Multiple 2 All

SECTION: 0 MEDICAL AND SURGICAL
BODY SYSTEM: C MOUTH AND THROAT
OPERATION: B EXCISION: Cutting out or off, without replacement, a portion of a body part

Body Part	Approach	Device	Qualifier
0 Upper Lip 1 Lower Lip 2 Hard Palate 3 Soft Palate 4 Buccal Mucosa 5 Upper Gingiva 6 Lower Gingiva 7 Tongue N Uvula P Tonsils Q Adenoids	0 Open 3 Percutaneous X External	Z No Device	X Diagnostic Z No Qualifier
8 Parotid Gland, Right 9 Parotid Gland, Left B Parotid Duct, Right C Parotid Duct, Left D Sublingual Gland, Right F Sublingual Gland, Left G Submaxillary Gland, Right H Submaxillary Gland, Left J Minor Salivary Gland	0 Open 3 Percutaneous	Z No Device	X Diagnostic Z No Qualifier
M Pharynx R Epiglottis S Larynx T Vocal Cord, Right V Vocal Cord, Left	0 Open 3 Percutaneous 4 Percutaneous Endoscopic 7 Via Natural or Artificial Opening 8 Via Natural or Artificial Opening Endoscopic	Z No Device	X Diagnostic Z No Qualifier
W Upper Tooth X Lower Tooth	0 Open X External	Z No Device	0 Single 1 Multiple 2 All

0: M/S

C: MOUTH AND THROAT

9: DRAINAGE   B: EXCISION

SECTION: **0 MEDICAL AND SURGICAL**

BODY SYSTEM: C MOUTH AND THROAT

OPERATION: C **EXTIRPATION:** Taking or cutting out solid matter from a body part

Body Part	Approach	Device	Qualifier
0 Upper Lip 1 Lower Lip 2 Hard Palate 3 Soft Palate 4 Buccal Mucosa 5 Upper Gingiva 6 Lower Gingiva 7 Tongue N Uvula P Tonsils Q Adenoids	0 Open 3 Percutaneous X External	Z No Device	Z No Qualifier
8 Parotid Gland, Right 9 Parotid Gland, Left B Parotid Duct, Right C Parotid Duct, Left D Sublingual Gland, Right F Sublingual Gland, Left G Submaxillary Gland, Right H Submaxillary Gland, Left J Minor Salivary Gland	0 Open 3 Percutaneous	Z No Device	Z No Qualifier
M Pharynx R Epiglottis S Larynx T Vocal Cord, Right V Vocal Cord, Left	0 Open 3 Percutaneous 4 Percutaneous Endoscopic 7 Via Natural or Artificial Opening 8 Via Natural or Artificial Opening Endoscopic	Z No Device	Z No Qualifier
W Upper Tooth X Lower Tooth	0 Open X External	Z No Device	0 Single 1 Multiple 2 All

SECTION: **0 MEDICAL AND SURGICAL**

BODY SYSTEM: C MOUTH AND THROAT

OPERATION: D **EXTRACTION:** Pulling or stripping out or off all or a portion of a body part by the use of force

Body Part	Approach	Device	Qualifier
T Vocal Cord, Right V Vocal Cord, Left	0 Open 3 Percutaneous 4 Percutaneous Endoscopic 7 Via Natural or Artificial Opening 8 Via Natural or Artificial Opening Endoscopic	Z No Device	Z No Qualifier
W Upper Tooth X Lower Tooth	X External	Z No Device	0 Single 1 Multiple 2 All

C: EXTIRPATION   D: EXTRACTION

C: MOUTH AND THROAT

0: M/S

◄ New　◄ⅢⅢ Revised　deleted Deleted　♀ Females Only　♂ Males Only
Ⓝ Noncovered　Ⓛ Limited Coverage　Ⓗ Hospital-Acquired Condition　**Coding Clinic**

SECTION: 0 MEDICAL AND SURGICAL
BODY SYSTEM: C MOUTH AND THROAT
OPERATION: F FRAGMENTATION: Breaking solid matter in a body part into pieces

Body Part	Approach	Device	Qualifier
B Parotid Duct, Right 🐾 C Parotid Duct, Left 🐾	0 Open 3 Percutaneous 7 Via Natural or Artificial Opening X External	Z No Device	Z No Qualifier

🐾 0CFBXZZ, 0CFCXZZ

SECTION: 0 MEDICAL AND SURGICAL
BODY SYSTEM: C MOUTH AND THROAT
OPERATION: H INSERTION: Putting in a nonbiological appliance that monitors, assists, performs, or prevents a physiological function but does not physically take the place of a body part

Body Part	Approach	Device	Qualifier
7 Tongue	0 Open 3 Percutaneous X External	1 Radioactive Element	Z No Qualifier
Y Mouth and Throat	7 Via Natural or Artificial Opening 8 Via Natural or Artificial Opening Endoscopic	B Intraluminal Device, Airway	Z No Qualifier

SECTION: 0 MEDICAL AND SURGICAL
BODY SYSTEM: C MOUTH AND THROAT
OPERATION: J INSPECTION: Visually and/or manually exploring a body part

Body Part	Approach	Device	Qualifier
A Salivary Gland	0 Open 3 Percutaneous X External	Z No Device	Z No Qualifier
S Larynx Y Mouth and Throat	0 Open 3 Percutaneous 4 Percutaneous Endoscopic 7 Via Natural or Artificial Opening 8 Via Natural or Artificial Opening Endoscopic X External	Z No Device	Z No Qualifier

◀ New   ◀▦ Revised   ~~deleted~~ Deleted   ♀ Females Only   ♂ Males Only
🐾 Noncovered   🐾 Limited Coverage   🐾 Hospital-Acquired Condition   **Coding Clinic**

209

SECTION: 0 MEDICAL AND SURGICAL
BODY SYSTEM: C MOUTH AND THROAT
OPERATION: L OCCLUSION: Completely closing an orifice or the lumen of a tubular body part

Body Part	Approach	Device	Qualifier
B Parotid Duct, Right C Parotid Duct, Left	0 Open 3 Percutaneous 4 Percutaneous Endoscopic	C Extraluminal Device D Intraluminal Device Z No Device	Z No Qualifier
B Parotid Duct, Right C Parotid Duct, Left	7 Via Natural or Artificial Opening 8 Via Natural or Artificial Opening Endoscopic	D Intraluminal Device Z No Device	Z No Qualifier

SECTION: 0 MEDICAL AND SURGICAL
BODY SYSTEM: C MOUTH AND THROAT
OPERATION: M REATTACHMENT: Putting back in or on all or a portion of a separated body part to its normal location or other suitable location

Body Part	Approach	Device	Qualifier
0 Upper Lip 1 Lower Lip 3 Soft Palate 7 Tongue N Uvula	0 Open	Z No Device	Z No Qualifier
W Upper Tooth X Lower Tooth	0 Open X External	Z No Device	0 Single 1 Multiple 2 All

Vertical side text: L: OCCLUSION   M: REATTACHMENT   C: MOUTH AND THROAT   0: M/S

SECTION: 0 MEDICAL AND SURGICAL
BODY SYSTEM: C MOUTH AND THROAT
OPERATION: N RELEASE: Freeing a body part from an abnormal physical constraint by cutting or by the use of force

Body Part	Approach	Device	Qualifier
0 Upper Lip 1 Lower Lip 2 Hard Palate 3 Soft Palate 4 Buccal Mucosa 5 Upper Gingiva 6 Lower Gingiva 7 Tongue N Uvula P Tonsils Q Adenoids	0 Open 3 Percutaneous X External	Z No Device	Z No Qualifier
8 Parotid Gland, Right 9 Parotid Gland, Left B Parotid Duct, Right C Parotid Duct, Left D Sublingual Gland, Right F Sublingual Gland, Left G Submaxillary Gland, Right H Submaxillary Gland, Left J Minor Salivary Gland	0 Open 3 Percutaneous	Z No Device	Z No Qualifier
M Pharynx R Epiglottis S Larynx T Vocal Cord, Right V Vocal Cord, Left	0 Open 3 Percutaneous 4 Percutaneous Endoscopic 7 Via Natural or Artificial Opening 8 Via Natural or Artificial Opening Endoscopic	Z No Device	Z No Qualifier
W Upper Tooth X Lower Tooth	0 Open X External	Z No Device	0 Single 1 Multiple 2 All

SECTION: 0 MEDICAL AND SURGICAL
BODY SYSTEM: C MOUTH AND THROAT
OPERATION: P REMOVAL: Taking out or off a device from a body part

Body Part	Approach	Device	Qualifier
A Salivary Gland	0 Open 3 Percutaneous	0 Drainage Device C Extraluminal Device	Z No Qualifier
S Larynx	0 Open 3 Percutaneous 7 Via Natural or Artificial Opening 8 Via Natural or Artificial Opening Endoscopic X External	0 Drainage Device 7 Autologous Tissue Substitute D Intraluminal Device J Synthetic Substitute K Nonautologous Tissue Substitute	Z No Qualifier
Y Mouth and Throat	0 Open 3 Percutaneous 7 Via Natural or Artificial Opening 8 Via Natural or Artificial Opening Endoscopic X External	0 Drainage Device 1 Radioactive Element 7 Autologous Tissue Substitute D Intraluminal Device J Synthetic Substitute K Nonautologous Tissue Substitute	Z No Qualifier

P: REMOVAL

C: MOUTH AND THROAT

0: M/S

◄ New   ◄ Revised   deleted Deleted   ♀ Females Only   ♂ Males Only
Noncovered   Limited Coverage   Hospital-Acquired Condition   **Coding Clinic**

SECTION: 0 MEDICAL AND SURGICAL

BODY SYSTEM: C MOUTH AND THROAT

OPERATION: Q REPAIR: Restoring, to the extent possible, a body part to its normal anatomic structure and function

Body Part	Approach	Device	Qualifier
0 Upper Lip 1 Lower Lip 2 Hard Palate 3 Soft Palate 4 Buccal Mucosa 5 Upper Gingiva 6 Lower Gingiva 7 Tongue N Uvula P Tonsils Q Adenoids	0 Open 3 Percutaneous X External	Z No Device	Z No Qualifier
8 Parotid Gland, Right 9 Parotid Gland, Left B Parotid Duct, Right C Parotid Duct, Left D Sublingual Gland, Right F Sublingual Gland, Left G Submaxillary Gland, Right H Submaxillary Gland, Left J Minor Salivary Gland	0 Open 3 Percutaneous	Z No Device	Z No Qualifier
M Pharynx R Epiglottis S Larynx T Vocal Cord, Right V Vocal Cord, Left	0 Open 3 Percutaneous 4 Percutaneous Endoscopic 7 Via Natural or Artificial Opening 8 Via Natural or Artificial Opening Endoscopic	Z No Device	Z No Qualifier
W Upper Tooth X Lower Tooth	0 Open X External	Z No Device	0 Single 1 Multiple 2 All

0: M/S

C: MOUTH AND THROAT

Q: REPAIR

◄ New ◄⠂⠂ Revised ~~deleted~~ Deleted ♀ Females Only ♂ Males Only
🚫 Noncovered 🚫 Limited Coverage 🚫 Hospital-Acquired Condition **Coding Clinic**

SECTION: 0 MEDICAL AND SURGICAL
BODY SYSTEM: C MOUTH AND THROAT
OPERATION: R REPLACEMENT: Putting in or on biological or synthetic material that physically takes the place and/or function of all or a portion of a body part

Body Part	Approach	Device	Qualifier
0 Upper Lip 1 Lower Lip 2 Hard Palate 3 Soft Palate 4 Buccal Mucosa 5 Upper Gingiva 6 Lower Gingiva 7 Tongue N Uvula	0 Open 3 Percutaneous X External	7 Autologous Tissue Substitute J Synthetic Substitute K Nonautologous Tissue Substitute	Z No Qualifier
B Parotid Duct, Right C Parotid Duct, Left	0 Open 3 Percutaneous	7 Autologous Tissue Substitute J Synthetic Substitute K Nonautologous Tissue Substitute	Z No Qualifier
M Pharynx R Epiglottis S Larynx T Vocal Cord, Right V Vocal Cord, Left	0 Open 7 Via Natural or Artificial Opening 8 Via Natural or Artificial Opening Endoscopic	7 Autologous Tissue Substitute J Synthetic Substitute K Nonautologous Tissue Substitute	Z No Qualifier
W Upper Tooth X Lower Tooth	0 Open X External	7 Autologous Tissue Substitute J Synthetic Substitute K Nonautologous Tissue Substitute	0 Single 1 Multiple 2 All

SECTION: 0 MEDICAL AND SURGICAL
BODY SYSTEM: C MOUTH AND THROAT
OPERATION: S REPOSITION: Moving to its normal location, or other suitable location, all or a portion of a body part

Body Part	Approach	Device	Qualifier
0 Upper Lip 1 Lower Lip 2 Hard Palate 3 Soft Palate 7 Tongue N Uvula	0 Open X External	Z No Device	Z No Qualifier
B Parotid Duct, Right C Parotid Duct, Left	0 Open 3 Percutaneous	Z No Device	Z No Qualifier
R Epiglottis T Vocal Cord, Right V Vocal Cord, Left	0 Open 7 Via Natural or Artificial Opening 8 Via Natural or Artificial Opening Endoscopic	Z No Device	Z No Qualifier
W Upper Tooth X Lower Tooth	0 Open X External	5 External Fixation Device Z No Device	0 Single 1 Multiple 2 All

◄ New   ◄ Revised   ~~deleted~~ Deleted   ♀ Females Only   ♂ Males Only
Noncovered   Limited Coverage   Hospital-Acquired Condition   **Coding Clinic**

SECTION: 0 MEDICAL AND SURGICAL

BODY SYSTEM: C MOUTH AND THROAT

OPERATION: T RESECTION: Cutting out or off, without replacement, all of a body part

Body Part	Approach	Device	Qualifier
0 Upper Lip 1 Lower Lip 2 Hard Palate 3 Soft Palate 7 Tongue N Uvula P Tonsils Q Adenoids	0 Open X External	Z No Device	Z No Qualifier
8 Parotid Gland, Right 9 Parotid Gland, Left B Parotid Duct, Right C Parotid Duct, Left D Sublingual Gland, Right F Sublingual Gland, Left G Submaxillary Gland, Right H Submaxillary Gland, Left J Minor Salivary Gland	0 Open	Z No Device	Z No Qualifier
M Pharynx R Epiglottis S Larynx T Vocal Cord, Right V Vocal Cord, Left	0 Open 4 Percutaneous Endoscopic 7 Via Natural or Artificial Opening 8 Via Natural or Artificial Opening Endoscopic	Z No Device	Z No Qualifier
W Upper Tooth X Lower Tooth	0 Open	Z No Device	0 Single 1 Multiple 2 All

SECTION: 0 MEDICAL AND SURGICAL

BODY SYSTEM: C MOUTH AND THROAT

OPERATION: U SUPPLEMENT: Putting in or on biological or synthetic material that physically reinforces and/or augments the function of a portion of a body part

Body Part	Approach	Device	Qualifier
0 Upper Lip 1 Lower Lip 2 Hard Palate 3 Soft Palate 4 Buccal Mucosa 5 Upper Gingiva 6 Lower Gingiva 7 Tongue N Uvula	0 Open 3 Percutaneous X External	7 Autologous Tissue Substitute J Synthetic Substitute K Nonautologous Tissue Substitute	Z No Qualifier
M Pharynx R Epiglottis S Larynx T Vocal Cord, Right V Vocal Cord, Left	0 Open 7 Via Natural or Artificial Opening 8 Via Natural or Artificial Opening Endoscopic	7 Autologous Tissue Substitute J Synthetic Substitute K Nonautologous Tissue Substitute	Z No Qualifier

0: M/S C: MOUTH AND THROAT T: RESECTION U: SUPPLEMENT

◀ New   ◀ Revised   deleted Deleted   ♀ Females Only   ♂ Males Only
🚫 Noncovered   🚫 Limited Coverage   🚫 Hospital-Acquired Condition   **Coding Clinic**

SECTION: 0 MEDICAL AND SURGICAL
BODY SYSTEM: C MOUTH AND THROAT
OPERATION: V **RESTRICTION:** Partially closing an orifice or the lumen of a tubular body part

Body Part	Approach	Device	Qualifier
B Parotid Duct, Right C Parotid Duct, Left	0 Open 3 Percutaneous	C Extraluminal Device D Intraluminal Device Z No Device	Z No Qualifier
B Parotid Duct, Right C Parotid Duct, Left	7 Via Natural or Artificial Opening 8 Via Natural or Artificial Opening Endoscopic	D Intraluminal Device Z No Device	Z No Qualifier

SECTION: 0 MEDICAL AND SURGICAL
BODY SYSTEM: C MOUTH AND THROAT
OPERATION: W **REVISION:** Correcting, to the extent possible, a portion of a malfunctioning device or the position of a displaced device

Body Part	Approach	Device	Qualifier
A Salivary Gland	0 Open 3 Percutaneous X External	0 Drainage Device C Extraluminal Device	Z No Qualifier
S Larynx	0 Open 3 Percutaneous 7 Via Natural or Artificial Opening 8 Via Natural or Artificial Opening Endoscopic X External	0 Drainage Device 7 Autologous Tissue Substitute D Intraluminal Device J Synthetic Substitute K Nonautologous Tissue Substitute	Z No Qualifier
Y Mouth and Throat	0 Open 3 Percutaneous 7 Via Natural or Artificial Opening 8 Via Natural or Artificial Opening Endoscopic X External	0 Drainage Device 1 Radioactive Element 7 Autologous Tissue Substitute D Intraluminal Device J Synthetic Substitute K Nonautologous Tissue Substitute	Z No Qualifier

◀ New　◀ Revised　deleted Deleted　♀ Females Only　♂ Males Only
Noncovered　Limited Coverage　Hospital-Acquired Condition　**Coding Clinic**

SECTION: 0 MEDICAL AND SURGICAL
BODY SYSTEM: C MOUTH AND THROAT
OPERATION: X TRANSFER: Moving, without taking out, all or a portion of a body part to another location to take over the function of all or a portion of a body part

Body Part	Approach	Device	Qualifier
0 Upper Lip 1 Lower Lip 3 Soft Palate 4 Buccal Mucosa 5 Upper Gingiva 6 Lower Gingiva 7 Tongue	0 Open X External	Z No Device	Z No Qualifier

◀ New ◀▥ Revised ~~deleted~~ Deleted ♀ Females Only ♂ Males Only
🅝 Noncovered 🅛 Limited Coverage 🅗 Hospital-Acquired Condition **Coding Clinic**

SECTION: 0 MEDICAL AND SURGICAL
BODY SYSTEM: D GASTROINTESTINAL SYSTEM
OPERATION: 1 BYPASS: *(on multiple pages)*
        Altering the route of passage of the contents of a tubular body part

Body Part	Approach	Device	Qualifier

1 Esophagus, Upper
2 Esophagus, Middle
3 Esophagus, Lower
5 Esophagus
	0 Open
	4 Percutaneous Endoscopic
	8 Via Natural or Artificial
	    Opening Endoscopic
		7 Autologous Tissue Substitute
		J Synthetic Substitute
		K Nonautologous Tissue
		    Substitute
		Z No Device
			4 Cutaneous
			6 Stomach
			9 Duodenum
			A Jejunum
			B Ileum

1 Esophagus, Upper 2 Esophagus, Middle 3 Esophagus, Lower 5 Esophagus	3 Percutaneous	J Synthetic Substitute	4 Cutaneous

6 Stomach 🚫
9 Duodenum
	0 Open
	4 Percutaneous Endoscopic
	8 Via Natural or Artificial
	    Opening Endoscopic
		7 Autologous Tissue Substitute
		J Synthetic Substitute
		K Nonautologous Tissue
		    Substitute
		Z No Device
			4 Cutaneous
			9 Duodenum
			A Jejunum
			B Ileum
			L Transverse Colon

6 Stomach 9 Duodenum	3 Percutaneous	J Synthetic Substitute	4 Cutaneous

A Jejunum	0 Open
	4 Percutaneous Endoscopic
	8 Via Natural or Artificial
	    Opening Endoscopic
		7 Autologous Tissue Substitute
		J Synthetic Substitute
		K Nonautologous Tissue
		    Substitute
		Z No Device
			4 Cutaneous
			A Jejunum
			B Ileum
			H Cecum
			K Ascending Colon
			L Transverse Colon
			M Descending Colon
			N Sigmoid Colon
			P Rectum
			Q Anus

A Jejunum	3 Percutaneous	J Synthetic Substitute	4 Cutaneous

B Ileum	0 Open
	4 Percutaneous Endoscopic
	8 Via Natural or Artificial
	    Opening Endoscopic
		7 Autologous Tissue Substitute
		J Synthetic Substitute
		K Nonautologous Tissue
		    Substitute
		Z No Device
			4 Cutaneous
			B Ileum
			H Cecum
			K Ascending Colon
			L Transverse Colon
			M Descending Colon
			N Sigmoid Colon
			P Rectum
			Q Anus

B Ileum	3 Percutaneous	J Synthetic Substitute	4 Cutaneous

H Cecum	0 Open
	4 Percutaneous Endoscopic
	8 Via Natural or Artificial
	    Opening Endoscopic
		7 Autologous Tissue Substitute
		J Synthetic Substitute
		K Nonautologous Tissue
		    Substitute
		Z No Device
			4 Cutaneous
			H Cecum
			K Ascending Colon
			L Transverse Colon
			M Descending Colon
			N Sigmoid Colon
			P Rectum

H Cecum	3 Percutaneous	J Synthetic Substitute	4 Cutaneous

0: M/S

D: GASTROINTESTINAL SYSTEM

1: BYPASS

◀ New   ◀▦ Revised   ~~deleted~~ Deleted   ♀ Females Only   ♂ Males Only
🚫 Noncovered   🚫 Limited Coverage   🚫 Hospital-Acquired Condition   **Coding Clinic**

SECTION: 0 MEDICAL AND SURGICAL

BODY SYSTEM: D GASTROINTESTINAL SYSTEM
OPERATION: 1 BYPASS: *(continued)*
Altering the route of passage of the contents of a tubular body part

Body Part	Approach	Device	Qualifier
K Ascending Colon	0 Open 4 Percutaneous Endoscopic 8 Via Natural or Artificial Opening Endoscopic	7 Autologous Tissue Substitute J Synthetic Substitute K Nonautologous Tissue Substitute Z No Device	4 Cutaneous K Ascending Colon L Transverse Colon M Descending Colon N Sigmoid Colon P Rectum
K Ascending Colon	3 Percutaneous	J Synthetic Substitute	4 Cutaneous
L Transverse Colon	0 Open 4 Percutaneous Endoscopic 8 Via Natural or Artificial Opening Endoscopic	7 Autologous Tissue Substitute J Synthetic Substitute K Nonautologous Tissue Substitute Z No Device	4 Cutaneous L Transverse Colon M Descending Colon N Sigmoid Colon P Rectum
L Transverse Colon	3 Percutaneous	J Synthetic Substitute	4 Cutaneous
M Descending Colon	0 Open 4 Percutaneous Endoscopic 8 Via Natural or Artificial Opening Endoscopic	7 Autologous Tissue Substitute J Synthetic Substitute K Nonautologous Tissue Substitute Z No Device	4 Cutaneous M Descending Colon N Sigmoid Colon P Rectum
M Descending Colon	3 Percutaneous	J Synthetic Substitute	4 Cutaneous
N Sigmoid Colon	0 Open 4 Percutaneous Endoscopic 8 Via Natural or Artificial Opening Endoscopic	7 Autologous Tissue Substitute J Synthetic Substitute K Nonautologous Tissue Substitute Z No Device	4 Cutaneous N Sigmoid Colon P Rectum
N Sigmoid Colon	3 Percutaneous	J Synthetic Substitute	4 Cutaneous

- 0D16079, 0D1607A, 0D1607B, 0D1607L
- 0D160J9, 0D160JA, 0D160JB, 0D160JL
- 0D160K9, 0D160KA, 0D160KB, 0D160KL
- 0D160Z9, 0D160ZA, 0D160ZB, 0D160ZL
- 0D16479, 0D1647A, 0D1647B, 0D1647L
- 0D164J9, 0D164JA, 0D164JB, 0D164JL

- 0D164K9, 0D164KA, 0D164KB, 0D164KL
- 0D164Z9, 0D164ZA, 0D164ZB, 0D164ZL
- 0D16879, 0D1687A, 0D1687B, 0D1687L
- 0D168J9, 0D168JA, 0D168JB, 0D168JL
- 0D168K9, 0D168KA, 0D168KB, 0D168KL
- 0D168Z9, 0D168ZA, 0D168ZB, 0D168ZL

SECTION: 0 MEDICAL AND SURGICAL

BODY SYSTEM: D GASTROINTESTINAL SYSTEM
OPERATION: 2 CHANGE: Taking out or off a device from a body part and putting back an identical or similar device in or on the same body part without cutting or puncturing the skin or a mucous membrane

Body Part	Approach	Device	Qualifier
0 Upper Intestinal Tract D Lower Intestinal Tract	X External	0 Drainage Device U Feeding Device Y Other Device	Z No Qualifier
U Omentum V Mesentery W Peritoneum	X External	0 Drainage Device Y Other Device	Z No Qualifier

◀ New　　◀▥ Revised　　deleted Deleted　　♀ Females Only　　♂ Males Only
Noncovered　　Limited Coverage　　Hospital-Acquired Condition　　**Coding Clinic**

SECTION: 0 MEDICAL AND SURGICAL
BODY SYSTEM: D GASTROINTESTINAL SYSTEM
OPERATION: 5 **DESTRUCTION:** Physical eradication of all or a portion of a body part by the direct use of energy, force, or a destructive agent

Body Part	Approach	Device	Qualifier
1 Esophagus, Upper 2 Esophagus, Middle 3 Esophagus, Lower 4 Esophagogastric Junction 5 Esophagus 6 Stomach 7 Stomach, Pylorus 8 Small Intestine 9 Duodenum A Jejunum B Ileum C Ileocecal Valve E Large Intestine F Large Intestine, Right G Large Intestine, Left H Cecum J Appendix K Ascending Colon L Transverse Colon M Descending Colon N Sigmoid Colon P Rectum	0 Open 3 Percutaneous 4 Percutaneous Endoscopic 7 Via Natural or Artificial Opening 8 Via Natural or Artificial Opening Endoscopic	Z No Device	Z No Qualifier
Q Anus	0 Open 3 Percutaneous 4 Percutaneous Endoscopic 7 Via Natural or Artificial Opening 8 Via Natural or Artificial Opening Endoscopic X External	Z No Device	Z No Qualifier
R Anal Sphincter S Greater Omentum T Lesser Omentum V Mesentery W Peritoneum	0 Open 3 Percutaneous 4 Percutaneous Endoscopic	Z No Device	Z No Qualifier

◄ New   ◄ Revised   deleted Deleted   ♀ Females Only   ♂ Males Only
⊘ Noncovered   ⊘ Limited Coverage   ⊘ Hospital-Acquired Condition   **Coding Clinic**

SECTION: 0 MEDICAL AND SURGICAL
BODY SYSTEM: D GASTROINTESTINAL SYSTEM
OPERATION: 7 DILATION: Expanding an orifice or the lumen of a tubular body part

Body Part	Approach	Device	Qualifier
1 Esophagus, Upper 2 Esophagus, Middle 3 Esophagus, Lower 4 Esophagogastric Junction 5 Esophagus 6 Stomach 7 Stomach, Pylorus 8 Small Intestine 9 Duodenum A Jejunum B Ileum C Ileocecal Valve E Large Intestine F Large Intestine, Right G Large Intestine, Left H Cecum K Ascending Colon L Transverse Colon M Descending Colon N Sigmoid Colon P Rectum Q Anus	0 Open 3 Percutaneous 4 Percutaneous Endoscopic 7 Via Natural or Artificial Opening 8 Via Natural or Artificial Opening Endoscopic	D Intraluminal Device Z No Device	Z No Qualifier

SECTION: 0 MEDICAL AND SURGICAL
BODY SYSTEM: D GASTROINTESTINAL SYSTEM
OPERATION: 8 DIVISION: Cutting into a body part, without draining fluids and/or gases from the body part, in order to separate or transect a body part

Body Part	Approach	Device	Qualifier
4 Esophagogastric Junction 7 Stomach, Pylorus	0 Open 3 Percutaneous 4 Percutaneous Endoscopic 7 Via Natural or Artificial Opening 8 Via Natural or Artificial Opening Endoscopic	Z No Device	Z No Qualifier
R Anal Sphincter	0 Open 3 Percutaneous	Z No Device	Z No Qualifier

◀ New ◀ Revised ~~deleted~~ Deleted ♀ Females Only ♂ Males Only
℞ Noncovered ℞ Limited Coverage ℞ Hospital-Acquired Condition **Coding Clinic**

SECTION: 0 MEDICAL AND SURGICAL
BODY SYSTEM: D GASTROINTESTINAL SYSTEM
OPERATION: 9 DRAINAGE: *(on multiple pages)*
Taking or letting out fluids and/or gases from a body part

Body Part	Approach	Device	Qualifier
1 Esophagus, Upper 2 Esophagus, Middle 3 Esophagus, Lower 4 Esophagogastric Junction 5 Esophagus 6 Stomach 7 Stomach, Pylorus 8 Small Intestine 9 Duodenum A Jejunum B Ileum C Ileocecal Valve E Large Intestine F Large Intestine, Right G Large Intestine, Left H Cecum J Appendix K Ascending Colon L Transverse Colon M Descending Colon N Sigmoid Colon P Rectum	0 Open 3 Percutaneous 4 Percutaneous Endoscopic 7 Via Natural or Artificial Opening 8 Via Natural or Artificial Opening Endoscopic	0 Drainage Device	Z No Qualifier
1 Esophagus, Upper 2 Esophagus, Middle 3 Esophagus, Lower 4 Esophagogastric Junction 5 Esophagus 6 Stomach 7 Stomach, Pylorus 8 Small Intestine 9 Duodenum A Jejunum B Ileum C Ileocecal Valve E Large Intestine F Large Intestine, Right G Large Intestine, Left H Cecum J Appendix K Ascending Colon L Transverse Colon M Descending Colon N Sigmoid Colon P Rectum	0 Open 3 Percutaneous 4 Percutaneous Endoscopic 7 Via Natural or Artificial Opening 8 Via Natural or Artificial Opening Endoscopic	Z No Device	X Diagnostic Z No Qualifier
Q Anus	0 Open 3 Percutaneous 4 Percutaneous Endoscopic 7 Via Natural or Artificial Opening 8 Via Natural or Artificial Opening Endoscopic X External	0 Drainage Device	Z No Qualifier

◀ New ◀‖‖ Revised ~~deleted~~ Deleted ♀ Females Only ♂ Males Only
🚫 Noncovered 🚫 Limited Coverage 🚫 Hospital-Acquired Condition **Coding Clinic**

SECTION: 0 MEDICAL AND SURGICAL
BODY SYSTEM: D GASTROINTESTINAL SYSTEM
OPERATION: 9 DRAINAGE: *(continued)*
Taking or letting out fluids and/or gases from a body part

Body Part	Approach	Device	Qualifier
Q Anus	0 Open 3 Percutaneous 4 Percutaneous Endoscopic 7 Via Natural or Artificial Opening 8 Via Natural or Artificial Opening Endoscopic X External	Z No Device	X Diagnostic Z No Qualifier
R Anal Sphincter S Greater Omentum T Lesser Omentum V Mesentery W Peritoneum	0 Open 3 Percutaneous 4 Percutaneous Endoscopic	0 Drainage Device	Z No Qualifier
R Anal Sphincter S Greater Omentum T Lesser Omentum V Mesentery W Peritoneum	0 Open 3 Percutaneous 4 Percutaneous Endoscopic	Z No Device	X Diagnostic Z No Qualifier

9: DRAINAGE

D: GASTROINTESTINAL SYSTEM

0: M/S

◀ New ◀ Revised ~~deleted~~ Deleted ♀ Females Only ♂ Males Only
Noncovered Limited Coverage Hospital-Acquired Condition **Coding Clinic**

SECTION: 0 MEDICAL AND SURGICAL
BODY SYSTEM: D GASTROINTESTINAL SYSTEM
OPERATION: B EXCISION: Cutting out or off, without replacement, a portion of a body part

Body Part	Approach	Device	Qualifier
1 Esophagus, Upper 2 Esophagus, Middle 3 Esophagus, Lower 4 Esophagogastric Junction 5 Esophagus 7 Stomach, Pylorus 8 Small Intestine 9 Duodenum A Jejunum B Ileum C Ileocecal Valve E Large Intestine F Large Intestine, Right G Large Intestine, Left H Cecum J Appendix K Ascending Colon L Transverse Colon M Descending Colon N Sigmoid Colon P Rectum	0 Open 3 Percutaneous 4 Percutaneous Endoscopic 7 Via Natural or Artificial Opening 8 Via Natural or Artificial Opening Endoscopic	Z No Device	X Diagnostic Z No Qualifier
6 Stomach	0 Open 3 Percutaneous 4 Percutaneous Endoscopic 7 Via Natural or Artificial Opening 8 Via Natural or Artificial Opening Endoscopic	Z No Device	3 Vertical X Diagnostic Z No Qualifier
Q Anus	0 Open 3 Percutaneous 4 Percutaneous Endoscopic 7 Via Natural or Artificial Opening 8 Via Natural or Artificial Opening Endoscopic X External	Z No Device	X Diagnostic Z No Qualifier
R Anal Sphincter S Greater Omentum T Lesser Omentum V Mesentery W Peritoneum	0 Open 3 Percutaneous 4 Percutaneous Endoscopic	Z No Device	X Diagnostic Z No Qualifier

0: M/S

D: GASTROINTESTINAL SYSTEM

B: EXCISION

◀ New ◀ Revised deleted Deleted ♀ Females Only ♂ Males Only
Ⓝ Noncovered Ⓛ Limited Coverage Ⓗ Hospital-Acquired Condition **Coding Clinic**

SECTION: 0 MEDICAL AND SURGICAL
BODY SYSTEM: D GASTROINTESTINAL SYSTEM
OPERATION: C EXTIRPATION: Taking or cutting out solid matter from a body part

C: EXTIRPATION

D: GASTROINTESTINAL SYSTEM

0: M/S

Body Part	Approach	Device	Qualifier
1 Esophagus, Upper 2 Esophagus, Middle 3 Esophagus, Lower 4 Esophagogastric Junction 5 Esophagus 6 Stomach 7 Stomach, Pylorus 8 Small Intestine 9 Duodenum A Jejunum B Ileum C Ileocecal Valve E Large Intestine F Large Intestine, Right G Large Intestine, Left H Cecum J Appendix K Ascending Colon L Transverse Colon M Descending Colon N Sigmoid Colon P Rectum	0 Open 3 Percutaneous 4 Percutaneous Endoscopic 7 Via Natural or Artificial Opening 8 Via Natural or Artificial Opening Endoscopic	Z No Device	Z No Qualifier
Q Anus	0 Open 3 Percutaneous 4 Percutaneous Endoscopic 7 Via Natural or Artificial Opening 8 Via Natural or Artificial Opening Endoscopic X External	Z No Device	Z No Qualifier
R Anal Sphincter S Greater Omentum T Lesser Omentum V Mesentery W Peritoneum	0 Open 3 Percutaneous 4 Percutaneous Endoscopic	Z No Device	Z No Qualifier

◀ New   ◀▥ Revised   ~~deleted~~ Deleted   ♀ Females Only   ♂ Males Only
🅝 Noncovered   🅛 Limited Coverage   🅗 Hospital-Acquired Condition   **Coding Clinic**

SECTION: 0 MEDICAL AND SURGICAL
BODY SYSTEM: D GASTROINTESTINAL SYSTEM
OPERATION: F FRAGMENTATION: Breaking solid matter in a body part into pieces

Body Part	Approach	Device	Qualifier
5 Esophagus 6 Stomach 8 Small Intestine 9 Duodenum A Jejunum B Ileum E Large Intestine F Large Intestine, Right G Large Intestine, Left H Cecum J Appendix K Ascending Colon L Transverse Colon M Descending Colon N Sigmoid Colon P Rectum Q Anus	0 Open 3 Percutaneous 4 Percutaneous Endoscopic 7 Via Natural or Artificial Opening 8 Via Natural or Artificial Opening Endoscopic X External ⊘	Z No Device	Z No Qualifier

◀ New ◀▬ Revised deleted Deleted ♀ Females Only ♂ Males Only
⊘ Noncovered ⊘ Limited Coverage ⊘ Hospital-Acquired Condition **Coding Clinic**

227

SECTION: 0 MEDICAL AND SURGICAL
BODY SYSTEM: D GASTROINTESTINAL SYSTEM
OPERATION: H INSERTION: Putting in a nonbiological appliance that monitors, assists, performs, or prevents a physiological function but does not physically take the place of a body part

Body Part	Approach	Device	Qualifier
5 Esophagus	0 Open 3 Percutaneous 4 Percutaneous Endoscopic	1 Radioactive Element 2 Monitoring Device 3 Infusion Device D Intraluminal Device U Feeding Device	Z No Qualifier
5 Esophagus	7 Via Natural or Artificial Opening 8 Via Natural or Artificial Opening Endoscopic	1 Radioactive Element 2 Monitoring Device 3 Infusion Device B Airway D Intraluminal Device U Feeding Device	Z No Qualifier
6 Stomach	0 Open 3 Percutaneous 4 Percutaneous Endoscopic	2 Monitoring Device 3 Infusion Device D Intraluminal Device M Stimulator Lead U Feeding Device	Z No Qualifier
6 Stomach	7 Via Natural or Artificial Opening 8 Via Natural or Artificial Opening Endoscopic	2 Monitoring Device 3 Infusion Device D Intraluminal Device U Feeding Device	Z No Qualifier
8 Small Intestine 9 Duodenum A Jejunum B Ileum	0 Open 3 Percutaneous 4 Percutaneous Endoscopic 7 Via Natural or Artificial Opening 8 Via Natural or Artificial Opening Endoscopic	2 Monitoring Device 3 Infusion Device D Intraluminal Device U Feeding Device	Z No Qualifier
E Large Intestine	0 Open 3 Percutaneous 4 Percutaneous Endoscopic 7 Via Natural or Artificial Opening 8 Via Natural or Artificial Opening Endoscopic	D Intraluminal Device	Z No Qualifier
P Rectum	0 Open 3 Percutaneous 4 Percutaneous Endoscopic 7 Via Natural or Artificial Opening 8 Via Natural or Artificial Opening Endoscopic	1 Radioactive Element D Intraluminal Device	Z No Qualifier
Q Anus	0 Open 3 Percutaneous 4 Percutaneous Endoscopic	D Intraluminal Device L Artificial Sphincter	Z No Qualifier
Q Anus	7 Via Natural or Artificial Opening 8 Via Natural or Artificial Opening Endoscopic	D Intraluminal Device	Z No Qualifier
R Anal Sphincter	0 Open 3 Percutaneous 4 Percutaneous Endoscopic	M Stimulator Lead	Z No Qualifier

◀ New ◀ Revised ~~deleted~~ Deleted ♀ Females Only ♂ Males Only Noncovered Limited Coverage Hospital-Acquired Condition **Coding Clinic**

SECTION: **0 MEDICAL AND SURGICAL**
BODY SYSTEM: D GASTROINTESTINAL SYSTEM
OPERATION: **J INSPECTION:** Visually and/or manually exploring a body part

Body Part	Approach	Device	Qualifier
0 Upper Intestinal Tract 6 Stomach D Lower Intestinal Tract	0 Open 3 Percutaneous 4 Percutaneous Endoscopic 7 Via Natural or Artificial Opening 8 Via Natural or Artificial Opening Endoscopic X External ⓝ	Z No Device	Z No Qualifier
U Omentum V Mesentery W Peritoneum	0 Open 3 Percutaneous 4 Percutaneous Endoscopic X External	Z No Device	Z No Qualifier

SECTION: 0 MEDICAL AND SURGICAL
BODY SYSTEM: D GASTROINTESTINAL SYSTEM
OPERATION: L OCCLUSION: Completely closing an orifice or the lumen of a tubular body part

L: OCCLUSION

D: GASTROINTESTINAL SYSTEM

0: M/S

Body Part	Approach	Device	Qualifier
1 Esophagus, Upper 2 Esophagus, Middle 3 Esophagus, Lower 4 Esophagogastric Junction 5 Esophagus 6 Stomach 7 Stomach, Pylorus 8 Small Intestine 9 Duodenum A Jejunum B Ileum C Ileocecal Valve E Large Intestine F Large Intestine, Right G Large Intestine, Left H Cecum K Ascending Colon L Transverse Colon M Descending Colon N Sigmoid Colon P Rectum	0 Open 3 Percutaneous 4 Percutaneous Endoscopic	C Extraluminal Device D Intraluminal Device Z No Device	Z No Qualifier
1 Esophagus, Upper 2 Esophagus, Middle 3 Esophagus, Lower 4 Esophagogastric Junction 5 Esophagus 6 Stomach 7 Stomach, Pylorus 8 Small Intestine 9 Duodenum A Jejunum B Ileum C Ileocecal Valve E Large Intestine F Large Intestine, Right G Large Intestine, Left H Cecum K Ascending Colon L Transverse Colon M Descending Colon N Sigmoid Colon P Rectum	7 Via Natural or Artificial Opening 8 Via Natural or Artificial Opening Endoscopic	D Intraluminal Device Z No Device	Z No Qualifier
Q Anus	0 Open 3 Percutaneous 4 Percutaneous Endoscopic X External	C Extraluminal Device D Intraluminal Device Z No Device	Z No Qualifier
Q Anus	7 Via Natural or Artificial Opening 8 Via Natural or Artificial Opening Endoscopic	D Intraluminal Device Z No Device	Z No Qualifier

◄ New ◀ Revised ~~deleted~~ Deleted ♀ Females Only ♂ Males Only
Noncovered Limited Coverage Hospital-Acquired Condition **Coding Clinic**

SECTION: 0 MEDICAL AND SURGICAL
BODY SYSTEM: D GASTROINTESTINAL SYSTEM
OPERATION: M REATTACHMENT: Putting back in or on all or a portion of a separated
body part to its normal location or other suitable location

Body Part	Approach	Device	Qualifier
5 Esophagus 6 Stomach 8 Small Intestine 9 Duodenum A Jejunum B Ileum E Large Intestine F Large Intestine, Right G Large Intestine, Left H Cecum K Ascending Colon L Transverse Colon M Descending Colon N Sigmoid Colon P Rectum	0 Open 4 Percutaneous Endoscopic	Z No Device	Z No Qualifier

◀ New   ◀ Revised   deleted Deleted   ♀ Females Only   ♂ Males Only
Noncovered   Limited Coverage   Hospital-Acquired Condition   **Coding Clinic**

231

0: M/S

D: GASTROINTESTINAL SYSTEM

M: REATTACHMENT

SECTION: 0 MEDICAL AND SURGICAL
BODY SYSTEM: D GASTROINTESTINAL SYSTEM
OPERATION: N RELEASE: Freeing a body part from an abnormal physical constraint by cutting or by the use of force

N: RELEASE

D: GASTROINTESTINAL SYSTEM

0: M/S

Body Part	Approach	Device	Qualifier
1 Esophagus, Upper 2 Esophagus, Middle 3 Esophagus, Lower 4 Esophagogastric Junction 5 Esophagus 6 Stomach 7 Stomach, Pylorus 8 Small Intestine 9 Duodenum A Jejunum B Ileum C Ileocecal Valve E Large Intestine F Large Intestine, Right G Large Intestine, Left H Cecum J Appendix K Ascending Colon L Transverse Colon M Descending Colon N Sigmoid Colon P Rectum	0 Open 3 Percutaneous 4 Percutaneous Endoscopic 7 Via Natural or Artificial Opening 8 Via Natural or Artificial Opening Endoscopic	Z No Device	Z No Qualifier
Q Anus	0 Open 3 Percutaneous 4 Percutaneous Endoscopic 7 Via Natural or Artificial Opening 8 Via Natural or Artificial Opening Endoscopic X External	Z No Device	Z No Qualifier
R Anal Sphincter S Greater Omentum T Lesser Omentum V Mesentery W Peritoneum	0 Open 3 Percutaneous 4 Percutaneous Endoscopic	Z No Device	Z No Qualifier

◀ New ◀▥ Revised ~~deleted~~ Deleted ♀ Females Only ♂ Males Only
🚫 Noncovered 🚫 Limited Coverage 🚫 Hospital-Acquired Condition **Coding Clinic**

SECTION: 0 MEDICAL AND SURGICAL
BODY SYSTEM: D GASTROINTESTINAL SYSTEM
OPERATION: P REMOVAL: *(on multiple pages)*
Taking out or off a device from a body part

Body Part	Approach	Device	Qualifier
0 Upper Intestinal Tract D Lower Intestinal Tract	0 Open 3 Percutaneous 4 Percutaneous Endoscopic 7 Via Natural or Artificial Opening 8 Via Natural or Artificial Opening Endoscopic	0 Drainage Device 2 Monitoring Device 3 Infusion Device 7 Autologous Tissue Substitute C Extraluminal Device D Intraluminal Device J Synthetic Substitute K Nonautologous Tissue Substitute U Feeding Device	Z No Qualifier
0 Upper Intestinal Tract D Lower Intestinal Tract	X External	0 Drainage Device 2 Monitoring Device 3 Infusion Device D Intraluminal Device U Feeding Device	Z No Qualifier
5 Esophagus	0 Open 3 Percutaneous 4 Percutaneous Endoscopic	1 Radioactive Element 2 Monitoring Device 3 Infusion Device U Feeding Device	Z No Qualifier
5 Esophagus	7 Via Natural or Artificial Opening 8 Via Natural or Artificial Opening Endoscopic	1 Radioactive Element B Airway	Z No Qualifier
5 Esophagus	X External	1 Radioactive Element 2 Monitoring Device 3 Infusion Device D Intraluminal Device U Feeding Device	Z No Qualifier
6 Stomach	0 Open 3 Percutaneous 4 Percutaneous Endoscopic	0 Drainage Device 2 Monitoring Device 3 Infusion Device 7 Autologous Tissue Substitute C Extraluminal Device D Intraluminal Device J Synthetic Substitute K Nonautologous Tissue Substitute M Stimulator Lead U Feeding Device	Z No Qualifier
6 Stomach	7 Via Natural or Artificial Opening 8 Via Natural or Artificial Opening Endoscopic	0 Drainage Device 2 Monitoring Device 3 Infusion Device 7 Autologous Tissue Substitute C Extraluminal Device D Intraluminal Device J Synthetic Substitute K Nonautologous Tissue Substitute U Feeding Device	Z No Qualifier

◀ New   ◀ Revised   ~~deleted~~ Deleted   ♀ Females Only   ♂ Males Only
NC Noncovered   LC Limited Coverage   HAC Hospital-Acquired Condition   **Coding Clinic**

233

SECTION: 0 MEDICAL AND SURGICAL
BODY SYSTEM: D GASTROINTESTINAL SYSTEM
OPERATION: P REMOVAL: *(Continued)*
Taking out or off a device from a body part

Body Part	Approach	Device	Qualifier
6 Stomach	X External	0 Drainage Device 2 Monitoring Device 3 Infusion Device D Intraluminal Device U Feeding Device	Z No Qualifier
P Rectum	0 Open 3 Percutaneous 4 Percutaneous Endoscopic 7 Via Natural or Artificial Opening 8 Via Natural or Artificial Opening Endoscopic X External	1 Radioactive Element	Z No Qualifier
Q Anus	0 Open 3 Percutaneous 4 Percutaneous Endoscopic 7 Via Natural or Artificial Opening 8 Via Natural or Artificial Opening Endoscopic	L Artificial Sphincter	Z No Qualifier
R Anal Sphincter	0 Open 3 Percutaneous 4 Percutaneous Endoscopic	M Stimulator Lead	Z No Qualifier
U Omentum V Mesentery W Peritoneum	0 Open 3 Percutaneous 4 Percutaneous Endoscopic	0 Drainage Device 1 Radioactive Element 7 Autologous Tissue Substitute J Synthetic Substitute K Nonautologous Tissue Substitute	Z No Qualifier

◀ New ◀ Revised ~~deleted~~ Deleted ♀ Females Only ♂ Males Only
Noncovered Limited Coverage Hospital-Acquired Condition **Coding Clinic**

SECTION: 0 MEDICAL AND SURGICAL
BODY SYSTEM: D GASTROINTESTINAL SYSTEM
OPERATION: Q REPAIR: Restoring, to the extent possible, a body part to its normal anatomic structure and function

Body Part	Approach	Device	Qualifier
1 Esophagus, Upper 2 Esophagus, Middle 3 Esophagus, Lower 4 Esophagogastric Junction 5 Esophagus 6 Stomach 7 Stomach, Pylorus 8 Small Intestine 9 Duodenum A Jejunum B Ileum C Ileocecal Valve E Large Intestine F Large Intestine, Right G Large Intestine, Left H Cecum J Appendix K Ascending Colon L Transverse Colon M Descending Colon N Sigmoid Colon P Rectum	0 Open 3 Percutaneous 4 Percutaneous Endoscopic 7 Via Natural or Artificial Opening 8 Via Natural or Artificial Opening Endoscopic	Z No Device	Z No Qualifier
Q Anus	0 Open 3 Percutaneous 4 Percutaneous Endoscopic 7 Via Natural or Artificial Opening 8 Via Natural or Artificial Opening Endoscopic X External	Z No Device	Z No Qualifier
R Anal Sphincter S Greater Omentum T Lesser Omentum V Mesentery W Peritoneum	0 Open 3 Percutaneous 4 Percutaneous Endoscopic	Z No Device	Z No Qualifier

◀ New ◀ Revised deleted Deleted ♀ Females Only ♂ Males Only
Noncovered Limited Coverage Hospital-Acquired Condition **Coding Clinic**

235

0: M/S

D: GASTROINTESTINAL SYSTEM

Q: REPAIR

SECTION: 0 MEDICAL AND SURGICAL
BODY SYSTEM: D GASTROINTESTINAL SYSTEM
OPERATION: R REPLACEMENT: Putting in or on biological or synthetic material that physically takes the place and/or function of all or a portion of a body part

Body Part	Approach	Device	Qualifier
5 Esophagus	0 Open 4 Percutaneous Endoscopic 7 Via Natural or Artificial Opening 8 Via Natural or Artificial Opening Endoscopic	7 Autologous Tissue Substitute J Synthetic Substitute K Nonautologous Tissue Substitute	Z No Qualifier
R Anal Sphincter S Greater Omentum T Lesser Omentum V Mesentery W Peritoneum	0 Open 4 Percutaneous Endoscopic	7 Autologous Tissue Substitute J Synthetic Substitute K Nonautologous Tissue Substitute	Z No Qualifier

SECTION: 0 MEDICAL AND SURGICAL
BODY SYSTEM: D GASTROINTESTINAL SYSTEM
OPERATION: S REPOSITION: Moving to its normal location, or other suitable location, all or a portion of a body part

Body Part	Approach	Device	Qualifier
5 Esophagus 6 Stomach 9 Duodenum A Jejunum B Ileum H Cecum K Ascending Colon L Transverse Colon M Descending Colon N Sigmoid Colon P Rectum Q Anus	0 Open 4 Percutaneous Endoscopic 7 Via Natural or Artificial Opening 8 Via Natural or Artificial Opening Endoscopic X External	Z No Device	Z No Qualifier

Side labels: R: REPLACEMENT S: REPOSITION D: GASTROINTESTINAL SYSTEM 0: M/S

◀ New ◀▥ Revised ~~deleted~~ Deleted ♀ Females Only ♂ Males Only
🔾 Noncovered 🔾 Limited Coverage 🔾 Hospital-Acquired Condition **Coding Clinic**

SECTION: 0 MEDICAL AND SURGICAL
BODY SYSTEM: D GASTROINTESTINAL SYSTEM
OPERATION: T RESECTION: Cutting out or off, without replacement, all of a body part

Body Part	Approach	Device	Qualifier
1 Esophagus, Upper 2 Esophagus, Middle 3 Esophagus, Lower 4 Esophagogastric Junction 5 Esophagus 6 Stomach 7 Stomach, Pylorus 8 Small Intestine 9 Duodenum A Jejunum B Ileum C Ileocecal Valve E Large Intestine F Large Intestine, Right G Large Intestine, Left H Cecum J Appendix K Ascending Colon L Transverse Colon M Descending Colon N Sigmoid Colon P Rectum Q Anus	0 Open 4 Percutaneous Endoscopic 7 Via Natural or Artificial Opening 8 Via Natural or Artificial Opening Endoscopic	Z No Device	Z No Qualifier
R Anal Sphincter S Greater Omentum T Lesser Omentum	0 Open 4 Percutaneous Endoscopic	Z No Device	Z No Qualifier

◀ New   ◀▥ Revised   ~~deleted~~ Deleted   ♀ Females Only   ♂ Males Only
Ⓝⓒ Noncovered   Ⓛⓒ Limited Coverage   Ⓗⓐⓒ Hospital-Acquired Condition   **Coding Clinic**

SECTION: 0 MEDICAL AND SURGICAL

BODY SYSTEM: D GASTROINTESTINAL SYSTEM

OPERATION: U SUPPLEMENT: Putting in or on biological or synthetic material that physically reinforces and/or augments the function of a portion of a body part

Body Part	Approach	Device	Qualifier
1 Esophagus, Upper 2 Esophagus, Middle 3 Esophagus, Lower 4 Esophagogastric Junction 5 Esophagus 6 Stomach 7 Stomach, Pylorus 8 Small Intestine 9 Duodenum A Jejunum B Ileum C Ileocecal Valve E Large Intestine F Large Intestine, Right G Large Intestine, Left H Cecum K Ascending Colon L Transverse Colon M Descending Colon N Sigmoid Colon P Rectum	0 Open 4 Percutaneous Endoscopic 7 Via Natural or Artificial Opening 8 Via Natural or Artificial Opening Endoscopic	7 Autologous Tissue Substitute J Synthetic Substitute K Nonautologous Tissue Substitute	Z No Qualifier
Q Anus	0 Open 4 Percutaneous Endoscopic 7 Via Natural or Artificial Opening 8 Via Natural or Artificial Opening Endoscopic X External	7 Autologous Tissue Substitute J Synthetic Substitute K Nonautologous Tissue Substitute	Z No Qualifier
R Anal Sphincter S Greater Omentum T Lesser Omentum V Mesentery W Peritoneum	0 Open 4 Percutaneous Endoscopic	7 Autologous Tissue Substitute J Synthetic Substitute K Nonautologous Tissue Substitute	Z No Qualifier

◄ New   ◄ Revised   deleted Deleted   ♀ Females Only   ♂ Males Only
◇ Noncovered   ◈ Limited Coverage   ◈ Hospital-Acquired Condition   **Coding Clinic**

SECTION: 0 MEDICAL AND SURGICAL
BODY SYSTEM: D GASTROINTESTINAL SYSTEM
OPERATION: V **RESTRICTION:** Partially closing an orifice or the lumen of a tubular body part

Body Part	Approach	Device	Qualifier
1 Esophagus, Upper 2 Esophagus, Middle 3 Esophagus, Lower 4 Esophagogastric Junction 5 Esophagus 6 Stomach 7 Stomach, Pylorus 8 Small Intestine 9 Duodenum A Jejunum B Ileum C Ileocecal Valve E Large Intestine F Large Intestine, Right G Large Intestine, Left H Cecum K Ascending Colon L Transverse Colon M Descending Colon N Sigmoid Colon P Rectum	0 Open 3 Percutaneous 4 Percutaneous Endoscopic	C Extraluminal Device D Intraluminal Device Z No Device	Z No Qualifier
1 Esophagus, Upper 2 Esophagus, Middle 3 Esophagus, Lower 4 Esophagogastric Junction 5 Esophagus 6 Stomach 7 Stomach, Pylorus 8 Small Intestine 9 Duodenum A Jejunum B Ileum C Ileocecal Valve E Large Intestine F Large Intestine, Right G Large Intestine, Left H Cecum K Ascending Colon L Colon M Descending Colon N Sigmoid Colon P Rectum	7 Via Natural or Artificial Opening 8 Via Natural or Artificial Opening Endoscopic	D Intraluminal Device Z No Device	Z No Qualifier
Q Anus	0 Open 3 Percutaneous 4 Percutaneous Endoscopic X External	C Extraluminal Device D Intraluminal Device Z No Device	Z No Qualifier
Q Anus	7 Via Natural or Artificial Opening 8 Via Natural or Artificial Opening Endoscopic	D Intraluminal Device Z No Device	Z No Qualifier

 0DV67DZ, 0DV68DZ
 0DV64CZ

◀ New ◀ Revised ~~deleted~~ Deleted ♀ Females Only ♂ Males Only
 Noncovered Limited Coverage Hospital-Acquired Condition **Coding Clinic**

0: M/S

D: GASTROINTESTINAL SYSTEM

V: RESTRICTION

SECTION: 0 MEDICAL AND SURGICAL
BODY SYSTEM: D GASTROINTESTINAL SYSTEM
OPERATION: W REVISION: Correcting, to the extent possible, a portion of a malfunctioning device or the position of a displaced device

W: REVISION

D: GASTROINTESTINAL SYSTEM

0: M/S

Body Part	Approach	Device	Qualifier
0 Upper Intestinal Tract D Lower Intestinal Tract	0 Open 3 Percutaneous 4 Percutaneous Endoscopic 7 Via Natural or Artificial Opening 8 Via Natural or Artificial Opening Endoscopic X External	0 Drainage Device 2 Monitoring Device 3 Infusion Device 7 Autologous Tissue Substitute C Extraluminal Device D Intraluminal Device J Synthetic Substitute K Nonautologous Tissue Substitute U Feeding Device	Z No Qualifier
5 Esophagus	7 Via Natural or Artificial Opening 8 Via Natural or Artificial Opening Endoscopic X External	D Intraluminal Device	Z No Qualifier
6 Stomach	0 Open 3 Percutaneous 4 Percutaneous Endoscopic	0 Drainage Device 2 Monitoring Device 3 Infusion Device 7 Autologous Tissue Substitute C Extraluminal Device D Intraluminal Device J Synthetic Substitute K Nonautologous Tissue Substitute M Stimulator Lead U Feeding Device	Z No Qualifier
6 Stomach	7 Via Natural or Artificial Opening 8 Via Natural or Artificial Opening Endoscopic X External	0 Drainage Device 2 Monitoring Device 3 Infusion Device 7 Autologous Tissue Substitute C Extraluminal Device D Intraluminal Device J Synthetic Substitute K Nonautologous Tissue Substitute U Feeding Device	Z No Qualifier
8 Small Intestine E Large Intestine	0 Open 4 Percutaneous Endoscopic 7 Via Natural or Artificial Opening 8 Via Natural or Artificial Opening Endoscopic	7 Autologous Tissue Substitute J Synthetic Substitute K Nonautologous Tissue Substitute	Z No Qualifier
Q Anus	0 Open 3 Percutaneous 4 Percutaneous Endoscopic 7 Via Natural or Artificial Opening 8 Via Natural or Artificial Opening Endoscopic	L Artificial Sphincter	Z No Qualifier
R Anal Sphincter	0 Open 3 Percutaneous 4 Percutaneous Endoscopic	M Stimulator Lead	Z No Qualifier
U Omentum V Mesentery W Peritoneum	0 Open 3 Percutaneous 4 Percutaneous Endoscopic	0 Drainage Device 7 Autologous Tissue Substitute J Synthetic Substitute K Nonautologous Tissue Substitute	Z No Qualifier

◀ New ◀ Revised ~~deleted~~ Deleted ♀ Females Only ♂ Males Only
🚫 Noncovered 🚫 Limited Coverage 🚫 Hospital-Acquired Condition **Coding Clinic**

SECTION: 0 MEDICAL AND SURGICAL
BODY SYSTEM: D GASTROINTESTINAL SYSTEM
OPERATION: X TRANSFER: Moving, without taking out, all or a portion of a body part to another location to take over the function of all or a portion of a body part

Body Part	Approach	Device	Qualifier
6 Stomach 8 Small Intestine E Large Intestine	0 Open 4 Percutaneous Endoscopic	Z No Device	5 Esophagus

SECTION: 0 MEDICAL AND SURGICAL
BODY SYSTEM: D GASTROINTESTINAL SYSTEM
OPERATION: Y TRANSPLANTATION: Putting in or on all or a portion of a living body part taken from another individual or animal to physically take the place and/or function of all or a portion of a similar body part

Body Part	Approach	Device	Qualifier
5 Esophagus 6 Stomach 8 Small Intestine 🦠 E Large Intestine 🦠	0 Open	Z No Device	0 Allogeneic 1 Syngeneic 2 Zooplastic

◀ New   ◀▥ Revised   ~~deleted~~ Deleted   ♀ Females Only   ♂ Males Only
🦠 Noncovered   🦠 Limited Coverage   🦠 Hospital-Acquired Condition   **Coding Clinic**

SECTION: 0 MEDICAL AND SURGICAL
BODY SYSTEM: F HEPATOBILIARY SYSTEM AND PANCREAS
OPERATION: 1 **BYPASS:** Altering the route of passage of the contents of a tubular body part

Body Part	Approach	Device	Qualifier
4 Gallbladder 5 Hepatic Duct, Right 6 Hepatic Duct, Left 8 Cystic Duct 9 Common Bile Duct	0 Open 4 Percutaneous Endoscopic	D Intraluminal Device Z No Device	3 Duodenum 4 Stomach 5 Hepatic Duct, Right 6 Hepatic Duct, Left 7 Hepatic Duct, Caudate 8 Cystic Duct 9 Common Bile Duct B Small Intestine
D Pancreatic Duct F Pancreatic Duct, Accessory G Pancreas	0 Open 4 Percutaneous Endoscopic	D Intraluminal Device Z No Device	3 Duodenum B Small Intestine C Large Intestine

SECTION: 0 MEDICAL AND SURGICAL
BODY SYSTEM: F HEPATOBILIARY SYSTEM AND PANCREAS
OPERATION: 2 **CHANGE:** Taking out or off a device from a body part and putting back an identical or similar device in or on the same body part without cutting or puncturing the skin or a mucous membrane

Body Part	Approach	Device	Qualifier
0 Liver 4 Gallbladder B Hepatobiliary Duct D Pancreatic Duct G Pancreas	X External	0 Drainage Device Y Other Device	Z No Qualifier

SECTION: 0 MEDICAL AND SURGICAL
BODY SYSTEM: F HEPATOBILIARY SYSTEM AND PANCREAS
OPERATION: 5 **DESTRUCTION:** Physical eradication of all or a portion of a body part by the direct use of energy, force, or a destructive agent

Body Part	Approach	Device	Qualifier
0 Liver 1 Liver, Right Lobe 2 Liver, Left Lobe 4 Gallbladder G Pancreas	0 Open 3 Percutaneous 4 Percutaneous Endoscopic	Z No Device	Z No Qualifier
5 Hepatic Duct, Right 6 Hepatic Duct, Left 8 Cystic Duct 9 Common Bile Duct C Ampulla of Vater D Pancreatic Duct F Pancreatic Duct, Accessory	0 Open 3 Percutaneous 4 Percutaneous Endoscopic 7 Via Natural or Artificial Opening 8 Via Natural or Artificial Opening Endoscopic	Z No Device	Z No Qualifier

◀ New   ◀◀ Revised   ~~deleted~~ Deleted   ♀ Females Only   ♂ Males Only
🚫 Noncovered   🔵 Limited Coverage   🚫 Hospital-Acquired Condition   **Coding Clinic**

243

SECTION: 0 MEDICAL AND SURGICAL
BODY SYSTEM: F HEPATOBILIARY SYSTEM AND PANCREAS
OPERATION: 7 DILATION: Expanding an orifice or the lumen of a tubular body part

Body Part	Approach	Device	Qualifier
5 Hepatic Duct, Right 6 Hepatic Duct, Left 8 Cystic Duct 9 Common Bile Duct C Ampulla of Vater D Pancreatic Duct F Pancreatic Duct, Accessory	0 Open 3 Percutaneous 4 Percutaneous Endoscopic 7 Via Natural or Artificial Opening 8 Via Natural or Artificial Opening Endoscopic	D Intraluminal Device Z No Device	Z No Qualifier

SECTION: 0 MEDICAL AND SURGICAL
BODY SYSTEM: F HEPATOBILIARY SYSTEM AND PANCREAS
OPERATION: 8 DIVISION: Cutting into a body part, without draining fluids and/or gases from the body part, in order to separate or transect a body part

Body Part	Approach	Device	Qualifier
G Pancreas	0 Open 3 Percutaneous 4 Percutaneous Endoscopic	Z No Device	Z No Qualifier

SECTION: 0 MEDICAL AND SURGICAL
BODY SYSTEM: F HEPATOBILIARY SYSTEM AND PANCREAS
OPERATION: 9 DRAINAGE: Taking or letting out fluids and/or gases from a body part

Body Part	Approach	Device	Qualifier
0 Liver 1 Liver, Right Lobe 2 Liver, Left Lobe 4 Gallbladder G Pancreas	0 Open 3 Percutaneous 4 Percutaneous Endoscopic	0 Drainage Device	Z No Qualifier
0 Liver 1 Liver, Right Lobe 2 Liver, Left Lobe 4 Gallbladder G Pancreas	0 Open 3 Percutaneous 4 Percutaneous Endoscopic	Z No Device	X Diagnostic Z No Qualifier
5 Hepatic Duct, Right 6 Hepatic Duct, Left 8 Cystic Duct 9 Common Bile Duct C Ampulla of Vater D Pancreatic Duct F Pancreatic Duct, Accessory	0 Open 3 Percutaneous 4 Percutaneous Endoscopic 7 Via Natural or Artificial Opening 8 Via Natural or Artificial Opening Endoscopic	0 Drainage Device	Z No Qualifier
5 Hepatic Duct, Right 6 Hepatic Duct, Left 8 Cystic Duct 9 Common Bile Duct C Ampulla of Vater D Pancreatic Duct F Pancreatic Duct, Accessory	0 Open 3 Percutaneous 4 Percutaneous Endoscopic 7 Via Natural or Artificial Opening 8 Via Natural or Artificial Opening Endoscopic	Z No Device	X Diagnostic Z No Qualifier

◀ New ◀ Revised ~~deleted~~ Deleted ♀ Females Only ♂ Males Only
Noncovered Limited Coverage Hospital-Acquired Condition **Coding Clinic**

SECTION: 0 MEDICAL AND SURGICAL
BODY SYSTEM: F HEPATOBILIARY SYSTEM AND PANCREAS
OPERATION: B EXCISION: Cutting out or off, without replacement, a portion of a body part

Body Part	Approach	Device	Qualifier
0 Liver 1 Liver, Right Lobe 2 Liver, Left Lobe 4 Gallbladder G Pancreas	0 Open 3 Percutaneous 4 Percutaneous Endoscopic	Z No Device	X Diagnostic Z No Qualifier
5 Hepatic Duct, Right 6 Hepatic Duct, Left 8 Cystic Duct 9 Common Bile Duct C Ampulla of Vater D Pancreatic Duct F Pancreatic Duct, Accessory	0 Open 3 Percutaneous 4 Percutaneous Endoscopic 7 Via Natural or Artificial Opening 8 Via Natural or Artificial Opening Endoscopic	Z No Device	X Diagnostic Z No Qualifier

SECTION: 0 MEDICAL AND SURGICAL
BODY SYSTEM: F HEPATOBILIARY SYSTEM AND PANCREAS
OPERATION: C EXTIRPATION: Taking or cutting out solid matter from a body part

Body Part	Approach	Device	Qualifier
0 Liver 1 Liver, Right Lobe 2 Liver, Left Lobe 4 Gallbladder G Pancreas	0 Open 3 Percutaneous 4 Percutaneous Endoscopic	Z No Device	Z No Qualifier
5 Hepatic Duct, Right 6 Hepatic Duct, Left 8 Cystic Duct 9 Common Bile Duct C Ampulla of Vater D Pancreatic Duct F Pancreatic Duct, Accessory	0 Open 3 Percutaneous 4 Percutaneous Endoscopic 7 Via Natural or Artificial Opening 8 Via Natural or Artificial Opening Endoscopic	Z No Device	Z No Qualifier

SECTION: 0 MEDICAL AND SURGICAL
BODY SYSTEM: F HEPATOBILIARY SYSTEM AND PANCREAS
OPERATION: F FRAGMENTATION: Breaking solid matter in a body part into pieces

Body Part	Approach	Device	Qualifier
4 Gallbladder 5 Hepatic Duct, Right 6 Hepatic Duct, Left 8 Cystic Duct 9 Common Bile Duct C Ampulla of Vater D Pancreatic Duct F Pancreatic Duct, Accessory	0 Open 3 Percutaneous 4 Percutaneous Endoscopic 7 Via Natural or Artificial Opening 8 Via Natural or Artificial Opening Endoscopic X External ⊘	Z No Device	Z No Qualifier

◀ New   ◀▥ Revised   ~~deleted~~ Deleted   ♀ Females Only   ♂ Males Only
⊘ Noncovered   ⊘ Limited Coverage   ⊘ Hospital-Acquired Condition   **Coding Clinic**

245

0: M/S

F: HEPATOBILIARY SYSTEM AND PANCREAS

B: EXCISION   C: EXTIRPATION   F: FRAGMENTATION

SECTION: 0 MEDICAL AND SURGICAL
BODY SYSTEM: F HEPATOBILIARY SYSTEM AND PANCREAS
OPERATION: H INSERTION: Putting in a nonbiological appliance that monitors, assists, performs, or prevents a physiological function but does not physically take the place of a body part

Body Part	Approach	Device	Qualifier
0 Liver 1 Liver, Right Lobe 2 Liver, Left Lobe 4 Gallbladder G Pancreas	0 Open 3 Percutaneous 4 Percutaneous Endoscopic	2 Monitoring Device 3 Infusion Device	Z No Qualifier
B Hepatobiliary Duct D Pancreatic Duct	0 Open 3 Percutaneous 4 Percutaneous Endoscopic 7 Via Natural or Artificial Opening 8 Via Natural or Artificial Opening Endoscopic	1 Radioactive Element 2 Monitoring Device 3 Infusion Device D Intraluminal Device	Z No Qualifier

SECTION: 0 MEDICAL AND SURGICAL
BODY SYSTEM: F HEPATOBILIARY SYSTEM AND PANCREAS
OPERATION: J INSPECTION: Visually and/or manually exploring a body part

Body Part	Approach	Device	Qualifier
0 Liver 4 Gallbladder G Pancreas	0 Open 3 Percutaneous 4 Percutaneous Endoscopic X External	Z No Device	Z No Qualifier
B Hepatobiliary Duct D Pancreatic Duct	0 Open 3 Percutaneous 4 Percutaneous Endoscopic 7 Via Natural or Artificial Opening 8 Via Natural or Artificial Opening Endoscopic	Z No Device	Z No Qualifier

◀ New   ◀▓ Revised   ~~deleted~~ Deleted   ♀ Females Only   ♂ Males Only
⊘ Noncovered   ⊘ Limited Coverage   ⊘ Hospital-Acquired Condition   **Coding Clinic**

SECTION: 0 MEDICAL AND SURGICAL
BODY SYSTEM: F HEPATOBILIARY SYSTEM AND PANCREAS
OPERATION: L OCCLUSION: Completely closing an orifice or the lumen of a tubular body part

Body Part	Approach	Device	Qualifier
5 Hepatic Duct, Right 6 Hepatic Duct, Left 8 Cystic Duct 9 Common Bile Duct C Ampulla of Vater D Pancreatic Duct F Pancreatic Duct, Accessory	0 Open 3 Percutaneous 4 Percutaneous Endoscopic	C Extraluminal Device D Intraluminal Device Z No Device	Z No Qualifier
5 Hepatic Duct, Right 6 Hepatic Duct, Left 8 Cystic Duct 9 Common Bile Duct C Ampulla of Vater D Pancreatic Duct F Pancreatic Duct, Accessory	7 Via Natural or Artificial Opening 8 Via Natural or Artificial Opening Endoscopic	D Intraluminal Device Z No Device	Z No Qualifier

SECTION: 0 MEDICAL AND SURGICAL
BODY SYSTEM: F HEPATOBILIARY SYSTEM AND PANCREAS
OPERATION: M REATTACHMENT: Putting back in or on all or a portion of a separated body part to its normal location or other suitable location

Body Part	Approach	Device	Qualifier
0 Liver 1 Liver, Right Lobe 2 Liver, Left Lobe 4 Gallbladder 5 Hepatic Duct, Right 6 Hepatic Duct, Left 8 Cystic Duct 9 Common Bile Duct C Ampulla of Vater D Pancreatic Duct F Pancreatic Duct, Accessory G Pancreas	0 Open 4 Percutaneous Endoscopic	Z No Device	Z No Qualifier

SECTION: 0 MEDICAL AND SURGICAL
BODY SYSTEM: F HEPATOBILIARY SYSTEM AND PANCREAS
OPERATION: N RELEASE: Freeing a body part from an abnormal physical constraint by cutting or by the use of force

Body Part	Approach	Device	Qualifier
0 Liver 1 Liver, Right Lobe 2 Liver, Left Lobe 4 Gallbladder G Pancreas	0 Open 3 Percutaneous 4 Percutaneous Endoscopic	Z No Device	Z No Qualifier
5 Hepatic Duct, Right 6 Hepatic Duct, Left 8 Cystic Duct 9 Common Bile Duct C Ampulla of Vater D Pancreatic Duct F Pancreatic Duct, Accessory	0 Open 3 Percutaneous 4 Percutaneous Endoscopic 7 Via Natural or Artificial Opening 8 Via Natural or Artificial Opening Endoscopic	Z No Device	Z No Qualifier

SECTION: 0 MEDICAL AND SURGICAL
BODY SYSTEM: F HEPATOBILIARY SYSTEM AND PANCREAS
OPERATION: P REMOVAL: Taking out or off a device from a body part

Body Part	Approach	Device	Qualifier
0 Liver	0 Open 3 Percutaneous 4 Percutaneous Endoscopic X External	0 Drainage Device 2 Monitoring Device 3 Infusion Device	Z No Qualifier
4 Gallbladder G Pancreas	0 Open 3 Percutaneous 4 Percutaneous Endoscopic X External	0 Drainage Device 2 Monitoring Device 3 Infusion Device D Intraluminal Device	Z No Qualifier
B Hepatobiliary Duct D Pancreatic Duct	0 Open 3 Percutaneous 4 Percutaneous Endoscopic 7 Via Natural or Artificial Opening 8 Via Natural or Artificial Opening Endoscopic	0 Drainage Device 1 Radioactive Element 2 Monitoring Device 3 Infusion Device 7 Autologous Tissue Substitute C Extraluminal Device D Intraluminal Device J Synthetic Substitute K Nonautologous Tissue Substitute	Z No Qualifier
B Hepatobiliary Duct D Pancreatic Duct	X External	0 Drainage Device 1 Radioactive Element 2 Monitoring Device 3 Infusion Device D Intraluminal Device	Z No Qualifier

◀ New ◀ Revised ~~deleted~~ Deleted ♀ Females Only ♂ Males Only
Noncovered Limited Coverage Hospital-Acquired Condition **Coding Clinic**

SECTION: 0 MEDICAL AND SURGICAL
BODY SYSTEM: F HEPATOBILIARY SYSTEM AND PANCREAS
OPERATION: Q REPAIR: Restoring, to the extent possible, a body part to its normal anatomic structure and function

Body Part	Approach	Device	Qualifier
0 Liver 1 Liver, Right Lobe 2 Liver, Left Lobe 4 Gallbladder G Pancreas	0 Open 3 Percutaneous 4 Percutaneous Endoscopic	Z No Device	Z No Qualifier
5 Hepatic Duct, Right 6 Hepatic Duct, Left 8 Cystic Duct 9 Common Bile Duct C Ampulla of Vater D Pancreatic Duct F Pancreatic Duct, Accessory	0 Open 3 Percutaneous 4 Percutaneous Endoscopic 7 Via Natural or Artificial Opening 8 Via Natural or Artificial Opening Endoscopic	Z No Device	Z No Qualifier

SECTION: 0 MEDICAL AND SURGICAL
BODY SYSTEM: F HEPATOBILIARY SYSTEM AND PANCREAS
OPERATION: R REPLACEMENT: Putting in or on biological or synthetic material that physically takes the place and/or function of all or a portion of a body part

Body Part	Approach	Device	Qualifier
5 Hepatic Duct, Right 6 Hepatic Duct, Left 8 Cystic Duct 9 Common Bile Duct C Ampulla of Vater D Pancreatic Duct F Pancreatic Duct, Accessory	0 Open 4 Percutaneous Endoscopic	7 Autologous Tissue Substitute J Synthetic Substitute K Nonautologous Tissue Substitute	Z No Qualifier

SECTION: 0 MEDICAL AND SURGICAL
BODY SYSTEM: F HEPATOBILIARY SYSTEM AND PANCREAS
OPERATION: S REPOSITION: Moving to its normal location, or other suitable location, all or a portion of a body part

Body Part	Approach	Device	Qualifier
0 Liver 4 Gallbladder 5 Hepatic Duct, Right 6 Hepatic Duct, Left 8 Cystic Duct 9 Common Bile Duct C Ampulla of Vater D Pancreatic Duct F Pancreatic Duct, Accessory G Pancreas	0 Open 4 Percutaneous Endoscopic	Z No Device	Z No Qualifier

SECTION: 0 MEDICAL AND SURGICAL
BODY SYSTEM: F **HEPATOBILIARY SYSTEM AND PANCREAS**
OPERATION: T **RESECTION:** Cutting out or off, without replacement, all of a body part

Body Part	Approach	Device	Qualifier
0 Liver 1 Liver, Right Lobe 2 Liver, Left Lobe 4 Gallbladder G Pancreas	0 Open 4 Percutaneous Endoscopic	Z No Device	Z No Qualifier

5 Hepatic Duct, Right
6 Hepatic Duct, Left
8 Cystic Duct
9 Common Bile Duct
C Ampulla of Vater
D Pancreatic Duct
F Pancreatic Duct, Accessory
	0 Open
	4 Percutaneous Endoscopic
	7 Via Natural or Artificial
	   Opening
	8 Via Natural or Artificial
	   Opening Endoscopic
		Z No Device	Z No Qualifier

Coding Clinic: 2012, Q4, P100 – 0FT00ZZ

SECTION: 0 MEDICAL AND SURGICAL
BODY SYSTEM: F **HEPATOBILIARY SYSTEM AND PANCREAS**
OPERATION: U **SUPPLEMENT:** Putting in or on biological or synthetic material that physically reinforces and/or augments the function of a portion of a body part

Body Part	Approach	Device	Qualifier
5 Hepatic Duct, Right 6 Hepatic Duct, Left 8 Cystic Duct 9 Common Bile Duct C Ampulla of Vater D Pancreatic Duct F Pancreatic Duct, Accessory	0 Open 3 Percutaneous 4 Percutaneous Endoscopic	7 Autologous Tissue Substitute J Synthetic Substitute K Nonautologous Tissue Substitute	Z No Qualifier

SECTION: 0 MEDICAL AND SURGICAL
BODY SYSTEM: F HEPATOBILIARY SYSTEM AND PANCREAS
OPERATION: V RESTRICTION: Partially closing an orifice or the lumen of a tubular body part

Body Part	Approach	Device	Qualifier
5 Hepatic Duct, Right 6 Hepatic Duct, Left 8 Cystic Duct 9 Common Bile Duct C Ampulla of Vater D Pancreatic Duct F Pancreatic Duct, Accessory	0 Open 3 Percutaneous 4 Percutaneous Endoscopic	C Extraluminal Device D Intraluminal Device Z No Device	Z No Qualifier
5 Hepatic Duct, Right 6 Hepatic Duct, Left 8 Cystic Duct 9 Common Bile Duct C Ampulla of Vater D Pancreatic Duct F Pancreatic Duct, Accessory	7 Via Natural or Artificial Opening 8 Via Natural or Artificial Opening Endoscopic	D Intraluminal Device Z No Device	Z No Qualifier

SECTION: 0 MEDICAL AND SURGICAL
BODY SYSTEM: F HEPATOBILIARY SYSTEM AND PANCREAS
OPERATION: W REVISION: Correcting, to the extent possible, a portion of a malfunctioning device or the position of a displaced device

Body Part	Approach	Device	Qualifier
0 Liver	0 Open 3 Percutaneous 4 Percutaneous Endoscopic X External	0 Drainage Device 2 Monitoring Device 3 Infusion Device	Z No Qualifier
4 Gallbladder G Pancreas	0 Open 3 Percutaneous 4 Percutaneous Endoscopic X External	0 Drainage Device 2 Monitoring Device 3 Infusion Device D Intraluminal Device	Z No Qualifier
B Hepatobiliary Duct D Pancreatic Duct	0 Open 3 Percutaneous 4 Percutaneous Endoscopic 7 Via Natural or Artificial Opening 8 Via Natural or Artificial Opening Endoscopic X External	0 Drainage Device 2 Monitoring Device 3 Infusion Device 7 Autologous Tissue Substitute C Extraluminal Device D Intraluminal Device J Synthetic Substitute K Nonautologous Tissue Substitute	Z No Qualifier

Y: TRANSPLANTATION

SECTION: 0 MEDICAL AND SURGICAL
BODY SYSTEM: F HEPATOBILIARY SYSTEM AND PANCREAS
OPERATION: Y TRANSPLANTATION: Putting in or on all or a portion of a living body part taken from another individual or animal to physically take the place and/or function of all or a portion of a similar body part

Body Part	Approach	Device	Qualifier
0 Liver 🔴 G Pancreas 🔴 🔴	0 Open	Z No Device	0 Allogeneic 1 Syngeneic 2 Zooplastic

🔴 0F4G0Z2: 0FYG0Z0, 0FYG0Z1 alone [without kidney transplant codes (0TY00Z0, 0TY00Z1, 0TY00Z2, 0TY10Z0, 0TY10Z1, 0TY10Z2)]. Except when 0FYG0Z0 or 0FYG0Z1 is combined with at least one principal or secondary diagnosis code from the following list:

E10.10	E10.321	E10.359	E10.44	E10.620	E10.649
E10.11	E10.329	E10.36	E10.49	E10.621	E10.65
E10.21	E10.331	E10.39	E10.51	E10.622	E10.69
E10.22	E10.339	E10.40	E10.52	E10.628	E10.8
E10.29	E10.341	E10.41	E10.59	E10.630	E10.9
E10.311	E10.349	E10.42	E10.610	E10.638	E89.1
E10.319	E10.351	E10.43	E10.618	E10.641	

🔴 0FYG0Z0, 0FYG0Z1

Coding Clinic: 2012, Q4, P100 – 0FY00Z0

F: HEPATOBILIARY SYSTEM AND PANCREAS   0: M/S

SECTION: 0 MEDICAL AND SURGICAL
BODY SYSTEM: G ENDOCRINE SYSTEM
OPERATION: 2 CHANGE: Taking out or off a device from a body part and putting back an identical or similar device in or on the same body part without cutting or puncturing the skin or a mucous membrane

Body Part	Approach	Device	Qualifier
0 Pituitary Gland 1 Pineal Body 5 Adrenal Gland K Thyroid Gland R Parathyroid Gland S Endocrine Gland	X External	0 Drainage Device Y Other Device	Z No Qualifier

SECTION: 0 MEDICAL AND SURGICAL
BODY SYSTEM: G ENDOCRINE SYSTEM
OPERATION: 5 DESTRUCTION: Physical eradication of all or a portion of a body part by the direct use of energy, force, or a destructive agent

Body Part	Approach	Device	Qualifier
0 Pituitary Gland 1 Pineal Body 2 Adrenal Gland, Left 3 Adrenal Gland, Right 4 Adrenal Glands, Bilateral 6 Carotid Body, Left 7 Carotid Body, Right 8 Carotid Bodies, Bilateral 9 Para-aortic Body B Coccygeal Glomus C Glomus Jugulare D Aortic Body F Paraganglion Extremity G Thyroid Gland Lobe, Left H Thyroid Gland Lobe, Right K Thyroid Gland L Superior Parathyroid Gland, Right M Superior Parathyroid Gland, Left N Inferior Parathyroid Gland, Right P Inferior Parathyroid Gland, Left Q Parathyroid Glands, Multiple R Parathyroid Gland	0 Open 3 Percutaneous 4 Percutaneous Endoscopic	Z No Device	Z No Qualifier

SECTION: 0 MEDICAL AND SURGICAL
BODY SYSTEM: G ENDOCRINE SYSTEM
OPERATION: 8 DIVISION: Cutting into a body part, without draining fluids and/or gases from the body part, in order to separate or transect a body part

Body Part	Approach	Device	Qualifier
0 Pituitary Gland J Thyroid Gland Isthmus	0 Open 3 Percutaneous 4 Percutaneous Endoscopic	Z No Device	Z No Qualifier

SECTION: 0 MEDICAL AND SURGICAL
BODY SYSTEM: G ENDOCRINE SYSTEM
OPERATION: 9 DRAINAGE: Taking or letting out fluids and/or gases from a body part

Body Part	Approach	Device	Qualifier
0 Pituitary Gland 1 Pineal Body 2 Adrenal Gland, Left 3 Adrenal Gland, Right 4 Adrenal Glands, Bilateral 6 Carotid Body, Left 7 Carotid Body, Right 8 Carotid Bodies, Bilateral 9 Para-aortic Body B Coccygeal Glomus C Glomus Jugulare D Aortic Body F Paraganglion Extremity G Thyroid Gland Lobe, Left H Thyroid Gland Lobe, Right K Thyroid Gland L Superior Parathyroid Gland, Right M Superior Parathyroid Gland, Left N Inferior Parathyroid Gland, Right P Inferior Parathyroid Gland, Left Q Parathyroid Glands, Multiple R Parathyroid Gland	0 Open 3 Percutaneous 4 Percutaneous Endoscopic	0 Drainage Device	Z No Qualifier
0 Pituitary Gland 1 Pineal Body 2 Adrenal Gland, Left 3 Adrenal Gland, Right 4 Adrenal Glands, Bilateral 6 Carotid Body, Left 7 Carotid Body, Right 8 Carotid Bodies, Bilateral 9 Para-aortic Body B Coccygeal Glomus C Glomus Jugulare D Aortic Body F Paraganglion Extremity G Thyroid Gland Lobe, Left H Thyroid Gland Lobe, Right K Thyroid Gland L Superior Parathyroid Gland, Right M Superior Parathyroid Gland, Left N Inferior Parathyroid Gland, Right P Inferior Parathyroid Gland, Left Q Parathyroid Glands, Multiple R Parathyroid Gland	0 Open 3 Percutaneous 4 Percutaneous Endoscopic	Z No Device	X Diagnostic Z No Qualifier

◀ New   ◀▥ Revised   ~~deleted~~ Deleted   ♀ Females Only   ♂ Males Only
 Noncovered   Limited Coverage   Hospital-Acquired Condition   **Coding Clinic**

255

SECTION: **0 MEDICAL AND SURGICAL**
BODY SYSTEM: G ENDOCRINE SYSTEM
OPERATION: **B EXCISION:** Cutting out or off, without replacement, a portion of a body part

Body Part	Approach	Device	Qualifier
0 Pituitary Gland 1 Pineal Body 2 Adrenal Gland, Left 3 Adrenal Gland, Right 4 Adrenal Glands, Bilateral 6 Carotid Body, Left 7 Carotid Body, Right 8 Carotid Bodies, Bilateral 9 Para-aortic Body B Coccygeal Glomus C Glomus Jugulare D Aortic Body F Paraganglion Extremity G Thyroid Gland Lobe, Left H Thyroid Gland Lobe, Right L Superior Parathyroid Gland, Right M Superior Parathyroid Gland, Left N Inferior Parathyroid Gland, Right P Inferior Parathyroid Gland, Left Q Parathyroid Glands, Multiple R Parathyroid Gland	0 Open 3 Percutaneous 4 Percutaneous Endoscopic	Z No Device	X Diagnostic Z No Qualifier

SECTION: **0 MEDICAL AND SURGICAL**
BODY SYSTEM: G ENDOCRINE SYSTEM
OPERATION: **C EXTIRPATION:** Taking or cutting out solid matter from a body part

Body Part	Approach	Device	Qualifier
0 Pituitary Gland 1 Pineal Body 2 Adrenal Gland, Left 3 Adrenal Gland, Right 4 Adrenal Glands, Bilateral 6 Carotid Body, Left 7 Carotid Body, Right 8 Carotid Bodies, Bilateral 9 Para-aortic Body B Coccygeal Glomus C Glomus Jugulare D Aortic Body F Paraganglion Extremity G Thyroid Gland Lobe, Left H Thyroid Gland Lobe, Right K Thyroid Gland L Superior Parathyroid Gland, Right M Superior Parathyroid Gland, Left N Inferior Parathyroid Gland, Right P Inferior Parathyroid Gland, Left Q Parathyroid Glands, Multiple R Parathyroid Gland	0 Open 3 Percutaneous 4 Percutaneous Endoscopic	Z No Device	Z No Qualifier

◀ New   ◀▦ Revised   deleted Deleted   ♀ Females Only   ♂ Males Only
Noncovered   Limited Coverage   Hospital-Acquired Condition   **Coding Clinic**

SECTION: 0 MEDICAL AND SURGICAL

BODY SYSTEM: G ENDOCRINE SYSTEM

OPERATION: H INSERTION: Putting in a nonbiological appliance that monitors, assists, performs, or prevents a physiological function but does not physically take the place of a body part

Body Part	Approach	Device	Qualifier
S Endocrine Gland	0 Open 3 Percutaneous 4 Percutaneous Endoscopic	2 Monitoring Device 3 Infusion Device	Z No Qualifier

SECTION: 0 MEDICAL AND SURGICAL

BODY SYSTEM: G ENDOCRINE SYSTEM

OPERATION: J INSPECTION: Visually and/or manually exploring a body part

Body Part	Approach	Device	Qualifier
0 Pituitary Gland 1 Pineal Body 5 Adrenal Gland K Thyroid Gland R Parathyroid Gland S Endocrine Gland	0 Open 3 Percutaneous 4 Percutaneous Endoscopic	Z No Device	Z No Qualifier

SECTION: 0 MEDICAL AND SURGICAL

BODY SYSTEM: G ENDOCRINE SYSTEM

OPERATION: M REATTACHMENT: Putting back in or on all or a portion of a separated body part to its normal location or other suitable location

Body Part	Approach	Device	Qualifier
2 Adrenal Gland, Left 3 Adrenal Gland, Right G Thyroid Gland Lobe, Left H Thyroid Gland Lobe, Right L Superior Parathyroid Gland, Right M Superior Parathyroid Gland, Left N Inferior Parathyroid Gland, Right P Inferior Parathyroid Gland, Left Q Parathyroid Glands, Multiple R Parathyroid Gland	0 Open 4 Percutaneous Endoscopic	Z No Device	Z No Qualifier

SECTION: 0 MEDICAL AND SURGICAL

BODY SYSTEM: G ENDOCRINE SYSTEM

OPERATION: N RELEASE: Freeing a body part from an abnormal physical constraint by cutting or by the use of force

Body Part	Approach	Device	Qualifier
0 Pituitary Gland 1 Pineal Body 2 Adrenal Gland, Left 3 Adrenal Gland, Right 4 Adrenal Glands, Bilateral 6 Carotid Body, Left 7 Carotid Body, Right 8 Carotid Bodies, Bilateral 9 Para-aortic Body B Coccygeal Glomus C Glomus Jugulare D Aortic Body F Paraganglion Extremity G Thyroid Gland Lobe, Left H Thyroid Gland Lobe, Right K Thyroid Gland L Superior Parathyroid Gland, Right M Superior Parathyroid Gland, Left N Inferior Parathyroid Gland, Right P Inferior Parathyroid Gland, Left Q Parathyroid Glands, Multiple R Parathyroid Gland	0 Open 3 Percutaneous 4 Percutaneous Endoscopic	Z No Device	Z No Qualifier

SECTION: 0 MEDICAL AND SURGICAL

BODY SYSTEM: G ENDOCRINE SYSTEM

OPERATION: P REMOVAL: Taking out or off a device from a body part

Body Part	Approach	Device	Qualifier
0 Pituitary Gland 1 Pineal Body 5 Adrenal Gland K Thyroid Gland R Parathyroid Gland	0 Open 3 Percutaneous 4 Percutaneous Endoscopic X External	0 Drainage Device	Z No Qualifier
S Endocrine Gland	0 Open 3 Percutaneous 4 Percutaneous Endoscopic X External	0 Drainage Device 2 Monitoring Device 3 Infusion Device	Z No Qualifier

◀ New   ◀ Revised   ~~deleted~~ Deleted   ♀ Females Only   ♂ Males Only
Ⓝⓒ Noncovered   Ⓛⓒ Limited Coverage   Hospital-Acquired Condition   **Coding Clinic**

SECTION: 0 MEDICAL AND SURGICAL

BODY SYSTEM: G ENDOCRINE SYSTEM

OPERATION: Q REPAIR: Restoring, to the extent possible, a body part to its normal anatomic structure and function

Body Part	Approach	Device	Qualifier
0 Pituitary Gland 1 Pineal Body 2 Adrenal Gland, Left 3 Adrenal Gland, Right 4 Adrenal Glands, Bilateral 6 Carotid Body, Left 7 Carotid Body, Right 8 Carotid Bodies, Bilateral 9 Para-aortic Body B Coccygeal Glomus C Glomus Jugulare D Aortic Body F Paraganglion Extremity G Thyroid Gland Lobe, Left H Thyroid Gland Lobe, Right J Thyroid Gland Isthmus K Thyroid Gland L Superior Parathyroid Gland, Right M Superior Parathyroid Gland, Left N Inferior Parathyroid Gland, Right P Inferior Parathyroid Gland, Left Q Parathyroid Glands, Multiple R Parathyroid Gland	0 Open 3 Percutaneous 4 Percutaneous Endoscopic	Z No Device	Z No Qualifier

SECTION: 0 MEDICAL AND SURGICAL

BODY SYSTEM: G ENDOCRINE SYSTEM

OPERATION: S REPOSITION: Moving to its normal location, or other suitable location, all or a portion of a body part

Body Part	Approach	Device	Qualifier
2 Adrenal Gland, Left 3 Adrenal Gland, Right G Thyroid Gland Lobe, Left H Thyroid Gland Lobe, Right L Superior Parathyroid Gland, Right M Superior Parathyroid Gland, Left N Inferior Parathyroid Gland, Right P Inferior Parathyroid Gland, Left Q Parathyroid Glands, Multiple R Parathyroid Gland	0 Open 4 Percutaneous Endoscopic	Z No Device	Z No Qualifier

0: M/S

G: ENDOCRINE SYSTEM

Q: REPAIR S: REPOSITION

◀ New   ◀▦ Revised   deleted Deleted   ♀ Females Only   ♂ Males Only
🅝ₒ Noncovered   🅛𝒸 Limited Coverage   🅗ₐ𝒸 Hospital-Acquired Condition   **Coding Clinic**

259

SECTION: 0 MEDICAL AND SURGICAL
BODY SYSTEM: G ENDOCRINE SYSTEM
OPERATION: T RESECTION: Cutting out or off, without replacement, all of a body part

Body Part	Approach	Device	Qualifier
0 Pituitary Gland 1 Pineal Body 2 Adrenal Gland, Left 3 Adrenal Gland, Right 4 Adrenal Glands, Bilateral 6 Carotid Body, Left 7 Carotid Body, Right 8 Carotid Bodies, Bilateral 9 Para-aortic Body B Coccygeal Glomus C Glomus Jugulare D Aortic Body F Paraganglion Extremity G Thyroid Gland Lobe, Left H Thyroid Gland Lobe, Right K Thyroid Gland L Superior Parathyroid Gland, Right M Superior Parathyroid Gland, Left N Inferior Parathyroid Gland, Right P Inferior Parathyroid Gland, Left Q Parathyroid Glands, Multiple R Parathyroid Gland	0 Open 4 Percutaneous Endoscopic	Z No Device	Z No Qualifier

SECTION: 0 MEDICAL AND SURGICAL
BODY SYSTEM: G ENDOCRINE SYSTEM
OPERATION: W REVISION: Correcting, to the extent possible, a portion of a malfunctioning device or the position of a displaced device

Body Part	Approach	Device	Qualifier
0 Pituitary Gland 1 Pineal Body 5 Adrenal Gland K Thyroid Gland R Parathyroid Gland	0 Open 3 Percutaneous 4 Percutaneous Endoscopic X External	0 Drainage Device	Z No Qualifier
S Endocrine Gland	0 Open 3 Percutaneous 4 Percutaneous Endoscopic X External	0 Drainage Device 2 Monitoring Device 3 Infusion Device	Z No Qualifier

◀ New　　◀▥ Revised　　~~deleted~~ Deleted　　♀ Females Only　　♂ Males Only
🅽🄲 Noncovered　　🄻🄲 Limited Coverage　　🄷🄰🄲 Hospital-Acquired Condition　　**Coding Clinic**

SECTION: 0 MEDICAL AND SURGICAL
BODY SYSTEM: **H SKIN AND BREAST**
OPERATION: **0 ALTERATION:** Modifying the anatomic structure of a body part without affecting the function of the body part

Body Part	Approach	Device	Qualifier
T Breast, Right U Breast, Left V Breast, Bilateral	0 Open 3 Percutaneous X External	7 Autologous Tissue Substitute J Synthetic Substitute K Nonautologous Tissue Substitute Z No Device	Z No Qualifier

SECTION: 0 MEDICAL AND SURGICAL
BODY SYSTEM: **H SKIN AND BREAST**
OPERATION: **2 CHANGE:** Taking out or off a device from a body part and putting back an identical or similar device in or on the same body part without cutting or puncturing the skin or a mucous membrane

Body Part	Approach	Device	Qualifier
P Skin T Breast, Right U Breast, Left	X External	0 Drainage Device Y Other Device	Z No Qualifier

◀ New ◀ Revised ~~deleted~~ Deleted ♀ Females Only ♂ Males Only
Noncovered Limited Coverage Hospital-Acquired Condition **Coding Clinic**

SECTION: 0 MEDICAL AND SURGICAL
BODY SYSTEM: H SKIN AND BREAST
OPERATION: 5 DESTRUCTION: Physical eradication of all or a portion of a body part by the direct use of energy, force, or a destructive agent

Body Part	Approach	Device	Qualifier
0 Skin, Scalp 1 Skin, Face 2 Skin, Right Ear 3 Skin, Left Ear 4 Skin, Neck 5 Skin, Chest 6 Skin, Back 7 Skin, Abdomen 8 Skin, Buttock 9 Skin, Perineum A Skin, Genitalia B Skin, Right Upper Arm C Skin, Left Upper Arm D Skin, Right Lower Arm E Skin, Left Lower Arm F Skin, Right Hand G Skin, Left Hand H Skin, Right Upper Leg J Skin, Left Upper Leg K Skin, Right Lower Leg L Skin, Left Lower Leg M Skin, Right Foot N Skin, Left Foot	X External	Z No Device	D Multiple Z No Qualifier
Q Finger Nail R Toe Nail	X External	Z No Device	Z No Qualifier
T Breast, Right U Breast, Left V Breast, Bilateral W Nipple, Right X Nipple, Left	0 Open 3 Percutaneous 7 Via Natural or Artificial Opening 8 Via Natural or Artificial Opening Endoscopic X External	Z No Device	Z No Qualifier

◀ New ◀◀ Revised ~~deleted~~ Deleted ♀ Females Only ♂ Males Only
⊗ Noncovered ⊗ Limited Coverage ⊗ Hospital-Acquired Condition **Coding Clinic**

263

SECTION: 0 MEDICAL AND SURGICAL
BODY SYSTEM: H SKIN AND BREAST
OPERATION: 8 **DIVISION:** Cutting into a body part, without draining fluids and/or gases from the body part, in order to separate or transect a body part

Body Part	Approach	Device	Qualifier
0 Skin, Scalp	X External	Z No Device	Z No Qualifier
1 Skin, Face			
2 Skin, Right Ear			
3 Skin, Left Ear			
4 Skin, Neck			
5 Skin, Chest			
6 Skin, Back			
7 Skin, Abdomen			
8 Skin, Buttock			
9 Skin, Perineum			
A Skin, Genitalia			
B Skin, Right Upper Arm			
C Skin, Left Upper Arm			
D Skin, Right Lower Arm			
E Skin, Left Lower Arm			
F Skin, Right Hand			
G Skin, Left Hand			
H Skin, Right Upper Leg			
J Skin, Left Upper Leg			
K Skin, Right Lower Leg			
L Skin, Left Lower Leg			
M Skin, Right Foot			
N Skin, Left Foot			

8: DIVISION

H: SKIN AND BREAST

0: M/S

◀ New   ◀▥ Revised   ~~deleted~~ Deleted   ♀ Females Only   ♂ Males Only
🦰 Noncovered   🦰 Limited Coverage   🦰 Hospital-Acquired Condition   **Coding Clinic**

SECTION: 0 MEDICAL AND SURGICAL
BODY SYSTEM: H SKIN AND BREAST
OPERATION: 9 DRAINAGE: *(on multiple pages)*
Taking or letting out fluids and/or gases from a body part

Body Part	Approach	Device	Qualifier
0 Skin, Scalp 1 Skin, Face 2 Skin, Right Ear 3 Skin, Left Ear 4 Skin, Neck 5 Skin, Chest 6 Skin, Back 7 Skin, Abdomen 8 Skin, Buttock 9 Skin, Perineum A Skin, Genitalia B Skin, Right Upper Arm C Skin, Left Upper Arm D Skin, Right Lower Arm E Skin, Left Lower Arm F Skin, Right Hand G Skin, Left Hand H Skin, Right Upper Leg J Skin, Left Upper Leg K Skin, Right Lower Leg L Skin, Left Lower Leg M Skin, Right Foot N Skin, Left Foot Q Finger Nail R Toe Nail	X External	0 Drainage Device	Z No Qualifier
0 Skin, Scalp 1 Skin, Face 2 Skin, Right Ear 3 Skin, Left Ear 4 Skin, Neck 5 Skin, Chest 6 Skin, Back 7 Skin, Abdomen 8 Skin, Buttock 9 Skin, Perineum A Skin, Genitalia B Skin, Right Upper Arm C Skin, Left Upper Arm D Skin, Right Lower Arm E Skin, Left Lower Arm F Skin, Right Hand G Skin, Left Hand H Skin, Right Upper Leg J Skin, Left Upper Leg K Skin, Right Lower Leg L Skin, Left Lower Leg M Skin, Right Foot N Skin, Left Foot Q Finger Nail R Toe Nail	X External	Z No Device	X Diagnostic Z No Qualifier

0: M/S

H: SKIN AND BREAST

9: DRAINAGE

◀ New   ◀▥ Revised   ~~deleted~~ Deleted   ♀ Females Only   ♂ Males Only
🅝 Noncovered   🅛 Limited Coverage   🅗 Hospital-Acquired Condition   **Coding Clinic**

265

SECTION: **0 MEDICAL AND SURGICAL**
BODY SYSTEM: H **SKIN AND BREAST**
OPERATION: 9 **DRAINAGE:** *(continued)*
Taking or letting out fluids and/or gases from a body part

Body Part	Approach	Device	Qualifier
T Breast, Right U Breast, Left V Breast, Bilateral W Nipple, Right X Nipple, Left	0 Open 3 Percutaneous 7 Via Natural or Artificial Opening 8 Via Natural or Artificial Opening Endoscopic X External	0 Drainage Device	Z No Qualifier
T Breast, Right U Breast, Left V Breast, Bilateral W Nipple, Right X Nipple, Left	0 Open 3 Percutaneous 7 Via Natural or Artificial Opening 8 Via Natural or Artificial Opening Endoscopic X External	Z No Device	X Diagnostic Z No Qualifier

SECTION: **0 MEDICAL AND SURGICAL**
BODY SYSTEM: H **SKIN AND BREAST**
OPERATION: B **EXCISION:** Cutting out or off, without replacement, a portion of a body part

Body Part	Approach	Device	Qualifier
0 Skin, Scalp 1 Skin, Face 2 Skin, Right Ear 3 Skin, Left Ear 4 Skin, Neck 5 Skin, Chest 6 Skin, Back 7 Skin, Abdomen 8 Skin, Buttock 9 Skin, Perineum A Skin, Genitalia B Skin, Right Upper Arm C Skin, Left Upper Arm D Skin, Right Lower Arm E Skin, Left Lower Arm F Skin, Right Hand G Skin, Left Hand H Skin, Right Upper Leg J Skin, Left Upper Leg K Skin, Right Lower Leg L Skin, Left Lower Leg M Skin, Right Foot N Skin, Left Foot Q Finger Nail R Toe Nail	X External	Z No Device	X Diagnostic Z No Qualifier
T Breast, Right U Breast, Left V Breast, Bilateral W Nipple, Right X Nipple, Left Y Supernumerary Breast	0 Open 3 Percutaneous 7 Via Natural or Artificial Opening 8 Via Natural or Artificial Opening Endoscopic X External	Z No Device	X Diagnostic Z No Qualifier

9: DRAINAGE   B: EXCISION   H: SKIN AND BREAST   0: M/S

◀ New   ◀◀◀ Revised   ~~deleted~~ Deleted   ♀ Females Only   ♂ Males Only
Noncovered   Limited Coverage   Hospital-Acquired Condition   **Coding Clinic**

SECTION: 0 MEDICAL AND SURGICAL
BODY SYSTEM: H SKIN AND BREAST
OPERATION: C EXTIRPATION: Taking or cutting out solid matter from a body part

Body Part	Approach	Device	Qualifier
0 Skin, Scalp 1 Skin, Face 2 Skin, Right Ear 3 Skin, Left Ear 4 Skin, Neck 5 Skin, Chest 6 Skin, Back 7 Skin, Abdomen 8 Skin, Buttock 9 Skin, Perineum A Skin, Genitalia B Skin, Right Upper Arm C Skin, Left Upper Arm D Skin, Right Lower Arm E Skin, Left Lower Arm F Skin, Right Hand G Skin, Left Hand H Skin, Right Upper Leg J Skin, Left Upper Leg K Skin, Right Lower Leg L Skin, Left Lower Leg M Skin, Right Foot N Skin, Left Foot Q Finger Nail R Toe Nail	X External	Z No Device	Z No Qualifier

T Breast, Right
U Breast, Left
V Breast, Bilateral
W Nipple, Right
X Nipple, Left
	0 Open
	3 Percutaneous
	7 Via Natural or Artificial
	   Opening
	8 Via Natural or Artificial
	   Opening Endoscopic
	X External
		Z No Device	Z No Qualifier

◀ New   ◀◀ Revised   deleted Deleted   ♀ Females Only   ♂ Males Only
Noncovered   Limited Coverage   Hospital-Acquired Condition   **Coding Clinic**

267

SECTION: 0 MEDICAL AND SURGICAL
BODY SYSTEM: H SKIN AND BREAST
OPERATION: D EXTRACTION: Pulling or stripping out or off all or a portion of a body part by the use of force

Body Part	Approach	Device	Qualifier
0 Skin, Scalp	X External	Z No Device	Z No Qualifier
1 Skin, Face			
2 Skin, Right Ear			
3 Skin, Left Ear			
4 Skin, Neck			
5 Skin, Chest			
6 Skin, Back			
7 Skin, Abdomen			
8 Skin, Buttock			
9 Skin, Perineum			
A Skin, Genitalia			
B Skin, Right Upper Arm			
C Skin, Left Upper Arm			
D Skin, Right Lower Arm			
E Skin, Left Lower Arm			
F Skin, Right Hand			
G Skin, Left Hand			
H Skin, Right Upper Leg			
J Skin, Left Upper Leg			
K Skin, Right Lower Leg			
L Skin, Left Lower Leg			
M Skin, Right Foot			
N Skin, Left Foot			
Q Finger Nail			
R Toe Nail			
S Hair			

SECTION: 0 MEDICAL AND SURGICAL
BODY SYSTEM: H SKIN AND BREAST
OPERATION: H INSERTION: Putting in a nonbiological appliance that monitors, assists, performs, or prevents a physiological function but does not physically take the place of a body part

Body Part	Approach	Device	Qualifier
T Breast, Right U Breast, Left V Breast, Bilateral W Nipple, Right X Nipple, Left	0 Open 3 Percutaneous 7 Via Natural or Artificial Opening 8 Via Natural or Artificial Opening Endoscopic	1 Radioactive Element N Tissue Expander	Z No Qualifier
T Breast, Right U Breast, Left V Breast, Bilateral W Nipple, Right X Nipple, Left	X External	1 Radioactive Element	Z No Qualifier

◀ New ◀ Revised deleted Deleted ♀ Females Only ♂ Males Only
Noncovered Limited Coverage Hospital-Acquired Condition Coding Clinic

SECTION: 0 MEDICAL AND SURGICAL
BODY SYSTEM: **H SKIN AND BREAST**
OPERATION: **J INSPECTION:** Visually and/or manually exploring a body part

Body Part	Approach	Device	Qualifier
P Skin Q Finger Nail R Toe Nail	X External	Z No Device	Z No Qualifier
T Breast, Right U Breast, Left	0 Open 3 Percutaneous 7 Via Natural or Artificial Opening 8 Via Natural or Artificial Opening Endoscopic X External	Z No Device	Z No Qualifier

SECTION: 0 MEDICAL AND SURGICAL
BODY SYSTEM: **H SKIN AND BREAST**
OPERATION: **M REATTACHMENT:** Putting back in or on all or a portion of a separated body part to its normal location or other suitable location

Body Part	Approach	Device	Qualifier
0 Skin, Scalp 1 Skin, Face 2 Skin, Right Ear 3 Skin, Left Ear 4 Skin, Neck 5 Skin, Chest 6 Skin, Back 7 Skin, Abdomen 8 Skin, Buttock 9 Skin, Perineum A Skin, Genitalia B Skin, Right Upper Arm C Skin, Left Upper Arm D Skin, Right Lower Arm E Skin, Left Lower Arm F Skin, Right Hand G Skin, Left Hand H Skin, Right Upper Leg J Skin, Left Upper Leg K Skin, Right Lower Leg L Skin, Left Lower Leg M Skin, Right Foot N Skin, Left Foot T Breast, Right U Breast, Left V Breast, Bilateral W Nipple, Right X Nipple, Left	X External	Z No Device	Z No Qualifier

◄ New ◄▥ Revised ~~deleted~~ Deleted ♀ Females Only ♂ Males Only
🔻 Noncovered 🔻 Limited Coverage 🔻 Hospital-Acquired Condition **Coding Clinic**

269

SECTION: 0 MEDICAL AND SURGICAL
BODY SYSTEM: H SKIN AND BREAST
OPERATION: N RELEASE: Freeing a body part from an abnormal physical constraint

Body Part	Approach	Device	Qualifier
0 Skin, Scalp 1 Skin, Face 2 Skin, Right Ear 3 Skin, Left Ear 4 Skin, Neck 5 Skin, Chest 6 Skin, Back 7 Skin, Abdomen 8 Skin, Buttock 9 Skin, Perineum A Skin, Genitalia B Skin, Right Upper Arm C Skin, Left Upper Arm D Skin, Right Lower Arm E Skin, Left Lower Arm F Skin, Right Hand G Skin, Left Hand H Skin, Right Upper Leg J Skin, Left Upper Leg K Skin, Right Lower Leg L Skin, Left Lower Leg M Skin, Right Foot N Skin, Left Foot Q Finger Nail R Toe Nail	X External	Z No Device	Z No Qualifier
T Breast, Right U Breast, Left V Breast, Bilateral W Nipple, Right X Nipple, Left	0 Open 3 Percutaneous 7 Via Natural or Artificial Opening 8 Via Natural or Artificial Opening Endoscopic X External	Z No Device	Z No Qualifier

◀ New ◀ Revised ~~deleted~~ Deleted ♀ Females Only ♂ Males Only
Noncovered Limited Coverage Hospital-Acquired Condition **Coding Clinic**

SECTION: 0 MEDICAL AND SURGICAL
BODY SYSTEM: H SKIN AND BREAST
OPERATION: P REMOVAL: Taking out or off a device from a body part

Body Part	Approach	Device	Qualifier
P Skin Q Finger Nail R Toe Nail	X External	0 Drainage Device 7 Autologous Tissue Substitute J Synthetic Substitute K Nonautologous Tissue Substitute	Z No Qualifier
S Hair	X External	7 Autologous Tissue Substitute J Synthetic Substitute K Nonautologous Tissue Substitute	Z No Qualifier
T Breast, Right U Breast, Left	0 Open 3 Percutaneous 7 Via Natural or Artificial Opening 8 Via Natural or Artificial Opening Endoscopic	0 Drainage Device 1 Radioactive Element 7 Autologous Tissue Substitute J Synthetic Substitute K Nonautologous Tissue Substitute N Tissue Expander	Z No Qualifier
T Breast, Right U Breast, Left	X External	0 Drainage Device 1 Radioactive Element 7 Autologous Tissue Substitute J Synthetic Substitute K Nonautologous Tissue Substitute	Z No Qualifier

◄ New ◄ Revised deleted Deleted ♀ Females Only ♂ Males Only
Noncovered Limited Coverage Hospital-Acquired Condition **Coding Clinic**

271

0: M/S

H: SKIN AND BREAST

P: REMOVAL

SECTION: 0 MEDICAL AND SURGICAL
BODY SYSTEM: H SKIN AND BREAST
OPERATION: Q REPAIR: Restoring, to the extent possible, a body part to its normal anatomic structure and function

Body Part	Approach	Device	Qualifier
0 Skin, Scalp 1 Skin, Face 2 Skin, Right Ear 3 Skin, Left Ear 4 Skin, Neck 5 Skin, Chest 6 Skin, Back 7 Skin, Abdomen 8 Skin, Buttock 9 Skin, Perineum A Skin, Genitalia B Skin, Right Upper Arm C Skin, Left Upper Arm D Skin, Right Lower Arm E Skin, Left Lower Arm F Skin, Right Hand G Skin, Left Hand H Skin, Right Upper Leg J Skin, Left Upper Leg K Skin, Right Lower Leg L Skin, Left Lower Leg M Skin, Right Foot N Skin, Left Foot Q Finger Nail R Toe Nail	X External	Z No Device	Z No Qualifier
T Breast, Right U Breast, Left V Breast, Bilateral W Nipple, Right X Nipple, Left Y Supernumerary Breast	0 Open 3 Percutaneous 7 Via Natural or Artificial Opening 8 Via Natural or Artificial Opening Endoscopic X External	Z No Device	Z No Qualifier

Q: REPAIR

H: SKIN AND BREAST

0: M/S

◀ New   ◀ Revised   ~~deleted~~ Deleted   ♀ Females Only   ♂ Males Only
Noncovered   Limited Coverage   Hospital-Acquired Condition   **Coding Clinic**

SECTION: 0 MEDICAL AND SURGICAL
BODY SYSTEM: H SKIN AND BREAST
OPERATION: R REPLACEMENT: *(on multiple pages)*
Putting in or on biological or synthetic material that physically takes the place and/or function of all or a portion of a body part

Body Part	Approach	Device	Qualifier
0 Skin, Scalp 1 Skin, Face 2 Skin, Right Ear 3 Skin, Left Ear 4 Skin, Neck 5 Skin, Chest 6 Skin, Back 7 Skin, Abdomen 8 Skin, Buttock 9 Skin, Perineum A Skin, Genitalia B Skin, Right Upper Arm C Skin, Left Upper Arm D Skin, Right Lower Arm E Skin, Left Lower Arm F Skin, Right Hand G Skin, Left Hand H Skin, Right Upper Leg J Skin, Left Upper Leg K Skin, Right Lower Leg L Skin, Left Lower Leg M Skin, Right Foot N Skin, Left Foot	X External	7 Autologous Tissue Substitute K Nonautologous Tissue Substitute	3 Full Thickness 4 Partial Thickness
0 Skin, Scalp 1 Skin, Face 2 Skin, Right Ear 3 Skin, Left Ear 4 Skin, Neck 5 Skin, Chest 6 Skin, Back 7 Skin, Abdomen 8 Skin, Buttock 9 Skin, Perineum A Skin, Genitalia B Skin, Right Upper Arm C Skin, Left Upper Arm D Skin, Right Lower Arm E Skin, Left Lower Arm F Skin, Right Hand G Skin, Left Hand H Skin, Right Upper Leg J Skin, Left Upper Leg K Skin, Right Lower Leg L Skin, Left Lower Leg M Skin, Right Foot N Skin, Left Foot	X External	J Synthetic Substitute	3 Full Thickness 4 Partial Thickness Z No Qualifier
Q Finger Nail R Toe Nail S Hair	X External	7 Autologous Tissue Substitute J Synthetic Substitute K Nonautologous Tissue Substitute	Z No Qualifier

◀ New ◀▬ Revised ~~deleted~~ Deleted ♀ Females Only ♂ Males Only
 Noncovered   Limited Coverage   Hospital-Acquired Condition   **Coding Clinic**

273

R: REPLACEMENT   S: REPOSITION

H: SKIN AND BREAST

0: M/S

SECTION: 0 MEDICAL AND SURGICAL
BODY SYSTEM: H SKIN AND BREAST
OPERATION: R REPLACEMENT: *(continued)*
Putting in or on biological or synthetic material that physically takes the place and/or function of all or a portion of a body part

Body Part	Approach	Device	Qualifier
T Breast, Right U Breast, Left V Breast, Bilateral	0 Open	7 Autologous Tissue Substitute	5 Latissimus Dorsi Myocutaneous Flap 6 Transverse Rectus Abdominis Myocutaneous Flap 7 Deep Inferior Epigastric Artery Perforator Flap 8 Superficial Inferior Epigastric Artery Flap 9 Gluteal Artery Perforator Flap Z No Qualifier
T Breast, Right U Breast, Left V Breast, Bilateral	0 Open	J Synthetic Substitute K Nonautologous Tissue Substitute	Z No Qualifier
T Breast, Right U Breast, Left V Breast, Bilateral	3 Percutaneous X External	7 Autologous Tissue Substitute J Synthetic Substitute K Nonautologous Tissue Substitute	Z No Qualifier
W Nipple, Right X Nipple, Left	0 Open 3 Percutaneous X External	7 Autologous Tissue Substitute J Synthetic Substitute K Nonautologous Tissue Substitute	Z No Qualifier

SECTION: 0 MEDICAL AND SURGICAL
BODY SYSTEM: H SKIN AND BREAST
OPERATION: S REPOSITION: Moving to its normal location, or other suitable location, all or a portion of a body part

Body Part	Approach	Device	Qualifier
S Hair W Nipple, Right X Nipple, Left	X External	Z No Device	Z No Qualifier
T Breast, Right U Breast, Left V Breast, Bilateral	0 Open	Z No Device	Z No Qualifier

◄ New   ◄ Revised   ~~deleted~~ Deleted   ♀ Females Only   ♂ Males Only
Ⓝ Noncovered   Ⓛ Limited Coverage   Ⓗ Hospital-Acquired Condition   **Coding Clinic**

SECTION: 0 MEDICAL AND SURGICAL
BODY SYSTEM: H SKIN AND BREAST
OPERATION: T RESECTION: Cutting out or off, without replacement, all of a body part

Body Part	Approach	Device	Qualifier
Q Finger Nail R Toe Nail W Nipple, Right X Nipple, Left	X External	Z No Device	Z No Qualifier
T Breast, Right U Breast, Left V Breast, Bilateral Y Supernumerary Breast	0 Open	Z No Device	Z No Qualifier

SECTION: 0 MEDICAL AND SURGICAL
BODY SYSTEM: H SKIN AND BREAST
OPERATION: U SUPPLEMENT: Putting in or on biological or synthetic material that physically reinforces and/or augments the function of a portion of a body part

Body Part	Approach	Device	Qualifier
T Breast, Right U Breast, Left V Breast, Bilateral W Nipple, Right X Nipple, Left	0 Open 3 Percutaneous 7 Via Natural of Artificial Opening 8 Via Natural or Artificial Opening Endoscopic X External	7 Autologous Tissue Substitute J Synthetic Substitute K Nonautologous Tissue Substitute	Z No Qualifier

◀ New   ◀▥ Revised   deleted Deleted   ♀ Females Only   ♂ Males Only
🚫 Noncovered   🚫 Limited Coverage   🚫 Hospital-Acquired Condition   **Coding Clinic**

275

SECTION: 0 MEDICAL AND SURGICAL
BODY SYSTEM: **H SKIN AND BREAST**
OPERATION: **W REVISION:** Correcting, to the extent possible, a portion of a malfunctioning device or the position of a displaced device

Body Part	Approach	Device	Qualifier
P Skin Q Finger Nail R Toe Nail	X External	0 Drainage Device 7 Autologous Tissue Substitute J Synthetic Substitute K Nonautologous Tissue Substitute	Z No Qualifier
S Hair	X External	7 Autologous Tissue Substitute J Synthetic Substitute K Nonautologous Tissue Substitute	Z No Qualifier
T Breast, Right U Breast, Left	0 Open 3 Percutaneous 7 Via Natural or Artificial Opening 8 Via Natural or Artificial Opening Endoscopic	0 Drainage Device 7 Autologous Tissue Substitute J Synthetic Substitute K Nonautologous Tissue Substitute N Tissue Expander	Z No Qualifier
T Breast, Right U Breast, Left	X External	0 Drainage Device 7 Autologous Tissue Substitute J Synthetic Substitute K Nonautologous Tissue Substitute	Z No Qualifier

SECTION: 0 MEDICAL AND SURGICAL
BODY SYSTEM: **H SKIN AND BREAST**
OPERATION: **X TRANSFER:** Moving, without taking out, all or a portion of a body part to another location to take over the function of all or a portion of a body part

Body Part	Approach	Device	Qualifier
0 Skin, Scalp 1 Skin, Face 2 Skin, Right Ear 3 Skin, Left Ear 4 Skin, Neck 5 Skin, Chest 6 Skin, Back 7 Skin, Abdomen 8 Skin, Buttock 9 Skin, Perineum A Skin, Genitalia B Skin, Right Upper Arm C Skin, Left Upper Arm D Skin, Right Lower Arm E Skin, Left Lower Arm F Skin, Right Hand G Skin, Left Hand H Skin, Right Upper Leg J Skin, Left Upper Leg K Skin, Right Lower Leg L Skin, Left Lower Leg M Skin, Right Foot N Skin, Left Foot	X External	Z No Device	Z No Qualifier

◀ New   ◀ Revised   ~~deleted~~ Deleted   ♀ Females Only   ♂ Males Only
Noncovered   Limited Coverage   Hospital-Acquired Condition   **Coding Clinic**

SECTION: 0 MEDICAL AND SURGICAL
BODY SYSTEM: J SUBCUTANEOUS TISSUE AND FASCIA
OPERATION: 0 **ALTERATION:** Modifying the anatomic structure of a body part without affecting the function of the body part

Body Part	Approach	Device	Qualifier
1 Subcutaneous Tissue and Fascia, Face	0 Open	Z No Device	Z No Qualifier
4 Subcutaneous Tissue and Fascia, Anterior Neck	3 Percutaneous		
5 Subcutaneous Tissue and Fascia, Posterior Neck			
6 Subcutaneous Tissue and Fascia, Chest			
7 Subcutaneous Tissue and Fascia, Back			
8 Subcutaneous Tissue and Fascia, Abdomen			
9 Subcutaneous Tissue and Fascia, Buttock			
D Subcutaneous Tissue and Fascia, Right Upper Arm			
F Subcutaneous Tissue and Fascia, Left Upper Arm			
G Subcutaneous Tissue and Fascia, Right Lower Arm			
H Subcutaneous Tissue and Fascia, Left Lower Arm			
L Subcutaneous Tissue and Fascia, Right Upper Leg			
M Subcutaneous Tissue and Fascia, Left Upper Leg			
N Subcutaneous Tissue and Fascia, Right Lower Leg			
P Subcutaneous Tissue and Fascia, Left Lower Leg			

SECTION: 0 MEDICAL AND SURGICAL
BODY SYSTEM: J SUBCUTANEOUS TISSUE AND FASCIA
OPERATION: 2 **CHANGE:** Taking out or off a device from a body part and putting back an identical or similar device in or on the same body part without cutting or puncturing the skin or a mucous membrane

Body Part	Approach	Device	Qualifier
S Subcutaneous Tissue and Fascia, Head and Neck	X External	0 Drainage Device	Z No Qualifier
T Subcutaneous Tissue and Fascia, Trunk		Y Other Device	
V Subcutaneous Tissue and Fascia, Upper Extremity			
W Subcutaneous Tissue and Fascia, Lower Extremity			

◀ New   ◀▥ Revised   ~~deleted~~ Deleted   ♀ Females Only   ♂ Males Only
🅝 Noncovered   🅛 Limited Coverage   🅗 Hospital-Acquired Condition   **Coding Clinic**

SECTION: 0 MEDICAL AND SURGICAL
BODY SYSTEM: J SUBCUTANEOUS TISSUE AND FASCIA
OPERATION: 5 **DESTRUCTION:** Physical eradication of all or a portion of a body part by the direct use of energy, force, or a destructive agent

Body Part	Approach	Device	Qualifier
0 Subcutaneous Tissue and Fascia, Scalp 1 Subcutaneous Tissue and Fascia, Face 4 Subcutaneous Tissue and Fascia, Anterior Neck 5 Subcutaneous Tissue and Fascia, Posterior Neck 6 Subcutaneous Tissue and Fascia, Chest 7 Subcutaneous Tissue and Fascia, Back 8 Subcutaneous Tissue and Fascia, Abdomen 9 Subcutaneous Tissue and Fascia, Buttock B Subcutaneous Tissue and Fascia, Perineum C Subcutaneous Tissue and Fascia, Pelvic Region D Subcutaneous Tissue and Fascia, Right Upper Arm F Subcutaneous Tissue and Fascia, Left Upper Arm G Subcutaneous Tissue and Fascia, Right Lower Arm H Subcutaneous Tissue and Fascia, Left Lower Arm J Subcutaneous Tissue and Fascia, Right Hand K Subcutaneous Tissue and Fascia, Left Hand L Subcutaneous Tissue and Fascia, Right Upper Leg M Subcutaneous Tissue and Fascia, Left Upper Leg N Subcutaneous Tissue and Fascia, Right Lower Leg P Subcutaneous Tissue and Fascia, Left Lower Leg Q Subcutaneous Tissue and Fascia, Right Foot R Subcutaneous Tissue and Fascia, Left Foot	0 Open 3 Percutaneous	Z No Device	Z No Qualifier

SECTION: 0 MEDICAL AND SURGICAL
BODY SYSTEM: J SUBCUTANEOUS TISSUE AND FASCIA
OPERATION: 8 **DIVISION:** Cutting into a body part, without draining fluids and/or gases from the body part, in order to separate or transect a body part

Body Part	Approach	Device	Qualifier
0 Subcutaneous Tissue and Fascia, Scalp	0 Open	Z No Device	Z No Qualifier
1 Subcutaneous Tissue and Fascia, Face	3 Percutaneous		
4 Subcutaneous Tissue and Fascia, Anterior Neck			
5 Subcutaneous Tissue and Fascia, Posterior Neck			
6 Subcutaneous Tissue and Fascia, Chest			
7 Subcutaneous Tissue and Fascia, Back			
8 Subcutaneous Tissue and Fascia, Abdomen			
9 Subcutaneous Tissue and Fascia, Buttock			
B Subcutaneous Tissue and Fascia, Perineum			
C Subcutaneous Tissue and Fascia, Pelvic Region			
D Subcutaneous Tissue and Fascia, Right Upper Arm			
F Subcutaneous Tissue and Fascia, Left Upper Arm			
G Subcutaneous Tissue and Fascia, Right Lower Arm			
H Subcutaneous Tissue and Fascia, Left Lower Arm			
J Subcutaneous Tissue and Fascia, Right Hand			
K Subcutaneous Tissue and Fascia, Left Hand			
L Subcutaneous Tissue and Fascia, Right Upper Leg			
M Subcutaneous Tissue and Fascia, Left Upper Leg			
N Subcutaneous Tissue and Fascia, Right Lower Leg			
P Subcutaneous Tissue and Fascia, Left Lower Leg			
Q Subcutaneous Tissue and Fascia, Right Foot			
R Subcutaneous Tissue and Fascia, Left Foot			
S Subcutaneous Tissue and Fascia, Head and Neck			
T Subcutaneous Tissue and Fascia, Trunk			
V Subcutaneous Tissue and Fascia, Upper Extremity			
W Subcutaneous Tissue and Fascia, Lower Extremity			

◀ New   ◀▥ Revised   ~~deleted~~ Deleted   ♀ Females Only   ♂ Males Only
⬚ Noncovered   ⬚ Limited Coverage   ⬚ Hospital-Acquired Condition   **Coding Clinic**

SECTION: 0 MEDICAL AND SURGICAL

BODY SYSTEM: J SUBCUTANEOUS TISSUE AND FASCIA
OPERATION: 9 DRAINAGE: *(on multiple pages)*
Taking or letting out fluids and/or gases from a body part

Body Part	Approach	Device	Qualifier
0 Subcutaneous Tissue and Fascia, Scalp	0 Open	0 Drainage Device	Z No Qualifier
1 Subcutaneous Tissue and Fascia, Face	3 Percutaneous		
4 Subcutaneous Tissue and Fascia, Anterior Neck			
5 Subcutaneous Tissue and Fascia, Posterior Neck			
6 Subcutaneous Tissue and Fascia, Chest			
7 Subcutaneous Tissue and Fascia, Back			
8 Subcutaneous Tissue and Fascia, Abdomen			
9 Subcutaneous Tissue and Fascia, Buttock			
B Subcutaneous Tissue and Fascia, Perineum			
C Subcutaneous Tissue and Fascia, Pelvic Region			
D Subcutaneous Tissue and Fascia, Right Upper Arm			
F Subcutaneous Tissue and Fascia, Left Upper Arm			
G Subcutaneous Tissue and Fascia, Right Lower Arm			
H Subcutaneous Tissue and Fascia, Left Lower Arm			
J Subcutaneous Tissue and Fascia, Right Hand			
K Subcutaneous Tissue and Fascia, Left Hand			
L Subcutaneous Tissue and Fascia, Right Upper Leg			
M Subcutaneous Tissue and Fascia, Left Upper Leg			
N Subcutaneous Tissue and Fascia, Right Lower Leg			
P Subcutaneous Tissue and Fascia, Left Lower Leg			
Q Subcutaneous Tissue and Fascia, Right Foot			
R Subcutaneous Tissue and Fascia, Left Foot			

0: M/S

J: SUBCUTANEOUS TISSUE AND FASCIA

9: DRAINAGE

◄ New　◄━ Revised　~~deleted~~ Deleted　♀ Females Only　♂ Males Only
🚱 Noncovered　🚱 Limited Coverage　🚱 Hospital-Acquired Condition　**Coding Clinic**

SECTION: 0 MEDICAL AND SURGICAL
BODY SYSTEM: J SUBCUTANEOUS TISSUE AND FASCIA
OPERATION: 9 DRAINAGE: *(continued)*
Taking or letting out fluids and/or gases from a body part

Body Part	Approach	Device	Qualifier
0 Subcutaneous Tissue and Fascia, Scalp	0 Open	Z No Device	X Diagnostic
1 Subcutaneous Tissue and Fascia, Face	3 Percutaneous		Z No Qualifier
4 Subcutaneous Tissue and Fascia, Anterior Neck			
5 Subcutaneous Tissue and Fascia, Posterior Neck			
6 Subcutaneous Tissue and Fascia, Chest			
7 Subcutaneous Tissue and Fascia, Back			
8 Subcutaneous Tissue and Fascia, Abdomen			
9 Subcutaneous Tissue and Fascia, Buttock			
B Subcutaneous Tissue and Fascia, Perineum			
C Subcutaneous Tissue and Fascia, Pelvic Region			
D Subcutaneous Tissue and Fascia, Right Upper Arm			
F Subcutaneous Tissue and Fascia, Left Upper Arm			
G Subcutaneous Tissue and Fascia, Right Lower Arm			
H Subcutaneous Tissue and Fascia, Left Lower Arm			
J Subcutaneous Tissue and Fascia, Right Hand			
K Subcutaneous Tissue and Fascia, Left Hand			
L Subcutaneous Tissue and Fascia, Right Upper Leg			
M Subcutaneous Tissue and Fascia, Left Upper Leg			
N Subcutaneous Tissue and Fascia, Right Lower Leg			
P Subcutaneous Tissue and Fascia, Left Lower Leg			
Q Subcutaneous Tissue and Fascia, Right Foot			
R Subcutaneous Tissue and Fascia, Left Foot			

◀ New ◀ Revised deleted Deleted ♀ Females Only ♂ Males Only
Noncovered Limited Coverage Hospital-Acquired Condition **Coding Clinic**

SECTION: 0 MEDICAL AND SURGICAL
BODY SYSTEM: J SUBCUTANEOUS TISSUE AND FASCIA
OPERATION: B EXCISION: Cutting out or off, without replacement, a portion of a body part

Body Part	Approach	Device	Qualifier
0 Subcutaneous Tissue and Fascia, Scalp	0 Open	Z No Device	X Diagnostic
1 Subcutaneous Tissue and Fascia, Face	3 Percutaneous		Z No Qualifier
4 Subcutaneous Tissue and Fascia, Anterior Neck			
5 Subcutaneous Tissue and Fascia, Posterior Neck			
6 Subcutaneous Tissue and Fascia, Chest			
7 Subcutaneous Tissue and Fascia, Back			
8 Subcutaneous Tissue and Fascia, Abdomen			
9 Subcutaneous Tissue and Fascia, Buttock			
B Subcutaneous Tissue and Fascia, Perineum			
C Subcutaneous Tissue and Fascia, Pelvic Region			
D Subcutaneous Tissue and Fascia, Right Upper Arm			
F Subcutaneous Tissue and Fascia, Left Upper Arm			
G Subcutaneous Tissue and Fascia, Right Lower Arm			
H Subcutaneous Tissue and Fascia, Left Lower Arm			
J Subcutaneous Tissue and Fascia, Right Hand			
K Subcutaneous Tissue and Fascia, Left Hand			
L Subcutaneous Tissue and Fascia, Right Upper Leg			
M Subcutaneous Tissue and Fascia, Left Upper Leg			
N Subcutaneous Tissue and Fascia, Right Lower Leg			
P Subcutaneous Tissue and Fascia, Left Lower Leg			
Q Subcutaneous Tissue and Fascia, Right Foot			
R Subcutaneous Tissue and Fascia, Left Foot			

◀ New ◀ Revised ~~deleted~~ Deleted ♀ Females Only ♂ Males Only
Noncovered Limited Coverage Hospital-Acquired Condition **Coding Clinic**

SECTION: 0 MEDICAL AND SURGICAL
BODY SYSTEM: J SUBCUTANEOUS TISSUE AND FASCIA
OPERATION: C EXTIRPATION: Taking or cutting out solid matter from a body part

Body Part	Approach	Device	Qualifier
0 Subcutaneous Tissue and Fascia, Scalp	0 Open	Z No Device	Z No Qualifier
1 Subcutaneous Tissue and Fascia, Face	3 Percutaneous		
4 Subcutaneous Tissue and Fascia, Anterior Neck			
5 Subcutaneous Tissue and Fascia, Posterior Neck			
6 Subcutaneous Tissue and Fascia, Chest			
7 Subcutaneous Tissue and Fascia, Back			
8 Subcutaneous Tissue and Fascia, Abdomen			
9 Subcutaneous Tissue and Fascia, Buttock			
B Subcutaneous Tissue and Fascia, Perineum			
C Subcutaneous Tissue and Fascia, Pelvic Region			
D Subcutaneous Tissue and Fascia, Right Upper Arm			
F Subcutaneous Tissue and Fascia, Left Upper Arm			
G Subcutaneous Tissue and Fascia, Right Lower Arm			
H Subcutaneous Tissue and Fascia, Left Lower Arm			
J Subcutaneous Tissue and Fascia, Right Hand			
K Subcutaneous Tissue and Fascia, Left Hand			
L Subcutaneous Tissue and Fascia, Right Upper Leg			
M Subcutaneous Tissue and Fascia, Left Upper Leg			
N Subcutaneous Tissue and Fascia, Right Lower Leg			
P Subcutaneous Tissue and Fascia, Left Lower Leg			
Q Subcutaneous Tissue and Fascia, Right Foot			
R Subcutaneous Tissue and Fascia, Left Foot			

◀ New   ◀▥ Revised   ~~deleted~~ Deleted   ♀ Females Only   ♂ Males Only
🅝 Noncovered   🅛 Limited Coverage   🅗 Hospital-Acquired Condition   **Coding Clinic**

SECTION: 0 MEDICAL AND SURGICAL
BODY SYSTEM: J SUBCUTANEOUS TISSUE AND FASCIA
OPERATION: D **EXTRACTION:** Pulling or stripping out or off all or a portion of a body part by the use of force

Body Part	Approach	Device	Qualifier
0 Subcutaneous Tissue and Fascia, Scalp	0 Open	Z No Device	Z No Qualifier
1 Subcutaneous Tissue and Fascia, Face	3 Percutaneous		
4 Subcutaneous Tissue and Fascia, Anterior Neck			
5 Subcutaneous Tissue and Fascia, Posterior Neck			
6 Subcutaneous Tissue and Fascia, Chest			
7 Subcutaneous Tissue and Fascia, Back			
8 Subcutaneous Tissue and Fascia, Abdomen			
9 Subcutaneous Tissue and Fascia, Buttock			
B Subcutaneous Tissue and Fascia, Perineum			
C Subcutaneous Tissue and Fascia, Pelvic Region			
D Subcutaneous Tissue and Fascia, Right Upper Arm			
F Subcutaneous Tissue and Fascia, Left Upper Arm			
G Subcutaneous Tissue and Fascia, Right Lower Arm			
H Subcutaneous Tissue and Fascia, Left Lower Arm			
J Subcutaneous Tissue and Fascia, Right Hand			
K Subcutaneous Tissue and Fascia, Left Hand			
L Subcutaneous Tissue and Fascia, Right Upper Leg			
M Subcutaneous Tissue and Fascia, Left Upper Leg			
N Subcutaneous Tissue and Fascia, Right Lower Leg			
P Subcutaneous Tissue and Fascia, Left Lower Leg			
Q Subcutaneous Tissue and Fascia, Right Foot			
R Subcutaneous Tissue and Fascia, Left Foot			

◀ New ◀▥ Revised ~~deleted~~ Deleted ♀ Females Only ♂ Males Only
🜹 Noncovered 🜹 Limited Coverage 🜹 Hospital-Acquired Condition **Coding Clinic**

SECTION: 0 MEDICAL AND SURGICAL
BODY SYSTEM: J SUBCUTANEOUS TISSUE AND FASCIA
OPERATION: H INSERTION: *(on multiple pages)*

Putting in a nonbiological appliance that monitors, assists, performs, or prevents a physiological function but does not physically take the place of a body part

Body Part	Approach	Device	Qualifier
0 Subcutaneous Tissue and Fascia, Scalp 1 Subcutaneous Tissue and Fascia, Face 4 Subcutaneous Tissue and Fascia, Anterior Neck 5 Subcutaneous Tissue and Fascia, Posterior Neck 9 Subcutaneous Tissue and Fascia, Buttock B Subcutaneous Tissue and Fascia, Perineum C Subcutaneous Tissue and Fascia, Pelvic Region J Subcutaneous Tissue and Fascia, Right Hand K Subcutaneous Tissue and Fascia, Left Hand Q Subcutaneous Tissue and Fascia, Right Foot R Subcutaneous Tissue and Fascia, Left Foot	0 Open 3 Percutaneous	N Tissue Expander	Z No Qualifer
6 Subcutaneous Tissue and Fascia, Chest 8 Subcutaneous Tissue and Fascia, Abdomen	0 Open 3 Percutaneous	0 Monitoring Device, Hemodynamic 2 Monitoring Device 4 Pacemaker, Single Chamber 🔹 5 Pacemaker, Single Chamber Rate Responsive 🔹 6 Pacemaker, Dual Chamber 🔹 7 Cardiac Resynchronization Pacemaker Pulse Generator 🔹 8 Defibrillator Generator 🔹 9 Cardiac Resynchronization Defibrillator Pulse Generator 🔹 A Contractility Modulation Device B Stimulator Generator, Single Array C Stimulator Generator, Single Array Rechargeable D Stimulator Generator, Multiple Array E Stimulator Generator, Multiple Array Rechargeable H Contraceptive Device M Stimulator Generator 🔹 N Tissue Expander P Cardiac Rhythm Related Device 🔹 V Infusion Device, Pump W Vascular Access Device, Reservoir X Vascular Access Device 🔹	Z No Qualifier

◀ New ◀ Revised ~~deleted~~ Deleted ♀ Females Only ♂ Males Only
🔹 Noncovered 🔹 Limited Coverage 🔹 Hospital-Acquired Condition **Coding Clinic**

SECTION: 0 MEDICAL AND SURGICAL
BODY SYSTEM: J SUBCUTANEOUS TISSUE AND FASCIA
OPERATION: H INSERTION: *(continued)*

Putting in a nonbiological appliance that monitors, assists, performs, or prevents a physiological function but does not physically take the place of a body part

Body Part	Approach	Device	Qualifier
7 Subcutaneous Tissue and Fascia, Back	0 Open 3 Percutaneous	B Stimulator Generator, Single Array C Stimulator Generator, Single Array Rechargeable D Stimulator Generator, Multiple Array E Stimulator Generator, Multiple Array Rechargeable M Stimulator Generator 🚫 N Tissue Expander V Infusion Device, Pump	Z No Qualifier
D Subcutaneous Tissue and Fascia, Right Upper Arm F Subcutaneous Tissue and Fascia, Left Upper Arm G Subcutaneous Tissue and Fascia, Right Lower Arm H Subcutaneous Tissue and Fascia, Left Lower Arm L Subcutaneous Tissue and Fascia, Right Upper Leg M Subcutaneous Tissue and Fascia, Left Upper Leg N Subcutaneous Tissue and Fascia, Right Lower Leg P Subcutaneous Tissue and Fascia, Left Lower Leg	0 Open 3 Percutaneous	H Contraceptive Device N Tissue Expander V Infusion Pump W Reservoir X Vascular Access Device	Z No Qualifier
S Subcutaneous Tissue and Fascia, Head and Neck V Subcutaneous Tissue and Fascia, Upper Extremity W Subcutaneous Tissue and Fascia, Lower Extremity	0 Open 3 Percutaneous	1 Radioactive Element 3 Infusion Device	Z No Qualifier
T Subcutaneous Tissue and Fascia, Trunk	0 Open 3 Percutaneous	1 Radioactive Element 3 Infusion Device V Infusion Pump	Z No Qualifier

Coding Clinic: 2012, Q4, P105 – 0JH608Z & 0JH60PZ

SECTION: 0 MEDICAL AND SURGICAL
BODY SYSTEM: J SUBCUTANEOUS TISSUE AND FASCIA
OPERATION: J INSPECTION: Visually and/or manually exploring a body part

Body Part	Approach	Device	Qualifier
S Subcutaneous Tissue and Fascia, Head and Neck T Subcutaneous Tissue and Fascia, Trunk V Subcutaneous Tissue and Fascia, Upper Extremity W Subcutaneous Tissue and Fascia, Lower Extremity	0 Open 3 Percutaneous X External	Z No Device	Z No Qualifier

◀ New   ◀▥ Revised   ~~deleted~~ Deleted   ♀ Females Only   ♂ Males Only
🚫 Noncovered   🚫 Limited Coverage   🚫 Hospital-Acquired Condition   **Coding Clinic**

SECTION: 0 MEDICAL AND SURGICAL
BODY SYSTEM: J SUBCUTANEOUS TISSUE AND FASCIA
OPERATION: N RELEASE: Freeing a body part from an abnormal physical constraint by cutting or by the use of force

Body Part	Approach	Device	Qualifier
0 Subcutaneous Tissue and Fascia, Scalp	0 Open	Z No Device	Z No Qualifier
1 Subcutaneous Tissue and Fascia, Face	3 Percutaneous		
4 Subcutaneous Tissue and Fascia, Anterior Neck	X External		
5 Subcutaneous Tissue and Fascia, Posterior Neck			
6 Subcutaneous Tissue and Fascia, Chest			
7 Subcutaneous Tissue and Fascia, Back			
8 Subcutaneous Tissue and Fascia, Abdomen			
9 Subcutaneous Tissue and Fascia, Buttock			
B Subcutaneous Tissue and Fascia, Perineum			
C Subcutaneous Tissue and Fascia, Pelvic Region			
D Subcutaneous Tissue and Fascia, Right Upper Arm			
F Subcutaneous Tissue and Fascia, Left Upper Arm			
G Subcutaneous Tissue and Fascia, Right Lower Arm			
H Subcutaneous Tissue and Fascia, Left Lower Arm			
J Subcutaneous Tissue and Fascia, Right Hand			
K Subcutaneous Tissue and Fascia, Left Hand			
L Subcutaneous Tissue and Fascia, Right Upper Leg			
M Subcutaneous Tissue and Fascia, Left Upper Leg			
N Subcutaneous Tissue and Fascia, Right Lower Leg			
P Subcutaneous Tissue and Fascia, Left Lower Leg			
Q Subcutaneous Tissue and Fascia, Right Foot			
R Subcutaneous Tissue and Fascia, Left Foot			

◀ New   ◀ Revised   ~~deleted~~ Deleted   ♀ Females Only   ♂ Males Only
Noncovered   Limited Coverage   Hospital-Acquired Condition   **Coding Clinic**

SECTION: 0 MEDICAL AND SURGICAL
BODY SYSTEM: J SUBCUTANEOUS TISSUE AND FASCIA
OPERATION: P REMOVAL: Taking out or off a device from a body part

Body Part	Approach	Device	Qualifier
S Subcutaneous Tissue and Fascia, Head and Neck	0 Open 3 Percutaneous	0 Drainage Device 1 Radioactive Element 3 Infusion Device 7 Autologous Tissue Substitute J Synthetic Substitute K Nonautologous Tissue Substitute N Tissue Expander	Z No Qualifier
S Subcutaneous Tissue and Fascia, Head and Neck	X External	0 Drainage Device 1 Radioactive Element 3 Infusion Device	Z No Qualifier
T Subcutaneous Tissue and Fascia, Trunk	0 Open 3 Percutaneous	0 Drainage Device 1 Radioactive Element 2 Monitoring Device 3 Infusion Device 7 Autologous Tissue Substitute H Contraceptive Device J Synthetic Substitute K Nonautologous Tissue Substitute M Stimulator Generator N Tissue Expander P Cardiac Rhythm Related Device V Infusion Device, Pump W Vascular Access Device, Reservoir X Vascular Access Device	Z No Qualifier
T Subcutaneous Tissue and Fascia, Trunk	X External	0 Drainage Device 1 Radioactive Element 2 Monitoring Device 3 Infusion Device H Contraceptive Device V Infusion Device, Pump X Vascular Access Device	Z No Qualifier
V Subcutaneous Tissue and Fascia, Upper Extremity W Subcutaneous Tissue and Fascia, Lower Extremity	0 Open 3 Percutaneous	0 Drainage Device 1 Radioactive Element 3 Infusion Device 7 Autologous Tissue Substitute H Contraceptive Device J Synthetic Substitute K Nonautologous Tissue Substitute N Tissue Expander V Infusion Device, Pump W Vascular Access Device, Reservoir X Vascular Access Device	Z No Qualifier
V Subcutaneous Tissue and Fascia, Upper Extremity W Subcutaneous Tissue and Fascia, Lower Extremity	X External	0 Drainage Device 1 Radioactive Element 3 Infusion Device H Contraceptive Device V Infusion Pump X Vascular Access Device	Z No Qualifier

Coding Clinic: 2012, Q4, P105 – 0JPT0PZ

◄ New   ◄▥ Revised   deleted Deleted   ♀ Females Only   ♂ Males Only
 Noncovered   Limited Coverage   Hospital-Acquired Condition   **Coding Clinic**

SECTION: 0 MEDICAL AND SURGICAL
BODY SYSTEM: J SUBCUTANEOUS TISSUE AND FASCIA
OPERATION: Q REPAIR: Restoring, to the extent possible, a body part to its normal anatomic structure and function

Body Part	Approach	Device	Qualifier
0 Subcutaneous Tissue and Fascia, Scalp	0 Open	Z No Device	Z No Qualifier
1 Subcutaneous Tissue and Fascia, Face	3 Percutaneous		
4 Subcutaneous Tissue and Fascia, Anterior Neck			
5 Subcutaneous Tissue and Fascia, Posterior Neck			
6 Subcutaneous Tissue and Fascia, Chest			
7 Subcutaneous Tissue and Fascia, Back			
8 Subcutaneous Tissue and Fascia, Abdomen			
9 Subcutaneous Tissue and Fascia, Buttock			
B Subcutaneous Tissue and Fascia, Perineum			
C Subcutaneous Tissue and Fascia, Pelvic Region			
D Subcutaneous Tissue and Fascia, Right Upper Arm			
F Subcutaneous Tissue and Fascia, Left Upper Arm			
G Subcutaneous Tissue and Fascia, Right Lower Arm			
H Subcutaneous Tissue and Fascia, Left Lower Arm			
J Subcutaneous Tissue and Fascia, Right Hand			
K Subcutaneous Tissue and Fascia, Left Hand			
L Subcutaneous Tissue and Fascia, Right Upper Leg			
M Subcutaneous Tissue and Fascia, Left Upper Leg			
N Subcutaneous Tissue and Fascia, Right Lower Leg			
P Subcutaneous Tissue and Fascia, Left Lower Leg			
Q Subcutaneous Tissue and Fascia, Right Foot			
R Subcutaneous Tissue and Fascia, Left Foot			

Q: REPAIR

J: SUBCUTANEOUS TISSUE AND FASCIA

0: M/S

◀ New ◀▥ Revised ~~deleted~~ Deleted ♀ Females Only ♂ Males Only
Ⓝ Noncovered Ⓛ Limited Coverage Ⓗ Hospital-Acquired Condition **Coding Clinic**

SECTION: 0 MEDICAL AND SURGICAL
BODY SYSTEM: J SUBCUTANEOUS TISSUE AND FASCIA
OPERATION: R REPLACEMENT: Putting in or on biological or synthetic material that physically takes the place and/or function of all or a portion of a body part

Body Part	Approach	Device	Qualifier
0 Subcutaneous Tissue and Fascia, Scalp	0 Open	7 Autologous Tissue Substitute	Z No Qualifier
1 Subcutaneous Tissue and Fascia, Face	3 Percutaneous	J Synthetic Substitute	
4 Subcutaneous Tissue and Fascia, Anterior Neck		K Nonautologous Tissue Substitute	
5 Subcutaneous Tissue and Fascia, Posterior Neck			
6 Subcutaneous Tissue and Fascia, Chest			
7 Subcutaneous Tissue and Fascia, Back			
8 Subcutaneous Tissue and Fascia, Abdomen			
9 Subcutaneous Tissue and Fascia, Buttock			
B Subcutaneous Tissue and Fascia, Perineum			
C Subcutaneous Tissue and Fascia, Pelvic Region			
D Subcutaneous Tissue and Fascia, Right Upper Arm			
F Subcutaneous Tissue and Fascia, Left Upper Arm			
G Subcutaneous Tissue and Fascia, Right Lower Arm			
H Subcutaneous Tissue and Fascia, Left Lower Arm			
J Subcutaneous Tissue and Fascia, Right Hand			
K Subcutaneous Tissue and Fascia, Left Hand			
L Subcutaneous Tissue and Fascia, Right Upper Leg			
M Subcutaneous Tissue and Fascia, Left Upper Leg			
N Subcutaneous Tissue and Fascia, Right Lower Leg			
P Subcutaneous Tissue and Fascia, Left Lower Leg			
Q Subcutaneous Tissue and Fascia, Right Foot			
R Subcutaneous Tissue and Fascia, Left Foot			

0: M/S

J: SUBCUTANEOUS TISSUE AND FASCIA

R: REPLACEMENT

SECTION: 0 MEDICAL AND SURGICAL
BODY SYSTEM: J SUBCUTANEOUS TISSUE AND FASCIA
OPERATION: U SUPPLEMENT: Putting in or on biological or synthetic material that physically reinforces and/or augments the function of a portion of a body part

Body Part	Approach	Device	Qualifier
0 Subcutaneous Tissue and Fascia, Scalp	0 Open	7 Autologous Tissue Substitute	Z No Qualifier
1 Subcutaneous Tissue and Fascia, Face	3 Percutaneous	J Synthetic Substitute	
4 Subcutaneous Tissue and Fascia, Anterior Neck		K Nonautologous Tissue Substitute	
5 Subcutaneous Tissue and Fascia, Posterior Neck			
6 Subcutaneous Tissue and Fascia, Chest			
7 Subcutaneous Tissue and Fascia, Back			
8 Subcutaneous Tissue and Fascia, Abdomen			
9 Subcutaneous Tissue and Fascia, Buttock			
B Subcutaneous Tissue and Fascia, Perineum			
C Subcutaneous Tissue and Fascia, Pelvic Region			
D Subcutaneous Tissue and Fascia, Right Upper Arm			
F Subcutaneous Tissue and Fascia, Left Upper Arm			
G Subcutaneous Tissue and Fascia, Right Lower Arm			
H Subcutaneous Tissue and Fascia, Left Lower Arm			
J Subcutaneous Tissue and Fascia, Right Hand			
K Subcutaneous Tissue and Fascia, Left Hand			
L Subcutaneous Tissue and Fascia, Right Upper Leg			
M Subcutaneous Tissue and Fascia, Left Upper Leg			
N Subcutaneous Tissue and Fascia, Right Lower Leg			
P Subcutaneous Tissue and Fascia, Left Lower Leg			
Q Subcutaneous Tissue and Fascia, Right Foot			
R Subcutaneous Tissue and Fascia, Left Foot			

◀ New ◀▥ Revised ~~deleted~~ Deleted ♀ Females Only ♂ Males Only
Noncovered Limited Coverage Hospital-Acquired Condition **Coding Clinic**

SECTION: 0 MEDICAL AND SURGICAL
BODY SYSTEM: J SUBCUTANEOUS TISSUE AND FASCIA
OPERATION: W REVISION: Correcting, to the extent possible, a portion of a malfunctioning device or the position of a displaced device

Body Part	Approach	Device	Qualifier
S Subcutaneous Tissue and Fascia, Head and Neck	0 Open 3 Percutaneous X External	0 Drainage Device 3 Infusion Device 7 Autologous Tissue Substitute J Synthetic Substitute K Nonautologous Tissue Substitute N Tissue Expander	Z No Qualifier
T Subcutaneous Tissue and Fascia, Trunk	0 Open 🐾 3 Percutaneous 🐾 X External	0 Drainage Device 2 Monitoring Device 3 Infusion Device 7 Autologous Tissue Substitute H Contraceptive Device J Synthetic Substitute K Nonautologous Tissue Substitute M Stimulator Generator N Tissue Expander P Cardiac Rhythm Related Device V Infusion Device, Pump W Vascular Access Device, Reservoir X Vascular Access Device	Z No Qualifier
V Subcutaneous Tissue and Fascia, Upper Extremity W Subcutaneous Tissue and Fascia, Lower Extremity	0 Open 3 Percutaneous X External	0 Drainage Device 3 Infusion Device 7 Autologous Tissue Substitute H Contraceptive Device J Synthetic Substitute K Nonautologous Tissue Substitute N Tissue Expander V Infusion Device, Pump W Vascular Access Device, Reservoir X Vascular Access Device	Z No Qualifier

🐾 0JWT0PZ, 0JWT3PZ

Coding Clinic: 2012, Q4, P106 – 0JWT0PZ

◀ New   ◀▥ Revised   ~~deleted~~ Deleted   ♀ Females Only   ♂ Males Only
🐾 Noncovered   🐾 Limited Coverage   🐾 Hospital-Acquired Condition   **Coding Clinic**

SECTION: 0 MEDICAL AND SURGICAL
BODY SYSTEM: J SUBCUTANEOUS TISSUE AND FASCIA
OPERATION: X TRANSFER: Moving, without taking out, all or a portion of a body part to another location to take over the function of all or a portion of a body part

Body Part	Approach	Device	Qualifier
0 Subcutaneous Tissue and Fascia, Scalp 1 Subcutaneous Tissue and Fascia, Face 4 Subcutaneous Tissue and Fascia, Anterior Neck 5 Subcutaneous Tissue and Fascia, Posterior Neck 6 Subcutaneous Tissue and Fascia, Chest 7 Subcutaneous Tissue and Fascia, Back 8 Subcutaneous Tissue and Fascia, Abdomen 9 Subcutaneous Tissue and Fascia, Buttock B Subcutaneous Tissue and Fascia, Perineum C Subcutaneous Tissue and Fascia, Pelvic Region D Subcutaneous Tissue and Fascia, Right Upper Arm F Subcutaneous Tissue and Fascia, Left Upper Arm G Subcutaneous Tissue and Fascia, Right Lower Arm H Subcutaneous Tissue and Fascia, Left Lower Arm J Subcutaneous Tissue and Fascia, Right Hand K Subcutaneous Tissue and Fascia, Left Hand L Subcutaneous Tissue and Fascia, Right Upper Leg M Subcutaneous Tissue and Fascia, Left Upper Leg N Subcutaneous Tissue and Fascia, Right Lower Leg P Subcutaneous Tissue and Fascia, Left Lower Leg Q Subcutaneous Tissue and Fascia, Right Foot R Subcutaneous Tissue and Fascia, Left Foot	0 Open 3 Percutaneous	Z No Device	B Skin and Subcutaneous Tissue C Skin, Subcutaneous Tissue and Fascia Z No Qualifier

◀ New   ◀▥ Revised   ~~deleted~~ Deleted   ♀ Females Only   ♂ Males Only
⬀ Noncovered   ⬀ Limited Coverage   ⬀ Hospital-Acquired Condition   **Coding Clinic**

SECTION: 0 MEDICAL AND SURGICAL

BODY SYSTEM: K MUSCLES

OPERATION: 2 CHANGE: Taking out or off a device from a body part and putting back an identical or similar device in or on the same body part without cutting or puncturing the skin or a mucous membrane

Body Part	Approach	Device	Qualifier
X Upper Muscle Y Lower Muscle	X External	0 Drainage Device Y Other Device	Z No Qualifier

SECTION: 0 MEDICAL AND SURGICAL

BODY SYSTEM: K MUSCLES

OPERATION: 5 DESTRUCTION: Physical eradication of all or a portion of a body part by the direct use of energy, force, or a destructive agent

Body Part	Approach	Device	Qualifier
0 Head Muscle 1 Facial Muscle 2 Neck Muscle, Right 3 Neck Muscle, Left 4 Tongue, Palate, Pharynx Muscle 5 Shoulder Muscle, Right 6 Shoulder Muscle, Left 7 Upper Arm Muscle, Right 8 Upper Arm Muscle, Left 9 Lower Arm and Wrist Muscle, Right B Lower Arm and Wrist Muscle, Left C Hand Muscle, Right D Hand Muscle, Left F Trunk Muscle, Right G Trunk Muscle, Left H Thorax Muscle, Right J Thorax Muscle, Left K Abdomen Muscle, Right L Abdomen Muscle, Left M Perineum Muscle N Hip Muscle, Right P Hip Muscle, Left Q Upper Leg Muscle, Right R Upper Leg Muscle, Left S Lower Leg Muscle, Right T Lower Leg Muscle, Left V Foot Muscle, Right W Foot Muscle, Left	0 Open 3 Percutaneous 4 Percutaneous Endoscopic	Z No Device	Z No Qualifier

New ◄ Revised deleted Deleted ♀ Females Only ♂ Males Only
Noncovered Limited Coverage Hospital-Acquired Condition Coding Clinic

SECTION: 0 MEDICAL AND SURGICAL
BODY SYSTEM: K MUSCLES
OPERATION: 8 DIVISION: Cutting into a body part, without draining fluids and/or gases from the body part, in order to separate or transect a body part

Body Part	Approach	Device	Qualifier
0 Head Muscle	0 Open	Z No Device	Z No Qualifier
1 Facial Muscle	3 Percutaneous		
2 Neck Muscle, Right	4 Percutaneous Endoscopic		
3 Neck Muscle, Left			
4 Tongue, Palate, Pharynx Muscle			
5 Shoulder Muscle, Right			
6 Shoulder Muscle, Left			
7 Upper Arm Muscle, Right			
8 Upper Arm Muscle, Left			
9 Lower Arm and Wrist Muscle, Right			
B Lower Arm and Wrist Muscle, Left			
C Hand Muscle, Right			
D Hand Muscle, Left			
F Trunk Muscle, Right			
G Trunk Muscle, Left			
H Thorax Muscle, Right			
J Thorax Muscle, Left			
K Abdomen Muscle, Right			
L Abdomen Muscle, Left			
M Perineum Muscle			
N Hip Muscle, Right			
P Hip Muscle, Left			
Q Upper Leg Muscle, Right			
R Upper Leg Muscle, Left			
S Lower Leg Muscle, Right			
T Lower Leg Muscle, Left			
V Foot Muscle, Right			
W Foot Muscle, Left			

0: M/S

K: MUSCLES

8: DIVISION

SECTION: 0 MEDICAL AND SURGICAL
BODY SYSTEM: K MUSCLES
OPERATION: 9 DRAINAGE: *(on multiple pages)*
　　　　　　　　Taking or letting out fluids and/or gases from a body part

Body Part	Approach	Device	Qualifier
0 Head Muscle	0 Open	0 Drainage Device	Z No Qualifier
1 Facial Muscle	3 Percutaneous		
2 Neck Muscle, Right	4 Percutaneous Endoscopic		
3 Neck Muscle, Left			
4 Tongue, Palate, Pharynx Muscle			
5 Shoulder Muscle, Right			
6 Shoulder Muscle, Left			
7 Upper Arm Muscle, Right			
8 Upper Arm Muscle, Left			
9 Lower Arm and Wrist Muscle, Right			
B Lower Arm and Wrist Muscle, Left			
C Hand Muscle, Right			
D Hand Muscle, Left			
F Trunk Muscle, Right			
G Trunk Muscle, Left			
H Thorax Muscle, Right			
J Thorax Muscle, Left			
K Abdomen Muscle, Right			
L Abdomen Muscle, Left			
M Perineum Muscle			
N Hip Muscle, Right			
P Hip Muscle, Left			
Q Upper Leg Muscle, Right			
R Upper Leg Muscle, Left			
S Lower Leg Muscle, Right			
T Lower Leg Muscle, Left			
V Foot Muscle, Right			
W Foot Muscle, Left			

9: DRAINAGE

K: MUSCLES

0: M/S

◀ New　　◀▥ Revised　　deleted Deleted　　♀ Females Only　　♂ Males Only
Ⓝ Noncovered　　Ⓛ Limited Coverage　　Ⓗ Hospital-Acquired Condition　　**Coding Clinic**

SECTION: 0 MEDICAL AND SURGICAL
BODY SYSTEM: K MUSCLES
OPERATION: 9 DRAINAGE: *(continued)*
Taking or letting out fluids and/or gases from a body part

Body Part	Approach	Device	Qualifier
0 Head Muscle	0 Open	Z No Device	X Diagnostic
1 Facial Muscle	3 Percutaneous		Z No Qualifier
2 Neck Muscle, Right	4 Percutaneous Endoscopic		
3 Neck Muscle, Left			
4 Tongue, Palate, Pharynx Muscle			
5 Shoulder Muscle, Right			
6 Shoulder Muscle, Left			
7 Upper Arm Muscle, Right			
8 Upper Arm Muscle, Left			
9 Lower Arm and Wrist Muscle, Right			
B Lower Arm and Wrist Muscle, Left			
C Hand Muscle, Right			
D Hand Muscle, Left			
F Trunk Muscle, Right			
G Trunk Muscle, Left			
H Thorax Muscle, Right			
J Thorax Muscle, Left			
K Abdomen Muscle, Right			
L Abdomen Muscle, Left			
M Perineum Muscle			
N Hip Muscle, Right			
P Hip Muscle, Left			
Q Upper Leg Muscle, Right			
R Upper Leg Muscle, Left			
S Lower Leg Muscle, Right			
T Lower Leg Muscle, Left			
V Foot Muscle, Right			
W Foot Muscle, Left			

SECTION: 0 MEDICAL AND SURGICAL
BODY SYSTEM: K MUSCLES
OPERATION: **B EXCISION:** Cutting out or off, without replacement, a portion of a body part

Body Part	Approach	Device	Qualifier
0 Head Muscle	0 Open	Z No Device	X Diagnostic
1 Facial Muscle	3 Percutaneous		Z No Qualifier
2 Neck Muscle, Right	4 Percutaneous Endoscopic		
3 Neck Muscle, Left			
4 Tongue, Palate, Pharynx Muscle			
5 Shoulder Muscle, Right			
6 Shoulder Muscle, Left			
7 Upper Arm Muscle, Right			
8 Upper Arm Muscle, Left			
9 Lower Arm and Wrist Muscle, Right			
B Lower Arm and Wrist Muscle, Left			
C Hand Muscle, Right			
D Hand Muscle, Left			
F Trunk Muscle, Right			
G Trunk Muscle, Left			
H Thorax Muscle, Right			
J Thorax Muscle, Left			
K Abdomen Muscle, Right			
L Abdomen Muscle, Left			
M Perineum Muscle			
N Hip Muscle, Right			
P Hip Muscle, Left			
Q Upper Leg Muscle, Right			
R Upper Leg Muscle, Left			
S Lower Leg Muscle, Right			
T Lower Leg Muscle, Left			
V Foot Muscle, Right			
W Foot Muscle, Left			

B: EXCISION

K: MUSCLES

0: M/S

◀ New   ◀▥ Revised   ~~deleted~~ Deleted   ♀ Females Only   ♂ Males Only
NC Noncovered   LC Limited Coverage   HAC Hospital-Acquired Condition   **Coding Clinic**

SECTION: 0 MEDICAL AND SURGICAL
BODY SYSTEM: K MUSCLES
OPERATION: C EXTIRPATION: Taking or cutting out solid matter from a body part

Body Part	Approach	Device	Qualifier
0 Head Muscle 1 Facial Muscle 2 Neck Muscle, Right 3 Neck Muscle, Left 4 Tongue, Palate, Pharynx Muscle 5 Shoulder Muscle, Right 6 Shoulder Muscle, Left 7 Upper Arm Muscle, Right 8 Upper Arm Muscle, Left 9 Lower Arm and Wrist Muscle, Right B Lower Arm and Wrist Muscle, Left C Hand Muscle, Right D Hand Muscle, Left F Trunk Muscle, Right G Trunk Muscle, Left H Thorax Muscle, Right J Thorax Muscle, Left K Abdomen Muscle, Right L Abdomen Muscle, Left M Perineum Muscle N Hip Muscle, Right P Hip Muscle, Left Q Upper Leg Muscle, Right R Upper Leg Muscle, Left S Lower Leg Muscle, Right T Lower Leg Muscle, Left V Foot Muscle, Right W Foot Muscle, Left	0 Open 3 Percutaneous 4 Percutaneous Endoscopic	Z No Device	Z No Qualifier

SECTION: 0 MEDICAL AND SURGICAL
BODY SYSTEM: K MUSCLES
OPERATION: H INSERTION: Putting in a nonbiological appliance that monitors, assists, performs, or prevents a physiological function but does not physically take the place of a body part

Body Part	Approach	Device	Qualifier
X Upper Muscle Y Lower Muscle	0 Open 3 Percutaneous 4 Percutaneous Endoscopic	M Stimulator Lead	Z No Qualifier

SECTION: 0 MEDICAL AND SURGICAL
BODY SYSTEM: K MUSCLES
OPERATION: J INSPECTION: Visually and/or manually exploring a body part

Body Part	Approach	Device	Qualifier
X Upper Muscle Y Lower Muscle	0 Open 3 Percutaneous 4 Percutaneous Endoscopic X External	Z No Device	Z No Qualifier

SECTION: 0 MEDICAL AND SURGICAL
BODY SYSTEM: K MUSCLES
OPERATION: M REATTACHMENT: Putting back in or on all or a portion of a separated body part to its normal location or other suitable location

Body Part	Approach	Device	Qualifier
0 Head Muscle 1 Facial Muscle 2 Neck Muscle, Right 3 Neck Muscle, Left 4 Tongue, Palate, Pharynx Muscle 5 Shoulder Muscle, Right 6 Shoulder Muscle, Left 7 Upper Arm Muscle, Right 8 Upper Arm Muscle, Left 9 Lower Arm and Wrist Muscle, Right B Lower Arm and Wrist Muscle, Left C Hand Muscle, Right D Hand Muscle, Left F Trunk Muscle, Right G Trunk Muscle, Left H Thorax Muscle, Right J Thorax Muscle, Left K Abdomen Muscle, Right L Abdomen Muscle, Left M Perineum Muscle N Hip Muscle, Right P Hip Muscle, Left Q Upper Leg Muscle, Right R Upper Leg Muscle, Left S Lower Leg Muscle, Right T Lower Leg Muscle, Left V Foot Muscle, Right W Foot Muscle, Left	0 Open 4 Percutaneous Endoscopic	Z No Device	Z No Qualifier

◀ New   ◀▥ Revised   ~~deleted~~ Deleted   ♀ Females Only   ♂ Males Only
🚫 Noncovered   🇱🇨 Limited Coverage   🚫 Hospital-Acquired Condition   **Coding Clinic**

SECTION: 0 MEDICAL AND SURGICAL
BODY SYSTEM: K MUSCLES
OPERATION: N RELEASE: Freeing a body part from an abnormal physical constraint by cutting or by the use of force

Body Part	Approach	Device	Qualifier
0 Head Muscle 1 Facial Muscle 2 Neck Muscle, Right 3 Neck Muscle, Left 4 Tongue, Palate, Pharynx Muscle 5 Shoulder Muscle, Right 6 Shoulder Muscle, Left 7 Upper Arm Muscle, Right 8 Upper Arm Muscle, Left 9 Lower Arm and Wrist Muscle, Right B Lower Arm and Wrist Muscle, Left C Hand Muscle, Right D Hand Muscle, Left F Trunk Muscle, Right G Trunk Muscle, Left H Thorax Muscle, Right J Thorax Muscle, Left K Abdomen Muscle, Right L Abdomen Muscle, Left M Perineum Muscle N Hip Muscle, Right P Hip Muscle, Left Q Upper Leg Muscle, Right R Upper Leg Muscle, Left S Lower Leg Muscle, Right T Lower Leg Muscle, Left V Foot Muscle, Right W Foot Muscle, Left	0 Open 3 Percutaneous 4 Percutaneous Endoscopic X External	Z No Device	Z No Qualifier

SECTION: 0 MEDICAL AND SURGICAL
BODY SYSTEM: K MUSCLES
OPERATION: P REMOVAL: Taking out or off a device from a body part

Body Part	Approach	Device	Qualifier
X Upper Muscle Y Lower Muscle	0 Open 3 Percutaneous 4 Percutaneous Endoscopic	0 Drainage Device 7 Autologous Tissue Substitute J Synthetic Substitute K Nonautologous Tissue Substitute M Stimulator Lead	Z No Qualifier
X Upper Muscle Y Lower Muscle	X External	0 Drainage Device M Stimulator Lead	Z No Qualifier

◀ New ◀ Revised ~~deleted~~ Deleted ♀ Females Only ♂ Males Only
Ⓝ Noncovered Ⓛ Limited Coverage Ⓗ Hospital-Acquired Condition **Coding Clinic**

303

SECTION: 0 MEDICAL AND SURGICAL
BODY SYSTEM: K MUSCLES
OPERATION: Q REPAIR: Restoring, to the extent possible, a body part to its normal anatomic structure and function

Body Part	Approach	Device	Qualifier
0 Head Muscle	0 Open	Z No Device	Z No Qualifier
1 Facial Muscle	3 Percutaneous		
2 Neck Muscle, Right	4 Percutaneous Endoscopic		
3 Neck Muscle, Left			
4 Tongue, Palate, Pharynx Muscle			
5 Shoulder Muscle, Right			
6 Shoulder Muscle, Left			
7 Upper Arm Muscle, Right			
8 Upper Arm Muscle, Left			
9 Lower Arm and Wrist Muscle, Right			
B Lower Arm and Wrist Muscle, Left			
C Hand Muscle, Right			
D Hand Muscle, Left			
F Trunk Muscle, Right			
G Trunk Muscle, Left			
H Thorax Muscle, Right			
J Thorax Muscle, Left			
K Abdomen Muscle, Right			
L Abdomen Muscle, Left			
M Perineum Muscle			
N Hip Muscle, Right			
P Hip Muscle, Left			
Q Upper Leg Muscle, Right			
R Upper Leg Muscle, Left			
S Lower Leg Muscle, Right			
T Lower Leg Muscle, Left			
V Foot Muscle, Right			
W Foot Muscle, Left			

SECTION: 0 MEDICAL AND SURGICAL
BODY SYSTEM: K MUSCLES
OPERATION: S REPOSITION: Moving to its normal location, or other suitable location, all or a portion of a body part

Body Part	Approach	Device	Qualifier
0 Head Muscle	0 Open	Z No Device	Z No Qualifier
1 Facial Muscle	4 Percutaneous Endoscopic		
2 Neck Muscle, Right			
3 Neck Muscle, Left			
4 Tongue, Palate, Pharynx Muscle			
5 Shoulder Muscle, Right			
6 Shoulder Muscle, Left			
7 Upper Arm Muscle, Right			
8 Upper Arm Muscle, Left			
9 Lower Arm and Wrist Muscle, Right			
B Lower Arm and Wrist Muscle, Left			
C Hand Muscle, Right			
D Hand Muscle, Left			
F Trunk Muscle, Right			
G Trunk Muscle, Left			
H Thorax Muscle, Right			
J Thorax Muscle, Left			
K Abdomen Muscle, Right			
L Abdomen Muscle, Left			
M Perineum Muscle			
N Hip Muscle, Right			
P Hip Muscle, Left			
Q Upper Leg Muscle, Right			
R Upper Leg Muscle, Left			
S Lower Leg Muscle, Right			
T Lower Leg Muscle, Left			
V Foot Muscle, Right			
W Foot Muscle, Left			

SECTION: 0 MEDICAL AND SURGICAL
BODY SYSTEM: K MUSCLES
OPERATION: T RESECTION: Cutting out or off, without replacement, all of a body part

Body Part	Approach	Device	Qualifier
0 Head Muscle 1 Facial Muscle 2 Neck Muscle, Right 3 Neck Muscle, Left 4 Tongue, Palate, Pharynx Muscle 5 Shoulder Muscle, Right 6 Shoulder Muscle, Left 7 Upper Arm Muscle, Right 8 Upper Arm Muscle, Left 9 Lower Arm and Wrist Muscle, Right B Lower Arm and Wrist Muscle, Left C Hand Muscle, Right D Hand Muscle, Left F Trunk Muscle, Right G Trunk Muscle, Left H Thorax Muscle, Right J Thorax Muscle, Left K Abdomen Muscle, Right L Abdomen Muscle, Left M Perineum Muscle N Hip Muscle, Right P Hip Muscle, Left Q Upper Leg Muscle, Right R Upper Leg Muscle, Left S Lower Leg Muscle, Right T Lower Leg Muscle, Left V Foot Muscle, Right W Foot Muscle, Left	0 Open 4 Percutaneous Endoscopic	Z No Device	Z No Qualifier

T: RESECTION

K: MUSCLES

0: M/S

◀ New   ◀ Revised   ~~deleted~~ Deleted   ♀ Females Only   ♂ Males Only
ⓃⒸ Noncovered   ⓁⒸ Limited Coverage   ⒽⒶⒸ Hospital-Acquired Condition   **Coding Clinic**

SECTION: 0 MEDICAL AND SURGICAL

BODY SYSTEM: K MUSCLES

OPERATION: U SUPPLEMENT: Putting in or on biological or synthetic material that physically reinforces and/or augments the function of a portion of a body part

Body Part	Approach	Device	Qualifier
0 Head Muscle 1 Facial Muscle 2 Neck Muscle, Right 3 Neck Muscle, Left 4 Tongue, Palate, Pharynx Muscle 5 Shoulder Muscle, Right 6 Shoulder Muscle, Left 7 Upper Arm Muscle, Right 8 Upper Arm Muscle, Left 9 Lower Arm and Wrist Muscle, Right B Lower Arm and Wrist Muscle, Left C Hand Muscle, Right D Hand Muscle, Left F Trunk Muscle, Right G Trunk Muscle, Left H Thorax Muscle, Right J Thorax Muscle, Left K Abdomen Muscle, Right L Abdomen Muscle, Left M Perineum Muscle N Hip Muscle, Right P Hip Muscle, Left Q Upper Leg Muscle, Right R Upper Leg Muscle, Left S Lower Leg Muscle, Right T Lower Leg Muscle, Left V Foot Muscle, Right W Foot Muscle, Left	0 Open 4 Percutaneous Endoscopic	7 Autologous Tissue Substitute J Synthetic Substitute K Nonautologous Tissue Substitute	Z No Qualifier

SECTION: 0 MEDICAL AND SURGICAL

BODY SYSTEM: K MUSCLES

OPERATION: W REVISION: Correcting, to the extent possible, a portion of a malfunctioning device or the position of a displaced device

Body Part	Approach	Device	Qualifier
X Upper Muscle Y Lower Muscle	0 Open 3 Percutaneous 4 Percutaneous Endoscopic X External	0 Drainage Device 7 Autologous Tissue Substitute J Synthetic Substitute K Nonautologous Tissue Substitute M Stimulator Lead	Z No Qualifier

SECTION: 0 MEDICAL AND SURGICAL
BODY SYSTEM: K MUSCLES
OPERATION: X TRANSFER: Moving, without taking out, all or a portion of a body part to another location to take over the function of all or a portion of a body part

Body Part	Approach	Device	Qualifier
0 Head Muscle 1 Facial Muscle 2 Neck Muscle, Right 3 Neck Muscle, Left 4 Tongue, Palate, Pharynx Muscle 5 Shoulder Muscle, Right 6 Shoulder Muscle, Left 7 Upper Arm Muscle, Right 8 Upper Arm Muscle, Left 9 Lower Arm and Wrist Muscle, Right B Lower Arm and Wrist Muscle, Left C Hand Muscle, Right D Hand Muscle, Left F Trunk Muscle, Right G Trunk Muscle, Left H Thorax Muscle, Right J Thorax Muscle, Left M Perineum Muscle N Hip Muscle, Right P Hip Muscle, Left Q Upper Leg Muscle, Right R Upper Leg Muscle, Left S Lower Leg Muscle, Right T Lower Leg Muscle, Left V Foot Muscle, Right W Foot Muscle, Left	0 Open 4 Percutaneous Endoscopic	Z No Device	0 Skin 1 Subcutaneous Tissue 2 Skin and Subcutaneous Tissue Z No Qualifier
K Abdomen Muscle, Right L Abdomen Muscle, Left	0 Open 4 Percutaneous Endoscopic	Z No Device	0 Skin 1 Subcutaneous Tissue 2 Skin and Subcutaneous Tissue 6 Transverse Rectus Abdominis Myocutaneous Flap Z No Qualifier

X: TRANSFER

K: MUSCLES

0: M/S

◄ New   ◄▥ Revised   ~~deleted~~ Deleted   ♀ Females Only   ♂ Males Only
⚕ Noncovered   ⚕ Limited Coverage   ⚕ Hospital-Acquired Condition   **Coding Clinic**

SECTION: 0 MEDICAL AND SURGICAL

BODY SYSTEM: L TENDONS

OPERATION: 2 CHANGE: Taking out or off a device from a body part and putting back an identical or similar device in or on the same body part without cutting or puncturing the skin or a mucous membrane

Body Part	Approach	Device	Qualifier
X Upper Tendon Y Lower Tendon	X External	0 Drainage Device Y Other Device	Z No Qualifier

SECTION: 0 MEDICAL AND SURGICAL

BODY SYSTEM: L TENDONS

OPERATION: 5 DESTRUCTION: Physical eradication of all or a portion of a body part by the direct use of energy, force, or a destructive agent

Body Part	Approach	Device	Qualifier
0 Head and Neck Tendon 1 Shoulder Tendon, Right 2 Shoulder Tendon, Left 3 Upper Arm Tendon, Right 4 Upper Arm Tendon, Left 5 Lower Arm and Wrist Tendon, Right 6 Lower Arm and Wrist Tendon, Left 7 Hand Tendon, Right 8 Hand Tendon, Left 9 Trunk Tendon, Right B Trunk Tendon, Left C Thorax Tendon, Right D Thorax Tendon, Left F Abdomen Tendon, Right G Abdomen Tendon, Left H Perineum Tendon J Hip Tendon, Right K Hip Tendon, Left L Upper Leg Tendon, Right M Upper Leg Tendon, Left N Lower Leg Tendon, Right P Lower Leg Tendon, Left Q Knee Tendon, Right R Knee Tendon, Left S Ankle Tendon, Right T Ankle Tendon, Left V Foot Tendon, Right W Foot Tendon, Left	0 Open 3 Percutaneous 4 Percutaneous Endoscopic	Z No Device	Z No Qualifier

L: TENDONS   0: M/S   2: CHANGE   5: DESTRUCTION

SECTION: 0 MEDICAL AND SURGICAL
BODY SYSTEM: L TENDONS
OPERATION: 8 DIVISION: Cutting into a body part, without draining fluids and/or gases from the body part, in order to separate or transect a body part

Body Part	Approach	Device	Qualifier
0 Head and Neck Tendon	0 Open	Z No Device	Z No Qualifier
1 Shoulder Tendon, Right	3 Percutaneous		
2 Shoulder Tendon, Left	4 Percutaneous Endoscopic		
3 Upper Arm Tendon, Right			
4 Upper Arm Tendon, Left			
5 Lower Arm and Wrist Tendon, Right			
6 Lower Arm and Wrist Tendon, Left			
7 Hand Tendon, Right			
8 Hand Tendon, Left			
9 Trunk Tendon, Right			
B Trunk Tendon, Left			
C Thorax Tendon, Right			
D Thorax Tendon, Left			
F Abdomen Tendon, Right			
G Abdomen Tendon, Left			
H Perineum Tendon			
J Hip Tendon, Right			
K Hip Tendon, Left			
L Upper Leg Tendon, Right			
M Upper Leg Tendon, Left			
N Lower Leg Tendon, Right			
P Lower Leg Tendon, Left			
Q Knee Tendon, Right			
R Knee Tendon, Left			
S Ankle Tendon, Right			
T Ankle Tendon, Left			
V Foot Tendon, Right			
W Foot Tendon, Left			

0: M/S L: TENDONS 8: DIVISION

◀ New   ◀ Revised   ~~deleted~~ Deleted   ♀ Females Only   ♂ Males Only
Noncovered   Limited Coverage   Hospital-Acquired Condition   **Coding Clinic**

311

SECTION: 0 MEDICAL AND SURGICAL
BODY SYSTEM: L TENDONS
OPERATION: 9 DRAINAGE: Taking or letting out fluids and/or gases from a body part

Body Part	Approach	Device	Qualifier
0 Head and Neck Tendon 1 Shoulder Tendon, Right 2 Shoulder Tendon, Left 3 Upper Arm Tendon, Right 4 Upper Arm Tendon, Left 5 Lower Arm and Wrist Tendon, Right 6 Lower Arm and Wrist Tendon, Left 7 Hand Tendon, Right 8 Hand Tendon, Left 9 Trunk Tendon, Right B Trunk Tendon, Left C Thorax Tendon, Right D Thorax Tendon, Left F Abdomen Tendon, Right G Abdomen Tendon, Left H Perineum Tendon J Hip Tendon, Right K Hip Tendon, Left L Upper Leg Tendon, Right M Upper Leg Tendon, Left N Lower Leg Tendon, Right P Lower Leg Tendon, Left Q Knee Tendon, Right R Knee Tendon, Left S Ankle Tendon, Right T Ankle Tendon, Left V Foot Tendon, Right W Foot Tendon, Left	0 Open 3 Percutaneous 4 Percutaneous Endoscopic	0 Drainage Device	Z No Qualifier
0 Head and Neck Tendon 1 Shoulder Tendon, Right 2 Shoulder Tendon, Left 3 Upper Arm Tendon, Right 4 Upper Arm Tendon, Left 5 Lower Arm and Wrist Tendon, Right 6 Lower Arm and Wrist Tendon, Left 7 Hand Tendon, Right 8 Hand Tendon, Left 9 Trunk Tendon, Right B Trunk Tendon, Left C Thorax Tendon, Right D Thorax Tendon, Left F Abdomen Tendon, Right G Abdomen Tendon, Left H Perineum Tendon J Hip Tendon, Right K Hip Tendon, Left L Upper Leg Tendon, Right M Upper Leg Tendon, Left N Lower Leg Tendon, Right P Lower Leg Tendon, Left Q Knee Tendon, Right R Knee Tendon, Left S Ankle Tendon, Right T Ankle Tendon, Left V Foot Tendon, Right W Foot Tendon, Left	0 Open 3 Percutaneous 4 Percutaneous Endoscopic	Z No Device	X Diagnostic Z No Qualifier

9: DRAINAGE

L: TENDONS

0: M/S

◀ New　　◀▥ Revised　　~~deleted~~ Deleted　　♀ Females Only　　♂ Males Only
 Noncovered　　Limited Coverage　　Hospital-Acquired Condition　　**Coding Clinic**

SECTION: 0 MEDICAL AND SURGICAL
BODY SYSTEM: L TENDONS
OPERATION: B EXCISION: Cutting out or off, without replacement, a portion of a body part

Body Part	Approach	Device	Qualifier
0 Head and Neck Tendon 1 Shoulder Tendon, Right 2 Shoulder Tendon, Left 3 Upper Arm Tendon, Right 4 Upper Arm Tendon, Left 5 Lower Arm and Wrist Tendon, Right 6 Lower Arm and Wrist Tendon, Left 7 Hand Tendon, Right 8 Hand Tendon, Left 9 Trunk Tendon, Right B Trunk Tendon, Left C Thorax Tendon, Right D Thorax Tendon, Left F Abdomen Tendon, Right G Abdomen Tendon, Left H Perineum Tendon J Hip Tendon, Right K Hip Tendon, Left L Upper Leg Tendon, Right M Upper Leg Tendon, Left N Lower Leg Tendon, Right P Lower Leg Tendon, Left Q Knee Tendon, Right R Knee Tendon, Left S Ankle Tendon, Right T Ankle Tendon, Left V Foot Tendon, Right W Foot Tendon, Left	0 Open 3 Percutaneous 4 Percutaneous Endoscopic	Z No Device	X Diagnostic Z No Qualifier

◄ New ◄ Revised deleted Deleted ♀ Females Only ♂ Males Only ⓝ Noncovered ⓛ Limited Coverage ⓗ Hospital-Acquired Condition **Coding Clinic**

313

SECTION: 0 MEDICAL AND SURGICAL
BODY SYSTEM: L TENDONS
OPERATION: C EXTIRPATION: Taking or cutting out solid matter from a body part

Body Part	Approach	Device	Qualifier
0 Head and Neck Tendon	0 Open	Z No Device	Z No Qualifier
1 Shoulder Tendon, Right	3 Percutaneous		
2 Shoulder Tendon, Left	4 Percutaneous Endoscopic		
3 Upper Arm Tendon, Right			
4 Upper Arm Tendon, Left			
5 Lower Arm and Wrist Tendon, Right			
6 Lower Arm and Wrist Tendon, Left			
7 Hand Tendon, Right			
8 Hand Tendon, Left			
9 Trunk Tendon, Right			
B Trunk Tendon, Left			
C Thorax Tendon, Right			
D Thorax Tendon, Left			
F Abdomen Tendon, Right			
G Abdomen Tendon, Left			
H Perineum Tendon			
J Hip Tendon, Right			
K Hip Tendon, Left			
L Upper Leg Tendon, Right			
M Upper Leg Tendon, Left			
N Lower Leg Tendon, Right			
P Lower Leg Tendon, Left			
Q Knee Tendon, Right			
R Knee Tendon, Left			
S Ankle Tendon, Right			
T Ankle Tendon, Left			
V Foot Tendon, Right			
W Foot Tendon, Left			

SECTION: 0 MEDICAL AND SURGICAL
BODY SYSTEM: L TENDONS
OPERATION: J INSPECTION: Visually and/or manually exploring a body part

Body Part	Approach	Device	Qualifier
X Upper Tendon	0 Open	Z No Device	Z No Qualifier
Y Lower Tendon	3 Percutaneous		
	4 Percutaneous Endoscopic		
	X External		

◀ New   ◀ Revised   deleted Deleted   ♀ Females Only   ♂ Males Only
Noncovered   Limited Coverage   Hospital-Acquired Condition   **Coding Clinic**

SECTION: 0 MEDICAL AND SURGICAL
BODY SYSTEM: L TENDONS
OPERATION: M REATTACHMENT: Putting back in or on all or a portion of a separated body part to its normal location or other suitable location

Body Part	Approach	Device	Qualifier
0 Head and Neck Tendon 1 Shoulder Tendon, Right 2 Shoulder Tendon, Left 3 Upper Arm Tendon, Right 4 Upper Arm Tendon, Left 5 Lower Arm and Wrist Tendon, Right 6 Lower Arm and Wrist Tendon, Left 7 Hand Tendon, Right 8 Hand Tendon, Left 9 Trunk Tendon, Right B Trunk Tendon, Left C Thorax Tendon, Right D Thorax Tendon, Left F Abdomen Tendon, Right G Abdomen Tendon, Left H Perineum Tendon J Hip Tendon, Right K Hip Tendon, Left L Upper Leg Tendon, Right M Upper Leg Tendon, Left N Lower Leg Tendon, Right P Lower Leg Tendon, Left Q Knee Tendon, Right R Knee Tendon, Left S Ankle Tendon, Right T Ankle Tendon, Left V Foot Tendon, Right W Foot Tendon, Left	0 Open 4 Percutaneous Endoscopic	Z No Device	Z No Qualifier

◀ New ◀ Revised deleted Deleted ♀ Females Only ♂ Males Only
⊘ Noncovered ⊘ Limited Coverage ⊘ Hospital-Acquired Condition **Coding Clinic**

315

SECTION: **0 MEDICAL AND SURGICAL**
BODY SYSTEM: **L TENDONS**
OPERATION: **N RELEASE:** Freeing a body part from an abnormal physical constraint by cutting or by the use of force

Body Part	Approach	Device	Qualifier
0 Head and Neck Tendon	0 Open	Z No Device	Z No Qualifier
1 Shoulder Tendon, Right	3 Percutaneous		
2 Shoulder Tendon, Left	4 Percutaneous Endoscopic		
3 Upper Arm Tendon, Right	X External		
4 Upper Arm Tendon, Left			
5 Lower Arm and Wrist Tendon, Right			
6 Lower Arm and Wrist Tendon, Left			
7 Hand Tendon, Right			
8 Hand Tendon, Left			
9 Trunk Tendon, Right			
B Trunk Tendon, Left			
C Thorax Tendon, Right			
D Thorax Tendon, Left			
F Abdomen Tendon, Right			
G Abdomen Tendon, Left			
H Perineum Tendon			
J Hip Tendon, Right			
K Hip Tendon, Left			
L Upper Leg Tendon, Right			
M Upper Leg Tendon, Left			
N Lower Leg Tendon, Right			
P Lower Leg Tendon, Left			
Q Knee Tendon, Right			
R Knee Tendon, Left			
S Ankle Tendon, Right			
T Ankle Tendon, Left			
V Foot Tendon, Right			
W Foot Tendon, Left			

SECTION: **0 MEDICAL AND SURGICAL**
BODY SYSTEM: **L TENDONS**
OPERATION: **P REMOVAL:** Taking out or off a device from a body part

Body Part	Approach	Device	Qualifier
X Upper Tendon Y Lower Tendon	0 Open 3 Percutaneous 4 Percutaneous Endoscopic	0 Drainage Device 7 Autologous Tissue Substitute J Synthetic Substitute K Nonautologous Tissue Substitute	Z No Qualifier
X Upper Tendon Y Lower Tendon	X External	0 Drainage Device	Z No Qualifier

N: RELEASE P: REMOVAL
L: TENDONS
0: M/S

SECTION: 0 MEDICAL AND SURGICAL
BODY SYSTEM: L TENDONS
OPERATION: **Q REPAIR:** Restoring, to the extent possible, a body part to its normal anatomic structure and function

Body Part	Approach	Device	Qualifier
0 Head and Neck Tendon 1 Shoulder Tendon, Right 2 Shoulder Tendon, Left 3 Upper Arm Tendon, Right 4 Upper Arm Tendon, Left 5 Lower Arm and Wrist Tendon, Right 6 Lower Arm and Wrist Tendon, Left 7 Hand Tendon, Right 8 Hand Tendon, Left 9 Trunk Tendon, Right B Trunk Tendon, Left C Thorax Tendon, Right D Thorax Tendon, Left F Abdomen Tendon, Right G Abdomen Tendon, Left H Perineum Tendon J Hip Tendon, Right K Hip Tendon, Left L Upper Leg Tendon, Right M Upper Leg Tendon, Left N Lower Leg Tendon, Right P Lower Leg Tendon, Left Q Knee Tendon, Right R Knee Tendon, Left S Ankle Tendon, Right T Ankle Tendon, Left V Foot Tendon, Right W Foot Tendon, Left	0 Open 3 Percutaneous 4 Percutaneous Endoscopic	Z No Device	Z No Qualifier

Coding Clinic: 2013, Q3, P21 – 0LQ14ZZ

SECTION: 0 MEDICAL AND SURGICAL
BODY SYSTEM: L TENDONS
OPERATION: R **REPLACEMENT:** Putting in or on biological or synthetic material that physically takes the place and/or function of all or a portion of a body part

Body Part	Approach	Device	Qualifier
0 Head and Neck Tendon	0 Open	7 Autologous Tissue Substitute	Z No Qualifier
1 Shoulder Tendon, Right	4 Percutaneous Endoscopic	J Synthetic Substitute	
2 Shoulder Tendon, Left		K Nonautologous Tissue Substitute	
3 Upper Arm Tendon, Right			
4 Upper Arm Tendon, Left			
5 Lower Arm and Wrist Tendon, Right			
6 Lower Arm and Wrist Tendon, Left			
7 Hand Tendon, Right			
8 Hand Tendon, Left			
9 Trunk Tendon, Right			
B Trunk Tendon, Left			
C Thorax Tendon, Right			
D Thorax Tendon, Left			
F Abdomen Tendon, Right			
G Abdomen Tendon, Left			
H Perineum Tendon			
J Hip Tendon, Right			
K Hip Tendon, Left			
L Upper Leg Tendon, Right			
M Upper Leg Tendon, Left			
N Lower Leg Tendon, Right			
P Lower Leg Tendon, Left			
Q Knee Tendon, Right			
R Knee Tendon, Left			
S Ankle Tendon, Right			
T Ankle Tendon, Left			
V Foot Tendon, Right			
W Foot Tendon, Left			

R: REPLACEMENT

L: TENDONS

0: M/S

◀ New ◀ Revised ~~deleted~~ Deleted ♀ Females Only ♂ Males Only
Noncovered Limited Coverage Hospital-Acquired Condition **Coding Clinic**

SECTION: 0 MEDICAL AND SURGICAL
BODY SYSTEM: L TENDONS
OPERATION: S REPOSITION: Moving to its normal location, or other suitable location, all or a portion of a body part

Body Part	Approach	Device	Qualifier
0 Head and Neck Tendon	0 Open	Z No Device	Z No Qualifier
1 Shoulder Tendon, Right	4 Percutaneous Endoscopic		
2 Shoulder Tendon, Left			
3 Upper Arm Tendon, Right			
4 Upper Arm Tendon, Left			
5 Lower Arm and Wrist Tendon, Right			
6 Lower Arm and Wrist Tendon, Left			
7 Hand Tendon, Right			
8 Hand Tendon, Left			
9 Trunk Tendon, Right			
B Trunk Tendon, Left			
C Thorax Tendon, Right			
D Thorax Tendon, Left			
F Abdomen Tendon, Right			
G Abdomen Tendon, Left			
H Perineum Tendon			
J Hip Tendon, Right			
K Hip Tendon, Left			
L Upper Leg Tendon, Right			
M Upper Leg Tendon, Left			
N Lower Leg Tendon, Right			
P Lower Leg Tendon, Left			
Q Knee Tendon, Right			
R Knee Tendon, Left			
S Ankle Tendon, Right			
T Ankle Tendon, Left			
V Foot Tendon, Right			
W Foot Tendon, Left			

0: M/S   L: TENDONS   S: REPOSITION

◀ New   ◀ Revised   ~~deleted~~ Deleted   ♀ Females Only   ♂ Males Only
Noncovered   Limited Coverage   Hospital-Acquired Condition   **Coding Clinic**

319

SECTION: 0 MEDICAL AND SURGICAL
BODY SYSTEM: L TENDONS
OPERATION: T RESECTION: Cutting out or off, without replacement, all of a body part

Body Part	Approach	Device	Qualifier
0 Head and Neck Tendon 1 Shoulder Tendon, Right 2 Shoulder Tendon, Left 3 Upper Arm Tendon, Right 4 Upper Arm Tendon, Left 5 Lower Arm and Wrist Tendon, Right 6 Lower Arm and Wrist Tendon, Left 7 Hand Tendon, Right 8 Hand Tendon, Left 9 Trunk Tendon, Right B Trunk Tendon, Left C Thorax Tendon, Right D Thorax Tendon, Left F Abdomen Tendon, Right G Abdomen Tendon, Left H Perineum Tendon J Hip Tendon, Right K Hip Tendon, Left L Upper Leg Tendon, Right M Upper Leg Tendon, Left N Lower Leg Tendon, Right P Lower Leg Tendon, Left Q Knee Tendon, Right R Knee Tendon, Left S Ankle Tendon, Right T Ankle Tendon, Left V Foot Tendon, Right W Foot Tendon, Left	0 Open 4 Percutaneous Endoscopic	Z No Device	Z No Qualifier

New, Revised, deleted Deleted, Females Only, Males Only, Noncovered, Limited Coverage, Hospital-Acquired Condition, Coding Clinic

SECTION: 0 MEDICAL AND SURGICAL
BODY SYSTEM: L TENDONS
OPERATION: U SUPPLEMENT: Putting in or on biological or synthetic material that physically reinforces and/or augments the function of a portion of a body part

Body Part	Approach	Device	Qualifier
0 Head and Neck Tendon 1 Shoulder Tendon, Right 2 Shoulder Tendon, Left 3 Upper Arm Tendon, Right 4 Upper Arm Tendon, Left 5 Lower Arm and Wrist Tendon, Right 6 Lower Arm and Wrist Tendon, Left 7 Hand Tendon, Right 8 Hand Tendon, Left 9 Trunk Tendon, Right B Trunk Tendon, Left C Thorax Tendon, Right D Thorax Tendon, Left F Abdomen Tendon, Right G Abdomen Tendon, Left H Perineum Tendon J Hip Tendon, Right K Hip Tendon, Left L Upper Leg Tendon, Right M Upper Leg Tendon, Left N Lower Leg Tendon, Right P Lower Leg Tendon, Left Q Knee Tendon, Right R Knee Tendon, Left S Ankle Tendon, Right T Ankle Tendon, Left V Foot Tendon, Right W Foot Tendon, Left	0 Open 4 Percutaneous Endoscopic	7 Autologous Tissue Substitute J Synthetic Substitute K Nonautologous Tissue Substitute	Z No Qualifier

SECTION: 0 MEDICAL AND SURGICAL
BODY SYSTEM: L TENDONS
OPERATION: W REVISION: Correcting, to the extent possible, a portion of a malfunctioning device or the position of a displaced device

Body Part	Approach	Device	Qualifier
X Upper Tendon Y Lower Tendon	0 Open 3 Percutaneous 4 Percutaneous Endoscopic X External	0 Drainage Device 7 Autologous Tissue Substitute J Synthetic Substitute K Nonautologous Tissue Substitute	Z No Qualifier

◄ New   ◄▬ Revised   ~~deleted~~ Deleted   ♀ Females Only   ♂ Males Only
⊘ Noncovered   ⊘ Limited Coverage   ⊘ Hospital-Acquired Condition   **Coding Clinic**

321

SECTION: 0 MEDICAL AND SURGICAL
BODY SYSTEM: L TENDONS
OPERATION: X **TRANSFER:** Moving, without taking out, all or a portion of a body part to another location to take over the function of all or a portion of a body part

Body Part	Approach	Device	Qualifier
0 Head and Neck Tendon	0 Open	Z No Device	Z No Qualifier
1 Shoulder Tendon, Right	4 Percutaneous Endoscopic		
2 Shoulder Tendon, Left			
3 Upper Arm Tendon, Right			
4 Upper Arm Tendon, Left			
5 Lower Arm and Wrist Tendon, Right			
6 Lower Arm and Wrist Tendon, Left			
7 Hand Tendon, Right			
8 Hand Tendon, Left			
9 Trunk Tendon, Right			
B Trunk Tendon, Left			
C Thorax Tendon, Right			
D Thorax Tendon, Left			
F Abdomen Tendon, Right			
G Abdomen Tendon, Left			
H Perineum Tendon			
J Hip Tendon, Right			
K Hip Tendon, Left			
L Upper Leg Tendon, Right			
M Upper Leg Tendon, Left			
N Lower Leg Tendon, Right			
P Lower Leg Tendon, Left			
Q Knee Tendon, Right			
R Knee Tendon, Left			
S Ankle Tendon, Right			
T Ankle Tendon, Left			
V Foot Tendon, Right			
W Foot Tendon, Left			

X: TRANSFER

L: TENDONS

0: M/S

◀ New   ◀▥ Revised   ~~deleted~~ Deleted   ♀ Females Only   ♂ Males Only
▨ Noncovered   ▨ Limited Coverage   ▨ Hospital-Acquired Condition   **Coding Clinic**

◀ New   ◀▥ Revised   ~~deleted~~ Deleted   ♀ Females Only   ♂ Males Only
🅝 Noncovered   🅛 Limited Coverage   🅗 Hospital-Acquired Condition   **Coding Clinic**

323

SECTION:　0　MEDICAL AND SURGICAL
BODY SYSTEM: M BURSAE AND LIGAMENTS
OPERATION:　2　CHANGE: Taking out or off a device from a body part and putting back an identical or similar device in or on the same body part without cutting or puncturing the skin or a mucous membrane

Body Part	Approach	Device	Qualifier
X Upper Bursa and Ligament Y Lower Bursa and Ligament	X External	0 Drainage Device Y Other Device	Z No Qualifier

SECTION:　0　MEDICAL AND SURGICAL
BODY SYSTEM: M BURSAE AND LIGAMENTS
OPERATION:　5　DESTRUCTION: Physical eradication of all or a portion of a body part by the direct use of energy, force, or a destructive agent

Body Part	Approach	Device	Qualifier
0 Head and Neck Bursa and Ligament 1 Shoulder Bursa and Ligament, Right 2 Shoulder Bursa and Ligament, Left 3 Elbow Bursa and Ligament, Right 4 Elbow Bursa and Ligament, Left 5 Wrist Bursa and Ligament, Right 6 Wrist Bursa and Ligament, Left 7 Hand Bursa and Ligament, Right 8 Hand Bursa and Ligament, Left 9 Upper Extremity Bursa and Ligament, Right B Upper Extremity Bursa and Ligament, Left C Trunk Bursa and Ligament, Right D Trunk Bursa and Ligament, Left F Thorax Bursa and Ligament, Right G Thorax Bursa and Ligament, Left H Abdomen Bursa and Ligament, Right J Abdomen Bursa and Ligament, Left K Perineum Bursa and Ligament L Hip Bursa and Ligament, Right M Hip Bursa and Ligament, Left N Knee Bursa and Ligament, Right P Knee Bursa and Ligament, Left Q Ankle Bursa and Ligament, Right R Ankle Bursa and Ligament, Left S Foot Bursa and Ligament, Right T Foot Bursa and Ligament, Left V Lower Extremity Bursa and Ligament, Right W Lower Extremity Bursa and Ligament, Left	0 Open 3 Percutaneous 4 Percutaneous Endoscopic	Z No Device	Z No Qualifier

SECTION: 0 MEDICAL AND SURGICAL
BODY SYSTEM: M BURSAE AND LIGAMENTS
OPERATION: 8 DIVISION: Cutting into a body part, without draining fluids and/or gases from the body part, in order to separate or transect a body part

Body Part	Approach	Device	Qualifier
0 Head and Neck Bursa and Ligament 1 Shoulder Bursa and Ligament, Right 2 Shoulder Bursa and Ligament, Left 3 Elbow Bursa and Ligament, Right 4 Elbow Bursa and Ligament, Left 5 Wrist Bursa and Ligament, Right 6 Wrist Bursa and Ligament, Left 7 Hand Bursa and Ligament, Right 8 Hand Bursa and Ligament, Left 9 Upper Extremity Bursa and Ligament, Right B Upper Extremity Bursa and Ligament, Left C Trunk Bursa and Ligament, Right D Trunk Bursa and Ligament, Left F Thorax Bursa and Ligament, Right G Thorax Bursa and Ligament, Left H Abdomen Bursa and Ligament, Right J Abdomen Bursa and Ligament, Left K Perineum Bursa and Ligament L Hip Bursa and Ligament, Right M Hip Bursa and Ligament, Left N Knee Bursa and Ligament, Right P Knee Bursa and Ligament, Left Q Ankle Bursa and Ligament, Right R Ankle Bursa and Ligament, Left S Foot Bursa and Ligament, Right T Foot Bursa and Ligament, Left V Lower Extremity Bursa and Ligament, Right W Lower Extremity Bursa and Ligament, Left	0 Open 3 Percutaneous 4 Percutaneous Endoscopic	Z No Device	Z No Qualifier

0: M/S

M: BURSAE AND LIGAMENTS

8: DIVISION

◄ New ◄ Revised ~~deleted~~ Deleted ♀ Females Only ♂ Males Only
Noncovered Limited Coverage Hospital-Acquired Condition **Coding Clinic**

325

SECTION: 0 MEDICAL AND SURGICAL
BODY SYSTEM: M BURSAE AND LIGAMENTS
OPERATION: 9 DRAINAGE: Taking or letting out fluids and/or gases from a body part

9: DRAINAGE

M: BURSAE AND LIGAMENTS

0: M/S

Body Part	Approach	Device	Qualifier
0 Head and Neck Bursa and Ligament 1 Shoulder Bursa and Ligament, Right 2 Shoulder Bursa and Ligament, Left 3 Elbow Bursa and Ligament, Right 4 Elbow Bursa and Ligament, Left 5 Wrist Bursa and Ligament, Right 6 Wrist Bursa and Ligament, Left 7 Hand Bursa and Ligament, Right 8 Hand Bursa and Ligament, Left 9 Upper Extremity Bursa and Ligament, Right B Upper Extremity Bursa and Ligament, Left C Trunk Bursa and Ligament, Right D Trunk Bursa and Ligament, Left F Thorax Bursa and Ligament, Right G Thorax Bursa and Ligament, Left H Abdomen Bursa and Ligament, Right J Abdomen Bursa and Ligament, Left K Perineum Bursa and Ligament L Hip Bursa and Ligament, Right M Hip Bursa and Ligament, Left N Knee Bursa and Ligament, Right P Knee Bursa and Ligament, Left Q Ankle Bursa and Ligament, Right R Ankle Bursa and Ligament, Left S Foot Bursa and Ligament, Right T Foot Bursa and Ligament, Left V Lower Extremity Bursa and Ligament, Right W Lower Extremity Bursa and Ligament, Left	0 Open 3 Percutaneous 4 Percutaneous Endoscopic	0 Drainage Device	Z No Qualifier
0 Head and Neck Bursa and Ligament 1 Shoulder Bursa and Ligament, Right 2 Shoulder Bursa and Ligament, Left 3 Elbow Bursa and Ligament, Right 4 Elbow Bursa and Ligament, Left 5 Wrist Bursa and Ligament, Right 6 Wrist Bursa and Ligament, Left 7 Hand Bursa and Ligament, Right 8 Hand Bursa and Ligament, Left 9 Upper Extremity Bursa and Ligament, Right B Upper Extremity Bursa and Ligament, Left C Trunk Bursa and Ligament, Right D Trunk Bursa and Ligament, Left F Thorax Bursa and Ligament, Right G Thorax Bursa and Ligament, Left H Abdomen Bursa and Ligament, Right J Abdomen Bursa and Ligament, Left K Perineum Bursa and Ligament L Hip Bursa and Ligament, Right M Hip Bursa and Ligament, Left N Knee Bursa and Ligament, Right P Knee Bursa and Ligament, Left Q Ankle Bursa and Ligament, Right R Ankle Bursa and Ligament, Left S Foot Bursa and Ligament, Right T Foot Bursa and Ligament, Left V Lower Extremity Bursa and Ligament, Right W Lower Extremity Bursa and Ligament, Left	0 Open 3 Percutaneous 4 Percutaneous Endoscopic	Z No Device	X Diagnostic Z No Qualifier

◄ New   ◄ Revised   deleted Deleted   ♀ Females Only   ♂ Males Only
Noncovered   Limited Coverage   Hospital-Acquired Condition   **Coding Clinic**

SECTION: 0 MEDICAL AND SURGICAL
BODY SYSTEM: M BURSAE AND LIGAMENTS
OPERATION: B **EXCISION:** Cutting out or off, without replacement, a portion of a body part

Body Part	Approach	Device	Qualifier
0 Head and Neck Bursa and Ligament	0 Open	Z No Device	X Diagnostic
1 Shoulder Bursa and Ligament, Right	3 Percutaneous		Z No Qualifier
2 Shoulder Bursa and Ligament, Left	4 Percutaneous Endoscopic		
3 Elbow Bursa and Ligament, Right			
4 Elbow Bursa and Ligament, Left			
5 Wrist Bursa and Ligament, Right			
6 Wrist Bursa and Ligament, Left			
7 Hand Bursa and Ligament, Right			
8 Hand Bursa and Ligament, Left			
9 Upper Extremity Bursa and Ligament, Right			
B Upper Extremity Bursa and Ligament, Left			
C Trunk Bursa and Ligament, Right			
D Trunk Bursa and Ligament, Left			
F Thorax Bursa and Ligament, Right			
G Thorax Bursa and Ligament, Left			
H Abdomen Bursa and Ligament, Right			
J Abdomen Bursa and Ligament, Left			
K Perineum Bursa and Ligament			
L Hip Bursa and Ligament, Right			
M Hip Bursa and Ligament, Left			
N Knee Bursa and Ligament, Right			
P Knee Bursa and Ligament, Left			
Q Ankle Bursa and Ligament, Right			
R Ankle Bursa and Ligament, Left			
S Foot Bursa and Ligament, Right			
T Foot Bursa and Ligament, Left			
V Lower Extremity Bursa and Ligament, Right			
W Lower Extremity Bursa and Ligament, Left			

SECTION: 0 MEDICAL AND SURGICAL
BODY SYSTEM: M BURSAE AND LIGAMENTS
OPERATION: C EXTIRPATION: Taking or cutting out solid matter from a body part

Body Part	Approach	Device	Qualifier
0 Head and Neck Bursa and Ligament 1 Shoulder Bursa and Ligament, Right 2 Shoulder Bursa and Ligament, Left 3 Elbow Bursa and Ligament, Right 4 Elbow Bursa and Ligament, Left 5 Wrist Bursa and Ligament, Right 6 Wrist Bursa and Ligament, Left 7 Hand Bursa and Ligament, Right 8 Hand Bursa and Ligament, Left 9 Upper Extremity Bursa and Ligament, Right B Upper Extremity Bursa and Ligament, Left C Trunk Bursa and Ligament, Right D Trunk Bursa and Ligament, Left F Thorax Bursa and Ligament, Right G Thorax Bursa and Ligament, Left H Abdomen Bursa and Ligament, Right J Abdomen Bursa and Ligament, Left K Perineum Bursa and Ligament L Hip Bursa and Ligament, Right M Hip Bursa and Ligament, Left N Knee Bursa and Ligament, Right P Knee Bursa and Ligament, Left Q Ankle Bursa and Ligament, Right R Ankle Bursa and Ligament, Left S Foot Bursa and Ligament, Right T Foot Bursa and Ligament, Left V Lower Extremity Bursa and Ligament, Right W Lower Extremity Bursa and Ligament, Left	0 Open 3 Percutaneous 4 Percutaneous Endoscopic	Z No Device	Z No Qualifier

◀ New ◀▥ Revised ~~deleted~~ Deleted ♀ Females Only ♂ Males Only
🔖 Noncovered 🔖 Limited Coverage 🔖 Hospital-Acquired Condition **Coding Clinic**

SECTION: 0 MEDICAL AND SURGICAL
BODY SYSTEM: M BURSAE AND LIGAMENTS
OPERATION: D **EXTRACTION:** Pulling or stripping out or off all or a portion of a body part by the use of force

Body Part	Approach	Device	Qualifier
0 Head and Neck Bursa and Ligament	0 Open	Z No Device	Z No Qualifier
1 Shoulder Bursa and Ligament, Right	3 Percutaneous		
2 Shoulder Bursa and Ligament, Left	4 Percutaneous Endoscopic		
3 Elbow Bursa and Ligament, Right			
4 Elbow Bursa and Ligament, Left			
5 Wrist Bursa and Ligament, Right			
6 Wrist Bursa and Ligament, Left			
7 Hand Bursa and Ligament, Right			
8 Hand Bursa and Ligament, Left			
9 Upper Extremity Bursa and Ligament, Right			
B Upper Extremity Bursa and Ligament, Left			
C Trunk Bursa and Ligament, Right			
D Trunk Bursa and Ligament, Left			
F Thorax Bursa and Ligament, Right			
G Thorax Bursa and Ligament, Left			
H Abdomen Bursa and Ligament, Right			
J Abdomen Bursa and Ligament, Left			
K Perineum Bursa and Ligament			
L Hip Bursa and Ligament, Right			
M Hip Bursa and Ligament, Left			
N Knee Bursa and Ligament, Right			
P Knee Bursa and Ligament, Left			
Q Ankle Bursa and Ligament, Right			
R Ankle Bursa and Ligament, Left			
S Foot Bursa and Ligament, Right			
T Foot Bursa and Ligament, Left			
V Lower Extremity Bursa and Ligament, Right			
W Lower Extremity Bursa and Ligament, Left			

SECTION: 0 MEDICAL AND SURGICAL
BODY SYSTEM: M BURSAE AND LIGAMENTS
OPERATION: J **INSPECTION:** Visually and/or manually exploring a body part

Body Part	Approach	Device	Qualifier
X Upper Bursa and Ligament	0 Open	Z No Device	Z No Qualifier
Y Lower Bursa and Ligament	3 Percutaneous		
	4 Percutaneous Endoscopic		
	X External		

0: M/S

M: BURSAE AND LIGAMENTS

D: EXTRACTION   J: INSPECTION

SECTION: 0 MEDICAL AND SURGICAL
BODY SYSTEM: M BURSAE AND LIGAMENTS
OPERATION: M REATTACHMENT: Putting back in or on all or a portion of a separated body part to its normal location or other suitable location

Body Part	Approach	Device	Qualifier
0 Head and Neck Bursa and Ligament 1 Shoulder Bursa and Ligament, Right 2 Shoulder Bursa and Ligament, Left 3 Elbow Bursa and Ligament, Right 4 Elbow Bursa and Ligament, Left 5 Wrist Bursa and Ligament, Right 6 Wrist Bursa and Ligament, Left 7 Hand Bursa and Ligament, Right 8 Hand Bursa and Ligament, Left 9 Upper Extremity Bursa and Ligament, Right B Upper Extremity Bursa and Ligament, Left C Trunk Bursa and Ligament, Right D Trunk Bursa and Ligament, Left F Thorax Bursa and Ligament, Right G Thorax Bursa and Ligament, Left H Abdomen Bursa and Ligament, Right J Abdomen Bursa and Ligament, Left K Perineum Bursa and Ligament L Hip Bursa and Ligament, Right M Hip Bursa and Ligament, Left N Knee Bursa and Ligament, Right P Knee Bursa and Ligament, Left Q Ankle Bursa and Ligament, Right R Ankle Bursa and Ligament, Left S Foot Bursa and Ligament, Right T Foot Bursa and Ligament, Left V Lower Extremity Bursa and Ligament, Right W Lower Extremity Bursa and Ligament, Left	0 Open 4 Percutaneous Endoscopic	Z No Device	Z No Qualifier

Coding Clinic: 2013, Q3, P22 – 0MM14ZZ

◀ New ◀▥ Revised ~~deleted~~ Deleted ♀ Females Only ♂ Males Only
℞ Noncovered ℞ Limited Coverage ℞ Hospital-Acquired Condition **Coding Clinic**

SECTION: 0 MEDICAL AND SURGICAL
BODY SYSTEM: M BURSAE AND LIGAMENTS
OPERATION: N **RELEASE:** Freeing a body part from an abnormal physical constraint by cutting or by the use of force

Body Part	Approach	Device	Qualifier
0 Head and Neck Bursa and Ligament	0 Open	Z No Device	Z No Qualifier
1 Shoulder Bursa and Ligament, Right	3 Percutaneous		
2 Shoulder Bursa and Ligament, Left	4 Percutaneous Endoscopic		
3 Elbow Bursa and Ligament, Right	X External		
4 Elbow Bursa and Ligament, Left			
5 Wrist Bursa and Ligament, Right			
6 Wrist Bursa and Ligament, Left			
7 Hand Bursa and Ligament, Right			
8 Hand Bursa and Ligament, Left			
9 Upper Extremity Bursa and Ligament, Right			
B Upper Extremity Bursa and Ligament, Left			
C Trunk Bursa and Ligament, Right			
D Trunk Bursa and Ligament, Left			
F Thorax Bursa and Ligament, Right			
G Thorax Bursa and Ligament, Left			
H Abdomen Bursa and Ligament, Right			
J Abdomen Bursa and Ligament, Left			
K Perineum Bursa and Ligament			
L Hip Bursa and Ligament, Right			
M Hip Bursa and Ligament, Left			
N Knee Bursa and Ligament, Right			
P Knee Bursa and Ligament, Left			
Q Ankle Bursa and Ligament, Right			
R Ankle Bursa and Ligament, Left			
S Foot Bursa and Ligament, Right			
T Foot Bursa and Ligament, Left			
V Lower Extremity Bursa and Ligament, Right			
W Lower Extremity Bursa and Ligament, Left			

SECTION: 0 MEDICAL AND SURGICAL
BODY SYSTEM: M BURSAE AND LIGAMENTS
OPERATION: P **REMOVAL:** Taking out or off a device from a body part

Body Part	Approach	Device	Qualifier
X Upper Bursa and Ligament Y Lower Bursa and Ligament	0 Open 3 Percutaneous 4 Percutaneous Endoscopic	0 Drainage Device 7 Autologous Tissue Substitute J Synthetic Substitute K Nonautologous Tissue Substitute	Z No Qualifier
X Upper Bursa and Ligament Y Lower Bursa and Ligament	X External	0 Drainage Device	Z No Qualifier

SECTION: 0 MEDICAL AND SURGICAL
BODY SYSTEM: **M BURSAE AND LIGAMENTS**
OPERATION: **Q REPAIR:** Restoring, to the extent possible, a body part to its normal anatomic structure and function

Body Part	Approach	Device	Qualifier
0 Head and Neck Bursa and Ligament 1 Shoulder Bursa and Ligament, Right 2 Shoulder Bursa and Ligament, Left 3 Elbow Bursa and Ligament, Right 4 Elbow Bursa and Ligament, Left 5 Wrist Bursa and Ligament, Right 6 Wrist Bursa and Ligament, Left 7 Hand Bursa and Ligament, Right 8 Hand Bursa and Ligament, Left 9 Upper Extremity Bursa and Ligament, Right B Upper Extremity Bursa and Ligament, Left C Trunk Bursa and Ligament, Right D Trunk Bursa and Ligament, Left F Thorax Bursa and Ligament, Right G Thorax Bursa and Ligament, Left H Abdomen Bursa and Ligament, Right J Abdomen Bursa and Ligament, Left K Perineum Bursa and Ligament L Hip Bursa and Ligament, Right M Hip Bursa and Ligament, Left N Knee Bursa and Ligament, Right P Knee Bursa and Ligament, Left Q Ankle Bursa and Ligament, Right R Ankle Bursa and Ligament, Left S Foot Bursa and Ligament, Right T Foot Bursa and Ligament, Left V Lower Extremity Bursa and Ligament, Right W Lower Extremity Bursa and Ligament, Left	0 Open 3 Percutaneous 4 Percutaneous Endoscopic	Z No Device	Z No Qualifier

Q: REPAIR

M: BURSAE AND LIGAMENTS

0: M/S

◀ New   ◀▥ Revised   ~~deleted~~ Deleted   ♀ Females Only   ♂ Males Only
   ⦸ Noncovered   ⦸ Limited Coverage   ⦸ Hospital-Acquired Condition   **Coding Clinic**

SECTION: 0 MEDICAL AND SURGICAL

BODY SYSTEM: M BURSAE AND LIGAMENTS

OPERATION: S REPOSITION: Moving to its normal location, or other suitable location, all or a portion of a body part

Body Part	Approach	Device	Qualifier
0 Head and Neck Bursa and Ligament	0 Open	Z No Device	Z No Qualifier
1 Shoulder Bursa and Ligament, Right	4 Percutaneous Endoscopic		
2 Shoulder Bursa and Ligament, Left			
3 Elbow Bursa and Ligament, Right			
4 Elbow Bursa and Ligament, Left			
5 Wrist Bursa and Ligament, Right			
6 Wrist Bursa and Ligament, Left			
7 Hand Bursa and Ligament, Right			
8 Hand Bursa and Ligament, Left			
9 Upper Extremity Bursa and Ligament, Right			
B Upper Extremity Bursa and Ligament, Left			
C Trunk Bursa and Ligament, Right			
D Trunk Bursa and Ligament, Left			
F Thorax Bursa and Ligament, Right			
G Thorax Bursa and Ligament, Left			
H Abdomen Bursa and Ligament, Right			
J Abdomen Bursa and Ligament, Left			
K Perineum Bursa and Ligament			
L Hip Bursa and Ligament, Right			
M Hip Bursa and Ligament, Left			
N Knee Bursa and Ligament, Right			
P Knee Bursa and Ligament, Left			
Q Ankle Bursa and Ligament, Right			
R Ankle Bursa and Ligament, Left			
S Foot Bursa and Ligament, Right			
T Foot Bursa and Ligament, Left			
V Lower Extremity Bursa and Ligament, Right			
W Lower Extremity Bursa and Ligament, Left			

0: M/S

M: BURSAE AND LIGAMENTS

S: REPOSITION

◀ New ◀ Revised ~~deleted~~ Deleted ♀ Females Only ♂ Males Only
⊘ Noncovered ⊘ Limited Coverage ⊘ Hospital-Acquired Condition **Coding Clinic**

333

SECTION: 0 MEDICAL AND SURGICAL
BODY SYSTEM: M BURSAE AND LIGAMENTS
OPERATION: T RESECTION: Cutting out or off, without replacement, all of a body part

Body Part	Approach	Device	Qualifier
0 Head and Neck Bursa and Ligament	0 Open	Z No Device	Z No Qualifier
1 Shoulder Bursa and Ligament, Right	4 Percutaneous Endoscopic		
2 Shoulder Bursa and Ligament, Left			
3 Elbow Bursa and Ligament, Right			
4 Elbow Bursa and Ligament, Left			
5 Wrist Bursa and Ligament, Right			
6 Wrist Bursa and Ligament, Left			
7 Hand Bursa and Ligament, Right			
8 Hand Bursa and Ligament, Left			
9 Upper Extremity Bursa and Ligament, Right			
B Upper Extremity Bursa and Ligament, Left			
C Trunk Bursa and Ligament, Right			
D Trunk Bursa and Ligament, Left			
F Thorax Bursa and Ligament, Right			
G Thorax Bursa and Ligament, Left			
H Abdomen Bursa and Ligament, Right			
J Abdomen Bursa and Ligament, Left			
K Perineum Bursa and Ligament			
L Hip Bursa and Ligament, Right			
M Hip Bursa and Ligament, Left			
N Knee Bursa and Ligament, Right			
P Knee Bursa and Ligament, Left			
Q Ankle Bursa and Ligament, Right			
R Ankle Bursa and Ligament, Left			
S Foot Bursa and Ligament, Right			
T Foot Bursa and Ligament, Left			
V Lower Extremity Bursa and Ligament, Right			
W Lower Extremity Bursa and Ligament, Left			

◀ New ◀ Revised deleted Deleted ♀ Females Only ♂ Males Only
Noncovered Limited Coverage Hospital-Acquired Condition **Coding Clinic**

SECTION: 0 MEDICAL AND SURGICAL
BODY SYSTEM: M BURSAE AND LIGAMENTS
OPERATION: U SUPPLEMENT: Putting in or on biological or synthetic material that physically reinforces and/or augments the function of a portion of a body part

Body Part	Approach	Device	Qualifier
0 Head and Neck Bursa and Ligament	0 Open	7 Autologous Tissue Substitute	Z No Qualifier
1 Shoulder Bursa and Ligament, Right	4 Percutaneous Endoscopic	J Synthetic Substitute	
2 Shoulder Bursa and Ligament, Left		K Nonautologous Tissue Substitute	
3 Elbow Bursa and Ligament, Right			
4 Elbow Bursa and Ligament, Left			
5 Wrist Bursa and Ligament, Right			
6 Wrist Bursa and Ligament, Left			
7 Hand Bursa and Ligament, Right			
8 Hand Bursa and Ligament, Left			
9 Upper Extremity Bursa and Ligament, Right			
B Upper Extremity Bursa and Ligament, Left			
C Trunk Bursa and Ligament, Right			
D Trunk Bursa and Ligament, Left			
F Thorax Bursa and Ligament, Right			
G Thorax Bursa and Ligament, Left			
H Abdomen Bursa and Ligament, Right			
J Abdomen Bursa and Ligament, Left			
K Perineum Bursa and Ligament			
L Hip Bursa and Ligament, Right			
M Hip Bursa and Ligament, Left			
N Knee Bursa and Ligament, Right			
P Knee Bursa and Ligament, Left			
Q Ankle Bursa and Ligament, Right			
R Ankle Bursa and Ligament, Left			
S Foot Bursa and Ligament, Right			
T Foot Bursa and Ligament, Left			
V Lower Extremity Bursa and Ligament, Right			
W Lower Extremity Bursa and Ligament, Left			

◀ New   ◀▥ Revised   ~~deleted~~ Deleted   ♀ Females Only   ♂ Males Only
🚫 Noncovered   🚫 Limited Coverage   🚫 Hospital-Acquired Condition   **Coding Clinic**

SECTION: 0 MEDICAL AND SURGICAL
BODY SYSTEM: M BURSAE AND LIGAMENTS
OPERATION: W REVISION: Correcting, to the extent possible, a portion of a malfunctioning device or the position of a displaced device

Body Part	Approach	Device	Qualifier
X Upper Bursa and Ligament Y Lower Bursa and Ligament	0 Open 3 Percutaneous 4 Percutaneous Endoscopic X External	0 Drainage Device 7 Autologous Tissue Substitute J Synthetic Substitute K Nonautologous Tissue Substitute	Z No Qualifier

SECTION: 0 MEDICAL AND SURGICAL
BODY SYSTEM: M BURSAE AND LIGAMENTS
OPERATION: X TRANSFER: Moving, without taking out, all or a portion of a body part to another location to take over the function of all or a portion of a body part

Body Part	Approach	Device	Qualifier
0 Head and Neck Bursa and Ligament 1 Shoulder Bursa and Ligament, Right 2 Shoulder Bursa and Ligament, Left 3 Elbow Bursa and Ligament, Right 4 Elbow Bursa and Ligament, Left 5 Wrist Bursa and Ligament, Right 6 Wrist Bursa and Ligament, Left 7 Hand Bursa and Ligament, Right 8 Hand Bursa and Ligament, Left 9 Upper Extremity Bursa and Ligament, Right B Upper Extremity Bursa and Ligament, Left C Trunk Bursa and Ligament, Right D Trunk Bursa and Ligament, Left F Thorax Bursa and Ligament, Right G Thorax Bursa and Ligament, Left H Abdomen Bursa and Ligament, Right J Abdomen Bursa and Ligament, Left K Perineum Bursa and Ligament L Hip Bursa and Ligament, Right M Hip Bursa and Ligament, Left N Knee Bursa and Ligament, Right P Knee Bursa and Ligament, Left Q Ankle Bursa and Ligament, Right R Ankle Bursa and Ligament, Left S Foot Bursa and Ligament, Right T Foot Bursa and Ligament, Left V Lower Extremity Bursa and Ligament, Right W Lower Extremity Bursa and Ligament, Left	0 Open 4 Percutaneous Endoscopic	Z No Device	Z No Qualifier

W: REVISION   X: TRANSFER

M: BURSAE AND LIGAMENTS   0: M/S

SECTION: 0 MEDICAL AND SURGICAL
BODY SYSTEM: N HEAD AND FACIAL BONES
OPERATION: 2 CHANGE: Taking out or off a device from a body part and putting back an identical or similar device in or on the same body part without cutting or puncturing the skin or a mucous membrane

Body Part	Approach	Device	Qualifier
0 Skull B Nasal Bone W Facial Bone	X External	0 Drainage Device Y Other Device	Z No Qualifier

SECTION: 0 MEDICAL AND SURGICAL
BODY SYSTEM: N HEAD AND FACIAL BONES
OPERATION: 5 DESTRUCTION: Physical eradication of all or a portion of a body part by the direct use of energy, force, or a destructive agent

Body Part	Approach	Device	Qualifier
0 Skull 1 Frontal Bone, Right 2 Frontal Bone, Left 3 Parietal Bone, Right 4 Parietal Bone, Left 5 Temporal Bone, Right 6 Temporal Bone, Left 7 Occipital Bone, Right 8 Occipital Bone, Left B Nasal Bone C Sphenoid Bone, Right D Sphenoid Bone, Left F Ethmoid Bone, Right G Ethmoid Bone, Left H Lacrimal Bone, Right J Lacrimal Bone, Left K Palatine Bone, Right L Palatine Bone, Left M Zygomatic Bone, Right N Zygomatic Bone, Left P Orbit, Right Q Orbit, Left R Maxilla, Right S Maxilla, Left T Mandible, Right V Mandible, Left X Hyoid Bone	0 Open 3 Percutaneous 4 Percutaneous Endoscopic	Z No Device	Z No Qualifier

SECTION: 0 MEDICAL AND SURGICAL
BODY SYSTEM: N HEAD AND FACIAL BONES
OPERATION: 8 **DIVISION:** Cutting into a body part, without draining fluids and/or gases from the body part, in order to separate or transect a body part

Body Part	Approach	Device	Qualifier
0 Skull	0 Open	Z No Device	Z No Qualifier
1 Frontal Bone, Right	3 Percutaneous		
2 Frontal Bone, Left	4 Percutaneous Endoscopic		
3 Parietal Bone, Right			
4 Parietal Bone, Left			
5 Temporal Bone, Right			
6 Temporal Bone, Left			
7 Occipital Bone, Right			
8 Occipital Bone, Left			
B Nasal Bone			
C Sphenoid Bone, Right			
D Sphenoid Bone, Left			
F Ethmoid Bone, Right			
G Ethmoid Bone, Left			
H Lacrimal Bone, Right			
J Lacrimal Bone, Left			
K Palatine Bone, Right			
L Palatine Bone, Left			
M Zygomatic Bone, Right			
N Zygomatic Bone, Left			
P Orbit, Right			
Q Orbit, Left			
R Maxilla, Right			
S Maxilla, Left			
T Mandible, Right			
V Mandible, Left			
X Hyoid Bone			

◄ New ◄ Revised deleted Deleted ♀ Females Only ♂ Males Only
Noncovered Limited Coverage Hospital-Acquired Condition **Coding Clinic**

SECTION: 0 MEDICAL AND SURGICAL
BODY SYSTEM: N HEAD AND FACIAL BONES
OPERATION: 9 DRAINAGE: Taking or letting out fluids and/or gases from a body part

Body Part	Approach	Device	Qualifier
0 Skull	0 Open	0 Drainage Device	Z No Qualifier
1 Frontal Bone, Right	3 Percutaneous		
2 Frontal Bone, Left	4 Percutaneous Endoscopic		
3 Parietal Bone, Right			
4 Parietal Bone, Left			
5 Temporal Bone, Right			
6 Temporal Bone, Left			
7 Occipital Bone, Right			
8 Occipital Bone, Left			
B Nasal Bone			
C Sphenoid Bone, Right			
D Sphenoid Bone, Left			
F Ethmoid Bone, Right			
G Ethmoid Bone, Left			
H Lacrimal Bone, Right			
J Lacrimal Bone, Left			
K Palatine Bone, Right			
L Palatine Bone, Left			
M Zygomatic Bone, Right			
N Zygomatic Bone, Left			
P Orbit, Right			
Q Orbit, Left			
R Maxilla, Right			
S Maxilla, Left			
T Mandible, Right			
V Mandible, Left			
X Hyoid Bone			
0 Skull	0 Open	Z No Device	X Diagnostic
1 Frontal Bone, Right	3 Percutaneous		Z No Qualifier
2 Frontal Bone, Left	4 Percutaneous Endoscopic		
3 Parietal Bone, Right			
4 Parietal Bone, Left			
5 Temporal Bone, Right			
6 Temporal Bone, Left			
7 Occipital Bone, Right			
8 Occipital Bone, Left			
B Nasal Bone			
C Sphenoid Bone, Right			
D Sphenoid Bone, Left			
F Ethmoid Bone, Right			
G Ethmoid Bone, Left			
H Lacrimal Bone, Right			
J Lacrimal Bone, Left			
K Palatine Bone, Right			
L Palatine Bone, Left			
M Zygomatic Bone, Right			
N Zygomatic Bone, Left			
P Orbit, Right			
Q Orbit, Left			
R Maxilla, Right			
S Maxilla, Left			
T Mandible, Right			
V Mandible, Left			
X Hyoid Bone			

◀ New ◀ Revised ~~deleted~~ Deleted ♀ Females Only ♂ Males Only
Noncovered Limited Coverage Hospital-Acquired Condition **Coding Clinic**

SECTION: 0 MEDICAL AND SURGICAL
BODY SYSTEM: N HEAD AND FACIAL BONES
OPERATION: B EXCISION: Cutting out or off, without replacement, a portion of a body part

Body Part	Approach	Device	Qualifier
0 Skull	0 Open	Z No Device	X Diagnostic
1 Frontal Bone, Right	3 Percutaneous		Z No Qualifier
2 Frontal Bone, Left	4 Percutaneous Endoscopic		
3 Parietal Bone, Right			
4 Parietal Bone, Left			
5 Temporal Bone, Right			
6 Temporal Bone, Left			
7 Occipital Bone, Right			
8 Occipital Bone, Left			
B Nasal Bone			
C Sphenoid Bone, Right			
D Sphenoid Bone, Left			
F Ethmoid Bone, Right			
G Ethmoid Bone, Left			
H Lacrimal Bone, Right			
J Lacrimal Bone, Left			
K Palatine Bone, Right			
L Palatine Bone, Left			
M Zygomatic Bone, Right			
N Zygomatic Bone, Left			
P Orbit, Right			
Q Orbit, Left			
R Maxilla, Right			
S Maxilla, Left			
T Mandible, Right			
V Mandible, Left			
X Hyoid Bone			

◀ New   ◀▥ Revised   ~~deleted~~ Deleted   ♀ Females Only   ♂ Males Only
🚱 Noncovered   🚱 Limited Coverage   🚱 Hospital-Acquired Condition   **Coding Clinic**

341

SECTION: 0 MEDICAL AND SURGICAL
BODY SYSTEM: N HEAD AND FACIAL BONES
OPERATION: C EXTIRPATION: Taking or cutting out solid matter from a body part

Body Part	Approach	Device	Qualifier
1 Frontal Bone, Right	0 Open	Z No Device	Z No Qualifier
2 Frontal Bone, Left	3 Percutaneous		
3 Parietal Bone, Right	4 Percutaneous Endoscopic		
4 Parietal Bone, Left			
5 Temporal Bone, Right			
6 Temporal Bone, Left			
7 Occipital Bone, Right			
8 Occipital Bone, Left			
B Nasal Bone			
C Sphenoid Bone, Right			
D Sphenoid Bone, Left			
F Ethmoid Bone, Right			
G Ethmoid Bone, Left			
H Lacrimal Bone, Right			
J Lacrimal Bone, Left			
K Palatine Bone, Right			
L Palatine Bone, Left			
M Zygomatic Bone, Right			
N Zygomatic Bone, Left			
P Orbit, Right			
Q Orbit, Left			
R Maxilla, Right			
S Maxilla, Left			
T Mandible, Right			
V Mandible, Left			
X Hyoid Bone			

◀ New ◀▥ Revised ~~deleted~~ Deleted ♀ Females Only ♂ Males Only
🅝 Noncovered 🅛 Limited Coverage 🅗 Hospital-Acquired Condition **Coding Clinic**

SECTION: 0 MEDICAL AND SURGICAL
BODY SYSTEM: N HEAD AND FACIAL BONES
OPERATION: H INSERTION: Putting in a nonbiological appliance that monitors, assists, performs, or prevents a physiological function but does not physically take the place of a body part

Body Part	Approach	Device	Qualifier
0 Skull	0 Open	4 Internal Fixation Device 5 External Fixation Device M Bone Growth Stimulator N Neurostimulator Generator	Z No Qualifier
0 Skull	3 Percutaneous 4 Percutaneous Endoscopic	4 Internal Fixation Device 5 External Fixation Device M Bone Growth Stimulator	Z No Qualifier
1 Frontal Bone, Right 2 Frontal Bone, Left 3 Parietal Bone, Right 4 Parietal Bone, Left 7 Occipital Bone, Right 8 Occipital Bone, Left C Sphenoid Bone, Right D Sphenoid Bone, Left F Ethmoid Bone, Right G Ethmoid Bone, Left H Lacrimal Bone, Right J Lacrimal Bone, Left K Palatine Bone, Right L Palatine Bone, Left M Zygomatic Bone, Right N Zygomatic Bone, Left P Orbit, Right Q Orbit, Left X Hyoid Bone	0 Open 3 Percutaneous 4 Percutaneous Endoscopic	4 Internal Fixation Device	Z No Qualifier
5 Temporal Bone, Right 6 Temporal Bone, Left	0 Open 3 Percutaneous 4 Percutaneous Endoscopic	4 Internal Fixation Device S Hearing Device	Z No Qualifier
B Nasal Bone	0 Open 3 Percutaneous 4 Percutaneous Endoscopic	4 Internal Fixation Device M Bone Growth Stimulator	Z No Qualifier
R Maxilla, Right S Maxilla, Left T Mandible, Right V Mandible, Left	0 Open 3 Percutaneous 4 Percutaneous Endoscopic	4 Internal Fixation Device 5 External Fixation Device	Z No Qualifier
W Facial Bone	0 Open 3 Percutaneous 4 Percutaneous Endoscopic	M Bone Growth Stimulator	Z No Qualifier

SECTION: 0 MEDICAL AND SURGICAL
BODY SYSTEM: N HEAD AND FACIAL BONES
OPERATION: J INSPECTION: Visually and/or manually exploring a body part

Body Part	Approach	Device	Qualifier
0 Skull	0 Open	Z No Device	Z No Qualifier
B Nasal Bone	3 Percutaneous		
W Facial Bone	4 Percutaneous Endoscopic		
	X External		

SECTION: 0 MEDICAL AND SURGICAL
BODY SYSTEM: N HEAD AND FACIAL BONES
OPERATION: N RELEASE: Freeing a body part from an abnormal physical constraint by cutting or by the use of force

Body Part	Approach	Device	Qualifier
1 Frontal Bone, Right	0 Open	Z No Device	Z No Qualifier
2 Frontal Bone, Left	3 Percutaneous		
3 Parietal Bone, Right	4 Percutaneous Endoscopic		
4 Parietal Bone, Left			
5 Temporal Bone, Right			
6 Temporal Bone, Left			
7 Occipital Bone, Right			
8 Occipital Bone, Left			
B Nasal Bone			
C Sphenoid Bone, Right			
D Sphenoid Bone, Left			
F Ethmoid Bone, Right			
G Ethmoid Bone, Left			
H Lacrimal Bone, Right			
J Lacrimal Bone, Left			
K Palatine Bone, Right			
L Palatine Bone, Left			
M Zygomatic Bone, Right			
N Zygomatic Bone, Left			
P Orbit, Right			
Q Orbit, Left			
R Maxilla, Right			
S Maxilla, Left			
T Mandible, Right			
V Mandible, Left			
X Hyoid Bone			

◀ New   ◀▥ Revised   ~~deleted~~ Deleted   ♀ Females Only   ♂ Males Only
🐾 Noncovered   🐾 Limited Coverage   🐾 Hospital-Acquired Condition   **Coding Clinic**

SECTION: 0 MEDICAL AND SURGICAL
BODY SYSTEM: N HEAD AND FACIAL BONES
OPERATION: P REMOVAL: Taking out or off a device from a body part

Body Part	Approach	Device	Qualifier
0 Skull	0 Open	0 Drainage Device 4 Internal Fixation Device 5 External Fixation Device 7 Autologous Tissue Substitute J Synthetic Substitute K Nonautologous Tissue Substitute M Bone Growth Stimulator N Neurostimulator Generator S Hearing Device	Z No Qualifier
0 Skull	3 Percutaneous 4 Percutaneous Endoscopic	0 Drainage Device 4 Internal Fixation Device 5 External Fixation Device 7 Autologous Tissue Substitute J Synthetic Substitute K Nonautologous Tissue Substitute M Bone Growth Stimulator S Hearing Device	Z No Qualifier
0 Skull	X External	0 Drainage Device 4 Internal Fixation Device 5 External Fixation Device M Bone Growth Stimulator S Hearing Device	Z No Qualifier
B Nasal Bone W Facial Bone	0 Open 3 Percutaneous 4 Percutaneous Endoscopic	0 Drainage Device 4 Internal Fixation Device 7 Autologous Tissue Substitute J Synthetic Substitute K Nonautologous Tissue Substitute M Bone Growth Stimulator	Z No Qualifier
B Nasal Bone W Facial Bone	X External	0 Drainage Device 4 Internal Fixation Device M Bone Growth Stimulator	Z No Qualifier

◄ New ◄▥ Revised ~~deleted~~ Deleted ♀ Females Only ♂ Males Only
🚫 Noncovered 🚫 Limited Coverage 🚫 Hospital-Acquired Condition **Coding Clinic**

SECTION: 0 MEDICAL AND SURGICAL
BODY SYSTEM: N HEAD AND FACIAL BONES
OPERATION: Q REPAIR: Restoring, to the extent possible, a body part to its normal anatomic structure and function

Body Part	Approach	Device	Qualifier
0 Skull	0 Open	Z No Device	Z No Qualifier
1 Frontal Bone, Right	3 Percutaneous		
2 Frontal Bone, Left	4 Percutaneous Endoscopic		
3 Parietal Bone, Right	X External		
4 Parietal Bone, Left			
5 Temporal Bone, Right			
6 Temporal Bone, Left			
7 Occipital Bone, Right			
8 Occipital Bone, Left			
B Nasal Bone			
C Sphenoid Bone, Right			
D Sphenoid Bone, Left			
F Ethmoid Bone, Right			
G Ethmoid Bone, Left			
H Lacrimal Bone, Right			
J Lacrimal Bone, Left			
K Palatine Bone, Right			
L Palatine Bone, Left			
M Zygomatic Bone, Right			
N Zygomatic Bone, Left			
P Orbit, Right			
Q Orbit, Left			
R Maxilla, Right			
S Maxilla, Left			
T Mandible, Right			
V Mandible, Left			
X Hyoid Bone			

◀ New   ◀▥ Revised   ~~deleted~~ Deleted   ♀ Females Only   ♂ Males Only
⚕ Noncovered   ⚕ Limited Coverage   ⚕ Hospital-Acquired Condition   **Coding Clinic**

SECTION: 0 MEDICAL AND SURGICAL

BODY SYSTEM: N HEAD AND FACIAL BONES

OPERATION: R REPLACEMENT: Putting in or on biological or synthetic material that physically takes the place and/or function of all or a portion of a body part

Body Part	Approach	Device	Qualifier
0 Skull 1 Frontal Bone, Right 2 Frontal Bone, Left 3 Parietal Bone, Right 4 Parietal Bone, Left 5 Temporal Bone, Right 6 Temporal Bone, Left 7 Occipital Bone, Right 8 Occipital Bone, Left B Nasal Bone C Sphenoid Bone, Right D Sphenoid Bone, Left F Ethmoid Bone, Right G Ethmoid Bone, Left H Lacrimal Bone, Right J Lacrimal Bone, Left K Palatine Bone, Right L Palatine Bone, Left M Zygomatic Bone, Right N Zygomatic Bone, Left P Orbit, Right Q Orbit, Left R Maxilla, Right S Maxilla, Left T Mandible, Right V Mandible, Left X Hyoid Bone	0 Open 3 Percutaneous 4 Percutaneous Endoscopic	7 Autologous Tissue Substitute J Synthetic Substitute K Nonautologous Tissue Substitute	Z No Qualifier

SECTION: 0 MEDICAL AND SURGICAL

BODY SYSTEM: N HEAD AND FACIAL BONES

OPERATION: S REPOSITION: *(on multiple pages)*
Moving to its normal location, or other suitable location, all or a portion of a body part

Body Part	Approach	Device	Qualifier
0 Skull R Maxilla, Right S Maxilla, Left T Mandible, Right V Mandible, Left	0 Open 3 Percutaneous 4 Percutaneous Endoscopic	4 Internal Fixation Device 5 External Fixation Device Z No Device	Z No Qualifier
0 Skull R Maxilla, Right S Maxilla, Left T Mandible, Right V Mandible, Left	X External	Z No Device	Z No Qualifier

◀ New ◀ Revised deleted Deleted ♀ Females Only ♂ Males Only
Noncovered Limited Coverage Hospital-Acquired Condition **Coding Clinic**

347

SECTION: 0 MEDICAL AND SURGICAL
BODY SYSTEM: N HEAD AND FACIAL BONES
OPERATION: S REPOSITION: *(continued)*
Moving to its normal location, or other suitable location, all or a portion of a body part

Body Part	Approach	Device	Qualifier
1 Frontal Bone, Right 2 Frontal Bone, Left 3 Parietal Bone, Right 4 Parietal Bone, Left 5 Temporal Bone, Right 6 Temporal Bone, Left 7 Occipital Bone, Right 8 Occipital Bone, Left B Nasal Bone C Sphenoid Bone, Right D Sphenoid Bone, Left F Ethmoid Bone, Right G Ethmoid Bone, Left H Lacrimal Bone, Right J Lacrimal Bone, Left K Palatine Bone, Right L Palatine Bone, Left M Zygomatic Bone, Right N Zygomatic Bone, Left P Orbit, Right Q Orbit, Left X Hyoid Bone	0 Open 3 Percutaneous 4 Percutaneous Endoscopic	4 Internal Fixation Device Z No Device	Z No Qualifier
1 Frontal Bone, Right 2 Frontal Bone, Left 3 Parietal Bone, Right 4 Parietal Bone, Left 5 Temporal Bone, Right 6 Temporal Bone, Left 7 Occipital Bone, Right 8 Occipital Bone, Left B Nasal Bone C Sphenoid Bone, Right D Sphenoid Bone, Left F Ethmoid Bone, Right G Ethmoid Bone, Left H Lacrimal Bone, Right J Lacrimal Bone, Left K Palatine Bone, Right L Palatine Bone, Left M Zygomatic Bone, Right N Zygomatic Bone, Left P Orbit, Right Q Orbit, Left X Hyoid Bone	X External	Z No Device	Z No Qualifier

Coding Clinic: 2013, Q3, P25 – 0NS005Z, 0NS104Z

◄ New ◄ Revised ~~deleted~~ Deleted ♀ Females Only ♂ Males Only
Noncovered Limited Coverage Hospital-Acquired Condition Coding Clinic

SECTION: 0 MEDICAL AND SURGICAL
BODY SYSTEM: N HEAD AND FACIAL BONES
OPERATION: T RESECTION: Cutting out or off, without replacement, all of a body part

Body Part	Approach	Device	Qualifier
1 Frontal Bone, Right	0 Open	Z No Device	Z No Qualifier
2 Frontal Bone, Left			
3 Parietal Bone, Right			
4 Parietal Bone, Left			
5 Temporal Bone, Right			
6 Temporal Bone, Left			
7 Occipital Bone, Right			
8 Occipital Bone, Left			
B Nasal Bone			
C Sphenoid Bone, Right			
D Sphenoid Bone, Left			
F Ethmoid Bone, Right			
G Ethmoid Bone, Left			
H Lacrimal Bone, Right			
J Lacrimal Bone, Left			
K Palatine Bone, Right			
L Palatine Bone, Left			
M Zygomatic Bone, Right			
N Zygomatic Bone, Left			
P Orbit, Right			
Q Orbit, Left			
R Maxilla, Right			
S Maxilla, Left			
T Mandible, Right			
V Mandible, Left			
X Hyoid Bone			

0: M/S

N: HEAD AND FACIAL BONES

T: RESECTION

SECTION: 0 MEDICAL AND SURGICAL
BODY SYSTEM: N HEAD AND FACIAL BONES
OPERATION: U SUPPLEMENT: Putting in or on biological or synthetic material that physically reinforces and/or augments the function of a portion of a body part

Body Part	Approach	Device	Qualifier
0 Skull 1 Frontal Bone, Right 2 Frontal Bone, Left 3 Parietal Bone, Right 4 Parietal Bone, Left 5 Temporal Bone, Right 6 Temporal Bone, Left 7 Occipital Bone, Right 8 Occipital Bone, Left B Nasal Bone C Sphenoid Bone, Right D Sphenoid Bone, Left F Ethmoid Bone, Right G Ethmoid Bone, Left H Lacrimal Bone, Right J Lacrimal Bone, Left K Palatine Bone, Right L Palatine Bone, Left M Zygomatic Bone, Right N Zygomatic Bone, Left P Orbit, Right Q Orbit, Left R Maxilla, Right S Maxilla, Left T Mandible, Right V Mandible, Left X Hyoid Bone	0 Open 3 Percutaneous 4 Percutaneous Endoscopic	7 Autologous Tissue Substitute J Synthetic Substitute K Nonautologous Tissue Substitute	Z No Qualifier

Coding Clinic: 2013, Q3, P25 – 0NU00JZ

◀ New   ◀▥ Revised   ~~deleted~~ Deleted   ♀ Females Only   ♂ Males Only
🅝🅒 Noncovered   🅛🅒 Limited Coverage   🅗🅐🅒 Hospital-Acquired Condition   **Coding Clinic**

SECTION: 0 MEDICAL AND SURGICAL
BODY SYSTEM: N HEAD AND FACIAL BONES
OPERATION: W REVISION: Correcting, to the extent possible, a portion of a malfunctioning device or the position of a displaced device

Body Part	Approach	Device	Qualifier
0 Skull	0 Open	0 Drainage Device 4 Internal Fixation Device 5 External Fixation Device 7 Autologous Tissue Substitute J Synthetic Substitute K Nonautologous Tissue Substitute M Bone Growth Stimulator N Neurostimulator Generator S Hearing Device	Z No Qualifier
0 Skull	3 Percutaneous 4 Percutaneous Endoscopic X External	0 Drainage Device 4 Internal Fixation Device 5 External Fixation Device 7 Autologous Tissue Substitute J Synthetic Substitute K Nonautologous Tissue Substitute M Bone Growth Stimulator S Hearing Device	Z No Qualifier
B Nasal Bone W Facial Bone	0 Open 3 Percutaneous 4 Percutaneous Endoscopic X External	0 Drainage Device 4 Internal Fixation Device 7 Autologous Tissue Substitute J Synthetic Substitute K Nonautologous Tissue Substitute M Bone Growth Stimulator	Z No Qualifier

0: M/S

N: HEAD AND FACIAL BONES

W: REVISION

◀ New   ◀ Revised   deleted Deleted   ♀ Females Only   ♂ Males Only
🚫 Noncovered   🚫 Limited Coverage   🚫 Hospital-Acquired Condition   **Coding Clinic**

351

◀ New　◀▥ Revised　~~deleted~~ Deleted　♀ Females Only　♂ Males Only
℞ Noncovered　℞ Limited Coverage　℞ Hospital-Acquired Condition　**Coding Clinic**

SECTION: 0 MEDICAL AND SURGICAL

BODY SYSTEM: P UPPER BONES

OPERATION: 2 **CHANGE:** Taking out or off a device from a body part and putting back an identical or similar device in or on the same body part without cutting or puncturing the skin or a mucous membrane

Body Part	Approach	Device	Qualifier
Y Upper Bone	X External	0 Drainage Device Y Other Device	Z No Qualifier

SECTION: 0 MEDICAL AND SURGICAL

BODY SYSTEM: P UPPER BONES

OPERATION: 5 **DESTRUCTION:** Physical eradication of all or a portion of a body part by the direct use of energy, force, or a destructive agent

Body Part	Approach	Device	Qualifier
0 Sternum 1 Rib, Right 2 Rib, Left 3 Cervical Vertebra 4 Thoracic Vertebra 5 Scapula, Right 6 Scapula, Left 7 Glenoid Cavity, Right 8 Glenoid Cavity, Left 9 Clavicle, Right B Clavicle, Left C Humeral Head, Right D Humeral Head, Left F Humeral Shaft, Right G Humeral Shaft, Left H Radius, Right J Radius, Left K Ulna, Right L Ulna, Left M Carpal, Right N Carpal, Left P Metacarpal, Right Q Metacarpal, Left R Thumb Phalanx, Right S Thumb Phalanx, Left T Finger Phalanx, Right V Finger Phalanx, Left	0 Open 3 Percutaneous 4 Percutaneous Endoscopic	Z No Device	Z No Qualifier

0: M/S   P: UPPER BONES   2: CHANGE   5: DESTRUCTION

SECTION: 0 MEDICAL AND SURGICAL
BODY SYSTEM: P UPPER BONES
OPERATION: 8 DIVISION: Cutting into a body part, without draining fluids and/or gases from the body part, in order to separate or transect a body part

Body Part	Approach	Device	Qualifier
0 Sternum 1 Rib, Right 2 Rib, Left 3 Cervical Vertebra 4 Thoracic Vertebra 5 Scapula, Right 6 Scapula, Left 7 Glenoid Cavity, Right 8 Glenoid Cavity, Left 9 Clavicle, Right B Clavicle, Left C Humeral Head, Right D Humeral Head, Left F Humeral Shaft, Right G Humeral Shaft, Left H Radius, Right J Radius, Left K Ulna, Right L Ulna, Left M Carpal, Right N Carpal, Left P Metacarpal, Right Q Metacarpal, Left R Thumb Phalanx, Right S Thumb Phalanx, Left T Finger Phalanx, Right V Finger Phalanx, Left	0 Open 3 Percutaneous 4 Percutaneous Endoscopic	Z No Device	Z No Qualifier

P: UPPER BONES

8: DIVISION

0: M/S

◀ New　◀▥ Revised　~~deleted~~ Deleted　♀ Females Only　♂ Males Only
🔾 Noncovered　🔾 Limited Coverage　🔾 Hospital-Acquired Condition　**Coding Clinic**

SECTION: 0 MEDICAL AND SURGICAL
BODY SYSTEM: P UPPER BONES
OPERATION: 9 DRAINAGE: Taking or letting out fluids and/or gases from a body part

Body Part	Approach	Device	Qualifier
0 Sternum 1 Rib, Right 2 Rib, Left 3 Cervical Vertebra 4 Thoracic Vertebra 5 Scapula, Right 6 Scapula, Left 7 Glenoid Cavity, Right 8 Glenoid Cavity, Left 9 Clavicle, Right B Clavicle, Left C Humeral Head, Right D Humeral Head, Left F Humeral Shaft, Right G Humeral Shaft, Left H Radius, Right J Radius, Left K Ulna, Right L Ulna, Left M Carpal, Right N Carpal, Left P Metacarpal, Right Q Metacarpal, Left R Thumb Phalanx, Right S Thumb Phalanx, Left T Finger Phalanx, Right V Finger Phalanx, Left	0 Open 3 Percutaneous 4 Percutaneous Endoscopic	0 Drainage Device	Z No Qualifier
0 Sternum 1 Rib, Right 2 Rib, Left 3 Cervical Vertebra 4 Thoracic Vertebra 5 Scapula, Right 6 Scapula, Left 7 Glenoid Cavity, Right 8 Glenoid Cavity, Left 9 Clavicle, Right B Clavicle, Left C Humeral Head, Right D Humeral Head, Left F Humeral Shaft, Right G Humeral Shaft, Left H Radius, Right J Radius, Left K Ulna, Right L Ulna, Left M Carpal, Right N Carpal, Left P Metacarpal, Right Q Metacarpal, Left R Thumb Phalanx, Right S Thumb Phalanx, Left T Finger Phalanx, Right V Finger Phalanx, Left	0 Open 3 Percutaneous 4 Percutaneous Endoscopic	Z No Device	X Diagnostic Z No Qualifier

◄ New   ◄ Revised   deleted Deleted   ♀ Females Only   ♂ Males Only
🚫 Noncovered   🔵 Limited Coverage   🔵 Hospital-Acquired Condition   **Coding Clinic**

SECTION: 0   MEDICAL AND SURGICAL
BODY SYSTEM: P   UPPER BONES
OPERATION: **B   EXCISION:** Cutting out or off, without replacement, a portion of a body part

Body Part	Approach	Device	Qualifier
0 Sternum	0 Open	Z No Device	X Diagnostic
1 Rib, Right	3 Percutaneous		Z No Qualifier
2 Rib, Left	4 Percutaneous Endoscopic		
3 Cervical Vertebra			
4 Thoracic Vertebra			
5 Scapula, Right			
6 Scapula, Left			
7 Glenoid Cavity, Right			
8 Glenoid Cavity, Left			
9 Clavicle, Right			
B Clavicle, Left			
C Humeral Head, Right			
D Humeral Head, Left			
F Humeral Shaft, Right			
G Humeral Shaft, Left			
H Radius, Right			
J Radius, Left			
K Ulna, Right			
L Ulna, Left			
M Carpal, Right			
N Carpal, Left			
P Metacarpal, Right			
Q Metacarpal, Left			
R Thumb Phalanx, Right			
S Thumb Phalanx, Left			
T Finger Phalanx, Right			
V Finger Phalanx, Left			

Coding Clinic: 2012, Q4, P101 – 0PB10ZZ

Coding Clinic: 2013, Q3, P22 – 0PB54ZZ

B: EXCISION

P: UPPER BONES

0: M/S

◀ New   ◀ Revised   ~~deleted~~ Deleted   ♀ Females Only   ♂ Males Only
Noncovered   Limited Coverage   Hospital-Acquired Condition   **Coding Clinic**

SECTION: 0 MEDICAL AND SURGICAL
BODY SYSTEM: P UPPER BONES
OPERATION: C EXTIRPATION: Taking or cutting out solid matter from a body part

Body Part	Approach	Device	Qualifier
0 Sternum	0 Open	Z No Device	Z No Qualifier
1 Rib, Right	3 Percutaneous		
2 Rib, Left	4 Percutaneous Endoscopic		
3 Cervical Vertebra			
4 Thoracic Vertebra			
5 Scapula, Right			
6 Scapula, Left			
7 Glenoid Cavity, Right			
8 Glenoid Cavity, Left			
9 Clavicle, Right			
B Clavicle, Left			
C Humeral Head, Right			
D Humeral Head, Left			
F Humeral Shaft, Right			
G Humeral Shaft, Left			
H Radius, Right			
J Radius, Left			
K Ulna, Right			
L Ulna, Left			
M Carpal, Right			
N Carpal, Left			
P Metacarpal, Right			
Q Metacarpal, Left			
R Thumb Phalanx, Right			
S Thumb Phalanx, Left			
T Finger Phalanx, Right			
V Finger Phalanx, Left			

◀ New ◀▥ Revised ~~deleted~~ Deleted ♀ Females Only ♂ Males Only
 Noncovered   Limited Coverage Hospital-Acquired Condition **Coding Clinic**

357

SECTION: 0 MEDICAL AND SURGICAL
BODY SYSTEM: P UPPER BONES
OPERATION: H INSERTION: Putting in a nonbiological appliance that monitors, assists, performs, or prevents a physiological function but does not physically take the place of a body part

SECTION: 0 MEDICAL
BODY SYSTEM: P UPPER BONES

H: INSERTION

P: UPPER BONES

0: M/S

Body Part	Approach	Device	Qualifier
0 Sternum	0 Open 3 Percutaneous 4 Percutaneous Endoscopic	0 Internal Fixation Device, Rigid Plate 4 Internal Fixation Device	Z No Qualifier
1 Rib, Right 2 Rib, Left 3 Cervical Vertebra 4 Thoracic Vertebra 5 Scapula, Right 6 Scapula, Left 7 Glenoid Cavity, Right 8 Glenoid Cavity, Left 9 Clavicle, Right B Clavicle, Left	0 Open 3 Percutaneous 4 Percutaneous Endoscopic	4 Internal Fixation Device	Z No Qualifier
C Humeral Head, Right D Humeral Head, Left F Humeral Shaft, Right G Humeral Shaft, Left H Radius, Right J Radius, Left K Ulna, Right L Ulna, Left	0 Open 3 Percutaneous 4 Percutaneous Endoscopic	4 Internal Fixation Device 5 External Fixation Device 6 Intramedullary Fixation Device 8 External Fixation Device, Limb Lengthening B External Fixation Device, Monoplanar C External Fixation Device, Ring D External Fixation Device, Hybrid	Z No Qualifier
M Carpal, Right N Carpal, Left P Metacarpal, Right Q Metacarpal, Left R Thumb Phalanx, Right S Thumb Phalanx, Left T Finger Phalanx, Right V Finger Phalanx, Left	0 Open 3 Percutaneous 4 Percutaneous Endoscopic	4 Internal Fixation Device 5 External Fixation Device	Z No Qualifier
Y Upper Bone	0 Open 3 Percutaneous 4 Percutaneous Endoscopic	M Bone Growth Stimulator	Z No Qualifier
Y Upper Bone	0 Open 3 Percutaneous 4 Percutaneous Endoscopic X External	Z No Device	Z No Qualifier

◀ New   ◀ Revised   deleted Deleted   ♀ Females Only   ♂ Males Only
Noncovered   Limited Coverage   Hospital-Acquired Condition   **Coding Clinic**

SECTION: 0 MEDICAL AND SURGICAL
BODY SYSTEM: P UPPER BONES
OPERATION: J INSPECTION: Visually and/or manually exploring a body part

Body Part	Approach	Device	Qualifier
Y Upper Bone	0 Open 3 Percutaneous 4 Percutaneous Endoscopic X External	Z No Device	Z No Qualifier

SECTION: 0 MEDICAL AND SURGICAL
BODY SYSTEM: P UPPER BONES
OPERATION: N RELEASE: Freeing a body part from an abnormal physical constraint by cutting or by the use of force

Body Part	Approach	Device	Qualifier
0 Sternum 1 Rib, Right 2 Rib, Left 3 Cervical Vertebra 4 Thoracic Vertebra 5 Scapula, Right 6 Scapula, Left 7 Glenoid Cavity, Right 8 Glenoid Cavity, Left 9 Clavicle, Right B Clavicle, Left C Humeral Head, Right D Humeral Head, Left F Humeral Shaft, Right G Humeral Shaft, Left H Radius, Right J Radius, Left K Ulna, Right L Ulna, Left M Carpal, Right N Carpal, Left P Metacarpal, Right Q Metacarpal, Left R Thumb Phalanx, Right S Thumb Phalanx, Left T Finger Phalanx, Right V Finger Phalanx, Left	0 Open 3 Percutaneous 4 Percutaneous Endoscopic	Z No Device	Z No Qualifier

0: M/S   P: UPPER BONES   J: INSPECTION   N: RELEASE

SECTION: 0 MEDICAL AND SURGICAL
BODY SYSTEM: P UPPER BONES
OPERATION: P REMOVAL: *(on multiple pages)*
Taking out or off a device from a body part

Body Part	Approach	Device	Qualifier
0 Sternum 1 Rib, Right 2 Rib, Left 3 Cervical Vertebra 4 Thoracic Vertebra 5 Scapula, Right 6 Scapula, Left 7 Glenoid Cavity, Right 8 Glenoid Cavity, Left 9 Clavicle, Right B Clavicle, Left	0 Open 3 Percutaneous 4 Percutaneous Endoscopic	4 Internal Fixation Device 7 Autologous Tissue Substitute J Synthetic Substitute K Nonautologous Tissue Substitute	Z No Qualifier
0 Sternum 1 Rib, Right 2 Rib, Left 3 Cervical Vertebra 4 Thoracic Vertebra 5 Scapula, Right 6 Scapula, Left 7 Glenoid Cavity, Right 8 Glenoid Cavity, Left 9 Clavicle, Right B Clavicle, Left	X External	4 Internal Fixation Device	Z No Qualifier
C Humeral Head, Right D Humeral Head, Left F Humeral Shaft, Right G Humeral Shaft, Left H Radius, Right J Radius, Left K Ulna, Right L Ulna, Left M Carpal, Right N Carpal, Left P Metacarpal, Right Q Metacarpal, Left R Thumb Phalanx, Right S Thumb Phalanx, Left T Finger Phalanx, Right V Finger Phalanx, Left	0 Open 3 Percutaneous 4 Percutaneous Endoscopic	4 Internal Fixation Device 5 External Fixation Device 7 Autologous Tissue Substitute J Synthetic Substitute K Nonautologous Tissue Substitute	Z No Qualifier

P: REMOVAL

P: UPPER BONES

0: M/S

◀ New ◀▥ Revised ~~deleted~~ Deleted ♀ Females Only ♂ Males Only
Nc Noncovered Lc Limited Coverage Hac Hospital-Acquired Condition **Coding Clinic**

SECTION: 0 MEDICAL AND SURGICAL
BODY SYSTEM: P UPPER BONES
OPERATION: P REMOVAL: *(continued)*
Taking out or off a device from a body part

Body Part	Approach	Device	Qualifier
C Humeral Head, Right D Humeral Head, Left F Humeral Shaft, Right G Humeral Shaft, Left H Radius, Right J Radius, Left K Ulna, Right L Ulna, Left M Carpal, Right N Carpal, Left P Metacarpal, Right Q Metacarpal, Left R Thumb Phalanx, Right S Thumb Phalanx, Left T Finger Phalanx, Right V Finger Phalanx, Left	X External	4 Internal Fixation Device 5 External Fixation Device	Z No Qualifier
M Carpal, Right N Carpal, Left P Metacarpal, Right Q Metacarpal, Left R Thumb Phalanx, Right S Thumb Phalanx, Left T Finger Phalanx, Right V Finger Phalanx, Left	0 Open 3 Percutaneous 4 Percutaneous Endoscopic	4 Internal Fixation Device 5 External Fixation Device 7 Autologous Tissue Substitute J Synthetic Substitute K Nonautologous Tissue Substitute	Z No Qualifier
Y Upper Bone	0 Open 3 Percutaneous 4 Percutaneous Endoscopic X External	0 Drainage Device M Bone Growth Stimulator	Z No Qualifier

◀ New   ◀▥ Revised   ~~deleted~~ Deleted   ♀ Females Only   ♂ Males Only
🅝🅒 Noncovered   🅛🅒 Limited Coverage   🅗🅒 Hospital-Acquired Condition   **Coding Clinic**

SECTION: 0 MEDICAL AND SURGICAL
BODY SYSTEM: P UPPER BONES
OPERATION: Q **REPAIR:** Restoring, to the extent possible, a body part to its normal anatomic structure and function

Body Part	Approach	Device	Qualifier
0 Sternum	0 Open	Z No Device	Z No Qualifier
1 Rib, Right	3 Percutaneous		
2 Rib, Left	4 Percutaneous Endoscopic		
3 Cervical Vertebra	X External		
4 Thoracic Vertebra			
5 Scapula, Right			
6 Scapula, Left			
7 Glenoid Cavity, Right			
8 Glenoid Cavity, Left			
9 Clavicle, Right			
B Clavicle, Left			
C Humeral Head, Right			
D Humeral Head, Left			
F Humeral Shaft, Right			
G Humeral Shaft, Left			
H Radius, Right			
J Radius, Left			
K Ulna, Right			
L Ulna, Left			
M Carpal, Right			
N Carpal, Left			
P Metacarpal, Right			
Q Metacarpal, Left			
R Thumb Phalanx, Right			
S Thumb Phalanx, Left			
T Finger Phalanx, Right			
V Finger Phalanx, Left			

Q: REPAIR   P: UPPER BONES   0: M/S

SECTION: 0 MEDICAL AND SURGICAL
BODY SYSTEM: P UPPER BONES
OPERATION: R REPLACEMENT: Putting in or on biological or synthetic material that physically takes the place and/or function of all or a portion of a body part

Body Part	Approach	Device	Qualifier
0 Sternum 1 Rib, Right 2 Rib, Left 3 Cervical Vertebra 4 Thoracic Vertebra 5 Scapula, Right 6 Scapula, Left 7 Glenoid Cavity, Right 8 Glenoid Cavity, Left 9 Clavicle, Right B Clavicle, Left C Humeral Head, Right D Humeral Head, Left F Humeral Shaft, Right G Humeral Shaft, Left H Radius, Right J Radius, Left K Ulna, Right L Ulna, Left M Carpal, Right N Carpal, Left P Metacarpal, Right Q Metacarpal, Left R Thumb Phalanx, Right S Thumb Phalanx, Left T Finger Phalanx, Right V Finger Phalanx, Left	0 Open 3 Percutaneous 4 Percutaneous Endoscopic	7 Autologous Tissue Substitute J Synthetic Substitute K Nonautologous Tissue Substitute	Z No Qualifier

SECTION: 0 MEDICAL AND SURGICAL
BODY SYSTEM: P UPPER BONES
OPERATION: S REPOSITION: *(on multiple pages)*
Moving to its normal location, or other suitable location, all or a portion of a body part

Body Part	Approach	Device	Qualifier
0 Sternum	0 Open 3 Percutaneous 4 Percutaneous Endoscopic	0 Internal Fixation Device, Rigid Plate 4 Internal Fixation Device Z No Device	Z No Qualifier
0 Sternum	X External	Z No Device	Z No Qualifier
1 Rib, Right 2 Rib, Left 3 Cervical Vertebra 4 Thoracic Vertebra 5 Scapula, Right 6 Scapula, Left 7 Glenoid Cavity, Right 8 Glenoid Cavity, Left 9 Clavicle, Right B Clavicle, Left	0 Open 3 Percutaneous 4 Percutaneous Endoscopic	4 Internal Fixation Device Z No Device	Z No Qualifier

◄ New   ◄▦ Revised   ~~deleted~~ Deleted   ♀ Females Only   ♂ Males Only
🅝🅒 Noncovered   🅛🅒 Limited Coverage   🆀🅒 Hospital-Acquired Condition   **Coding Clinic**

SECTION: 0 MEDICAL AND SURGICAL
BODY SYSTEM: P UPPER BONES
OPERATION: S REPOSITION: *(continued)*

Moving to its normal location, or other suitable location, all or a portion of a body part

Body Part	Approach	Device	Qualifier
1 Rib, Right 2 Rib, Left 3 Cervical Vertebra 4 Thoracic Vertebra 5 Scapula, Right 6 Scapula, Left 7 Glenoid Cavity, Right 8 Glenoid Cavity, Left 9 Clavicle, Right B Clavicle, Left	X External	Z No Device	Z No Qualifier
C Humeral Head, Right D Humeral Head, Left F Humeral Shaft, Right G Humeral Shaft, Left H Radius, Right J Radius, Left K Ulna, Right L Ulna, Left	0 Open 3 Percutaneous 4 Percutaneous Endoscopic	4 Internal Fixation Device 5 External Fixation Device 6 Intramedullary Fixation Device B External Fixation Device, Monoplanar C External Fixation Device, Ring D External Fixation Device, Hybrid Z No Device	Z No Qualifier
C Humeral Head, Right D Humeral Head, Left F Humeral Shaft, Right G Humeral Shaft, Left H Radius, Right J Radius, Left K Ulna, Right L Ulna, Left	X External	Z No Device	Z No Qualifier
M Carpal, Right N Carpal, Left P Metacarpal, Right Q Metacarpal, Left R Thumb Phalanx, Right S Thumb Phalanx, Left T Finger Phalanx, Right V Finger Phalanx, Left	0 Open 3 Percutaneous 4 Percutaneous Endoscopic	4 Internal Fixation Device 5 External Fixation Device Z No Device	Z No Qualifier
M Carpal, Right N Carpal, Left P Metacarpal, Right Q Metacarpal, Left R Thumb Phalanx, Right S Thumb Phalanx, Left T Finger Phalanx, Right V Finger Phalanx, Left	X External	Z No Device	Z No Qualifier

S: REPOSITION

P: UPPER BONES

0: M/S

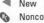 New Revised ~~deleted~~ Deleted ♀ Females Only ♂ Males Only
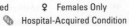 Noncovered 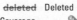 Limited Coverage Hospital-Acquired Condition **Coding Clinic**

SECTION: 0 MEDICAL AND SURGICAL
BODY SYSTEM: P UPPER BONES
OPERATION: T RESECTION: Cutting out or off, without replacement, all of a body part

Body Part	Approach	Device	Qualifier
0 Sternum	0 Open	Z No Device	Z No Qualifier
1 Rib, Right			
2 Rib, Left			
5 Scapula, Right			
6 Scapula, Left			
7 Glenoid Cavity, Right			
8 Glenoid Cavity, Left			
9 Clavicle, Right			
B Clavicle, Left			
C Humeral Head, Right			
D Humeral Head, Left			
F Humeral Shaft, Right			
G Humeral Shaft, Left			
H Radius, Right			
J Radius, Left			
K Ulna, Right			
L Ulna, Left			
M Carpal, Right			
N Carpal, Left			
P Metacarpal, Right			
Q Metacarpal, Left			
R Thumb Phalanx, Right			
S Thumb Phalanx, Left			
T Finger Phalanx, Right			
V Finger Phalanx, Left			

0: M/S

P: UPPER BONES

T: RESECTION

◀ New ◀▦ Revised ~~deleted~~ Deleted ♀ Females Only ♂ Males Only
🚫 Noncovered 🚫 Limited Coverage 🚫 Hospital-Acquired Condition **Coding Clinic**

365

SECTION: 0 MEDICAL AND SURGICAL
BODY SYSTEM: P UPPER BONES
OPERATION: **U SUPPLEMENT:** Putting in or on biological or synthetic material that physically reinforces and/or augments the function of a portion of a body part

Body Part	Approach	Device	Qualifier
0 Sternum	0 Open	7 Autologous Tissue Substitute	Z No Qualifier
1 Rib, Right	3 Percutaneous	J Synthetic Substitute	
2 Rib, Left	4 Percutaneous Endoscopic	K Nonautologous Tissue Substitute	
3 Cervical Vertebra			
4 Thoracic Vertebra			
5 Scapula, Right			
6 Scapula, Left			
7 Glenoid Cavity, Right			
8 Glenoid Cavity, Left			
9 Clavicle, Right			
B Clavicle, Left			
C Humeral Head, Right			
D Humeral Head, Left			
F Humeral Shaft, Right			
G Humeral Shaft, Left			
H Radius, Right			
J Radius, Left			
K Ulna, Right			
L Ulna, Left			
M Carpal, Right			
N Carpal, Left			
P Metacarpal, Right			
Q Metacarpal, Left			
R Thumb Phalanx, Right			
S Thumb Phalanx, Left			
T Finger Phalanx, Right			
V Finger Phalanx, Left			

◀ New　◀ Revised　deleted Deleted　♀ Females Only　♂ Males Only
Noncovered　Limited Coverage　Hospital-Acquired Condition　**Coding Clinic**

SECTION: 0 MEDICAL AND SURGICAL
BODY SYSTEM: P UPPER BONES
OPERATION: W REVISION: Correcting, to the extent possible, a portion of a malfunctioning device or the position of a displaced device

Body Part	Approach	Device	Qualifier
0 Sternum 1 Rib, Right 2 Rib, Left 3 Cervical Vertebra 4 Thoracic Vertebra 5 Scapula, Right 6 Scapula, Left 7 Glenoid Cavity, Right 8 Glenoid Cavity, Left 9 Clavicle, Right B Clavicle, Left	0 Open 3 Percutaneous 4 Percutaneous Endoscopic X External	4 Internal Fixation Device 7 Autologous Tissue Substitute J Synthetic Substitute K Nonautologous Tissue Substitute	Z No Qualifier
C Humeral Head, Right D Humeral Head, Left F Humeral Shaft, Right G Humeral Shaft, Left H Radius, Right J Radius, Left K Ulna, Right L Ulna, Left M Carpal, Right N Carpal, Left P Metacarpal, Right Q Metacarpal, Left R Thumb Phalanx, Right S Thumb Phalanx, Left T Finger Phalanx, Right V Finger Phalanx, Left	0 Open 3 Percutaneous 4 Percutaneous Endoscopic X External	4 Internal Fixation Device 5 External Fixation Device 7 Autologous Tissue Substitute J Synthetic Substitute K Nonautologous Tissue Substitute	Z No Qualifier
Y Upper Bone	0 Open 3 Percutaneous 4 Percutaneous Endoscopic X External	0 Drainage Device M Bone Growth Stimulator	Z No Qualifier

◀ New   ◀▥ Revised   ~~deleted~~ Deleted   ♀ Females Only   ♂ Males Only
◔ Noncovered   ◔ Limited Coverage   ◔ Hospital-Acquired Condition   **Coding Clinic**

367

SECTION: 0 MEDICAL AND SURGICAL
BODY SYSTEM: Q LOWER BONES
OPERATION: 2 CHANGE: Taking out or off a device from a body part and putting back an identical or similar device in or on the same body part without cutting or puncturing the skin or a mucous membrane

Body Part	Approach	Device	Qualifier
Y Lower Bone	X External	0 Drainage Device Y Other Device	Z No Qualifier

SECTION: 0 MEDICAL AND SURGICAL
BODY SYSTEM: Q LOWER BONES
OPERATION: 5 DESTRUCTION: Physical eradication of all or a portion of a body part by the direct use of energy, force, or a destructive agent

Body Part	Approach	Device	Qualifier
0 Lumbar Vertebra 1 Sacrum 2 Pelvic Bone, Right 3 Pelvic Bone, Left 4 Acetabulum, Right 5 Acetabulum, Left 6 Upper Femur, Right 7 Upper Femur, Left 8 Femoral Shaft, Right 9 Femoral Shaft, Left B Lower Femur, Right C Lower Femur, Left D Patella, Right F Patella, Left G Tibia, Right H Tibia, Left J Fibula, Right K Fibula, Left L Tarsal, Right M Tarsal, Left N Metatarsal, Right P Metatarsal, Left Q Toe Phalanx, Right R Toe Phalanx, Left S Coccyx	0 Open 3 Percutaneous 4 Percutaneous Endoscopic	Z No Device	Z No Qualifier

SECTION: 0 MEDICAL AND SURGICAL
BODY SYSTEM: Q LOWER BONES
OPERATION: 8 DIVISION: Cutting into a body part, without draining fluids and/or gases from the body part, in order to separate or transect a body part

Body Part	Approach	Device	Qualifier
0 Lumbar Vertebra	0 Open	Z No Device	Z No Qualifier
1 Sacrum	3 Percutaneous		
2 Pelvic Bone, Right	4 Percutaneous Endoscopic		
3 Pelvic Bone, Left			
4 Acetabulum, Right			
5 Acetabulum, Left			
6 Upper Femur, Right			
7 Upper Femur, Left			
8 Femoral Shaft, Right			
9 Femoral Shaft, Left			
B Lower Femur, Right			
C Lower Femur, Left			
D Patella, Right			
F Patella, Left			
G Tibia, Right			
H Tibia, Left			
J Fibula, Right			
K Fibula, Left			
L Tarsal, Right			
M Tarsal, Left			
N Metatarsal, Right			
P Metatarsal, Left			
Q Toe Phalanx, Right			
R Toe Phalanx, Left			
S Coccyx			

8: DIVISION

Q: LOWER BONES

0: M/S

◀ New ◀ Revised ~~deleted~~ Deleted ♀ Females Only ♂ Males Only
⊘ Noncovered ⊘ Limited Coverage ⊘ Hospital-Acquired Condition **Coding Clinic**

SECTION: 0 MEDICAL AND SURGICAL
BODY SYSTEM: Q LOWER BONES
OPERATION: 9 DRAINAGE: Taking or letting out fluids and/or gases from a body part

Body Part	Approach	Device	Qualifier
0 Lumbar Vertebra	0 Open	0 Drainage Device	Z No Qualifier
1 Sacrum	3 Percutaneous		
2 Pelvic Bone, Right	4 Percutaneous Endoscopic		
3 Pelvic Bone, Left			
4 Acetabulum, Right			
5 Acetabulum, Left			
6 Upper Femur, Right			
7 Upper Femur, Left			
8 Femoral Shaft, Right			
9 Femoral Shaft, Left			
B Lower Femur, Right			
C Lower Femur, Left			
D Patella, Right			
F Patella, Left			
G Tibia, Right			
H Tibia, Left			
J Fibula, Right			
K Fibula, Left			
L Tarsal, Right			
M Tarsal, Left			
N Metatarsal, Right			
P Metatarsal, Left			
Q Toe Phalanx, Right			
R Toe Phalanx, Left			
S Coccyx			
0 Lumbar Vertebra	0 Open	Z No Device	X Diagnostic
1 Sacrum	3 Percutaneous		Z No Qualifier
2 Pelvic Bone, Right	4 Percutaneous Endoscopic		
3 Pelvic Bone, Left			
4 Acetabulum, Right			
5 Acetabulum, Left			
6 Upper Femur, Right			
7 Upper Femur, Left			
8 Femoral Shaft, Right			
9 Femoral Shaft, Left			
B Lower Femur, Right			
C Lower Femur, Left			
D Patella, Right			
F Patella, Left			
G Tibia, Right			
H Tibia, Left			
J Fibula, Right			
K Fibula, Left			
L Tarsal, Right			
M Tarsal, Left			
N Metatarsal, Right			
P Metatarsal, Left			
Q Toe Phalanx, Right			
R Toe Phalanx, Left			
S Coccyx			

◀ New   ◀ Revised   deleted Deleted   ♀ Females Only   ♂ Males Only
 Noncovered   Limited Coverage   Hospital-Acquired Condition   **Coding Clinic**

SECTION: 0 MEDICAL AND SURGICAL
BODY SYSTEM: Q LOWER BONES
OPERATION: B EXCISION: Cutting out or off, without replacement, a portion of a body part

Body Part	Approach	Device	Qualifier
0 Lumbar Vertebra	0 Open	Z No Device	X Diagnostic
1 Sacrum	3 Percutaneous		Z No Qualifier
2 Pelvic Bone, Right	4 Percutaneous Endoscopic		
3 Pelvic Bone, Left			
4 Acetabulum, Right			
5 Acetabulum, Left			
6 Upper Femur, Right			
7 Upper Femur, Left			
8 Femoral Shaft, Right			
9 Femoral Shaft, Left			
B Lower Femur, Right			
C Lower Femur, Left			
D Patella, Right			
F Patella, Left			
G Tibia, Right			
H Tibia, Left			
J Fibula, Right			
K Fibula, Left			
L Tarsal, Right			
M Tarsal, Left			
N Metatarsal, Right			
P Metatarsal, Left			
Q Toe Phalanx, Right			
R Toe Phalanx, Left			
S Coccyx			

Coding Clinic: 2013, Q2, P40 – 0QBK0ZZ

◄ New   ◄ Revised   ~~deleted~~ Deleted   ♀ Females Only   ♂ Males Only
⚕ Noncovered   ⚕ Limited Coverage   ⚕ Hospital-Acquired Condition   **Coding Clinic**

SECTION: 0 MEDICAL AND SURGICAL
BODY SYSTEM: Q LOWER BONES
OPERATION: C EXTIRPATION: Taking or cutting out solid matter from a body part

Body Part	Approach	Device	Qualifier
0 Lumbar Vertebra	0 Open	Z No Device	Z No Qualifier
1 Sacrum	3 Percutaneous		
2 Pelvic Bone, Right	4 Percutaneous Endoscopic		
3 Pelvic Bone, Left			
4 Acetabulum, Right			
5 Acetabulum, Left			
6 Upper Femur, Right			
7 Upper Femur, Left			
8 Femoral Shaft, Right			
9 Femoral Shaft, Left			
B Lower Femur, Right			
C Lower Femur, Left			
D Patella, Right			
F Patella, Left			
G Tibia, Right			
H Tibia, Left			
J Fibula, Right			
K Fibula, Left			
L Tarsal, Right			
M Tarsal, Left			
N Metatarsal, Right			
P Metatarsal, Left			
Q Toe Phalanx, Right			
R Toe Phalanx, Left			
S Coccyx			

SECTION: 0 MEDICAL AND SURGICAL
BODY SYSTEM: Q LOWER BONES
OPERATION: H **INSERTION:** Putting in a nonbiological appliance that monitors, assists, performs, or prevents a physiological function but does not physically take the place of a body part

Body Part	Approach	Device	Qualifier
0 Lumbar Vertebra 1 Sacrum 2 Pelvic Bone, Right 3 Pelvic Bone, Left 4 Acetabulum, Right 5 Acetabulum, Left D Patella, Right F Patella, Left L Tarsal, Right M Tarsal, Left N Metatarsal, Right P Metatarsal, Left Q Toe Phalanx, Right R Toe Phalanx, Left S Coccyx	0 Open 3 Percutaneous 4 Percutaneous Endoscopic	4 Internal Fixation Device 5 External Fixation Device	Z No Qualifier
6 Upper Femur, Right 7 Upper Femur, Left 8 Femoral Shaft, Right 9 Femoral Shaft, Left B Lower Femur, Right C Lower Femur, Left G Tibia, Right H Tibia, Left J Fibula, Right K Fibula, Left	0 Open 3 Percutaneous 4 Percutaneous Endoscopic	4 Internal Fixation Device 5 External Fixation Device 6 Internal Fixation Device, Intramedullary 8 External Fixation Device, Limb Lengthening B External Fixation Device, Monoplanar C External Fixation Device, Ring D External Fixation Device, Hybrid	Z No Qualifier
Y Lower Bone	0 Open 3 Percutaneous 4 Percutaneous Endoscopic	M Bone Growth Stimulator	Z No Qualifier

H: INSERTION

Q: LOWER BONES

0: M/S

◀ New   ◀▬ Revised   ~~deleted~~ Deleted   ♀ Females Only   ♂ Males Only
🅝 Noncovered   🅛 Limited Coverage   🅗 Hospital-Acquired Condition   **Coding Clinic**

SECTION: 0 MEDICAL AND SURGICAL
BODY SYSTEM: Q LOWER BONES
OPERATION: J INSPECTION: Visually and/or manually exploring a body part

Body Part	Approach	Device	Qualifier
Y Lower Bone	0 Open 3 Percutaneous 4 Percutaneous Endoscopic X External	Z No Device	Z No Qualifier

SECTION: 0 MEDICAL AND SURGICAL
BODY SYSTEM: Q LOWER BONES
OPERATION: N RELEASE: Freeing a body part from an abnormal physical constraint by cutting or by the use of force

Body Part	Approach	Device	Qualifier
0 Lumbar Vertebra 1 Sacrum 2 Pelvic Bone, Right 3 Pelvic Bone, Left 4 Acetabulum, Right 5 Acetabulum, Left 6 Upper Femur, Right 7 Upper Femur, Left 8 Femoral Shaft, Right 9 Femoral Shaft, Left B Lower Femur, Right C Lower Femur, Left D Patella, Right F Patella, Left G Tibia, Right H Tibia, Left J Fibula, Right K Fibula, Left L Tarsal, Right M Tarsal, Left N Metatarsal, Right P Metatarsal, Left Q Toe Phalanx, Right R Toe Phalanx, Left S Coccyx	0 Open 3 Percutaneous 4 Percutaneous Endoscopic	Z No Device	Z No Qualifier

◄ New   ◄ Revised   deleted Deleted   ♀ Females Only   ♂ Males Only
 Noncovered   Limited Coverage   Hospital-Acquired Condition   **Coding Clinic**

375

SECTION: 0 MEDICAL AND SURGICAL
BODY SYSTEM: Q LOWER BONES
OPERATION: P REMOVAL: *(on multiple pages)*
Taking out or off a device from a body part

Body Part	Approach	Device	Qualifier
0 Lumbar Vertebra 1 Sacrum 4 Acetabulum, Right 5 Acetabulum, Left S Coccyx	0 Open 3 Percutaneous 4 Percutaneous Endoscopic	4 Internal Fixation Device 7 Autologous Tissue Substitute J Synthetic Substitute K Nonautologous Tissue Substitute	Z No Qualifier
0 Lumbar Vertebra 1 Sacrum 4 Acetabulum, Right 5 Acetabulum, Left S Coccyx	X External	4 Internal Fixation Device	Z No Qualifier
2 Pelvic Bone, Right 3 Pelvic Bone, Left 6 Upper Femur, Right 7 Upper Femur, Left 8 Femoral Shaft, Right 9 Femoral Shaft, Left B Lower Femur, Right C Lower Femur, Left D Patella, Right F Patella, Left G Tibia, Right H Tibia, Left J Fibula, Right K Fibula, Left L Tarsal, Right M Tarsal, Left N Metatarsal, Right P Metatarsal, Left Q Toe Phalanx, Right R Toe Phalanx, Left	0 Open 3 Percutaneous 4 Percutaneous Endoscopic	4 Internal Fixation Device 5 External Fixation Device 7 Autologous Tissue Substitute J Synthetic Substitute K Nonautologous Tissue Substitute	Z No Qualifier
2 Pelvic Bone, Right 3 Pelvic Bone, Left 6 Upper Femur, Right 7 Upper Femur, Left 8 Femoral Shaft, Right 9 Femoral Shaft, Left B Lower Femur, Right C Lower Femur, Left D Patella, Right F Patella, Left L Tarsal, Right M Tarsal, Left N Metatarsal, Right P Metatarsal, Left Q Toe Phalanx, Right R Toe Phalanx, Left	X External	4 Internal Fixation Device 5 External Fixation Device	Z No Qualifier

◀ New ◀ Revised deleted Deleted ♀ Females Only ♂ Males Only
Noncovered Limited Coverage Hospital-Acquired Condition **Coding Clinic**

SECTION: 0 MEDICAL AND SURGICAL
BODY SYSTEM: Q LOWER BONES
OPERATION: P REMOVAL: *(continued)*
Taking out or off a device from a body part

Body Part	Approach	Device	Qualifier
Y Lower Bone	0 Open 3 Percutaneous 4 Percutaneous Endoscopic X External	0 Drainage Device M Bone Growth Stimulator	Z No Qualifier

SECTION: 0 MEDICAL AND SURGICAL
BODY SYSTEM: Q LOWER BONES
OPERATION: Q REPAIR: Restoring, to the extent possible, a body part to its normal anatomic structure and function

Body Part	Approach	Device	Qualifier
0 Lumbar Vertebra 1 Sacrum 2 Pelvic Bone, Right 3 Pelvic Bone, Left 4 Acetabulum, Right 5 Acetabulum, Left 6 Upper Femur, Right 7 Upper Femur, Left 8 Femoral Shaft, Right 9 Femoral Shaft, Left B Lower Femur, Right C Lower Femur, Left D Patella, Right F Patella, Left G Tibia, Right H Tibia, Left J Fibula, Right K Fibula, Left L Tarsal, Right M Tarsal, Left N Metatarsal, Right P Metatarsal, Left Q Toe Phalanx, Right R Toe Phalanx, Left S Coccyx	0 Open 3 Percutaneous 4 Percutaneous Endoscopic X External	Z No Device	Z No Qualifier

◀ New   ◀▬ Revised   ~~deleted~~ Deleted   ♀ Females Only   ♂ Males Only
🚫 Noncovered   🚫 Limited Coverage   🚫 Hospital-Acquired Condition   **Coding Clinic**

377

SECTION: **0 MEDICAL AND SURGICAL**
BODY SYSTEM: Q LOWER BONES
OPERATION: R REPLACEMENT: Putting in or on biological or synthetic material that physically takes the place and/or function of all or a portion of a body part

Body Part	Approach	Device	Qualifier
0 Lumbar Vertebra 1 Sacrum 2 Pelvic Bone, Right 3 Pelvic Bone, Left 4 Acetabulum, Right 5 Acetabulum, Left 6 Upper Femur, Right 7 Upper Femur, Left 8 Femoral Shaft, Right 9 Femoral Shaft, Left B Lower Femur, Right C Lower Femur, Left D Patella, Right F Patella, Left G Tibia, Right H Tibia, Left J Fibula, Right K Fibula, Left L Tarsal, Right M Tarsal, Left N Metatarsal, Right P Metatarsal, Left Q Toe Phalanx, Right R Toe Phalanx, Left S Coccyx	0 Open 3 Percutaneous 4 Percutaneous Endoscopic	7 Autologous Tissue Substitute J Synthetic Substitute K Nonautologous Tissue Substitute	Z No Qualifier

R: REPLACEMENT

Q: LOWER BONES

0: M/S

◀ New ◀▥ Revised ~~deleted~~ Deleted ♀ Females Only ♂ Males Only
Ⓝc Noncovered Ⓛc Limited Coverage Ⓗ Hospital-Acquired Condition **Coding Clinic**

SECTION: 0 MEDICAL AND SURGICAL
BODY SYSTEM: Q LOWER BONES
OPERATION: S REPOSITION: *(on multiple pages)*
Moving to its normal location, or other suitable location, all or a portion of a body part

Body Part	Approach	Device	Qualifier
0 Lumbar Vertebra 1 Sacrum 4 Acetabulum, Right 5 Acetabulum, Left S Coccyx	0 Open 3 Percutaneous 4 Percutaneous Endoscopic	4 Internal Fixation Device Z No Device	Z No Qualifier
0 Lumbar Vertebra 1 Sacrum 4 Acetabulum, Right 5 Acetabulum, Left S Coccyx	X External	Z No Device	Z No Qualifier
2 Pelvic Bone, Right 3 Pelvic Bone, Left D Patella, Right F Patella, Left L Tarsal, Right M Tarsal, Left N Metatarsal, Right P Metatarsal, Left Q Toe Phalanx, Right R Toe Phalanx, Left	0 Open 3 Percutaneous 4 Percutaneous Endoscopic	4 Internal Fixation Device 5 External Fixation Device Z No Device	Z No Qualifier
2 Pelvic Bone, Right 3 Pelvic Bone, Left D Patella, Right F Patella, Left L Tarsal, Right M Tarsal, Left N Metatarsal, Right P Metatarsal, Left Q Toe Phalanx, Right R Toe Phalanx, Left	X External	Z No Device	Z No Qualifier
6 Upper Femur, Right 7 Upper Femur, Left 8 Femoral Shaft, Right 9 Femoral Shaft, Left B Lower Femur, Right C Lower Femur, Left G Tibia, Right H Tibia, Left J Fibula, Right K Fibula, Left	0 Open 3 Percutaneous 4 Percutaneous Endoscopic	4 Internal Fixation Device 5 External Fixation Device 6 Intramedullary Fixation Device B External Fixation Device, Monoplanar C External Fixation Device, Ring D External Fixation Device, Hybrid Z No Device	Z No Qualifier

SECTION: 0 MEDICAL AND SURGICAL
BODY SYSTEM: Q LOWER BONES
OPERATION: S REPOSITION: *(continued)*
Moving to its normal location, or other suitable location, all or a portion of a body part

Body Part	Approach	Device	Qualifier
6 Upper Femur, Right 7 Upper Femur, Left 8 Femoral Shaft, Right 9 Femoral Shaft, Left B Lower Femur, Right C Lower Femur, Left G Tibia, Right H Tibia, Left J Fibula, Right K Fibula, Left	X External	Z No Device	Z No Qualifier

SECTION: 0 MEDICAL AND SURGICAL
BODY SYSTEM: Q LOWER BONES
OPERATION: T RESECTION: Cutting out or off, without replacement, all of a body part

Body Part	Approach	Device	Qualifier
2 Pelvic Bone, Right 3 Pelvic Bone, Left 4 Acetabulum, Right 5 Acetabulum, Left 6 Upper Femur, Right 7 Upper Femur, Left 8 Femoral Shaft, Right 9 Femoral Shaft, Left B Lower Femur, Right C Lower Femur, Left D Patella, Right F Patella, Left G Tibia, Right H Tibia, Left J Fibula, Right K Fibula, Left L Tarsal, Right M Tarsal, Left N Metatarsal, Right P Metatarsal, Left Q Toe Phalanx, Right R Toe Phalanx, Left S Coccyx	0 Open	Z No Device	Z No Qualifier

◀ New   ◀▥ Revised   ~~deleted~~ Deleted   ♀ Females Only   ♂ Males Only
🜹 Noncovered   🜹 Limited Coverage   🜹 Hospital-Acquired Condition   **Coding Clinic**

Side tab: T: RESECTION   S: REPOSITION   Q: LOWER BONES   0: M/S

SECTION: 0 MEDICAL AND SURGICAL
BODY SYSTEM: Q LOWER BONES
OPERATION: U SUPPLEMENT: Putting in or on biological or synthetic material that physically reinforces and/or augments the function of a portion of a body part

Body Part	Approach	Device	Qualifier
0 Lumbar Vertebra	0 Open	7 Autologous Tissue Substitute	Z No Qualifier
1 Sacrum	3 Percutaneous	J Synthetic Substitute	
2 Pelvic Bone, Right	4 Percutaneous Endoscopic	K Nonautologous Tissue Substitute	
3 Pelvic Bone, Left			
4 Acetabulum, Right			
5 Acetabulum, Left			
6 Upper Femur, Right			
7 Upper Femur, Left			
8 Femoral Shaft, Right			
9 Femoral Shaft, Left			
B Lower Femur, Right			
C Lower Femur, Left			
D Patella, Right			
F Patella, Left			
G Tibia, Right			
H Tibia, Left			
J Fibula, Right			
K Fibula, Left			
L Tarsal, Right			
M Tarsal, Left			
N Metatarsal, Right			
P Metatarsal, Left			
Q Toe Phalanx, Right			
R Toe Phalanx, Left			
S Coccyx			

Coding Clinic: 2013, Q2, P36 – 0QU20JZ

◀ New   ◀━ Revised   ~~deleted~~ Deleted   ♀ Females Only   ♂ Males Only
Ⓝc Noncovered   Ⓛc Limited Coverage   Ⓗc Hospital-Acquired Condition   **Coding Clinic**

381

SECTION: 0 MEDICAL AND SURGICAL
BODY SYSTEM: Q LOWER BONES
OPERATION: W REVISION: Correcting, to the extent possible, a portion of a malfunctioning device or the position of a displaced device

Body Part	Approach	Device	Qualifier
0 Lumbar Vertebra 1 Sacrum 4 Acetabulum, Right 5 Acetabulum, Left S Coccyx	0 Open 3 Percutaneous 4 Percutaneous Endoscopic X External	4 Internal Fixation Device 7 Autologous Tissue Substitute J Synthetic Substitute K Nonautologous Tissue Substitute	Z No Qualifier
2 Pelvic Bone, Right 3 Pelvic Bone, Left 6 Upper Femur, Right 7 Upper Femur, Left 8 Femoral Shaft, Right 9 Femoral Shaft, Left B Lower Femur, Right C Lower Femur, Left D Patella, Right F Patella, Left L Tarsal, Right M Tarsal, Left N Metatarsal, Right P Metatarsal, Left Q Toe Phalanx, Right R Toe Phalanx, Left	0 Open 3 Percutaneous 4 Percutaneous Endoscopic X External	4 Internal Fixation Device 5 External Fixation Device 7 Autologous Tissue Substitute J Synthetic Substitute K Nonautologous Tissue Substitute	Z No Qualifier
Y Lower Bone	0 Open 3 Percutaneous 4 Percutaneous Endoscopic X External	0 Drainage Device M Bone Growth Stimulator	Z No Qualifier

◀ New ◀ Revised ~~deleted~~ Deleted ♀ Females Only ♂ Males Only
Noncovered Limited Coverage Hospital-Acquired Condition **Coding Clinic**

SECTION: 0 MEDICAL AND SURGICAL

BODY SYSTEM: R UPPER JOINTS

OPERATION: 2 CHANGE: Taking out or off a device from a body part and putting back an identical or similar device in or on the same body part without cutting or puncturing the skin or a mucous membrane

Body Part	Approach	Device	Qualifier
Y Upper Joint	X External	0 Drainage Device Y Other Device	Z No Qualifier

SECTION: 0 MEDICAL AND SURGICAL

BODY SYSTEM: R UPPER JOINTS

OPERATION: 5 DESTRUCTION: Physical eradication of all or a portion of a body part by the direct use of energy, force, or destructive agent

Body Part	Approach	Device	Qualifier
0 Occipital-cervical Joint 1 Cervical Vertebral Joint 3 Cervical Vertebral Disc 4 Cervicothoracic Vertebral Joint 5 Cervicothoracic Vertebral Disc 6 Thoracic Vertebral Joint 9 Thoracic Vertebral Disc A Thoracolumbar Vertebral Joint B Thoracolumbar Vertebral Disc C Temporomandibular Joint, Right D Temporomandibular Joint, Left E Sternoclavicular Joint, Right F Sternoclavicular Joint, Left G Acromioclavicular Joint, Right H Acromioclavicular Joint, Left J Shoulder Joint, Right K Shoulder Joint, Left L Elbow Joint, Right M Elbow Joint, Left N Wrist Joint, Right P Wrist Joint, Left Q Carpal Joint, Right R Carpal Joint, Left S Metacarpocarpal Joint, Right T Metacarpocarpal Joint, Left U Metacarpophalangeal Joint, Right V Metacarpophalangeal Joint, Left W Finger Phalangeal Joint, Right X Finger Phalangeal Joint, Left	0 Open 3 Percutaneous 4 Percutaneous Endoscopic	Z No Device	Z No Qualifier

◀ New　◀▥ Revised　~~deleted~~ Deleted　♀ Females Only　♂ Males Only
Ⓝ Noncovered　Ⓛ Limited Coverage　Ⓗ Hospital-Acquired Condition　**Coding Clinic**

SECTION: 0 MEDICAL AND SURGICAL
BODY SYSTEM: R UPPER JOINTS
OPERATION: 9 DRAINAGE: *(on multiple pages)*
Taking or letting out fluids and/or gases from a body part

Body Part	Approach	Device	Qualifier
0 Occipital-cervical Joint	0 Open	0 Drainage Device	Z No Qualifier
1 Cervical Vertebral Joint	3 Percutaneous		
3 Cervical Vertebral Disc	4 Percutaneous Endoscopic		
4 Cervicothoracic Vertebral Joint			
5 Cervicothoracic Vertebral Disc			
6 Thoracic Vertebral Joint			
9 Thoracic Vertebral Disc			
A Thoracolumbar Vertebral Joint			
B Thoracolumbar Vertebral Disc			
C Temporomandibular Joint, Right			
D Temporomandibular Joint, Left			
E Sternoclavicular Joint, Right			
F Sternoclavicular Joint, Left			
G Acromioclavicular Joint, Right			
H Acromioclavicular Joint, Left			
J Shoulder Joint, Right			
K Shoulder Joint, Left			
L Elbow Joint, Right			
M Elbow Joint, Left			
N Wrist Joint, Right			
P Wrist Joint, Left			
Q Carpal Joint, Right			
R Carpal Joint, Left			
S Metacarpocarpal Joint, Right			
T Metacarpocarpal Joint, Left			
U Metacarpophalangeal Joint, Right			
V Metacarpophalangeal Joint, Left			
W Finger Phalangeal Joint, Right			
X Finger Phalangeal Joint, Left			

◄ New ◄ Revised ~~deleted~~ Deleted ♀ Females Only ♂ Males Only
🅝 Noncovered 🅛 Limited Coverage 🅗 Hospital-Acquired Condition **Coding Clinic**

385

SECTION: 0 MEDICAL AND SURGICAL
BODY SYSTEM: R UPPER JOINTS
OPERATION: 9 DRAINAGE: *(continued)*
Taking or letting out fluids and/or gases from a body part

Body Part	Approach	Device	Qualifier
0 Occipital-cervical Joint 1 Cervical Vertebral Joint 3 Cervical Vertebral Disc 4 Cervicothoracic Vertebral Joint 5 Cervicothoracic Vertebral Disc 6 Thoracic Vertebral Joint 9 Thoracic Vertebral Disc A Thoracolumbar Vertebral Joint B Thoracolumbar Vertebral Disc C Temporomandibular Joint, Right D Temporomandibular Joint, Left E Sternoclavicular Joint, Right F Sternoclavicular Joint, Left G Acromioclavicular Joint, Right H Acromioclavicular Joint, Left J Shoulder Joint, Right K Shoulder Joint, Left L Elbow Joint, Right M Elbow Joint, Left N Wrist Joint, Right P Wrist Joint, Left Q Carpal Joint, Right R Carpal Joint, Left S Metacarpocarpal Joint, Right T Metacarpocarpal Joint, Left U Metacarpophalangeal Joint, Right V Metacarpophalangeal Joint, Left W Finger Phalangeal Joint, Right X Finger Phalangeal Joint, Left	0 Open 3 Percutaneous 4 Percutaneous Endoscopic	Z No Device	X Diagnostic Z No Qualifier

9: DRAINAGE

R: UPPER JOINTS

0: M/S

◀ New   ◀▥ Revised   ~~deleted~~ Deleted   ♀ Females Only   ♂ Males Only
🅝 Noncovered   🅛 Limited Coverage   🅗 Hospital-Acquired Condition   **Coding Clinic**

SECTION: 0 MEDICAL AND SURGICAL

BODY SYSTEM: R UPPER JOINTS

OPERATION: B EXCISION: Cutting out or off, without replacement, a portion of a body part

Body Part	Approach	Device	Qualifier
0 Occipital-cervical Joint	0 Open	Z No Device	X Diagnostic
1 Cervical Vertebral Joint	3 Percutaneous		Z No Qualifier
3 Cervical Vertebral Disc	4 Percutaneous Endoscopic		
4 Cervicothoracic Vertebral Joint			
5 Cervicothoracic Vertebral Disc			
6 Thoracic Vertebral Joint			
9 Thoracic Vertebral Disc			
A Thoracolumbar Vertebral Joint			
B Thoracolumbar Vertebral Disc			
C Temporomandibular Joint, Right			
D Temporomandibular Joint, Left			
E Sternoclavicular Joint, Right			
F Sternoclavicular Joint, Left			
G Acromioclavicular Joint, Right			
H Acromioclavicular Joint, Left			
J Shoulder Joint, Right			
K Shoulder Joint, Left			
L Elbow Joint, Right			
M Elbow Joint, Left			
N Wrist Joint, Right			
P Wrist Joint, Left			
Q Carpal Joint, Right			
R Carpal Joint, Left			
S Metacarpocarpal Joint, Right			
T Metacarpocarpal Joint, Left			
U Metacarpophalangeal Joint, Right			
V Metacarpophalangeal Joint, Left			
W Finger Phalangeal Joint, Right			
X Finger Phalangeal Joint, Left			

0: M/S

R: UPPER JOINTS

B: EXCISION

◀ New ◀ Revised ~~deleted~~ Deleted ♀ Females Only ♂ Males Only
🅝 Noncovered 🅛 Limited Coverage 🅗 Hospital-Acquired Condition **Coding Clinic**

387

SECTION: 0 MEDICAL AND SURGICAL
BODY SYSTEM: R UPPER JOINTS
OPERATION: C EXTIRPATION: Taking or cutting out solid matter from a body part

Body Part	Approach	Device	Qualifier
0 Occipital-cervical Joint	0 Open	Z No Device	Z No Qualifier
1 Cervical Vertebral Joint	3 Percutaneous		
3 Cervical Vertebral Disc	4 Percutaneous Endoscopic		
4 Cervicothoracic Vertebral Joint			
5 Cervicothoracic Vertebral Disc			
6 Thoracic Vertebral Joint			
9 Thoracic Vertebral Disc			
A Thoracolumbar Vertebral Joint			
B Thoracolumbar Vertebral Disc			
C Temporomandibular Joint, Right			
D Temporomandibular Joint, Left			
E Sternoclavicular Joint, Right			
F Sternoclavicular Joint, Left			
G Acromioclavicular Joint, Right			
H Acromioclavicular Joint, Left			
J Shoulder Joint, Right			
K Shoulder Joint, Left			
L Elbow Joint, Right			
M Elbow Joint, Left			
N Wrist Joint, Right			
P Wrist Joint, Left			
Q Carpal Joint, Right			
R Carpal Joint, Left			
S Metacarpocarpal Joint, Right			
T Metacarpocarpal Joint, Left			
U Metacarpophalangeal Joint, Right			
V Metacarpophalangeal Joint, Left			
W Finger Phalangeal Joint, Right			
X Finger Phalangeal Joint, Left			

C: EXTIRPATION

R: UPPER JOINTS

0: M/S

◀ New　◀ Revised　~~deleted~~ Deleted　♀ Females Only　♂ Males Only
Noncovered　Limited Coverage　Hospital-Acquired Condition　**Coding Clinic**

SECTION: 0 MEDICAL AND SURGICAL

BODY SYSTEM: R UPPER JOINTS

OPERATION: G FUSION: Joining together portions of an articular body part, rendering the articular body part immobile

Body Part	Approach	Device	Qualifier
0 Occipital-cervical Joint ⊘ᵤ 1 Cervical Vertebral Joint ⊘ᵤ 2 Cervical Vertebral Joints, 2 or more ⊘ᵤ 4 Cervicothoracic Vertebral Joint ⊘ᵤ 6 Thoracic Vertebral Joint ⊘ᵤ 7 Thoracic Vertebral Joint, 2 to 7 ⊘ᵤ 8 Thoracic Vertebral Joint, 8 or more ⊘ᵤ A Thoracolumbar Vertebral Joint ⊘ᵤ	0 Open 3 Percutaneous 4 Percutaneous Endoscopic	7 Autologous Tissue Substitute A Interbody Fusion Device J Synthetic Substitute K Nonautologous Tissue Substitute Z No Device	0 Anterior Approach, Anterior Column 1 Posterior Approach, Posterior Column J Posterior Approach, Anterior Column
C Temporomandibular Joint, Right D Temporomandibular Joint, Left E Sternoclavicular Joint, Right ⊘ᵤ F Sternoclavicular Joint, Left ⊘ᵤ G Acromioclavicular Joint, Right ⊘ᵤ H Acromioclavicular Joint, Left ⊘ᵤ J Shoulder Joint, Right ⊘ᵤ K Shoulder Joint, Left ⊘ᵤ	0 Open 3 Percutaneous 4 Percutaneous Endoscopic	4 Internal Fixation Device 7 Autologous Tissue Substitute J Synthetic Substitute K Nonautologous Tissue Substitute Z No Device	Z No Qualifier
L Elbow Joint, Right ⊘ᵤ M Elbow Joint, Left ⊘ᵤ N Wrist Joint, Right P Wrist Joint, Left Q Carpal Joint, Right R Carpal Joint, Left S Metacarpocarpal Joint, Right T Metacarpocarpal Joint, Left U Metacarpophalangeal Joint, Right V Metacarpophalangeal Joint, Left W Finger Phalangeal Joint, Right X Finger Phalangeal Joint, Left	0 Open 3 Percutaneous 4 Percutaneous Endoscopic	4 Internal Fixation Device 5 External Fixation Device 7 Autologous Tissue Substitute J Synthetic Substitute K Nonautologous Tissue Substitute Z No Device	Z No Qualifier

Coding Clinic: 2013, Q1, P29 – 0RG40A0

Coding Clinic: 2013, Q1, P22 – 0RG7071, 0RGA071

◀ New   ◀ Revised   deleted Deleted   ♀ Females Only   ♂ Males Only
⊘ᵤ Noncovered   ⊘ᵤ Limited Coverage   ⊘ᵤ Hospital-Acquired Condition   **Coding Clinic**

SECTION: 0 MEDICAL AND SURGICAL
BODY SYSTEM: R UPPER JOINTS
OPERATION: H INSERTION: Putting in a nonbiological appliance that monitors, assists, performs, or prevents a physiological function but does not physically take the place of a body part

Body Part	Approach	Device	Qualifier
0 Occipital-cervical Joint 1 Cervical Vertebral Joint 4 Cervicothoracic Vertebral Joint 6 Thoracic Vertebral Joint A Thoracolumbar Vertebral Joint	0 Open 3 Percutaneous 4 Percutaneous Endoscopic	3 Infusion Device 4 Internal Fixation Device 8 Spacer B Spinal Stabilization Device, Interspinous Process C Spinal Stabilization Device, Pedicle-Based D Spinal Stabilization Device, Facet Replacement	Z No Qualifier
3 Cervical Vertebral Disc 5 Cervicothoracic Vertebral Disc 9 Thoracic Vertebral Disc B Thoracolumbar Vertebral Disc	0 Open 3 Percutaneous 4 Percutaneous Endoscopic	3 Infusion Device	Z No Qualifier
C Temporomandibular Joint, Right D Temporomandibular Joint, Left E Sternoclavicular Joint, Right F Sternoclavicular Joint, Left G Acromioclavicular Joint, Right H Acromioclavicular Joint, Left J Shoulder Joint, Right K Shoulder Joint, Left	0 Open 3 Percutaneous 4 Percutaneous Endoscopic	3 Infusion Device 4 Internal Fixation Device 8 Spacer	Z No Qualifier
L Elbow Joint, Right M Elbow Joint, Left N Wrist Joint, Right P Wrist Joint, Left Q Carpal Joint, Right R Carpal Joint, Left S Metacarpocarpal Joint, Right T Metacarpocarpal Joint, Left U Metacarpophalangeal Joint, Right V Metacarpophalangeal Joint, Left W Finger Phalangeal Joint, Right X Finger Phalangeal Joint, Left	0 Open 3 Percutaneous 4 Percutaneous Endoscopic	3 Infusion Device 4 Internal Fixation Device 5 External Fixation Device 8 Spacer	Z No Qualifier

◀ New ◀▥ Revised ~~deleted~~ Deleted ♀ Females Only ♂ Males Only
Ⓝ Noncovered Ⓛ Limited Coverage Ⓗ Hospital-Acquired Condition **Coding Clinic**

SECTION: 0 MEDICAL AND SURGICAL
BODY SYSTEM: R UPPER JOINTS
OPERATION: J INSPECTION: Visually and/or manually exploring a body part

Body Part	Approach	Device	Qualifier
0 Occipital-cervical Joint	0 Open	Z No Device	Z No Qualifier
1 Cervical Vertebral Joint	3 Percutaneous		
3 Cervical Vertebral Disc	4 Percutaneous Endoscopic		
4 Cervicothoracic Vertebral Joint	X External		
5 Cervicothoracic Vertebral Disc			
6 Thoracic Vertebral Joint			
9 Thoracic Vertebral Disc			
A Thoracolumbar Vertebral Joint			
B Thoracolumbar Vertebral Disc			
C Temporomandibular Joint, Right			
D Temporomandibular Joint, Left			
E Sternoclavicular Joint, Right			
F Sternoclavicular Joint, Left			
G Acromioclavicular Joint, Right			
H Acromioclavicular Joint, Left			
J Shoulder Joint, Right			
K Shoulder Joint, Left			
L Elbow Joint, Right			
M Elbow Joint, Left			
N Wrist Joint, Right			
P Wrist Joint, Left			
Q Carpal Joint, Right			
R Carpal Joint, Left			
S Metacarpocarpal Joint, Right			
T Metacarpocarpal Joint, Left			
U Metacarpophalangeal Joint, Right			
V Metacarpophalangeal Joint, Left			
W Finger Phalangeal Joint, Right			
X Finger Phalangeal Joint, Left			

◀ New ◀▥ Revised deleted Deleted ♀ Females Only ♂ Males Only
🚫 Noncovered 🚫 Limited Coverage 🚫 Hospital-Acquired Condition Coding Clinic

391

SECTION: 0 MEDICAL AND SURGICAL
BODY SYSTEM: R UPPER JOINTS
OPERATION: N RELEASE: Freeing a body part from an abnormal physical constraint by cutting or by the use of force

Body Part	Approach	Device	Qualifier
0 Occipital-cervical Joint 1 Cervical Vertebral Joint 3 Cervical Vertebral Disc 4 Cervicothoracic Vertebral Joint 5 Cervicothoracic Vertebral Disc 6 Thoracic Vertebral Joint 9 Thoracic Vertebral Disc A Thoracolumbar Vertebral Joint B Thoracolumbar Vertebral Disc C Temporomandibular Joint, Right D Temporomandibular Joint, Left E Sternoclavicular Joint, Right F Sternoclavicular Joint, Left G Acromioclavicular Joint, Right H Acromioclavicular Joint, Left J Shoulder Joint, Right K Shoulder Joint, Left L Elbow Joint, Right M Elbow Joint, Left N Wrist Joint, Right P Wrist Joint, Left Q Carpal Joint, Right R Carpal Joint, Left S Metacarpocarpal Joint, Right T Metacarpocarpal Joint, Left U Metacarpophalangeal Joint, Right V Metacarpophalangeal Joint, Left W Finger Phalangeal Joint, Right X Finger Phalangeal Joint, Left	0 Open 3 Percutaneous 4 Percutaneous Endoscopic X External	Z No Device	Z No Qualifier

N: RELEASE

R: UPPER JOINTS

0: M/S

◄ New   ◄▥ Revised   ~~deleted~~ Deleted   ♀ Females Only   ♂ Males Only

℞ Noncovered   ℞ Limited Coverage   ℞ Hospital-Acquired Condition   **Coding Clinic**

SECTION: 0 MEDICAL AND SURGICAL
BODY SYSTEM: R UPPER JOINTS
OPERATION: P REMOVAL: *(on multiple pages)*
Taking out or off a device from a body part

Body Part	Approach	Device	Qualifier
0 Occipital-cervical Joint 1 Cervical Vertebral Joint 4 Cervicothoracic Vertebral Joint 6 Thoracic Vertebral Joint A Thoracolumbar Vertebral Joint	0 Open 3 Percutaneous 4 Percutaneous Endoscopic	0 Drainage Device 3 Infusion Device 4 Internal Fixation Device 7 Autologous Tissue Substitute 8 Spacer A Interbody Fusion Device J Synthetic Substitute K Nonautologous Tissue Substitute	Z No Qualifier
0 Occipital-cervical Joint 1 Cervical Vertebral Joint 4 Cervicothoracic Vertebral Joint 6 Thoracic Vertebral Joint A Thoracolumbar Vertebral Joint	X External	0 Drainage Device 3 Infusion Device 4 Internal Fixation Device	Z No Qualifier
3 Cervical Vertebral Disc 5 Cervicothoracic Vertebral Disc 9 Thoracic Vertebral Disc B Thoracolumbar Vertebral Disc	0 Open 3 Percutaneous 4 Percutaneous Endoscopic	0 Drainage Device 3 Infusion Device 7 Autologous Tissue Substitute J Synthetic Substitute K Nonautologous Tissue Substitute	Z No Qualifier
3 Cervical Vertebral Disc 5 Cervicothoracic Vertebral Disc 9 Thoracic Vertebral Disc B Thoracolumbar Vertebral Disc	X External	0 Drainage Device 3 Infusion Device	Z No Qualifier
C Temporomandibular Joint, Right D Temporomandibular Joint, Left E Sternoclavicular Joint, Right F Sternoclavicular Joint, Left G Acromioclavicular Joint, Right H Acromioclavicular Joint, Left J Shoulder Joint, Right K Shoulder Joint, Left	0 Open 3 Percutaneous 4 Percutaneous Endoscopic	0 Drainage Device 3 Infusion Device 4 Internal Fixation Device 7 Autologous Tissue Substitute 8 Spacer J Synthetic Substitute K Nonautologous Tissue Substitute	Z No Qualifier
C Temporomandibular Joint, Right D Temporomandibular Joint, Left E Sternoclavicular Joint, Right F Sternoclavicular Joint, Left G Acromioclavicular Joint, Right H Acromioclavicular Joint, Left J Shoulder Joint, Right K Shoulder Joint, Left	X External	0 Drainage Device 3 Infusion Device 4 Internal Fixation Device	Z No Qualifier
L Elbow Joint, Right M Elbow Joint, Left N Wrist Joint, Right P Wrist Joint, Left Q Carpal Joint, Right R Carpal Joint, Left S Metacarpocarpal Joint, Right T Metacarpocarpal Joint, Left U Metacarpophalangeal Joint, Right V Metacarpophalangeal Joint, Left W Finger Phalangeal Joint, Right X Finger Phalangeal Joint, Left	0 Open 3 Percutaneous 4 Percutaneous Endoscopic	0 Drainage Device 3 Infusion Device 4 Internal Fixation Device 5 External Fixation Device 7 Autologous Tissue Substitute 8 Spacer J Synthetic Substitute K Nonautologous Tissue Substitute	Z No Qualifier

◀ New   ◀ Revised   ~~deleted~~ Deleted   ♀ Females Only   ♂ Males Only
🚫 Noncovered   🚫 Limited Coverage   🚫 Hospital-Acquired Condition   **Coding Clinic**

0: M/S

R: UPPER JOINTS

P: REMOVAL

P: REMOVAL   Q: REPAIR

R: UPPER JOINTS

0: M/S

SECTION: 0 MEDICAL AND SURGICAL
BODY SYSTEM: R UPPER JOINTS
OPERATION: P REMOVAL: (continued)
Taking out or off a device from a body part

Body Part	Approach	Device	Qualifier
L Elbow Joint, Right	X External	0 Drainage Device	Z No Qualifier
M Elbow Joint, Left		3 Infusion Device	
N Wrist Joint, Right		4 Internal Fixation Device	
P Wrist Joint, Left		5 External Fixation Device	
Q Carpal Joint, Right			
R Carpal Joint, Left			
S Metacarpocarpal Joint, Right			
T Metacarpocarpal Joint, Left			
U Metacarpophalangeal Joint, Right			
V Metacarpophalangeal Joint, Left			
W Finger Phalangeal Joint, Right			
X Finger Phalangeal Joint, Left			

SECTION: 0 MEDICAL AND SURGICAL
BODY SYSTEM: R UPPER JOINTS
OPERATION: Q REPAIR: Restoring, to the extent possible, a body part to its normal anatomic structure and function

Body Part	Approach	Device	Qualifier
0 Occipital-cervical Joint	0 Open	Z No Device	Z No Qualifier
1 Cervical Vertebral Joint	3 Percutaneous		
3 Cervical Vertebral Disc	4 Percutaneous Endoscopic		
4 Cervicothoracic Vertebral Joint	X External		
5 Cervicothoracic Vertebral Disc			
6 Thoracic Vertebral Joint			
9 Thoracic Vertebral Disc			
A Thoracolumbar Vertebral Joint			
B Thoracolumbar Vertebral Disc			
C Temporomandibular Joint, Right			
D Temporomandibular Joint, Left			
E Sternoclavicular Joint, Right ⚕			
F Sternoclavicular Joint, Left ⚕			
G Acromioclavicular Joint, Right ⚕			
H Acromioclavicular Joint, Left ⚕			
J Shoulder Joint, Right ⚕			
K Shoulder Joint, Left ⚕			
L Elbow Joint, Right ⚕			
M Elbow Joint, Left ⚕			
N Wrist Joint, Right			
P Wrist Joint, Left			
Q Carpal Joint, Right			
R Carpal Joint, Left			
S Metacarpocarpal Joint, Right			
T Metacarpocarpal Joint, Left			
U Metacarpophalangeal Joint, Right			
V Metacarpophalangeal Joint, Left			
W Finger Phalangeal Joint, Right			
X Finger Phalangeal Joint, Left			

◀ New ⬅ Revised ~~deleted~~ Deleted ♀ Females Only ♂ Males Only
⚕ Noncovered ⚕ Limited Coverage ⚕ Hospital-Acquired Condition **Coding Clinic**

SECTION: 0 MEDICAL AND SURGICAL
BODY SYSTEM: R UPPER JOINTS
OPERATION: R REPLACEMENT: Putting in or on biological or synthetic material that physically takes the place and/or function of all or a portion of a body part

Body Part	Approach	Device	Qualifier
0 Occipital-cervical Joint 1 Cervical Vertebral Joint 3 Cervical Vertebral Disc 4 Cervicothoracic Vertebral Joint 5 Cervicothoracic Vertebral Disc 6 Thoracic Vertebral Joint 9 Thoracic Vertebral Disc A Thoracolumbar Vertebral Joint B Thoracolumbar Vertebral Disc C Temporomandibular Joint, Right D Temporomandibular Joint, Left E Sternoclavicular Joint, Right F Sternoclavicular Joint, Left G Acromioclavicular Joint, Right H Acromioclavicular Joint, Left L Elbow Joint, Right M Elbow Joint, Left N Wrist Joint, Right P Wrist Joint, Left Q Carpal Joint, Right R Carpal Joint, Left S Metacarpocarpal Joint, Right T Metacarpocarpal Joint, Left U Metacarpophalangeal Joint, Right V Metacarpophalangeal Joint, Left W Finger Phalangeal Joint, Right X Finger Phalangeal Joint, Left	0 Open	7 Autologous Tissue Substitute J Synthetic Substitute K Nonautologous Tissue Substitute	Z No Qualifier
J Should Joint, Right K Shoulder Joint, Left	0 Open	0 Synthetic Substitute, Reverse Ball and Socket 7 Autologous Tissue Substitute K Nonautologous Tissue Substitute	Z No Qualifier
J Should Joint, Right K Shoulder Joint, Left	0 Open	J Synthetic Substitute	6 Humeral Surface 7 Glenoid Surface Z No Qualifier

SECTION: 0 MEDICAL AND SURGICAL

BODY SYSTEM: R UPPER JOINTS

OPERATION: S REPOSITION: Moving to its normal location, or other suitable location, all or a portion of a body part

Body Part	Approach	Device	Qualifier
0 Occipital-cervical Joint 1 Cervical Vertebral Joint 4 Cervicothoracic Vertebral Joint 6 Thoracic Vertebral Joint A Thoracolumbar Vertebral Joint C Temporomandibular Joint, Right D Temporomandibular Joint, Left E Sternoclavicular Joint, Right F Sternoclavicular Joint, Left G Acromioclavicular Joint, Right H Acromioclavicular Joint, Left J Shoulder Joint, Right K Shoulder Joint, Left	0 Open 3 Percutaneous 4 Percutaneous Endoscopic X External	4 Internal Fixation Device Z No Device	Z No Qualifier
L Elbow Joint, Right M Elbow Joint, Left N Wrist Joint, Right P Wrist Joint, Left Q Carpal Joint, Right R Carpal Joint, Left S Metacarpocarpal Joint, Right T Metacarpocarpal Joint, Left U Metacarpophalangeal Joint, Right V Metacarpophalangeal Joint, Left W Finger Phalangeal Joint, Right X Finger Phalangeal Joint, Left	0 Open 3 Percutaneous 4 Percutaneous Endoscopic X External	4 Internal Fixation Device 5 External Fixation Device Z No Device	Z No Qualifier

Coding Clinic: 2013, Q2, P39 – 0RS1XZZ

S: REPOSITION

R: UPPER JOINTS

0: M/S

◀ New   ◀▥ Revised   ~~deleted~~ Deleted   ♀ Females Only   ♂ Males Only
🝚 Noncovered   🝚 Limited Coverage   🝚 Hospital-Acquired Condition   **Coding Clinic**

SECTION: 0 MEDICAL AND SURGICAL

BODY SYSTEM: R UPPER JOINTS

OPERATION: T RESECTION: Cutting out or off, without replacement, all of a body part

Body Part	Approach	Device	Qualifier
3 Cervical Vertebral Disc 4 Cervicothoracic Vertebral Joint 5 Cervicothoracic Vertebral Disc 9 Thoracic Vertebral Disc B Thoracolumbar Vertebral Disc C Temporomandibular Joint, Right D Temporomandibular Joint, Left E Sternoclavicular Joint, Right F Sternoclavicular Joint, Left G Acromioclavicular Joint, Right H Acromioclavicular Joint, Left J Shoulder Joint, Right K Shoulder Joint, Left L Elbow Joint, Right M Elbow Joint, Left N Wrist Joint, Right P Wrist Joint, Left Q Carpal Joint, Right R Carpal Joint, Left S Metacarpocarpal Joint, Right T Metacarpocarpal Joint, Left U Metacarpophalangeal Joint, Right V Metacarpophalangeal Joint, Left W Finger Phalangeal Joint, Right X Finger Phalangeal Joint, Left	0 Open	Z No Device	Z No Qualifier

0: M/S

R: UPPER JOINTS

T: RESECTION

SECTION: 0 MEDICAL AND SURGICAL

BODY SYSTEM: R UPPER JOINTS

OPERATION: U SUPPLEMENT: Putting in or on biological or synthetic material that physically reinforces and/or augments the function of a portion of a body part

Body Part	Approach	Device	Qualifier
0 Occipital-cervical Joint	0 Open	7 Autologous Tissue Substitute	Z No Qualifier
1 Cervical Vertebral Joint	3 Percutaneous	J Synthetic Substitute	
3 Cervical Vertebral Disc	4 Percutaneous Endoscopic	K Nonautologous Tissue	
4 Cervicothoracic Vertebral Joint		Substitute	
5 Cervicothoracic Vertebral Disc			
6 Thoracic Vertebral Joint			
9 Thoracic Vertebral Disc			
A Thoracolumbar Vertebral Joint			
B Thoracolumbar Vertebral Disc			
C Temporomandibular Joint, Right			
D Temporomandibular Joint, Left			
E Sternoclavicular Joint, Right ⚕			
F Sternoclavicular Joint, Left ⚕			
G Acromioclavicular Joint, Right ⚕			
H Acromioclavicular Joint, Left ⚕			
J Shoulder Joint, Right ⚕			
K Shoulder Joint, Left ⚕			
L Elbow Joint, Right ⚕			
M Elbow Joint, Left ⚕			
N Wrist Joint, Right			
P Wrist Joint, Left			
Q Carpal Joint, Right			
R Carpal Joint, Left			
S Metacarpocarpal Joint, Right			
T Metacarpocarpal Joint, Left			
U Metacarpophalangeal Joint, Right			
V Metacarpophalangeal Joint, Left			
W Finger Phalangeal Joint, Right			
X Finger Phalangeal Joint, Left			

U: SUPPLEMENT

R: UPPER JOINTS

0: M/S

◀ New ◀ Revised deleted Deleted ♀ Females Only ♂ Males Only
⚕ Noncovered ⚕ Limited Coverage ⚕ Hospital-Acquired Condition **Coding Clinic**

SECTION: 0 MEDICAL AND SURGICAL
BODY SYSTEM: R UPPER JOINTS
OPERATION: W REVISION: Correcting, to the extent possible, a portion of a malfunctioning device or the position of a displaced device

Body Part	Approach	Device	Qualifier
0 Occipital-cervical Joint 1 Cervical Vertebral Joint 4 Cervicothoracic Vertebral Joint 6 Thoracic Vertebral Joint A Thoracolumbar Vertebral Joint	0 Open 3 Percutaneous 4 Percutaneous Endoscopic X External	0 Drainage Device 3 Infusion Device 4 Internal Fixation Device 7 Autologous Tissue Substitute 8 Spacer J Synthetic Substitute K Nonautologous Tissue Substitute	Z No Qualifier
3 Cervical Vertebral Disc 5 Cervicothoracic Vertebral Disc 9 Thoracic Vertebral Disc B Thoracolumbar Vertebral Disc	0 Open 3 Percutaneous 4 Percutaneous Endoscopic X External	0 Drainage Device 3 Infusion Device 7 Autologous Tissue Substitute J Synthetic Substitute K Nonautologous Tissue Substitute	Z No Qualifier
C Temporomandibular Joint, Right D Temporomandibular Joint, Left E Sternoclavicular Joint, Right F Sternoclavicular Joint, Left G Acromioclavicular Joint, Right H Acromioclavicular Joint, Left J Shoulder Joint, Right K Shoulder Joint, Left	0 Open 3 Percutaneous 4 Percutaneous Endoscopic X External	0 Drainage Device 3 Infusion Device 4 Internal Fixation Device 7 Autologous Tissue Substitute 8 Spacer J Synthetic Substitute K Nonautologous Tissue Substitute	Z No Qualifier
L Elbow Joint, Right M Elbow Joint, Left N Wrist Joint, Right P Wrist Joint, Left Q Carpal Joint, Right R Carpal Joint, Left S Metacarpocarpal Joint, Right T Metacarpocarpal Joint, Left U Metacarpophalangeal Joint, Right V Metacarpophalangeal Joint, Left W Finger Phalangeal Joint, Right X Finger Phalangeal Joint, Left	0 Open 3 Percutaneous 4 Percutaneous Endoscopic X External	0 Drainage Device 3 Infusion Device 4 Internal Fixation Device 5 External Fixation Device 7 Autologous Tissue Substitute 8 Spacer J Synthetic Substitute K Nonautologous Tissue Substitute	Z No Qualifier

0: M/S

R: UPPER JOINTS

W: REVISION

◀ New   ◀▥ Revised   ~~deleted~~ Deleted   ♀ Females Only   ♂ Males Only
Ⓝc Noncovered   Ⓛc Limited Coverage   Ⓗac Hospital-Acquired Condition   **Coding Clinic**

SECTION: 0 MEDICAL AND SURGICAL
BODY SYSTEM: S LOWER JOINTS
OPERATION: 2 **CHANGE:** Taking out or off a device from a body part and putting back an identical or similar device in or on the same body part without cutting or puncturing the skin or a mucous membrane

Body Part	Approach	Device	Qualifier
Y Lower Joint	X External	0 Drainage Device Y Other Device	Z No Qualifier

SECTION: 0 MEDICAL AND SURGICAL
BODY SYSTEM: S LOWER JOINTS
OPERATION: 5 **DESTRUCTION:** Physical eradication of all or a portion of a body part by the direct use of energy, force, or destructive agent

Body Part	Approach	Device	Qualifier
0 Lumbar Vertebral Joint 2 Lumbar Vertebral Disc 3 Lumbosacral Joint 4 Lumbosacral Disc 5 Sacrococcygeal Joint 6 Coccygeal Joint 7 Sacroiliac Joint, Right 8 Sacroiliac Joint, Left 9 Hip Joint, Right B Hip Joint, Left C Knee Joint, Right D Knee Joint, Left F Ankle Joint, Right G Ankle Joint, Left H Tarsal Joint, Right J Tarsal Joint, Left K Metatarsal-Tarsal Joint, Right L Metatarsal-Tarsal Joint, Left M Metatarsal-Phalangeal Joint, Right N Metatarsal-Phalangeal Joint, Left P Toe Phalangeal Joint, Right Q Toe Phalangeal Joint, Left	0 Open 3 Percutaneous 4 Percutaneous Endoscopic	Z No Device	Z No Qualifier

SECTION: 0 MEDICAL AND SURGICAL
BODY SYSTEM: S LOWER JOINTS
OPERATION: 9 DRAINAGE: Taking or letting out fluids and/or gases from a body part

9: DRAINAGE

S: LOWER JOINTS

0: M/S

Body Part	Approach	Device	Qualifier
0 Lumbar Vertebral Joint 2 Lumbar Vertebral Disc 3 Lumbosacral Joint 4 Lumbosacral Disc 5 Sacrococcygeal Joint 6 Coccygeal Joint 7 Sacroiliac Joint, Right 8 Sacroiliac Joint, Left 9 Hip Joint, Right B Hip Joint, Left C Knee Joint, Right D Knee Joint, Left F Ankle Joint, Right G Ankle Joint, Left H Tarsal Joint, Right J Tarsal Joint, Left K Metatarsal-Tarsal Joint, Right L Metatarsal-Tarsal Joint, Left M Metatarsal-Phalangeal Joint, Right N Metatarsal-Phalangeal Joint, Left P Toe Phalangeal Joint, Right Q Toe Phalangeal Joint, Left	0 Open 3 Percutaneous 4 Percutaneous Endoscopic	0 Drainage Device	Z No Qualifier
0 Lumbar Vertebral Joint 2 Lumbar Vertebral Disc 3 Lumbosacral Joint 4 Lumbosacral Disc 5 Sacrococcygeal Joint 6 Coccygeal Joint 7 Sacroiliac Joint, Right 8 Sacroiliac Joint, Left 9 Hip Joint, Right B Hip Joint, Left C Knee Joint, Right D Knee Joint, Left F Ankle Joint, Right G Ankle Joint, Left H Tarsal Joint, Right J Tarsal Joint, Left K Metatarsal-Tarsal Joint, Right L Metatarsal-Tarsal Joint, Left M Metatarsal-Phalangeal Joint, Right N Metatarsal-Phalangeal Joint, Left P Toe Phalangeal Joint, Right Q Toe Phalangeal Joint, Left	0 Open 3 Percutaneous 4 Percutaneous Endoscopic	Z No Device	X Diagnostic Z No Qualifier

◀ New   ◀|||| Revised   ~~deleted~~ Deleted   ♀ Females Only   ♂ Males Only
⬡ Noncovered   ⬡ Limited Coverage   ⬡ Hospital-Acquired Condition   **Coding Clinic**

SECTION: 0 MEDICAL AND SURGICAL

BODY SYSTEM: S LOWER JOINTS
OPERATION: B EXCISION: Cutting out or off, without replacement, a portion of a body part

Body Part	Approach	Device	Qualifier
0 Lumbar Vertebral Joint 2 Lumbar Vertebral Disc 3 Lumbosacral Joint 4 Lumbosacral Disc 5 Sacrococcygeal Joint 6 Coccygeal Joint 7 Sacroiliac Joint, Right 8 Sacroiliac Joint, Left 9 Hip Joint, Right B Hip Joint, Left C Knee Joint, Right D Knee Joint, Left F Ankle Joint, Right G Ankle Joint, Left H Tarsal Joint, Right J Tarsal Joint, Left K Metatarsal-Tarsal Joint, Right L Metatarsal-Tarsal Joint, Left M Metatarsal-Phalangeal Joint, Right N Metatarsal-Phalangeal Joint, Left P Toe Phalangeal Joint, Right Q Toe Phalangeal Joint, Left	0 Open 3 Percutaneous 4 Percutaneous Endoscopic	Z No Device	X Diagnostic Z No Qualifier

SECTION: 0 MEDICAL AND SURGICAL

BODY SYSTEM: S LOWER JOINTS
OPERATION: C EXTIRPATION: Taking or cutting out solid matter from a body part

Body Part	Approach	Device	Qualifier
0 Lumbar Vertebral Joint 2 Lumbar Vertebral Disc 3 Lumbosacral Joint 4 Lumbosacral Disc 5 Sacrococcygeal Joint 6 Coccygeal Joint 7 Sacroiliac Joint, Right 8 Sacroiliac Joint, Left 9 Hip Joint, Right B Hip Joint, Left C Knee Joint, Right D Knee Joint, Left F Ankle Joint, Right G Ankle Joint, Left H Tarsal Joint, Right J Tarsal Joint, Left K Metatarsal-Tarsal Joint, Right L Metatarsal-Tarsal Joint, Left M Metatarsal-Phalangeal Joint, Right N Metatarsal-Phalangeal Joint, Left P Toe Phalangeal Joint, Right Q Toe Phalangeal Joint, Left	0 Open 3 Percutaneous 4 Percutaneous Endoscopic	Z No Device	Z No Qualifier

◀ New   ◀‖ Revised   ~~deleted~~ Deleted   ♀ Females Only   ♂ Males Only
🝆 Noncovered   🝆 Limited Coverage   🝆 Hospital-Acquired Condition   **Coding Clinic**

SECTION: 0 MEDICAL AND SURGICAL

BODY SYSTEM: S LOWER JOINTS

OPERATION: G FUSION: Joining together portions of an articular body part, rendering the articular body part immobile

Body Part	Approach	Device	Qualifier
0 Lumbar Vertebral Joint 🦠 1 Lumbar Vertebral Joints, 2 or more 🦠 3 Lumbosacral Joint 🦠	0 Open 3 Percutaneous 4 Percutaneous Endoscopic	7 Autologous Tissue Substitute A Interbody Fusion Device J Synthetic Substitute K Nonautologous Tissue Substitute Z No Device	0 Anterior Approach, Anterior Column 1 Posterior Approach, Posterior Column J Posterior Approach, Anterior Column
5 Sacrococcygeal Joint 6 Coccygeal Joint 7 Sacroiliac Joint, Right 🦠 8 Sacroiliac Joint, Left 🦠	0 Open 3 Percutaneous 4 Percutaneous Endoscopic	4 Internal Fixation Device 7 Autologous Tissue Substitute J Synthetic Substitute K Nonautologous Tissue Substitute Z No Device	Z No Qualifier
9 Hip Joint, Right B Hip Joint, Left C Knee Joint, Right D Knee Joint, Left F Ankle Joint, Right G Ankle Joint, Left H Tarsal Joint, Right J Tarsal Joint, Left K Metatarsal-Tarsal Joint, Right L Metatarsal-Tarsal Joint, Left M Metatarsal-Phalangeal Joint, Right N Metatarsal-Phalangeal Joint, Left P Toe Phalangeal Joint, Right Q Toe Phalangeal Joint, Left	0 Open 3 Percutaneous 4 Percutaneous Endoscopic	4 Internal Fixation Device 5 External Fixation Device 7 Autologous Tissue Substitute J Synthetic Substitute K Nonautologous Tissue Substitute Z No Device	Z No Qualifier

Coding Clinic: 2013, Q3, P26, Q1, P23 – 0SG0071

Coding Clinic: 2013, Q3, P26 – 0SG00AJ

Coding Clinic: 2013, Q2, P40 – 0SGG04Z, 0SGG07Z

G: FUSION

S: LOWER JOINTS

0: M/S

◀ New   ◀▥ Revised   ~~deleted~~ Deleted   ♀ Females Only   ♂ Males Only
🦠 Noncovered   🦠 Limited Coverage   🦠 Hospital-Acquired Condition   **Coding Clinic**

SECTION: 0 MEDICAL AND SURGICAL
BODY SYSTEM: S LOWER JOINTS
OPERATION: H INSERTION: Putting in a nonbiological appliance that monitors, assists, performs, or prevents a physiological function but does not physically take the place of a body part

Body Part	Approach	Device	Qualifier
0 Lumbar Vertebral Joint 3 Lumbosacral Joint	0 Open 3 Percutaneous 4 Percutaneous Endoscopic	3 Infusion Device 4 Internal Fixation Device 8 Spacer B Spinal Stabilization Device, Interspinous Process C Spinal Stabilization Device, Pedicle-Based D Spinal Stabilization Device, Facet Replacement	Z No Qualifier
2 Lumbar Vertebral Disc 4 Lumbosacral Disc	0 Open 3 Percutaneous 4 Percutaneous Endoscopic	3 Infusion Device 8 Spacer	Z No Qualifier
5 Sacrococcygeal Joint 6 Coccygeal Joint 7 Sacroiliac Joint, Right 8 Sacroiliac Joint, Left	0 Open 3 Percutaneous 4 Percutaneous Endoscopic	3 Infusion Device 4 Internal Fixation Device 8 Spacer	Z No Qualifier
9 Hip Joint, Right B Hip Joint, Left C Knee Joint, Right D Knee Joint, Left F Ankle Joint, Right G Ankle Joint, Left H Tarsal Joint, Right J Tarsal Joint, Left K Metatarsal-Tarsal Joint, Right L Metatarsal-Tarsal Joint, Left M Metatarsal-Phalangeal Joint, Right N Metatarsal-Phalangeal Joint, Left P Toe Phalangeal Joint, Right Q Toe Phalangeal Joint, Left	0 Open 3 Percutaneous 4 Percutaneous Endoscopic	3 Infusion Device 4 Internal Fixation Device 5 External Fixation Device 8 Spacer	Z No Qualifier

0: M/S

S: LOWER JOINTS

H: INSERTION

◀ New ◀ Revised ~~deleted~~ Deleted ♀ Females Only ♂ Males Only
 Noncovered   Limited Coverage   Hospital-Acquired Condition **Coding Clinic**

405

SECTION: 0 MEDICAL AND SURGICAL
BODY SYSTEM: S LOWER JOINTS
OPERATION: J INSPECTION: Visually and/or manually exploring a body part

Body Part	Approach	Device	Qualifier
0 Lumbar Vertebral Joint	0 Open	Z No Device	Z No Qualifier
2 Lumbar Vertebral Disc	3 Percutaneous		
3 Lumbosacral Joint	4 Percutaneous Endoscopic		
4 Lumbosacral Disc	X External		
5 Sacrococcygeal Joint			
6 Coccygeal Joint			
7 Sacroiliac Joint, Right			
8 Sacroiliac Joint, Left			
9 Hip Joint, Right			
B Hip Joint, Left			
C Knee Joint, Right			
D Knee Joint, Left			
F Ankle Joint, Right			
G Ankle Joint, Left			
H Tarsal Joint, Right			
J Tarsal Joint, Left			
K Metatarsal-Tarsal Joint, Right			
L Metatarsal-Tarsal Joint, Left			
M Metatarsal-Phalangeal Joint, Right			
N Metatarsal-Phalangeal Joint, Left			
P Toe Phalangeal Joint, Right			
Q Toe Phalangeal Joint, Left			

SECTION: 0 MEDICAL AND SURGICAL
BODY SYSTEM: S LOWER JOINTS
OPERATION: N RELEASE: Freeing a body part from an abnormal physical constraint by cutting or by the use of force

Body Part	Approach	Device	Qualifier
0 Lumbar Vertebral Joint	0 Open	Z No Device	Z No Qualifier
2 Lumbar Vertebral Disc	3 Percutaneous		
3 Lumbosacral Joint	4 Percutaneous Endoscopic		
4 Lumbosacral Disc	X External		
5 Sacrococcygeal Joint			
6 Coccygeal Joint			
7 Sacroiliac Joint, Right			
8 Sacroiliac Joint, Left			
9 Hip Joint, Right			
B Hip Joint, Left			
C Knee Joint, Right			
D Knee Joint, Left			
F Ankle Joint, Right			
G Ankle Joint, Left			
H Tarsal Joint, Right			
J Tarsal Joint, Left			
K Metatarsal-Tarsal Joint, Right			
L Metatarsal-Tarsal Joint, Left			
M Metatarsal-Phalangeal Joint, Right			
N Metatarsal-Phalangeal Joint, Left			
P Toe Phalangeal Joint, Right			
Q Toe Phalangeal Joint, Left			

SECTION: 0 MEDICAL AND SURGICAL
BODY SYSTEM: S LOWER JOINTS
OPERATION: P REMOVAL: *(on multiple pages)*
Taking out or off a device from a body part

Body Part	Approach	Device	Qualifier
0 Lumbar Vertebral Joint 3 Lumbosacral Joint	0 Open 3 Percutaneous 4 Percutaneous Endoscopic	0 Drainage Device 3 Infusion Device 4 Internal Fixation Device 7 Autologous Tissue Substitute 8 Spacer A Interbody Fusion Device J Synthetic Substitute K Nonautologous Tissue Substitute	Z No Qualifier
0 Lumbar Vertebral Joint 3 Lumbosacral Joint	X External	0 Drainage Device 3 Infusion Device 4 Internal Fixation Device	Z No Qualifier
2 Lumbar Vertebral Disc 4 Lumbosacral Disc	0 Open 3 Percutaneous 4 Percutaneous Endoscopic	0 Drainage Device 3 Infusion Device 7 Autologous Tissue Substitute J Synthetic Substitute K Nonautologous Tissue Substitute	Z No Qualifier
2 Lumbar Vertebral Disc 4 Lumbosacral Disc	X External	0 Drainage Device 3 Infusion Device	Z No Qualifier
5 Sacrococcygeal Joint 6 Coccygeal Joint 7 Sacroiliac Joint, Right 8 Sacroiliac Joint, Left	0 Open 3 Percutaneous 4 Percutaneous Endoscopic	0 Drainage Device 3 Infusion Device 4 Internal Fixation Device 7 Autologous Tissue Substitute 8 Spacer J Synthetic Substitute K Nonautologous Tissue Substitute	Z No Qualifier
5 Sacrococcygeal Joint 6 Coccygeal Joint 7 Sacroiliac Joint, Right 8 Sacroiliac Joint, Left	X External	0 Drainage Device 3 Infusion Device 4 Internal Fixation Device	Z No Qualifier
9 Hip Joint, Right B Hip Joint, Left	0 Open	0 Drainage Device 3 Infusion Device 4 Internal Fixation Device 5 External Fixation Device 7 Autologous Tissue Substitute 8 Spacer 9 Liner B Resurfacing Device J Synthetic Substitute K Nonautologous Tissue Substitute	Z No Qualifier
9 Hip Joint, Right B Hip Joint, Left	3 Percutaneous 4 Percutaneous Endoscopic	0 Drainage Device 3 Infusion Device 4 Internal Fixation Device 5 External Fixation Device 7 Autologous Tissue Substitute 8 Spacer J Synthetic Substitute K Nonautologous Tissue Substitute	Z No Qualifier

◄ New ◄▥ Revised ~~deleted~~ Deleted ♀ Females Only ♂ Males Only
▧ Noncovered ▧ Limited Coverage ▧ Hospital-Acquired Condition **Coding Clinic**

0: M/S

S: LOWER JOINTS

P: REMOVAL

SECTION: 0 MEDICAL AND SURGICAL
BODY SYSTEM: S LOWER JOINTS
OPERATION: P REMOVAL: *(continued)*
Taking out or off a device from a body part

Body Part	Approach	Device	Qualifier
9 Hip Joint, Right B Hip Joint, Left	X External	0 Drainage Device 3 Infusion Device 4 Internal Fixation Device 5 External Fixation Device	Z No Qualifier
C Knee Joint, Right D Knee Joint, Left	0 Open	0 Drainage Device 3 Infusion Device 4 Internal Fixation Device 5 External Fixation Device 7 Autologous Tissue Substitute 8 Spacer 9 Liner J Synthetic Substitute K Nonautologous Tissue Substitute	Z No Qualifier
C Knee Joint, Right D Knee Joint, Left	3 Percutaneous 4 Percutaneous Endoscopic	0 Drainage Device 3 Infusion Device 4 Internal Fixation Device 5 External Fixation Device 7 Autologous Tissue Substitute 8 Spacer J Synthetic Substitute K Nonautologous Tissue Substitute	Z No Qualifier
C Knee Joint, Right D Knee Joint, Left	X External	0 Drainage Device 3 Infusion Device 4 Internal Fixation Device 5 External Fixation Device	Z No Qualifier
F Ankle Joint, Right G Ankle Joint, Left H Tarsal Joint, Right J Tarsal Joint, Left K Metatarsal-Tarsal Joint, Right L Metatarsal-Tarsal Joint, Left M Metatarsal-Phalangeal Joint, Right N Metatarsal-Phalangeal Joint, Left P Toe Phalangeal Joint, Right Q Toe Phalangeal Joint, Left	0 Open 3 Percutaneous 4 Percutaneous Endoscopic	0 Drainage Device 3 Infusion Device 4 Internal Fixation Device 5 External Fixation Device 7 Autologous Tissue Substitute 8 Spacer J Synthetic Substitute K Nonautologous Tissue Substitute	Z No Qualifier
F Ankle Joint, Right G Ankle Joint, Left H Tarsal Joint, Right J Tarsal Joint, Left K Metatarsal-Tarsal Joint, Right L Metatarsal-Tarsal Joint, Left M Metatarsal-Phalangeal Joint, Right N Metatarsal-Phalangeal Joint, Left P Toe Phalangeal Joint, Right Q Toe Phalangeal Joint, Left	X External	0 Drainage Device 3 Infusion Device 4 Internal Fixation Device 5 External Fixation Device	Z No Qualifier

Coding Clinic: 2013, Q2, P40 – 0SPG04Z

P: REMOVAL
S: LOWER JOINTS
0: M/S

◀ New ◀ Revised ~~deleted~~ Deleted ♀ Females Only ♂ Males Only
Noncovered Limited Coverage Hospital-Acquired Condition **Coding Clinic**

SECTION: 0 MEDICAL AND SURGICAL

BODY SYSTEM: S LOWER JOINTS
OPERATION: Q REPAIR: Restoring, to the extent possible, a body part to its normal anatomic structure and function

Body Part	Approach	Device	Qualifier
0 Lumbar Vertebral Joint	0 Open	Z No Device	Z No Qualifier
2 Lumbar Vertebral Disc	3 Percutaneous		
3 Lumbosacral Joint	4 Percutaneous Endoscopic		
4 Lumbosacral Disc	X External		
5 Sacrococcygeal Joint			
6 Coccygeal Joint			
7 Sacroiliac Joint, Right			
8 Sacroiliac Joint, Left			
9 Hip Joint, Right			
B Hip Joint, Left			
C Knee Joint, Right			
D Knee Joint, Left			
F Ankle Joint, Right			
G Ankle Joint, Left			
H Tarsal Joint, Right			
J Tarsal Joint, Left			
K Metatarsal-Tarsal Joint, Right			
L Metatarsal-Tarsal Joint, Left			
M Metatarsal-Phalangeal Joint, Right			
N Metatarsal-Phalangeal Joint, Left			
P Toe Phalangeal Joint, Right			
Q Toe Phalangeal Joint, Left			

SECTION: 0 MEDICAL AND SURGICAL

BODY SYSTEM: S LOWER JOINTS
OPERATION: R REPLACEMENT: *(on multiple pages)*
Putting in or on biological or synthetic material that physically takes the place and/or function of all or a portion of a body part

Body Part	Approach	Device	Qualifier
0 Lumbar Vertebral Joint	0 Open	7 Autologous Tissue Substitute	Z No Qualifier
2 Lumbar Vertebral Disc 🝖		J Synthetic Substitute	
3 Lumbosacral Joint		K Nonautologous Tissue Substitute	
4 Lumbosacral Disc 🝖			
5 Sacrococcygeal Joint			
6 Coccygeal Joint			
7 Sacroiliac Joint, Right			
8 Sacroiliac Joint, Left			
H Tarsal Joint, Right			
J Tarsal Joint, Left			
K Metatarsal-Tarsal Joint, Right			
L Metatarsal-Tarsal Joint, Left			
M Metatarsal-Phalangeal Joint, Right			
N Metatarsal-Phalangeal Joint, Left			
P Toe Phalangeal Joint, Right			
Q Toe Phalangeal Joint, Left			

◀ New　◀ Revised　deleted Deleted　♀ Females Only　♂ Males Only
🝖 Noncovered　🝖 Limited Coverage　🝖 Hospital-Acquired Condition　**Coding Clinic**

SECTION: 0 MEDICAL AND SURGICAL
BODY SYSTEM: S LOWER JOINTS
OPERATION: R REPLACEMENT: *(continued)*
Putting in or on biological or synthetic material that physically takes the place and/or function of all or a portion of a body part

R: REPLACEMENT

S: LOWER JOINTS

0: M/S

Body Part	Approach	Device	Qualifier
9 Hip Joint, Right ⚭ B Hip Joint, Left ⚭	0 Open	1 Synthetic Substitute, Metal 2 Synthetic Substitute, Metal on Polyethylene 3 Synthetic Substitute, Ceramic 4 Synthetic Substitute, Ceramic on Polyethylene J Synthetic Substitute	9 Cemented A Uncemented Z No Qualifier
9 Hip Joint, Right ⚭ B Hip Joint, Left ⚭	0 Open	7 Autologous Tissue Substitute K Nonautologous Tissue Substitute	Z No Qualifier
A Hip Joint, Acetabular Surface, Right ⚭ E Hip Joint, Acetabular Surface, Left ⚭	0 Open	0 Synthetic Substitute, Polyethylene 1 Synthetic Substitute, Metal 3 Synthetic Substitute, Ceramic J Synthetic Substitute	9 Cemented A Uncemented Z No Qualifier
A Hip Joint, Acetabular Surface, Right ⚭ E Hip Joint, Acetabular Surface, Left ⚭	0 Open	7 Autologous Tissue Substitute K Nonautologous Tissue Substitute	Z No Qualifier
C Knee Joint, Right ⚭ D Knee Joint, Left ⚭ F Ankle Joint, Right G Ankle Joint, Left T Knee Joint, Femoral Surface, Right ⚭ U Knee Joint, Femoral Surface, Left ⚭ V Knee Joint, Tibial Surface, Right ⚭ W Knee Joint, Tibial Surface, Left ⚭	0 Open	7 Autologous Tissue Substitute K Nonautologous Tissue Substitute	Z No Qualifier
C Knee Joint, Right ⚭ D Knee Joint, Left ⚭ F Ankle Joint, Right G Ankle Joint, Left T Knee Joint, Femoral Surface, Right ⚭ U Knee Joint, Femoral Surface, Left ⚭ V Knee Joint, Tibial Surface, Right ⚭ W Knee Joint, Tibial Surface, Left ⚭	0 Open	J Synthetic Substitute	9 Cemented A Uncemented Z No Qualifier
R Hip Joint, Femoral Surface, Right ⚭ S Hip Joint, Femoral Surface, Left ⚭	0 Open	1 Synthetic Substitute, Metal 3 Synthetic Substitute, Ceramic J Synthetic Substitute	9 Cemented A Uncemented Z No Qualifier
R Hip Joint, Femoral Surface, Right ⚭ S Hip Joint, Femoral Surface, Left ⚭	0 Open	7 Autologous Tissue Substitute K Nonautologous Tissue Substitute	Z No Qualifier

⚭ 0SR20JZ, 0SR40Z: when beneficiary is over age 60

◀ New ◀ Revised ~~deleted~~ Deleted ♀ Females Only ♂ Males Only
⚭ Noncovered ⚭ Limited Coverage ⚭ Hospital-Acquired Condition **Coding Clinic**

SECTION: 0 MEDICAL AND SURGICAL
BODY SYSTEM: S LOWER JOINTS
OPERATION: S REPOSITION: Moving to its normal location, or other suitable location, all or a portion of a body part

Body Part	Approach	Device	Qualifier
0 Lumbar Vertebral Joint 3 Lumbosacral Joint 5 Sacrococcygeal Joint 6 Coccygeal Joint 7 Sacroiliac Joint, Right 8 Sacroiliac Joint, Left	0 Open 3 Percutaneous 4 Percutaneous Endoscopic X External	4 Internal Fixation Device Z No Device	Z No Qualifier
9 Hip Joint, Right B Hip Joint, Left C Knee Joint, Right D Knee Joint, Left F Ankle Joint, Right G Ankle Joint, Left H Tarsal Joint, Right J Tarsal Joint, Left K Metatarsal-Tarsal Joint, Right L Metatarsal-Tarsal Joint, Left M Metatarsal-Phalangeal Joint, Right N Metatarsal-Phalangeal Joint, Left P Toe Phalangeal Joint, Right Q Toe Phalangeal Joint, Left	0 Open 3 Percutaneous 4 Percutaneous Endoscopic X External	4 Internal Fixation Device 5 External Fixation Device Z No Device	Z No Qualifier

SECTION: 0 MEDICAL AND SURGICAL
BODY SYSTEM: S LOWER JOINTS
OPERATION: T RESECTION: Cutting out or off, without replacement, all of a body part

Body Part	Approach	Device	Qualifier
2 Lumbar Vertebral Disc 4 Lumbosacral Disc 5 Sacrococcygeal Joint 6 Coccygeal Joint 7 Sacroiliac Joint, Right 8 Sacroiliac Joint, Left 9 Hip Joint, Right B Hip Joint, Left C Knee Joint, Right D Knee Joint, Left F Ankle Joint, Right G Ankle Joint, Left H Tarsal Joint, Right J Tarsal Joint, Left K Metatarsal-Tarsal Joint, Right L Metatarsal-Tarsal Joint, Left M Metatarsal-Phalangeal Joint, Right N Metatarsal-Phalangeal Joint, Left P Toe Phalangeal Joint, Right Q Toe Phalangeal Joint, Left	0 Open	Z No Device	Z No Qualifier

0: M/S

S: LOWER JOINTS

S: REPOSITION   T: RESECTION

SECTION: 0 MEDICAL AND SURGICAL
BODY SYSTEM: S LOWER JOINTS
OPERATION: U **SUPPLEMENT:** Putting in or on biological or synthetic material that physically reinforces and/or augments the function of a portion of a body part

Body Part	Approach	Device	Qualifier
2 Lumbar Vertebral Joint 4 Lumbosacral Disc 5 Sacrococcygeal Joint 6 Coccygeal Joint 7 Sacroiliac Joint, Right 8 Sacroiliac Joint, Left F Ankle Joint, Right G Ankle Joint, Left H Tarsal Joint, Right J Tarsal Joint, Left K Metatarsal-Tarsal Joint, Right L Metatarsal-Tarsal Joint, Left M Metatarsal-Phalangeal Joint, Right N Metatarsal-Phalangeal Joint, Left P Toe Phalangeal Joint, Right Q Toe Phalangeal Joint, Left	0 Open 3 Percutaneous 4 Percutaneous Endoscopic	7 Autologous Tissue Substitute J Synthetic Substitute K Nonautologous Tissue Substitute	Z No Qualifier
9 Hip Joint, Right 🖎 B Hip Joint, Left 🖎	0 Open	7 Autologous Tissue Substitute 9 Liner B Resurfacing Device J Synthetic Substitute K Nonautologous Tissue Substitute	Z No Qualifier
9 Hip Joint, Right B Hip Joint, Left	3 Percutaneous 4 Percutaneous Endoscopic	7 Autologous Tissue Substitute J Synthetic Substitute K Nonautologous Tissue Substitute	Z No Qualifier
A Hip Joint, Acetabular Surface, Right 🖎 E Hip Joint, Acetabular Surface, Left 🖎 R Hip Joint, Femoral Surface, Right 🖎 S Hip Joint, Femoral Surface, Left 🖎	0 Open	9 Liner B Resurfacing Device	Z No Qualifier
C Knee Joint, Right D Knee Joint, Left	0 Open	7 Autologous Tissue Substitute J Synthetic Substitute K Nonautologous Tissue Substitute	Z No Qualifier
C Knee Joint, Right D Knee Joint, Left	0 Open	9 Liner	C Patellar Surface Z No Qualifier
C Knee Joint, Right D Knee Joint, Left	3 Percutaneous 4 Percutaneous Endoscopic	7 Autologous Tissue Substitute J Synthetic Substitute K Nonautologous Tissue Substitute	Z No Qualifier
T Knee Joint, Femoral Surface, Right U Knee Joint, Femoral Surface, Left V Knee Joint, Tibial Surface, Right W Knee Joint, Tibial Surface, Left	0 Open	9 Liner	Z No Qualifier

🖎 0SU90BZ, 0SUA0BZ, 0SUB0BZ, 0SUE0BZ, 0SUR0BZ, 0SUS0BZ

◀ New   ◀▥ Revised   ~~deleted~~ Deleted   ♀ Females Only   ♂ Males Only
🖎 Noncovered   🖎 Limited Coverage   🖎 Hospital-Acquired Condition   **Coding Clinic**

U: SUPPLEMENT   S: LOWER JOINTS   0: M/S

SECTION: 0 MEDICAL AND SURGICAL
BODY SYSTEM: S LOWER JOINTS
OPERATION: W REVISION: *(on multiple pages)*
Correcting, to the extent possible, a portion of a malfunctioning device or the position of a displaced device

Body Part	Approach	Device	Qualifier
0 Lumbar Vertebral Joint 3 Lumbosacral Joint	0 Open 3 Percutaneous 4 Percutaneous Endoscopic X External	0 Drainage Device 3 Infusion Device 4 Internal Fixation Device 7 Autologous Tissue Substitute 8 Spacer A Interbody Fusion Device J Synthetic Substitute K Nonautologous Tissue Substitute	Z No Qualifier
2 Lumbar Vertebral Disc 4 Lumbosacral Disc	0 Open 3 Percutaneous 4 Percutaneous Endoscopic X External	0 Drainage Device 3 Infusion Device 7 Autologous Tissue Substitute J Synthetic Substitute K Nonautologous Tissue Substitute	Z No Qualifier
5 Sacrococcygeal Joint 6 Coccygeal Joint 7 Sacroiliac Joint, Right 8 Sacroiliac Joint, Left	0 Open 3 Percutaneous 4 Percutaneous Endoscopic X External	0 Drainage Device 3 Infusion Device 4 Internal Fixation Device 7 Autologous Tissue Substitute 8 Spacer J Synthetic Substitute K Nonautologous Tissue Substitute	Z No Qualifier
9 Hip Joint, Right B Hip Joint, Left	0 Open	0 Drainage Device 3 Infusion Device 4 Internal Fixation Device 5 External Fixation Device 7 Autologous Tissue Substitute 8 Spacer 9 Liner B Resurfacing Device J Synthetic Substitute K Nonautologous Tissue Substitute	Z No Qualifier
9 Hip Joint, Right B Hip Joint, Left	3 Percutaneous 4 Percutaneous Endoscopic X External	0 Drainage Device 3 Infusion Device 4 Internal Fixation Device 5 External Fixation Device 7 Autologous Tissue Substitute 8 Spacer J Synthetic Substitute K Nonautologous Tissue Substitute	Z No Qualifier

0: M/S

S: LOWER JOINTS

W: REVISION

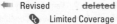 New ◀ Revised ~~deleted~~ Deleted ♀ Females Only ♂ Males Only
Noncovered Limited Coverage Hospital-Acquired Condition **Coding Clinic**

413

SECTION: 0 MEDICAL AND SURGICAL
BODY SYSTEM: S LOWER JOINTS
OPERATION: W REVISION: *(continued)*
Correcting, to the extent possible, a portion of a malfunctioning device or the position of a displaced device

Body Part	Approach	Device	Qualifier
C Knee Joint, Right D Knee Joint, Left	0 Open	0 Drainage Device 3 Infusion Device 4 Internal Fixation Device 5 External Fixation Device 7 Autologous Tissue Substitute 8 Spacer 9 Liner J Synthetic Substitute K Nonautologous Tissue Substitute	Z No Qualifier
C Knee Joint, Right D Knee Joint, Left	3 Percutaneous 4 Percutaneous Endoscopic X External	0 Drainage Device 3 Infusion Device 4 Internal Fixation Device 5 External Fixation Device 7 Autologous Tissue Substitute 8 Spacer J Synthetic Substitute K Nonautologous Tissue Substitute	Z No Qualifier
F Ankle Joint, Right G Ankle Joint, Left H Tarsal Joint, Right J Tarsal Joint, Left K Metatarsal-Tarsal Joint, Right L Metatarsal-Tarsal Joint, Left M Metatarsal-Phalangeal Joint, Right N Metatarsal-Phalangeal Joint, Left P Toe Phalangeal Joint, Right Q Toe Phalangeal Joint, Lef	0 Open 3 Percutaneous 4 Percutaneous Endoscopic X External	0 Drainage Device 3 Infusion Device 4 Internal Fixation Device 5 External Fixation Device 7 Autologous Tissue Substitute 8 Spacer J Synthetic Substitute K Nonautologous Tissue Substitute	Z No Qualifier

W: REVISION

S: LOWER JOINTS

0: M/S

◀ New ◀ Revised ~~deleted~~ Deleted ♀ Females Only ♂ Males Only
Noncovered Limited Coverage Hospital-Acquired Condition **Coding Clinic**

SECTION: 0 MEDICAL AND SURGICAL

BODY SYSTEM: T URINARY SYSTEM

OPERATION: 1 BYPASS: Altering the route of passage of the contents of a tubular body part

Body Part	Approach	Device	Qualifier
3 Kidney Pelvis, Right 4 Kidney Pelvis, Left	0 Open 4 Percutaneous Endoscopic	7 Autologous Tissue Substitute J Synthetic Substitute K Nonautologous Tissue Substitute Z No Device	3 Kidney Pelvis, Right 4 Kidney Pelvis, Left 6 Ureter, Right 7 Ureter, Left 8 Colon 9 Colocutaneous A Ileum B Bladder C Ileocutaneous D Cutaneous
3 Kidney Pelvis, Right 4 Kidney Pelvis, Left	3 Percutaneous	J Synthetic Substitute	D Cutaneous
6 Ureter, Right 7 Ureter, Left 8 Ureters, Bilateral	0 Open 4 Percutaneous Endoscopic	7 Autologous Tissue Substitute J Synthetic Substitute K Nonautologous Tissue Substitute Z No Device	6 Ureter, Right 7 Ureter, Left 8 Colon 9 Colocutaneous A Ileum B Bladder C Ileocutaneous D Cutaneous
6 Ureter, Right 7 Ureter, Left 8 Ureters, Bilateral	3 Percutaneous	J Synthetic Substitute	D Cutaneous
B Bladder	0 Open 4 Percutaneous Endoscopic	7 Autologous Tissue Substitute J Synthetic Substitute K Nonautologous Tissue Substitute Z No Device	9 Colocutaneous C Ileocutaneous D Cutaneous
B Bladder	3 Percutaneous	J Synthetic Substitute	D Cutaneous

SECTION: 0 MEDICAL AND SURGICAL

BODY SYSTEM: T URINARY SYSTEM

OPERATION: 2 CHANGE: Taking out or off a device from a body part and putting back an identical or similar device in or on the same body part without cutting or puncturing the skin or a mucous membrane

Body Part	Approach	Device	Qualifier
5 Kidney 9 Ureter B Bladder D Urethra	X External	0 Drainage Device Y Other Device	Z No Qualifier

1: BYPASS 2: CHANGE

T: URINARY SYSTEM

0: M/S

SECTION: 0 MEDICAL AND SURGICAL
BODY SYSTEM: T URINARY SYSTEM
OPERATION: 5 DESTRUCTION: Physical eradication of all or a portion of a body part by the direct use of energy, force, or a destructive agent

Body Part	Approach	Device	Qualifier
0 Kidney, Right 1 Kidney, Left 3 Kidney Pelvis, Right 4 Kidney Pelvis, Left 6 Ureter, Right 7 Ureter, Left B Bladder C Bladder Neck	0 Open 3 Percutaneous 4 Percutaneous Endoscopic 7 Via Natural or Artificial Opening 8 Via Natural or Artificial Opening Endoscopic	Z No Device	Z No Qualifier
D Urethra	0 Open 3 Percutaneous 4 Percutaneous Endoscopic 7 Via Natural or Artificial Opening 8 Via Natural or Artificial Opening Endoscopic X External	Z No Device	Z No Qualifier

SECTION: 0 MEDICAL AND SURGICAL
BODY SYSTEM: T URINARY SYSTEM
OPERATION: 7 DILATION: Expanding an orifice or the lumen of a tubular body part

Body Part	Approach	Device	Qualifier
3 Kidney Pelvis, Right 4 Kidney Pelvis, Left 6 Ureter, Right 7 Ureter, Left 8 Ureters, Bilateral B Bladder C Bladder Neck D Urethra	0 Open 3 Percutaneous 4 Percutaneous Endoscopic 7 Via Natural or Artificial Opening 8 Via Natural or Artificial Opening Endoscopic	D Intraluminal Device Z No Device	Z No Qualifier

SECTION: 0 MEDICAL AND SURGICAL
BODY SYSTEM: T URINARY SYSTEM
OPERATION: 8 DIVISION: Cutting into a body part, without draining fluids and/or gases from the body part, in order to separate or transect a body part

Body Part	Approach	Device	Qualifier
2 Kidneys, Bilateral C Bladder Neck	0 Open 3 Percutaneous 4 Percutaneous Endoscopic	Z No Device	Z No Qualifier

◀ New　◀ Revised　deleted Deleted　♀ Females Only　♂ Males Only
Ⓝⓒ Noncovered　Ⓛⓒ Limited Coverage　ⒽⓐⒸ Hospital-Acquired Condition　**Coding Clinic**

417

C: M/S

T: URINARY SYSTEM

5: DESTRUCTION 7: DILATION 8: DIVISION

SECTION: 0 MEDICAL AND SURGICAL
BODY SYSTEM: T URINARY SYSTEM
OPERATION: 9 DRAINAGE: Taking or letting out fluids and/or gases from a body part

Body Part	Approach	Device	Qualifier
0 Kidney, Right 1 Kidney, Left 3 Kidney Pelvis, Right 4 Kidney Pelvis, Left 6 Ureter, Right 7 Ureter, Left 8 Ureters, Bilateral B Bladder C Bladder Neck	0 Open 3 Percutaneous 4 Percutaneous Endoscopic 7 Via Natural or Artificial Opening 8 Via Natural or Artificial Opening Endoscopic	0 Drainage Device	Z No Qualifier
0 Kidney, Right 1 Kidney, Left 3 Kidney Pelvis, Right 4 Kidney Pelvis, Left 6 Ureter, Right 7 Ureter, Left 8 Ureters, Bilateral B Bladder C Bladder Neck	0 Open 3 Percutaneous 4 Percutaneous Endoscopic 7 Via Natural or Artificial Opening 8 Via Natural or Artificial Opening Endoscopic	Z No Device	X Diagnostic Z No Qualifier
D Urethra	0 Open 3 Percutaneous 4 Percutaneous Endoscopic 7 Via Natural or Artificial Opening 8 Via Natural or Artificial Opening Endoscopic X External	0 Drainage Device	Z No Qualifier
D Urethra	0 Open 3 Percutaneous 4 Percutaneous Endoscopic 7 Via Natural or Artificial Opening 8 Via Natural or Artificial Opening Endoscopic X External	Z No Device	X Diagnostic Z No Qualifier

SECTION: 0 MEDICAL AND SURGICAL
BODY SYSTEM: T URINARY SYSTEM
OPERATION: B EXCISION: Cutting out or off, without replacement, a portion of a body part

Body Part	Approach	Device	Qualifier
0 Kidney, Right 1 Kidney, Left 3 Kidney Pelvis, Right 4 Kidney Pelvis, Left 6 Ureter, Right 7 Ureter, Left B Bladder C Bladder Neck	0 Open 3 Percutaneous 4 Percutaneous Endoscopic 7 Via Natural or Artificial Opening 8 Via Natural or Artificial Opening Endoscopic	Z No Device	X Diagnostic Z No Qualifier
D Urethra	0 Open 3 Percutaneous 4 Percutaneous Endoscopic 7 Via Natural or Artificial Opening 8 Via Natural or Artificial Opening Endoscopic X External	Z No Device	X Diagnostic Z No Qualifier

Side margin: 9: DRAINAGE   B: EXCISION   T: URINARY SYSTEM   0: M/S

◀ New   ◀ Revised   ~~deleted~~ Deleted   ♀ Females Only   ♂ Males Only
Ⓝⓒ Noncovered   Ⓛⓒ Limited Coverage   Ⓗⓐⓒ Hospital-Acquired Condition   **Coding Clinic**

SECTION: 0 MEDICAL AND SURGICAL
BODY SYSTEM: T URINARY SYSTEM
OPERATION: C EXTIRPATION: Taking or cutting out solid matter from a body part

Body Part	Approach	Device	Qualifier
0 Kidney, Right 1 Kidney, Left 3 Kidney Pelvis, Right 4 Kidney Pelvis, Left 6 Ureter, Right 7 Ureter, Left B Bladder C Bladder Neck	0 Open 3 Percutaneous 4 Percutaneous Endoscopic 7 Via Natural or Artificial Opening 8 Via Natural or Artificial Opening Endoscopic	Z No Device	Z No Qualifier
D Urethra	0 Open 3 Percutaneous 4 Percutaneous Endoscopic 7 Via Natural or Artificial Opening 8 Via Natural or Artificial Opening Endoscopic X External	Z No Device	Z No Qualifier

SECTION: 0 MEDICAL AND SURGICAL
BODY SYSTEM: T URINARY SYSTEM
OPERATION: D EXTRACTION: Pulling or stripping out or off all or a portion of a body part by the use of force

Body Part	Approach	Device	Qualifier
0 Kidney, Right 1 Kidney, Left	0 Open 3 Percutaneous 4 Percutaneous Endoscopic	Z No Device	Z No Qualifier

SECTION: 0 MEDICAL AND SURGICAL
BODY SYSTEM: T URINARY SYSTEM
OPERATION: F FRAGMENTATION: Breaking solid matter in a body part into pieces

Body Part	Approach	Device	Qualifier
3 Kidney Pelvis, Right 4 Kidney Pelvis, Left 6 Ureter, Right 7 Ureter, Left B Bladder C Bladder Neck D Urethra ⍦	0 Open 3 Percutaneous 4 Percutaneous Endoscopic 7 Via Natural or Artificial Opening 8 Via Natural or Artificial Opening Endoscopic X External	Z No Device	Z No Qualifier

⍦ 0TFDXZZ

◀ New ◀ Revised deleted Deleted ♀ Females Only ♂ Males Only
⍦ Noncovered ⍦ Limited Coverage ⍦ Hospital-Acquired Condition **Coding Clinic**

419

0: M/S T: URINARY SYSTEM C: EXTIRPATION D: EXTRACTION F: FRAGMENTATION

SECTION: 0 MEDICAL AND SURGICAL
BODY SYSTEM: T URINARY SYSTEM
OPERATION: H INSERTION: Putting in a nonbiological appliance that monitors, assists, performs, or prevents a physiological function but does not physically take the place of a body part

Body Part	Approach	Device	Qualifier
5 Kidney	0 Open 3 Percutaneous 4 Percutaneous Endoscopic 7 Via Natural or Artificial Opening 8 Via Natural or Artificial Opening Endoscopic	2 Monitoring Device 3 Infusion Device	Z No Qualifier
9 Ureter	0 Open 3 Percutaneous 4 Percutaneous Endoscopic 7 Via Natural or Artificial Opening 8 Via Natural or Artificial Opening Endoscopic	2 Monitoring Device 3 Infusion Device M Stimulator Lead	Z No Qualifier
B Bladder	0 Open 3 Percutaneous 4 Percutaneous Endoscopic 7 Via Natural or Artificial Opening 8 Via Natural or Artificial Opening Endoscopic	2 Monitoring Device 3 Infusion Device L Artificial Sphincter M Stimulator Lead ⊗	Z No Qualifier
C Bladder Neck	0 Open 3 Percutaneous 4 Percutaneous Endoscopic 7 Via Natural or Artificial Opening 8 Via Natural or Artificial Opening Endoscopic	L Artificial Sphincter	Z No Qualifier
D Urethra	0 Open 3 Percutaneous 4 Percutaneous Endoscopic 7 Via Natural or Artificial Opening 8 Via Natural or Artificial Opening Endoscopic X External	2 Monitoring Device 3 Infusion Device L Artificial Sphincter	Z No Qualifier

H: INSERTION

T: URINARY SYSTEM

0: M/S

◀ New   ◀ Revised   ~~deleted~~ Deleted   ♀ Females Only   ♂ Males Only
⊗ Noncovered   ⊗ Limited Coverage   ⊗ Hospital-Acquired Condition   **Coding Clinic**

SECTION: 0 MEDICAL AND SURGICAL
BODY SYSTEM: T URINARY SYSTEM
OPERATION: J INSPECTION: Visually and/or manually exploring a body part

Body Part	Approach	Device	Qualifier

5 Kidney
9 Ureter
B Bladder
D Urethra
	0 Open
	3 Percutaneous
	4 Percutaneous Endoscopic
	7 Via Natural or Artificial
	   Opening
	8 Via Natural or Artificial
	   Opening Endoscopic
	X External
		Z No Device	Z No Qualifier

SECTION: 0 MEDICAL AND SURGICAL
BODY SYSTEM: T URINARY SYSTEM
OPERATION: L OCCLUSION: Completely closing an orifice or the lumen of a tubular body part

Body Part	Approach	Device	Qualifier
3 Kidney Pelvis, Right 4 Kidney Pelvis, Left 6 Ureter, Right 7 Ureter, Left B Bladder C Bladder Neck	0 Open 3 Percutaneous 4 Percutaneous Endoscopic	C Extraluminal Device D Intraluminal Device Z No Device	Z No Qualifier

3 Kidney Pelvis, Right
4 Kidney Pelvis, Left
6 Ureter, Right
7 Ureter, Left
B Bladder
C Bladder Neck
	7 Via Natural or Artificial
	   Opening
	8 Via Natural or Artificial
	   Opening Endoscopic
		D Intraluminal Device
		Z No Device
			Z No Qualifier

D Urethra	0 Open 3 Percutaneous 4 Percutaneous Endoscopic X External	C Extraluminal Device D Intraluminal Device Z No Device	Z No Qualifier

D Urethra	7 Via Natural or Artificial
	   Opening
	8 Via Natural or Artificial
	   Opening Endoscopic
		D Intraluminal Device
		Z No Device
			Z No Qualifier

0: M/S   T: URINARY SYSTEM   J: INSPECTION   L: OCCLUSION

M: REATTACHMENT   N: RELEASE

T: URINARY SYSTEM

0: M/S

SECTION: 0 MEDICAL AND SURGICAL
BODY SYSTEM: T URINARY SYSTEM
OPERATION: M **REATTACHMENT:** Putting back in or on all or a portion of a separated body part to its normal location or other suitable location

Body Part	Approach	Device	Qualifier
0 Kidney, Right 1 Kidney, Left 2 Kidneys, Bilateral 3 Kidney Pelvis, Right 4 Kidney Pelvis, Left 6 Ureter, Right 7 Ureter, Left 8 Ureters, Bilateral B Bladder C Bladder Neck D Urethra	0 Open 4 Percutaneous Endoscopic	Z No Device	Z No Qualifier

SECTION: 0 MEDICAL AND SURGICAL
BODY SYSTEM: T URINARY SYSTEM
OPERATION: N **RELEASE:** Freeing a body part from an abnormal physical constraint by cutting or by the use of force

Body Part	Approach	Device	Qualifier
0 Kidney, Right 1 Kidney, Left 3 Kidney Pelvis, Right 4 Kidney Pelvis, Left 6 Ureter, Right 7 Ureter, Left B Bladder C Bladder Neck	0 Open 3 Percutaneous 4 Percutaneous Endoscopic 7 Via Natural or Artificial Opening 8 Via Natural or Artificial Opening Endoscopic	Z No Device	Z No Qualifier
D Urethra	0 Open 3 Percutaneous 4 Percutaneous Endoscopic 7 Via Natural or Artificial Opening 8 Via Natural or Artificial Opening Endoscopic X External	Z No Device	Z No Qualifier

◀ New   ◀ Revised   deleted Deleted   ♀ Females Only   ♂ Males Only
Ⓝ Noncovered   Ⓛ Limited Coverage   Ⓗ Hospital-Acquired Condition   **Coding Clinic**

SECTION: 0 MEDICAL AND SURGICAL
BODY SYSTEM: T URINARY SYSTEM
OPERATION: P REMOVAL: *(on multiple pages)*
Taking out or off a device from a body part

Body Part	Approach	Device	Qualifier
5 Kidney	0 Open 3 Percutaneous 4 Percutaneous Endoscopic 7 Via Natural or Artificial Opening 8 Via Natural or Artificial Opening Endoscopic	0 Drainage Device 2 Monitoring Device 3 Infusion Device 7 Autologous Tissue Substitute C Extraluminal Device D Intraluminal Device J Synthetic Substitute K Nonautologous Tissue Substitute	Z No Qualifier
5 Kidney	X External	0 Drainage Device 2 Monitoring Device 3 Infusion Device D Intraluminal Device	Z No Qualifier
9 Ureter	0 Open 3 Percutaneous 4 Percutaneous Endoscopic 7 Via Natural or Artificial Opening 8 Via Natural or Artificial Opening Endoscopic	0 Drainage Device 2 Monitoring Device 3 Infusion Device 7 Autologous Tissue Substitute C Extraluminal Device D Intraluminal Device J Synthetic Substitute K Nonautologous Tissue Substitute M Stimulator Lead	Z No Qualifier
9 Ureter	X External	0 Drainage Device 2 Monitoring Device 3 Infusion Device D Intraluminal Device M Stimulator Lead	Z No Qualifier
B Bladder	0 Open 3 Percutaneous 4 Percutaneous Endoscopic 7 Via Natural or Artificial Opening 8 Via Natural or Artificial Opening Endoscopic	0 Drainage Device 2 Monitoring Device 3 Infusion Device 7 Autologous Tissue Substitute C Extraluminal Device D Intraluminal Device J Synthetic Substitute K Nonautologous Tissue Substitute L Artificial Sphincter M Stimulator Lead	Z No Qualifier
B Bladder	X External	0 Drainage Device 2 Monitoring Device 3 Infusion Device D Intraluminal Device L Artificial Sphincter M Stimulator Lead	Z No Qualifier

SECTION: 0 MEDICAL AND SURGICAL
BODY SYSTEM: T URINARY SYSTEM
OPERATION: P REMOVAL: *(continued)*
Taking out or off a device from a body part

Body Part	Approach	Device	Qualifier
D Urethra	0 Open 3 Percutaneous 4 Percutaneous Endoscopic 7 Via Natural or Artificial Opening 8 Via Natural or Artificial Opening Endoscopic	0 Drainage Device 2 Monitoring Device 3 Infusion Device 7 Autologous Tissue Substitute C Extraluminal Device D Intraluminal Device J Synthetic Substitute K Nonautologous Tissue Substitute L Artificial Sphincter	Z No Qualifier
D Urethra	X External	0 Drainage Device 2 Monitoring Device 3 Infusion Device D Intraluminal Device L Artificial Sphincter	Z No Qualifier

SECTION: 0 MEDICAL AND SURGICAL
BODY SYSTEM: T URINARY SYSTEM
OPERATION: Q REPAIR: Restoring, to the extent possible, a body part to its normal anatomic structure and function

Body Part	Approach	Device	Qualifier
0 Kidney, Right 1 Kidney, Left 3 Kidney Pelvis, Right 4 Kidney Pelvis, Left 6 Ureter, Right 7 Ureter, Left B Bladder C Bladder Neck	0 Open 3 Percutaneous 4 Percutaneous Endoscopic 7 Via Natural or Artificial Opening 8 Via Natural or Artificial Opening Endoscopic	Z No Device	Z No Qualifier
D Urethra	0 Open 3 Percutaneous 4 Percutaneous Endoscopic 7 Via Natural or Artificial Opening 8 Via Natural or Artificial Opening Endoscopic X External	Z No Device	Z No Qualifier

◀ New ⬅ Revised ~~deleted~~ Deleted ♀ Females Only ♂ Males Only
Ⓝ Noncovered Ⓛ Limited Coverage Ⓗ Hospital-Acquired Condition **Coding Clinic**

P: REMOVAL Q: REPAIR
T: URINARY SYSTEM
0: M/S

SECTION: 0 MEDICAL AND SURGICAL
BODY SYSTEM: T URINARY SYSTEM
OPERATION: R REPLACEMENT: Putting in or on biological or synthetic material that physically takes the place and/or function of all or a portion of a body part

Body Part	Approach	Device	Qualifier
3 Kidney Pelvis, Right 4 Kidney Pelvis, Left 6 Ureter, Right 7 Ureter, Left B Bladder C Bladder Neck	0 Open 4 Percutaneous Endoscopic 7 Via Natural or Artificial Opening 8 Via Natural or Artificial Opening Endoscopic	7 Autologous Tissue Substitute J Synthetic Substitute K Nonautologous Tissue Substitute	Z No Qualifier
D Urethra	0 Open 4 Percutaneous Endoscopic 7 Via Natural or Artificial Opening 8 Via Natural or Artificial Opening Endoscopic X External	7 Autologous Tissue Substitute J Synthetic Substitute K Nonautologous Tissue Substitute	Z No Qualifier

SECTION: 0 MEDICAL AND SURGICAL
BODY SYSTEM: T URINARY SYSTEM
OPERATION: S REPOSITION: Moving to its normal location, or other suitable location, all or a portion of a body part

Body Part	Approach	Device	Qualifier
0 Kidney, Right 1 Kidney, Left 2 Kidneys, Bilateral 3 Kidney Pelvis, Right 4 Kidney Pelvis, Left 6 Ureter, Right 7 Ureter, Left 8 Ureters, Bilateral B Bladder C Bladder Neck D Urethra	0 Open 4 Percutaneous Endoscopic	Z No Device	Z No Qualifier

SECTION: 0 MEDICAL AND SURGICAL
BODY SYSTEM: T URINARY SYSTEM
OPERATION: T RESECTION: Cutting out or off, without replacement, all of a body part

Body Part	Approach	Device	Qualifier
0 Kidney, Right 1 Kidney, Left 2 Kidneys, Bilateral	0 Open 4 Percutaneous Endoscopic	Z No Device	Z No Qualifier
3 Kidney Pelvis, Right 4 Kidney Pelvis, Left 6 Ureter, Right 7 Ureter, Left B Bladder C Bladder Neck D Urethra	0 Open 4 Percutaneous Endoscopic 7 Via Natural or Artificial Opening 8 Via Natural or Artificial Opening Endoscopic	Z No Device	Z No Qualifier

◀ New ◀ Revised ~~deleted~~ Deleted ♀ Females Only ♂ Males Only
ⓃⒸ Noncovered ⓁⒸ Limited Coverage ⒽⒶⒸ Hospital-Acquired Condition **Coding Clinic**

425

0: M/S

T: URINARY SYSTEM

R: REPLACEMENT S: REPOSITION T: RESECTION

SECTION: 0 MEDICAL AND SURGICAL
BODY SYSTEM: T URINARY SYSTEM
OPERATION: U SUPPLEMENT: Putting in or on biological or synthetic material that physically reinforces and/or augments the function of a portion of a body part

Body Part	Approach	Device	Qualifier
3 Kidney Pelvis, Right 4 Kidney Pelvis, Left 6 Ureter, Right 7 Ureter, Left B Bladder C Bladder Neck	0 Open 4 Percutaneous Endoscopic 7 Via Natural or Artificial Opening 8 Via Natural or Artificial Opening Endoscopic	7 Autologous Tissue Substitute J Synthetic Substitute K Nonautologous Tissue Substitute	Z No Qualifier
D Urethra	0 Open 4 Percutaneous Endoscopic 7 Via Natural or Artificial Opening 8 Via Natural or Artificial Opening Endoscopic X External	7 Autologous Tissue Substitute J Synthetic Substitute K Nonautologous Tissue Substitute	Z No Qualifier

SECTION: 0 MEDICAL AND SURGICAL
BODY SYSTEM: T URINARY SYSTEM
OPERATION: V RESTRICTION: Partially closing an orifice or the lumen of a tubular body part

Body Part	Approach	Device	Qualifier
3 Kidney Pelvis, Right 4 Kidney Pelvis, Left 6 Ureter, Right 7 Ureter, Left B Bladder C Bladder Neck	0 Open 3 Percutaneous 4 Percutaneous Endoscopic	C Extraluminal Device D Intraluminal Device Z No Device	Z No Qualifier
3 Kidney Pelvis, Right 4 Kidney Pelvis, Left 6 Ureter, Right 7 Ureter, Left B Bladder C Bladder Neck	7 Via Natural or Artificial Opening 8 Via Natural or Artificial Opening Endoscopic	D Intraluminal Device Z No Device	Z No Qualifier
D Urethra	0 Open 3 Percutaneous 4 Percutaneous Endoscopic	C Extraluminal Device D Intraluminal Device Z No Device	Z No Qualifier
D Urethra	7 Via Natural or Artificial Opening 8 Via Natural or Artificial Opening Endoscopic	D Intraluminal Device Z No Device	Z No Qualifier
D Urethra	X External	Z No Device	Z No Qualifier

◀ New   ◀ Revised   ~~deleted~~ Deleted   ♀ Females Only   ♂ Males Only
⊘ Noncovered   ⊘ Limited Coverage   ⊘ Hospital-Acquired Condition   **Coding Clinic**

SECTION: 0 MEDICAL AND SURGICAL
BODY SYSTEM: T URINARY SYSTEM
OPERATION: W REVISION: Correcting, to the extent possible, a portion of a malfunctioning device or the position of a displaced device

Body Part	Approach	Device	Qualifier
5 Kidney	0 Open 3 Percutaneous 4 Percutaneous Endoscopic 7 Via Natural or Artificial Opening 8 Via Natural or Artificial Opening Endoscopic X External	0 Drainage Device 2 Monitoring Device 3 Infusion Device 7 Autologous Tissue Substitute C Extraluminal Device D Intraluminal Device J Synthetic Substitute K Nonautologous Tissue Substitute	Z No Qualifier
9 Ureter	0 Open 3 Percutaneous 4 Percutaneous Endoscopic 7 Via Natural or Artificial Opening 8 Via Natural or Artificial Opening Endoscopic X External	0 Drainage Device 2 Monitoring Device 3 Infusion Device 7 Autologous Tissue Substitute C Extraluminal Device D Intraluminal Device J Synthetic Substitute K Nonautologous Tissue Substitute M Stimulator Lead	Z No Qualifier
B Bladder	0 Open 3 Percutaneous 4 Percutaneous Endoscopic 7 Via Natural or Artificial Opening 8 Via Natural or Artificial Opening Endoscopic X External	0 Drainage Device 2 Monitoring Device 3 Infusion Device 7 Autologous Tissue Substitute C Extraluminal Device D Intraluminal Device J Synthetic Substitute K Nonautologous Tissue Substitute L Artificial Sphincter M Stimulator Lead	Z No Qualifier
D Urethra	0 Open 3 Percutaneous 4 Percutaneous Endoscopic 7 Via Natural or Artificial Opening 8 Via Natural or Artificial Opening Endoscopic X External	0 Drainage Device 2 Monitoring Device 3 Infusion Device 7 Autologous Tissue Substitute C Extraluminal Device D Intraluminal Device J Synthetic Substitute K Nonautologous Tissue Substitute L Artificial Sphincter	Z No Qualifier

SECTION: 0 MEDICAL AND SURGICAL
BODY SYSTEM: T URINARY SYSTEM
OPERATION: Y TRANSPLANTATION: Putting in or on all or a portion of a living body part taken from another individual or animal to physically take the place and/or function of all or a portion of a similar body part

Body Part	Approach	Device	Qualifier
0 Kidney, Right 🜲 1 Kidney, Left 🜲	0 Open	Z No Device	0 Allogeneic 1 Syngeneic 2 Zooplastic

(left margin) Y: TRANSPLANTATION   T: URINARY SYSTEM   0: M/S

SECTION: 0 MEDICAL AND SURGICAL
BODY SYSTEM: U FEMALE REPRODUCTIVE SYSTEM
OPERATION: 1 **BYPASS:** Altering the route of passage of the contents of a tubular body part

Body Part	Approach	Device	Qualifier
5 Fallopian Tube, Right ♀ 6 Fallopian Tube, Left ♀	0 Open 4 Percutaneous Endoscopic	7 Autologous Tissue Substitute J Synthetic Substitute K Nonautologous Tissue Substitute Z No Device	5 Fallopian Tube, Right 6 Fallopian Tube, Left 9 Uterus

SECTION: 0 MEDICAL AND SURGICAL
BODY SYSTEM: U FEMALE REPRODUCTIVE SYSTEM
OPERATION: 2 **CHANGE:** Taking out or off a device from a body part and putting back an identical or similar device in or on the same body part without cutting or puncturing the skin or a mucous membrane

Body Part	Approach	Device	Qualifier
3 Ovary ♀ 8 Fallopian Tube ♀ M Vulva ♀	X External	0 Drainage Device Y Other Device	Z No Qualifier
D Uterus and Cervix ♀	X External	0 Drainage Device H Contraceptive Device Y Other Device	Z No Qualifier
H Vagina and Cul-de-sac ♀	X External	0 Drainage Device G Intraluminal Device, Pessary Y Other Device	Z No Qualifier

◀ New   ◀▥ Revised   ~~deleted~~ Deleted   ♀ Females Only   ♂ Males Only
℞ₒ Noncovered   ℞ₒ Limited Coverage   ℞ₒ Hospital-Acquired Condition   **Coding Clinic**

SECTION: 0 MEDICAL AND SURGICAL
BODY SYSTEM: U FEMALE REPRODUCTIVE SYSTEM
OPERATION: 5 DESTRUCTION: Physical eradication of all or a portion of a body part by the direct use of energy, force, or a destructive agent

Body Part	Approach	Device	Qualifier
0 Ovary, Right ♀ 1 Ovary, Left ♀ 2 Ovaries, Bilateral ♀ 4 Uterine Supporting Structure ♀	0 Open 3 Percutaneous 4 Percutaneous Endoscopic	Z No Device	Z No Qualifier
5 Fallopian Tube, Right ♀ 6 Fallopian Tube, Left ♀ 7 Fallopian Tubes, Bilateral ♀ ⓠ 9 Uterus ♀ B Endometrium ♀ C Cervix ♀ F Cul-de-sac ♀	0 Open 3 Percutaneous 4 Percutaneous Endoscopic 7 Via Natural or Artificial Opening 8 Via Natural or Artificial Opening Endoscopic	Z No Device	Z No Qualifier
G Vagina ♀ K Hymen ♀	0 Open 3 Percutaneous 4 Percutaneous Endoscopic 7 Via Natural or Artificial Opening 8 Via Natural or Artificial Opening Endoscopic X External	Z No Device	Z No Qualifier
J Clitoris ♀ L Vestibular Gland ♀ M Vulva ♀	0 Open X External	Z No Device	Z No Qualifier

◀ New   ◀▥ Revised   deleted Deleted   ♀ Females Only   ♂ Males Only
ⓠ Noncovered   ⓠ Limited Coverage   ⓠ Hospital-Acquired Condition   **Coding Clinic**

SECTION: 0 MEDICAL AND SURGICAL
BODY SYSTEM: U FEMALE REPRODUCTIVE SYSTEM
OPERATION: 7 DILATION: Expanding an orifice or the lumen of a tubular body part

Body Part	Approach	Device	Qualifier
5 Fallopian Tube, Right ♀ 6 Fallopian Tube, Left ♀ 7 Fallopian Tubes, Bilateral ♀ 9 Uterus ♀ C Cervix ♀ G Vagina ♀	0 Open 3 Percutaneous 4 Percutaneous Endoscopic 7 Via Natural or Artificial Opening 8 Via Natural or Artificial Opening Endoscopic	D Intraluminal Device Z No Device	Z No Qualifier
K Hymen ♀	0 Open 3 Percutaneous 4 Percutaneous Endoscopic 7 Via Natural or Artificial Opening 8 Via Natural or Artificial Opening Endoscopic X External	D Intraluminal Device Z No Device	Z No Qualifier

SECTION: 0 MEDICAL AND SURGICAL
BODY SYSTEM: U FEMALE REPRODUCTIVE SYSTEM
OPERATION: 8 DIVISION: Cutting into a body part, without draining fluids and/or gases from the body part, in order to separate or transect a body part

Body Part	Approach	Device	Qualifier
0 Ovary, Right ♀ 1 Ovary, Left ♀ 2 Ovaries, Bilateral ♀ 4 Uterine Supporting Structure ♀	0 Open 3 Percutaneous 4 Percutaneous Endoscopic	Z No Device	Z No Qualifier
K Hymen ♀	7 Via Natural or Artificial Opening 8 Via Natural or Artificial Opening Endoscopic X External	Z No Device	Z No Qualifier

◄ New   ◄▪ Revised   deleted Deleted   ♀ Females Only   ♂ Males Only
Noncovered   Limited Coverage   Hospital-Acquired Condition   **Coding Clinic**

SECTION: 0 MEDICAL AND SURGICAL
BODY SYSTEM: U FEMALE REPRODUCTIVE SYSTEM
OPERATION: 9 DRAINAGE: *(on multiple pages)*
Taking or letting out fluids and/or gases from a body part

Body Part	Approach	Device	Qualifier
0 Ovary, Right ♀ 1 Ovary, Left ♀ 2 Ovaries, Bilateral ♀	0 Open 3 Percutaneous 4 Percutaneous Endoscopic	0 Drainage Device	Z No Qualifier
0 Ovary, Right ♀ 1 Ovary, Left ♀ 2 Ovaries, Bilateral ♀	0 Open 3 Percutaneous 4 Percutaneous Endoscopic	Z No Device	X Diagnostic Z No Qualifier
0 Ovary, Right ♀ 1 Ovary, Left ♀ 2 Ovaries, Bilateral ♀	X External	Z No Device	Z No Qualifier
4 Uterine Supporting Structure ♀	0 Open 3 Percutaneous 4 Percutaneous Endoscopic	0 Drainage Device	Z No Qualifier
4 Uterine Supporting Structure ♀	0 Open 3 Percutaneous 4 Percutaneous Endoscopic	Z No Device	X Diagnostic Z No Qualifier
5 Fallopian Tube, Right ♀ 6 Fallopian Tube, Left ♀ 7 Fallopian Tubes, Bilateral ♀ 9 Uterus ♀ C Cervix ♀ F Cul-de-sac ♀	0 Open 3 Percutaneous 4 Percutaneous Endoscopic 7 Via Natural or Artificial Opening 8 Via Natural or Artificial Opening Endoscopic	0 Drainage Device	Z No Qualifier
5 Fallopian Tube, Right ♀ 6 Fallopian Tube, Left ♀ 7 Fallopian Tubes, Bilateral ♀ 9 Uterus ♀ C Cervix ♀ F Cul-de-sac ♀	0 Open 3 Percutaneous 4 Percutaneous Endoscopic 7 Via Natural or Artificial Opening 8 Via Natural or Artificial Opening Endoscopic	Z No Device	X Diagnostic Z No Qualifier
G Vagina ♀ K Hymen ♀	0 Open 3 Percutaneous 4 Percutaneous Endoscopic 7 Via Natural or Artificial Opening 8 Via Natural or Artificial Opening Endoscopic X External	0 Drainage Device	Z No Qualifier
G Vagina ♀ K Hymen ♀	0 Open 3 Percutaneous 4 Percutaneous Endoscopic 7 Via Natural or Artificial Opening 8 Via Natural or Artificial Opening Endoscopic X External	Z No Device	X Diagnostic Z No Qualifier

◀ New   ◀ Revised   ~~deleted~~ Deleted   ♀ Females Only   ♂ Males Only
Noncovered   Limited Coverage   Hospital-Acquired Condition   **Coding Clinic**

433

SECTION: 0 MEDICAL AND SURGICAL

BODY SYSTEM: U FEMALE REPRODUCTIVE SYSTEM
OPERATION: 9 DRAINAGE: *(continued)*
Taking or letting out fluids and/or gases from a body part

Body Part	Approach	Device	Qualifier
J Clitoris ♀ L Vestibular Gland ♀ M Vulva ♀	0 Open X External	0 Drainage Device	Z No Qualifier
J Clitoris ♀ L Vestibular Gland ♀ M Vulva ♀	0 Open X External	Z No Device	X Diagnostic Z No Qualifier

SECTION: 0 MEDICAL AND SURGICAL

BODY SYSTEM: U FEMALE REPRODUCTIVE SYSTEM
OPERATION: B EXCISION: Cutting out or off, without replacement, a portion of a body part

Body Part	Approach	Device	Qualifier
0 Ovary, Right ♀ 1 Ovary, Left ♀ 2 Ovaries, Bilateral ♀ 4 Uterine Supporting Structure ♀ 5 Fallopian Tube, Right ♀ 6 Fallopian Tube, Left ♀ 7 Fallopian Tubes, Bilateral ♀ 9 Uterus ♀ C Cervix ♀ F Cul-de-sac ♀	0 Open 3 Percutaneous 4 Percutaneous Endoscopic 7 Via Natural or Artificial Opening 8 Via Natural or Artificial Opening Endoscopic	Z No Device	X Diagnostic Z No Qualifier
G Vagina ♀ K Hymen ♀	0 Open 3 Percutaneous 4 Percutaneous Endoscopic 7 Via Natural or Artificial Opening 8 Via Natural or Artificial Opening Endoscopic X External	Z No Device	X Diagnostic Z No Qualifier
J Clitoris ♀ L Vestibular Gland ♀ M Vulva ♀	0 Open X External	Z No Device	X Diagnostic Z No Qualifier

SECTION: 0 MEDICAL AND SURGICAL
BODY SYSTEM: U FEMALE REPRODUCTIVE SYSTEM
OPERATION: C **EXTIRPATION:** Taking or cutting out solid matter from a body part

Body Part	Approach	Device	Qualifier
0 Ovary, Right ♀ 1 Ovary, Left ♀ 2 Ovaries, Bilateral ♀ 4 Uterine Supporting Structure ♀	0 Open 3 Percutaneous 4 Percutaneous Endoscopic	Z No Device	Z No Qualifier
5 Fallopian Tube, Right ♀ 6 Fallopian Tube, Left ♀ 7 Fallopian Tubes, Bilateral ♀ 9 Uterus ♀ B Endometrium ♀ C Cervix ♀ F Cul-de-sac ♀	0 Open 3 Percutaneous 4 Percutaneous Endoscopic 7 Via Natural or Artificial Opening 8 Via Natural or Artificial Opening Endoscopic	Z No Device	Z No Qualifier
G Vagina ♀ K Hymen ♀	0 Open 3 Percutaneous 4 Percutaneous Endoscopic 7 Via Natural or Artificial Opening 8 Via Natural or Artificial Opening Endoscopic X External	Z No Device	Z No Qualifier
J Clitoris ♀ L Vestibular Gland ♀ M Vulva ♀	0 Open X External	Z No Device	Z No Qualifier

Coding Clinic: 2013, Q2, P38 – 0UC97ZZ

◀ New ◀▥ Revised ~~deleted~~ Deleted ♀ Females Only ♂ Males Only
Ⓝ Noncovered Ⓛ Limited Coverage Ⓗ Hospital-Acquired Condition **Coding Clinic**

435

SECTION: 0 MEDICAL AND SURGICAL

BODY SYSTEM: U FEMALE REPRODUCTIVE SYSTEM

OPERATION: D EXTRACTION: Pulling or stripping out or off all or a portion of a body part by the use of force

Body Part	Approach	Device	Qualifier
B Endometrium ♀	7 Via Natural or Artificial Opening 8 Via Natural or Artificial Opening Endoscopic	Z No Device	X Diagnostic Z No Qualifier
N Ova ♀	0 Open 3 Percutaneous 4 Percutaneous Endoscopic	Z No Device	Z No Qualifier

SECTION: 0 MEDICAL AND SURGICAL

BODY SYSTEM: U FEMALE REPRODUCTIVE SYSTEM

OPERATION: F FRAGMENTATION: Breaking solid matter in a body part into pieces

Body Part	Approach	Device	Qualifier
5 Fallopian Tube, Right ♀ 6 Fallopian Tube, Left ♀ 7 Fallopian Tubes, Bilateral ♀ 9 Uterus ♀	0 Open 3 Percutaneous 4 Percutaneous Endoscopic 7 Via Natural or Artificial Opening 8 Via Natural or Artificial Opening Endoscopic X External 🏥	Z No Device	Z No Qualifier

SECTION: 0 MEDICAL AND SURGICAL

BODY SYSTEM: U FEMALE REPRODUCTIVE SYSTEM

OPERATION: H INSERTION: Putting in a nonbiological appliance that monitors, assists, performs, or prevents a physiological function but does not physically take the place of a body part

Body Part	Approach	Device	Qualifier
3 Ovary ♀	0 Open 3 Percutaneous 4 Percutaneous Endoscopic	3 Infusion Device	Z No Qualifier
8 Fallopian Tube ♀ D Uterus and Cervix ♀ H Vagina and Cul-de-sac ♀	0 Open 3 Percutaneous 4 Percutaneous Endoscopic 7 Via Natural or Artificial Opening 8 Via Natural or Artificial Opening Endoscopic	3 Infusion Device	Z No Qualifier
9 Uterus ♀	7 Via Natural or Artificial Opening 8 Via Natural or Artificial Opening Endoscopic	H Contraceptive Device	Z No Qualifier
C Cervix ♀	0 Open 3 Percutaneous 4 Percutaneous Endoscopic	1 Radioactive Element	Z No Qualifier
C Cervix ♀	7 Via Natural or Artificial Opening 8 Via Natural or Artificial Opening Endoscopic	1 Radioactive Element H Contraceptive Device	Z No Qualifier
F Cul-de-sac ♀	7 Via Natural or Artificial Opening 8 Via Natural or Artificial Opening Endoscopic	G Intraluminal Device, Pessary	Z No Qualifier
G Vagina ♀	0 Open 3 Percutaneous 4 Percutaneous Endoscopic X External	1 Radioactive Element	Z No Qualifier
G Vagina ♀	7 Via Natural or Artificial Opening 8 Via Natural or Artificial Opening Endoscopic	1 Radioactive Element G Pessary	Z No Qualifier

Coding Clinic: 2013, Q2, P34 – 0UH97HZ

SECTION: 0 MEDICAL AND SURGICAL
BODY SYSTEM: U FEMALE REPRODUCTIVE SYSTEM
OPERATION: J INSPECTION: Visually and/or manually exploring a body part

Body Part	Approach	Device	Qualifier
3 Ovary ♀	0 Open 3 Percutaneous 4 Percutaneous Endoscopic X External	Z No Device	Z No Qualifier
8 Fallopian Tube ♀ D Uterus and Cervix ♀ H Vagina and Cul-de-sac ♀	0 Open 3 Percutaneous 4 Percutaneous Endoscopic 7 Via Natural or Artificial Opening 8 Via Natural or Artificial Opening Endoscopic X External	Z No Device	Z No Qualifier
M Vulva ♀	0 Open X External	Z No Device	Z No Qualifier

SECTION: 0 MEDICAL AND SURGICAL
BODY SYSTEM: U FEMALE REPRODUCTIVE SYSTEM
OPERATION: L OCCLUSION: Completely closing an orifice or the lumen of a tubular body part

Body Part	Approach	Device	Qualifier
5 Fallopian Tube, Right ♀ 6 Fallopian Tube, Left ♀ 7 Fallopian Tubes, Bilateral ♀	0 Open 3 Percutaneous 4 Percutaneous Endoscopic	C Extraluminal Device D Intraluminal Device Z No Device	Z No Qualifier
5 Fallopian Tube, Right ♀ 6 Fallopian Tube, Left ♀ 7 Fallopian Tubes, Bilateral ♀	7 Via Natural or Artificial Opening 8 Via Natural or Artificial Opening Endoscopic	D Intraluminal Device Z No Device	Z No Qualifier
F Cul-de-sac ♀ G Vagina ♀	7 Via Natural or Artificial Opening 8 Via Natural or Artificial Opening Endoscopic	D Intraluminal Device Z No Device	Z No Qualifier

◀ New ◀ Revised deleted Deleted ♀ Females Only ♂ Males Only
Noncovered Limited Coverage Hospital-Acquired Condition Coding Clinic

SECTION: 0 MEDICAL AND SURGICAL
BODY SYSTEM: U FEMALE REPRODUCTIVE SYSTEM
OPERATION: M REATTACHMENT: Putting back in or on all or a portion of a separated body part to its normal location or other suitable location

Body Part	Approach	Device	Qualifier
0 Ovary, Right ♀ 1 Ovary, Left ♀ 2 Ovaries, Bilateral ♀ 4 Uterine Supporting Structure ♀ 5 Fallopian Tube, Right ♀ 6 Fallopian Tube, Left ♀ 7 Fallopian Tubes, Bilateral ♀ 9 Uterus ♀ C Cervix ♀ F Cul-de-sac ♀ G Vagina ♀	0 Open 4 Percutaneous Endoscopic	Z No Device	Z No Qualifier
J Clitoris ♀ M Vulva ♀	X External	Z No Device	Z No Qualifier
K Hymen ♀	0 Open 4 Percutaneous Endoscopic X External	Z No Device	Z No Qualifier

SECTION: 0 MEDICAL AND SURGICAL
BODY SYSTEM: U FEMALE REPRODUCTIVE SYSTEM
OPERATION: N RELEASE: Freeing a body part from an abnormal physical constraint by cutting or by the use of force

Body Part	Approach	Device	Qualifier
0 Ovary, Right ♀ 1 Ovary, Left ♀ 2 Ovaries, Bilateral ♀ 4 Uterine Supporting Structure ♀	0 Open 3 Percutaneous 4 Percutaneous Endoscopic	Z No Device	Z No Qualifier
5 Fallopian Tube, Right ♀ 6 Fallopian Tube, Left ♀ 7 Fallopian Tubes, Bilateral ♀ 9 Uterus ♀ C Cervix ♀ F Cul-de-sac ♀	0 Open 3 Percutaneous 4 Percutaneous Endoscopic 7 Via Natural or Artificial Opening 8 Via Natural or Artificial Opening Endoscopic	Z No Device	Z No Qualifier
G Vagina ♀ K Hymen ♀	0 Open 3 Percutaneous 4 Percutaneous Endoscopic 7 Via Natural or Artificial Opening 8 Via Natural or Artificial Opening Endoscopic X External	Z No Device	Z No Qualifier
J Clitoris ♀ L Vestibular Gland ♀ M Vulva ♀	0 Open X External	Z No Device	Z No Qualifier

SECTION: 0 MEDICAL AND SURGICAL
BODY SYSTEM: U FEMALE REPRODUCTIVE SYSTEM
OPERATION: P REMOVAL: Taking out or off a device from a body part

Body Part	Approach	Device	Qualifier
3 Ovary ♀	0 Open 3 Percutaneous 4 Percutaneous Endoscopic X External	0 Drainage Device 3 Infusion Device	Z No Qualifier
8 Fallopian Tube ♀	0 Open 3 Percutaneous 4 Percutaneous Endoscopic 7 Via Natural or Artificial Opening 8 Via Natural or Artificial Opening Endoscopic	0 Drainage Device 3 Infusion Device 7 Autologous Tissue Substitute C Extraluminal Device D Intraluminal Device J Synthetic Substitute K Nonautologous Tissue Substitute	Z No Qualifier
8 Fallopian Tube ♀	X External	0 Drainage Device 3 Infusion Device D Intraluminal Device	Z No Qualifier
D Uterus and Cervix ♀	0 Open 3 Percutaneous 4 Percutaneous Endoscopic 7 Via Natural or Artificial Opening 8 Via Natural or Artificial Opening Endoscopic	0 Drainage Device 1 Radioactive Element 3 Infusion Device 7 Autologous Tissue Substitute C Extraluminal Device D Intraluminal Device H Contraceptive Device J Synthetic Substitute K Nonautologous Tissue Substitute	Z No Qualifier
D Uterus and Cervix ♀	X External	0 Drainage Device 3 Infusion Device D Intraluminal Device H Contraceptive Device	Z No Qualifier
H Vagina and Cul-de-sac ♀	0 Open 3 Percutaneous 4 Percutaneous Endoscopic 7 Via Natural or Artificial Opening 8 Via Natural or Artificial Opening Endoscopic	0 Drainage Device 1 Radioactive Element 3 Infusion Device 7 Autologous Tissue Substitute D Intraluminal Device J Synthetic Substitute K Nonautologous Tissue Substitute	Z No Qualifier
H Vagina and Cul-de-sac ♀	X External	0 Drainage Device 1 Radioactive Element 3 Infusion Device D Intraluminal Device	Z No Qualifier
M Vulva ♀	0 Open	0 Drainage Device 7 Autologous Tissue Substitute J Synthetic Substitute K Nonautologous Tissue Substitute	Z No Qualifier
M Vulva ♀	X External	0 Drainage Device	Z No Qualifier

SECTION: 0 MEDICAL AND SURGICAL

BODY SYSTEM: U FEMALE REPRODUCTIVE SYSTEM

OPERATION: Q REPAIR: Restoring, to the extent possible, a body part to its normal anatomic structure and function

Body Part	Approach	Device	Qualifier
0 Ovary, Right ♀ 1 Ovary, Left ♀ 2 Ovaries, Bilateral ♀ 4 Uterine Supporting Structure ♀	0 Open 3 Percutaneous 4 Percutaneous Endoscopic	Z No Device	Z No Qualifier
5 Fallopian Tube, Right ♀ 6 Fallopian Tube, Left ♀ 7 Fallopian Tubes, Bilateral ♀ 9 Uterus ♀ C Cervix ♀ F Cul-de-sac ♀	0 Open 3 Percutaneous 4 Percutaneous Endoscopic 7 Via Natural or Artificial Opening 8 Via Natural or Artificial Opening Endoscopic	Z No Device	Z No Qualifier
G Vagina ♀ K Hymen ♀	0 Open 3 Percutaneous 4 Percutaneous Endoscopic 7 Via Natural or Artificial Opening 8 Via Natural or Artificial Opening Endoscopic X External	Z No Device	Z No Qualifier
J Clitoris ♀ L Vestibular Gland ♀ M Vulva ♀	0 Open X External	Z No Device	Z No Qualifier

SECTION: 0 MEDICAL AND SURGICAL

BODY SYSTEM: U FEMALE REPRODUCTIVE SYSTEM

OPERATION: S REPOSITION: Moving to its normal location, or other suitable location, all or a portion of a body part

Body Part	Approach	Device	Qualifier
0 Ovary, Right ♀ 1 Ovary, Left ♀ 2 Ovaries, Bilateral ♀ 4 Uterine Supporting Structure ♀ 5 Fallopian Tube, Right ♀ 6 Fallopian Tube, Left ♀ 7 Fallopian Tubes, Bilateral ♀ C Cervix ♀ F Cul-de-sac ♀	0 Open 4 Percutaneous Endoscopic	Z No Device	Z No Qualifier
9 Uterus ♀ G Vagina ♀	0 Open 4 Percutaneous Endoscopic X External	Z No Device	Z No Qualifier

SECTION: 0 MEDICAL AND SURGICAL
BODY SYSTEM: U FEMALE REPRODUCTIVE SYSTEM
OPERATION: T RESECTION: Cutting out or off, without replacement, all of a body part

Body Part	Approach	Device	Qualifier
0 Ovary, Right ♀ 1 Ovary, Left ♀ 2 Ovaries, Bilateral ♀ 5 Fallopian Tube, Right ♀ 6 Fallopian Tube, Left ♀ 7 Fallopian Tubes, Bilateral ♀ 9 Uterus ♀	0 Open 4 Percutaneous Endoscopic 7 Via Natural or Artificial Opening 8 Via Natural or Artificial Opening Endoscopic F Via Natural or Artificial Opening With Percutaneous Endoscopic Assistance	Z No Device	Z No Qualifier
4 Uterine Supporting Structure ♀ C Cervix ♀ F Cul-de-sac ♀ G Vagina ♀	0 Open 4 Percutaneous Endoscopic 7 Via Natural or Artificial Opening 8 Via Natural or Artificial Opening Endoscopic	Z No Device	Z No Qualifier
J Clitoris ♀ L Vestibular Gland ♀ M Vulva ♀	0 Open X External	Z No Device	Z No Qualifier
K Hymen ♀	0 Open 4 Percutaneous Endoscopic 7 Via Natural or Artificial Opening 8 Via Natural or Artificial Opening Endoscopic X External	Z No Device	Z No Qualifier

Coding Clinic: 2013, Q3, P28 – 0UT90ZZ, 0UTC0ZZ

Coding Clinic: 2013, Q1, P24 – 0UT00ZZ

SECTION: 0 MEDICAL AND SURGICAL
BODY SYSTEM: U FEMALE REPRODUCTIVE SYSTEM
OPERATION: U SUPPLEMENT: Putting in or on biological or synthetic material that physically reinforces and/or augments the function of a portion of a body part

Body Part	Approach	Device	Qualifier
4 Uterine Supporting Structure ♀	0 Open 4 Percutaneous Endoscopic	7 Autologous Tissue Substitute J Synthetic Substitute K Nonautologous Tissue Substitute	Z No Qualifier
5 Fallopian Tube Right ♀ 6 Fallopian Tube, Left ♀ 7 Fallopian Tubes, Bilateral ♀ F Cul-de-sac ♀	0 Open 4 Percutaneous Endoscopic 7 Via Natural or Artificial Opening 8 Via Natural or Artificial Opening Endoscopic	7 Autologous Tissue Substitute J Synthetic Substitute K Nonautologous Tissue Substitute	Z No Qualifier
G Vagina ♀ K Hymen ♀	0 Open 4 Percutaneous Endoscopic 7 Via Natural or Artificial Opening 8 Via Natural or Artificial Opening Endoscopic X External	7 Autologous Tissue Substitute J Synthetic Substitute K Nonautologous Tissue Substitute	Z No Qualifier
J Clitoris ♀ M Vulva ♀	0 Open X External	7 Autologous Tissue Substitute J Synthetic Substitute K Nonautologous Tissue Substitute	Z No Qualifier

◀ New   ◀▥ Revised   ~~deleted~~ Deleted   ♀ Females Only   ♂ Males Only
🄝c Noncovered   🄛c Limited Coverage   🄗c Hospital-Acquired Condition   **Coding Clinic**

SECTION: 0 MEDICAL AND SURGICAL
BODY SYSTEM: U FEMALE REPRODUCTIVE SYSTEM
OPERATION: V RESTRICTION: Partially closing an orifice or the lumen of a tubular body part

Body Part	Approach	Device	Qualifier
C Cervix ♀	0 Open 3 Percutaneous 4 Percutaneous Endoscopic	C Extraluminal Device D Intraluminal Device Z No Device	Z No Qualifier
C Cervix ♀	7 Via Natural or Artificial Opening 8 Via Natural or Artificial Opening Endoscopic	D Intraluminal Device Z No Device	Z No Qualifier

SECTION: 0 MEDICAL AND SURGICAL
BODY SYSTEM: U FEMALE REPRODUCTIVE SYSTEM
OPERATION: W REVISION: *(on multiple pages)*
Correcting, to the extent possible, a portion of a malfunctioning device or the position of a displaced device

Body Part	Approach	Device	Qualifier
3 Ovary ♀	0 Open 3 Percutaneous 4 Percutaneous Endoscopic X External	0 Drainage Device 3 Infusion Device	Z No Qualifier
8 Fallopian Tube ♀	0 Open 3 Percutaneous 4 Percutaneous Endoscopic 7 Via Natural or Artificial Opening 8 Via Natural or Artificial Opening Endoscopic X External	0 Drainage Device 3 Infusion Device 7 Autologous Tissue Substitute C Extraluminal Device D Intraluminal Device J Synthetic Substitute K Nonautologous Tissue Substitute	Z No Qualifier
D Uterus and Cervix ♀	0 Open 3 Percutaneous 4 Percutaneous Endoscopic 7 Via Natural or Artificial Opening 8 Via Natural or Artificial Opening Endoscopic	0 Drainage Device 1 Radioactive Element 3 Infusion Device 7 Autologous Tissue Substitute C Extraluminal Device D Intraluminal Device H Contraceptive Device J Synthetic Substitute K Nonautologous Tissue Substitute	Z No Qualifier
D Uterus and Cervix ♀	X External	0 Drainage Device 3 Infusion Device 7 Autologous Tissue Substitute C Extraluminal Device D Intraluminal Device H Contraceptive Device J Synthetic Substitute K Nonautologous Tissue Substitute	Z No Qualifier

SECTION: 0 MEDICAL AND SURGICAL
BODY SYSTEM: U FEMALE REPRODUCTIVE SYSTEM
OPERATION: W REVISION: *(continued)*
Correcting, to the extent possible, a portion of a malfunctioning device or the position of a displaced device

Body Part	Approach	Device	Qualifier
H Vagina and Cul-de-sac ♀	0 Open 3 Percutaneous 4 Percutaneous Endoscopic 7 Via Natural or Artificial Opening 8 Via Natural or Artificial Opening Endoscopic	0 Drainage Device 1 Radioactive Element 3 Infusion Device 7 Autologous Tissue Substitute D Intraluminal Device J Synthetic Substitute K Nonautologous Tissue Substitute	Z No Qualifier
H Vagina and Cul-de-sac ♀	X External	0 Drainage Device 3 Infusion Device 7 Autologous Tissue Substitute D Intraluminal Device J Synthetic Substitute K Nonautologous Tissue Substitute	Z No Qualifier
M Vulva ♀	0 Open X External	0 Drainage Device 7 Autologous Tissue Substitute J Synthetic Substitute K Nonautologous Tissue Substitute	Z No Qualifier

SECTION: 0 MEDICAL AND SURGICAL
BODY SYSTEM: U FEMALE REPRODUCTIVE SYSTEM
OPERATION: Y TRANSPLANTATION: Putting in or on all or a portion of a living body part taken from another individual or animal to physically take the place and/or function of all or a portion of a similar body part

Body Part	Approach	Device	Qualifier
0 Ovary, Right ♀ 1 Ovary, Left ♀	0 Open	Z No Device	0 Allogeneic 1 Syngeneic 2 Zooplastic

◀ New   ◀▥ Revised   ~~deleted~~ Deleted   ♀ Females Only   ♂ Males Only
🅝 Noncovered   🅛 Limited Coverage   🅗 Hospital-Acquired Condition   **Coding Clinic**

◀ New ◀▥ Revised ~~deleted~~ Deleted ♀ Females Only ♂ Males Only
🄽 Noncovered 🄻 Limited Coverage 🄷 Hospital-Acquired Condition **Coding Clinic**

445

SECTION: 0 MEDICAL AND SURGICAL
BODY SYSTEM: V MALE REPRODUCTIVE SYSTEM
OPERATION: 1 BYPASS: Altering the route of passage of the contents of a tubular body part

Body Part	Approach	Device	Qualifier
N Vas Deferens, Right ♂	0 Open	7 Autologous Tissue Substitute	J Epididymis, Right
P Vas Deferens, Left ♂	4 Percutaneous Endoscopic	J Synthetic Substitute	K Epididymis, Left
Q Vas Deferens, Bilateral ♂		K Nonautologous Tissue Substitute	N Vas Deferens, Right
		Z No Device	P Vas Deferens, Left

SECTION: 0 MEDICAL AND SURGICAL
BODY SYSTEM: V MALE REPRODUCTIVE SYSTEM
OPERATION: 2 CHANGE: Taking out or off a device from a body part and putting back an identical or similar device in or on the same body part without cutting or puncturing the skin or a mucous membrane

Body Part	Approach	Device	Qualifier
4 Prostate and Seminal Vesicles ♂	X External	0 Drainage Device	Z No Qualifier
8 Scrotum and Tunica Vaginalis ♂		Y Other Device	
D Testis ♂			
M Epididymis and Spermatic Cord ♂			
R Vas Deferens ♂			
S Penis ♂			

◀ New   ◀▥ Revised   ~~deleted~~ Deleted   ♀ Females Only   ♂ Males Only
🚳 Noncovered   🚳 Limited Coverage   🚳 Hospital-Acquired Condition   **Coding Clinic**

SECTION: 0 MEDICAL AND SURGICAL
BODY SYSTEM: V MALE REPRODUCTIVE SYSTEM
OPERATION: 5 **DESTRUCTION:** Physical eradication of all or a portion of a body part by the direct use of energy, force, or a destructive agent

Body Part	Approach	Device	Qualifier
0 Prostate ♂	0 Open 3 Percutaneous 4 Percutaneous Endoscopic 7 Via Natural or Artificial Opening 8 Via Natural or Artificial Opening Endoscopic	Z No Device	Z No Qualifier
1 Seminal Vesicle, Right ♂ 2 Seminal Vesicle, Left ♂ 3 Seminal Vesicles, Bilateral ♂ 6 Tunica Vaginalis, Right ♂ 7 Tunica Vaginalis, Left ♂ 9 Testis, Right ♂ B Testis, Left ♂ C Testes, Bilateral ♂ F Spermatic Cord, Right ♂ G Spermatic Cord, Left ♂ H Spermatic Cords, Bilateral ♂ J Epididymis, Right ♂ K Epididymis, Left ♂ L Epididymis, Bilateral ♂ N Vas Deferens, Right ♂ 🔾 P Vas Deferens, Left ♂ 🔾 Q Vas Deferens, Bilateral ♂ 🔾	0 Open 3 Percutaneous 4 Percutaneous Endoscopic	Z No Device	Z No Qualifier
5 Scrotum ♂ S Penis ♂ T Prepuce ♂	0 Open 3 Percutaneous 4 Percutaneous Endoscopic X External	Z No Device	Z No Qualifier

SECTION: 0 MEDICAL AND SURGICAL
BODY SYSTEM: V MALE REPRODUCTIVE SYSTEM
OPERATION: 7 **DILATION:** Expanding an orifice or the lumen of a tubular body part

Body Part	Approach	Device	Qualifier
N Vas Deferens, Right ♂ P Vas Deferens, Left ♂ Q Vas Deferens, Bilateral ♂	0 Open 3 Percutaneous 4 Percutaneous Endoscopic	D Intraluminal Device Z No Device	Z No Qualifier

SECTION: 0 MEDICAL AND SURGICAL
BODY SYSTEM: V MALE REPRODUCTIVE SYSTEM
OPERATION: 9 DRAINAGE: *(on multiple pages)*
Taking or letting out fluids and/or gases from a body part

Body Part	Approach	Device	Qualifier
0 Prostate ♂	0 Open 3 Percutaneous 4 Percutaneous Endoscopic 7 Via Natural or Artificial Opening 8 Via Natural or Artificial Opening Endoscopic	0 Drainage Device	Z No Qualifier
0 Prostate ♂	0 Open 3 Percutaneous 4 Percutaneous Endoscopic 7 Via Natural or Artificial Opening 8 Via Natural or Artificial Opening Endoscopic	Z No Device	X Diagnostic Z No Qualifier
1 Seminal Vesicle, Right ♂ 2 Seminal Vesicle, Left ♂ 3 Seminal Vesicles, Bilateral ♂ 6 Tunica Vaginalis, Right ♂ 7 Tunica Vaginalis, Left ♂ 9 Testis, Right ♂ B Testis, Left ♂ C Testes, Bilateral ♂ F Spermatic Cord, Right ♂ G Spermatic Cord, Left ♂ H Spermatic Cords, Bilateral ♂ J Epididymis, Right ♂ K Epididymis, Left ♂ L Epididymis, Bilateral ♂ N Vas Deferens, Right ♂ P Vas Deferens, Left ♂ Q Vas Deferens, Bilateral ♂	0 Open 3 Percutaneous 4 Percutaneous Endoscopic	0 Drainage Device	Z No Qualifier
1 Seminal Vesicle, Right ♂ 2 Seminal Vesicle, Left ♂ 3 Seminal Vesicles, Bilateral ♂ 6 Tunica Vaginalis, Right ♂ 7 Tunica Vaginalis, Left ♂ 9 Testis, Right ♂ B Testis, Left ♂ C Testes, Bilateral ♂ F Spermatic Cord, Right ♂ G Spermatic Cord, Left ♂ H Spermatic Cords, Bilateral ♂ J Epididymis, Right ♂ K Epididymis, Left ♂ L Epididymis, Bilateral ♂ N Vas Deferens, Right ♂ P Vas Deferens, Left ♂ Q Vas Deferens, Bilateral ♂	0 Open 3 Percutaneous 4 Percutaneous Endoscopic	Z No Device	X Diagnostic Z No Qualifier
5 Scrotum ♂ S Penis ♂ T Prepuce ♂	0 Open 3 Percutaneous 4 Percutaneous Endoscopic X External	0 Drainage Device	Z No Qualifier

◀ New   ◀ Revised   ~~deleted~~ Deleted   ♀ Females Only   ♂ Males Only
ⓃⒸ Noncovered   ⒧Ⓒ Limited Coverage   ⒽⒶⒸ Hospital-Acquired Condition   **Coding Clinic**

SECTION: 0 MEDICAL AND SURGICAL
BODY SYSTEM: V MALE REPRODUCTIVE SYSTEM
OPERATION: 9 DRAINAGE: *(continued)*
Taking or letting out fluids and/or gases from a body part

Body Part	Approach	Device	Qualifier
5 Scrotum ♂ S Penis ♂ T Prepuce ♂	0 Open 3 Percutaneous 4 Percutaneous Endoscopic X External	Z No Device	X Diagnostic Z No Qualifier

SECTION: 0 MEDICAL AND SURGICAL
BODY SYSTEM: V MALE REPRODUCTIVE SYSTEM
OPERATION: B EXCISION: Cutting out or off, without replacement, a portion of a body part

Body Part	Approach	Device	Qualifier
0 Prostate ♂	0 Open 3 Percutaneous 4 Percutaneous Endoscopic 7 Via Natural or Artificial Opening 8 Via Natural or Artificial Opening Endoscopic	Z No Device	X Diagnostic Z No Qualifier
1 Seminal Vesicle, Right ♂ 2 Seminal Vesicle, Left ♂ 3 Seminal Vesicles, Bilateral ♂ 6 Tunica Vaginalis, Right ♂ 7 Tunica Vaginalis, Left ♂ 9 Testis, Right ♂ B Testis, Left ♂ C Testes, Bilateral ♂ F Spermatic Cord, Right ♂ G Spermatic Cord, Left ♂ H Spermatic Cords, Bilateral ♂ J Epididymis, Right ♂ K Epididymis, Left ♂ L Epididymis, Bilateral ♂ N Vas Deferens, Right ♂ ⓝⓒ P Vas Deferens, Left ♂ ⓝⓒ Q Vas Deferens, Bilateral ♂ ⓝⓒ	0 Open 3 Percutaneous 4 Percutaneous Endoscopic	Z No Device	X Diagnostic Z No Qualifier
5 Scrotum ♂ S Penis ♂ T Prepuce ♂	0 Open 3 Percutaneous 4 Percutaneous Endoscopic X External	Z No Device	X Diagnostic Z No Qualifier

SECTION: 0 MEDICAL AND SURGICAL
BODY SYSTEM: V MALE REPRODUCTIVE SYSTEM
OPERATION: C EXTIRPATION: Taking or cutting out solid matter from a body part

Body Part	Approach	Device	Qualifier
0 Prostate ♂	0 Open 3 Percutaneous 4 Percutaneous Endoscopic 7 Via Natural or Artificial Opening 8 Via Natural or Artificial Opening Endoscopic	Z No Device	Z No Qualifier
1 Seminal Vesicle, Right ♂ 2 Seminal Vesicle, Left ♂ 3 Seminal Vesicles, Bilateral ♂ 6 Tunica Vaginalis, Right ♂ 7 Tunica Vaginalis, Left ♂ 9 Testis, Right ♂ B Testis, Left ♂ C Testes, Bilateral ♂ F Spermatic Cord, Right ♂ G Spermatic Cord, Left ♂ H Spermatic Cords, Bilateral ♂ J Epididymis, Right ♂ K Epididymis, Left ♂ L Epididymis, Bilateral ♂ N Vas Deferens, Right ♂ P Vas Deferens, Left ♂ Q Vas Deferens, Bilateral ♂	0 Open 3 Percutaneous 4 Percutaneous Endoscopic	Z No Device	Z No Qualifier
5 Scrotum ♂ S Penis ♂ T Prepuce ♂	0 Open 3 Percutaneous 4 Percutaneous Endoscopic X External	Z No Device	Z No Qualifier

SECTION: 0 MEDICAL AND SURGICAL
BODY SYSTEM: V MALE REPRODUCTIVE SYSTEM
OPERATION: H INSERTION: Putting in a nonbiological appliance that monitors, assists, performs, or prevents a physiological function but does not physically take the place of a body part

Body Part	Approach	Device	Qualifier
0 Prostate ♂	0 Open 3 Percutaneous 4 Percutaneous Endoscopic 7 Via Natural or Artificial Opening 8 Via Natural or Artificial Opening Endoscopic	1 Radioactive Element	Z No Qualifier
4 Prostate and Seminal Vesicles ♂ 8 Scrotum and Tunica Vaginalis ♂ D Testis ♂ M Epididymis and Spermatic Cord ♂ R Vas Deferens ♂	0 Open 3 Percutaneous 4 Percutaneous Endoscopic 7 Via Natural or Artificial Opening 8 Via Natural or Artificial Opening Endoscopic	3 Infusion Device	Z No Qualifier
S Penis ♂	0 Open 3 Percutaneous 4 Percutaneous Endoscopic X External	3 Infusion Device	Z No Qualifier

SECTION: 0 MEDICAL AND SURGICAL
BODY SYSTEM: V MALE REPRODUCTIVE SYSTEM
OPERATION: J INSPECTION: Visually and/or manually exploring a body part

Body Part	Approach	Device	Qualifier
4 Prostate and Seminal Vesicles ♂ 8 Scrotum and Tunica Vaginalis ♂ D Testis ♂ M Epididymis and Spermatic Cord ♂ R Vas Deferens ♂ S Penis ♂	0 Open 3 Percutaneous 4 Percutaneous Endoscopic X External	Z No Device	Z No Qualifier

◀ New   ◀▥ Revised   deleted Deleted   ♀ Females Only   ♂ Males Only
Ⓝ Noncovered   Ⓛ Limited Coverage   Ⓗ Hospital-Acquired Condition   **Coding Clinic**

451

SECTION: 0   MEDICAL AND SURGICAL
BODY SYSTEM: V   MALE REPRODUCTIVE SYSTEM
OPERATION: L   OCCLUSION: Completely closing an orifice or the lumen of a tubular body part

Body Part	Approach	Device	Qualifier
F Spermatic Cord, Right ♂ 🔵 G Spermatic Cord, Left ♂ 🔵 H Spermatic Cords, Bilateral ♂ 🔵 N Vas Deferens, Right ♂ 🔵 P Vas Deferens, Left ♂ 🔵 Q Vas Deferens, Bilateral ♂ 🔵	0 Open 3 Percutaneous 4 Percutaneous Endoscopic	C Extraluminal Device D Intraluminal Device Z No Device	Z No Qualifier

🔵 0VLN0CZ, 0VLN0ZZ   🔵 0VLP0CZ, 0VLP0ZZ   🔵 0VLQ0CZ, 0VLQ0ZZ
🔵 0VLN3CZ, 0VLN3ZZ   🔵 0VLP3CZ, 0VLP3ZZ   🔵 0VLQ3CZ, 0VLQ3ZZ
🔵 0VLN4CZ, 0VLN4ZZ   🔵 0VLP4CZ, 0VLP4ZZ   🔵 0VLQ4CZ, 0VLQ4ZZ

SECTION: 0   MEDICAL AND SURGICAL
BODY SYSTEM: V   MALE REPRODUCTIVE SYSTEM
OPERATION: M   REATTACHMENT: Putting back in or on all or a portion of a separated body part to its normal location or other suitable location

Body Part	Approach	Device	Qualifier
5 Scrotum ♂ S Penis ♂	X External	Z No Device	Z No Qualifier
6 Tunica Vaginalis, Right ♂ 7 Tunica Vaginalis, Left ♂ 9 Testis, Right ♂ B Testis, Left ♂ C Testes, Bilateral ♂ F Spermatic Cord, Right ♂ G Spermatic Cord, Left ♂ H Spermatic Cords, Bilateral ♂	0 Open 4 Percutaneous Endoscopic	Z No Device	Z No Qualifier

L: OCCLUSION   M: REATTACHMENT

V: MALE REPRODUCTIVE SYSTEM

0: M/S

◀ New   ◀ Revised   ~~deleted~~ Deleted   ♀ Females Only   ♂ Males Only
🔵 Noncovered   🔵 Limited Coverage   🔵 Hospital-Acquired Condition   **Coding Clinic**

SECTION: 0 MEDICAL AND SURGICAL
BODY SYSTEM: V MALE REPRODUCTIVE SYSTEM
OPERATION: N RELEASE: Freeing a body part from an abnormal physical restraint by cutting or by the use of force

Body Part	Approach	Device	Qualifier
0 Prostate ♂	0 Open 3 Percutaneous 4 Percutaneous Endoscopic 7 Via Natural or Artificial Opening 8 Via Natural or Artificial Opening Endoscopic	Z No Device	Z No Qualifier
1 Seminal Vesicle, Right ♂ 2 Seminal Vesicle, Left ♂ 3 Seminal Vesicles, Bilateral ♂ 6 Tunica Vaginalis, Right ♂ 7 Tunica Vaginalis, Left ♂ 9 Testis, Right ♂ B Testis, Left ♂ C Testes, Bilateral ♂ F Spermatic Cord, Right ♂ G Spermatic Cord, Left ♂ H Spermatic Cords, Bilateral ♂ J Epididymis, Right ♂ K Epididymis, Left ♂ L Epididymis, Bilateral ♂ N Vas Deferens, Right ♂ P Vas Deferens, Left ♂ Q Vas Deferens, Bilateral ♂	0 Open 3 Percutaneous 4 Percutaneous Endoscopic	Z No Device	Z No Qualifier
5 Scrotum ♂ S Penis ♂ T Prepuce ♂	0 Open 3 Percutaneous 4 Percutaneous Endoscopic X External	Z No Device	Z No Qualifier

◀ New ◀ Revised deleted Deleted ♀ Females Only ♂ Males Only
Noncovered Limited Coverage Hospital-Acquired Condition **Coding Clinic**

453

SECTION: 0 MEDICAL AND SURGICAL
BODY SYSTEM: V MALE REPRODUCTIVE SYSTEM
OPERATION: P REMOVAL: Taking out or off a device from a body part

Body Part	Approach	Device	Qualifier
4 Prostate and Seminal Vesicles ♂	0 Open 3 Percutaneous 4 Percutaneous Endoscopic 7 Via Natural or Artificial Opening 8 Via Natural or Artificial Opening Endoscopic	0 Drainage Device 1 Radioactive Element 3 Infusion Device 7 Autologous Tissue Substitute J Synthetic Substitute K Nonautologous Tissue Substitute	Z No Qualifier
4 Prostate and Seminal Vesicles ♂	X External	0 Drainage Device 1 Radioactive Element 3 Infusion Device	Z No Qualifier
8 Scrotum and Tunica Vaginalis ♂ D Testis ♂ S Penis ♂	0 Open 3 Percutaneous 4 Percutaneous Endoscopic 7 Via Natural or Artificial Opening 8 Via Natural or Artificial Opening Endoscopic	0 Drainage Device 3 Infusion Device 7 Autologous Tissue Substitute J Synthetic Substitute K Nonautologous Tissue Substitute	Z No Qualifier
8 Scrotum and Tunica Vaginalis ♂ D Testis ♂ S Penis ♂	X External	0 Drainage Device 3 Infusion Device	Z No Qualifier
M Epididymis and Spermatic Cord ♂	0 Open 3 Percutaneous 4 Percutaneous Endoscopic 7 Via Natural or Artificial Opening 8 Via Natural or Artificial Opening Endoscopic	0 Drainage Device 3 Infusion Device 7 Autologous Tissue Substitute C Extraluminal Device J Synthetic Substitute K Nonautologous Tissue Substitute	Z No Qualifier
M Epididymis and Spermatic Cord ♂	X External	0 Drainage Device 3 Infusion Device	Z No Qualifier
R Vas Deferens ♂	0 Open 3 Percutaneous 4 Percutaneous Endoscopic 7 Via Natural or Artificial Opening 8 Via Natural or Artificial Opening Endoscopic	0 Drainage Device 3 Infusion Device 7 Autologous Tissue Substitute C Extraluminal Device D Intraluminal Device J Synthetic Substitute K Nonautologous Tissue Substitute	Z No Qualifier
R Vas Deferens ♂	X External	0 Drainage Device 3 Infusion Device D Intraluminal Device	Z No Qualifier

◄ New   ◄ Revised   ~~deleted~~ Deleted   ♀ Females Only   ♂ Males Only
Noncovered   Limited Coverage   Hospital-Acquired Condition   **Coding Clinic**

SECTION: 0 MEDICAL AND SURGICAL
BODY SYSTEM: V MALE REPRODUCTIVE SYSTEM
OPERATION: Q REPAIR: Restoring, to the extent possible, a body part to its normal anatomic structure and function

Body Part	Approach	Device	Qualifier
0 Prostate ♂	0 Open 3 Percutaneous 4 Percutaneous Endoscopic 7 Via Natural or Artificial Opening 8 Via Natural or Artificial Opening Endoscopic	Z No Device	Z No Qualifier
1 Seminal Vesicle, Right ♂ 2 Seminal Vesicle, Left ♂ 3 Seminal Vesicles, Bilateral ♂ 6 Tunica Vaginalis, Right ♂ 7 Tunica Vaginalis, Left ♂ 9 Testis, Right ♂ B Testis, Left ♂ C Testes, Bilateral ♂ F Spermatic Cord, Right ♂ G Spermatic Cord, Left ♂ H Spermatic Cords, Bilateral ♂ J Epididymis, Right ♂ K Epididymis, Left ♂ L Epididymis, Bilateral ♂ N Vas Deferens, Right ♂ P Vas Deferens, Left ♂ Q Vas Deferens, Bilateral ♂	0 Open 3 Percutaneous 4 Percutaneous Endoscopic	Z No Device	Z No Qualifier
5 Scrotum ♂ S Penis ♂ T Prepuce ♂	0 Open 3 Percutaneous 4 Percutaneous Endoscopic X External	Z No Device	Z No Qualifier

SECTION: 0 MEDICAL AND SURGICAL
BODY SYSTEM: V MALE REPRODUCTIVE SYSTEM
OPERATION: R REPLACEMENT: Putting in or on biological or synthetic material that physically takes the place and/or function of all or a portion of a body part

Body Part	Approach	Device	Qualifier
9 Testis, Right ♂ B Testis, Left ♂ C Testis, Bilateral ♂	0 Open	J Synthetic Substitute	Z No Qualifier

◀ New   ◀ Revised   deleted Deleted   ♀ Females Only   ♂ Males Only
🚫 Noncovered   🚫 Limited Coverage   🚫 Hospital-Acquired Condition   **Coding Clinic**

SECTION: 0 MEDICAL AND SURGICAL
BODY SYSTEM: V MALE REPRODUCTIVE SYSTEM
OPERATION: S REPOSITION: Moving to its normal location or other suitable location all or a portion of a body part

Body Part	Approach	Device	Qualifier
9 Testis, Right ♂ B Testis, Left ♂ C Testes, Bilateral ♂ F Spermatic Cord, Right ♂ G Spermatic Cord, Left ♂ H Spermatic Cords, Bilateral ♂	0 Open 3 Percutaneous 4 Percutaneous Endoscopic	Z No Device	Z No Qualifier

SECTION: 0 MEDICAL AND SURGICAL
BODY SYSTEM: V MALE REPRODUCTIVE SYSTEM
OPERATION: T RESECTION: Cutting out or off, without replacement, all of a body part

Body Part	Approach	Device	Qualifier
0 Prostate ♂	0 Open 4 Percutaneous Endoscopic 7 Via Natural or Artificial Opening 8 Via Natural or Artificial Opening Endoscopic	Z No Device	Z No Qualifier
1 Seminal Vesicle, Right ♂ 2 Seminal Vesicle, Left ♂ 3 Seminal Vesicles, Bilateral ♂ 6 Tunica Vaginalis, Right ♂ 7 Tunica Vaginalis, Left ♂ 9 Testis, Right ♂ B Testis, Left ♂ C Testes, Bilateral ♂ F Spermatic Cord, Right ♂ G Spermatic Cord, Left ♂ H Spermatic Cords, Bilateral ♂ J Epididymis, Right ♂ K Epididymis, Left ♂ L Epididymis, Bilateral ♂ N Vas Deferens, Right ♂ ⊛ P Vas Deferens, Left ♂ ⊛ Q Vas Deferens, Bilateral ♂ ⊛	0 Open 4 Percutaneous Endoscopic	Z No Device	Z No Qualifier
5 Scrotum ♂ S Penis ♂ T Prepuce ♂	0 Open 4 Percutaneous Endoscopic X External	Z No Device	Z No Qualifier

◄ New   ◄▥ Revised   ~~deleted~~ Deleted   ♀ Females Only   ♂ Males Only
⊛ Noncovered   ⊛ Limited Coverage   ⊛ Hospital-Acquired Condition   **Coding Clinic**

SECTION: 0 MEDICAL AND SURGICAL
BODY SYSTEM: V MALE REPRODUCTIVE SYSTEM
OPERATION: U SUPPLEMENT: Putting in or on biological or synthetic material that physically reinforces and/or augments the function of a portion of a body part

Body Part	Approach	Device	Qualifier
1 Seminal Vesicle, Right ♂ 2 Seminal Vesicle, Left ♂ 3 Seminal Vesicles, Bilateral ♂ 6 Tunica Vaginalis, Right ♂ 7 Tunica Vaginalis, Left ♂ F Spermatic Cord, Right ♂ G Spermatic Cord, Left ♂ H Spermatic Cords, Bilateral ♂ J Epididymis, Right ♂ K Epididymis, Left ♂ L Epididymis, Bilateral ♂ N Vas Deferens, Right ♂ P Vas Deferens, Left ♂ Q Vas Deferens, Bilateral ♂	0 Open 4 Percutaneous Endoscopic	7 Autologous Tissue Substitute J Synthetic Substitute K Nonautologous Tissue Substitute	Z No Qualifier
5 Scrotum ♂ S Penis ♂ T Prepuce ♂	0 Open 4 Percutaneous Endoscopic X External	7 Autologous Tissue Substitute J Synthetic Substitute K Nonautologous Tissue Substitute	Z No Qualifier
9 Testis, Right ♂ B Testis, Left ♂ C Testis, Bilateral ♂	0 Open	7 Autologous Tissue Substitute J Synthetic Substitute K Nonautologous Tissue Substitute	Z No Qualifier

◀ New   ◀ Revised   ~~deleted~~ Deleted   ♀ Females Only   ♂ Males Only
🅝🅒 Noncovered   🅛🅒 Limited Coverage   🅗🅐🅒 Hospital-Acquired Condition   **Coding Clinic**

SECTION: 0 MEDICAL AND SURGICAL
BODY SYSTEM: V MALE REPRODUCTIVE SYSTEM
OPERATION: W REVISION: Correcting, to the extent possible, a portion of a malfunctioning device or the position of a displaced device

Body Part	Approach	Device	Qualifier
4 Prostate and Seminal Vesicles ♂ 8 Scrotum and Tunica Vaginalis ♂ D Testis ♂ S Penis ♂	0 Open 3 Percutaneous 4 Percutaneous Endoscopic 7 Via Natural or Artificial Opening 8 Via Natural or Artificial Opening Endoscopic X External	0 Drainage Device 3 Infusion Device 7 Autologous Tissue Substitute J Synthetic Substitute K Nonautologous Tissue Substitute	Z No Qualifier
M Epididymis and Spermatic Cord ♂	0 Open 3 Percutaneous 4 Percutaneous Endoscopic 7 Via Natural or Artificial Opening 8 Via Natural or Artificial Opening Endoscopic X External	0 Drainage Device 3 Infusion Device 7 Autologous Tissue Substitute C Extraluminal Device J Synthetic Substitute K Nonautologous Tissue Substitute	Z No Qualifier
R Vas Deferens ♂	0 Open 3 Percutaneous 4 Percutaneous Endoscopic 7 Via Natural or Artificial Opening 8 Via Natural or Artificial Opening Endoscopic X External	0 Drainage Device 3 Infusion Device 7 Autologous Tissue Substitute C Extraluminal Device D Intraluminal Device J Synthetic Substitute K Nonautologous Tissue Substitute	Z No Qualifier

W: REVISION

V: MALE REPRODUCTIVE SYSTEM

0: M/S

◀ New ◀ Revised deleted Deleted ♀ Females Only ♂ Males Only
Noncovered Limited Coverage Hospital-Acquired Condition **Coding Clinic**

SECTION: 0 MEDICAL AND SURGICAL
BODY SYSTEM: W ANATOMICAL REGIONS, GENERAL
OPERATION: 0 **ALTERATION:** Modifying the anatomic structure of a body part without affecting the function of the body part

Body Part	Approach	Device	Qualifier
0 Head 2 Face 4 Upper Jaw 5 Lower Jaw 6 Neck 8 Chest Wall F Abdominal Wall K Upper Back L Lower Back M Perineum, Male ♂ N Perineum, Female ♀	0 Open 3 Percutaneous 4 Percutaneous Endoscopic	7 Autologous Tissue Substitute J Synthetic Substitute K Nonautologous Tissue Substitute Z No Device	Z No Qualifier

SECTION: 0 MEDICAL AND SURGICAL
BODY SYSTEM: W ANATOMICAL REGIONS, GENERAL
OPERATION: 1 **BYPASS:** Altering the route of passage of the contents of a tubular body part

Body Part	Approach	Device	Qualifier
1 Cranial Cavity	0 Open	J Synthetic Substitute	9 Pleural Cavity, Right B Pleural Cavity, Left G Peritoneal Cavity J Pelvic Cavity
9 Pleural Cavity, Right B Pleural Cavity, Left G Peritoneal Cavity J Pelvic Cavity ♀	0 Open 4 Percutaneous Endoscopic	J Synthetic Substitute	4 Cutaneous 9 Pleural Cavity, Right B Pleural Cavity, Left G Peritoneal Cavity J Pelvic Cavity Y Lower Vein
9 Pleural Cavity, Right B Pleural Cavity, Left G Peritoneal Cavity J Pelvic Cavity	3 Percutaneous	J Synthetic Substitute	4 Cutaneous

SECTION: 0 MEDICAL AND SURGICAL
BODY SYSTEM: W ANATOMICAL REGIONS, GENERAL
OPERATION: 2 CHANGE: Taking out or off a device from a body part and putting back an identical or similar device in or on the same body part without cutting or puncturing the skin or a mucous membrane

Body Part	Approach	Device	Qualifier
0 Head	X External	0 Drainage Device	Z No Qualifier
1 Cranial Cavity		Y Other Device	
2 Face			
4 Upper Jaw			
5 Lower Jaw			
8 Chest Wall			
9 Pleural Cavity, Right			
B Pleural Cavity, Left			
C Mediastinum			
D Pericardial Cavity			
F Abdominal Wall			
G Peritoneal Cavity			
H Retroperitoneum			
J Pelvic Cavity			
K Upper Back			
L Lower Back			
M Perineum, Male			
N Perineum, Female			

SECTION: 0 MEDICAL AND SURGICAL
BODY SYSTEM: W ANATOMICAL REGIONS, GENERAL
OPERATION: 3 CONTROL: *(on multiple pages)*
Stopping, or attempting to stop, postprocedure bleeding

Body Part	Approach	Device	Qualifier
0 Head	0 Open	Z No Device	Z No Qualifier
1 Cranial Cavity	3 Percutaneous		
2 Face	4 Percutaneous Endoscopic		
3 Oral Cavity and Throat			
4 Upper Jaw			
5 Lower Jaw			
6 Neck			
8 Chest Wall			
9 Pleural Cavity, Right			
B Pleural Cavity, Left			
C Mediastinum			
D Pericardial Cavity			
F Abdominal Wall			
G Peritoneal Cavity			
H Retroperitoneum			
J Pelvic Cavity			
K Upper Back			
L Lower Back			
M Perineum, Male			
N Perineum, Female			

0: M/S   W: ANATOMICAL REGIONS, GENERAL   2: CHANGE   3: CONTROL

3: CONTROL   4: CREATION   8: DIVISION

W: ANATOMICAL REGIONS, GENERAL

0: M/S

SECTION: 0 MEDICAL AND SURGICAL
BODY SYSTEM: W ANATOMICAL REGIONS, GENERAL
OPERATION: 3 CONTROL: *(continued)*
Stopping, or attempting to stop, postprocedure bleeding

Body Part	Approach	Device	Qualifier
3 Oral Cavity and Throat	0 Open 3 Percutaneous 4 Percutaneous Endoscopic 7 Via Natural or Artificial Opening 8 Via Natural or Artificial Opening Endoscopic X External	Z No Device	Z No Qualifier
P Gastrointestinal Tract Q Respiratory Tract R Genitourinary Tract	0 Open 3 Percutaneous 4 Percutaneous Endoscopic 7 Via Natural or Artificial Opening 8 Via Natural or Artificial Opening Endoscopic	Z No Device	Z No Qualifier

SECTION: 0 MEDICAL AND SURGICAL
BODY SYSTEM: W ANATOMICAL REGIONS, GENERAL
OPERATION: 4 CREATION: Making a new structure that does not take over the function of a body part

Body Part	Approach	Device	Qualifier
M Perineum, Male ♂ ⦸	0 Open	7 Autologous Tissue Substitute J Synthetic Substitute K Nonautologous Tissue Substitute Z No Device	0 Vagina
N Perineum, Female ♀ ⦸	0 Open	7 Autologous Tissue Substitute J Synthetic Substitute K Nonautologous Tissue Substitute Z No Device	1 Penis

SECTION: 0 MEDICAL AND SURGICAL
BODY SYSTEM: W ANATOMICAL REGIONS, GENERAL
OPERATION: 8 DIVISION: Cutting into a body part, without draining fluids and/or gases from the body part, in order to separate or transect a body part

Body Part	Approach	Device	Qualifier
N Perineum, Female ♀	X External	Z No Device	Z No Qualifier

◀ New   ◀▥ Revised   ~~deleted~~ Deleted   ♀ Females Only   ♂ Males Only
⦸ Noncovered   ⦸ Limited Coverage   ⦸ Hospital-Acquired Condition   **Coding Clinic**

SECTION: 0 MEDICAL AND SURGICAL
BODY SYSTEM: W ANATOMICAL REGIONS, GENERAL
OPERATION: 9 DRAINAGE: Taking or letting out fluids and/or gases from a body part

Body Part	Approach	Device	Qualifier
0 Head 1 Cranial Cavity 2 Face 3 Oral Cavity and Throat 4 Upper Jaw 5 Lower Jaw 6 Neck 8 Chest Wall 9 Pleural Cavity, Right B Pleural Cavity, Left C Mediastinum D Pericardial Cavity F Abdominal Wall G Peritoneal Cavity H Retroperitoneum J Pelvic Cavity K Upper Back L Lower Back M Perineum, Male ♂ N Perineum, Female ♀	0 Open 3 Percutaneous 4 Percutaneous Endoscopic	0 Drainage Device	Z No Qualifier
0 Head 1 Cranial Cavity 2 Face 3 Oral Cavity and Throat 4 Upper Jaw 5 Lower Jaw 6 Neck 8 Chest Wall 9 Pleural Cavity, Right B Pleural Cavity, Left C Mediastinum D Pericardial Cavity F Abdominal Wall G Peritoneal Cavity H Retroperitoneum J Pelvic Cavity K Upper Back L Lower Back M Perineum, Male ♂ N Perineum, Female ♀	0 Open 3 Percutaneous 4 Percutaneous Endoscopic	Z No Device	X Diagnostic Z No Qualifier

SECTION: **0 MEDICAL AND SURGICAL**
BODY SYSTEM: **W ANATOMICAL REGIONS, GENERAL**
OPERATION: **B EXCISION:** Cutting out or off, without replacement, a portion of a body part

Body Part	Approach	Device	Qualifier
0 Head 2 Face 4 Upper Jaw 5 Lower Jaw 8 Chest Wall K Upper Back L Lower Back M Perineum, Male ♂ N Perineum, Female ♀	0 Open 3 Percutaneous 4 Percutaneous Endoscopic X External	Z No Device	X Diagnostic Z No Qualifier
6 Neck F Abdominal Wall	0 Open 3 Percutaneous 4 Percutaneous Endoscopic	Z No Device	X Diagnostic Z No Qualifier
6 Neck F Abdominal Wall	X External	Z No Device	2 Stoma X Diagnostic Z No Qualifier
C Mediastinum H Retroperitoneum	0 Open 3 Percutaneous 4 Percutaneous Endoscopic	Z No Device	X Diagnostic Z No Qualifier

SECTION: **0 MEDICAL AND SURGICAL**
BODY SYSTEM: **W ANATOMICAL REGIONS, GENERAL**
OPERATION: **C EXTIRPATION:** Taking or cutting out solid matter from a body part

Body Part	Approach	Device	Qualifier
1 Cranial Cavity 3 Oral Cavity and Throat 9 Pleural Cavity, Right B Pleural Cavity, Left C Mediastinum D Pericardial Cavity G Peritoneal Cavity J Pelvic Cavity	0 Open 3 Percutaneous 4 Percutaneous Endoscopic X External	Z No Device	Z No Qualifier
P Gastrointestinal Tract Q Respiratory Tract R Genitourinary Tract	0 Open 3 Percutaneous 4 Percutaneous Endoscopic 7 Via Natural or Artificial Opening 8 Via Natural or Artificial Opening Endoscopic X External	Z No Device	Z No Qualifier

◀ New ◀ Revised ~~deleted~~ Deleted ♀ Females Only ♂ Males Only
🅝 Noncovered 🅛 Limited Coverage 🅗 Hospital-Acquired Condition **Coding Clinic**

B: EXCISION   C: EXTIRPATION

W: ANATOMICAL REGIONS, GENERAL

0: M/S

SECTION:　0 MEDICAL AND SURGICAL
BODY SYSTEM: W ANATOMICAL REGIONS, GENERAL
OPERATION:　F FRAGMENTATION: Breaking solid matter in a body part into pieces

Body Part	Approach	Device	Qualifier
1 Cranial Cavity ⊘ 3 Oral Cavity and Throat ⊘ 9 Pleural Cavity, Right ⊘ B Pleural Cavity, Left ⊘ C Mediastinum ⊘ D Pericardial Cavity G Peritoneal Cavity ⊘ J Pelvic Cavity ⊘	0 Open 3 Percutaneous 4 Percutaneous Endoscopic X External	Z No Device	Z No Qualifier
P Gastrointestinal Tract ⊘ Q Respiratory Tract ⊘ R Genitourinary Tract	0 Open 3 Percutaneous 4 Percutaneous Endoscopic 7 Via Natural or Artificial 　Opening 8 Via Natural or Artificial 　Opening Endoscopic X External	Z No Device	Z No Qualifier

⊘ 0WF1XZZ, 0WF3XZZ, 0WF9XZZ, 0WFBXZZ, 0WFCXZZ, 0WFGXZZ, 0WFJXZZ, 0WFPXZZ, 0WFQXZZ

◀ New　◀▭ Revised　~~deleted~~ Deleted　♀ Females Only　♂ Males Only
⊘ Noncovered　⊘ Limited Coverage　⊘ Hospital-Acquired Condition　**Coding Clinic**

W: ANATOMICAL REGIONS, GENERAL   0: M/S   H: INSERTION   J: INSPECTION

SECTION: 0 MEDICAL AND SURGICAL
BODY SYSTEM: W ANATOMICAL REGIONS, GENERAL
OPERATION: H INSERTION: Putting in a nonbiological appliance that monitors, assists, performs, or prevents a physiological function but does not physically take the place of a body part

Body Part	Approach	Device	Qualifier
0 Head 1 Cranial Cavity 2 Face 3 Oral Cavity and Throat 4 Upper Jaw 5 Lower Jaw 6 Neck 8 Chest Wall 9 Pleural Cavity, Right B Pleural Cavity, Left C Mediastinum D Pericardial Cavity F Abdominal Wall G Peritoneal Cavity H Retroperitoneum J Pelvic Cavity K Upper Back L Lower Back M Perineum, Male ♂ N Perineum, Female ♀	0 Open 3 Percutaneous 4 Percutaneous Endoscopic	1 Radioactive Element 3 Infusion Device Y Other Device	Z No Qualifier
P Gastrointestinal Tract Q Respiratory Tract R Genitourinary Tract	0 Open 3 Percutaneous 4 Percutaneous Endoscopic 7 Via Natural or Artificial Opening 8 Via Natural or Artificial Opening Endoscopic	1 Radioactive Element 3 Infusion Device Y Other Device	Z No Qualifier

SECTION: 0 MEDICAL AND SURGICAL
BODY SYSTEM: W ANATOMICAL REGIONS, GENERAL
OPERATION: J INSPECTION: (on multiple pages)
Visually and/or manually exploring a body part

Body Part	Approach	Device	Qualifier
0 Head 2 Face 3 Oral Cavity and Throat 4 Upper Jaw 5 Lower Jaw 6 Neck 8 Chest Wall F Abdominal Wall K Upper Back L Lower Back M Perineum, Male ♂ N Perineum, Female ♀	0 Open 3 Percutaneous 4 Percutaneous Endoscopic X External	Z No Device	Z No Qualifier

◀ New   ◀◀ Revised   ~~deleted~~ Deleted   ♀ Females Only   ♂ Males Only
Ⓝ Noncovered   Ⓛ Limited Coverage   Ⓗ Hospital-Acquired Condition   **Coding Clinic**

SECTION: 0 MEDICAL AND SURGICAL
BODY SYSTEM: W ANATOMICAL REGIONS, GENERAL
OPERATION: J INSPECTION: *(continued)*
Visually and/or manually exploring a body part

Body Part	Approach	Device	Qualifier
0 Head 2 Face 3 Oral Cavity and Throat 4 Upper Jaw 5 Lower Jaw 6 Neck 8 Chest Wall F Abdominal Wall K Upper Back L Lower Back M Perineum, Male ♂ N Perineum, Female ♀	0 Open 3 Percutaneous 4 Percutaneous Endoscopic X External	Z No Device	Z No Qualifier
1 Cranial Cavity 9 Pleural Cavity, Right B Pleural Cavity, Left C Mediastinum D Pericardial Cavity G Peritoneal Cavity H Retroperitoneum J Pelvic Cavity	0 Open 3 Percutaneous 4 Percutaneous Endoscopic	Z No Device	Z No Qualifier
P Gastrointestinal Tract Q Respiratory Tract R Genitourinary Tract	0 Open 3 Percutaneous 4 Percutaneous Endoscopic 7 Via Natural or Artificial Opening 8 Via Natural or Artificial Opening Endoscopic	Z No Device	Z No Qualifier

Coding Clinic: 2013, Q2, P37 – 0WJG4ZZ

SECTION: 0 MEDICAL AND SURGICAL
BODY SYSTEM: W ANATOMICAL REGIONS, GENERAL
OPERATION: M REATTACHMENT: Putting back in or on all or a portion of a separated body part to its normal location or other suitable location

Body Part	Approach	Device	Qualifier
2 Face 4 Upper Jaw 5 Lower Jaw 6 Neck 8 Chest Wall F Abdominal Wall K Upper Back L Lower Back M Perineum, Male ♂ N Perineum, Female ♀	0 Open	Z No Device	Z No Qualifier

SECTION: 0 MEDICAL AND SURGICAL

BODY SYSTEM: W ANATOMICAL REGIONS, GENERAL
OPERATION: P REMOVAL: Taking out or off a device from a body part

P: REMOVAL

W: ANATOMICAL REGIONS, GENERAL

0: M/S

Body Part	Approach	Device	Qualifier
0 Head 2 Face 4 Upper Jaw 5 Lower Jaw 6 Neck 8 Chest Wall C Mediastinum F Abdominal Wall K Upper Back L Lower Back M Perineum, Male ♂ N Perineum, Female ♀	0 Open 3 Percutaneous 4 Percutaneous Endoscopic X External	0 Drainage Device 1 Radioactive Element 3 Infusion Device 7 Autologous Tissue Substitute J Synthetic Substitute K Nonautologous Tissue 　Substitute Y Other Device	Z No Qualifier
1 Cranial Cavity 9 Pleural Cavity, Right B Pleural Cavity, Left G Peritoneal Cavity J Pelvic Cavity	0 Open 3 Percutaneous 4 Percutaneous Endoscopic	0 Drainage Device 1 Radioactive Element 3 Infusion Device J Synthetic Substitute Y Other Device	Z No Qualifier
1 Cranial Cavity 9 Pleural Cavity, Right B Pleural Cavity, Left G Peritoneal Cavity J Pelvic Cavity	X External	0 Drainage Device 1 Radioactive Element 3 Infusion Device	Z No Qualifier
D Pericardial Cavity H Retroperitoneum	0 Open 3 Percutaneous 4 Percutaneous Endoscopic	0 Drainage Device 1 Radioactive Element 3 Infusion Device Y Other Device	Z No Qualifier
D Pericardial Cavity H Retroperitoneum	X External	0 Drainage Device 1 Radioactive Element 3 Infusion Device	Z No Qualifier
P Gastrointestinal Tract Q Respiratory Tract R Genitourinary Tract	0 Open 3 Percutaneous 4 Percutaneous Endoscopic 7 Via Natural or Artificial 　Opening 8 Via Natural or Artificial 　Opening Endoscopic X External	1 Radioactive Element 3 Infusion Device Y Other Device	Z No Qualifier

◀ New　◀ Revised　deleted Deleted　♀ Females Only　♂ Males Only
℞ Noncovered　℞ Limited Coverage　℞ Hospital-Acquired Condition　**Coding Clinic**

SECTION: 0 MEDICAL AND SURGICAL

BODY SYSTEM: W ANATOMICAL REGIONS, GENERAL

OPERATION: Q REPAIR: Restoring, to the extent possible, a body part to its normal anatomic structure and function

Body Part	Approach	Device	Qualifier
0 Head 2 Face 4 Upper Jaw 5 Lower Jaw 8 Chest Wall K Upper Back L Lower Back M Perineum, Male ♂ N Perineum, Female ♀	0 Open 3 Percutaneous 4 Percutaneous Endoscopic X External	Z No Device	Z No Qualifier
6 Neck F Abdominal Wall	0 Open 3 Percutaneous 4 Percutaneous Endoscopic	Z No Device	Z No Qualifier
6 Neck F Abdominal Wall	X External	Z No Device	2 Stoma Z No Qualifier
C Mediastinum	0 Open 3 Percutaneous 4 Percutaneous Endoscopic	Z No Device	Z No Qualifier

SECTION: 0 MEDICAL AND SURGICAL

BODY SYSTEM: W ANATOMICAL REGIONS, GENERAL

OPERATION: U SUPPLEMENT: Putting in or on biological or synthetic material that physically reinforces and/or augments the function of a portion of a body part

Body Part	Approach	Device	Qualifier
0 Head 2 Face 4 Upper Jaw 5 Lower Jaw 6 Neck 8 Chest Wall C Mediastinum F Abdominal Wall K Upper Back L Lower Back M Perineum, Male ♂ N Perineum, Female ♀	0 Open 4 Percutaneous Endoscopic	7 Autologous Tissue Substitute J Synthetic Substitute K Nonautologous Tissue Substitute	Z No Qualifier

Coding Clinic: 2012, Q4, P101 – 0WU80JZ

SECTION: 0 MEDICAL AND SURGICAL
BODY SYSTEM: W ANATOMICAL REGIONS, GENERAL
OPERATION: W REVISION: Correcting, to the extent possible, a portion of a malfunctioning device or the position of a displaced device

W: REVISION · W: ANATOMICAL REGIONS, GENERAL · 0: M/S

Body Part	Approach	Device	Qualifier
0 Head 2 Face 4 Upper Jaw 5 Lower Jaw 6 Neck 8 Chest Wall C Mediastinum F Abdominal Wall K Upper Back L Lower Back M Perineum, Male ♂ N Perineum, Female ♀	0 Open 3 Percutaneous 4 Percutaneous Endoscopic X External	0 Drainage Device 1 Radioactive Element 3 Infusion Device 7 Autologous Tissue Substitute J Synthetic Substitute K Nonautologous Tissue Substitute Y Other Device	Z No Qualifier
1 Cranial Cavity 9 Pleural Cavity, Right B Pleural Cavity, Left G Peritoneal Cavity J Pelvic Cavity	0 Open 3 Percutaneous 4 Percutaneous Endoscopic X External	0 Drainage Device 1 Radioactive Element 3 Infusion Device J Synthetic Substitute Y Other Device	Z No Qualifier
D Pericardial Cavity H Retroperitoneum	0 Open 3 Percutaneous 4 Percutaneous Endoscopic X External	0 Drainage Device 1 Radioactive Element 3 Infusion Device Y Other Device	Z No Qualifier
P Gastrointestinal Tract Q Respiratory Tract R Genitourinary Tract	0 Open 3 Percutaneous 4 Percutaneous Endoscopic 7 Via Natural or Artificial Opening 8 Via Natural or Artificial Opening Endoscopic X External	1 Radioactive Element 3 Infusion Device Y Other Device	Z No Qualifier

◄ New ◄ Revised deleted Deleted ♀ Females Only ♂ Males Only Noncovered Limited Coverage Hospital-Acquired Condition Coding Clinic

◀ New   ◀▥ Revised   ~~deleted~~ Deleted   ♀ Females Only   ♂ Males Only
🝙 Noncovered   🝙 Limited Coverage   🝙 Hospital-Acquired Condition   **Coding Clinic**

471

SECTION: 0 MEDICAL AND SURGICAL
BODY SYSTEM: X ANATOMICAL REGIONS, UPPER EXTREMITIES
OPERATION: 0 **ALTERATION:** Modifying the anatomic structure of a body part without affecting the function of the body part

Body Part	Approach	Device	Qualifier
2 Shoulder Region, Right 3 Shoulder Region, Left 4 Axilla, Right 5 Axilla, Left 6 Upper Extremity, Right 7 Upper Extremity, Left 8 Upper Arm, Right 9 Upper Arm, Left B Elbow Region, Right C Elbow Region, Left D Lower Arm, Right F Lower Arm, Left G Wrist Region, Right H Wrist Region, Left	0 Open 3 Percutaneous 4 Percutaneous Endoscopic	7 Autologous Tissue Substitute J Synthetic Substitute K Nonautologous Tissue Substitute Z No Device	Z No Qualifier

SECTION: 0 MEDICAL AND SURGICAL
BODY SYSTEM: X ANATOMICAL REGIONS, UPPER EXTREMITIES
OPERATION: 2 **CHANGE:** Taking out or off a device from a body part and putting back an identical or similar device in or on the same body part without cutting or puncturing the skin or a mucous membrane

Body Part	Approach	Device	Qualifier
6 Upper Extremity, Right 7 Upper Extremity, Left	X External	0 Drainage Device Y Other Device	Z No Qualifier

SECTION: 0 MEDICAL AND SURGICAL
BODY SYSTEM: X ANATOMICAL REGIONS, UPPER EXTREMITIES
OPERATION: 3 **CONTROL:** Stopping, or attempting to stop, postprocedure bleeding

Body Part	Approach	Device	Qualifier
2 Shoulder Region, Right 3 Shoulder Region, Left 4 Axilla, Right 5 Axilla, Left 6 Upper Extremity, Right 7 Upper Extremity, Left 8 Upper Arm, Right 9 Upper Arm, Left B Elbow Region, Right C Elbow Region, Left D Lower Arm, Right F Lower Arm, Left G Wrist Region, Right H Wrist Region, Left J Hand, Right K Hand, Left	0 Open 3 Percutaneous 4 Percutaneous Endoscopic	Z No Device	Z No Qualifier

◀ New   ◀꟱ Revised   ~~deleted~~ Deleted   ♀ Females Only   ♂ Males Only
🔾 Noncovered   🔾 Limited Coverage   🔾 Hospital-Acquired Condition   **Coding Clinic**

Side tab: 0: ALTERATION   2: CHANGE   3: CONTROL

Side tab: X: ANATOMICAL REGIONS, UPPER EXTREMITIES   0: M/S

SECTION: 0 MEDICAL AND SURGICAL
BODY SYSTEM: X ANATOMICAL REGIONS, UPPER EXTREMITIES
OPERATION: 6 **DETACHMENT:** Cutting off all or a portion of the upper or lower extremities

Body Part	Approach	Device	Qualifier
0 Forequarter, Right 1 Forequarter, Left 2 Shoulder Region, Right 3 Shoulder Region, Left B Elbow Region, Right C Elbow Region, Left	0 Open	Z No Device	Z No Qualifier
8 Upper Arm, Right 9 Upper Arm, Left D Lower Arm, Right F Lower Arm, Left	0 Open	Z No Device	1 High 2 Mid 3 Low
J Hand, Right K Hand, Left	0 Open	Z No Device	0 Complete 4 Complete 1st Ray 5 Complete 2nd Ray 6 Complete 3rd Ray 7 Complete 4th Ray 8 Complete 5th Ray 9 Partial 1st Ray B Partial 2nd Ray C Partial 3rd Ray D Partial 4th Ray F Partial 5th Ray
L Thumb, Right M Thumb, Left N Index Finger, Right P Index Finger, Left Q Middle Finger, Right R Middle Finger, Left S Ring Finger, Right T Ring Finger, Left V Little Finger, Right W Little Finger, Left	0 Open	Z No Device	0 Complete 1 High 2 Mid 3 Low

◀ New   ◀▥ Revised   ~~deleted~~ Deleted   ♀ Females Only   ♂ Males Only
 Noncovered   Limited Coverage   Hospital-Acquired Condition   **Coding Clinic**

473

SECTION: 0 MEDICAL AND SURGICAL
BODY SYSTEM: X ANATOMICAL REGIONS, UPPER EXTREMITIES
OPERATION: 9 DRAINAGE: Taking or letting out fluids and/or gases from a body part

Body Part	Approach	Device	Qualifier
2 Shoulder Region, Right 3 Shoulder Region, Left 4 Axilla, Right 5 Axilla, Left 6 Upper Extremity, Right 7 Upper Extremity, Left 8 Upper Arm, Right 9 Upper Arm, Left B Elbow Region, Right C Elbow Region, Left D Lower Arm, Right F Lower Arm, Left G Wrist Region, Right H Wrist Region, Left J Hand, Right K Hand, Left	0 Open 3 Percutaneous 4 Percutaneous Endoscopic	0 Drainage Device	Z No Qualifier
2 Shoulder Region, Right 3 Shoulder Region, Left 4 Axilla, Right 5 Axilla, Left 6 Upper Extremity, Right 7 Upper Extremity, Left 8 Upper Arm, Right 9 Upper Arm, Left B Elbow Region, Right C Elbow Region, Left D Lower Arm, Right F Lower Arm, Left G Wrist Region, Right H Wrist Region, Left J Hand, Right K Hand, Left	0 Open 3 Percutaneous 4 Percutaneous Endoscopic	Z No Device	X Diagnostic Z No Qualifier

9: DRAINAGE

X: ANATOMICAL REGIONS, UPPER EXTREMITIES

0: M/S

◀ New ◀ Revised ~~deleted~~ Deleted ♀ Females Only ♂ Males Only
Noncovered Limited Coverage Hospital-Acquired Condition **Coding Clinic**

SECTION: 0 MEDICAL AND SURGICAL
BODY SYSTEM: X ANATOMICAL REGIONS, UPPER EXTREMITIES
OPERATION: B EXCISION: Cutting out or off, without replacement, a portion of a body part

Body Part	Approach	Device	Qualifier
2　Shoulder Region, Right 3　Shoulder Region, Left 4　Axilla, Right 5　Axilla, Left 6　Upper Extremity, Right 7　Upper Extremity, Left 8　Upper Arm, Right 9　Upper Arm, Left B　Elbow Region, Right C　Elbow Region, Left D　Lower Arm, Right F　Lower Arm, Left G　Wrist Region, Right H　Wrist Region, Left J　Hand, Right K　Hand, Left	0　Open 3　Percutaneous 4　Percutaneous Endoscopic	Z　No Device	X　Diagnostic Z　No Qualifier

SECTION: 0 MEDICAL AND SURGICAL
BODY SYSTEM: X ANATOMICAL REGIONS, UPPER EXTREMITIES
OPERATION: H INSERTION: Putting in a nonbiological appliance that monitors, assists, performs, or prevents a physiological function but does not physically take the place of a body part

Body Part	Approach	Device	Qualifier
2　Shoulder Region, Right 3　Shoulder Region, Left 4　Axilla, Right 5　Axilla, Left 6　Upper Extremity, Right 7　Upper Extremity, Left 8　Upper Arm, Right 9　Upper Arm, Left B　Elbow Region, Right C　Elbow Region, Left D　Lower Arm, Right F　Lower Arm, Left G　Wrist Region, Right H　Wrist Region, Left J　Hand, Right K　Hand, Left	0　Open 3　Percutaneous 4　Percutaneous Endoscopic	1　Radioactive Element 3　Infusion Device Y　Other Device	Z　No Qualifier

New　　Revised　　deleted Deleted　　♀ Females Only　　♂ Males Only
Noncovered　　Limited Coverage　　Hospital-Acquired Condition　　**Coding Clinic**

J: INSPECTION   M: REATTACHMENT

X: ANATOMICAL REGIONS, UPPER EXTREMITIES

0: M/S

SECTION: 0 MEDICAL AND SURGICAL
BODY SYSTEM: X ANATOMICAL REGIONS, UPPER EXTREMITIES
OPERATION: J INSPECTION: Visually and/or manually exploring a body part

Body Part	Approach	Device	Qualifier
2 Shoulder Region, Right 3 Shoulder Region, Left 4 Axilla, Right 5 Axilla, Left 6 Upper Extremity, Right 7 Upper Extremity, Left 8 Upper Arm, Right 9 Upper Arm, Left B Elbow Region, Right C Elbow Region, Left D Lower Arm, Right F Lower Arm, Left G Wrist Region, Right H Wrist Region, Left J Hand, Right K Hand, Left	0 Open 3 Percutaneous 4 Percutaneous Endoscopic X External	Z No Device	Z No Qualifier

SECTION: 0 MEDICAL AND SURGICAL
BODY SYSTEM: X ANATOMICAL REGIONS, UPPER EXTREMITIES
OPERATION: M REATTACHMENT: Putting back in or on all or a portion of a separated body part to its normal location or other suitable location

Body Part	Approach	Device	Qualifier
0 Forequarter, Right 1 Forequarter, Left 2 Shoulder Region, Right 3 Shoulder Region, Left 4 Axilla, Right 5 Axilla, Left 6 Upper Extremity, Right 7 Upper Extremity, Left 8 Upper Arm, Right 9 Upper Arm, Left B Elbow Region, Right C Elbow Region, Left D Lower Arm, Right F Lower Arm, Left G Wrist Region, Right H Wrist Region, Left J Hand, Right K Hand, Left L Thumb, Right M Thumb, Left N Index Finger, Right P Index Finger, Left Q Middle Finger, Right R Middle Finger, Left S Ring Finger, Right T Ring Finger, Left V Little Finger, Right W Little Finger, Left	0 Open	Z No Device	Z No Qualifier

◄ New ◄ Revised ~~deleted~~ Deleted ♀ Females Only ♂ Males Only
Noncovered Limited Coverage Hospital-Acquired Condition **Coding Clinic**

SECTION: 0 MEDICAL AND SURGICAL
BODY SYSTEM: X ANATOMICAL REGIONS, UPPER EXTREMITIES
OPERATION: P REMOVAL: Taking out or off a device from a body part

Body Part	Approach	Device	Qualifier
6 Upper Extremity, Right 7 Upper Extremity, Left	0 Open 3 Percutaneous 4 Percutaneous Endoscopic X External	0 Drainage Device 1 Radioactive Element 3 Infusion Device 7 Autologous Tissue Substitute J Synthetic Substitute K Nonautologous Tissue Substitute Y Other Device	Z No Qualifier

SECTION: 0 MEDICAL AND SURGICAL
BODY SYSTEM: X ANATOMICAL REGIONS, UPPER EXTREMITIES
OPERATION: Q REPAIR: Restoring, to the extent possible, a body part to its normal anatomic structure and function

Body Part	Approach	Device	Qualifier
2 Shoulder Region, Right 3 Shoulder Region, Left 4 Axilla, Right 5 Axilla, Left 6 Upper Extremity, Right 7 Upper Extremity, Left 8 Upper Arm, Right 9 Upper Arm, Left B Elbow Region, Right C Elbow Region, Left D Lower Arm, Right F Lower Arm, Left G Wrist Region, Right H Wrist Region, Left J Hand, Right K Hand, Left L Thumb, Right M Thumb, Left N Index Finger, Right P Index Finger, Left Q Middle Finger, Right R Middle Finger, Left S Ring Finger, Right T Ring Finger, Left V Little Finger, Right W Little Finger, Left	0 Open 3 Percutaneous 4 Percutaneous Endoscopic X External	Z No Device	Z No Qualifier

0: M/S

X: ANATOMICAL REGIONS, UPPER EXTREMITIES

P: REMOVAL   Q: REPAIR

◀ New   ◀ Revised   deleted Deleted   ♀ Females Only   ♂ Males Only
 Noncovered   Limited Coverage   Hospital-Acquired Condition   **Coding Clinic**

477

SECTION: 0 MEDICAL AND SURGICAL
BODY SYSTEM: X ANATOMICAL REGIONS, UPPER EXTREMITIES
OPERATION: R REPLACEMENT: Putting in or on biological or synthetic material that physically takes the place and/or function of all or a portion of a body part

Body Part	Approach	Device	Qualifier
L Thumb, Right M Thumb, Left	0 Open 4 Percutaneous Endoscopic	7 Autologous Tissue Substitute	N Toe, Right P Toe, Left

SECTION: 0 MEDICAL AND SURGICAL
BODY SYSTEM: X ANATOMICAL REGIONS, UPPER EXTREMITIES
OPERATION: U SUPPLEMENT: Putting in or on biological or synthetic material that physically reinforces and/or augments the function of a portion of a body part

Body Part	Approach	Device	Qualifier
2 Shoulder Region, Right 3 Shoulder Region, Left 4 Axilla, Right 5 Axilla, Left 6 Upper Extremity, Right 7 Upper Extremity, Left 8 Upper Arm, Right 9 Upper Arm, Left B Elbow Region, Right C Elbow Region, Left D Lower Arm, Right F Lower Arm, Left G Wrist Region, Right H Wrist Region, Left J Hand, Right K Hand, Left L Thumb, Right M Thumb, Left N Index Finger, Right P Index Finger, Left Q Middle Finger, Right R Middle Finger, Left S Ring Finger, Right T Ring Finger, Left V Little Finger, Right W Little Finger, Left	0 Open 4 Percutaneous Endoscopic	7 Autologous Tissue Substitute J Synthetic Substitute K Nonautologous Tissue Substitute	Z No Qualifier

◀ New   ◀▥ Revised   ~~deleted~~ Deleted   ♀ Females Only   ♂ Males Only
🅝 Noncovered   🅛 Limited Coverage   🅗 Hospital-Acquired Condition   **Coding Clinic**

SECTION: 0 MEDICAL AND SURGICAL

BODY SYSTEM: X ANATOMICAL REGIONS, UPPER EXTREMITIES
OPERATION: W REVISION: Correcting, to the extent possible, a portion of a malfunctioning device or the position of displaced device

Body Part	Approach	Device	Qualifier
6 Upper Extremity, Right 7 Upper Extremity, Left	0 Open 3 Percutaneous 4 Percutaneous Endoscopic X External	0 Drainage Device 3 Infusion Device 7 Autologous Tissue Substitute J Synthetic Substitute K Nonautologous Tissue Substitute Y Other Device	Z No Qualifier

SECTION: 0 MEDICAL AND SURGICAL

BODY SYSTEM: X ANATOMICAL REGIONS, UPPER EXTREMITIES
OPERATION: X TRANSFER: Moving, without taking out, all or a portion of a body part to another location to take over the function of all or a portion of a body part

Body Part	Approach	Device	Qualifier
N Index Finger, Right	0 Open	Z No Device	L Thumb, Right
P Index Finger, Left	0 Open	Z No Device	M Thumb, Left

SECTION: 0 MEDICAL AND SURGICAL
BODY SYSTEM: Y ANATOMICAL REGIONS, LOWER EXTREMITIES
OPERATION: 0 ALTERATION: Modifying the anatomic structure of a body part without affecting the function of the body part

Body Part	Approach	Device	Qualifier
0 Buttock, Right 1 Buttock, Left 9 Lower Extremity, Right B Lower Extremity, Left C Upper Leg, Right D Upper Leg, Left F Knee Region, Right G Knee Region, Left H Lower Leg, Right J Lower Leg, Left K Ankle Region, Right L Ankle Region, Left	0 Open 3 Percutaneous 4 Percutaneous Endoscopic	7 Autologous Tissue Substitute J Synthetic Substitute K Nonautologous Tissue Substitute Z No Device	Z No Qualifier

SECTION: 0 MEDICAL AND SURGICAL
BODY SYSTEM: Y ANATOMICAL REGIONS, LOWER EXTREMITIES
OPERATION: 2 CHANGE: Taking out or off a device from a body part and putting back an identical or similar device in or on the same body part without cutting or puncturing the skin or a mucous membrane

Body Part	Approach	Device	Qualifier
9 Lower Extremity, Right B Lower Extremity, Left	X External	0 Drainage Device Y Other Device	Z No Qualifier

SECTION: 0 MEDICAL AND SURGICAL
BODY SYSTEM: Y ANATOMICAL REGIONS, LOWER EXTREMITIES
OPERATION: 3 CONTROL: Stopping, or attempting to stop, postprocedure bleeding

Body Part	Approach	Device	Qualifier
0 Buttock, Right 1 Buttock, Left 5 Inguinal Region, Right 6 Inguinal Region, Left 7 Femoral Region, Right 8 Femoral Region, Left 9 Lower Extremity, Right B Lower Extremity, Left C Upper Leg, Right D Upper Leg, Left F Knee Region, Right G Knee Region, Left H Lower Leg, Right J Lower Leg, Left K Ankle Region, Right L Ankle Region, Left M Foot, Right N Foot, Left	0 Open 3 Percutaneous 4 Percutaneous Endoscopic	Z No Device	Z No Qualifier

SECTION: 0 MEDICAL AND SURGICAL
BODY SYSTEM: Y ANATOMICAL REGIONS, LOWER EXTREMITIES
OPERATION: 6 DETACHMENT: Cutting off all or a portion of the upper or lower extremities

Body Part	Approach	Device	Qualifier
2 Hindquarter, Right 3 Hindquarter, Left 4 Hindquarter, Bilateral 7 Femoral Region, Right 8 Femoral Region, Left F Knee Region, Right G Knee Region, Left	0 Open	Z No Device	Z No Qualifier
C Upper Leg, Right D Upper Leg, Left H Lower Leg, Right J Lower Leg, Left	0 Open	Z No Device	1 High 2 Mid 3 Low
M Foot, Right N Foot, Left	0 Open	Z No Device	0 Complete 4 Complete 1st Ray 5 Complete 2nd Ray 6 Complete 3rd Ray 7 Complete 4th Ray 8 Complete 5th Ray 9 Partial 1st Ray B Partial 2nd Ray C Partial 3rd Ray D Partial 4th Ray F Partial 5th Ray
P 1st Toe, Right Q 1st Toe, Left R 2nd Toe, Right S 2nd Toe, Left T 3rd Toe, Right U 3rd Toe, Left V 4th Toe, Right W 4th Toe, Left X 5th Toe, Right Y 5th Toe, Left	0 Open	Z No Device	0 Complete 1 High 2 Mid 3 Low

SECTION: 0 MEDICAL AND SURGICAL

BODY SYSTEM: Y ANATOMICAL REGIONS, LOWER EXTREMITIES
OPERATION: 9 DRAINAGE: Taking or letting out fluids and/or gases from a body part

Body Part	Approach	Device	Qualifier
0 Buttock, Right 1 Buttock, Left 5 Inguinal Region, Right 6 Inguinal Region, Left 7 Femoral Region, Right 8 Femoral Region, Left 9 Lower Extremity, Right B Lower Extremity, Left C Upper Leg, Right D Upper Leg, Left F Knee Region, Right G Knee Region, Left H Lower Leg, Right J Lower Leg, Left K Ankle Region, Right L Ankle Region, Left M Foot, Right N Foot, Left	0 Open 3 Percutaneous 4 Percutaneous Endoscopic	0 Drainage Device	Z No Qualifier
0 Buttock, Right 1 Buttock, Left 5 Inguinal Region, Right 6 Inguinal Region, Left 7 Femoral Region, Right 8 Femoral Region, Left 9 Lower Extremity, Right B Lower Extremity, Left C Upper Leg, Right D Upper Leg, Left F Knee Region, Right G Knee Region, Left H Lower Leg, Right J Lower Leg, Left K Ankle Region, Right L Ankle Region, Left M Foot, Right N Foot, Left	0 Open 3 Percutaneous 4 Percutaneous Endoscopic	Z No Device	X Diagnostic Z No Qualifier

SECTION: **0 MEDICAL AND SURGICAL**
BODY SYSTEM: Y ANATOMICAL REGIONS, LOWER EXTREMITIES
OPERATION: **B EXCISION:** Cutting out or off, without replacement, a portion of a body part

Body Part	Approach	Device	Qualifier
0 Buttock, Right	0 Open	Z No Device	X Diagnostic
1 Buttock, Left	3 Percutaneous		Z No Qualifier
5 Inguinal Region, Right	4 Percutaneous Endoscopic		
6 Inguinal Region, Left			
7 Femoral Region, Right			
8 Femoral Region, Left			
9 Lower Extremity, Right			
B Lower Extremity, Left			
C Upper Leg, Right			
D Upper Leg, Left			
F Knee Region, Right			
G Knee Region, Left			
H Lower Leg, Right			
J Lower Leg, Left			
K Ankle Region, Right			
L Ankle Region, Left			
M Foot, Right			
N Foot, Left			

SECTION: **0 MEDICAL AND SURGICAL**
BODY SYSTEM: Y ANATOMICAL REGIONS, LOWER EXTREMITIES
OPERATION: **H INSERTION:** Putting in a nonbiological appliance that monitors, assists, performs, or prevents a physiological function but does not physically take the place of a body part

Body Part	Approach	Device	Qualifier
0 Buttock, Right	0 Open	1 Radioactive Element	Z No Qualifier
1 Buttock, Left	3 Percutaneous	3 Infusion Device	
5 Inguinal Region, Right	4 Percutaneous Endoscopic	Y Other Device	
6 Inguinal Region, Left			
7 Femoral Region, Right			
8 Femoral Region, Left			
9 Lower Extremity, Right			
B Lower Extremity, Left			
C Upper Leg, Right			
D Upper Leg, Left			
F Knee Region, Right			
G Knee Region, Left			
H Lower Leg, Right			
J Lower Leg, Left			
K Ankle Region, Right			
L Ankle Region, Left			
M Foot, Right			
N Foot, Left			

◀ New   ◀▥ Revised   ~~deleted~~ Deleted   ♀ Females Only   ♂ Males Only
℞꜀ Noncovered   ℞꜀ Limited Coverage   ℞꜀ Hospital-Acquired Condition   **Coding Clinic**

SECTION: 0 MEDICAL AND SURGICAL
BODY SYSTEM: Y ANATOMICAL REGIONS, LOWER EXTREMITIES
OPERATION: J INSPECTION: Visually and/or manually exploring a body part

Body Part	Approach	Device	Qualifier
0 Buttock, Right	0 Open	Z No Device	Z No Qualifier
1 Buttock, Left	3 Percutaneous		
5 Inguinal Region, Right	4 Percutaneous Endoscopic		
6 Inguinal Region, Left	X External		
7 Femoral Region, Right			
8 Femoral Region, Left			
9 Lower Extremity, Right			
A Inguinal Region, Bilateral			
B Lower Extremity, Left			
C Upper Leg, Right			
D Upper Leg, Left			
E Femoral Region, Bilateral			
F Knee Region, Right			
G Knee Region, Left			
H Lower Leg, Right			
J Lower Leg, Left			
K Ankle Region, Right			
L Ankle Region, Left			
M Foot, Right			
N Foot, Left			

SECTION: 0 MEDICAL AND SURGICAL
BODY SYSTEM: Y ANATOMICAL REGIONS, LOWER EXTREMITIES
OPERATION: M REATTACHMENT: Putting back in or on all or a portion of a separated body part to its normal location or other suitable location

Body Part	Approach	Device	Qualifier
0 Buttock, Right	0 Open	Z No Device	Z No Qualifier
1 Buttock, Left			
2 Hindquarter, Right			
3 Hindquarter, Left			
4 Hindquarter, Bilateral			
5 Inguinal Region, Right			
6 Inguinal Region, Left			
7 Femoral Region, Right			
8 Femoral Region, Left			
9 Lower Extremity, Right			
B Lower Extremity, Left			
C Upper Leg, Right			
D Upper Leg, Left			
F Knee Region, Right			
G Knee Region, Left			
H Lower Leg, Right			
J Lower Leg, Left			
K Ankle Region, Right			
L Ankle Region, Left			
M Foot, Right			
N Foot, Left			
P 1st Toe, Right			
Q 1st Toe, Left			
R 2nd Toe, Right			
S 2nd Toe, Left			
T 3rd Toe, Right			
U 3rd Toe, Left			
V 4th Toe, Right			
W 4th Toe, Left			
X 5th Toe, Right			
Y 5th Toe, Left			

SECTION: 0 MEDICAL AND SURGICAL
BODY SYSTEM: Y ANATOMICAL REGIONS, LOWER EXTREMITIES
OPERATION: P REMOVAL: Taking out or off a device from a body part

Body Part	Approach	Device	Qualifier
9 Lower Extremity, Right	0 Open	0 Drainage Device	Z No Qualifier
B Lower Extremity, Left	3 Percutaneous	1 Radioactive Element	
	4 Percutaneous Endoscopic	3 Infusion Device	
	X External	7 Autologous Tissue Substitute	
		J Synthetic Substitute	
		K Nonautologous Tissue Substitute	
		Y Other Device	

◀ New   ◀ Revised   deleted Deleted   ♀ Females Only   ♂ Males Only
Noncovered   Limited Coverage   Hospital-Acquired Condition   **Coding Clinic**

SECTION: 0 MEDICAL AND SURGICAL

BODY SYSTEM: Y ANATOMICAL REGIONS, LOWER EXTREMITIES

OPERATION: Q REPAIR: Restoring, to the extent possible, a body part to its normal anatomic structure and function

Body Part	Approach	Device	Qualifier
0 Buttock, Right	0 Open	Z No Device	Z No Qualifier
1 Buttock, Left	3 Percutaneous		
5 Inguinal Region, Right	4 Percutaneous Endoscopic		
6 Inguinal Region, Left	X External		
7 Femoral Region, Right			
8 Femoral Region, Left			
9 Lower Extremity, Right			
A Inguinal Region, Bilateral			
B Lower Extremity, Left			
C Upper Leg, Right			
D Upper Leg, Left			
E Femoral Region, Bilateral			
F Knee Region, Right			
G Knee Region, Left			
H Lower Leg, Right			
J Lower Leg, Left			
K Ankle Region, Right			
L Ankle Region, Left			
M Foot, Right			
N Foot, Left			
P 1st Toe, Right			
Q 1st Toe, Left			
R 2nd Toe, Right			
S 2nd Toe, Left			
T 3rd Toe, Right			
U 3rd Toe, Left			
V 4th Toe, Right			
W 4th Toe, Left			
X 5th Toe, Right			
Y 5th Toe, Left			

◀ New ◀ Revised ~~deleted~~ Deleted ♀ Females Only ♂ Males Only
 Noncovered 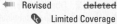 Limited Coverage ⬡ Hospital-Acquired Condition **Coding Clinic**

SECTION: 0 MEDICAL AND SURGICAL
BODY SYSTEM: Y ANATOMICAL REGIONS, LOWER EXTREMITIES
OPERATION: U SUPPLEMENT: Putting in or on biological or synthetic material that physically reinforces and/or augments the function of a portion of a body part

Body Part	Approach	Device	Qualifier
0 Buttock, Right 1 Buttock, Left 5 Inguinal Region, Right 6 Inguinal Region, Left 7 Femoral Region, Right 8 Femoral Region, Left 9 Lower Extremity, Right A Inguinal Region, Bilateral B Lower Extremity, Left C Upper Leg, Right D Upper Leg, Left E Femoral Region, Bilateral F Knee Region, Right G Knee Region, Left H Lower Leg, Right J Lower Leg, Left K Ankle Region, Right L Ankle Region, Left M Foot, Right N Foot, Left P 1st Toe, Right Q 1st Toe, Left R 2nd Toe, Right S 2nd Toe, Left T 3rd Toe, Right U 3rd Toe, Left V 4th Toe, Right W 4th Toe, Left X 5th Toe, Right Y 5th Toe, Left	0 Open 4 Percutaneous Endoscopic	7 Autologous Tissue Substitute J Synthetic Substitute K Nonautologous Tissue Substitute	Z No Qualifier

SECTION: 0 MEDICAL AND SURGICAL
BODY SYSTEM: Y ANATOMICAL REGIONS, LOWER EXTREMITIES
OPERATION: W REVISION: Correcting, to the extent possible, a portion of a malfunctioning device or the position of a displaced device

Body Part	Approach	Device	Qualifier
9 Lower Extremity, Right B Lower Extremity, Left	0 Open 3 Percutaneous 4 Percutaneous Endoscopic X External	0 Drainage Device 3 Infusion Device 7 Autologous Tissue Substitute J Synthetic Substitute K Nonautologous Tissue Substitute Y Other Device	Z No Qualifier

◀ New ◀ Revised ~~deleted~~ Deleted ♀ Females Only ♂ Males Only
Noncovered Limited Coverage Hospital-Acquired Condition **Coding Clinic**

ICD-10-PCS Coding Guidelines

Obstetric Section Guidelines (section 1)

C. Obstetrics Section

Products of conception

C1

Procedures performed on the products of conception are coded to the Obstetrics section. Procedures performed on the pregnant female other than the products of conception are coded to the appropriate root operation in the Medical and Surgical section.

Example: Amniocentesis is coded to the products of conception body part in the Obstetrics section. Repair of obstetric urethral laceration is coded to the urethra body part in the Medical and Surgical section.

Procedures following delivery or abortion

C2

Procedures performed following a delivery or abortion for curettage of the endometrium or evacuation of retained products of conception are all coded in the Obstetrics section, to the root operation Extraction and the body part Products of Conception, Retained. Diagnostic or therapeutic dilation and curettage performed during times other than the postpartum or post-abortion period are all coded in the Medical and Surgical section, to the root operation Extraction and the body part Endometrium.

SECTION: 1 OBSTETRICS
BODY SYSTEM: 0 PREGNANCY
OPERATION: 2 **CHANGE:** Taking out or off a device from a body part and putting back an identical or similar device in or on the same body part without cutting or puncturing the skin or a mucous membrane

Body Part	Approach	Device	Qualifier
0 Products of Conception ♀	7 Via Natural or Artificial Opening	3 Monitoring Electrode Y Other Device	Z No Qualifier

SECTION: 1 OBSTETRICS
BODY SYSTEM: 0 PREGNANCY
OPERATION: 9 **DRAINAGE:** Taking or letting out fluids and/or gases from a body part

Body Part	Approach	Device	Qualifier
0 Products of Conception ♀	0 Open 3 Percutaneous 4 Percutaneous Endoscopic 7 Via Natural or Artificial Opening 8 Via Natural or Artificial Opening Endoscopic	Z No Device	9 Fetal Blood A Fetal Cerebrospinal Fluid B Fetal Fluid, Other C Amniotic Fluid, Therapeutic D Fluid, Other U Amniotic Fluid, Diagnostic

SECTION: 1 OBSTETRICS
BODY SYSTEM: 0 PREGNANCY
OPERATION: A **ABORTION:** Artificially terminating a pregnancy

Body Part	Approach	Device	Qualifier
0 Products of Conception ♀	0 Open 3 Percutaneous 4 Percutaneous Endoscopic 8 Via Natural or Artificial Opening Endoscopic	Z No Device	Z No Qualifier
0 Products of Conception ♀	7 Via Natural or Artificial Opening	Z No Device	6 Vacuum W Laminaria X Abortifacient Z No Qualifier

◄ New   ◄ Revised   ~~deleted~~ Deleted   ♀ Females Only   ♂ Males Only
Noncovered   Limited Coverage   Hospital-Acquired Condition   **Coding Clinic**

SECTION: 1 OBSTETRICS
BODY SYSTEM: 0 PREGNANCY
OPERATION: D EXTRACTION: Pulling or stripping out or off all or a portion of a body part by the use of force

Body Part	Approach	Device	Qualifier
0 Products of Conception ♀	0 Open	Z No Device	0 Classical 1 Low Cervical 2 Extraperitoneal
0 Products of Conception ♀	7 Via Natural or Artificial Opening	Z No Device	3 Low Forceps 4 Mid Forceps 5 High Forceps 6 Vacuum 7 Internal Version 8 Other
1 Products of Conception, Retained ♀ 2 Products of Conception, Ectopic ♀	7 Via Natural or Artificial Opening 8 Via Natural or Artificial Opening Endoscopic	Z No Device	Z No Qualifier

SECTION: 1 OBSTETRICS
BODY SYSTEM: 0 PREGNANCY
OPERATION: E DELIVERY: Assisting the passage of the products of conception from the genital canal

Body Part	Approach	Device	Qualifier
0 Products of Conception ♀	X External	Z No Device	Z No Qualifier

SECTION: 1 OBSTETRICS
BODY SYSTEM: 0 PREGNANCY
OPERATION: H INSERTION: Putting in a nonbiological appliance that monitors, assists, performs, or prevents a physiological function but does not physically take the place of a body part

Body Part	Approach	Device	Qualifier
0 Products of Conception ♀	0 Open 7 Via Natural or Artificial Opening	3 Monitoring Electrode Y Other Device	Z No Qualifier

Coding Clinic: 2013, Q2, P36 – 10H07YZ

◄ New ◄≡ Revised ~~deleted~~ Deleted ♀ Females Only ♂ Males Only
🚫 Noncovered 🔵 Limited Coverage 🏥 Hospital-Acquired Condition **Coding Clinic**

491

SECTION: 1 OBSTETRICS
BODY SYSTEM: 0 PREGNANCY
OPERATION: J INSPECTION: Visually and/or manually exploring a body part

Body Part	Approach	Device	Qualifier
0 Products of Conception ♀ 1 Products of Conception, Retained ♀ 2 Products of Conception, Ectopic ♀	0 Open 3 Percutaneous 4 Percutaneous Endoscopic 7 Via Natural or Artificial Opening 8 Via Natural or Artificial Opening Endoscopic X External	Z No Device	Z No Qualifier

SECTION: 1 OBSTETRICS
BODY SYSTEM: 0 PREGNANCY
OPERATION: P REMOVAL: Taking out or off a device from a body part, region or orifice

Body Part	Approach	Device	Qualifier
0 Products of Conception ♀	0 Open 7 Via Natural or Artificial Opening	3 Monitoring Electrode Y Other Device	Z No Qualifier

SECTION: 1 OBSTETRICS
BODY SYSTEM: 0 PREGNANCY
OPERATION: Q REPAIR: Restoring, to the extent possible, a body part to its normal anatomic structure and function

Body Part	Approach	Device	Qualifier
0 Products of Conception ♀	0 Open 3 Percutaneous 4 Percutaneous Endoscopic 7 Via Natural or Artificial Opening 8 Via Natural or Artificial Opening Endoscopic	Y Other Device Z No Device	E Nervous System F Cardiovascular System G Lymphatics and Hemic H Eye J Ear, Nose, and Sinus K Respiratory System L Mouth and Throat M Gastrointestinal System N Hepatobiliary and Pancreas P Endocrine System Q Skin R Musculoskeletal System S Urinary System T Female Reproductive System V Male Reproductive System Y Other Body System

Side tab: J: INSPECTION P: REMOVAL Q: REPAIR 0: PREGNANCY 1: OBSTETRICS

◀ New   ◀ Revised   ~~deleted~~ Deleted   ♀ Females Only   ♂ Males Only
🚫 Noncovered   🚫 Limited Coverage   🚫 Hospital-Acquired Condition   **Coding Clinic**

SECTION: 1 OBSTETRICS
BODY SYSTEM: 0 PREGNANCY
OPERATION: S REPOSITION: Moving to its normal location or other suitable location all or a portion of a body part

Body Part	Approach	Device	Qualifier
0 Products of Conception ♀	7 Via Natural or Artificial Opening X External	Z No Device	Z No Qualifier
2 Products of Conception, Ectopic ♀	0 Open 3 Percutaneous 4 Percutaneous Endoscopic 7 Via Natural or Artificial Opening 8 Via Natural or Artificial Opening Endoscopic	Z No Device	Z No Qualifier

SECTION: 1 OBSTETRICS
BODY SYSTEM: 0 PREGNANCY
OPERATION: T RESECTION: Cutting out or off, without replacement, all of a body part

Body Part	Approach	Device	Qualifier
2 Products of Conception, Ectopic ♀	0 Open 3 Percutaneous 4 Percutaneous Endoscopic 7 Via Natural or Artificial Opening 8 Via Natural or Artificial Opening Endoscopic	Z No Device	Z No Qualifier

SECTION: 1 OBSTETRICS
BODY SYSTEM: 0 PREGNANCY
OPERATION: Y TRANSPLANTATION: Putting in or on all or a portion of a living body part taken from another individual or animal to physically take the place and/or function of all or a portion of a similar body part

Body Part	Approach	Device	Qualifier
0 Products of Conception ♀	3 Percutaneous 4 Percutaneous Endoscopic 7 Via Natural or Artificial Opening	Z No Device	E Nervous System F Cardiovascular System G Lymphatics and Hemic H Eye J Ear, Nose, and Sinus K Respiratory System L Mouth and Throat M Gastrointestinal System N Hepatobiliary and Pancreas P Endocrine System Q Skin R Musculoskeletal System S Urinary System T Female Reproductive System V Male Reproductive System Y Other Body System

◀ New   ◀▪▪ Revised   ~~deleted~~ Deleted   ♀ Females Only   ♂ Males Only
🚱 Noncovered   🚱 Limited Coverage   🚱 Hospital-Acquired Condition   **Coding Clinic**

493

SECTION: 2 PLACEMENT
BODY SYSTEM: W ANATOMICAL REGIONS
OPERATION: 0 CHANGE: Taking out or off a device from a body part and putting back an identical or similar device in or on the same body part without cutting or puncturing the skin or a mucous membrane

Body Region	Approach	Device	Qualifier
0 Head 2 Neck 3 Abdominal Wall 4 Chest Wall 5 Back 6 Inguinal Region, Right 7 Inguinal Region, Left 8 Upper Extremity, Right 9 Upper Extremity, Left A Upper Arm, Right B Upper Arm, Left C Lower Arm, Right D Lower Arm, Left E Hand, Right F Hand, Left G Thumb, Right H Thumb, Left J Finger, Right K Finger, Left L Lower Extremity, Right M Lower Extremity, Left N Upper Leg, Right P Upper Leg, Left Q Lower Leg, Right R Lower Leg, Left S Foot, Right T Foot, Left U Toe, Right V Toe, Left	X External	0 Traction Apparatus 1 Splint 2 Cast 3 Brace 4 Bandage 5 Packing Material 6 Pressure Dressing 7 Intermittent Pressure Device Y Other Device	Z No Qualifier
1 Face	X External	0 Traction Apparatus 1 Splint 2 Cast 3 Brace 4 Bandage 5 Packing Material 6 Pressure Dressing 7 Intermittent Pressure Device 9 Wire Y Other Device	Z No Qualifier

◀ New   ◀█ Revised   ~~deleted~~ Deleted   ♀ Females Only   ♂ Males Only
🔖 Noncovered   🔖 Limited Coverage   🔖 Hospital-Acquired Condition   **Coding Clinic**

495

SECTION: 2 PLACEMENT
BODY SYSTEM: W ANATOMICAL REGIONS
OPERATION: 1 COMPRESSION: Putting pressure on a body region

Body Region	Approach	Device	Qualifier
0 Head	X External	6 Pressure Dressing	Z No Qualifier
1 Face		7 Intermittent Pressure Device	
2 Neck			
3 Abdominal Wall			
4 Chest Wall			
5 Back			
6 Inguinal Region, Right			
7 Inguinal Region, Left			
8 Upper Extremity, Right			
9 Upper Extremity, Left			
A Upper Arm, Right			
B Upper Arm, Left			
C Lower Arm, Right			
D Lower Arm, Left			
E Hand, Right			
F Hand, Left			
G Thumb, Right			
H Thumb, Left			
J Finger, Right			
K Finger, Left			
L Lower Extremity, Right			
M Lower Extremity, Left			
N Upper Leg, Right			
P Upper Leg, Left			
Q Lower Leg, Right			
R Lower Leg, Left			
S Foot, Right			
T Foot, Left			
U Toe, Right			
V Toe, Left			

1: COMPRESSION

W: ANATOMICAL REGIONS

2: PLACEMENT

◄ New   ◄▥ Revised   deleted Deleted   ♀ Females Only   ♂ Males Only
Ⓝⓒ Noncovered   Ⓛⓒ Limited Coverage   ⒽⒶⓒ Hospital-Acquired Condition   **Coding Clinic**

SECTION: 2 PLACEMENT
BODY SYSTEM: W ANATOMICAL REGIONS
OPERATION: 2 DRESSING: Putting material on a body region for protection

Body Region	Approach	Device	Qualifier
0 Head	X External	4 Bandage	Z No Qualifier
1 Face			
2 Neck			
3 Abdominal Wall			
4 Chest Wall			
5 Back			
6 Inguinal Region, Right			
7 Inguinal Region, Left			
8 Upper Extremity, Right			
9 Upper Extremity, Left			
A Upper Arm, Right			
B Upper Arm, Left			
C Lower Arm, Right			
D Lower Arm, Left			
E Hand, Right			
F Hand, Left			
G Thumb, Right			
H Thumb, Left			
J Finger, Right			
K Finger, Left			
L Lower Extremity, Right			
M Lower Extremity, Left			
N Upper Leg, Right			
P Upper Leg, Left			
Q Lower Leg, Right			
R Lower Leg, Left			
S Foot, Right			
T Foot, Left			
U Toe, Right			
V Toe, Left			

2: PLACEMENT

W: ANATOMICAL REGIONS

2: DRESSING

◀ New   ◀▦ Revised   ~~deleted~~ Deleted   ♀ Females Only   ♂ Males Only
🐾 Noncovered   🐾 Limited Coverage   🐾 Hospital-Acquired Condition   **Coding Clinic**

SECTION: 2 PLACEMENT
BODY SYSTEM: W ANATOMICAL REGIONS
OPERATION: 3 **IMMOBILIZATION:** Limiting or preventing motion of a body region

Body Region	Approach	Device	Qualifier
0 Head 2 Neck 3 Abdominal Wall 4 Chest Wall 5 Back 6 Inguinal Region, Right 7 Inguinal Region, Left 8 Upper Extremity, Right 9 Upper Extremity, Left A Upper Arm, Right B Upper Arm, Left C Lower Arm, Right D Lower Arm, Left E Hand, Right F Hand, Left G Thumb, Right H Thumb, Left J Finger, Right K Finger, Left L Lower Extremity, Right M Lower Extremity, Left N Upper Leg, Right P Upper Leg, Left Q Lower Leg, Right R Lower Leg, Left S Foot, Right T Foot, Left U Toe, Right V Toe, Left	X External	1 Splint 2 Cast 3 Brace Y Other Device	Z No Qualifier
1 Face	X External	1 Splint 2 Cast 3 Brace 9 Wire Y Other Device	Z No Qualifier

3: IMMOBILIZATION
W: ANATOMICAL REGIONS
2: PLACEMENT

◀ New　◀ Revised　~~deleted~~ Deleted　♀ Females Only　♂ Males Only
Noncovered　Limited Coverage　Hospital-Acquired Condition　**Coding Clinic**

SECTION: 2 PLACEMENT

BODY SYSTEM: W ANATOMICAL REGIONS

OPERATION: 4 PACKING: Putting material in a body region or orifice

Body Region	Approach	Device	Qualifier
0 Head	X External	5 Packing Material	Z No Qualifier
1 Face			
2 Neck			
3 Abdominal Wall			
4 Chest Wall			
5 Back			
6 Inguinal Region, Right			
7 Inguinal Region, Left			
8 Upper Extremity, Right			
9 Upper Extremity, Left			
A Upper Arm, Right			
B Upper Arm, Left			
C Lower Arm, Right			
D Lower Arm, Left			
E Hand, Right			
F Hand, Left			
G Thumb, Right			
H Thumb, Left			
J Finger, Right			
K Finger, Left			
L Lower Extremity, Right			
M Lower Extremity, Left			
N Upper Leg, Right			
P Upper Leg, Left			
Q Lower Leg, Right			
R Lower Leg, Left			
S Foot, Right			
T Foot, Left			
U Toe, Right			
V Toe, Left			

SECTION: 2 PLACEMENT
BODY SYSTEM: W ANATOMICAL REGIONS
OPERATION: 5 REMOVAL: Taking out or off a device from a body part

Body Region	Approach	Device	Qualifier
0 Head 2 Neck 3 Abdominal Wall 4 Chest Wall 5 Back 6 Inguinal Region, Right 7 Inguinal Region, Left 8 Upper Extremity, Right 9 Upper Extremity, Left A Upper Arm, Right B Upper Arm, Left C Lower Arm, Right D Lower Arm, Left E Hand, Right F Hand, Left G Thumb, Right H Thumb, Left J Finger, Right K Finger, Left L Lower Extremity, Right M Lower Extremity, Left N Upper Leg, Right P Upper Leg, Left Q Lower Leg, Right R Lower Leg, Left S Foot, Right T Foot, Left U Toe, Right V Toe, Left	X External	0 Traction Apparatus 1 Splint 2 Cast 3 Brace 4 Bandage 5 Packing Material 6 Pressure Dressing 7 Intermittent Pressure Device Y Other Device	Z No Qualifier
1 Face	X External	0 Traction Apparatus 1 Splint 2 Cast 3 Brace 4 Bandage 5 Packing Material 6 Pressure Dressing 7 Intermittent Pressure Device 9 Wire Y Other Device	Z No Qualifier

(left margin) 5: REMOVAL   W: ANATOMICAL REGIONS   2: PLACEMENT

◀ New   ◀▥ Revised   ~~deleted~~ Deleted   ♀ Females Only   ♂ Males Only
🖉 Noncovered   🖉 Limited Coverage   🖉 Hospital-Acquired Condition   **Coding Clinic**

SECTION: 2 PLACEMENT
BODY SYSTEM: W ANATOMICAL REGIONS
OPERATION: 6 TRACTION: Exerting a pulling force on a body region in a distal direction

Body Region	Approach	Device	Qualifier
0 Head	X External	0 Traction Apparatus	Z No Qualifier
1 Face		Z No Device	
2 Neck			
3 Abdominal Wall			
4 Chest Wall			
5 Back			
6 Inguinal Region, Right			
7 Inguinal Region, Left			
8 Upper Extremity, Right			
9 Upper Extremity, Left			
A Upper Arm, Right			
B Upper Arm, Left			
C Lower Arm, Right			
D Lower Arm, Left			
E Hand, Right			
F Hand, Left			
G Thumb, Right			
H Thumb, Left			
J Finger, Right			
K Finger, Left			
L Lower Extremity, Right			
M Lower Extremity, Left			
N Upper Leg, Right			
P Upper Leg, Left			
Q Lower Leg, Right			
R Lower Leg, Left			
S Foot, Right			
T Foot, Left			
U Toe, Right			
V Toe, Left			

Coding Clinic: 2013, Q2, P39 – 2W60X0Z

2: PLACEMENT W: ANATOMICAL REGIONS 6: TRACTION

SECTION: **2 PLACEMENT**

BODY SYSTEM: Y ANATOMICAL ORIFICES

OPERATION: **0 CHANGE:** Taking out or off a device from a body part and putting back an identical or similar device in or on the same body part without cutting or puncturing the skin or a mucous membrane

Body Region	Approach	Device	Qualifier
0 Mouth and Pharynx 1 Nasal 2 Ear 3 Anorectal 4 Female Genital Tract ♀ 5 Urethra	X External	5 Packing Material	Z No Qualifier

SECTION: **2 PLACEMENT**

BODY SYSTEM: Y ANATOMICAL ORIFICES

OPERATION: **4 PACKING:** Putting material in a body region or orifice

Body Region	Approach	Device	Qualifier
0 Mouth and Pharynx 1 Nasal 2 Ear 3 Anorectal 4 Female Genital Tract ♀ 5 Urethra	X External	5 Packing Material	Z No Qualifier

SECTION: **2 PLACEMENT**

BODY SYSTEM: Y ANATOMICAL ORIFICES

OPERATION: **5 REMOVAL:** Taking out or off a device from a body part

Body Region	Approach	Device	Qualifier
0 Mouth and Pharynx 1 Nasal 2 Ear 3 Anorectal 4 Female Genital Tract ♀ 5 Urethra	X External	5 Packing Material	Z No Qualifier

◀ New   ◀▬ Revised   ~~deleted~~ Deleted   ♀ Females Only   ♂ Males Only
Ⓝ Noncovered   Ⓛ Limited Coverage   Ⓗ Hospital-Acquired Condition   **Coding Clinic**

SECTION: 3 ADMINISTRATION
BODY SYSTEM: 0 CIRCULATORY
OPERATION: 2 TRANSFUSION: *(on multiple pages)*
Putting in blood or blood products

Body System / Region	Approach	Substance	Qualifier
3 Peripheral Vein 4 Central Vein	0 Open 3 Percutaneous	A Stem Cells, Embryonic ⓝ	Z No Qualifier
3 Peripheral Vein 4 Central Vein	0 Open 3 Percutaneous	G Bone Marrow ⓝ H Whole Blood J Serum Albumin K Frozen Plasma L Fresh Plasma M Plasma Cryoprecipitate N Red Blood Cells P Frozen Red Cells Q White Cells R Platelets S Globulin T Fibrinogen V Antihemophilic Factors W Factor IX X Stem Cells, Cord Blood Y Stem Cells, Hematopoietic ⓝ	0 Autologous 1 Nonautologous
5 Peripheral Artery 6 Central Artery	0 Open 3 Percutaneous	G Bone Marrow ⓝ H Whole Blood J Serum Albumin K Frozen Plasma L Fresh Plasma M Plasma Cryoprecipitate N Red Blood Cells P Frozen Red Cells Q White Cells R Platelets S Globulin T Fibrinogen V Antihemophilic Factors W Factor IX X Stem Cells, Cord Blood Y Stem Cells, Hematopoietic ⓝ	0 Autologous 1 Nonautologous

2: TRANSFUSION

0: CIRCULATORY

3: ADMINISTRATION

◀ New ◀▥ Revised ~~deleted~~ Deleted ♀ Females Only ♂ Males Only
ⓝ Noncovered ⓝ Limited Coverage ⓗ Hospital-Acquired Condition **Coding Clinic**

SECTION: 3 ADMINISTRATION
BODY SYSTEM: 0 CIRCULATORY
OPERATION: 2 TRANSFUSION: *(continued)*
Putting in blood or blood products

Body System / Region	Approach	Substance	Qualifier
7 Products of Conception, Circulatory ♀	3 Percutaneous 7 Via Natural or Artificial Opening	H Whole Blood J Serum Albumin K Frozen Plasma L Fresh Plasma M Plasma Cryoprecipitate N Red Blood Cells P Frozen Red Cells Q White Cells R Platelets S Globulin T Fibrinogen V Antihemophilic Factors W Factor IX	1 Nonautologous
8 Vein	0 Open 3 Percutaneous	B 4-Factor Prothrombin Complex Concentrate	1 Nonautologous

🦚 Codes with Qualifier 0: are only noncovered when a code from the diagnosis list below is present as a principal or secondary diagnosis

C9100	C9240	C9300
C9200	C9250	C9400
C9210	C9260	C9500
C9211	C92A0	

🦚 Codes with Qualifier 1: are only noncovered when C90.00 or C90.01 are present as a principal or secondary diagnosis

30263Y1
30230Y1

SECTION: 3 ADMINISTRATION
BODY SYSTEM: C INDWELLING DEVICE
OPERATION: 1 IRRIGATION: Putting in or on a cleansing substance

Body System / Region	Approach	Substance	Qualifier
Z None	X External	8 Irrigating Substance	Z No Qualifier

SECTION: 3 ADMINISTRATION
BODY SYSTEM: E PHYSIOLOGICAL SYSTEMS AND ANATOMICAL REGIONS
OPERATION: 0 INTRODUCTION: *(on multiple pages)*

Putting in or on a therapeutic, diagnostic, nutritional, physiological, or prophylactic substance except blood or blood products

Body System / Region	Approach	Substance	Qualifier
0 Skin and Mucous Membranes	X External	0 Antineoplastic	5 Other Antineoplastic M Monoclonal Antibody
0 Skin and Mucous Membranes	X External	2 Anti-infective	8 Oxazolidinones 9 Other Anti-infective
0 Skin and Mucous Membranes	X External	3 Anti-inflammatory 4 Serum, Toxoid, and Vaccine B Local Anesthetic K Other Diagnostic Substance M Pigment N Analgesics, Hypnotics, Sedatives T Destructive Agent	Z No Qualifier
0 Skin and Mucous Membranes	X External	G Other Therapeutic Substance	C Other Substance
1 Subcutaneous Tissue	0 Open	2 Anti-infective	A Anti-Infective Envelope
1 Subcutaneous Tissue	3 Percutaneous	0 Antineoplastic	5 Other Antineoplastic M Monoclonal Antibody
1 Subcutaneous Tissue	3 Percutaneous	2 Anti-infective	8 Oxazolidinones 9 Other Anti-infective A Anti-Infective Envelope
1 Subcutaneous Tissue	3 Percutaneous	3 Anti-inflammatory 4 Serum, Toxoid, and Vaccine 6 Nutritional Substance 7 Electrolytic and Water Balance Substance B Local Anesthetic H Radioactive Substance K Other Diagnostic Substance N Analgesics, Hypnotics, Sedatives T Destructive Agent	Z No Qualifier
1 Subcutaneous Tissue	3 Percutaneous	G Other Therapeutic Substance	C Other Substance
1 Subcutaneous Tissue	3 Percutaneous	V Hormone	G Insulin J Other Hormone
2 Muscle	3 Percutaneous	0 Antineoplastic	5 Other Antineoplastic M Monoclonal Antibody

◀ New   ◀ Revised   ~~deleted~~ Deleted   ♀ Females Only   ♂ Males Only
Noncovered   Limited Coverage   Hospital-Acquired Condition   **Coding Clinic**

SECTION: 3 ADMINISTRATION

BODY SYSTEM: E PHYSIOLOGICAL SYSTEMS AND ANATOMICAL REGIONS

OPERATION: 0 INTRODUCTION: *(continued)*

Putting in or on a therapeutic, diagnostic, nutritional, physiological, or prophylactic substance except blood or blood products

Body System / Region	Approach	Substance	Qualifier
2 Muscle	3 Percutaneous	2 Anti-infective	8 Oxazolidinones 9 Other Anti-infective
2 Muscle	3 Percutaneous	3 Anti-inflammatory 4 Serum, Toxoid, and Vaccine 6 Nutritional Substance 7 Electrolytic and Water Balance Substance B Local Anesthetic H Radioactive Substance K Other Diagnostic Substance N Analgesics, Hypnotics, Sedatives T Destructive Agent	Z No Qualifier
2 Muscle	3 Percutaneous	G Other Therapeutic Substance	C Other Substance
3 Peripheral Vein	0 Open	0 Antineoplastic	2 High-dose Interleukin-2 3 Low-dose Interleukin-2 5 Other Antineoplastic M Monoclonal Antibody P Clofarabine
3 Peripheral Vein	0 Open	1 Thrombolytic	6 Recombinant Human-activated Protein C 7 Other Thrombolytic
3 Peripheral Vein	0 Open	2 Anti-infective	8 Oxazolidinones 9 Other Anti-infective
3 Peripheral Vein	0 Open	3 Anti-inflammatory 4 Serum, Toxoid and Vaccine 6 Nutritional Substance 7 Electrolytic and Water Balance Substance F Intracirculatory Anesthetic H Radioactive Substance K Other Diagnostic Substance N Analgesics, Hypnotics, Sedatives P Platelet Inhibitor R Antiarrhythmic T Destructive Agent X Vasopressor	Z No Qualifier
3 Peripheral Vein	0 Open	G Other Therapeutic Substance	C Other Substance N Blood Brain Barrier Disruption
3 Peripheral Vein	0 Open	U Pancreatic Islet Cells	0 Autologous 1 Nonautologous
3 Peripheral Vein	0 Open	V Hormone	G Insulin H Human B-type Natriuretic Peptide J Other Hormone
3 Peripheral Vein	0 Open	W Immunotherapeutic	K Immunostimulator L Immunosuppressive

◀ New   ◀ Revised   ~~deleted~~ Deleted   ♀ Females Only   ♂ Males Only
 Noncovered   Limited Coverage   Hospital-Acquired Condition   **Coding Clinic**

507

SECTION: 3 ADMINISTRATION
BODY SYSTEM: E PHYSIOLOGICAL SYSTEMS AND ANATOMICAL REGIONS
OPERATION: 0 INTRODUCTION: *(continued)*

Putting in or on a therapeutic, diagnostic, nutritional, physiological, or prophylactic substance except blood or blood products

Body System / Region	Approach	Substance	Qualifier
3 Peripheral Vein	3 Percutaneous	0 Antineoplastic	2 High-dose Interleukin-2 3 Low-dose Interleukin-2 5 Other Antineoplastic M Monoclonal Antibody P Clofarabine
3 Peripheral Vein	3 Percutaneous	1 Thrombolytic	6 Recombinant Human-activated Protein C 7 Other Thrombolytic
3 Peripheral Vein	3 Percutaneous	2 Anti-infective	8 Oxazolidinones 9 Other Anti-infective
3 Peripheral Vein	3 Percutaneous	3 Anti-inflammatory 4 Serum, Toxoid and Vaccine 6 Nutritional Substance 7 Electrolytic and Water Balance Substance F Intracirculatory Anesthetic H Radioactive Substance K Other Diagnostic Substance N Analgesics, Hypnotics, Sedatives P Platelet Inhibitor R Antiarrhythmic T Destructive Agent X Vasopressor	Z No Qualifier
3 Peripheral Vein	3 Percutaneous	G Other Therapeutic Substance	C Other Substance N Blood Brain Barrier Disruption Q Glucarpidase
3 Peripheral Vein	3 Percutaneous	U Pancreatic Islet Cells	0 Autologous 1 Nonautologous
3 Peripheral Vein	3 Percutaneous	V Hormone	G Insulin H Human B-type Natriuretic Peptide J Other Hormone
3 Peripheral Vein	3 Percutaneous	W Immunotherapeutic	K Immunostimulator L Immunosuppressive
4 Central Vein	0 Open	0 Antineoplastic	2 High-dose Interleukin-2 3 Low-dose Interleukin-2 5 Other Antineoplastic M Monoclonal Antibody P Clofarabine
4 Central Vein	0 Open	1 Thrombolytic	6 Recombinant Human-activated Protein C 7 Other Thrombolytic
4 Central Vein	0 Open	2 Anti-infective	8 Oxazolidinones 9 Other Anti-infective

◀ New ◀ Revised ~~deleted~~ Deleted ♀ Females Only ♂ Males Only
Ⓝ Noncovered Ⓛ Limited Coverage Hospital-Acquired Condition **Coding Clinic**

SECTION: 3 ADMINISTRATION

BODY SYSTEM: E PHYSIOLOGICAL SYSTEMS AND ANATOMICAL REGIONS
OPERATION: 0 INTRODUCTION: *(continued)*

Putting in or on a therapeutic, diagnostic, nutritional, physiological, or prophylactic substance except blood or blood products

Body System / Region	Approach	Substance	Qualifier
4 Central Vein	0 Open	3 Anti-inflammatory 4 Serum, Toxoid and Vaccine 6 Nutritional Substance 7 Electrolytic and Water Balance Substance F Intracirculatory Anesthetic H Radioactive Substance K Other Diagnostic Substance N Analgesics, Hypnotics, Sedatives P Platelet Inhibitor R Antiarrhythmic T Destructive Agent X Vasopressor	Z No Qualifier
4 Central Vein	0 Open	G Other Therapeutic Substance	C Other Substance N Blood Brain Barrier Disruption
4 Central Vein	0 Open	V Hormone	G Insulin H Human B-type Natriuretic Peptide J Other Hormone
4 Central Vein	0 Open	W Immunotherapeutic	K Immunostimulator L Immunosuppressive
4 Central Vein	3 Percutaneous	0 Antineoplastic	2 High-dose Interleukin-2 3 Low-dose Interleukin-2 5 Other Antineoplastic M Monoclonal Antibody P Clofarabine
4 Central Vein	3 Percutaneous	1 Thrombolytic	6 Recombinant Human-activated Protein C 7 Other Thrombolytic
4 Central Vein	3 Percutaneous	2 Anti-infective	8 Oxazolidinones 9 Other Anti-infective
4 Central Vein	3 Percutaneous	3 Anti-inflammatory 4 Serum, Toxoid and Vaccine 6 Nutritional Substance 7 Electrolytic and Water Balance Substance F Intracirculatory Anesthetic H Radioactive Substance K Other Diagnostic Substance N Analgesics, Hypnotics, Sedatives P Platelet Inhibitor R Antiarrhythmic T Destructive Agent X Vasopressor	Z No Qualifier
4 Central Vein	3 Percutaneous	G Other Therapeutic Substance	C Other Substance N Blood Brain Barrier Disruption Q Glucarpidase
4 Central Vein	3 Percutaneous	V Hormone	G Insulin H Human B-type Natriuretic Peptide J Other Hormone

SECTION: 3 ADMINISTRATION
BODY SYSTEM: E PHYSIOLOGICAL SYSTEMS AND ANATOMICAL REGIONS
OPERATION: 0 INTRODUCTION: *(continued)*
Putting in or on a therapeutic, diagnostic, nutritional, physiological, or prophylactic substance except blood or blood products

Body System / Region	Approach	Substance	Qualifier
4 Central Vein	3 Percutaneous	W Immunotherapeutic	K Immunostimulator L Immunosuppressive
5 Peripheral Artery 6 Central Artery	0 Open 3 Percutaneous	0 Antineoplastic	2 High-dose Interleukin-2 3 Low-dose Interleukin-2 5 Other Antineoplastic M Monoclonal Antibody P Clofarabine
5 Peripheral Artery 6 Central Artery	0 Open 3 Percutaneous	1 Thrombolytic	6 Recombinant Human-activated Protein C 7 Other Thrombolytic
5 Peripheral Artery 6 Central Artery	0 Open 3 Percutaneous	2 Anti-infective	8 Oxazolidinones 9 Other Anti-infective
5 Peripheral Artery 6 Central Artery	0 Open 3 Percutaneous	3 Anti-inflammatory 4 Serum, Toxoid and Vaccine 6 Nutritional Substance 7 Electrolytic and Water Balance Substance F Intracirculatory Anesthetic H Radioactive Substance K Other Diagnostic Substance N Analgesics, Hypnotics, Sedatives P Platelet Inhibitor R Antiarrhythmic T Destructive Agent X Vasopressor	Z No Qualifier
5 Peripheral Artery 6 Central Artery	0 Open 3 Percutaneous	G Other Therapeutic Substance	C Other Substance N Blood Brain Barrier Disruption
5 Peripheral Artery 6 Central Artery	0 Open 3 Percutaneous	V Hormone	G Insulin H Human B-type Natriuretic Peptide J Other Hormone
5 Peripheral Artery 6 Central Artery	0 Open 3 Percutaneous	W Immunotherapeutic	K Immunostimulator L Immunosuppressive
7 Coronary Artery 8 Heart	0 Open 3 Percutaneous	1 Thrombolytic	6 Recombinant Human-activated Protein C 7 Other Thrombolytic
7 Coronary Artery 8 Heart	0 Open 3 Percutaneous	G Other Therapeutic Substance	C Other Substance
7 Coronary Artery 8 Heart	0 Open 3 Percutaneous	K Other Diagnostic Substance P Platelet Inhibitor	Z No Qualifier
9 Nose	3 Percutaneous 7 Via Natural or Artificial Opening X External	0 Antineoplastic	5 Other Antineoplastic M Monoclonal Antibody
9 Nose	3 Percutaneous 7 Via Natural or Artificial Opening X External	2 Anti-infective	8 Oxazolidinones 9 Other Anti-infective

◀ New   ◀ Revised   ~~deleted~~ Deleted   ♀ Females Only   ♂ Males Only
℞ Noncovered   ℞ Limited Coverage   ℞ Hospital-Acquired Condition   **Coding Clinic**

SECTION: 3 ADMINISTRATION
BODY SYSTEM: E PHYSIOLOGICAL SYSTEMS AND ANATOMICAL REGIONS
OPERATION: 0 INTRODUCTION: *(continued)*

Putting in or on a therapeutic, diagnostic, nutritional, physiological, or prophylactic substance except blood or blood products

Body System / Region	Approach	Substance	Qualifier
9 Nose	3 Percutaneous 7 Via Natural or Artificial Opening X External	3 Anti-inflammatory 4 Serum, Toxoid and Vaccine B Local Anesthetic H Radioactive Substance K Other Diagnostic Substance N Analgesics, Hypnotics, Sedatives T Destructive Agent	Z No Qualifier
9 Nose	3 Percutaneous 7 Via Natural or Artificial Opening X External	G Other Therapeutic Substance	C Other Substance
A Bone Marrow	3 Percutaneous	0 Antineoplastic	5 Other Antineoplastic M Monoclonal Antibody
A Bone Marrow	3 Percutaneous	G Other Therapeutic Substance	C Other Substance
B Ear	3 Percutaneous 7 Via Natural or Artificial Opening X External	0 Antineoplastic	4 Liquid Brachytherapy Radioisotope 5 Other Antineoplastic M Monoclonal Antibody
B Ear	3 Percutaneous 7 Via Natural or Artificial Opening X External	2 Anti-infective	8 Oxazolidinones 9 Other Anti-infective
B Ear	3 Percutaneous 7 Via Natural or Artificial Opening X External	3 Anti-inflammatory B Local Anesthetic H Radioactive Substance K Other Diagnostic Substance N Analgesics, Hypnotics, Sedatives T Destructive Agent	Z No Qualifier
B Ear	3 Percutaneous 7 Via Natural or Artificial Opening X External	G Other Therapeutic Substance	C Other Substance
C Eye	3 Percutaneous 7 Via Natural or Artificial Opening X External	0 Antineoplastic	4 Liquid Brachytherapy Radioisotope 5 Other Antineoplastic M Monoclonal Antibody
C Eye	3 Percutaneous 7 Via Natural or Artificial Opening X External	2 Anti-infective	8 Oxazolidinones 9 Other Anti-infective
C Eye	3 Percutaneous 7 Via Natural or Artificial Opening X External	3 Anti-inflammatory B Local Anesthetic H Radioactive Substance K Other Diagnostic Substance M Pigment N Analgesics, Hypnotics, Sedatives T Destructive Agent	Z No Qualifier
C Eye	3 Percutaneous 7 Via Natural or Artificial Opening X External	G Other Therapeutic Substance	C Other Substance
C Eye	3 Percutaneous 7 Via Natural or Artificial Opening X External	S Gas	F Other Gas

SECTION: 3 ADMINISTRATION
BODY SYSTEM: E PHYSIOLOGICAL SYSTEMS AND ANATOMICAL REGIONS
OPERATION: 0 INTRODUCTION: *(continued)*

Putting in or on a therapeutic, diagnostic, nutritional, physiological, or prophylactic substance except blood or blood products

Body System / Region	Approach	Substance	Qualifier
D Mouth and Pharynx	3 Percutaneous 7 Via Natural or Artificial Opening X External	0 Antineoplastic	4 Liquid Brachytherapy Radioisotope 5 Other Antineoplastic M Monoclonal Antibody
D Mouth and Pharynx	3 Percutaneous 7 Via Natural or Artificial Opening X External	2 Anti-infective	8 Oxazolidinones 9 Other Anti-infective
D Mouth and Pharynx	3 Percutaneous 7 Via Natural or Artificial Opening X External	3 Anti-inflammatory 4 Serum, Toxoid and Vaccine 6 Nutritional Substance 7 Electrolytic and Water Balance Substance B Local Anesthetic H Radioactive Substance K Other Diagnostic Substance N Analgesics, Hypnotics, Sedatives R Antiarrhythmic T Destructive Agent	Z No Qualifier
D Mouth and Pharynx	3 Percutaneous 7 Via Natural or Artificial Opening X External	G Other Therapeutic Substance	C Other Substance
E Products of Conception ♀ G Upper GI H Lower GI K Genitourinary Tract N Male Reproductive ♂	3 Percutaneous 7 Via Natural or Artificial Opening 8 Via Natural or Artificial Opening Endoscopic	0 Antineoplastic	4 Liquid Brachytherapy Radioisotope 5 Other Antineoplastic M Monoclonal Antibody
E Products of Conception ♀ G Upper GI H Lower GI K Genitourinary Tract N Male Reproductive ♂	3 Percutaneous 7 Via Natural or Artificial Opening 8 Via Natural or Artificial Opening Endoscopic	2 Anti-infective	8 Oxazolidinones 9 Other Anti-infective
E Products of Conception ♀ G Upper GI H Lower GI K Genitourinary Tract N Male Reproductive ♂	3 Percutaneous 7 Via Natural or Artificial Opening 8 Via Natural or Artificial Opening Endoscopic	3 Anti-inflammatory 6 Nutritional Substance 7 Electrolytic and Water Balance Substance B Local Anesthetic H Radioactive Substance K Other Diagnostic Substance N Analgesics, Hypnotics, Sedatives T Destructive Agent	Z No Qualifier
E Products of Conception ♀ G Upper GI H Lower GI K Genitourinary Tract N Male Reproductive ♂	3 Percutaneous 7 Via Natural or Artificial Opening 8 Via Natural or Artificial Opening Endoscopic	G Other Therapeutic Substance	C Other Substance
E Products of Conception ♀ G Upper GI H Lower GI K Genitourinary Tract N Male Reproductive ♂	3 Percutaneous 7 Via Natural or Artificial Opening 8 Via Natural or Artificial Opening Endoscopic	S Gas	F Other Gas

New　Revised　deleted Deleted　♀ Females Only　♂ Males Only
Noncovered　Limited Coverage　Hospital-Acquired Condition　**Coding Clinic**

SECTION: 3 ADMINISTRATION
BODY SYSTEM: E PHYSIOLOGICAL SYSTEMS AND ANATOMICAL REGIONS
OPERATION: 0 INTRODUCTION: *(continued)*

Putting in or on a therapeutic, diagnostic, nutritional, physiological, or prophylactic substance except blood or blood products

Body System / Region	Approach	Substance	Qualifier
F Respiratory Tract	3 Percutaneous	0 Antineoplastic	4 Liquid Brachytherapy Radioisotope 5 Other Antineoplastic M Monoclonal Antibody
F Respiratory Tract	3 Percutaneous	2 Anti-infective	8 Oxazolidinones 9 Other Anti-infective
F Respiratory Tract	3 Percutaneous	3 Anti-inflammatory 6 Nutritional Substance 7 Electrolytic and Water Balance Substance B Local Anesthetic H Radioactive Substance K Other Diagnostic Substance N Analgesics, Hypnotics, Sedatives T Destructive Agent	Z No Qualifier
F Respiratory Tract	3 Percutaneous	G Other Therapeutic Substance	C Other Substance
F Respiratory Tract	3 Percutaneous	S Gas	D Nitric Oxide F Other Gas
F Respiratory Tract	7 Via Natural or Artificial Opening 8 Via Natural or Artificial Opening Endoscopic	0 Antineoplastic	4 Liquid Brachytherapy Radioisotope 5 Other Antineoplastic M Monoclonal Antibody
F Respiratory Tract	7 Via Natural or Artificial Opening 8 Via Natural or Artificial Opening Endoscopic	2 Anti-infective	8 Oxazolidinones 9 Other Anti-infective
F Respiratory Tract	7 Via Natural or Artificial Opening 8 Via Natural or Artificial Opening Endoscopic	3 Anti-inflammatory 6 Nutritional Substance 7 Electrolytic and Water Balance Substance B Local Anesthetic D Inhalation Anesthetic H Radioactive Substance K Other Diagnostic Substance N Analgesics, Hypnotics, Sedatives T Destructive Agent	Z No Qualifier
F Respiratory Tract	7 Via Natural or Artificial Opening 8 Via Natural or Artificial Opening Endoscopic	G Other Therapeutic Substance	C Other Substance
F Respiratory Tract	7 Via Natural or Artificial Opening 8 Via Natural or Artificial Opening Endoscopic	S Gas	D Nitric Oxide F Other Gas
J Biliary and Pancreatic Tract	3 Percutaneous 7 Via Natural or Artificial Opening 8 Via Natural or Artificial Opening Endoscopic	0 Antineoplastic	4 Liquid Brachytherapy Radioisotope 5 Other Antineoplastic M Monoclonal Antibody
J Biliary and Pancreatic Tract	3 Percutaneous 7 Via Natural or Artificial Opening 8 Via Natural or Artificial Opening Endoscopic	2 Anti-infective	8 Oxazolidinones 9 Other Anti-infective

◀ New   ◀▥ Revised   ~~deleted~~ Deleted   ♀ Females Only   ♂ Males Only
🅝 Noncovered   🅛 Limited Coverage   🅗 Hospital-Acquired Condition   **Coding Clinic**

513

0: INTRODUCTION

E: PHYSIOLOGICAL SYSTEMS AND ANATOMICAL REGIONS

3: ADMINISTRATION

SECTION: 3 ADMINISTRATION
BODY SYSTEM: E PHYSIOLOGICAL SYSTEMS AND ANATOMICAL REGIONS
OPERATION: 0 INTRODUCTION: *(continued)*

Putting in or on a therapeutic, diagnostic, nutritional, physiological, or prophylactic substance except blood or blood products

Body System / Region	Approach	Substance	Qualifier
J Biliary and Pancreatic Tract	3 Percutaneous 7 Via Natural or Artificial Opening 8 Via Natural or Artificial Opening Endoscopic	3 Anti-inflammatory 6 Nutritional Substance 7 Electrolytic and Water Balance Substance B Local Anesthetic H Radioactive Substance K Other Diagnostic Substance N Analgesics, Hypnotics, Sedatives T Destructive Agent	Z No Qualifier
J Biliary and Pancreatic Tract	3 Percutaneous 7 Via Natural or Artificial Opening 8 Via Natural or Artificial Opening Endoscopic	G Other Therapeutic Substance	C Other Substance
J Biliary and Pancreatic Tract	3 Percutaneous 7 Via Natural or Artificial Opening 8 Via Natural or Artificial Opening Endoscopic	S Gas	F Other Gas
J Biliary and Pancreatic Tract	3 Percutaneous 7 Via Natural or Artificial Opening 8 Via Natural or Artificial Opening Endoscopic	U Pancreatic Islet Cells	0 Autologous 1 Nonautologous
L Pleural Cavity M Peritoneal Cavity	0 Open	5 Adhesion Barrier	Z No Qualifier
L Pleural Cavity M Peritoneal Cavity	3 Percutaneous	0 Antineoplastic	4 Liquid Brachytherapy Radioisotope 5 Other Antineoplastic M Monoclonal Antibody
L Pleural Cavity M Peritoneal Cavity	3 Percutaneous	2 Anti-infective	8 Oxazolidinones 9 Other Anti-infective
L Pleural Cavity M Peritoneal Cavity	3 Percutaneous	3 Anti-inflammatory 6 Nutritional Substance 7 Electrolytic and Water Balance Substance B Local Anesthetic H Radioactive Substance K Other Diagnostic Substance N Analgesics, Hypnotics, Sedatives T Destructive Agent	Z No Qualifier
L Pleural Cavity M Peritoneal Cavity	3 Percutaneous	G Other Therapeutic Substance	C Other Substance
L Pleural Cavity M Peritoneal Cavity	3 Percutaneous	S Gas	F Other Gas
L Pleural Cavity M Peritoneal Cavity	7 Via Natural or Artificial Opening	0 Antineoplastic	4 Liquid Brachytherapy Radioisotope 5 Other Antineoplastic M Monoclonal Antibody
L Pleural Cavity M Peritoneal Cavity	7 Via Natural or Artificial Opening	S Gas	F Other Gas
P Female Reproductive ♀	0 Open	5 Adhesion Barrier	Z No Qualifier

SECTION: 3 ADMINISTRATION
BODY SYSTEM: E PHYSIOLOGICAL SYSTEMS AND ANATOMICAL REGIONS
OPERATION: 0 INTRODUCTION: *(continued)*
Putting in or on a therapeutic, diagnostic, nutritional, physiological, or prophylactic substance except blood or blood products

Body System / Region	Approach	Substance	Qualifier
P Female Reproductive ♀	3 Percutaneous 7 Via Natural or Artificial Opening	0 Antineoplastic	4 Liquid Brachytherapy Radioisotope 5 Other Antineoplastic M Monoclonal Antibody
P Female Reproductive ♀	3 Percutaneous 7 Via Natural or Artificial Opening	2 Anti-infective	8 Oxazolidinones 9 Other Anti-infective
P Female Reproductive ♀	3 Percutaneous 7 Via Natural or Artificial Opening	3 Anti-inflammatory 6 Nutritional Substance 7 Electrolytic and Water Balance Substance B Local Anesthetic H Radioactive Substance K Other Diagnostic Substance L Sperm N Analgesics, Hypnotics, Sedatives T Destructive Agent	Z No Qualifier
P Female Reproductive ♀	3 Percutaneous 7 Via Natural or Artificial Opening	G Other Therapeutic Substance	C Other Substance
P Female Reproductive ♀	3 Percutaneous 7 Via Natural or Artificial Opening	Q Fertilized Ovum	0 Autologous 1 Nonautologous
P Female Reproductive ♀	3 Percutaneous 7 Via Natural or Artificial Opening	S Gas	F Other Gas
P Female Reproductive ♀	8 Via Natural or Artificial Opening Endoscopic	0 Antineoplastic	4 Liquid Brachytherapy Radioisotope 5 Other Antineoplastic M Monoclonal Antibody
P Female Reproductive ♀	8 Via Natural or Artificial Opening Endoscopic	2 Anti-infective	8 Oxazolidinones 9 Other Anti-infective
P Female Reproductive ♀	8 Via Natural or Artificial Opening Endoscopic	3 Anti-inflammatory 6 Nutritional Substance 7 Electrolytic and Water Balance Substance B Local Anesthetic H Radioactive Substance K Other Diagnostic Substance N Analgesics, Hypnotics, Sedatives T Destructive Agent	Z No Qualifier
P Female Reproductive ♀	8 Via Natural or Artificial Opening Endoscopic	G Other Therapeutic Substance	C Other Substance
P Female Reproductive ♀	8 Via Natural or Artificial Opening Endoscopic	S Gas	F Other Gas
Q Cranial Cavity and Brain	0 Open	A Stem Cells, Embryonic	Z No Qualifier
Q Cranial Cavity and Brain	0 Open	E Stem Cells, Somatic	0 Autologous 1 Nonautologous
Q Cranial Cavity and Brain	3 Percutaneous	0 Antineoplastic	4 Liquid Brachytherapy Radioisotope 5 Other Antineoplastic M Monoclonal Antibody
Q Cranial Cavity and Brain	3 Percutaneous	2 Anti-infective	8 Oxazolidinones 9 Other Anti-infective

◀ New ◀▮ Revised ~~deleted~~ Deleted ♀ Females Only ♂ Males Only
🚫 Noncovered 🔒 Limited Coverage ⬢ Hospital-Acquired Condition **Coding Clinic**

515

SECTION: 3 ADMINISTRATION
BODY SYSTEM: E **PHYSIOLOGICAL SYSTEMS AND ANATOMICAL REGIONS**
OPERATION: 0 **INTRODUCTION:** *(continued)*

Putting in or on a therapeutic, diagnostic, nutritional, physiological, or prophylactic substance except blood or blood products

Body System / Region	Approach	Substance	Qualifier
Q Cranial Cavity and Brain	3 Percutaneous	3 Anti-inflammatory 6 Nutritional Substance 7 Electrolytic and Water Balance Substance A Stem Cells, Embryonic B Local Anesthetic H Radioactive Substance K Other Diagnostic Substance N Analgesics, Hypnotics, Sedatives T Destructive Agent	Z No Qualifier
Q Cranial Cavity and Brain	3 Percutaneous	E Stem Cells, Somatic	0 Autologous 1 Nonautologous
Q Cranial Cavity and Brain	3 Percutaneous	G Other Therapeutic Substance	C Other Substance
Q Cranial Cavity and Brain	3 Percutaneous	S Gas	F Other Gas
Q Cranial Cavity and Brain	7 Via Natural or Artificial Opening	0 Antineoplastic	4 Liquid Brachytherapy Radioisotope 5 Other Antineoplastic M Monoclonal Antibody
Q Cranial Cavity and Brain	7 Via Natural or Artificial Opening	S Gas	F Other Gas
R Spinal Canal	0 Open	A Stem Cells, Embryonic	Z No Qualifier
R Spinal Canal	0 Open	A Stem Cells, Somatic	0 Autologous 1 Nonautologous
R Spinal Canal	3 Percutaneous	0 Antineoplastic	2 High-dose Interleukin-2 3 Low-dose Interleukin-2 4 Liquid Brachytherapy Radioisotope 5 Other Antineoplastic M Monoclonal Antibody
R Spinal Canal	3 Percutaneous	2 Anti-infective	8 Oxazolidinones 9 Other Anti-infective
R Spinal Canal	3 Percutaneous	3 Anti-inflammatory 6 Nutritional Substance 7 Electrolytic and Water Balance Substance A Stem Cells, Embryonic B Local Anesthetic C Regional Anesthetic H Radioactive Substance K Other Diagnostic Substance N Analgesics, Hypnotics, Sedatives T Destructive Agent	Z No Qualifier
R Spinal Canal	3 Percutaneous	E Stem Cells, Somatic	0 Autologous 1 Nonautologous
R Spinal Canal	3 Percutaneous	G Other Therapeutic Substance	C Other Substance
R Spinal Canal	3 Percutaneous	S Gas	F Other Gas
R Spinal Canal	7 Via Natural or Artificial Opening	S Gas	F Other Gas

◀ New   ◀ Revised   ~~deleted~~ Deleted   ♀ Females Only   ♂ Males Only
Noncovered   Limited Coverage   Hospital-Acquired Condition   **Coding Clinic**

SECTION: 3 ADMINISTRATION

BODY SYSTEM: E PHYSIOLOGICAL SYSTEMS AND ANATOMICAL REGIONS

OPERATION: 0 INTRODUCTION: *(continued)*

Putting in or on a therapeutic, diagnostic, nutritional, physiological, or prophylactic substance except blood or blood products

Body System / Region	Approach	Substance	Qualifier
S Epidural Space	3 Percutaneous	0 Antineoplastic	2 High-dose Interleukin-2 3 Low-dose Interleukin-2 4 Liquid Brachytherapy Radioisotope 5 Other Antineoplastic M Monoclonal Antibody
S Epidural Space	3 Percutaneous	2 Anti-infective	8 Oxazolidinones 9 Other Anti-infective
S Epidural Space	3 Percutaneous	3 Anti-inflammatory 6 Nutritional Substance 7 Electrolytic and Water Balance Substance B Local Anesthetic C Regional Anesthetic H Radioactive Substance K Other Diagnostic Substance N Analgesics, Hypnotics, Sedatives T Destructive Agent	Z No Qualifier
S Epidural Space	3 Percutaneous	G Other Therapeutic Substance	C Other Substance
S Epidural Space	3 Percutaneous	S Gas	F Other Gas
S Epidural Space	7 Via Natural or Artificial Opening	S Gas	F Other Gas
T Peripheral Nerves and Plexi X Cranial Nerves	3 Percutaneous	3 Anti-inflammatory B Local Anesthetic C Regional Anesthetic T Destructive Agent	Z No Qualifier
T Peripheral Nerves and Plexi X Cranial Nerves	3 Percutaneous	G Other Therapeutic Substance	C Other Substance
U Joints	0 Open	2 Anti-infective	8 Oxazolidinones 9 Other Anti-infective
U Joints	0 Open	G Other Therapeutic Substance	B Recombinant Bone Morphogenetic Protein
U Joints	3 Percutaneous	0 Antineoplastic	4 Liquid Brachytherapy Radioisotope 5 Other Antineoplastic M Monoclonal Antibody
U Joints	3 Percutaneous	2 Anti-infective	8 Oxazolidinones 9 Other Anti-infective
U Joints	3 Percutaneous	3 Anti-inflammatory 6 Nutritional Substance 7 Electrolytic and Water Balance Substance B Local Anesthetic H Radioactive Substance K Other Diagnostic Substance N Analgesics, Hypnotics, Sedatives T Destructive Agent	Z No Qualifier
U Joints	3 Percutaneous	G Other Therapeutic Substance	B Recombinant Bone Morphogenetic Protein C Other Substance

0: INTRODUCTION

E: PHYSIOLOGICAL SYSTEMS AND ANATOMICAL REGIONS

3: ADMINISTRATION

SECTION: 3 ADMINISTRATION
BODY SYSTEM: E PHYSIOLOGICAL SYSTEMS AND ANATOMICAL REGIONS
OPERATION: 0 INTRODUCTION: *(continued)*

Putting in or on a therapeutic, diagnostic, nutritional, physiological, or prophylactic substance except blood or blood products

Body System / Region	Approach	Substance	Qualifier
U Joints	3 Percutaneous	S Gas	F Other Gas
V Bones	0 Open	G Other Therapeutic Substance	B Recombinant Bone Morphogenetic Protein
V Bones	3 Percutaneous	0 Antineoplastic	5 Other Antineoplastic M Monoclonal Antibody
V Bones	3 Percutaneous	2 Anti-infective	8 Oxazolidinones 9 Other Anti-infective
V Bones	3 Percutaneous	3 Anti-inflammatory 6 Nutritional Substance 7 Electrolytic and Water Balance Substance B Local Anesthetic H Radioactive Substance K Other Diagnostic Substance N Analgesics, Hypnotics, Sedatives T Destructive Agent	Z No Qualifier
V Bones	3 Percutaneous	G Other Therapeutic Substance	B Recombinant Bone Morphogenetic Protein C Other Substance
W Lymphatics	3 Percutaneous	0 Antineoplastic	5 Other Antineoplastic M Monoclonal Antibody
W Lymphatics	3 Percutaneous	2 Anti-infective	8 Oxazolidinones 9 Other Anti-infective
W Lymphatics	3 Percutaneous	3 Anti-inflammatory 6 Nutritional Substance 7 Electrolytic and Water Balance Substance B Local Anesthetic H Radioactive Substance K Other Diagnostic Substance N Analgesics, Hypnotics, Sedatives T Destructive Agent	Z No Qualifier

◀ New   ◀ Revised   deleted Deleted   ♀ Females Only   ♂ Males Only
Noncovered   Limited Coverage   Hospital-Acquired Condition   **Coding Clinic**

SECTION: 3 ADMINISTRATION
BODY SYSTEM: E PHYSIOLOGICAL SYSTEMS AND ANATOMICAL REGIONS
OPERATION: 0 INTRODUCTION: *(continued)*

Putting in or on a therapeutic, diagnostic, nutritional, physiological, or prophylactic substance except blood or blood products

Body System / Region	Approach	Substance	Qualifier
W Lymphatics	3 Percutaneous	G Other Therapeutic Substance	C Other Substance
Y Pericardial Cavity	3 Percutaneous	0 Antineoplastic	4 Liquid Brachytherapy Radioisotope 5 Other Antineoplastic M Monoclonal Antibody
Y Pericardial Cavity	3 Percutaneous	2 Anti-infective	8 Oxazolidinones 9 Other Anti-infective
Y Pericardial Cavity	3 Percutaneous	3 Anti-inflammatory 6 Nutritional Substance 7 Electrolytic and Water Balance Substance B Local Anesthetic H Radioactive Substance K Other Diagnostic Substance N Analgesics, Hypnotics, Sedatives T Destructive Agent	Z No Qualifier
Y Pericardial Cavity	3 Percutaneous	G Other Therapeutic Substance	C Other Substance
Y Pericardial Cavity	3 Percutaneous	S Gas	F Other Gas
Y Pericardial Cavity	7 Via Natural or Artificial Opening	0 Antineoplastic	4 Liquid Brachytherapy Radioisotope 5 Other Antineoplastic M Monoclonal Antibody
Y Pericardial Cavity	7 Via Natural or Artificial Opening	S Gas	F Other Gas

Coding Clinic: 2013, Q1, P27 – 3E0G8TZ

◀ New   ◀ Revised   deleted Deleted   ♀ Females Only   ♂ Males Only
ⓃⒸ Noncovered   ⓁⒸ Limited Coverage   ⒽⒶⒸ Hospital-Acquired Condition   **Coding Clinic**

SECTION: 3 ADMINISTRATION
BODY SYSTEM: E PHYSIOLOGICAL SYSTEMS AND ANATOMICAL REGIONS
OPERATION: 1 IRRIGATION: Putting in or on a cleansing substance

Body System / Region	Approach	Substance	Qualifier
0 Skin and Mucous Membranes C Eye	3 Percutaneous X External	8 Irrigating Substance	X Diagnostic Z No Qualifier
9 Nose B Ear F Respiratory Tract G Upper GI H Lower GI J Biliary and Pancreatic Tract K Genitourinary Tract N Male Reproductive ♂ P Female Reproductive ♀	3 Percutaneous 7 Via Natural or Artificial Opening 8 Via Natural or Artificial Opening Endoscopic	8 Irrigating Substance	X Diagnostic Z No Qualifier
L Pleural Cavity Q Cranial Cavity and Brain R Spinal Canal S Epidural Space U Joints Y Pericardial Cavity	3 Percutaneous	8 Irrigating Substance	X Diagnostic Z No Qualifier
M Peritoneal Cavity	3 Percutaneous	8 Irrigating Substance	X Diagnostic Z No Qualifier
M Peritoneal Cavity	3 Percutaneous	9 Dialysate	Z No Qualifier

◀ New   ◀▥ Revised   d̶e̶l̶e̶t̶e̶d̶ Deleted   ♀ Females Only   ♂ Males Only
🆀 Noncovered   🆀 Limited Coverage   🆀 Hospital-Acquired Condition   **Coding Clinic**

SECTION: 4 MEASUREMENT AND MONITORING
BODY SYSTEM: A PHYSIOLOGICAL SYSTEMS
OPERATION: 0 MEASUREMENT: *(on multiple pages)*
Determining the level of a physiological or physical function at a point in time

0: MEASUREMENT

A: PHYSIOLOGICAL SYSTEMS

4: MEASUREMENT AND MONITORING

Body System	Approach	Function / Device	Qualifier
0 Central Nervous	0 Open	2 Conductivity 4 Electrical Activity B Pressure	Z No Qualifier
0 Central Nervous	3 Percutaneous	4 Electrical Activity	Z No Qualifier
0 Central Nervous	3 Percutaneous	B Pressure K Temperature R Saturation	D Intracranial
0 Central Nervous	7 Via Natural or Artificial Opening	B Pressure K Temperature R Saturation	D Intracranial
0 Central Nervous	X External	2 Conductivity 4 Electrical Activity	Z No Qualifier
1 Peripheral Nervous	0 Open 3 Percutaneous X External	2 Conductivity	9 Sensory B Motor
1 Peripheral Nervous	0 Open 3 Percutaneous X External	4 Electrical Activity	Z No Qualifier
2 Cardiac	0 Open 3 Percutaneous	4 Electrical Activity 9 Output C Rate F Rhythm H Sound P Action Currents	Z No Qualifier
2 Cardiac	0 Open 3 Percutaneous	N Sampling and Pressure	6 Right Heart 7 Left Heart 8 Bilateral
2 Cardiac	X External	4 Electrical Activity	A Guidance Z No Qualifier
2 Cardiac	X External	9 Output C Rate F Rhythm H Sound P Action Currents	Z No Qualifier
2 Cardiac	X External	M Total Activity	4 Stress
3 Arterial	0 Open 3 Percutaneous	5 Flow J Pulse	1 Peripheral 3 Pulmonary C Coronary
3 Arterial	0 Open 3 Percutaneous	B Pressure	1 Peripheral 3 Pulmonary C Coronary F Other Thoracic
3 Arterial	0 Open 3 Percutaneous	H Sound R Saturation	1 Peripheral

◀ New ◀ Revised ~~deleted~~ Deleted ♀ Females Only ♂ Males Only
Nc Noncovered Lc Limited Coverage Hospital-Acquired Condition **Coding Clinic**

SECTION: 4 MEASUREMENT AND MONITORING
BODY SYSTEM: A PHYSIOLOGICAL SYSTEMS
OPERATION: 0 MEASUREMENT: *(continued)*
Determining the level of a physiological or physical function
at a point in time

Body System	Approach	Function / Device	Qualifier
3 Arterial	X External	5 Flow B Pressure H Sound J Pulse R Saturation	1 Peripheral
4 Venous	0 Open 3 Percutaneous	5 Flow B Pressure J Pulse	0 Central 1 Peripheral 2 Portal 3 Pulmonary
4 Venous	0 Open 3 Percutaneous	R Saturation	1 Peripheral
4 Venous	X External	5 Flow B Pressure J Pulse R Saturation	1 Peripheral
5 Circulatory	X External	L Volume	Z No Qualifier
6 Lymphatic	0 Open 3 Percutaneous	5 Flow B Pressure	Z No Qualifier
7 Visual	X External	0 Acuity 7 Mobility B Pressure	Z No Qualifier
8 Olfactory	X External	0 Acuity	Z No Qualifier
9 Respiratory	7 Via Natural or Artificial Opening 8 Via Natural or Artificial Opening Endoscopic X External	1 Capacity 5 Flow C Rate D Resistance L Volume M Total Activity	Z No Qualifier
B Gastrointestinal	7 Via Natural or Artificial Opening 8 Via Natural or Artificial Opening Endoscopic	8 Motility B Pressure G Secretion	Z No Qualifier
C Biliary	3 Percutaneous 4 Percutaneous Endoscopic 7 Via Natural or Artificial Opening 8 Via Natural or Artificial Opening Endoscopic	5 Flow B Pressure	Z No Qualifier
D Urinary	7 Via Natural or Artificial Opening	3 Contractility 5 Flow B Pressure D Resistance L Volume	Z No Qualifier
F Musculoskeletal	3 Percutaneous X External	3 Contractility	Z No Qualifier
H Products of Conception, Cardiac ♀	7 Via Natural or Artificial Opening 8 Via Natural or Artificial Opening Endoscopic X External	4 Electrical Activity C Rate F Rhythm H Sound	Z No Qualifier

◀ New   ◀▥ Revised   deleted Deleted   ♀ Females Only   ♂ Males Only
Ⓝⓒ Noncovered   Ⓛⓒ Limited Coverage   Ⓗⓐ Hospital-Acquired Condition   **Coding Clinic**

523

SECTION: 4 MEASUREMENT AND MONITORING

BODY SYSTEM: A PHYSIOLOGICAL SYSTEMS

OPERATION: 0 MEASUREMENT: *(continued)*
Determining the level of a physiological or physical function at a point in time

Body System	Approach	Function / Device	Qualifier
J Products of Conception, Nervous ♀	7 Via Natural or Artificial Opening 8 Via Natural or Artificial Opening Endoscopic X External	2 Conductivity 4 Electrical Activity B Pressure	Z No Qualifier
Z None	7 Via Natural or Artificial Opening	6 Metabolism K Temperature	Z No Qualifier
Z None	X External	6 Metabolism K Temperature Q Sleep	Z No Qualifier

SECTION: 4 MEASUREMENT AND MONITORING

BODY SYSTEM: A PHYSIOLOGICAL SYSTEMS

OPERATION: 1 MONITORING: *(on multiple pages)*
Determining the level of a physiological or physical function repetitively over a period of time

Body System	Approach	Function / Device	Qualifier
0 Central Nervous	0 Open	2 Conductivity B Pressure	Z No Qualifier
0 Central Nervous	0 Open	4 Electrical Activity	G Intraoperative Z No Qualifier
0 Central Nervous	3 Percutaneous	4 Electrical Activity	G Intraoperative Z No Qualifier
0 Central Nervous	3 Percutaneous	B Pressure K Temperature R Saturation	D Intracranial
0 Central Nervous	7 Via Natural or Artificial Opening	B Pressure K Temperature R Saturation	D Intracranial
0 Central Nervous	X External	2 Conductivity	Z No Qualifier
0 Central Nervous	X External	4 Electrical Activity	G Intraoperative Z No Qualifier
1 Peripheral Nervous	0 Open 3 Percutaneous X External	2 Conductivity	9 Sensory B Motor
1 Peripheral Nervous	0 Open 3 Percutaneous X External	4 Electrical Activity	G Intraoperative Z No Qualifier

◀ New　　◀ Revised　　deleted Deleted　　♀ Females Only　　♂ Males Only
℞ Noncovered　　℞ Limited Coverage　　℞ Hospital-Acquired Condition　　**Coding Clinic**

SECTION: 4 MEASUREMENT AND MONITORING
BODY SYSTEM: A PHYSIOLOGICAL SYSTEMS
OPERATION: 1 MONITORING: *(continued)*
Determining the level of a physiological or physical function repetitively over a period of time

Body System	Approach	Function / Device	Qualifier
2 Cardiac	0 Open 3 Percutaneous	4 Electrical Activity 9 Output C Rate F Rhythm H Sound	Z No Qualifier
2 Cardiac	X External	4 Electrical Activity	5 Ambulatory Z No Qualifier
2 Cardiac	X External	9 Output C Rate F Rhythm H Sound	Z No Qualifier
2 Cardiac	X External	M Total Activity	4 Stress
3 Arterial	0 Open 3 Percutaneous	5 Flow B Pressure J Pulse	1 Peripheral 3 Pulmonary C Coronary
3 Arterial	0 Open 3 Percutaneous	H Sound R Saturation	1 Peripheral
3 Arterial	X External	5 Flow B Pressure H Sound J Pulse R Saturation	1 Peripheral
4 Venous	0 Open 3 Percutaneous	5 Flow B Pressure J Pulse	0 Central 1 Peripheral 2 Portal 3 Pulmonary
4 Venous	0 Open 3 Percutaneous	R Saturation	0 Central 2 Portal 3 Pulmonary
4 Venous	X External	5 Flow B Pressure J Pulse	1 Peripheral
6 Lymphatic	0 Open 3 Percutaneous	5 Flow B Pressure	Z No Qualifier
9 Respiratory	7 Via Natural or Artificial Opening X External	1 Capacity 5 Flow C Rate D Resistance L Volume	Z No Qualifier
B Gastrointestinal	7 Via Natural or Artificial Opening 8 Via Natural or Artificial Opening Endoscopic	8 Motility B Pressure G Secretion	Z No Qualifier

◄ New　◄ Revised　~~deleted~~ Deleted　♀ Females Only　♂ Males Only
🚫 Noncovered　🚫 Limited Coverage　🚫 Hospital-Acquired Condition　**Coding Clinic**

525

SECTION: 4 MEASUREMENT AND MONITORING
BODY SYSTEM: A **PHYSIOLOGICAL SYSTEMS**
OPERATION: 1 **MONITORING:** *(continued)*
Determining the level of a physiological or physical function repetitively over a period of time

Body System	Approach	Function / Device	Qualifier
D Urinary	7 Via Natural or Artificial Opening	3 Contractility 5 Flow B Pressure D Resistance L Volume	Z No Qualifier
H Products of Conception, Cardiac ♀	7 Via Natural or Artificial Opening 8 Via Natural or Artificial Opening Endoscopic X External	4 Electrical Activity C Rate F Rhythm H Sound	Z No Qualifier
J Products of Conception, Nervous ♀	7 Via Natural or Artificial Opening 8 Via Natural or Artificial Opening Endoscopic X External	2 Conductivity 4 Electrical Activity B Pressure	Z No Qualifier
Z None	7 Via Natural or Artificial Opening	K Temperature	Z No Qualifier
Z None	X External	K Temperature Q Sleep	Z No Qualifier

SECTION: 4 MEASUREMENT AND MONITORING
BODY SYSTEM: B **PHYSIOLOGICAL DEVICES**
OPERATION: 0 **MEASUREMENT:** Determining the level of a physiological or physical function at a point in time

Body System	Approach	Function / Device	Qualifier
0 Central Nervous 1 Peripheral Nervous F Musculoskeletal	X External	V Stimulator	Z No Qualifier
2 Cardiac	X External	S Pacemaker T Defibrillator	Z No Qualifier
9 Respiratory	X External	S Pacemaker	Z No Qualifier

◄ New   ◄ Revised   ~~deleted~~ Deleted   ♀ Females Only   ♂ Males Only
Noncovered   Limited Coverage   Hospital-Acquired Condition   **Coding Clinic**

◀ New   ◀Ⅲ Revised   ~~deleted~~ Deleted   ♀ Females Only   ♂ Males Only
◐ₒ Noncovered   ◐ₒ Limited Coverage   ◐ₒ Hospital-Acquired Condition   **Coding Clinic**

527

SECTION: 5 EXTRACORPOREAL ASSISTANCE AND PERFORMANCE

BODY SYSTEM: A PHYSIOLOGICAL SYSTEMS

OPERATION: 0 ASSISTANCE: Taking over a portion of a physiological function by extracorporeal means

Body System	Duration	Function	Qualifier
2 Cardiac	1 Intermittent 2 Continuous	1 Output	0 Balloon Pump 5 Pulsatile Compression 6 Pump D Impeller Pump
5 Circulatory	1 Intermittent 2 Continuous	2 Oxygenation	1 Hyperbaric C Supersaturated
9 Respiratory	3 Less than 24 Consecutive Hours 4 24-96 Consecutive Hours 5 Greater than 96 Consecutive Hours	5 Ventilation	7 Continuous Positive Airway Pressure 8 Intermittent Positive Airway Pressure 9 Continuous Negative Airway Pressure B Intermittent Negative Airway Pressure Z No Qualifier

Coding Clinic: 2013, Q3, P19 – 5A02210

◀ New   ◀ Revised   deleted Deleted   ♀ Females Only   ♂ Males Only
Noncovered   Limited Coverage   Hospital-Acquired Condition   **Coding Clinic**

SECTION: 5 EXTRACORPOREAL ASSISTANCE AND PERFORMANCE

BODY SYSTEM: A PHYSIOLOGICAL SYSTEMS
OPERATION: 1 PERFORMANCE: Completely taking over a physiological function by extracorporeal means

Body System	Duration	Function	Qualifier
2 Cardiac	0 Single	1 Output	2 Manual
2 Cardiac	1 Intermittent	3 Pacing	Z No Qualifier
2 Cardiac	2 Continuous	1 Output 3 Pacing	Z No Qualifier
5 Circulatory	2 Continuous	2 Oxygenation	3 Membrane
9 Respiratory	0 Single	5 Ventilation	4 Nonmechanical
9 Respiratory	3 Less than 24 Consecutive Hours 4 24-96 Consecutive Hours 5 Greater than 96 Consecutive Hours	5 Ventilation	Z No Qualifier
C Biliary D Urinary	0 Single 6 Multiple	0 Filtration	Z No Qualifier

Coding Clinic: 2013, Q3, P19 – 5A1221Z, 5A1223Z

SECTION: 5 EXTRACORPOREAL ASSISTANCE AND PERFORMANCE

BODY SYSTEM: A PHYSIOLOGICAL SYSTEMS
OPERATION: 2 RESTORATION: Returning, or attempting to return, a physiological function to its original state by extracorporeal means

Body System	Duration	Function	Qualifier
2 Cardiac	0 Single	4 Rhythm	Z No Qualifier

◀ New   ◀▥ Revised   ~~deleted~~ Deleted   ♀ Females Only   ♂ Males Only
🅝 Noncovered   🅛 Limited Coverage   🅗 Hospital-Acquired Condition   **Coding Clinic**

SECTION: 6 EXTRACORPOREAL THERAPIES

BODY SYSTEM: A PHYSIOLOGICAL SYSTEMS
OPERATION: 0 **ATMOSPHERIC CONTROL:** Extracorporeal control of atmospheric pressure and composition

Body System	Duration	Qualifier	Qualifier
Z None	0 Single 1 Multiple	Z No Qualifier	Z No Qualifier

SECTION: 6 EXTRACORPOREAL THERAPIES

BODY SYSTEM: A PHYSIOLOGICAL SYSTEMS
OPERATION: 1 **DECOMPRESSION:** Extracorporeal elimination of undissolved gas from body fluids

Body System	Duration	Qualifier	Qualifier
5 Circulatory	0 Single 1 Multiple	Z No Qualifier	Z No Qualifier

SECTION: 6 EXTRACORPOREAL THERAPIES

BODY SYSTEM: A PHYSIOLOGICAL SYSTEMS
OPERATION: 2 **ELECTROMAGNETIC THERAPY:** Extracorporeal treatment by electromagnetic rays

Body System	Duration	Qualifier	Qualifier
1 Urinary 2 Central Nervous	0 Single 1 Multiple	Z No Qualifier	Z No Qualifier

SECTION: 6 EXTRACORPOREAL THERAPIES

BODY SYSTEM: A PHYSIOLOGICAL SYSTEMS
OPERATION: 3 **HYPERTHERMIA:** Extracorporeal raising of body temperature

Body System	Duration	Qualifier	Qualifier
Z None	0 Single 1 Multiple	Z No Qualifier	Z No Qualifier

SECTION: 6 EXTRACORPOREAL THERAPIES

BODY SYSTEM: A PHYSIOLOGICAL SYSTEMS
OPERATION: 4 **HYPOTHERMIA:** Extracorporeal lowering of body temperature

Body System	Duration	Qualifier	Qualifier
Z None	0 Single 1 Multiple	Z No Qualifier	Z No Qualifier

◀ New   ◀▥ Revised   ~~deleted~~ Deleted   ♀ Females Only   ♂ Males Only
🅝 Noncovered   🅛 Limited Coverage   🅗 Hospital-Acquired Condition   **Coding Clinic**

SECTION: 6 EXTRACORPOREAL THERAPIES
BODY SYSTEM: A PHYSIOLOGICAL SYSTEMS
OPERATION: 5 PHERESIS: Extracorporeal separation of blood products

Body System	Duration	Qualifier	Qualifier
5 Circulatory	0 Single 1 Multiple	Z No Qualifier	0 Erythrocytes 1 Leukocytes 2 Platelets 3 Plasma T Stem Cells, Cord Blood V Stem Cells, Hematopoietic

SECTION: 6 EXTRACORPOREAL THERAPIES
BODY SYSTEM: A PHYSIOLOGICAL SYSTEMS
OPERATION: 6 PHOTOTHERAPY: Extracorporeal treatment by light rays

Body System	Duration	Qualifier	Qualifier
0 Skin 5 Circulatory	0 Single 1 Multiple	Z No Qualifier	Z No Qualifier

SECTION: 6 EXTRACORPOREAL THERAPIES
BODY SYSTEM: A PHYSIOLOGICAL SYSTEMS
OPERATION: 7 ULTRASOUND THERAPY: Extracorporeal treatment by ultrasound

Body System	Duration	Qualifier	Qualifier
5 Circulatory	0 Single 1 Multiple	Z No Qualifier	4 Head and Neck Vessels 5 Heart 6 Peripheral Vessels 7 Other Vessels Z No Qualifier

SECTION: 6 EXTRACORPOREAL THERAPIES
BODY SYSTEM: A PHYSIOLOGICAL SYSTEMS
OPERATION: 8 ULTRAVIOLET LIGHT THERAPY: Extracorporeal treatment by ultraviolet light

Body System	Duration	Qualifier	Qualifier
0 Skin	0 Single 1 Multiple	Z No Qualifier	Z No Qualifier

SECTION: 6 EXTRACORPOREAL THERAPIES
BODY SYSTEM: A PHYSIOLOGICAL SYSTEMS
OPERATION: 9 SHOCK WAVE THERAPY: Extracorporeal treatment by shock waves

Body System	Duration	Qualifier	Qualifier
3 Musculoskeletal	0 Single 1 Multiple	Z No Qualifier	Z No Qualifier

SECTION: 7 OSTEOPATHIC
BODY SYSTEM: W ANATOMICAL REGIONS
OPERATION: 0 TREATMENT: Manual treatment to eliminate or alleviate somatic dysfunction and related disorders

Body Region	Approach	Method	Qualifier
0 Head	X External	0 Articulatory-Raising	Z None
1 Cervical		1 Fascial Release	
2 Thoracic		2 General Mobilization	
3 Lumbar		3 High Velocity-Low Amplitude	
4 Sacrum		4 Indirect	
5 Pelvis		5 Low Velocity-High Amplitude	
6 Lower Extremities		6 Lymphatic Pump	
7 Upper Extremities		7 Muscle Energy-Isometric	
8 Rib Cage		8 Muscle Energy-Isotonic	
9 Abdomen		9 Other Method	

0: TREATMENT
W: ANATOMICAL REGIONS
7: OSTEOPATHIC

SECTION: 8 OTHER PROCEDURES

BODY SYSTEM: C INDWELLING DEVICE

OPERATION: 0 **OTHER PROCEDURES:** Methodologies which attempt to remediate or cure a disorder or disease

Body Region	Approach	Method	Qualifier
1 Nervous System	X External	6 Collection	J Cerebrospinal Fluid L Other Fluid
2 Circulatory System	X External	6 Collection	K Blood L Other Fluid

◀ New　　◀▥ Revised　　deleted Deleted　　♀ Females Only　　♂ Males Only
🅝 Noncovered　　🅛 Limited Coverage　　🅗 Hospital-Acquired Condition　　**Coding Clinic**

SECTION: 8 OTHER PROCEDURES
BODY SYSTEM: E PHYSIOLOGICAL SYSTEMS AND ANATOMICAL REGIONS
OPERATION: 0 OTHER PROCEDURES: Methodologies which attempt to remediate or cure a disorder or disease

Body Region	Approach	Method	Qualifier
1 Nervous System U Female Reproductive System ♀	X External	Y Other Method	7 Examination
2 Circulatory System	3 Percutaneous	D Near Infrared Spectroscopy	Z No Qualifier
9 Head and Neck Region W Trunk Region	0 Open 3 Percutaneous 4 Percutaneous Endoscopic 7 Via Natural or Artificial Opening 8 Via Natural or Artificial Opening Endoscopic	C Robotic Assisted Procedure	Z No Qualifier
9 Head and Neck Region W Trunk Region	X External	B Computer Assisted Procedure	F With Fluoroscopy G With Computerized Tomography H With Magnetic Resonance Imaging Z No Qualifier
9 Head and Neck Region W Trunk Region	X External	C Robotic Assisted Procedure	Z No Qualifier
9 Head and Neck Region W Trunk Region	X External	Y Other Method	8 Suture Removal
H Integumentary System and Breast	3 Percutaneous	0 Acupuncture	0 Anesthesia Z No Qualifier
H Integumentary System and Breast	X External	6 Collection	2 Breast Milk ♀
H Integumentary System and Breast	X External	Y Other Method	9 Piercing
K Musculoskeletal System	X External	1 Therapeutic Massage	Z No Qualifier
K Musculoskeletal System	X External	Y Other Method	7 Examination
V Male Reproductive System ♂	X External	1 Therapeutic Massage	C Prostate D Rectum
V Male Reproductive System ♂	X External	6 Collection	3 Sperm
X Upper Extremity Y Lower Extremity	0 Open 3 Percutaneous 4 Percutaneous Endoscopic	C Robotic Assisted Procedure	Z No Qualifier
X Upper Extremity Y Lower Extremity	X External	B Computer Assisted Procedure	F With Fluoroscopy G With Computerized Tomography H With Magnetic Resonance Imaging Z No Qualifier
X Upper Extremity Y Lower Extremity	X External	C Robotic Assisted Procedure	Z No Qualifier
X Upper Extremity Y Lower Extremity	X External	Y Other Method	8 Suture Removal
Z None	X External	Y Other Method	1 In Vitro Fertilization 4 Yoga Therapy 5 Meditation 6 Isolation

◀ New ◀◀ Revised deleted Deleted ♀ Females Only ♂ Males Only
⬮ Noncovered ⬮ Limited Coverage ⬮ Hospital-Acquired Condition Coding Clinic

537

◀ New   ◀ Revised   deleted Deleted   ♀ Females Only   ♂ Males Only
🚫 Noncovered   🚫 Limited Coverage   🚫 Hospital-Acquired Condition   **Coding Clinic**

SECTION: 9 CHIROPRACTIC
BODY SYSTEM: W ANATOMICAL REGIONS
OPERATION: B **MANIPULATION:** Manual procedure that involves a directed thrust to move a joint past the physiological range of motion, without exceeding the anatomical limit

Body Region	Approach	Method	Qualifier
0 Head 1 Cervical 2 Thoracic 3 Lumbar 4 Sacrum 5 Pelvis 6 Lower Extremities 7 Upper Extremities 8 Rib Cage 9 Abdomen	X External	B Non-Manual C Indirect Visceral D Extra-Articular F Direct Visceral G Long Lever Specific Contact H Short Lever Specific Contact J Long and Short Lever Specific Contact K Mechanically Assisted L Other Method	Z None

◀ New ◀ Revised ~~deleted~~ Deleted ♀ Females Only ♂ Males Only
🅝 Noncovered 🅛 Limited Coverage 🅗 Hospital-Acquired Condition **Coding Clinic**

539

◀ New   ◀ Revised   ~~deleted~~ Deleted   ♀ Females Only   ♂ Males Only

🟢 Noncovered   🟢 Limited Coverage   🟢 Hospital-Acquired Condition   **Coding Clinic**

SECTION: B IMAGING
BODY SYSTEM: 0 CENTRAL NERVOUS SYSTEM
TYPE: 0 **PLAIN RADIOGRAPHY:** Planar display of an image developed from the capture of external ionizing radiation on photographic or photoconductive plate

Body Part	Contrast	Qualifier	Qualifier
B Spinal Cord	0 High Osmolar 1 Low Osmolar Y Other Contrast Z None	Z None	Z None

SECTION: B IMAGING
BODY SYSTEM: 0 CENTRAL NERVOUS SYSTEM
TYPE: 1 **FLUOROSCOPY:** Single plane or bi-plane real time display of an image developed from the capture of external ionizing radiation on a fluorescent screen. The image may also be stored by either digital or analog means

Body Part	Contrast	Qualifier	Qualifier
B Spinal Cord	0 High Osmolar 1 Low Osmolar Y Other Contrast Z None	Z None	Z None

SECTION: B IMAGING
BODY SYSTEM: 0 CENTRAL NERVOUS SYSTEM
TYPE: 2 **COMPUTERIZED TOMOGRAPHY (CT SCAN):** Computer reformatted digital display of multiplanar images developed from the capture of multiple exposures of external ionizing radiation

Body Part	Contrast	Qualifier	Qualifier
0 Brain 7 Cisterna 8 Cerebral Ventricle(s) 9 Sella Turcica/Pituitary Gland B Spinal Cord	0 High Osmolar 1 Low Osmolar Y Other Contrast	0 Unenhanced and Enhanced Z None	Z None
0 Brain 7 Cisterna 8 Cerebral Ventricle(s) 9 Sella Turcica/Pituitary Gland B Spinal Cord	Z None	Z None	Z None

Left margin: 0; 1; 2 **0: CENTRAL NERVOUS SYSTEM** **B: IMAGING**

◀ New   ◀ Revised   ~~deleted~~ Deleted   ♀ Females Only   ♂ Males Only
🅝 Noncovered   🅛 Limited Coverage   🅗 Hospital-Acquired Condition   **Coding Clinic**

SECTION: B IMAGING
BODY SYSTEM: 0 CENTRAL NERVOUS SYSTEM
TYPE: 3 **MAGNETIC RESONANCE IMAGING (MRI):** Computer reformatted digital display of multiplanar images developed from the capture of radiofrequency signals emitted by nuclei in a body site excited within a magnetic field

Body Part	Contrast	Qualifier	Qualifier
0 Brain 9 Sella Turcica/Pituitary Gland B Spinal Cord C Acoustic Nerves	Y Other Contrast	0 Unenhanced and Enhanced Z None	Z None
0 Brain 9 Sella Turcica/Pituitary Gland B Spinal Cord C Acoustic Nerves	Z None	Z None	Z None

SECTION: B IMAGING
BODY SYSTEM: 0 CENTRAL NERVOUS SYSTEM
TYPE: 4 **ULTRASONOGRAPHY:** Real time display of images of anatomy or flow information developed from the capture of reflected and attenuated high frequency sound waves

Body Part	Contrast	Qualifier	Qualifier
0 Brain B Spinal Cord	Z None	Z None	Z None

◀ New   ◀ Revised   ~~deleted~~ Deleted   ♀ Females Only   ♂ Males Only
Noncovered   Limited Coverage   Hospital-Acquired Condition   **Coding Clinic**

0: PLAIN RADIOGRAPHY   1: FLUOROSCOPY

2: HEART

B: IMAGING

SECTION: B IMAGING
BODY SYSTEM: 2 HEART
TYPE: 0 **PLAIN RADIOGRAPHY:** Planar display of an image developed from the capture of external ionizing radiation on photographic or photoconductive plate

Body Part	Contrast	Qualifier	Qualifier
0 Coronary Artery, Single 1 Coronary Arteries, Multiple 2 Coronary Artery Bypass Graft, Single 3 Coronary Artery Bypass Grafts, Multiple 4 Heart, Right 5 Heart, Left 6 Heart, Right and Left 7 Internal Mammary Bypass Graft, Right 8 Internal Mammary Bypass Graft, Left F Bypass Graft, Other	0 High Osmolar 1 Low Osmolar Y Other Contrast	Z None	Z None

SECTION: B IMAGING
BODY SYSTEM: 2 HEART
TYPE: 1 **FLUOROSCOPY:** Single plane or bi-plane real time display of an image developed from the capture of external ionizing radiation on a fluorescent screen. The image may also be stored by either digital or analog means

Body Part	Contrast	Qualifier	Qualifier
0 Coronary Artery, Single 1 Coronary Arteries, Multiple 2 Coronary Artery Bypass Graft, Single 3 Coronary Artery Bypass Grafts, Multiple	0 High Osmolar 1 Low Osmolar Y Other Contrast	1 Laser	0 Intraoperative
0 Coronary Artery, Single 1 Coronary Arteries, Multiple 2 Coronary Artery Bypass Graft, Single 3 Coronary Artery Bypass Grafts, Multiple	0 High Osmolar 1 Low Osmolar Y Other Contrast	Z None	Z None
4 Heart, Right 5 Heart, Left 6 Heart, Right and Left 7 Internal Mammary Bypass Graft, Right 8 Internal Mammary Bypass Graft, Left F Bypass Graft, Other	0 High Osmolar 1 Low Osmolar Y Other Contrast	Z None	Z None

◀ New   ◀▥ Revised   ~~deleted~~ Deleted   ♀ Females Only   ♂ Males Only
⊘ Noncovered   ⊘ Limited Coverage   ⊘ Hospital-Acquired Condition   **Coding Clinic**

SECTION: B IMAGING
BODY SYSTEM: 2 HEART
TYPE: 2 **COMPUTERIZED TOMOGRAPHY (CT SCAN):** Computer reformatted digital display of multiplanar images developed from the capture of multiple exposures of external ionizing radiation

Body Part	Contrast	Qualifier	Qualifier
1 Coronary Arteries, Multiple 3 Coronary Artery Bypass Grafts, Multiple 6 Heart, Right and Left	0 High Osmolar 1 Low Osmolar Y Other Contrast	0 Unenhanced and Enhanced Z None	Z None
1 Coronary Arteries, Multiple 3 Coronary Artery Bypass Grafts, Multiple 6 Heart, Right and Left	Z None	2 Intravascular Optical Coherence Z None	Z None

SECTION: B IMAGING
BODY SYSTEM: 2 HEART
TYPE: 3 **MAGNETIC RESONANCE IMAGING (MRI):** Computer reformatted digital display of multiplanar images developed from the capture of radiofrequency signals emitted by nuclei in a body site excited within a magnetic field

Body Part	Contrast	Qualifier	Qualifier
1 Coronary Arteries, Multiple 3 Coronary Artery Bypass Grafts, Multiple 6 Heart, Right and Left	Y Other Contrast	0 Unenhanced and Enhanced Z None	Z None
1 Coronary Arteries, Multiple 3 Coronary Artery Bypass Grafts, Multiple 6 Heart, Right and Left	Z None	Z None	Z None

◄ New   ◄ Revised   ~~deleted~~ Deleted   ♀ Females Only   ♂ Males Only
Ⓝⓒ Noncovered   Ⓛⓒ Limited Coverage   Ⓗⓐⓒ Hospital-Acquired Condition   **Coding Clinic**

545

SECTION: B IMAGING
BODY SYSTEM: 2 HEART
TYPE: 4 **ULTRASONOGRAPHY:** Real time display of images of anatomy or flow information developed from the capture of reflected and attenuated high frequency sound waves

Body Part	Contrast	Qualifier	Qualifier
0 Coronary Artery, Single 1 Coronary Arteries, Multiple 4 Heart, Right 5 Heart, Left 6 Heart, Right and Left B Heart with Aorta C Pericardium D Pediatric Heart	Y Other Contrast	Z None	Z None
0 Coronary Artery, Single 1 Coronary Arteries, Multiple 4 Heart, Right 5 Heart, Left 6 Heart, Right and Left B Heart with Aorta C Pericardium D Pediatric Heart	Z None	Z None	3 Intravascular 4 Transesophageal Z None

4: ULTRASONOGRAPHY

2: HEART

B: IMAGING

◄ New   ◄▥ Revised   ~~deleted~~ Deleted   ♀ Females Only   ♂ Males Only
🅝 Noncovered   🅛 Limited Coverage   🅗 Hospital-Acquired Condition   **Coding Clinic**

SECTION: B IMAGING
BODY SYSTEM: 3 UPPER ARTERIES
TYPE: 0 **PLAIN RADIOGRAPHY:** Planar display of an image developed from the capture of external ionizing radiation on photographic or photoconductive plate

Body Part	Contrast	Qualifier	Qualifier
0 Thoracic Aorta	0 High Osmolar	Z None	Z None
1 Brachiocephalic-Subclavian Artery, Right	1 Low Osmolar		
2 Subclavian Artery, Left	Y Other Contrast		
3 Common Carotid Artery, Right	Z None		
4 Common Carotid Artery, Left			
5 Common Carotid Arteries, Bilateral			
6 Internal Carotid Artery, Right			
7 Internal Carotid Artery, Left			
8 Internal Carotid Arteries, Bilateral			
9 External Carotid Artery, Right			
B External Carotid Artery, Left			
C External Carotid Arteries, Bilateral			
D Vertebral Artery, Right			
F Vertebral Artery, Left			
G Vertebral Arteries, Bilateral			
H Upper Extremity Arteries, Right			
J Upper Extremity Arteries, Left			
K Upper Extremity Arteries, Bilateral			
L Intercostal and Bronchial Arteries			
M Spinal Arteries			
N Upper Arteries, Other			
P Thoraco-Abdominal Aorta			
Q Cervico-Cerebral Arch			
R Intracranial Arteries			
S Pulmonary Artery, Right			
T Pulmonary Artery, Left			

B: IMAGING

3: UPPER ARTERIES

0: PLAIN RADIOGRAPHY

SECTION: B IMAGING
BODY SYSTEM: 3 UPPER ARTERIES
TYPE: 1 FLUOROSCOPY: *(on multiple pages)*

Single plane or bi-plane real time display of an image developed from the capture of external ionizing radiation on a fluorescent screen. The image may also be stored by either digital or analog means

Body Part	Contrast	Qualifier	Qualifier
0 Thoracic Aorta	0 High Osmolar	1 Laser	0 Intraoperative
1 Brachiocephalic-Subclavian Artery, Right	1 Low Osmolar		
2 Subclavian Artery, Left	Y Other Contrast		
3 Common Carotid Artery, Right			
4 Common Carotid Artery, Left			
5 Common Carotid Arteries, Bilateral			
6 Internal Carotid Artery, Right			
7 Internal Carotid Artery, Left			
8 Internal Carotid Arteries, Bilateral			
9 External Carotid Artery, Right			
B External Carotid Artery, Left			
C External Carotid Arteries, Bilateral			
D Vertebral Artery, Right			
F Vertebral Artery, Left			
G Vertebral Arteries, Bilateral			
H Upper Extremity Arteries, Right			
J Upper Extremity Arteries, Left			
K Upper Extremity Arteries, Bilateral			
L Intercostal and Bronchial Arteries			
M Spinal Arteries			
N Upper Arteries, Other			
P Thoraco-Abdominal Aorta			
Q Cervico-Cerebral Arch			
R Intracranial Arteries			
S Pulmonary Artery, Right			
T Pulmonary Artery, Left			

1: FLUOROSCOPY

3: UPPER ARTERIES

B: IMAGING

◀ New   ◀▥ Revised   ~~deleted~~ Deleted   ♀ Females Only   ♂ Males Only
🅝 Noncovered   🅛 Limited Coverage   🅗 Hospital-Acquired Condition   **Coding Clinic**

SECTION: B IMAGING
BODY SYSTEM: 3 UPPER ARTERIES
TYPE: 1 FLUOROSCOPY: *(continued)*

Single plane or bi-plane real time display of an image developed from the capture of external ionizing radiation on a fluorescent screen. The image may also be stored by either digital or analog means

Body Part	Contrast	Qualifier	Qualifier
0 Thoracic Aorta	0 High Osmolar	Z None	Z None
1 Brachiocephalic-Subclavian Artery, Right	1 Low Osmolar		
2 Subclavian Artery, Left	Y Other Contrast		
3 Common Carotid Artery, Right			
4 Common Carotid Artery, Left			
5 Common Carotid Arteries, Bilateral			
6 Internal Carotid Artery, Right			
7 Internal Carotid Artery, Left			
8 Internal Carotid Arteries, Bilateral			
9 External Carotid Artery, Right			
B External Carotid Artery, Left			
C External Carotid Arteries, Bilateral			
D Vertebral Artery, Right			
F Vertebral Artery, Left			
G Vertebral Arteries, Bilateral			
H Upper Extremity Arteries, Right			
J Upper Extremity Arteries, Left			
K Upper Extremity Arteries, Bilateral			
L Intercostal and Bronchial Arteries			
M Spinal Arteries			
N Upper Arteries, Other			
P Thoraco-Abdominal Aorta			
Q Cervico-Cerebral Arch			
R Intracranial Arteries			
S Pulmonary Artery, Right			
T Pulmonary Artery, Left			

SECTION: B IMAGING
BODY SYSTEM: 3 UPPER ARTERIES
TYPE: 1 **FLUOROSCOPY:** (continued)

Single plane or bi-plane real time display of an image developed from the capture of external ionizing radiation on a fluorescent screen. The image may also be stored by either digital or analog means

Body Part	Contrast	Qualifier	Qualifier
0 Thoracic Aorta 1 Brachiocephalic-Subclavian Artery, Right 2 Subclavian Artery, Left 3 Common Carotid Artery, Right 4 Common Carotid Artery, Left 5 Common Carotid Arteries, Bilateral 6 Internal Carotid Artery, Right 7 Internal Carotid Artery, Left 8 Internal Carotid Arteries, Bilateral 9 External Carotid Artery, Right B External Carotid Artery, Left C External Carotid Arteries, Bilateral D Vertebral Artery, Right F Vertebral Artery, Left G Vertebral Arteries, Bilateral H Upper Extremity Arteries, Right J Upper Extremity Arteries, Left K Upper Extremity Arteries, Bilateral L Intercostal and Bronchial Arteries M Spinal Arteries N Upper Arteries, Other P Thoraco-Abdominal Aorta Q Cervico-Cerebral Arch R Intracranial Arteries S Pulmonary Artery, Right T Pulmonary Artery, Left	Z None	Z None	Z None

SECTION: B IMAGING
BODY SYSTEM: 3 UPPER ARTERIES
TYPE: 2 **COMPUTERIZED TOMOGRAPHY (CT SCAN):** Computer reformatted digital display of multiplanar images developed from the capture of multiple exposures of external ionizing radiation

Body Part	Contrast	Qualifier	Qualifier
0 Thoracic Aorta 5 Common Carotid Arteries, Bilateral 8 Internal Carotid Arteries, Bilateral G Vertebral Arteries, Bilateral R Intracranial Arteries S Pulmonary Artery, Right T Pulmonary Artery, Left	0 High Osmolar 1 Low Osmolar Y Other Contrast	Z None	Z None
0 Thoracic Aorta 5 Common Carotid Arteries, Bilateral 8 Internal Carotid Arteries, Bilateral G Vertebral Arteries, Bilateral R Intracranial Arteries S Pulmonary Artery, Right T Pulmonary Artery, Left	Z None	2 Intravascular Optical Coherence Z None	Z None

1: FLUOROSCOPY 2: COMPUTERIZED TOMOGRAPHY (CT SCAN)

3: UPPER ARTERIES

B: IMAGING

◀ New ◀▥ Revised ~~deleted~~ Deleted ♀ Females Only ♂ Males Only
Ⓝc Noncovered Ⓛc Limited Coverage Ⓗ Hospital-Acquired Condition **Coding Clinic**

SECTION: B IMAGING

BODY SYSTEM: 3 UPPER ARTERIES

TYPE: 3 **MAGNETIC RESONANCE IMAGING (MRI):** Computer reformatted digital display of multiplanar images developed from the capture of radiofrequency signals emitted by nuclei in a body site excited within a magnetic field

Body Part	Contrast	Qualifier	Qualifier
0 Thoracic Aorta 5 Common Carotid Arteries, Bilateral 8 Internal Carotid Arteries, Bilateral G Vertebral Arteries, Bilateral H Upper Extremity Arteries, Right J Upper Extremity Arteries, Left K Upper Extremity Arteries, Bilateral M Spinal Arteries Q Cervico-Cerebral Arch R Intracranial Arteries	Y Other Contrast	0 Unenhanced and Enhanced Z None	Z None
0 Thoracic Aorta 5 Common Carotid Arteries, Bilateral 8 Internal Carotid Arteries, Bilateral G Vertebral Arteries, Bilateral H Upper Extremity Arteries, Right J Upper Extremity Arteries, Left K Upper Extremity Arteries, Bilateral M Spinal Arteries Q Cervico-Cerebral Arch R Intracranial Arteries	Z None	Z None	Z None

SECTION: B IMAGING

BODY SYSTEM: 3 UPPER ARTERIES

TYPE: 4 **ULTRASONOGRAPHY:** Real time display of images of anatomy or flow information developed from the capture of reflected and attenuated high frequency sound waves

Body Part	Contrast	Qualifier	Qualifier
0 Thoracic Aorta 1 Brachiocephalic-Subclavian Artery, Right 2 Subclavian Artery, Left 3 Common Carotid Artery, Right 4 Common Carotid Artery, Left 5 Common Carotid Arteries, Bilateral 6 Internal Carotid Artery, Right 7 Internal Carotid Artery, Left 8 Internal Carotid Arteries, Bilateral H Upper Extremity Arteries, Right J Upper Extremity Arteries, Left K Upper Extremity Arteries, Bilateral R Intracranial Arteries S Pulmonary Artery, Right T Pulmonary Artery, Left V Ophthalmic Arteries	Z None	Z None	3 Intravascular Z None

SECTION: B IMAGING
BODY SYSTEM: 4 LOWER ARTERIES
TYPE: 0 **PLAIN RADIOGRAPHY:** Planar display of an image developed from the capture of external ionizing radiation on photographic or photoconductive plate

Body Part	Contrast	Qualifier	Qualifier
0 Abdominal Aorta 2 Hepatic Artery 3 Splenic Arteries 4 Superior Mesenteric Artery 5 Inferior Mesenteric Artery 6 Renal Artery, Right 7 Renal Artery, Left 8 Renal Arteries, Bilateral 9 Lumbar Arteries B Intra-Abdominal Arteries, Other C Pelvic Arteries D Aorta and Bilateral Lower Extremity Arteries F Lower Extremity Arteries, Right G Lower Extremity Arteries, Left J Lower Arteries, Other M Renal Artery Transplant	0 High Osmolar 1 Low Osmolar Y Other Contrast	Z None	Z None

◄ New   ◄ Revised   ~~deleted~~ Deleted   ♀ Females Only   ♂ Males Only
🄽🄲 Noncovered   🄻🄲 Limited Coverage   🄷🄰🄲 Hospital-Acquired Condition   **Coding Clinic**

0: PLAIN RADIOGRAPHY

4: LOWER ARTERIES

B: IMAGING

SECTION: B IMAGING
BODY SYSTEM: 4 LOWER ARTERIES
TYPE: 1 **FLUOROSCOPY:** Single plane or bi-plane real time display of an image developed from the capture of external ionizing radiation on a fluorescent screen. The image may also be stored by either digital or analog means

Body Part	Contrast	Qualifier	Qualifier
0 Abdominal Aorta 2 Hepatic Artery 3 Splenic Arteries 4 Superior Mesenteric Artery 5 Inferior Mesenteric Artery 6 Renal Artery, Right 7 Renal Artery, Left 8 Renal Arteries, Bilateral 9 Lumbar Arteries B Intra-Abdominal Arteries, Other C Pelvic Arteries D Aorta and Bilateral Lower Extremity Arteries F Lower Extremity Arteries, Right G Lower Extremity Arteries, Left J Lower Arteries, Other	0 High Osmolar 1 Low Osmolar Y Other Contrast	1 Laser	0 Intraoperative
0 Abdominal Aorta 2 Hepatic Artery 3 Splenic Arteries 4 Superior Mesenteric Artery 5 Inferior Mesenteric Artery 6 Renal Artery, Right 7 Renal Artery, Left 8 Renal Arteries, Bilateral 9 Lumbar Arteries B Intra-Abdominal Arteries, Other C Pelvic Arteries D Aorta and Bilateral Lower Extremity Arteries F Lower Extremity Arteries, Right G Lower Extremity Arteries, Left J Lower Arteries, Other	0 High Osmolar 1 Low Osmolar Y Other Contrast	Z None	Z None
0 Abdominal Aorta 2 Hepatic Artery 3 Splenic Arteries 4 Superior Mesenteric Artery 5 Inferior Mesenteric Artery 6 Renal Artery, Right 7 Renal Artery, Left 8 Renal Arteries, Bilateral 9 Lumbar Arteries B Intra-Abdominal Arteries, Other C Pelvic Arteries D Aorta and Bilateral Lower Extremity Arteries F Lower Extremity Arteries, Right G Lower Extremity Arteries, Left J Lower Arteries, Other	Z None	Z None	Z None

B: IMAGING 4: LOWER ARTERIES 1: FLUOROSCOPY

◀ New ◀ Revised ~~deleted~~ Deleted ♀ Females Only ♂ Males Only
 Noncovered Limited Coverage Hospital-Acquired Condition **Coding Clinic**

553

2: COMPUTERIZED TOMOGRAPHY   3: MAGNETIC RESONANCE IMAGING

4: LOWER ARTERIES

B: IMAGING

SECTION: B IMAGING

BODY SYSTEM: 4 LOWER ARTERIES
TYPE: 2 **COMPUTERIZED TOMOGRAPHY (CT SCAN):** Computer reformatted digital display of multiplanar images developed from the capture of multiple exposures of external ionizing radiation

Body Part	Contrast	Qualifier	Qualifier
0 Abdominal Aorta 1 Celiac Artery 4 Superior Mesenteric Artery 8 Renal Arteries, Bilateral C Pelvic Arteries F Lower Extremity Arteries, Right G Lower Extremity Arteries, Left H Lower Extremity Arteries, Bilateral M Renal Artery Transplant	0 High Osmolar 1 Low Osmolar Y Other Contrast	Z None	Z None
0 Abdominal Aorta 1 Celiac Artery 4 Superior Mesenteric Artery 8 Renal Arteries, Bilateral C Pelvic Arteries F Lower Extremity Arteries, Right G Lower Extremity Arteries, Left H Lower Extremity Arteries, Bilateral M Renal Artery Transplant	Z None	2 Intravascular Optical Coherence Z None	Z None

SECTION: B IMAGING

BODY SYSTEM: 4 LOWER ARTERIES
TYPE: 3 **MAGNETIC RESONANCE IMAGING (MRI):** Computer reformatted digital display of multiplanar images developed from the capture of radiofrequency signals emitted by nuclei in a body site excited within a magnetic field

Body Part	Contrast	Qualifier	Qualifier
0 Abdominal Aorta 1 Celiac Artery 4 Superior Mesenteric Artery 8 Renal Arteries, Bilateral C Pelvic Arteries F Lower Extremity Arteries, Right G Lower Extremity Arteries, Left H Lower Extremity Arteries, Bilateral	Y Other Contrast	0 Unenhanced and Enhanced Z None	Z None
0 Abdominal Aorta 1 Celiac Artery 4 Superior Mesenteric Artery 8 Renal Arteries, Bilateral C Pelvic Arteries F Lower Extremity Arteries, Right G Lower Extremity Arteries, Left H Lower Extremity Arteries, Bilateral	Z None	Z None	Z None

◀ New	◀▥ Revised	~~deleted~~ Deleted	♀ Females Only	♂ Males Only
Noncovered	Limited Coverage	Hospital-Acquired Condition	**Coding Clinic**	

SECTION: B IMAGING
BODY SYSTEM: 4 LOWER ARTERIES
TYPE: 4 ULTRASONOGRAPHY: Real time display of images of anatomy or flow information developed from the capture of reflected and attenuated high frequency sound waves

Body Part	Contrast	Qualifier	Qualifier
0 Abdominal Aorta 4 Superior Mesenteric Artery 5 Inferior Mesenteric Artery 6 Renal Artery, Right 7 Renal Artery, Left 8 Renal Arteries, Bilateral B Intra-Abdominal Arteries, Other F Lower Extremity Arteries, Right G Lower Extremity Arteries, Left H Lower Extremity Arteries, Bilateral K Celiac and Mesenteric Arteries L Femoral Artery N Penile Arteries	Z None	Z None	3 Intravascular Z None

◄ New   ◄ Revised   ~~deleted~~ Deleted   ♀ Females Only   ♂ Males Only
Ⓝⓒ Noncovered   Ⓛⓒ Limited Coverage   Ⓗⓐⓒ Hospital-Acquired Condition   Coding Clinic

555

SECTION: B IMAGING
BODY SYSTEM: 5 VEINS
TYPE: 0 **PLAIN RADIOGRAPHY:** Planar display of an image developed from the capture of external ionizing radiation on photographic or photoconductive plate

Body Part	Contrast	Qualifier	Qualifier
0 Epidural Veins	0 High Osmolar	Z None	Z None
1 Cerebral and Cerebellar Veins	1 Low Osmolar		
2 Intracranial Sinuses	Y Other Contrast		
3 Jugular Veins, Right			
4 Jugular Veins, Left			
5 Jugular Veins, Bilateral			
6 Subclavian Vein, Right			
7 Subclavian Vein, Left			
8 Superior Vena Cava			
9 Inferior Vena Cava			
B Lower Extremity Veins, Right			
C Lower Extremity Veins, Left			
D Lower Extremity Veins, Bilateral			
F Pelvic (Iliac) Veins, Right			
G Pelvic (Iliac) Veins, Left			
H Pelvic (Iliac) Veins, Bilateral			
J Renal Vein, Right			
K Renal Vein, Left			
L Renal Veins, Bilateral			
M Upper Extremity Veins, Right			
N Upper Extremity Veins, Left			
P Upper Extremity Veins, Bilateral			
Q Pulmonary Vein, Right			
R Pulmonary Vein, Left			
S Pulmonary Veins, Bilateral			
T Portal and Splanchnic Veins			
V Veins, Other			
W Dialysis Shunt/Fistula			

0: PLAIN RADIOGRAPHY

5: VEINS

B: IMAGING

◀ New   ◀▥ Revised   ~~deleted~~ Deleted   ♀ Females Only   ♂ Males Only
℞ Noncovered   ℞ Limited Coverage   ℞ Hospital-Acquired Condition   **Coding Clinic**

SECTION: B IMAGING
BODY SYSTEM: 5 VEINS
TYPE: 1 **FLUOROSCOPY:** Single plane or bi-plane real time display of an image developed from the capture of external ionizing radiation on a fluorescent screen. The image may also be stored by either digital or analog means

Body Part	Contrast	Qualifier	Qualifier
0 Epidural Veins	0 High Osmolar	Z None	A Guidance
1 Cerebral and Cerebellar Veins	1 Low Osmolar		Z None
2 Intracranial Sinuses	Y Other Contrast		
3 Jugular Veins, Right	Z None		
4 Jugular Veins, Left			
5 Jugular Veins, Bilateral			
6 Subclavian Vein, Right			
7 Subclavian Vein, Left			
8 Superior Vena Cava			
9 Inferior Vena Cava			
B Lower Extremity Veins, Right			
C Lower Extremity Veins, Left			
D Lower Extremity Veins, Bilateral			
F Pelvic (Iliac) Veins, Right			
G Pelvic (Iliac) Veins, Left			
H Pelvic (Iliac) Veins, Bilateral			
J Renal Vein, Right			
K Renal Vein, Left			
L Renal Veins, Bilateral			
M Upper Extremity Veins, Right			
N Upper Extremity Veins, Left			
P Upper Extremity Veins, Bilateral			
Q Pulmonary Vein, Right			
R Pulmonary Vein, Left			
S Pulmonary Veins, Bilateral			
T Portal and Splanchnic Veins			
V Veins, Other			
W Dialysis Shunt/Fistula			

B: IMAGING 5: VEINS 1: FLUOROSCOPY

SECTION: B IMAGING
BODY SYSTEM: 5 VEINS
TYPE: 2 **COMPUTERIZED TOMOGRAPHY (CT SCAN):** Computer reformatted digital display of multiplanar images developed from the capture of multiple exposures of external ionizing radiation

Body Part	Contrast	Qualifier	Qualifier
2 Intracranial Sinuses 8 Superior Vena Cava 9 Inferior Vena Cava F Pelvic (Iliac) Veins, Right G Pelvic (Iliac) Veins, Left H Pelvic (Iliac) Veins, Bilateral J Renal Vein, Right K Renal Vein, Left L Renal Veins, Bilateral Q Pulmonary Vein, Right R Pulmonary Vein, Left S Pulmonary Veins, Bilateral T Portal and Splanchnic Veins	0 High Osmolar 1 Low Osmolar Y Other Contrast	0 Unenhanced and Enhanced Z None	Z None
2 Intracranial Sinuses 8 Superior Vena Cava 9 Inferior Vena Cava F Pelvic (Iliac) Veins, Right G Pelvic (Iliac) Veins, Left H Pelvic (Iliac) Veins, Bilateral J Renal Vein, Right K Renal Vein, Left L Renal Veins, Bilateral Q Pulmonary Vein, Right R Pulmonary Vein, Left S Pulmonary Veins, Bilateral T Portal and Splanchnic Veins	Z None	2 Intravascular Optical Coherence Z None	Z None

2: COMPUTERIZED TOMOGRAPHY (CT SCAN)

5: VEINS

B: IMAGING

◀ New   ◀▥ Revised   ~~deleted~~ Deleted   ♀ Females Only   ♂ Males Only
Ⓝ Noncovered   Ⓛ Limited Coverage   Ⓗ Hospital-Acquired Condition   **Coding Clinic**

SECTION: B IMAGING
BODY SYSTEM: 5 VEINS
TYPE: 3 **MAGNETIC RESONANCE IMAGING (MRI):** Computer reformatted digital display of multiplanar images developed from the capture of radiofrequency signals emitted by nuclei in a body site excited within a magnetic field

Body Part	Contrast	Qualifier	Qualifier
1 Cerebral and Cerebellar Veins 2 Intracranial Sinuses 5 Jugular Veins, Bilateral 8 Superior Vena Cava 9 Inferior Vena Cava B Lower Extremity Veins, Right C Lower Extremity Veins, Left D Lower Extremity Veins, Bilateral H Pelvic (Iliac) Veins, Bilateral L Renal Veins, Bilateral M Upper Extremity Veins, Right N Upper Extremity Veins, Left P Upper Extremity Veins, Bilateral S Pulmonary Veins, Bilateral T Portal and Splanchnic Veins V Veins, Other	Y Other Contrast	0 Unenhanced and Enhanced Z None	Z None
1 Cerebral and Cerebellar Veins 2 Intracranial Sinuses 5 Jugular Veins, Bilateral 8 Superior Vena Cava 9 Inferior Vena Cava B Lower Extremity Veins, Right C Lower Extremity Veins, Left D Lower Extremity Veins, Bilateral H Pelvic (Iliac) Veins, Bilateral L Renal Veins, Bilateral M Upper Extremity Veins, Right N Upper Extremity Veins, Left P Upper Extremity Veins, Bilateral S Pulmonary Veins, Bilateral T Portal and Splanchnic Veins V Veins, Other	Z None	Z None	Z None

◀ New   ◀▦ Revised   ~~deleted~~ Deleted   ♀ Females Only   ♂ Males Only
🚫 Noncovered   🚫 Limited Coverage   🚫 Hospital-Acquired Condition   **Coding Clinic**

559

SECTION: B IMAGING
BODY SYSTEM: 5 VEINS
TYPE: 4 **ULTRASONOGRAPHY:** Real time display of images of anatomy or flow information developed from the capture of reflected and attenuated high frequency sound waves

Body Part	Contrast	Qualifier	Qualifier
3 Jugular Veins, Right 4 Jugular Veins, Left 6 Subclavian Vein, Right 7 Subclavian Vein, Left 9 Inferior Vena Cava B Lower Extremity Veins, Right C Lower Extremity Veins, Left D Lower Extremity Veins, Bilateral J Renal Vein, Right K Renal Vein, Left L Renal Veins, Bilateral M Upper Extremity Veins, Right N Upper Extremity Veins, Left P Upper Extremity Veins, Bilateral T Portal and Splanchnic Veins	Z None	Z None	3 Intravascular A Guidance Z None

4: ULTRASONOGRAPHY

5: VEINS

B: IMAGING

◀ New ◀▥ Revised ~~deleted~~ Deleted ♀ Females Only ♂ Males Only
Ⓝ Noncovered Ⓛ Limited Coverage Ⓗ Hospital-Acquired Condition **Coding Clinic**

SECTION: B IMAGING
BODY SYSTEM: 7 LYMPHATIC SYSTEM
TYPE: 0 **PLAIN RADIOGRAPHY:** Planar display of an image developed from the capture of external ionizing radiation on photographic or photoconductive plate

Body Part	Contrast	Qualifier	Qualifier
0 Abdominal/Retroperitoneal Lymphatics, Unilateral 1 Abdominal/Retroperitoneal Lymphatics, Bilateral 4 Lymphatics, Head and Neck 5 Upper Extremity Lymphatics, Right 6 Upper Extremity Lymphatics, Left 7 Upper Extremity Lymphatics, Bilateral 8 Lower Extremity Lymphatics, Right 9 Lower Extremity Lymphatics, Left B Lower Extremity Lymphatics, Bilateral C Lymphatics, Pelvic	0 High Osmolar 1 Low Osmolar Y Other Contrast	Z None	Z None

◀ New ◀ Revised ~~deleted~~ Deleted ♀ Females Only ♂ Males Only
Ⓝ Noncovered Ⓛ Limited Coverage Ⓗ Hospital-Acquired Condition **Coding Clinic**

561

0: PLAIN RADIOGRAPHY   2: COMPUTERIZED TOMOGRAPHY (CT SCAN)

8: EYE

B: IMAGING

SECTION: B IMAGING

BODY SYSTEM: 8 EYE

TYPE: 0 **PLAIN RADIOGRAPHY:** Planar display of an image developed from the capture of external ionizing radiation on photographic or photoconductive plate

Body Part	Contrast	Qualifier	Qualifier
0 Lacrimal Duct, Right 1 Lacrimal Duct, Left 2 Lacrimal Ducts, Bilateral	0 High Osmolar 1 Low Osmolar Y Other Contrast	Z None	Z None
3 Optic Foramina, Right 4 Optic Foramina, Left 5 Eye, Right 6 Eye, Left 7 Eyes, Bilateral	Z None	Z None	Z None

SECTION: B IMAGING

BODY SYSTEM: 8 EYE

TYPE: 2 **COMPUTERIZED TOMOGRAPHY (CT SCAN):** Computer reformatted digital display of multiplanar images developed from the capture of multiple exposures of external ionizing radiation

Body Part	Contrast	Qualifier	Qualifier
5 Eye, Right 6 Eye, Left 7 Eyes, Bilateral	0 High Osmolar 1 Low Osmolar Y Other Contrast	0 Unenhanced and Enhanced Z None	Z None
5 Eye, Right 6 Eye, Left 7 Eyes, Bilateral	Z None	Z None	Z None

◀ New   ◀ Revised   ~~deleted~~ Deleted   ♀ Females Only   ♂ Males Only
Ⓝc Noncovered   Ⓛc Limited Coverage   Ⓗc Hospital-Acquired Condition   **Coding Clinic**

SECTION: B IMAGING
BODY SYSTEM: 8 EYE
TYPE: 3 **MAGNETIC RESONANCE IMAGING (MRI):** Computer reformatted digital display of multiplanar images developed from the capture of radiofrequency signals emitted by nuclei in a body site excited within a magnetic field

Body Part	Contrast	Qualifier	Qualifier
5 Eye, Right 6 Eye, Left 7 Eyes, Bilateral	Y Other Contrast	0 Unenhanced and Enhanced Z None	Z None
5 Eye, Right 6 Eye, Left 7 Eyes, Bilateral	Z None	Z None	Z None

SECTION: B IMAGING
BODY SYSTEM: 8 EYE
TYPE: 4 **ULTRASONOGRAPHY:** Real time display of images of anatomy or flow information developed from the capture of reflected and attenuated high frequency sound waves

Body Part	Contrast	Qualifier	Qualifier
5 Eye, Right 6 Eye, Left 7 Eyes, Bilateral	Z None	Z None	Z None

SECTION: B IMAGING

BODY SYSTEM: 9 **EAR, NOSE, MOUTH, AND THROAT**

TYPE: 0 **PLAIN RADIOGRAPHY:** Planar display of an image developed from the capture of external ionizing radiation on photographic or photoconductive plate

Body Part	Contrast	Qualifier	Qualifier
2 Paranasal Sinuses F Nasopharynx/Oropharynx H Mastoids	Z None	Z None	Z None
4 Parotid Gland, Right 5 Parotid Gland, Left 6 Parotid Glands, Bilateral 7 Submandibular Gland, Right 8 Submandibular Gland, Left 9 Submandibular Glands, Bilateral B Salivary Gland, Right C Salivary Gland, Left D Salivary Glands, Bilateral	0 High Osmolar 1 Low Osmolar Y Other Contrast	Z None	Z None

SECTION: B IMAGING

BODY SYSTEM: 9 **EAR, NOSE, MOUTH, AND THROAT**

TYPE: 1 **FLUOROSCOPY:** Single plane or bi-plane real time display of an image developed from the capture of external ionizing radiation on a fluorescent screen. The image may also be stored by either digital or analog means

Body Part	Contrast	Qualifier	Qualifier
G Pharynx and Epiglottis J Larynx	Y Other Contrast Z None	Z None	Z None

SECTION: B IMAGING
BODY SYSTEM: 9 **EAR, NOSE, MOUTH, AND THROAT**
TYPE: 2 **COMPUTERIZED TOMOGRAPHY (CT SCAN):** Computer reformatted digital display of multiplanar images developed from the capture of multiple exposures of external ionizing radiation

Body Part	Contrast	Qualifier	Qualifier
0 Ear 2 Paranasal Sinuses 6 Parotid Glands, Bilateral 9 Submandibular Glands, Bilateral D Salivary Glands, Bilateral F Nasopharynx/Oropharynx J Larynx	0 High Osmolar 1 Low Osmolar Y Other Contrast	0 Unenhanced and Enhanced Z None	Z None
0 Ear 2 Paranasal Sinuses 6 Parotid Glands, Bilateral 9 Submandibular Glands, Bilateral D Salivary Glands, Bilateral F Nasopharynx/Oropharynx J Larynx	Z None	Z None	Z None

SECTION: B IMAGING
BODY SYSTEM: 9 **EAR, NOSE, MOUTH, AND THROAT**
TYPE: 3 **MAGNETIC RESONANCE IMAGING (MRI):** Computer reformatted digital display of multiplanar images developed from the capture of radiofrequency signals emitted by nuclei in a body site excited within a magnetic field

Body Part	Contrast	Qualifier	Qualifier
0 Ear 2 Paranasal Sinuses 6 Parotid Glands, Bilateral 9 Submandibular Glands, Bilateral D Salivary Glands, Bilateral F Nasopharynx/Oropharynx J Larynx	Y Other Contrast	0 Unenhanced and Enhanced Z None	Z None
0 Ear 2 Paranasal Sinuses 6 Parotid Glands, Bilateral 9 Submandibular Glands, Bilateral D Salivary Glands, Bilateral F Nasopharynx/Oropharynx J Larynx	Z None	Z None	Z None

SECTION: B IMAGING
BODY SYSTEM: B RESPIRATORY SYSTEM
TYPE: 0 **PLAIN RADIOGRAPHY:** Planar display of an image developed from the capture of external ionizing radiation on photographic or photoconductive plate

Body Part	Contrast	Qualifier	Qualifier
7 Tracheobronchial Tree, Right 8 Tracheobronchial Tree, Left 9 Tracheobronchial Trees, Bilateral	Y Other Contrast	Z None	Z None
D Upper Airways	Z None	Z None	Z None

SECTION: B IMAGING
BODY SYSTEM: B RESPIRATORY SYSTEM
TYPE: 1 **FLUOROSCOPY:** Single plane or bi-plane real time display of an image developed from the capture of external ionizing radiation on a fluorescent screen. The image may also be stored by either digital or analog means

Body Part	Contrast	Qualifier	Qualifier
2 Lung, Right 3 Lung, Left 4 Lungs, Bilateral 6 Diaphragm C Mediastinum D Upper Airways	Z None	Z None	Z None
7 Tracheobronchial Tree, Right 8 Tracheobronchial Tree, Left 9 Tracheobronchial Trees, Bilateral	Y Other Contrast	Z None	Z None

SECTION: B IMAGING
BODY SYSTEM: B RESPIRATORY SYSTEM
TYPE: 2 **COMPUTERIZED TOMOGRAPHY (CT SCAN):** Computer reformatted digital display of multiplanar images developed from the capture of multiple exposures of external ionizing radiation

Body Part	Contrast	Qualifier	Qualifier
4 Lungs, Bilateral 7 Tracheobronchial Tree, Right 8 Tracheobronchial Tree, Left 9 Tracheobronchial Trees, Bilateral F Trachea/Airways	0 High Osmolar 1 Low Osmolar Y Other Contrast	0 Unenhanced and Enhanced Z None	Z None
4 Lungs, Bilateral 7 Tracheobronchial Tree, Right 8 Tracheobronchial Tree, Left 9 Tracheobronchial Trees, Bilateral F Trachea/Airways	Z None	Z None	Z None

◀ New ◀▨ Revised ~~deleted~~ Deleted ♀ Females Only ♂ Males Only
Ⓝⓒ Noncovered Ⓛⓒ Limited Coverage Ⓗⓒ Hospital-Acquired Condition **Coding Clinic**

SECTION: B IMAGING
BODY SYSTEM: B RESPIRATORY SYSTEM
TYPE: 3 **MAGNETIC RESONANCE IMAGING (MRI):** Computer reformatted digital display of multiplanar images developed from the capture of radiofrequency signals emitted by nuclei in a body site excited within a magnetic field

Body Part	Contrast	Qualifier	Qualifier
G Lung Apices	Y Other Contrast	0 Unenhanced and Enhanced Z None	Z None
G Lung Apices	Z None	Z None	Z None

SECTION: B IMAGING
BODY SYSTEM: B RESPIRATORY SYSTEM
TYPE: 4 **ULTRASONOGRAPHY:** Real time display of images of anatomy or flow information developed from the capture of reflected and attenuated high frequency sound waves

Body Part	Contrast	Qualifier	Qualifier
B Pleura C Mediastinum	Z None	Z None	Z None

◀ New ◀▥ Revised ~~deleted~~ Deleted ♀ Females Only ♂ Males Only
℞ Noncovered ℞ Limited Coverage Hospital-Acquired Condition **Coding Clinic**

567

SECTION: B IMAGING
BODY SYSTEM: D GASTROINTESTINAL SYSTEM
TYPE: **1 FLUOROSCOPY:** Single plane or bi-plane real time display of an image developed from the capture of external ionizing radiation on a fluorescent screen. The image may also be stored by either digital or analog means

Body Part	Contrast	Qualifier	Qualifier
1 Esophagus 2 Stomach 3 Small Bowel 4 Colon 5 Upper GI 6 Upper GI and Small Bowel 9 Duodenum B Mouth/Oropharynx	Y Other Contrast Z None	Z None	Z None

SECTION: B IMAGING
BODY SYSTEM: D GASTROINTESTINAL SYSTEM
TYPE: **2 COMPUTERIZED TOMOGRAPHY (CT SCAN):** Computer reformatted digital display of multiplanar images developed from the capture of multiple exposures of external ionizing radiation

Body Part	Contrast	Qualifier	Qualifier
4 Colon	0 High Osmolar 1 Low Osmolar Y Other Contrast	0 Unenhanced and Enhanced Z None	Z None
4 Colon	Z None	Z None	Z None

SECTION: B IMAGING
BODY SYSTEM: D GASTROINTESTINAL SYSTEM
TYPE: **4 ULTRASONOGRAPHY:** Real time display of images of anatomy or flow information developed from the capture of reflected and attenuated high frequency sound waves

Body Part	Contrast	Qualifier	Qualifier
1 Esophagus 2 Stomach 7 Gastrointestinal Tract 8 Appendix 9 Duodenum C Rectum	Z None	Z None	Z None

◄ New   ◄ Revised   ~~deleted~~ Deleted   ♀ Females Only   ♂ Males Only
Ⓝ Noncovered   Ⓛ Limited Coverage   Ⓗ Hospital-Acquired Condition   **Coding Clinic**

SECTION: B IMAGING

BODY SYSTEM: F HEPATOBILIARY SYSTEM AND PANCREAS

TYPE: 0 **PLAIN RADIOGRAPHY:** Planar display of an image developed from the capture of external ionizing radiation on photographic or photoconductive plate

Body Part	Contrast	Qualifier	Qualifier
0 Bile Ducts 3 Gallbladder and Bile Ducts C Hepatobiliary System, All	0 High Osmolar 1 Low Osmolar Y Other Contrast	Z None	Z None

SECTION: B IMAGING

BODY SYSTEM: F HEPATOBILIARY SYSTEM AND PANCREAS

TYPE: 1 **FLUOROSCOPY:** Single plane or bi-plane real time display of an image developed from the capture of external ionizing radiation on a fluorescent screen. The image may also be stored by either digital or analog means

Body Part	Contrast	Qualifier	Qualifier
0 Bile Ducts 1 Biliary and Pancreatic Ducts 2 Gallbladder 3 Gallbladder and Bile Ducts 4 Gallbladder, Bile Ducts, and Pancreatic Ducts 8 Pancreatic Ducts	0 High Osmolar 1 Low Osmolar Y Other Contrast	Z None	Z None

SECTION: B IMAGING
BODY SYSTEM: F HEPATOBILIARY SYSTEM AND PANCREAS
TYPE: 2 **COMPUTERIZED TOMOGRAPHY (CT SCAN):** Computer reformatted digital display of multiplanar images developed from the capture of multiple exposures of external ionizing radiation

Body Part	Contrast	Qualifier	Qualifier
5 Liver 6 Liver and Spleen 7 Pancreas C Hepatobiliary System, All	0 High Osmolar 1 Low Osmolar Y Other Contrast	0 Unenhanced and Enhanced Z None	Z None
5 Liver 6 Liver and Spleen 7 Pancreas C Hepatobiliary System, All	Z None	Z None	Z None

SECTION: B IMAGING
BODY SYSTEM: F HEPATOBILIARY SYSTEM AND PANCREAS
TYPE: 3 **MAGNETIC RESONANCE IMAGING (MRI):** Computer reformatted digital display of multiplanar images developed from the capture of radiofrequency signals emitted by nuclei in a body site excited within a magnetic field

Body Part	Contrast	Qualifier	Qualifier
5 Liver 6 Liver and Spleen 7 Pancreas	Y Other Contrast	0 Unenhanced and Enhanced Z None	Z None
5 Liver 6 Liver and Spleen 7 Pancreas	Z None	Z None	Z None

SECTION: B IMAGING
BODY SYSTEM: F HEPATOBILIARY SYSTEM AND PANCREAS
TYPE: 4 **ULTRASONOGRAPHY:** Real time display of images of anatomy or flow information developed from the capture of reflected and attenuated high frequency sound waves

Body Part	Contrast	Qualifier	Qualifier
0 Bile Ducts 2 Gallbladder 3 Gallbladder and Bile Ducts 5 Liver 6 Liver and Spleen 7 Pancreas C Hepatobiliary System, All	Z None	Z None	Z None

◀ New   ◀ Revised   ~~deleted~~ Deleted   ♀ Females Only   ♂ Males Only
🝝 Noncovered   🝝 Limited Coverage   🝝 Hospital-Acquired Condition   **Coding Clinic**

SECTION: B IMAGING
BODY SYSTEM: G ENDOCRINE SYSTEM
TYPE: 2 **COMPUTERIZED TOMOGRAPHY (CT SCAN):** Computer reformatted digital display of multiplanar images developed from the capture of multiple exposures of external ionizing radiation

Body Part	Contrast	Qualifier	Qualifier
2 Adrenal Glands, Bilateral 3 Parathyroid Glands 4 Thyroid Gland	0 High Osmolar 1 Low Osmolar Y Other Contrast	0 Unenhanced and Enhanced Z None	Z None
2 Adrenal Glands, Bilateral 3 Parathyroid Glands 4 Thyroid Gland	Z None	Z None	Z None

SECTION: B IMAGING
BODY SYSTEM: G ENDOCRINE SYSTEM
TYPE: 3 **MAGNETIC RESONANCE IMAGING (MRI):** Computer reformatted digital display of multiplanar images developed from the capture of radiofrequency signals emitted by nuclei in a body site excited within a magnetic field

Body Part	Contrast	Qualifier	Qualifier
2 Adrenal Glands, Bilateral 3 Parathyroid Glands 4 Thyroid Gland	Y Other Contrast	0 Unenhanced and Enhanced Z None	Z None
2 Adrenal Glands, Bilateral 3 Parathyroid Glands 4 Thyroid Gland	Z None	Z None	Z None

SECTION: B IMAGING
BODY SYSTEM: G ENDOCRINE SYSTEM
TYPE: 4 **ULTRASONOGRAPHY:** Real time display of images of anatomy or flow information developed from the capture of reflected and attenuated high frequency sound waves

Body Part	Contrast	Qualifier	Qualifier
0 Adrenal Gland, Right 1 Adrenal Gland, Left 2 Adrenal Glands, Bilateral 3 Parathyroid Glands 4 Thyroid Gland	Z None	Z None	Z None

◀ New ◀ Revised deleted Deleted ♀ Females Only ♂ Males Only
◐ Noncovered ◐ Limited Coverage ◐ Hospital-Acquired Condition **Coding Clinic**

571

SECTION: **B IMAGING**

BODY SYSTEM: **H SKIN, SUBCUTANEOUS TISSUE AND BREAST**

TYPE: **0 PLAIN RADIOGRAPHY:** Planar display of an image developed from the capture of external ionizing radiation on photographic or photoconductive plate

Body Part	Contrast	Qualifier	Qualifier
0 Breast, Right 1 Breast, Left 2 Breasts, Bilateral	Z None	Z None	Z None
3 Single Mammary Duct, Right 4 Single Mammary Duct, Left 5 Multiple Mammary Ducts, Right 6 Multiple Mammary Ducts, Left	0 High Osmolar 1 Low Osmolar Y Other Contrast Z None	Z None	Z None

SECTION: **B IMAGING**

BODY SYSTEM: **H SKIN, SUBCUTANEOUS TISSUE AND BREAST**

TYPE: **3 MAGNETIC RESONANCE IMAGING (MRI):** Computer reformatted digital display of multiplanar images developed from the capture of radiofrequency signals emitted by nuclei in a body site excited within a magnetic field

Body Part	Contrast	Qualifier	Qualifier
0 Breast, Right 1 Breast, Left 2 Breasts, Bilateral D Subcutaneous Tissue, Head/Neck F Subcutaneous Tissue, Upper Extremity G Subcutaneous Tissue, Thorax H Subcutaneous Tissue, Abdomen and Pelvis J Subcutaneous Tissue, Lower Extremity	Y Other Contrast	0 Unenhanced and Enhanced Z None	Z None
0 Breast, Right 1 Breast, Left 2 Breasts, Bilateral D Subcutaneous Tissue, Head/Neck F Subcutaneous Tissue, Upper Extremity G Subcutaneous Tissue, Thorax H Subcutaneous Tissue, Abdomen and Pelvis J Subcutaneous Tissue, Lower Extremity	Z None	Z None	Z None

◀ New   ◀◀ Revised   ~~deleted~~ Deleted   ♀ Females Only   ♂ Males Only
Ⓝⓒ Noncovered   Ⓛⓒ Limited Coverage   Ⓗⓐⓒ Hospital-Acquired Condition   **Coding Clinic**

SECTION: B IMAGING
BODY SYSTEM: H SKIN, SUBCUTANEOUS TISSUE AND BREAST
TYPE: 4 ULTRASONOGRAPHY: Real time display of images of anatomy or flow information developed from the capture of reflected and attenuated high frequency sound waves

Body Part	Contrast	Qualifier	Qualifier
0 Breast, Right 1 Breast, Left 2 Breasts, Bilateral 7 Extremity, Upper 8 Extremity, Lower 9 Abdominal Wall B Chest Wall C Head and Neck	Z None	Z None	Z None

SECTION: B IMAGING

BODY SYSTEM: L CONNECTIVE TISSUE

TYPE: 3 **MAGNETIC RESONANCE IMAGING (MRI):** Computer reformatted digital display of multiplanar images developed from the capture of radiofrequency signals emitted by nuclei in a body site excited within a magnetic field

Body Part	Contrast	Qualifier	Qualifier
0 Connective Tissue, Upper Extremity 1 Connective Tissue, Lower Extremity 2 Tendons, Upper Extremity 3 Tendons, Lower Extremity	Y Other Contrast	0 Unenhanced and Enhanced Z None	Z None
0 Connective Tissue, Upper Extremity 1 Connective Tissue, Lower Extremity 2 Tendons, Upper Extremity 3 Tendons, Lower Extremity	Z None	Z None	Z None

SECTION: B IMAGING

BODY SYSTEM: L CONNECTIVE TISSUE

TYPE: 4 **ULTRASONOGRAPHY:** Real time display of images of anatomy or flow information developed from the capture of reflected and attenuated high frequency sound waves

Body Part	Contrast	Qualifier	Qualifier
0 Connective Tissue, Upper Extremity 1 Connective Tissue, Lower Extremity 2 Tendons, Upper Extremity 3 Tendons, Lower Extremity	Z None	Z None	Z None

◀ New ◀▥ Revised ~~deleted~~ Deleted ♀ Females Only ♂ Males Only
Ⓝ Noncovered Ⓛ Limited Coverage Ⓗ Hospital-Acquired Condition **Coding Clinic**

SECTION: **B IMAGING**
BODY SYSTEM: N **SKULL AND FACIAL BONES**
TYPE: 0 **PLAIN RADIOGRAPHY:** Planar display of an image developed from the capture of external ionizing radiation on photographic or photoconductive plate

Body Part	Contrast	Qualifier	Qualifier
0 Skull 1 Orbit, Right 2 Orbit, Left 3 Orbits, Bilateral 4 Nasal Bones 5 Facial Bones 6 Mandible B Zygomatic Arch, Right C Zygomatic Arch, Left D Zygomatic Arches, Bilateral G Tooth, Single H Teeth, Multiple J Teeth, All	Z None	Z None	Z None
7 Temporomandibular Joint, Right 8 Temporomandibular Joint, Left 9 Temporomandibular Joints, Bilateral	0 High Osmolar 1 Low Osmolar Y Other Contrast Z None	Z None	Z None

SECTION: **B IMAGING**
BODY SYSTEM: N **SKULL AND FACIAL BONES**
TYPE: 1 **FLUOROSCOPY:** Single plane or bi-plane real time display of an image developed from the capture of external ionizing radiation on a fluorescent screen. The image may also be stored by either digital or analog means

Body Part	Contrast	Qualifier	Qualifier
7 Temporomandibular Joint, Right 8 Temporomandibular Joint, Left 9 Temporomandibular Joints, Bilateral	0 High Osmolar 1 Low Osmolar Y Other Contrast Z None	Z None	Z None

B: IMAGING

N: SKULL AND FACIAL BONES

0: PLAIN RADIOGRAPHY   1: FLUOROSCOPY

SECTION: B IMAGING
BODY SYSTEM: N SKULL AND FACIAL BONES
TYPE: 2 **COMPUTERIZED TOMOGRAPHY (CT SCAN):** Computer reformatted digital display of multiplanar images developed from the capture of multiple exposures of external ionizing radiation

Body Part	Contrast	Qualifier	Qualifier
0 Skull 3 Orbits, Bilateral 5 Facial Bones 6 Mandible 9 Temporomandibular Joints, Bilateral F Temporal Bones	0 High Osmolar 1 Low Osmolar Y Other Contrast Z None	Z None	Z None

SECTION: B IMAGING
BODY SYSTEM: N SKULL AND FACIAL BONES
TYPE: 3 **MAGNETIC RESONANCE IMAGING (MRI):** Computer reformatted digital display of multiplanar images developed from the capture of radiofrequency signals emitted by nuclei in a body site excited within a magnetic field

Body Part	Contrast	Qualifier	Qualifier
9 Temporomandibular Joints, Bilateral	Y Other Contrast Z None	Z None	Z None

SECTION: B IMAGING
BODY SYSTEM: P NON-AXIAL UPPER BONES
TYPE: 0 **PLAIN RADIOGRAPHY:** Planar display of an image developed from the capture of external ionizing radiation on photographic or photoconductive plate

Body Part	Contrast	Qualifier	Qualifier
0 Sternoclavicular Joint, Right 1 Sternoclavicular Joint, Left 2 Sternoclavicular Joints, Bilateral 3 Acromioclavicular Joints, Bilateral 4 Clavicle, Right 5 Clavicle, Left 6 Scapula, Right 7 Scapula, Left A Humerus, Right B Humerus, Left E Upper Arm, Right F Upper Arm, Left J Forearm, Right K Forearm, Left N Hand, Right P Hand, Left R Finger(s), Right S Finger(s), Left X Ribs, Right Y Ribs, Left	Z None	Z None	Z None
8 Shoulder, Right 9 Shoulder, Left C Hand/Finger Joint, Right D Hand/Finger Joint, Left G Elbow, Right H Elbow, Left L Wrist, Right M Wrist, Left	0 High Osmolar 1 Low Osmolar Y Other Contrast Z None	Z None	Z None

◄ New   ◄ Revised   deleted Deleted   ♀ Females Only   ♂ Males Only
🐾 Noncovered   🐾 Limited Coverage   🐾 Hospital-Acquired Condition   **Coding Clinic**

577

SECTION: B IMAGING
BODY SYSTEM: P NON-AXIAL UPPER BONES
TYPE: 1 **FLUOROSCOPY:** Single plane or bi-plane real time display of an image developed from the capture of external ionizing radiation on a fluorescent screen. The image may also be stored by either digital or analog means

Body Part	Contrast	Qualifier	Qualifier
0 Sternoclavicular Joint, Right 1 Sternoclavicular Joint, Left 2 Sternoclavicular Joints, Bilateral 3 Acromioclavicular Joints, Bilateral 4 Clavicle, Right 5 Clavicle, Left 6 Scapula, Right 7 Scapula, Left A Humerus, Right B Humerus, Left E Upper Arm, Right F Upper Arm, Left J Forearm, Right K Forearm, Left N Hand, Right P Hand, Left R Finger(s), Right S Finger(s), Left X Ribs, Right Y Ribs, Left	Z None	Z None	Z None
8 Shoulder, Right 9 Shoulder, Left L Wrist, Right M Wrist, Left	0 High Osmolar 1 Low Osmolar Y Other Contrast Z None	Z None	Z None
C Hand/Finger Joint, Right D Hand/Finger Joint, Left G Elbow, Right H Elbow, Left	0 High Osmolar 1 Low Osmolar Y Other Contrast	Z None	Z None

SECTION: B IMAGING
BODY SYSTEM: P NON-AXIAL UPPER BONES
TYPE: 2 **COMPUTERIZED TOMOGRAPHY (CT SCAN):** Computer reformatted digital display of multiplanar images developed from the capture of multiple exposures of external ionizing radiation

Body Part	Contrast	Qualifier	Qualifier
0 Sternoclavicular Joint, Right 1 Sternoclavicular Joint, Left W Thorax	0 High Osmolar 1 Low Osmolar Y Other Contrast	Z None	Z None
2 Sternoclavicular Joints, Bilateral 3 Acromioclavicular Joints, Bilateral 4 Clavicle, Right 5 Clavicle, Left 6 Scapula, Right 7 Scapula, Left 8 Shoulder, Right 9 Shoulder, Left A Humerus, Right B Humerus, Left E Upper Arm, Right F Upper Arm, Left G Elbow, Right H Elbow, Left J Forearm, Right K Forearm, Left L Wrist, Right M Wrist, Left N Hand, Right P Hand, Left Q Hands and Wrists, Bilateral R Finger(s), Right S Finger(s), Left T Upper Extremity, Right U Upper Extremity, Left V Upper Extremities, Bilateral X Ribs, Right Y Ribs, Left	0 High Osmolar 1 Low Osmolar Y Other Contrast Z None	Z None	Z None
C Hand/Finger Joint, Right D Hand/Finger Joint, Left	Z None	Z None	Z None

◄ New ◄ Revised ~~deleted~~ Deleted ♀ Females Only ♂ Males Only
🅝🅒 Noncovered 🅛🅒 Limited Coverage 🅗🅐🅒 Hospital-Acquired Condition **Coding Clinic**

SECTION: B IMAGING
BODY SYSTEM: P NON-AXIAL UPPER BONES
TYPE: 3 **MAGNETIC RESONANCE IMAGING (MRI):** Computer reformatted digital display of multiplanar images developed from the capture of radiofrequency signals emitted by nuclei in a body site excited within a magnetic field

3: MRI   4: ULTRASONOGRAPHY

P: NON-AXIAL UPPER BONES

B: IMAGING

Body Part	Contrast	Qualifier	Qualifier
8 Shoulder, Right 9 Shoulder, Left C Hand/Finger Joint, Right D Hand/Finger Joint, Left E Upper Arm, Right F Upper Arm, Left G Elbow, Right H Elbow, Left J Forearm, Right K Forearm, Left L Wrist, Right M Wrist, Left	Y Other Contrast	0 Unenhanced and Enhanced Z None	Z None
8 Shoulder, Right 9 Shoulder, Left C Hand/Finger Joint, Right D Hand/Finger Joint, Left E Upper Arm, Right F Upper Arm, Left G Elbow, Right H Elbow, Left J Forearm, Right K Forearm, Left L Wrist, Right M Wrist, Left	Z None	Z None	Z None

SECTION: B IMAGING
BODY SYSTEM: P NON-AXIAL UPPER BONES
TYPE: 4 **ULTRASONOGRAPHY:** Real time display of images of anatomy or flow information developed from the capture of reflected and attenuated high frequency sound waves

Body Part	Contrast	Qualifier	Qualifier
8 Shoulder, Right 9 Shoulder, Left G Elbow, Right H Elbow, Left L Wrist, Right M Wrist, Left N Hand, Right P Hand, Left	Z None	Z None	1 Densitometry Z None

◀ New   ◀▮ Revised   ~~deleted~~ Deleted   ♀ Females Only   ♂ Males Only
⟲ Noncovered   ⟲ Limited Coverage   ⟲ Hospital-Acquired Condition   **Coding Clinic**

SECTION: B IMAGING
BODY SYSTEM: Q NON-AXIAL LOWER BONES
TYPE: 0 PLAIN RADIOGRAPHY: Planar display of an image developed from the capture of external ionizing radiation on photographic or photoconductive plate

Body Part	Contrast	Qualifier	Qualifier
0 Hip, Right 1 Hip, Left	0 High Osmolar 1 Low Osmolar Y Other Contrast	Z None	Z None
0 Hip, Right 1 Hip, Left	Z None	Z None	1 Densitometry Z None
3 Femur, Right 4 Femur, Left	Z None	Z None	1 Densitometry Z None
7 Knee, Right 8 Knee, Left G Ankle, Right H Ankle, Left	0 High Osmolar 1 Low Osmolar Y Other Contrast Z None	Z None	Z None
D Lower Leg, Right F Lower Leg, Left J Calcaneus, Right K Calcaneus, Left L Foot, Right M Foot, Left P Toe(s), Right Q Toe(s), Left V Patella, Right W Patella, Left	Z None	Z None	Z None
X Foot/Toe Joint, Right Y Foot/Toe Joint, Left	0 High Osmolar 1 Low Osmolar Y Other Contrast	Z None	Z None

B: IMAGING

Q: NON-AXIAL LOWER BONES

0: PLAIN RADIOGRAPHY

SECTION: B IMAGING
BODY SYSTEM: Q NON-AXIAL LOWER BONES
TYPE: 1 **FLUOROSCOPY:** Single plane or bi-plane real time display of an image developed from the capture of external ionizing radiation on a fluorescent screen. The image may also be stored by either digital or analog means

Body Part	Contrast	Qualifier	Qualifier
0 Hip, Right 1 Hip, Left 7 Knee, Right 8 Knee, Left G Ankle, Right H Ankle, Left X Foot/Toe Joint, Right Y Foot/Toe Joint, Left	0 High Osmolar 1 Low Osmolar Y Other Contrast Z None	Z None	Z None
3 Femur, Right 4 Femur, Left D Lower Leg, Right F Lower Leg, Left J Calcaneus, Right K Calcaneus, Left L Foot, Right M Foot, Left P Toe(s), Right Q Toe(s), Left V Patella, Right W Patella, Left	Z None	Z None	Z None

1: FLUOROSCOPY

Q: NON-AXIAL LOWER BONES

B: IMAGING

◀ New ◀ Revised ~~deleted~~ Deleted ♀ Females Only ♂ Males Only
Ⓝⓒ Noncovered Ⓛⓒ Limited Coverage Ⓗⓐⓒ Hospital-Acquired Condition **Coding Clinic**

SECTION: B IMAGING
BODY SYSTEM: Q NON-AXIAL LOWER BONES
TYPE: 2 **COMPUTERIZED TOMOGRAPHY (CT SCAN):** Computer reformatted digital display of multiplanar images developed from the capture of multiple exposures of external ionizing radiation

Body Part	Contrast	Qualifier	Qualifier
0 Hip, Right 1 Hip, Left 3 Femur, Right 4 Femur, Left 7 Knee, Right 8 Knee, Left D Lower Leg, Right F Lower Leg, Left G Ankle, Right H Ankle, Left J Calcaneus, Right K Calcaneus, Left L Foot, Right M Foot, Left P Toe(s), Right Q Toe(s), Left R Lower Extremity, Right S Lower Extremity, Left V Patella, Right W Patella, Left X Foot/Toe Joint, Right Y Foot/Toe Joint, Left	0 High Osmolar 1 Low Osmolar Y Other Contrast Z None	Z None	Z None
B Tibia/Fibula, Right C Tibia/Fibula, Left	0 High Osmolar 1 Low Osmolar Y Other Contrast	Z None	Z None

◀ New ◀ Revised ~~deleted~~ Deleted ♀ Females Only ♂ Males Only
Noncovered Limited Coverage Hospital-Acquired Condition **Coding Clinic**

583

SECTION: B IMAGING

BODY SYSTEM: Q NON-AXIAL LOWER BONES

TYPE: 3 **MAGNETIC RESONANCE IMAGING (MRI):** Computer reformatted digital display of multiplanar images developed from the capture of radiofrequency signals emitted by nuclei in a body site excited within a magnetic field

3: MAGNETIC RESONANCE IMAGING (MRI)

Q: NON-AXIAL LOWER BONES

B: IMAGING

Body Part	Contrast	Qualifier	Qualifier
0 Hip, Right 1 Hip, Left 3 Femur, Right 4 Femur, Left 7 Knee, Right 8 Knee, Left D Lower Leg, Right F Lower Leg, Left G Ankle, Right H Ankle, Left J Calcaneus, Right K Calcaneus, Left L Foot, Right M Foot, Left P Toe(s), Right Q Toe(s), Left V Patella, Right W Patella, Left	Y Other Contrast	0 Unenhanced and Enhanced Z None	Z None
0 Hip, Right 1 Hip, Left 3 Femur, Right 4 Femur, Left 7 Knee, Right 8 Knee, Left D Lower Leg, Right F Lower Leg, Left G Ankle, Right H Ankle, Left J Calcaneus, Right K Calcaneus, Left L Foot, Right M Foot, Left P Toe(s), Right Q Toe(s), Left V Patella, Right W Patella, Left	Z None	Z None	Z None

◀ New ◀▥ Revised ~~deleted~~ Deleted ♀ Females Only ♂ Males Only
Ⓝⓒ Noncovered Ⓛⓒ Limited Coverage Ⓗⓐⓒ Hospital-Acquired Condition **Coding Clinic**

SECTION: B IMAGING
BODY SYSTEM: Q NON-AXIAL LOWER BONES
TYPE: 4 **ULTRASONOGRAPHY:** Real time display of images of anatomy or flow information developed from the capture of reflected and attenuated high frequency sound waves

Body Part	Contrast	Qualifier	Qualifier
0 Hip, Right 1 Hip, Left 2 Hips, Bilateral 7 Knee, Right 8 Knee, Left 9 Knees, Bilateral	Z None	Z None	Z None

◀ New ◀ Revised deleted Deleted ♀ Females Only ♂ Males Only
NC Noncovered LC Limited Coverage HAC Hospital-Acquired Condition **Coding Clinic**

585

SECTION: B IMAGING

BODY SYSTEM: R AXIAL SKELETON, EXCEPT SKULL AND FACIAL BONES

TYPE: 0 **PLAIN RADIOGRAPHY:** Planar display of an image developed from the capture of external ionizing radiation on photographic or photoconductive plate

Body Part	Contrast	Qualifier	Qualifier
0 Cervical Spine 7 Thoracic Spine 9 Lumbar Spine G Whole Spine	Z None	Z None	1 Densitometry Z None
1 Cervical Disc(s) 2 Thoracic Disc(s) 3 Lumbar Disc(s) 4 Cervical Facet Joint(s) 5 Thoracic Facet Joint(s) 6 Lumbar Facet Joint(s) D Sacroiliac Joints	0 High Osmolar 1 Low Osmolar Y Other Contrast Z None	Z None	Z None
8 Thoracolumbar Joint B Lumbosacral Joint C Pelvis F Sacrum and Coccyx H Sternum	Z None	Z None	Z None

SECTION: B IMAGING

BODY SYSTEM: R AXIAL SKELETON, EXCEPT SKULL AND FACIAL BONES

TYPE: 1 **FLUOROSCOPY:** Single plane or bi-plane real time display of an image developed from the capture of external ionizing radiation on a fluorescent screen. The image may also be stored by either digital or analog means

Body Part	Contrast	Qualifier	Qualifier
0 Cervical Spine 1 Cervical Disc(s) 2 Thoracic Disc(s) 3 Lumbar Disc(s) 4 Cervical Facet Joint(s) 5 Thoracic Facet Joint(s) 6 Lumbar Facet Joint(s) 7 Thoracic Spine 8 Thoracolumbar Joint 9 Lumbar Spine B Lumbosacral Joint C Pelvis D Sacroiliac Joints F Sacrum and Coccyx G Whole Spine H Sternum	0 High Osmolar 1 Low Osmolar Y Other Contrast Z None	Z None	Z None

◄ New   ◄ Revised   ~~deleted~~ Deleted   ♀ Females Only   ♂ Males Only
Noncovered   Limited Coverage   Hospital-Acquired Condition   **Coding Clinic**

SECTION: B IMAGING
BODY SYSTEM: R AXIAL SKELETON, EXCEPT SKULL AND FACIAL BONES
TYPE: 2 **COMPUTERIZED TOMOGRAPHY (CT SCAN):** Computer reformatted digital display of multiplanar images developed from the capture of multiple exposures of external ionizing radiation

Body Part	Contrast	Qualifier	Qualifier
0 Cervical Spine 7 Thoracic Spine 9 Lumbar Spine C Pelvis D Sacroiliac Joints F Sacrum and Coccyx	0 High Osmolar 1 Low Osmolar Y Other Contrast Z None	Z None	Z None

SECTION: B IMAGING
BODY SYSTEM: R AXIAL SKELETON, EXCEPT SKULL AND FACIAL BONES
TYPE: 3 **MAGNETIC RESONANCE IMAGING (MRI):** Computer reformatted digital display of multiplanar images developed from the capture of radiofrequency signals emitted by nuclei in a body site excited within a magnetic field

Body Part	Contrast	Qualifier	Qualifier
0 Cervical Spine 1 Cervical Disc(s) 2 Thoracic Disc(s) 3 Lumbar Disc(s) 7 Thoracic Spine 9 Lumbar Spine C Pelvis F Sacrum and Coccyx	Y Other Contrast	0 Unenhanced and Enhanced Z None	Z None
0 Cervical Spine 1 Cervical Disc(s) 2 Thoracic Disc(s) 3 Lumbar Disc(s) 7 Thoracic Spine 9 Lumbar Spine C Pelvis F Sacrum and Coccyx	Z None	Z None	Z None

SECTION: B IMAGING
BODY SYSTEM: R AXIAL SKELETON, EXCEPT SKULL AND FACIAL BONES
TYPE: 4 **ULTRASONOGRAPHY:** Real time display of images of anatomy or flow information developed from the capture of reflected and attenuated high frequency sound waves

Body Part	Contrast	Qualifier	Qualifier
0 Cervical Spine 7 Thoracic Spine 9 Lumbar Spine F Sacrum and Coccyx	Z None	Z None	Z None

◀ New   ◀▭ Revised   deleted Deleted   ♀ Females Only   ♂ Males Only
🅝 Noncovered   🅛 Limited Coverage   🅗 Hospital-Acquired Condition   **Coding Clinic**

587

B: IMAGING

R: AXIAL SKELETON, EXCEPT SKULL AND FACIAL BONES

2; 3; 4

SECTION: B IMAGING
BODY SYSTEM: T URINARY SYSTEM
TYPE: 0 PLAIN RADIOGRAPHY: Planar display of an image developed from the capture of external ionizing radiation on photographic or photoconductive plate

Body Part	Contrast	Qualifier	Qualifier
0 Bladder 1 Kidney, Right 2 Kidney, Left 3 Kidneys, Bilateral 4 Kidneys, Ureters, and Bladder 5 Urethra 6 Ureter, Right 7 Ureter, Left 8 Ureters, Bilateral B Bladder and Urethra C Ileal Diversion Loop	0 High Osmolar 1 Low Osmolar Y Other Contrast Z None	Z None	Z None

SECTION: B IMAGING
BODY SYSTEM: T URINARY SYSTEM
TYPE: 1 FLUOROSCOPY: Single plane or bi-plane real time display of an image developed from the capture of external ionizing radiation on a fluorescent screen. The image may also be stored by either digital or analog means

Body Part	Contrast	Qualifier	Qualifier
0 Bladder 1 Kidney, Right 2 Kidney, Left 3 Kidneys, Bilateral 4 Kidneys, Ureters, and Bladder 5 Urethra 6 Ureter, Right 7 Ureter, Left B Bladder and Urethra C Ileal Diversion Loop D Kidney, Ureter, and Bladder, Right F Kidney, Ureter, and Bladder, Left G Ileal Loop, Ureters, and Kidneys	0 High Osmolar 1 Low Osmolar Y Other Contrast Z None	Z None	Z None

◀ New　◀▥ Revised　~~deleted~~ Deleted　♀ Females Only　♂ Males Only
🦶 Noncovered　🦶 Limited Coverage　🦶 Hospital-Acquired Condition　**Coding Clinic**

SECTION: B IMAGING

BODY SYSTEM: T URINARY SYSTEM

TYPE: 2 **COMPUTERIZED TOMOGRAPHY (CT SCAN):** Computer reformatted digital display of multiplanar images developed from the capture of multiple exposures of external ionizing radiation

Body Part	Contrast	Qualifier	Qualifier
0 Bladder 1 Kidney, Right 2 Kidney, Left 3 Kidneys, Bilateral 9 Kidney Transplant	0 High Osmolar 1 Low Osmolar Y Other Contrast	0 Unenhanced and Enhanced Z None	Z None
0 Bladder 1 Kidney, Right 2 Kidney, Left 3 Kidneys, Bilateral 9 Kidney Transplant	Z None	Z None	Z None

SECTION: B IMAGING

BODY SYSTEM: T URINARY SYSTEM

TYPE: 3 **MAGNETIC RESONANCE IMAGING (MRI):** Computer reformatted digital display of multiplanar images developed from the capture of radiofrequency signals emitted by nuclei in a body site excited within a magnetic field

Body Part	Contrast	Qualifier	Qualifier
0 Bladder 1 Kidney, Right 2 Kidney, Left 3 Kidneys, Bilateral 9 Kidney Transplant	Y Other Contrast	0 Unenhanced and Enhanced Z None	Z None
0 Bladder 1 Kidney, Right 2 Kidney, Left 3 Kidneys, Bilateral 9 Kidney Transplant	Z None	Z None	Z None

◀ New   ◀ Revised   ~~deleted~~ Deleted   ♀ Females Only   ♂ Males Only
℞ℴ Noncovered   ℞ℴ Limited Coverage   ℞ℴ Hospital-Acquired Condition   **Coding Clinic**

SECTION: B IMAGING
BODY SYSTEM: T URINARY SYSTEM
TYPE: 4 ULTRASONOGRAPHY: Real time display of images of anatomy or flow information developed from the capture of reflected and attenuated high frequency sound waves

Body Part	Contrast	Qualifier	Qualifier
0 Bladder 1 Kidney, Right 2 Kidney, Left 3 Kidneys, Bilateral 5 Urethra 6 Ureter, Right 7 Ureter, Left 8 Ureters, Bilateral 9 Kidney Transplant J Kidneys and Bladder	Z None	Z None	Z None

4: ULTRASONOGRAPHY

T: URINARY SYSTEM

B: IMAGING

◀ New   ◀▥ Revised   ~~deleted~~ Deleted   ♀ Females Only   ♂ Males Only
🇳 Noncovered   🇱 Limited Coverage   🇭 Hospital-Acquired Condition   **Coding Clinic**

SECTION: B IMAGING

BODY SYSTEM: U FEMALE REPRODUCTIVE SYSTEM

TYPE: 0 **PLAIN RADIOGRAPHY:** Planar display of an image developed from the capture of external ionizing radiation on photographic or photoconductive plate

Body Part	Contrast	Qualifier	Qualifier
0 Fallopian Tube, Right ♀ 1 Fallopian Tube, Left ♀ 2 Fallopian Tubes, Bilateral ♀ 6 Uterus ♀ 8 Uterus and Fallopian Tubes ♀ 9 Vagina ♀	0 High Osmolar 1 Low Osmolar Y Other Contrast	Z None	Z None

SECTION: B IMAGING

BODY SYSTEM: U FEMALE REPRODUCTIVE SYSTEM

TYPE: 1 **FLUOROSCOPY:** Single plane or bi-plane real time display of an image developed from the capture of external ionizing radiation on a fluorescent screen. The image may also be stored by either digital or analog means

Body Part	Contrast	Qualifier	Qualifier
0 Fallopian Tube, Right ♀ 1 Fallopian Tube, Left ♀ 2 Fallopian Tubes, Bilateral ♀ 6 Uterus ♀ 8 Uterus and Fallopian Tubes ♀ 9 Vagina ♀	0 High Osmolar 1 Low Osmolar Y Other Contrast Z None	Z None	Z None

◀ New   ◀▥ Revised   ~~deleted~~ Deleted   ♀ Females Only   ♂ Males Only
⊘ Noncovered   ⊘ Limited Coverage   ⊘ Hospital-Acquired Condition   **Coding Clinic**

591

SECTION: B IMAGING
BODY SYSTEM: U FEMALE REPRODUCTIVE SYSTEM
TYPE: 3 **MAGNETIC RESONANCE IMAGING (MRI):** Computer reformatted digital display of multiplanar images developed from the capture of radiofrequency signals emitted by nuclei in a body site excited within a magnetic field

Body Part	Contrast	Qualifier	Qualifier
3 Ovary, Right ♀ 4 Ovary, Left ♀ 5 Ovaries, Bilateral ♀ 6 Uterus ♀ 9 Vagina ♀ B Pregnant Uterus ♀ C Uterus and Ovaries ♀	Y Other Contrast	0 Unenhanced and Enhanced Z None	Z None
3 Ovary, Right ♀ 4 Ovary, Left ♀ 5 Ovaries, Bilateral ♀ 6 Uterus ♀ 9 Vagina ♀ B Pregnant Uterus ♀ C Uterus and Ovaries ♀	Z None	Z None	Z None

SECTION: B IMAGING
BODY SYSTEM: U FEMALE REPRODUCTIVE SYSTEM
TYPE: 4 **ULTRASONOGRAPHY:** Real time display of images of anatomy or flow information developed from the capture of reflected and attenuated high frequency sound waves

Body Part	Contrast	Qualifier	Qualifier
0 Fallopian Tube, Right ♀ 1 Fallopian Tube, Left ♀ 2 Fallopian Tubes, Bilateral ♀ 3 Ovary, Right ♀ 4 Ovary, Left ♀ 5 Ovaries, Bilateral ♀ 6 Uterus ♀ C Uterus and Ovaries ♀	Y Other Contrast Z None	Z None	Z None

◀ New   ◀▦ Revised   ~~deleted~~ Deleted   ♀ Females Only   ♂ Males Only
Ⓝ Noncovered   Ⓛ Limited Coverage   Ⓗ Hospital-Acquired Condition   **Coding Clinic**

SECTION: B IMAGING
BODY SYSTEM: V MALE REPRODUCTIVE SYSTEM
TYPE: 0 PLAIN RADIOGRAPHY: Planar display of an image developed from the capture of external ionizing radiation on photographic or photoconductive plate

Body Part	Contrast	Qualifier	Qualifier
0 Corpora Cavernosa ♂ 1 Epididymis, Right ♂ 2 Epididymis, Left ♂ 3 Prostate ♂ 5 Testicle, Right ♂ 6 Testicle, Left ♂ 8 Vasa Vasorum ♂	0 High Osmolar 1 Low Osmolar Y Other Contrast	Z None	Z None

SECTION: B IMAGING
BODY SYSTEM: V MALE REPRODUCTIVE SYSTEM
TYPE: 1 FLUOROSCOPY: Single plane or bi-plane real time display of an image developed from the capture of external ionizing radiation on a fluorescent screen. The image may also be stored by either digital or analog means

Body Part	Contrast	Qualifier	Qualifier
0 Corpora Cavernosa ♂ 8 Vasa Vasorum ♂	0 High Osmolar 1 Low Osmolar Y Other Contrast Z None	Z None	Z None

2: CT SCAN   3: MRI   4: ULTRASONOGRAPHY

V: MALE REPRODUCTIVE SYSTEM

B: IMAGING

SECTION: B IMAGING

BODY SYSTEM: V MALE REPRODUCTIVE SYSTEM

TYPE: 2 COMPUTERIZED TOMOGRAPHY (CT SCAN): Computer reformatted digital display of multiplanar images developed from the capture of multiple exposures of external ionizing radiation

Body Part	Contrast	Qualifier	Qualifier
3 Prostate ♂	0 High Osmolar 1 Low Osmolar Y Other Contrast	0 Unenhanced and Enhanced Z None	Z None
3 Prostate ♂	Z None	Z None	Z None

SECTION: B IMAGING

BODY SYSTEM: V MALE REPRODUCTIVE SYSTEM

TYPE: 3 MAGNETIC RESONANCE IMAGING (MRI): Computer reformatted digital display of multiplanar images developed from the capture of radiofrequency signals emitted by nuclei in a body site excited within a magnetic field

Body Part	Contrast	Qualifier	Qualifier
0 Corpora Cavernosa ♂ 3 Prostate ♂ 4 Scrotum ♂ 5 Testicle, Right ♂ 6 Testicle, Left ♂ 7 Testicles, Bilateral ♂	Y Other Contrast	0 Unenhanced and Enhanced Z None	Z None
0 Corpora Cavernosa ♂ 3 Prostate ♂ 4 Scrotum ♂ 5 Testicle, Right ♂ 6 Testicle, Left ♂ 7 Testicles, Bilateral ♂	Z None	Z None	Z None

SECTION: B IMAGING

BODY SYSTEM: V MALE REPRODUCTIVE SYSTEM

TYPE: 4 ULTRASONOGRAPHY: Real time display of images of anatomy or flow information developed from the capture of reflected and attenuated high frequency sound waves

Body Part	Contrast	Qualifier	Qualifier
4 Scrotum ♂ 9 Prostate and Seminal Vesicles ♂ B Penis ♂	Z None	Z None	Z None

◀ New   ◀▥ Revised   ~~deleted~~ Deleted   ♀ Females Only   ♂ Males Only
🅝 Noncovered   🅛 Limited Coverage   🅗 Hospital-Acquired Condition   **Coding Clinic**

SECTION:　**B IMAGING**
BODY SYSTEM: W ANATOMICAL REGIONS
TYPE:　　　　　**0　PLAIN RADIOGRAPHY:** Planar display of an image developed from the capture of external ionizing radiation on photographic or photoconductive plate

Body Part	Contrast	Qualifier	Qualifier
0 Abdomen 1 Abdomen and Pelvis 3 Chest B Long Bones, All C Lower Extremity J Upper Extremity K Whole Body L Whole Skeleton M Whole Body, Infant	Z None	Z None	Z None

SECTION:　**B IMAGING**
BODY SYSTEM: W ANATOMICAL REGIONS
TYPE:　　　　　**1　FLUOROSCOPY:** Single plane or bi-plane real time display of an image developed from the capture of external ionizing radiation on a fluorescent screen. The image may also be stored by either digital or analog means

Body Part	Contrast	Qualifier	Qualifier
1 Abdomen and Pelvis 9 Head and Neck C Lower Extremity J Upper Extremity	0 High Osmolar 1 Low Osmolar Y Other Contrast Z None	Z None	Z None

SECTION:　**B IMAGING**
BODY SYSTEM: W ANATOMICAL REGIONS
TYPE:　　　　　**2　COMPUTERIZED TOMOGRAPHY (CT SCAN):** Computer reformatted digital display of multiplanar images developed from the capture of multiple exposures of external ionizing radiation

Body Part	Contrast	Qualifier	Qualifier
0 Abdomen 1 Abdomen and Pelvis 4 Chest and Abdomen 5 Chest, Abdomen, and Pelvis 8 Head 9 Head and Neck F Neck G Pelvic Region	0 High Osmolar 1 Low Osmolar Y Other Contrast	0 Unenhanced and Enhanced Z None	Z None
0 Abdomen 1 Abdomen and Pelvis 4 Chest and Abdomen 5 Chest, Abdomen, and Pelvis 8 Head 9 Head and Neck F Neck G Pelvic Region	Z None	Z None	Z None

4: ULTRASONOGRAPHY

3: MAGNETIC RESONANCE IMAGING (MRI)

SECTION: B IMAGING
BODY SYSTEM: W ANATOMICAL REGIONS
TYPE: 3 **MAGNETIC RESONANCE IMAGING (MRI):** Computer reformatted digital display of multiplanar images developed from the capture of radiofrequency signals emitted by nuclei in a body site excited within a magnetic field

Body Part	Contrast	Qualifier	Qualifier
0 Abdomen 8 Head F Neck G Pelvic Region H Retroperitoneum P Brachial Plexus	Y Other Contrast	0 Unenhanced and Enhanced Z None	Z None
0 Abdomen 8 Head F Neck G Pelvic Region H Retroperitoneum P Brachial Plexus	Z None	Z None	Z None
3 Chest	Y Other Contrast	0 Unenhanced and Enhanced Z None	Z None

SECTION: B IMAGING
BODY SYSTEM: W ANATOMICAL REGIONS
TYPE: 4 **ULTRASONOGRAPHY:** Real time display of images of anatomy or flow information developed from the capture of reflected and attenuated high frequency sound waves

Body Part	Contrast	Qualifier	Qualifier
0 Abdomen 1 Abdomen and Pelvis F Neck G Pelvic Region	Z None	Z None	Z None

W: ANATOMICAL REGIONS

B: IMAGING

◀ New	◀▥ Revised	~~deleted~~ Deleted	♀ Females Only	♂ Males Only
🅝ₒ Noncovered	🅛ₒ Limited Coverage	🅗ₐ Hospital-Acquired Condition	**Coding Clinic**

SECTION: B IMAGING
BODY SYSTEM: Y FETUS AND OBSTETRICAL
TYPE: 3 MAGNETIC RESONANCE IMAGING (MRI): Computer reformatted digital display of multiplanar images developed from the capture of radiofrequency signals emitted by nuclei in a body site excited within a magnetic field

Body Part	Contrast	Qualifier	Qualifier
0 Fetal Head ♀ 1 Fetal Heart ♀ 2 Fetal Thorax ♀ 3 Fetal Abdomen ♀ 4 Fetal Spine ♀ 5 Fetal Extremities ♀ 6 Whole Fetus ♀	Y Other Contrast	0 Unenhanced and Enhanced Z None	Z None
0 Fetal Head ♀ 1 Fetal Heart ♀ 2 Fetal Thorax ♀ 3 Fetal Abdomen ♀ 4 Fetal Spine ♀ 5 Fetal Extremities ♀ 6 Whole Fetus ♀	Z None	Z None	Z None

SECTION: B IMAGING
BODY SYSTEM: Y FETUS AND OBSTETRICAL
TYPE: 4 ULTRASONOGRAPHY: Real time display of images of anatomy or flow information developed from the capture of reflected and attenuated high frequency sound waves

Body Part	Contrast	Qualifier	Qualifier
7 Fetal Umbilical Cord ♀ 8 Placenta ♀ 9 First Trimester, Single Fetus ♀ B First Trimester, Multiple Gestation ♀ C Second Trimester, Single Fetus ♀ D Second Trimester, Multiple Gestation ♀ F Third Trimester, Single Fetus ♀ G Third Trimester, Multiple Gestation ♀	Z None	Z None	Z None

◀ New   ◀ Revised   ~~deleted~~ Deleted   ♀ Females Only   ♂ Males Only
Ⓝ Noncovered   Ⓛ Limited Coverage   Ⓗ Hospital-Acquired Condition   **Coding Clinic**

B: IMAGING   Y: FETUS AND OBSTETRICAL   3: MRI   4: ULTRASONOGRAPHY

◀ New   ◀▥ Revised   deleted Deleted   ♀ Females Only   ♂ Males Only
🅝 Noncovered   🅛 Limited Coverage   🅗 Hospital-Acquired Condition   **Coding Clinic**

SECTION: C NUCLEAR MEDICINE
BODY SYSTEM: 0 CENTRAL NERVOUS SYSTEM
TYPE: **1 PLANAR NUCLEAR MEDICINE IMAGING:** Introduction of radioactive materials into the body for single plane display of images developed from the capture of radioactive emissions

Body Part	Radionuclide	Qualifier	Qualifier
0 Brain	1 Technetium 99m (Tc-99m) Y Other Radionuclide	Z None	Z None
5 Cerebrospinal Fluid	D Indium 111 (In-111) Y Other Radionuclide	Z None	Z None
Y Central Nervous System	Y Other Radionuclide	Z None	Z None

SECTION: C NUCLEAR MEDICINE
BODY SYSTEM: 0 CENTRAL NERVOUS SYSTEM
TYPE: **2 TOMOGRAPHIC (TOMO) NUCLEAR MEDICINE IMAGING:** Introduction of radioactive materials into the body for three dimensional display of images developed from the capture of radioactive emissions

Body Part	Radionuclide	Qualifier	Qualifier
0 Brain	1 Technetium 99m (Tc-99m) F Iodine 123 (I-123) S Thallium 201 (Tl-201) Y Other Radionuclide	Z None	Z None
5 Cerebrospinal Fluid	D Indium 111 (In-111) Y Other Radionuclide	Z None	Z None
Y Central Nervous System	Y Other Radionuclide	Z None	Z None

C: NUCLEAR MEDICINE

0: CENTRAL NERVOUS SYSTEM

1; 2

SECTION: C NUCLEAR MEDICINE
BODY SYSTEM: 0 CENTRAL NERVOUS SYSTEM
TYPE: 3 **POSITRON EMISSION TOMOGRAPHIC (PET) IMAGING:** Introduction of radioactive materials into the body for three dimensional display of images developed from the simultaneous capture, 180 degrees apart, of radioactive emissions

Body Part	Radionuclide	Qualifier	Qualifier
0 Brain	B Carbon 11 (C-11) K Fluorine 18 (F-18) M Oxygen 15 (O-15) Y Other Radionuclide	Z None	Z None
Y Central Nervous System	Y Other Radionuclide	Z None	Z None

SECTION: C NUCLEAR MEDICINE
BODY SYSTEM: 0 CENTRAL NERVOUS SYSTEM
TYPE: 5 **NONIMAGING NUCLEAR MEDICINE PROBE:** Introduction of radioactive materials into the body for the study of distribution and fate of certain substances by the detection of radioactive emissions; or, alternatively, measurement of absorption of radioactive emissions from an external source

Body Part	Radionuclide	Qualifier	Qualifier
0 Brain	V Xenon 133 (Xe-133) Y Other Radionuclide	Z None	Z None
Y Central Nervous System	Y Other Radionuclide	Z None	Z None

◀ New   ◀▥ Revised   ~~deleted~~ Deleted   ♀ Females Only   ♂ Males Only
🅝 Noncovered   🅛 Limited Coverage   🅗 Hospital-Acquired Condition   **Coding Clinic**

SECTION: C NUCLEAR MEDICINE
BODY SYSTEM: 2 HEART

TYPE: **1 PLANAR NUCLEAR MEDICINE IMAGING:** Introduction of radioactive materials into the body for single plane display of images developed from the capture of radioactive emissions

Body Part	Radionuclide	Qualifier	Qualifier
6 Heart, Right and Left	1 Technetium 99m (Tc-99m) Y Other Radionuclide	Z None	Z None
G Myocardium	1 Technetium 99m (Tc-99m) D Indium 111 (In-111) S Thallium 201 (Tl-201) Y Other Radionuclide Z None	Z None	Z None
Y Heart	Y Other Radionuclide	Z None	Z None

SECTION: C NUCLEAR MEDICINE
BODY SYSTEM: 2 HEART

TYPE: **2 TOMOGRAPHIC (TOMO) NUCLEAR MEDICINE IMAGING:** Introduction of radioactive materials into the body for three dimensional display of images developed from the capture of radioactive emissions

Body Part	Radionuclide	Qualifier	Qualifier
6 Heart, Right and Left	1 Technetium 99m (Tc-99m) Y Other Radionuclide	Z None	Z None
G Myocardium	1 Technetium 99m (Tc-99m) D Indium 111 (In-111) K Fluorine 18 (F-18) S Thallium 201 (Tl-201) Y Other Radionuclide Z None	Z None	Z None
Y Heart	Y Other Radionuclide	Z None	Z None

◀ New ◀ Revised ~~deleted~~ Deleted ♀ Females Only ♂ Males Only
🅝🅒 Noncovered 🅛🅒 Limited Coverage 🅗🅐🅒 Hospital-Acquired Condition **Coding Clinic**

601

SECTION: C NUCLEAR MEDICINE
BODY SYSTEM: 2 HEART
TYPE: 3 **POSITRON EMISSION TOMOGRAPHIC (PET) IMAGING:** Introduction of radioactive materials into the body for three dimensional display of images developed from the simultaneous capture, 180 degrees apart, of radioactive emissions

Body Part	Radionuclide	Qualifier	Qualifier
G Myocardium	K Fluorine 18 (F-18) M Oxygen 15 (O-15) Q Rubidium 82 (Rb-82) R Nitrogen 13 (N-13) Y Other Radionuclide	Z None	Z None
Y Heart	Y Other Radionuclide	Z None	Z None

SECTION: C NUCLEAR MEDICINE
BODY SYSTEM: 2 HEART
TYPE: 5 **NONIMAGING NUCLEAR MEDICINE PROBE:** Introduction of radioactive materials into the body for the study of distribution and fate of certain substances by the detection of radioactive emissions; or, alternatively, measurement of absorption of radioactive emissions from an external source

Body Part	Radionuclide	Qualifier	Qualifier
6 Heart, Right and Left	1 Technetium 99m (Tc-99m) Y Other Radionuclide	Z None	Z None
Y Heart	Y Other Radionuclide	Z None	Z None

SECTION: C NUCLEAR MEDICINE
BODY SYSTEM: 5 VEINS
TYPE: 1 **PLANAR NUCLEAR MEDICINE IMAGING:** Introduction of radioactive materials into the body for single plane display of images developed from the capture of radioactive emissions

Body Part	Radionuclide	Qualifier	Qualifier
B Lower Extremity Veins, Right C Lower Extremity Veins, Left D Lower Extremity Veins, Bilateral N Upper Extremity Veins, Right P Upper Extremity Veins, Left Q Upper Extremity Veins, Bilateral R Central Veins	1 Technetium 99m (Tc-99m) Y Other Radionuclide	Z None	Z None
Y Veins	Y Other Radionuclide	Z None	Z None

◀ New   ◀▥ Revised   ~~deleted~~ Deleted   ♀ Females Only   ♂ Males Only
▨ Noncovered   ▨ Limited Coverage   ▨ Hospital-Acquired Condition   **Coding Clinic**

603

SECTION: C NUCLEAR MEDICINE

BODY SYSTEM: 7 LYMPHATIC AND HEMATOLOGIC SYSTEM

TYPE: 1 **PLANAR NUCLEAR MEDICINE IMAGING:** Introduction of radioactive materials into the body for single plane display of images developed from the capture of radioactive emissions

Body Part	Radionuclide	Qualifier	Qualifier
0 Bone Marrow	1 Technetium 99m (Tc-99m) D Indium 111 (In-111) Y Other Radionuclide	Z None	Z None
2 Spleen 5 Lymphatics, Head and Neck D Lymphatics, Pelvic J Lymphatics, Head K Lymphatics, Neck L Lymphatics, Upper Chest M Lymphatics, Trunk N Lymphatics, Upper Extremity P Lymphatics, Lower Extremity	1 Technetium 99m (Tc-99m) Y Other Radionuclide	Z None	Z None
3 Blood	D Indium 111 (In-111) Y Other Radionuclide	Z None	Z None
Y Lymphatic and Hematologic System	Y Other Radionuclide	Z None	Z None

SECTION: C NUCLEAR MEDICINE

BODY SYSTEM: 7 LYMPHATIC AND HEMATOLOGIC SYSTEM

TYPE: 2 **TOMOGRAPHIC (TOMO) NUCLEAR MEDICINE IMAGING:** Introduction of radioactive materials into the body for three dimensional display of images developed from the capture of radioactive emissions

Body Part	Radionuclide	Qualifier	Qualifier
2 Spleen	1 Technetium 99m (Tc-99m) Y Other Radionuclide	Z None	Z None
Y Lymphatic and Hematologic System	Y Other Radionuclide	Z None	Z None

7: LYMPHATIC AND HEMATOLOGIC SYSTEM

1; 2

C: NUCLEAR MEDICINE

◀ New ◀ Revised ~~deleted~~ Deleted ♀ Females Only ♂ Males Only
Noncovered Limited Coverage Hospital-Acquired Condition **Coding Clinic**

SECTION: C NUCLEAR MEDICINE

BODY SYSTEM: 7 LYMPHATIC AND HEMATOLOGIC SYSTEM

TYPE: 5 **NONIMAGING NUCLEAR MEDICINE PROBE:** Introduction of radioactive materials into the body for the study of distribution and fate of certain substances by the detection of radioactive emissions; or, alternatively, measurement of absorption of radioactive emissions from an external source

Body Part	Radionuclide	Qualifier	Qualifier
5 Lymphatics, Head and Neck D Lymphatics, Pelvic J Lymphatics, Head K Lymphatics, Neck L Lymphatics, Upper Chest M Lymphatics, Trunk N Lymphatics, Upper Extremity P Lymphatics, Lower Extremity	1 Technetium 99m (Tc-99m) Y Other Radionuclide	Z None	Z None
Y Lymphatic and Hematologic System	Y Other Radionuclide	Z None	Z None

SECTION: C NUCLEAR MEDICINE

BODY SYSTEM: 7 LYMPHATIC AND HEMATOLOGIC SYSTEM

TYPE: 6 **NONIMAGING NUCLEAR MEDICINE ASSAY:** Introduction of radioactive materials into the body for the study of body fluids and blood elements, by the detection of radioactive emissions

Body Part	Radionuclide	Qualifier	Qualifier
3 Blood	1 Technetium 99m (Tc-99m) 7 Cobalt 58 (Co-58) C Cobalt 57 (Co-57) D Indium 111 (In-111) H Iodine 125 (I-125) W Chromium (Cr-51) Y Other Radionuclide	Z None	Z None
Y Lymphatic and Hematologic System	Y Other Radionuclide	Z None	Z None

SECTION: C NUCLEAR MEDICINE
BODY SYSTEM: 8 EYE
TYPE: 1 **PLANAR NUCLEAR MEDICINE IMAGING:** Introduction of radioactive materials into the body for single plane display of images developed from the capture of radioactive emissions

Body Part	Radionuclide	Qualifier	Qualifier
9 Lacrimal Ducts, Bilateral	1 Technetium 99m (Tc-99m) Y Other Radionuclide	Z None	Z None
Y Eye	Y Other Radionuclide	Z None	Z None

SECTION: C NUCLEAR MEDICINE
BODY SYSTEM: 9 EAR, NOSE, MOUTH, AND THROAT

TYPE: 1 PLANAR NUCLEAR MEDICINE IMAGING: Introduction of radioactive materials into the body for single plane display of images developed from the capture of radioactive emissions

Body Part	Radionuclide	Qualifier	Qualifier
B Salivary Glands, Bilateral	1 Technetium 99m (Tc-99m) Y Other Radionuclide	Z None	Z None
Y Ear, Nose, Mouth and Throat	Y Other Radionuclide	Z None	Z None

SECTION: C NUCLEAR MEDICINE

BODY SYSTEM: B RESPIRATORY SYSTEM

TYPE: **1 PLANAR NUCLEAR MEDICINE IMAGING:** Introduction of radioactive materials into the body for single plane display of images developed from the capture of radioactive emissions

Body Part	Radionuclide	Qualifier	Qualifier
2 Lungs and Bronchi	1 Technetium 99m (Tc-99m) 9 Krypton (Kr-81m) T Xenon 127 (Xe-127) V Xenon 133 (Xe-133) Y Other Radionuclide	Z None	Z None
Y Respiratory System	Y Other Radionuclide	Z None	Z None

SECTION: C NUCLEAR MEDICINE

BODY SYSTEM: B RESPIRATORY SYSTEM

TYPE: **2 TOMOGRAPHIC (TOMO) NUCLEAR MEDICINE IMAGING:** Introduction of radioactive materials into the body for three dimensional display of images developed from the capture of radioactive emissions

Body Part	Radionuclide	Qualifier	Qualifier
2 Lungs and Bronchi	1 Technetium 99m (Tc-99m) 9 Krypton (Kr-81m) Y Other Radionuclide	Z None	Z None
Y Respiratory System	Y Other Radionuclide	Z None	Z None

SECTION: C NUCLEAR MEDICINE

BODY SYSTEM: B RESPIRATORY SYSTEM

TYPE: **3 POSITRON EMISSION TOMOGRAPHIC (PET) IMAGING:** Introduction of radioactive materials into the body for three dimensional display of images developed from the simultaneous capture, 180 degrees apart, of radioactive emissions

Body Part	Radionuclide	Qualifier	Qualifier
2 Lungs and Bronchi	K Fluorine 18 (F-18) Y Other Radionuclide	Z None	Z None
Y Respiratory System	Y Other Radionuclide	Z None	Z None

B: RESPIRATORY SYSTEM

C: NUCLEAR MEDICINE

1; 2; 3

◀ New   ◀ Revised   ~~deleted~~ Deleted   ♀ Females Only   ♂ Males Only
  Noncovered   Limited Coverage   Hospital-Acquired Condition   **Coding Clinic**

SECTION: C NUCLEAR MEDICINE
BODY SYSTEM: D GASTROINTESTINAL SYSTEM
TYPE: **1 PLANAR NUCLEAR MEDICINE IMAGING:** Introduction of radioactive materials into the body for single plane display of images developed from the capture of radioactive emissions

Body Part	Radionuclide	Qualifier	Qualifier
5 Upper Gastrointestinal Tract 7 Gastrointestinal Tract	1 Technetium 99m (Tc-99m) D Indium 111 (In-111) Y Other Radionuclide	Z None	Z None
Y Digestive System	Y Other Radionuclide	Z None	Z None

SECTION: C NUCLEAR MEDICINE
BODY SYSTEM: D GASTROINTESTINAL SYSTEM
TYPE: **2 TOMOGRAPHIC (TOMO) NUCLEAR MEDICINE IMAGING:** Introduction of radioactive materials into the body for three dimensional display of images developed from the capture of radioactive emissions

Body Part	Radionuclide	Qualifier	Qualifier
7 Gastrointestinal Tract	1 Technetium 99m (Tc-99m) D Indium 111 (In-111) Y Other Radionuclide	Z None	Z None
Y Digestive System	Y Other Radionuclide	Z None	Z None

SECTION: C NUCLEAR MEDICINE
BODY SYSTEM: F HEPATOBILIARY SYSTEM AND PANCREAS
TYPE: 1 **PLANAR NUCLEAR MEDICINE IMAGING:** Introduction of radioactive materials into the body for single plane display of images developed from the capture of radioactive emissions

Body Part	Radionuclide	Qualifier	Qualifier
4 Gallbladder 5 Liver 6 Liver and Spleen C Hepatobiliary System, All	1 Technetium 99m (Tc-99m) Y Other Radionuclide	Z None	Z None
Y Hepatobiliary System and Pancreas	Y Other Radionuclide	Z None	Z None

SECTION: C NUCLEAR MEDICINE
BODY SYSTEM: F HEPATOBILIARY SYSTEM AND PANCREAS
TYPE: 2 **TOMOGRAPHIC (TOMO) NUCLEAR MEDICINE IMAGING:** Introduction of radioactive materials into the body for three dimensional display of images developed from the capture of radioactive emissions

Body Part	Radionuclide	Qualifier	Qualifier
4 Gallbladder 5 Liver 6 Liver and Spleen	1 Technetium 99m (Tc-99m) Y Other Radionuclide	Z None	Z None
Y Hepatobiliary System and Pancreas	Y Other Radionuclide	Z None	Z None

◀ New   ◀▥ Revised   ~~deleted~~ Deleted   ♀ Females Only   ♂ Males Only
🅝 Noncovered   🅛 Limited Coverage   🅗 Hospital-Acquired Condition   **Coding Clinic**

F: HEPATOBILIARY SYSTEM AND PANCREAS

C: NUCLEAR MEDICINE

1; 2

SECTION: C NUCLEAR MEDICINE
BODY SYSTEM: G ENDOCRINE SYSTEM
TYPE: **1 PLANAR NUCLEAR MEDICINE IMAGING:** Introduction of radioactive materials into the body for single plane display of images developed from the capture of radioactive emissions

Body Part	Radionuclide	Qualifier	Qualifier
1 Parathyroid Glands	1 Technetium 99m (Tc-99m) S Thallium 201 (Tl-201) Y Other Radionuclide	Z None	Z None
2 Thyroid Gland	1 Technetium 99m (Tc-99m) F Iodine 123 (I-123) G Iodine 131 (I-131) Y Other Radionuclide	Z None	Z None
4 Adrenal Glands, Bilateral	G Iodine 131 (I-131) Y Other Radionuclide	Z None	Z None
Y Endocrine System	Y Other Radionuclide	Z None	Z None

SECTION: C NUCLEAR MEDICINE
BODY SYSTEM: G ENDOCRINE SYSTEM
TYPE: **2 TOMOGRAPHIC (TOMO) NUCLEAR MEDICINE IMAGING:** Introduction of radioactive materials into the body for three dimensional display of images developed from the capture of radioactive emissions

Body Part	Radionuclide	Qualifier	Qualifier
1 Parathyroid Glands	1 Technetium 99m (Tc-99m) S Thallium 201 (Tl-201) Y Other Radionuclide	Z None	Z None
Y Endocrine System	Y Other Radionuclide	Z None	Z None

SECTION: C NUCLEAR MEDICINE
BODY SYSTEM: G ENDOCRINE SYSTEM
TYPE: **4 NONIMAGING NUCLEAR MEDICINE UPTAKE:** Introduction of radioactive materials into the body for measurements of organ function, from the detection of radioactive emissions

Body Part	Radionuclide	Qualifier	Qualifier
2 Thyroid Gland	1 Technetium 99m (Tc-99m) F Iodine 123 (I-123) G Iodine 131 (I-131) Y Other Radionuclide	Z None	Z None
Y Endocrine System	Y Other Radionuclide	Z None	Z None

SECTION: C NUCLEAR MEDICINE

BODY SYSTEM: H SKIN, SUBCUTANEOUS TISSUE AND BREAST

TYPE: 1 **PLANAR NUCLEAR MEDICINE IMAGING:** Introduction of radioactive materials into the body for single plane display of images developed from the capture of radioactive emissions

Body Part	Radionuclide	Qualifier	Qualifier
0 Breast, Right 1 Breast, Left 2 Breasts, Bilateral	1 Technetium 99m (Tc-99m) S Thallium 201 (Tl-201) Y Other Radionuclide	Z None	Z None
Y Skin, Subcutaneous Tissue, and Breast	Y Other Radionuclide	Z None	Z None

SECTION: C NUCLEAR MEDICINE

BODY SYSTEM: H SKIN, SUBCUTANEOUS TISSUE AND BREAST

TYPE: 2 **TOMOGRAPHIC (TOMO) NUCLEAR MEDICINE IMAGING:** Introduction of radioactive materials into the body for three dimensional display of images developed from the capture of radioactive emissions

Body Part	Radionuclide	Qualifier	Qualifier
0 Breast, Right 1 Breast, Left 2 Breasts, Bilateral	1 Technetium 99m (Tc-99m) S Thallium 201 (Tl-201) Y Other Radionuclide	Z None	Z None
Y Skin, Subcutaneous Tissue, and Breast	Y Other Radionuclide	Z None	Z None

SECTION: C NUCLEAR MEDICINE
BODY SYSTEM: P MUSCULOSKELETAL SYSTEM
TYPE: 1 **PLANAR NUCLEAR MEDICINE IMAGING:** Introduction of radioactive materials into the body for single plane display of images developed from the capture of radioactive emissions

Body Part	Radionuclide	Qualifier	Qualifier
1 Skull 4 Thorax 5 Spine 6 Pelvis 7 Spine and Pelvis 8 Upper Extremity, Right 9 Upper Extremity, Left B Upper Extremities, Bilateral C Lower Extremity, Right D Lower Extremity, Left F Lower Extremities, Bilateral Z Musculoskeletal System, All	1 Technetium 99m (Tc-99m) Y Other Radionuclide	Z None	Z None
Y Musculoskeletal System, Other	Y Other Radionuclide	Z None	Z None

SECTION: C NUCLEAR MEDICINE
BODY SYSTEM: P MUSCULOSKELETAL SYSTEM
TYPE: 2 **TOMOGRAPHIC (TOMO) NUCLEAR MEDICINE IMAGING:** Introduction of radioactive materials into the body for three dimensional display of images developed from the capture of radioactive emissions

Body Part	Radionuclide	Qualifier	Qualifier
1 Skull 2 Cervical Spine 3 Skull and Cervical Spine 4 Thorax 6 Pelvis 7 Spine and Pelvis 8 Upper Extremity, Right 9 Upper Extremity, Left B Upper Extremities, Bilateral C Lower Extremity, Right D Lower Extremity, Left F Lower Extremities, Bilateral G Thoracic Spine H Lumbar Spine J Thoracolumbar Spine	1 Technetium 99m (Tc-99m) Y Other Radionuclide	Z None	Z None
Y Musculoskeletal System, Other	Y Other Radionuclide	Z None	Z None

◀ New ◀▥ Revised ~~deleted~~ Deleted ♀ Females Only ♂ Males Only
🦚 Noncovered 🦚 Limited Coverage 🦚 Hospital-Acquired Condition **Coding Clinic**

613

SECTION: C NUCLEAR MEDICINE
BODY SYSTEM: P MUSCULOSKELETAL SYSTEM
TYPE: 5 **NONIMAGING NUCLEAR MEDICINE PROBE:** Introduction of radioactive materials into the body for the study of distribution and fate of certain substances by the detection of radioactive emissions; or, alternatively, measurement of absorption of radioactive emissions from an external source

Body Part	Radionuclide	Qualifier	Qualifier
5 Spine N Upper Extremities P Lower Extremities	Z None	Z None	Z None
Y Musculoskeletal System, Other	Y Other Radionuclide	Z None	Z None

SECTION: C NUCLEAR MEDICINE
BODY SYSTEM: T URINARY SYSTEM
TYPE: **1 PLANAR NUCLEAR MEDICINE IMAGING:** Introduction of radioactive materials into the body for single plane display of images developed from the capture of radioactive emissions

Body Part	Radionuclide	Qualifier	Qualifier
3 Kidneys, Ureters, and Bladder	1 Technetium 99m (Tc-99m) F Iodine 123 (I-123) G Iodine 131 (I-131) Y Other Radionuclide	Z None	Z None
H Bladder and Ureters	1 Technetium 99m (Tc-99m) Y Other Radionuclide	Z None	Z None
Y Urinary System	Y Other Radionuclide	Z None	Z None

SECTION: C NUCLEAR MEDICINE
BODY SYSTEM: T URINARY SYSTEM
TYPE: **2 TOMOGRAPHIC (TOMO) NUCLEAR MEDICINE IMAGING:** Introduction of radioactive materials into the body for three dimensional display of images developed from the capture of radioactive emissions

Body Part	Radionuclide	Qualifier	Qualifier
3 Kidneys, Ureters, and Bladder	1 Technetium 99m (Tc-99m) Y Other Radionuclide	Z None	Z None
Y Urinary System	Y Other Radionuclide	Z None	Z None

SECTION: C NUCLEAR MEDICINE
BODY SYSTEM: T URINARY SYSTEM
TYPE: **6 NONIMAGING NUCLEAR MEDICINE ASSAY:** Introduction of radioactive materials into the body for the study of body fluids and blood elements, by the detection of radioactive emissions

Body Part	Radionuclide	Qualifier	Qualifier
3 Kidneys, Ureters, and Bladder	1 Technetium 99m (Tc-99m) F Iodine 123 (I-123) G Iodine 131 (I-131) H Iodine 125 (I-125) Y Other Radionuclide	Z None	Z None
Y Urinary System	Y Other Radionuclide	Z None	Z None

C: NUCLEAR MEDICINE

T: URINARY SYSTEM

1; 2; 6

SECTION: **C NUCLEAR MEDICINE**
BODY SYSTEM: V   MALE REPRODUCTIVE SYSTEM
TYPE: **1 PLANAR NUCLEAR MEDICINE IMAGING:** Introduction of radioactive materials into the body for single plane display of images developed from the capture of radioactive emissions

Body Part	Radionuclide	Qualifier	Qualifier
9 Testicles, Bilateral	1 Technetium 99m (Tc-99m) Y Other Radionuclide	Z None	Z None
Y Male Reproductive System	Y Other Radionuclide	Z None	Z None

SECTION: C NUCLEAR MEDICINE
BODY SYSTEM: W ANATOMICAL REGIONS
TYPE: **1 PLANAR NUCLEAR MEDICINE IMAGING:** Introduction of radioactive materials into the body for single plane display of images developed from the capture of radioactive emissions

Body Part	Radionuclide	Qualifier	Qualifier
0 Abdomen 1 Abdomen and Pelvis 4 Chest and Abdomen 6 Chest and Neck B Head and Neck D Lower Extremity J Pelvic Region M Upper Extremity N Whole Body	1 Technetium 99m (Tc-99m) D Indium 111 (In-111) F Iodine 123 (I-123) G Iodine 131 (I-131) L Gallium 67 (Ga-67) S Thallium 201 (Tl-201) Y Other Radionuclide	Z None	Z None
3 Chest	1 Technetium 99m (Tc-99m) D Indium 111 (In-111) F Iodine 123 (I-123) G Iodine 131 (I-131) K Fluorine 18 (F-18) L Gallium 67 (Ga-67) S Thallium 201 (Tl-201) Y Other Radionuclide	Z None	Z None
Y Anatomical Regions, Multiple	Y Other Radionuclide	Z None	Z None
Z Anatomical Region, Other	Z None	Z None	Z None

SECTION: C NUCLEAR MEDICINE
BODY SYSTEM: W ANATOMICAL REGIONS
TYPE: **2 TOMOGRAPHIC (TOMO) NUCLEAR MEDICINE IMAGING:** Introduction of radioactive materials into the body for three dimensional display of images developed from the capture of radioactive emissions

Body Part	Radionuclide	Qualifier	Qualifier
0 Abdomen 1 Abdomen and Pelvis 3 Chest 4 Chest and Abdomen 6 Chest and Neck B Head and Neck D Lower Extremity J Pelvic Region M Upper Extremity	1 Technetium 99m (Tc-99m) D Indium 111 (In-111) F Iodine 123 (I-123) G Iodine 131 (I-131) K Fluorine 18 (F-18) L Gallium 67 (Ga-67) S Thallium 201 (Tl-201) Y Other Radionuclide	Z None	Z None
Y Anatomical Regions, Multiple	Y Other Radionuclide	Z None	Z None

◀ New ◀▥ Revised ~~deleted~~ Deleted ♀ Females Only ♂ Males Only
Ⓝ Noncovered Ⓛ Limited Coverage Ⓗ Hospital-Acquired Condition **Coding Clinic**

617

SECTION: C NUCLEAR MEDICINE
BODY SYSTEM: W ANATOMICAL REGIONS
TYPE: **3 POSITRON EMISSION TOMOGRAPHIC (PET) IMAGING:** Introduction of radioactive materials into the body for three dimensional display of images developed from the simultaneous capture, 180 degrees apart, of radioactive emissions

Body Part	Radionuclide	Qualifier	Qualifier
N Whole Body	Y Other Radionuclide	Z None	Z None

SECTION: C NUCLEAR MEDICINE
BODY SYSTEM: W ANATOMICAL REGIONS
TYPE: **5 NONIMAGING NUCLEAR MEDICINE PROBE:** Introduction of radioactive materials into the body for the study of distribution and fate of certain substances by the detection of radioactive emissions; or, alternatively, measurement of absorption of radioactive emissions from an external source

Body Part	Radionuclide	Qualifier	Qualifier
0 Abdomen 1 Abdomen and Pelvis 3 Chest 4 Chest and Abdomen 6 Chest and Neck B Head and Neck D Lower Extremity J Pelvic Region M Upper Extremity	1 Technetium 99m (Tc-99m) D Indium 111 (In-111) Y Other Radionuclide	Z None	Z None

SECTION: C NUCLEAR MEDICINE
BODY SYSTEM: W ANATOMICAL REGIONS
TYPE: **7 SYSTEMIC NUCLEAR MEDICINE THERAPY:** Introduction of unsealed radioactive materials into the body for treatment

Body Part	Radionuclide	Qualifier	Qualifier
0 Abdomen 3 Chest	N Phosphorus 32 (P-32) Y Other Radionuclide	Z None	Z None
G Thyroid	G Iodine 131 (I-131) Y Other Radionuclide	Z None	Z None
N Whole Body	8 Samarium 153 (Sm-153) G Iodine 131 (I-131) N Phosphorus 32 (P-32) P Strontium 89 (Sr-89) Y Other Radionuclide	Z None	Z None
Y Anatomical Regions, Multiple	Y Other Radionuclide	Z None	Z None

W: ANATOMICAL REGIONS

C: NUCLEAR MEDICINE

3; 5; 7

◀ New   ◀▥ Revised   ~~deleted~~ Deleted   ♀ Females Only   ♂ Males Only
🔾 Noncovered   🔾 Limited Coverage   🔾 Hospital-Acquired Condition   **Coding Clinic**

◀ New   ◀ Revised   ~~deleted~~ Deleted   ♀ Females Only   ♂ Males Only
🅝 Noncovered   🅛 Limited Coverage   🅗 Hospital-Acquired Condition   **Coding Clinic**

◀ New   ◀▥ Revised   ~~deleted~~ Deleted   ♀ Females Only   ♂ Males Only
🝆 Noncovered   🝆 Limited Coverage   🝆 Hospital-Acquired Condition   **Coding Clinic**

SECTION: D RADIATION ONCOLOGY
BODY SYSTEM: 0 CENTRAL AND PERIPHERAL NERVOUS SYSTEM
MODALITY: 0 BEAM RADIATION

Treatment Site	Modality Qualifier	Isotope	Qualifier
0 Brain 1 Brain Stem 6 Spinal Cord 7 Peripheral Nerve	0 Photons <1 MeV 1 Photons 1 - 10 MeV 2 Photons >10 MeV 4 Heavy Particles (Protons, Ions) 5 Neutrons 6 Neutron Capture	Z None	Z None
0 Brain 1 Brain Stem 6 Spinal Cord 7 Peripheral Nerve	3 Electrons	Z None	0 Intraoperative Z None

SECTION: D RADIATION ONCOLOGY
BODY SYSTEM: 0 CENTRAL AND PERIPHERAL NERVOUS SYSTEM
MODALITY: 1 BRACHYTHERAPY

Treatment Site	Modality Qualifier	Isotope	Qualifier
0 Brain 1 Brain Stem 6 Spinal Cord 7 Peripheral Nerve	9 High Dose Rate (HDR) B Low Dose Rate (LDR)	7 Cesium 137 (Cs-137) 8 Iridium 192 (Ir-192) 9 Iodine 125 (I-125) B Palladium 103 (Pd-103) C Californium 252 (Cf-252) Y Other Isotope	Z None

SECTION: D RADIATION ONCOLOGY
BODY SYSTEM: 0 CENTRAL AND PERIPHERAL NERVOUS SYSTEM
MODALITY: 2 STEREOTACTIC RADIOSURGERY

Treatment Site	Modality Qualifier	Isotope	Qualifier
0 Brain 1 Brain Stem 6 Spinal Cord 7 Peripheral Nerve	D Stereotactic Other Photon Radiosurgery H Stereotactic Particulate Radiosurgery J Stereotactic Gamma Beam Radiosurgery	Z None	Z None

SECTION: D RADIATION ONCOLOGY
BODY SYSTEM: 0 CENTRAL AND PERIPHERAL NERVOUS SYSTEM
MODALITY: Y OTHER RADIATION

Treatment Site	Modality Qualifier	Isotope	Qualifier
0 Brain 1 Brain Stem 6 Spinal Cord 7 Peripheral Nerve	7 Contact Radiation 8 Hyperthermia F Plaque Radiation K Laser Interstitial Thermal Therapy	Z None	Z None

◀ New ◀ Revised ~~deleted~~ Deleted ♀ Females Only ♂ Males Only
Ⓝ Noncovered Ⓛ Limited Coverage Ⓗ Hospital-Acquired Condition **Coding Clinic**

621

SECTION: D RADIATION ONCOLOGY

BODY SYSTEM: 7 LYMPHATIC AND HEMATOLOGIC SYSTEM

MODALITY: 0 BEAM RADIATION

Treatment Site	Modality Qualifier	Isotope	Qualifier
0 Bone Marrow 1 Thymus 2 Spleen 3 Lymphatics, Neck 4 Lymphatics, Axillary 5 Lymphatics, Thorax 6 Lymphatics, Abdomen 7 Lymphatics, Pelvis 8 Lymphatics, Inguinal	0 Photons <1 MeV 1 Photons 1 - 10 MeV 2 Photons >10 MeV 4 Heavy Particles (Protons, Ions) 5 Neutrons 6 Neutron Capture	Z None	Z None
0 Bone Marrow 1 Thymus 2 Spleen 3 Lymphatics, Neck 4 Lymphatics, Axillary 5 Lymphatics, Thorax 6 Lymphatics, Abdomen 7 Lymphatics, Pelvis 8 Lymphatics, Inguinal	3 Electrons	Z None	0 Intraoperative Z None

SECTION: D RADIATION ONCOLOGY

BODY SYSTEM: 7 LYMPHATIC AND HEMATOLOGIC SYSTEM

MODALITY: 1 BRACHYTHERAPY

Treatment Site	Modality Qualifier	Isotope	Qualifier
0 Bone Marrow 1 Thymus 2 Spleen 3 Lymphatics, Neck 4 Lymphatics, Axillary 5 Lymphatics, Thorax 6 Lymphatics, Abdomen 7 Lymphatics, Pelvis 8 Lymphatics, Inguinal	9 High Dose Rate (HDR) B Low Dose Rate (LDR)	7 Cesium 137 (Cs-137) 8 Iridium 192 (Ir-192) 9 Iodine 125 (I-125) B Palladium 103 (Pd-103) C Californium 252 (Cf-252) Y Other Isotope	Z None

Side tab: 0; 1 — 7: LYMPHATIC AND HEMATOLOGIC SYSTEM — D: RADIATION ONCOLOGY

◀ New   ◀▮▮ Revised   ~~deleted~~ Deleted   ♀ Females Only   ♂ Males Only
🅝 Noncovered   🅛 Limited Coverage   🅗 Hospital-Acquired Condition   **Coding Clinic**

SECTION: D RADIATION ONCOLOGY

BODY SYSTEM: 7 LYMPHATIC AND HEMATOLOGIC SYSTEM
MODALITY: 2 STEREOTACTIC RADIOSURGERY

Treatment Site	Modality Qualifier	Isotope	Qualifier

0 Bone Marrow
1 Thymus
2 Spleen
3 Lymphatics, Neck
4 Lymphatics, Axillary
5 Lymphatics, Thorax
6 Lymphatics, Abdomen
7 Lymphatics, Pelvis
8 Lymphatics, Inguinal
	D Stereotactic Other Photon
	  Radiosurgery
	H Stereotactic Particulate
	  Radiosurgery
	J Stereotactic Gamma Beam
	  Radiosurgery
		Z None	Z None

SECTION: D RADIATION ONCOLOGY

BODY SYSTEM: 7 LYMPHATIC AND HEMATOLOGIC SYSTEM
MODALITY: Y OTHER RADIATION

Treatment Site	Modality Qualifier	Isotope	Qualifier
0 Bone Marrow 1 Thymus 2 Spleen 3 Lymphatics, Neck 4 Lymphatics, Axillary 5 Lymphatics, Thorax 6 Lymphatics, Abdomen 7 Lymphatics, Pelvis 8 Lymphatics, Inguinal	8 Hyperthermia F Plaque Radiation	Z None	Z None

◀ New ◀═ Revised ~~deleted~~ Deleted ♀ Females Only ♂ Males Only
Noncovered Limited Coverage Hospital-Acquired Condition **Coding Clinic**

623

SECTION: D RADIATION ONCOLOGY
BODY SYSTEM: 8 EYE
MODALITY: 0 BEAM RADIATION

Treatment Site	Modality Qualifier	Isotope	Qualifier
0 Eye	0 Photons <1 MeV 1 Photons 1 - 10 MeV 2 Photons >10 MeV 4 Heavy Particles (Protons, Ions) 5 Neutrons 6 Neutron Capture	Z None	Z None
0 Eye	3 Electrons	Z None	0 Intraoperative Z None

SECTION: D RADIATION ONCOLOGY
BODY SYSTEM: 8 EYE
MODALITY: 1 BRACHYTHERAPY

Treatment Site	Modality Qualifier	Isotope	Qualifier
0 Eye	9 High Dose Rate (HDR) B Low Dose Rate (LDR)	7 Cesium 137 (Cs-137) 8 Iridium 192 (Ir-192) 9 Iodine 125 (I-125) B Palladium 103 (Pd-103) C Californium 252 (Cf-252) Y Other Isotope	Z None

SECTION: D RADIATION ONCOLOGY
BODY SYSTEM: 8 EYE
MODALITY: 2 STEREOTACTIC RADIOSURGERY

Treatment Site	Modality Qualifier	Isotope	Qualifier
0 Eye	D Stereotactic Other Photon Radiosurgery H Stereotactic Particulate Radiosurgery J Stereotactic Gamma Beam Radiosurgery	Z None	Z None

SECTION: D RADIATION ONCOLOGY
BODY SYSTEM: 8 EYE
MODALITY: Y OTHER RADIATION

Treatment Site	Modality Qualifier	Isotope	Qualifier
0 Eye	7 Contact Radiation 8 Hyperthermia F Plaque Radiation	Z None	Z None

◀ New   ◀▦ Revised   ~~deleted~~ Deleted   ♀ Females Only   ♂ Males Only
🔾 Noncovered   🔾 Limited Coverage   🔾 Hospital-Acquired Condition   **Coding Clinic**

SECTION: D RADIATION ONCOLOGY
BODY SYSTEM: 9 EAR, NOSE, MOUTH, AND THROAT
MODALITY: 0 BEAM RADIATION

Treatment Site	Modality Qualifier	Isotope	Qualifier
0 Ear 1 Nose 3 Hypopharynx 4 Mouth 5 Tongue 6 Salivary Glands 7 Sinuses 8 Hard Palate 9 Soft Palate B Larynx D Nasopharynx F Oropharynx	0 Photons <1 MeV 1 Photons 1 - 10 MeV 2 Photons >10 MeV 4 Heavy Particles (Protons, Ions) 5 Neutrons 6 Neutron Capture	Z None	Z None
0 Ear 1 Nose 3 Hypopharynx 4 Mouth 5 Tongue 6 Salivary Glands 7 Sinuses 8 Hard Palate 9 Soft Palate B Larynx D Nasopharynx F Oropharynx	3 Electrons	Z None	0 Intraoperative Z None

SECTION: D RADIATION ONCOLOGY
BODY SYSTEM: 9 EAR, NOSE, MOUTH, AND THROAT
MODALITY: 1 BRACHYTHERAPY

Treatment Site	Modality Qualifier	Isotope	Qualifier
0 Ear 1 Nose 3 Hypopharynx 4 Mouth 5 Tongue 6 Salivary Glands 7 Sinuses 8 Hard Palate 9 Soft Palate B Larynx D Nasopharynx F Oropharynx	9 High Dose Rate (HDR) B Low Dose Rate (LDR)	7 Cesium 137 (Cs-137) 8 Iridium 192 (Ir-192) 9 Iodine 125 (I-125) B Palladium 103 (Pd-103) C Californium 252 (Cf-252) Y Other Isotope	Z None

SECTION: D RADIATION ONCOLOGY
BODY SYSTEM: 9 EAR, NOSE, MOUTH, AND THROAT
MODALITY: 2 STEREOTACTIC RADIOSURGERY

Treatment Site	Modality Qualifier	Isotope	Qualifier

0 Ear
1 Nose
4 Mouth
5 Tongue
6 Salivary Glands
7 Sinuses
8 Hard Palate
9 Soft Palate
B Larynx
C Pharynx
D Nasopharynx
	D Stereotactic Other Photon
	  Radiosurgery
	H Stereotactic Particulate
	  Radiosurgery
	J Stereotactic Gamma Beam
	  Radiosurgery
		Z None	Z None

SECTION: D RADIATION ONCOLOGY
BODY SYSTEM: 9 EAR, NOSE, MOUTH, AND THROAT
MODALITY: Y OTHER RADIATION

Treatment Site	Modality Qualifier	Isotope	Qualifier
0 Ear 1 Nose 5 Tongue 6 Salivary Glands 7 Sinuses 8 Hard Palate 9 Soft Palate	7 Contact Radiation 8 Hyperthermia F Plaque Radiation	Z None	Z None
3 Hypopharynx F Oropharynx	7 Contact Radiation 8 Hyperthermia	Z None	Z None
4 Mouth B Larynx D Nasopharynx	7 Contact Radiation 8 Hyperthermia C Intraoperative Radiation Therapy (IORT) F Plaque Radiation	Z None	Z None
C Pharynx	C Intraoperative Radiation Therapy (IORT) F Plaque Radiation	Z None	Z None

◀ New ◀▥ Revised ~~deleted~~ Deleted ♀ Females Only ♂ Males Only
Ⓝⓒ Noncovered Ⓛⓒ Limited Coverage Ⓗⓐⓒ Hospital-Acquired Condition **Coding Clinic**

2; Y

9: EAR, NOSE, MOUTH, AND THROAT

D: RADIATION ONCOLOGY

SECTION: D RADIATION ONCOLOGY
BODY SYSTEM: B RESPIRATORY SYSTEM
MODALITY: 0 BEAM RADIATION

Treatment Site	Modality Qualifier	Isotope	Qualifier
0 Trachea 1 Bronchus 2 Lung 5 Pleura 6 Mediastinum 7 Chest Wall 8 Diaphragm	0 Photons <1 MeV 1 Photons 1 - 10 MeV 2 Photons >10 MeV 4 Heavy Particles (Protons, Ions) 5 Neutrons 6 Neutron Capture	Z None	Z None
0 Trachea 1 Bronchus 2 Lung 5 Pleura 6 Mediastinum 7 Chest Wall 8 Diaphragm	3 Electrons	Z None	0 Intraoperative Z None

SECTION: D RADIATION ONCOLOGY
BODY SYSTEM: B RESPIRATORY SYSTEM
MODALITY: 1 BRACHYTHERAPY

Treatment Site	Modality Qualifier	Isotope	Qualifier
0 Trachea 1 Bronchus 2 Lung 5 Pleura 6 Mediastinum 7 Chest Wall 8 Diaphragm	9 High Dose Rate (HDR) B Low Dose Rate (LDR)	7 Cesium 137 (Cs-137) 8 Iridium 192 (Ir-192) 9 Iodine 125 (I-125) B Palladium 103 (Pd-103) C Californium 252 (Cf-252) Y Other Isotope	Z None

◀ New   ◀▥ Revised   ~~deleted~~ Deleted   ♀ Females Only   ♂ Males Only
◈ Noncovered   ◈ Limited Coverage   ◈ Hospital-Acquired Condition   **Coding Clinic**

627

SECTION: D RADIATION ONCOLOGY
BODY SYSTEM: B RESPIRATORY SYSTEM
MODALITY: 2 STEREOTACTIC RADIOSURGERY

Treatment Site	Modality Qualifier	Isotope	Qualifier
0 Trachea	D Stereotactic Other Photon Radiosurgery	Z None	Z None
1 Bronchus	H Stereotactic Particulate Radiosurgery		
2 Lung	J Stereotactic Gamma Beam Radiosurgery		
5 Pleura			
6 Mediastinum			
7 Chest Wall			
8 Diaphragm			

SECTION: D RADIATION ONCOLOGY
BODY SYSTEM: B RESPIRATORY SYSTEM
MODALITY: Y OTHER RADIATION

Treatment Site	Modality Qualifier	Isotope	Qualifier
0 Trachea	7 Contact Radiation	Z None	Z None
1 Bronchus	8 Hyperthermia		
2 Lung	F Plaque Radiation		
5 Pleura	K Laser Interstitial Thermal Therapy		
6 Mediastinum			
7 Chest Wall			
8 Diaphragm			

SECTION: D RADIATION ONCOLOGY
BODY SYSTEM: D GASTROINTESTINAL SYSTEM
MODALITY: 0 BEAM RADIATION

Treatment Site	Modality Qualifier	Isotope	Qualifier
0 Esophagus 1 Stomach 2 Duodenum 3 Jejunum 4 Ileum 5 Colon 7 Rectum	0 Photons <1 MeV 1 Photons 1 - 10 MeV 2 Photons >10 MeV 4 Heavy Particles (Protons, Ions) 5 Neutrons 6 Neutron Capture	Z None	Z None
0 Esophagus 1 Stomach 2 Duodenum 3 Jejunum 4 Ileum 5 Colon 7 Rectum	3 Electrons	Z None	0 Intraoperative Z None

SECTION: D RADIATION ONCOLOGY
BODY SYSTEM: D GASTROINTESTINAL SYSTEM
MODALITY: 1 BRACHYTHERAPY

Treatment Site	Modality Qualifier	Isotope	Qualifier
0 Esophagus 1 Stomach 2 Duodenum 3 Jejunum 4 Ileum 5 Colon 7 Rectum	9 High Dose Rate (HDR) B Low Dose Rate (LDR)	7 Cesium 137 (Cs-137) 8 Iridium 192 (Ir-192) 9 Iodine 125 (I-125) B Palladium 103 (Pd-103) C Californium 252 (Cf-252) Y Other Isotope	Z None

◄ New　◄▥ Revised　~~deleted~~ Deleted　♀ Females Only　♂ Males Only
Ⓝ Noncovered　Ⓛ Limited Coverage　Ⓗ Hospital-Acquired Condition　**Coding Clinic**

629

SECTION: D RADIATION ONCOLOGY
BODY SYSTEM: D GASTROINTESTINAL SYSTEM
MODALITY: 2 STEREOTACTIC RADIOSURGERY

Treatment Site	Modality Qualifier	Isotope	Qualifier
0 Esophagus 1 Stomach 2 Duodenum 3 Jejunum 4 Ileum 5 Colon 7 Rectum	D Stereotactic Other Photon Radiosurgery H Stereotactic Particulate Radiosurgery J Stereotactic Gamma Beam Radiosurgery	Z None	Z None

SECTION: D RADIATION ONCOLOGY
BODY SYSTEM: D GASTROINTESTINAL SYSTEM
MODALITY: Y OTHER RADIATION

Treatment Site	Modality Qualifier	Isotope	Qualifier
0 Esophagus	7 Contact Radiation 8 Hyperthermia F Plaque Radiation K Laser Interstitial Thermal Therapy	Z None	Z None
1 Stomach 2 Duodenum 3 Jejunum 4 Ileum 5 Colon 7 Rectum	7 Contact Radiation 8 Hyperthermia C Intraoperative Radiation Therapy (IORT) F Plaque Radiation K Laser Interstitial Thermal Therapy	Z None	Z None
8 Anus	C Intraoperative Radiation Therapy (IORT) F Plaque Radiation K Laser Interstitial Thermal Therapy	Z None	Z None

◄ New ◄ Revised ~~deleted~~ Deleted ♀ Females Only ♂ Males Only
Noncovered Limited Coverage Hospital-Acquired Condition **Coding Clinic**

SECTION: D RADIATION ONCOLOGY
BODY SYSTEM: F HEPATOBILIARY SYSTEM AND PANCREAS
MODALITY: 0 BEAM RADIATION

Treatment Site	Modality Qualifier	Isotope	Qualifier
0 Liver 1 Gallbladder 2 Bile Ducts 3 Pancreas	0 Photons <1 MeV 1 Photons 1 - 10 MeV 2 Photons >10 MeV 4 Heavy Particles (Protons, Ions) 5 Neutrons 6 Neutron Capture	Z None	Z None
0 Liver 1 Gallbladder 2 Bile Ducts 3 Pancreas	3 Electrons	Z None	0 Intraoperative Z None

SECTION: D RADIATION ONCOLOGY
BODY SYSTEM: F HEPATOBILIARY SYSTEM AND PANCREAS
MODALITY: 1 BRACHYTHERAPY

Treatment Site	Modality Qualifier	Isotope	Qualifier
0 Liver 1 Gallbladder 2 Bile Ducts 3 Pancreas	9 High Dose Rate (HDR) B Low Dose Rate (LDR)	7 Cesium 137 (Cs-137) 8 Iridium 192 (Ir-192) 9 Iodine 125 (I-125) B Palladium 103 (Pd-103) C Californium 252 (Cf-252) Y Other Isotope	Z None

SECTION: D RADIATION ONCOLOGY
BODY SYSTEM: F HEPATOBILIARY SYSTEM AND PANCREAS
MODALITY: 2 STEREOTACTIC RADIOSURGERY

Treatment Site	Modality Qualifier	Isotope	Qualifier
0 Liver 1 Gallbladder 2 Bile Ducts 3 Pancreas	D Stereotactic Other Photon Radiosurgery H Stereotactic Particulate Radiosurgery J Stereotactic Gamma Beam Radiosurgery	Z None	Z None

SECTION: D RADIATION ONCOLOGY
BODY SYSTEM: F HEPATOBILIARY SYSTEM AND PANCREAS
MODALITY: Y OTHER RADIATION

Treatment Site	Modality Qualifier	Isotope	Qualifier
0 Liver 1 Gallbladder 2 Bile Ducts 3 Pancreas	7 Contact Radiation 8 Hyperthermia C Intraoperative Radiation Therapy (IORT) F Plaque Radiation K Laser Interstitial Thermal Therapy	Z None	Z None

◀ New   ◀ Revised   ~~deleted~~ Deleted   ♀ Females Only   ♂ Males Only
🇶 Noncovered   🇶 Limited Coverage   🇶 Hospital-Acquired Condition   **Coding Clinic**

SECTION: D RADIATION ONCOLOGY
BODY SYSTEM: G ENDOCRINE SYSTEM
MODALITY: 0 BEAM RADIATION

Treatment Site	Modality Qualifier	Isotope	Qualifier
0 Pituitary Gland 1 Pineal Body 2 Adrenal Glands 4 Parathyroid Glands 5 Thyroid	0 Photons <1 MeV 1 Photons 1 - 10 MeV 2 Photons >10 MeV 5 Neutrons 6 Neutron Capture	Z None	Z None
0 Pituitary Gland 1 Pineal Body 2 Adrenal Glands 4 Parathyroid Glands 5 Thyroid	3 Electrons	Z None	0 Intraoperative Z None

SECTION: D RADIATION ONCOLOGY
BODY SYSTEM: G ENDOCRINE SYSTEM
MODALITY: 1 BRACHYTHERAPY

Treatment Site	Modality Qualifier	Isotope	Qualifier
0 Pituitary Gland 1 Pineal Body 2 Adrenal Glands 4 Parathyroid Glands 5 Thyroid	9 High Dose Rate (HDR) B Low Dose Rate (LDR)	7 Cesium 137 (Cs-137) 8 Iridium 192 (Ir-192) 9 Iodine 125 (I-125) B Palladium 103 (Pd-103) C Californium 252 (Cf-252) Y Other Isotope	Z None

SECTION: D RADIATION ONCOLOGY
BODY SYSTEM: G ENDOCRINE SYSTEM
MODALITY: 2 STEREOTACTIC RADIOSURGERY

Treatment Site	Modality Qualifier	Isotope	Qualifier
0 Pituitary Gland 1 Pineal Body 2 Adrenal Glands 4 Parathyroid Glands 5 Thyroid	D Stereotactic Other Photon 　Radiosurgery H Stereotactic Particulate 　Radiosurgery J Stereotactic Gamma Beam 　Radiosurgery	Z None	Z None

SECTION: D RADIATION ONCOLOGY
BODY SYSTEM: G ENDOCRINE SYSTEM
MODALITY: Y OTHER RADIATION

Treatment Site	Modality Qualifier	Isotope	Qualifier
0 Pituitary Gland 1 Pineal Body 2 Adrenal Glands 4 Parathyroid Glands 5 Thyroid	7 Contact Radiation 8 Hyperthermia F Plaque Radiation K Laser Interstitial Thermal 　Therapy	Z None	Z None

◀ New　◀||||| Revised　deleted Deleted　♀ Females Only　♂ Males Only
🚫 Noncovered　🔾 Limited Coverage　🔾 Hospital-Acquired Condition　**Coding Clinic**

SECTION: **D RADIATION ONCOLOGY**
BODY SYSTEM: **H SKIN**
MODALITY: **0   BEAM RADIATION**

Treatment Site	Modality Qualifier	Isotope	Qualifier
2 Skin, Face 3 Skin, Neck 4 Skin, Arm 6 Skin, Chest 7 Skin, Back 8 Skin, Abdomen 9 Skin, Buttock B Skin, Leg	0 Photons <1 MeV 1 Photons 1 - 10 MeV 2 Photons >10 MeV 4 Heavy Particles (Protons, Ions) 5 Neutrons 6 Neutron Capture	Z None	Z None
2 Skin, Face 3 Skin, Neck 4 Skin, Arm 6 Skin, Chest 7 Skin, Back 8 Skin, Abdomen 9 Skin, Buttock B Skin, Leg	3 Electrons	Z None	0 Intraoperative Z None

SECTION: **D RADIATION ONCOLOGY**
BODY SYSTEM: **H SKIN**
MODALITY: **Y   OTHER RADIATION**

Treatment Site	Modality Qualifier	Isotope	Qualifier
2 Skin, Face 3 Skin, Neck 4 Skin, Arm 6 Skin, Chest 7 Skin, Back 8 Skin, Abdomen 9 Skin, Buttock B Skin, Leg	7 Contact Radiation 8 Hyperthermia F Plaque Radiation	Z None	Z None
5 Skin, Hand C Skin, Foot	F Plaque Radiation	Z None	Z None

D: RADIATION ONCOLOGY   H: SKIN   0; Y

SECTION: D RADIATION ONCOLOGY
BODY SYSTEM: M BREAST
MODALITY: 0 BEAM RADIATION

Treatment Site	Modality Qualifier	Isotope	Qualifier
0 Breast, Left 1 Breast, Right	0 Photons <1 MeV 1 Photons 1 - 10 MeV 2 Photons >10 MeV 4 Heavy Particles (Protons, Ions) 5 Neutrons 6 Neutron Capture	Z None	Z None
0 Breast, Left 1 Breast, Right	3 Electrons	Z None	0 Intraoperative Z None

SECTION: D RADIATION ONCOLOGY
BODY SYSTEM: M BREAST
MODALITY: 1 BRACHYTHERAPY

Treatment Site	Modality Qualifier	Isotope	Qualifier
0 Breast, Left 1 Breast, Right	9 High Dose Rate (HDR) B Low Dose Rate (LDR)	7 Cesium 137 (Cs-137) 8 Iridium 192 (Ir-192) 9 Iodine 125 (I-125) B Palladium 103 (Pd-103) C Californium 252 (Cf-252) Y Other Isotope	Z None

SECTION: D RADIATION ONCOLOGY
BODY SYSTEM: M BREAST
MODALITY: 2 STEREOTACTIC RADIOSURGERY

Treatment Site	Modality Qualifier	Isotope	Qualifier
0 Breast, Left 1 Breast, Right	D Stereotactic Other Photon Radiosurgery H Stereotactic Particulate Radiosurgery J Stereotactic Gamma Beam Radiosurgery	Z None	Z None

SECTION: D RADIATION ONCOLOGY
BODY SYSTEM: M BREAST
MODALITY: Y OTHER RADIATION

Treatment Site	Modality Qualifier	Isotope	Qualifier
0 Breast, Left 1 Breast, Right	7 Contact Radiation 8 Hyperthermia F Plaque Radiation K Laser Interstitial Thermal Therapy	Z None	Z None

New ◀   Revised ◀   ~~deleted~~ Deleted   ♀ Females Only   ♂ Males Only   Noncovered   Limited Coverage   Hospital-Acquired Condition   **Coding Clinic**

SECTION: D RADIATION ONCOLOGY
BODY SYSTEM: P MUSCULOSKELETAL SYSTEM
MODALITY: 0 BEAM RADIATION

Treatment Site	Modality Qualifier	Isotope	Qualifier
0 Skull 2 Maxilla 3 Mandible 4 Sternum 5 Rib(s) 6 Humerus 7 Radius/Ulna 8 Pelvic Bones 9 Femur B Tibia/Fibula C Other Bone	0 Photons <1 MeV 1 Photons 1 - 10 MeV 2 Photons >10 MeV 4 Heavy Particles (Protons, Ions) 5 Neutrons 6 Neutron Capture	Z None	Z None
0 Skull 2 Maxilla 3 Mandible 4 Sternum 5 Rib(s) 6 Humerus 7 Radius/Ulna 8 Pelvic Bones 9 Femur B Tibia/Fibula C Other Bone	3 Electrons	Z None	0 Intraoperative Z None

SECTION: D RADIATION ONCOLOGY
BODY SYSTEM: P MUSCULOSKELETAL SYSTEM
MODALITY: Y OTHER RADIATION

Treatment Site	Modality Qualifier	Isotope	Qualifier
0 Skull 2 Maxilla 3 Mandible 4 Sternum 5 Rib(s) 6 Humerus 7 Radius/Ulna 8 Pelvic Bones 9 Femur B Tibia/Fibula C Other Bone	7 Contact Radiation 8 Hyperthermia F Plaque Radiation	Z None	Z None

D: RADIATION ONCOLOGY

P: MUSCULOSKELETAL SYSTEM

0; Y

◀ New ◀ Revised ~~deleted~~ Deleted ♀ Females Only ♂ Males Only
℞c Noncovered ℞c Limited Coverage ℞c Hospital-Acquired Condition **Coding Clinic**

635

SECTION: D RADIATION ONCOLOGY
BODY SYSTEM: T URINARY SYSTEM
MODALITY: 0 BEAM RADIATION

Treatment Site	Modality Qualifier	Isotope	Qualifier
0 Kidney 1 Ureter 2 Bladder 3 Urethra	0 Photons <1 MeV 1 Photons 1 - 10 MeV 2 Photons >10 MeV 4 Heavy Particles (Protons, Ions) 5 Neutrons 6 Neutron Capture	Z None	Z None
0 Kidney 1 Ureter 2 Bladder 3 Urethra	3 Electrons	Z None	0 Intraoperative Z None

SECTION: D RADIATION ONCOLOGY
BODY SYSTEM: T URINARY SYSTEM
MODALITY: 1 BRACHYTHERAPY

Treatment Site	Modality Qualifier	Isotope	Qualifier
0 Kidney 1 Ureter 2 Bladder 3 Urethra	9 High Dose Rate (HDR) B Low Dose Rate (LDR)	7 Cesium 137 (Cs-137) 8 Iridium 192 (Ir-192) 9 Iodine 125 (I-125) B Palladium 103 (Pd-103) C Californium 252 (Cf-252) Y Other Isotope	Z None

SECTION: D RADIATION ONCOLOGY
BODY SYSTEM: T URINARY SYSTEM
MODALITY: 2 STEREOTACTIC RADIOSURGERY

Treatment Site	Modality Qualifier	Isotope	Qualifier
0 Kidney 1 Ureter 2 Bladder 3 Urethra	D Stereotactic Other Photon Radiosurgery H Stereotactic Particulate Radiosurgery J Stereotactic Gamma Beam Radiosurgery	Z None	Z None

SECTION: D RADIATION ONCOLOGY
BODY SYSTEM: T URINARY SYSTEM
MODALITY: Y OTHER RADIATION

Treatment Site	Modality Qualifier	Isotope	Qualifier
0 Kidney 1 Ureter 2 Bladder 3 Urethra	7 Contact Radiation 8 Hyperthermia C Intraoperative Radiation Therapy (IORT) F Plaque Radiation	Z None	Z None

D: RADIATION ONCOLOGY — T: URINARY SYSTEM — 0; 1; 2; Y

◀ New   ◀ Revised   ~~deleted~~ Deleted   ♀ Females Only   ♂ Males Only
Nc Noncovered   Lc Limited Coverage   HAc Hospital-Acquired Condition   **Coding Clinic**

SECTION: D RADIATION ONCOLOGY
BODY SYSTEM: U FEMALE REPRODUCTIVE SYSTEM
MODALITY: 0 BEAM RADIATION

Treatment Site	Modality Qualifier	Isotope	Qualifier
0 Ovary ♀ 1 Cervix ♀ 2 Uterus ♀	0 Photons <1 MeV 1 Photons 1 - 10 MeV 2 Photons >10 MeV 4 Heavy Particles (Protons, Ions) 5 Neutrons 6 Neutron Capture	Z None	Z None
0 Ovary ♀ 1 Cervix ♀ 2 Uterus ♀	3 Electrons	Z None	0 Intraoperative Z None

SECTION: D RADIATION ONCOLOGY
BODY SYSTEM: U FEMALE REPRODUCTIVE SYSTEM
MODALITY: 1 BRACHYTHERAPY

Treatment Site	Modality Qualifier	Isotope	Qualifier
0 Ovary ♀ 1 Cervix ♀ 2 Uterus ♀	9 High Dose Rate (HDR) B Low Dose Rate (LDR)	7 Cesium 137 (Cs-137) 8 Iridium 192 (Ir-192) 9 Iodine 125 (I-125) B Palladium 103 (Pd-103) C Californium 252 (Cf-252) Y Other Isotope	Z None

D: RADIATION ONCOLOGY

U: FEMALE REPRODUCTIVE SYSTEM

0; 1

◀ New   ◀▥ Revised   ~~deleted~~ Deleted   ♀ Females Only   ♂ Males Only
ⓃⒸ Noncovered   ⓁⒸ Limited Coverage   ⒽⒶⒸ Hospital-Acquired Condition   **Coding Clinic**

637

2; Y

U: FEMALE REPRODUCTIVE SYSTEM

D: RADIATION ONCOLOGY

SECTION: D RADIATION ONCOLOGY
BODY SYSTEM: U FEMALE REPRODUCTIVE SYSTEM
MODALITY: 2 STEREOTACTIC RADIOSURGERY

Treatment Site	Modality Qualifier	Isotope	Qualifier

0 Ovary ♀
1 Cervix ♀
2 Uterus ♀
	D Stereotactic Other Photon
	   Radiosurgery
	H Stereotactic Particulate
	   Radiosurgery
	J Stereotactic Gamma Beam
	   Radiosurgery
		Z None	Z None

SECTION: D RADIATION ONCOLOGY
BODY SYSTEM: U FEMALE REPRODUCTIVE SYSTEM
MODALITY: Y OTHER RADIATION

Treatment Site	Modality Qualifier	Isotope	Qualifier
0 Ovary ♀ 1 Cervix ♀ 2 Uterus ♀	7 Contact Radiation 8 Hyperthermia C Intraoperative Radiation Therapy (IORT) F Plaque Radiation	Z None	Z None

◀ New   ◀ Revised   ~~deleted~~ Deleted   ♀ Females Only   ♂ Males Only
℞ Noncovered   ℞ Limited Coverage   ℞ Hospital-Acquired Condition   **Coding Clinic**

SECTION: **D RADIATION ONCOLOGY**
BODY SYSTEM: V MALE REPRODUCTIVE SYSTEM
MODALITY: 0 BEAM RADIATION

Treatment Site	Modality Qualifier	Isotope	Qualifier
0 Prostate ♂ 1 Testis ♂	0 Photons <1 MeV 1 Photons 1 - 10 MeV 2 Photons >10 MeV 4 Heavy Particles (Protons, Ions) 5 Neutrons 6 Neutron Capture	Z None	Z None
0 Prostate ♂ 1 Testis ♂	3 Electrons	Z None	0 Intraoperative Z None

SECTION: **D RADIATION ONCOLOGY**
BODY SYSTEM: V MALE REPRODUCTIVE SYSTEM
MODALITY: 1 BRACHYTHERAPY

Treatment Site	Modality Qualifier	Isotope	Qualifier
0 Prostate ♂ 1 Testis ♂	9 High Dose Rate (HDR) B Low Dose Rate (LDR)	7 Cesium 137 (Cs-137) 8 Iridium 192 (Ir-192) 9 Iodine 125 (I-125) B Palladium 103 (Pd-103) C Californium 252 (Cf-252) Y Other Isotope	Z None

◀ New   ◀▥ Revised   ~~deleted~~ Deleted   ♀ Females Only   ♂ Males Only
🝆 Noncovered   🝆 Limited Coverage   🝆 Hospital-Acquired Condition   **Coding Clinic**

SECTION: D RADIATION ONCOLOGY
BODY SYSTEM: V MALE REPRODUCTIVE SYSTEM
MODALITY: 2 STEREOTACTIC RADIOSURGERY

Treatment Site	Modality Qualifier	Isotope	Qualifier
0 Prostate ♂ 1 Testis ♂	D Stereotactic Other Photon Radiosurgery H Stereotactic Particulate Radiosurgery J Stereotactic Gamma Beam Radiosurgery	Z None	Z None

SECTION: D RADIATION ONCOLOGY
BODY SYSTEM: V MALE REPRODUCTIVE SYSTEM
MODALITY: Y OTHER RADIATION

Treatment Site	Modality Qualifier	Isotope	Qualifier
0 Prostate ♂	7 Contact Radiation 8 Hyperthermia C Intraoperative Radiation Therapy (IORT) F Plaque Radiation K Laser Interstitial Thermal Therapy	Z None	Z None
1 Testis ♂	7 Contact Radiation 8 Hyperthermia F Plaque Radiation	Z None	Z None

◀ New   ◀ Revised   ~~deleted~~ Deleted   ♀ Females Only   ♂ Males Only
 Noncovered   Limited Coverage   Hospital-Acquired Condition   **Coding Clinic**

V: MALE REPRODUCTIVE SYSTEM

D: RADIATION ONCOLOGY

2; Y

SECTION: D RADIATION ONCOLOGY
BODY SYSTEM: W ANATOMICAL REGIONS
MODALITY: 0 BEAM RADIATION

Treatment Site	Modality Qualifier	Isotope	Qualifier
1 Head and Neck 2 Chest 3 Abdomen 4 Hemibody 5 Whole Body 6 Pelvic Region	0 Photons <1 MeV 1 Photons 1 - 10 MeV 2 Photons >10 MeV 4 Heavy Particles (Protons, Ions) 5 Neutrons 6 Neutron Capture	Z None	Z None
1 Head and Neck 2 Chest 3 Abdomen 4 Hemibody 5 Whole Body 6 Pelvic Region	3 Electrons	Z None	0 Intraoperative Z None

SECTION: D RADIATION ONCOLOGY
BODY SYSTEM: W ANATOMICAL REGIONS
MODALITY: 1 BRACHYTHERAPY

Treatment Site	Modality Qualifier	Isotope	Qualifier
1 Head and Neck 2 Chest 3 Abdomen 6 Pelvic Region	9 High Dose Rate (HDR) B Low Dose Rate (LDR)	7 Cesium 137 (Cs-137) 8 Iridium 192 (Ir-192) 9 Iodine 125 (I-125) B Palladium 103 (Pd-103) C Californium 252 (Cf-252) Y Other Isotope	Z None

◄ New   ◄ Revised   ~~deleted~~ Deleted   ♀ Females Only   ♂ Males Only
Noncovered   Limited Coverage   Hospital-Acquired Condition   **Coding Clinic**

641

SECTION: D RADIATION ONCOLOGY
BODY SYSTEM: W ANATOMICAL REGIONS
MODALITY: 2 STEREOTACTIC RADIOSURGERY

Treatment Site	Modality Qualifier	Isotope	Qualifier
1 Head and Neck 2 Chest 3 Abdomen 6 Pelvic Region	D Stereotactic Other Photon Radiosurgery H Stereotactic Particulate Radiosurgery J Stereotactic Gamma Beam Radiosurgery	Z None	Z None

SECTION: D RADIATION ONCOLOGY
BODY SYSTEM: W ANATOMICAL REGIONS
MODALITY: Y OTHER RADIATION

Treatment Site	Modality Qualifier	Isotope	Qualifier
1 Head and Neck 2 Chest 3 Abdomen 4 Hemibody 6 Pelvic Region	7 Contact Radiation 8 Hyperthermia F Plaque Radiation	Z None	Z None
5 Whole Body	7 Contact Radiation 8 Hyperthermia F Plaque Radiation	Z None	Z None
5 Whole Body	G Isotope Administration	D Iodine 131 (I-131) F Phosphorus 32 (P-32) G Strontium 89 (Sr-89) H Strontium 90 (Sr-90) Y Other Isotope	Z None

W: ANATOMICAL REGIONS

2; Y

D: RADIATION ONCOLOGY

◀ New   ◀||| Revised   deleted Deleted   ♀ Females Only   ♂ Males Only
⊘ Noncovered   ⊘ Limited Coverage   ⊘ Hospital-Acquired Condition   **Coding Clinic**

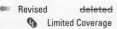

SECTION: F PHYSICAL REHABILITATION AND DIAGNOSTIC AUDIOLOGY

SECTION QUALIFIER: 0 **REHABILITATION**

TYPE: 0 **SPEECH ASSESSMENT:** *(on multiple pages)*
Measurement of speech and related functions

Body System – Body Region	Type Qualifier	Equipment	Qualifier
3 Neurological System - Whole Body	G Communicative/Cognitive Integration Skills	K Audiovisual M Augmentative/Alternative Communication P Computer Y Other Equipment Z None	Z None
Z None	0 Filtered Speech 3 Staggered Spondaic Word Q Performance Intensity Phonetically Balanced Speech Discrimination R Brief Tone Stimuli S Distorted Speech T Dichotic Stimuli V Temporal Ordering of Stimuli W Masking Patterns	1 Audiometer 2 Sound Field/Booth K Audiovisual Z None	Z None
Z None	1 Speech Threshold 2 Speech/Word Recognition	1 Audiometer 2 Sound Field/Booth 9 Cochlear Implant K Audiovisual Z None	Z None
Z None	4 Sensorineural Acuity Level	1 Audiometer 2 Sound Field/Booth Z None	Z None
Z None	5 Synthetic Sentence Identification	1 Audiometer 2 Sound Field/Booth 9 Cochlear Implant K Audiovisual	Z None
Z None	6 Speech and/or Language Screening 7 Nonspoken Language 8 Receptive/Expressive Language C Aphasia G Communicative/Cognitive Integration Skills L Augmentative/Alternative Communication System	K Audiovisual M Augmentative/Alternative Communication P Computer Y Other Equipment Z None	Z None
Z None	9 Articulation/Phonology	K Audiovisual P Computer Q Speech Analysis Y Other Equipment Z None	Z None
Z None	B Motor Speech	K Audiovisual N Biosensory Feedback P Computer Q Speech Analysis T Aerodynamic Function Y Other Equipment Z None	Z None

Sidebar: **F: PHYSICAL REHABILITATION AND DIAGNOSTIC AUDIOLOGY   0: REHABILITATION   0: SPEECH ASSESSMENT**

◀ New   ⬅ Revised   deleted Deleted   ♀ Females Only   ♂ Males Only
Nc Noncovered   Limited Coverage   Hospital-Acquired Condition   **Coding Clinic**

SECTION: F PHYSICAL REHABILITATION AND DIAGNOSTIC AUDIOLOGY

SECTION QUALIFIER: 0 REHABILITATION

TYPE: 0 SPEECH ASSESSMENT: *(continued)*

Measurement of speech and related functions

Body System – Body Region	Type Qualifier	Equipment	Qualifier
Z None	D Fluency	K Audiovisual N Biosensory Feedback P Computer Q Speech Analysis S Voice Analysis T Aerodynamic Function Y Other Equipment Z None	Z None
Z None	F Voice	K Audiovisual N Biosensory Feedback P Computer S Voice Analysis T Aerodynamic Function Y Other Equipment Z None	Z None
Z None	H Bedside Swallowing and Oral Function P Oral Peripheral Mechanism	Y Other Equipment Z None	Z None
Z None	J Instrumental Swallowing and Oral Function	T Aerodynamic Function W Swallowing Y Other Equipment	Z None
Z None	K Orofacial Myofunctional	K Audiovisual P Computer Y Other Equipment Z None	Z None
Z None	M Voice Prosthetic	K Audiovisual P Computer S Voice Analysis V Speech Prosthesis Y Other Equipment Z None	Z None
Z None	N Non-invasive Instrumental Status	N Biosensory Feedback P Computer Q Speech Analysis S Voice Analysis T Aerodynamic Function Y Other Equipment	Z None
Z None	X Other Specified Central Auditory Processing	Z None	Z None

◀ New ◀▥ Revised ~~deleted~~ Deleted ♀ Females Only ♂ Males Only
🅝 Noncovered 🅛 Limited Coverage 🅗 Hospital-Acquired Condition **Coding Clinic**

SECTION: F PHYSICAL REHABILITATION AND DIAGNOSTIC AUDIOLOGY

SECTION QUALIFIER: 0 REHABILITATION
TYPE: 1 MOTOR AND/OR NERVE FUNCTION ASSESSMENT: *(on multiple pages)*
Measurement of motor, nerve, and related functions

Body System – Body Region	Type Qualifier	Equipment	Qualifier
0 Neurological System - Head and Neck 1 Neurological System - Upper Back/Upper Extremity 2 Neurological System - Lower Back/Lower Extremity 3 Neurological System - Whole Body	0 Muscle Performance	E Orthosis F Assistive, Adaptive, Supportive or Protective U Prosthesis Y Other Equipment Z None	Z None
0 Neurological System - Head and Neck 1 Neurological System - Upper Back/Upper Extremity 2 Neurological System - Lower Back/Lower Extremity 3 Neurological System - Whole Body	1 Integumentary Integrity 3 Coordination/Dexterity 4 Motor Function G Reflex Integrity	Z None	Z None
0 Neurological System - Head and Neck 1 Neurological System - Upper Back/Upper Extremity 2 Neurological System - Lower Back/Lower Extremity 3 Neurological System - Whole Body	5 Range of Motion and Joint Integrity 6 Sensory Awareness/ Processing/Integrity	Y Other Equipment Z None	Z None
D Integumentary System - Head and Neck F Integumentary System - Upper Back/Upper Extremity G Integumentary System - Lower Back/Lower Extremity H Integumentary System - Whole Body J Musculoskeletal System - Head and Neck K Musculoskeletal System - Upper Back/Upper Extremity L Musculoskeletal System - Lower Back/Lower Extremity M Musculoskeletal System - Whole Body	0 Muscle Performance	E Orthosis F Assistive, Adaptive, Supportive or Protective U Prosthesis Y Other Equipment Z None	Z None
D Integumentary System - Head and Neck F Integumentary System - Upper Back/Upper Extremity G Integumentary System - Lower Back/Lower Extremity H Integumentary System - Whole Body J Musculoskeletal System - Head and Neck K Musculoskeletal System - Upper Back/Upper Extremity L Musculoskeletal System - Lower Back/Lower Extremity M Musculoskeletal System - Whole Body	1 Integumentary Integrity	Z None	Z None
D Integumentary System - Head and Neck F Integumentary System - Upper Back/Upper Extremity G Integumentary System - Lower Back/Lower Extremity H Integumentary System - Whole Body J Musculoskeletal System - Head and Neck K Musculoskeletal System - Upper Back/Upper Extremity L Musculoskeletal System - Lower Back/Lower Extremity M Musculoskeletal System - Whole Body	5 Range of Motion and Joint Integrity 6 Sensory Awareness/ Processing/Integrity	Y Other Equipment Z None	Z None

◀ New   ◀▥ Revised   ~~deleted~~ Deleted   ♀ Females Only   ♂ Males Only
🆖 Noncovered   🆖 Limited Coverage   🆖 Hospital-Acquired Condition   **Coding Clinic**

SECTION: F PHYSICAL REHABILITATION AND DIAGNOSTIC AUDIOLOGY

SECTION QUALIFIER: 0 REHABILITATION
TYPE: 1 MOTOR AND/OR NERVE FUNCTION
ASSESSMENT: *(continued)*
Measurement of motor, nerve, and related functions

Body System – Body Region	Type Qualifier	Equipment	Qualifier
N Genitourinary System	0 Muscle Performance	E Orthosis F Assistive, Adaptive, Supportive or Protective U Prosthesis Y Other Equipment Z None	Z None
Z None	2 Visual Motor Integration	K Audiovisual M Augmentative/Alternative Communication N Biosensory Feedback P Computer Q Speech Analysis S Voice Analysis Y Other Equipment Z None	Z None
Z None	7 Facial Nerve Function	7 Electrophysiologic	Z None
Z None	9 Somatosensory Evoked Potentials	J Somatosensory	Z None
Z None	B Bed Mobility C Transfer F Wheelchair Mobility	E Orthosis F Assistive, Adaptive, Supportive or Protective U Prosthesis Z None	Z None
Z None	D Gait and/or Balance	E Orthosis F Assistive, Adaptive, Supportive or Protective U Prosthesis Y Other Equipment Z None	Z None

◄ New ◄ Revised deleted Deleted ♀ Females Only ♂ Males Only
℞ Noncovered ℞ Limited Coverage ℞ Hospital-Acquired Condition **Coding Clinic**

647

SECTION: F PHYSICAL REHABILITATION AND DIAGNOSTIC AUDIOLOGY

SECTION QUALIFIER: 0 **REHABILITATION**

TYPE: 2 **ACTIVITIES OF DAILY LIVING ASSESSMENT:** *(on multiple pages)*

Measurement of functional level for activities of daily living

Body System – Body Region	Type Qualifier	Equipment	Qualifier
0 Neurological System - Head and Neck	9 Cranial Nerve Integrity D Neuromotor Development	Y Other Equipment Z None	Z None
1 Neurological System - Upper Back/Upper Extremity 2 Neurological System - Lower Back/Lower Extremity 3 Neurological System - Whole Body	D Neuromotor Development	Y Other Equipment Z None	Z None
4 Circulatory System - Head and Neck 5 Circulatory System - Upper Back/Upper Extremity 6 Circulatory System - Lower Back/Lower Extremity 8 Respiratory System - Head and Neck 9 Respiratory System - Upper Back/Upper Extremity B Respiratory System - Lower Back/Lower Extremity	G Ventilation, Respiration and Circulation	C Mechanical G Aerobic Endurance and Conditioning Y Other Equipment Z None	Z None
7 Circulatory System - Whole Body C Respiratory System - Whole Body	7 Aerobic Capacity and Endurance	E Orthosis G Aerobic Endurance and Conditioning U Prosthesis Y Other Equipment Z None	Z None
7 Circulatory System - Whole Body C Respiratory System - Whole Body	G Ventilation, Respiration and Circulation	C Mechanical G Aerobic Endurance and Conditioning Y Other Equipment Z None	Z None

◀ New ◀▥ Revised ~~deleted~~ Deleted ♀ Females Only ♂ Males Only
Ⓝⓒ Noncovered Ⓛⓒ Limited Coverage Ⓗⓐⓒ Hospital-Acquired Condition **Coding Clinic**

2

0: REHABILITATION

F: PHYSICAL REHABILITATION AND DIAGNOSTIC AUDIOLOGY

SECTION:

F PHYSICAL REHABILITATION AND DIAGNOSTIC AUDIOLOGY

SECTION QUALIFIER: 0   **REHABILITATION**

TYPE: 2   **ACTIVITIES OF DAILY LIVING ASSESSMENT:** *(continued)*

Measurement of functional level for activities of daily living

Body System – Body Region	Type Qualifier	Equipment	Qualifier
Z None	0 Bathing/Showering 1 Dressing 3 Grooming/Personal Hygiene 4 Home Management	E Orthosis F Assistive, Adaptive, Supportive or Protective U Prosthesis Z None	Z None
Z None	2 Feeding/Eating 8 Anthropometric Characteristics F Pain	Y Other Equipment Z None	Z None
Z None	5 Perceptual Processing	K Audiovisual M Augmentative/Alternative Communication N Biosensory Feedback P Computer Q Speech Analysis S Voice Analysis Y Other Equipment Z None	Z None
Z None	6 Psychosocial Skills	Z None	Z None
Z None	B Environmental, Home and Work Barriers C Ergonomics and Body Mechanics	E Orthosis F Assistive, Adaptive, Supportive or Protective U Prosthesis Y Other Equipment Z None	Z None
Z None	H Vocational Activities and Functional Community or Work Reintegration Skills	E Orthosis F Assistive, Adaptive, Supportive or Protective G Aerobic Endurance and Conditioning U Prosthesis Y Other Equipment Z None	Z None

◀ New   ◀ Revised   deleted Deleted   ♀ Females Only   ♂ Males Only
Noncovered   Limited Coverage   Hospital-Acquired Condition   **Coding Clinic**

649

SECTION: **F PHYSICAL REHABILITATION AND DIAGNOSTIC AUDIOLOGY**

SECTION QUALIFIER: 0 **REHABILITATION**

TYPE: 6 **SPEECH TREATMENT:** *(on multiple pages)*

Application of techniques to improve, augment, or compensate for speech and related functional impairment

Body System – Body Region	Type Qualifier	Equipment	Qualifier
3 Neurological System - Whole Body	6 Communicative/Cognitive Integration Skills	K Audiovisual M Augmentative/Alternative Communication P Computer Y Other Equipment Z None	Z None
Z None	0 Nonspoken Language 3 Aphasia 6 Communicative/Cognitive Integration Skills	K Audiovisual M Augmentative/Alternative Communication P Computer Y Other Equipment Z None	Z None
Z None	1 Speech-Language Pathology and Related Disorders Counseling 2 Speech-Language Pathology and Related Disorders Prevention	K Audiovisual Z None	Z None
Z None	4 Articulation/Phonology	K Audiovisual P Computer Q Speech Analysis T Aerodynamic Function Y Other Equipment Z None	Z None
Z None	5 Aural Rehabilitation	K Audiovisual L Assistive Listening M Augmentative/Alternative Communication N Biosensory Feedback P Computer Q Speech Analysis S Voice Analysis Y Other Equipment Z None	Z None
Z None	7 Fluency	4 Electroacoustic Immittance/Acoustic Reflex K Audiovisual N Biosensory Feedback Q Speech Analysis S Voice Analysis T Aerodynamic Function Y Other Equipment Z None	Z None

◄ New   ◄▌ Revised   ~~deleted~~ Deleted   ♀ Females Only   ♂ Males Only
℞̸ Noncovered   ℞̸ Limited Coverage   ℞̸ Hospital-Acquired Condition   **Coding Clinic**

SECTION: F PHYSICAL REHABILITATION AND DIAGNOSTIC AUDIOLOGY

SECTION QUALIFIER: 0 REHABILITATION

TYPE: 6 SPEECH TREATMENT: *(continued)*

Application of techniques to improve, augment, or compensate for speech and related functional impairment

Body System – Body Region	Type Qualifier	Equipment	Qualifier
Z None	8 Motor Speech	K Audiovisual N Biosensory Feedback P Computer Q Speech Analysis S Voice Analysis T Aerodynamic Function Y Other Equipment Z None	Z None
Z None	9 Orofacial Myofunctional	K Audiovisual P Computer Y Other Equipment Z None	Z None
Z None	B Receptive/Expressive Language	K Audiovisual L Assistive Listening M Augmentative/Alternative Communication P Computer Y Other Equipment Z None	Z None
Z None	C Voice	K Audiovisual N Biosensory Feedback P Computer S Voice Analysis T Aerodynamic Function V Speech Prosthesis Y Other Equipment Z None	Z None
Z None	D Swallowing Dysfunction	M Augmentative/Alternative Communication T Aerodynamic Function V Speech Prosthesis Y Other Equipment Z None	Z None

SECTION: F PHYSICAL REHABILITATION AND DIAGNOSTIC AUDIOLOGY

SECTION QUALIFIER: 0 REHABILITATION

TYPE: 7 MOTOR TREATMENT: *(on multiple pages)*

Exercise or activities to increase or facilitate motor function

Body System – Body Region	Type Qualifier	Equipment	Qualifier
0 Neurological System - Head and Neck 1 Neurological System - Upper Back/Upper Extremity 2 Neurological System - Lower Back/Lower Extremity 3 Neurological System - Whole Body D Integumentary System - Head and Neck F Integumentary System - Upper Back/Upper Extremity G Integumentary System - Lower Back/Lower Extremity H Integumentary System - Whole Body J Musculoskeletal System - Head and Neck K Musculoskeletal System - Upper Back/Upper Extremity L Musculoskeletal System - Lower Back/Lower Extremity M Musculoskeletal System - Whole Body	0 Range of Motion and Joint Mobility 1 Muscle Performance 2 Coordination/Dexterity 3 Motor Function	E Orthosis F Assistive, Adaptive, Supportive or Protective U Prosthesis Y Other Equipment Z None	Z None
0 Neurological System - Head and Neck 1 Neurological System - Upper Back/Upper Extremity 2 Neurological System - Lower Back/Lower Extremity 3 Neurological System - Whole Body D Integumentary System - Head and Neck F Integumentary System - Upper Back/Upper Extremity G Integumentary System - Lower Back/Lower Extremity H Integumentary System - Whole Body J Musculoskeletal System - Head and Neck K Musculoskeletal System - Upper Back/Upper Extremity L Musculoskeletal System - Lower Back/Lower Extremity M Musculoskeletal System - Whole Body	6 Therapeutic Exercise	B Physical Agents C Mechanical D Electrotherapeutic E Orthosis F Assistive, Adaptive, Supportive or Protective G Aerobic Endurance and Conditioning H Mechanical or Electromechanical U Prosthesis Y Other Equipment Z None	Z None
0 Neurological System - Head and Neck 1 Neurological System - Upper Back/Upper Extremity 2 Neurological System - Lower Back/Lower Extremity 3 Neurological System - Whole Body D Integumentary System - Head and Neck F Integumentary System - Upper Back/Upper Extremity G Integumentary System - Lower Back/Lower Extremity H Integumentary System - Whole Body J Musculoskeletal System - Head and Neck K Musculoskeletal System - Upper Back/Upper Extremity L Musculoskeletal System - Lower Back/Lower Extremity M Musculoskeletal System - Whole Body	7 Manual Therapy Techniques	Z None	Z None

SECTION: F PHYSICAL REHABILITATION AND DIAGNOSTIC AUDIOLOGY

SECTION QUALIFIER: 0 REHABILITATION
TYPE: 7 MOTOR TREATMENT: *(continued)*
Exercise or activities to increase or facilitate motor function

Body System – Body Region	Type Qualifier	Equipment	Qualifier
4 Circulatory System - Head and Neck 5 Circulatory System - Upper Back/Upper Extremity 6 Circulatory System - Lower Back/Lower Extremity 7 Circulatory System - Whole Body 8 Respiratory System - Head and Neck 9 Respiratory System - Upper Back/Upper Extremity B Respiratory System - Lower Back/Lower Extremity C Respiratory System - Whole Body	6 Therapeutic Exercise	B Physical Agents C Mechanical D Electrotherapeutic E Orthosis F Assistive, Adaptive, Supportive or Protective G Aerobic Endurance and Conditioning H Mechanical or Electromechanical U Prosthesis Y Other Equipment Z None	Z None
N Genitourinary System	1 Muscle Performance	E Orthosis F Assistive, Adaptive, Supportive or Protective U Prosthesis Y Other Equipment Z None	Z None
N Genitourinary System	6 Therapeutic Exercise	B Physical Agents C Mechanical D Electrotherapeutic E Orthosis F Assistive, Adaptive, Supportive or Protective G Aerobic Endurance and Conditioning H Mechanical or Electromechanical U Prosthesis Y Other Equipment Z None	Z None
Z None	4 Wheelchair Mobility	D Electrotherapeutic E Orthosis F Assistive, Adaptive, Supportive or Protective U Prosthesis Y Other Equipment Z None	Z None
Z None	5 Bed Mobility	C Mechanical E Orthosis F Assistive, Adaptive, Supportive or Protective U Prosthesis Y Other Equipment Z None	Z None
Z None	8 Transfer Training	C Mechanical D Electrotherapeutic E Orthosis F Assistive, Adaptive, Supportive or Protective U Prosthesis Y Other Equipment Z None	Z None
Z None	9 Gait Training/Functional Ambulation	C Mechanical D Electrotherapeutic E Orthosis F Assistive, Adaptive, Supportive or Protective G Aerobic Endurance and Conditioning U Prosthesis Y Other Equipment Z None	Z None

SECTION: F PHYSICAL REHABILITATION AND DIAGNOSTIC AUDIOLOGY

SECTION QUALIFIER: 0 REHABILITATION

TYPE: 8 ACTIVITIES OF DAILY LIVING TREATMENT: Exercise or activities to facilitate functional competence for activities of daily living

Body System – Body Region	Type Qualifier	Equipment	Qualifier
D Integumentary System - Head and Neck F Integumentary System - Upper Back/Upper Extremity G Integumentary System - Lower Back/Lower Extremity H Integumentary System - Whole Body J Musculoskeletal System - Head and Neck K Musculoskeletal System - Upper Back/Upper Extremity L Musculoskeletal System - Lower Back/Lower Extremity M Musculoskeletal System - Whole Body	5 Wound Management	B Physical Agents C Mechanical D Electrotherapeutic E Orthosis F Assistive, Adaptive, Supportive or Protective U Prosthesis Y Other Equipment Z None	Z None
Z None	0 Bathing/Showering Techniques 1 Dressing Techniques 2 Grooming/Personal Hygiene	E Orthosis F Assistive, Adaptive, Supportive or Protective U Prosthesis Y Other Equipment Z None	Z None
Z None	3 Feeding/Eating	C Mechanical D Electrotherapeutic E Orthosis F Assistive, Adaptive, Supportive or Protective U Prosthesis Y Other Equipment Z None	Z None
Z None	4 Home Management	D Electrotherapeutic E Orthosis F Assistive, Adaptive, Supportive or Protective U Prosthesis Y Other Equipment Z None	Z None
Z None	6 Psychosocial Skills	Z None	Z None
Z None	7 Vocational Activities and Functional Community or Work Reintegration Skills	B Physical Agents C Mechanical D Electrotherapeutic E Orthosis F Assistive, Adaptive, Supportive or Protective G Aerobic Endurance and Conditioning U Prosthesis Y Other Equipment Z None	Z None

◀ New ◀ Revised ~~deleted~~ Deleted ♀ Females Only ♂ Males Only
Ⓝ Noncovered Ⓛ Limited Coverage Ⓗ Hospital-Acquired Condition **Coding Clinic**

F: PHYSICAL REHABILITATION AND DIAGNOSTIC AUDIOLOGY

0: REHABILITATION

8

SECTION: **F PHYSICAL REHABILITATION AND DIAGNOSTIC AUDIOLOGY**

SECTION QUALIFIER: **0 REHABILITATION**

TYPE: **9 HEARING TREATMENT:** Application of techniques to improve, augment, or compensate for hearing and related functional impairment

Body System – Body Region	Type Qualifier	Equipment	Qualifier
Z None	0 Hearing and Related Disorders Counseling 1 Hearing and Related Disorders Prevention	K Audiovisual Z None	Z None
Z None	2 Auditory Processing	K Audiovisual L Assistive Listening P Computer Y Other Equipment Z None	Z None
Z None	3 Cerumen Management	X Cerumen Management Z None	Z None

SECTION: **F PHYSICAL REHABILITATION AND DIAGNOSTIC AUDIOLOGY**

SECTION QUALIFIER: **0 REHABILITATION**

TYPE: **B COCHLEAR IMPLANT TREATMENT:** Application of techniques to improve the communication abilities of individuals with cochlear implant

Body System – Body Region	Type Qualifier	Equipment	Qualifier
Z None	0 Cochlear Implant Rehabilitation	1 Audiometer 2 Sound Field/Booth 9 Cochlear Implant K Audiovisual P Computer Y Other Equipment	Z None

SECTION: F PHYSICAL REHABILITATION AND DIAGNOSTIC AUDIOLOGY

SECTION QUALIFIER: 0 **REHABILITATION**

TYPE: C **VESTIBULAR TREATMENT:** Application of techniques to improve, augment, or compensate for vestibular and related functional impairment

Body System – Body Region	Type Qualifier	Equipment	Qualifier
3 Neurological System - Whole Body H Integumentary System - Whole Body M Musculoskeletal System - Whole Body	3 Postural Control	E Orthosis F Assistive, Adaptive, Supportive or Protective U Prosthesis Y Other Equipment Z None	Z None
Z None	0 Vestibular	8 Vestibular/Balance Z None	Z None
Z None	1 Perceptual Processing 2 Visual Motor Integration	K Audiovisual L Assistive Listening N Biosensory Feedback P Computer Q Speech Analysis S Voice Analysis T Aerodynamic Function Y Other Equipment Z None	Z None

SECTION: F PHYSICAL REHABILITATION AND DIAGNOSTIC AUDIOLOGY

SECTION QUALIFIER: 0 **REHABILITATION**

TYPE: D **DEVICE FITTING:** Fitting of a device designed to facilitate or support achievement of a higher level of function

Body System – Body Region	Type Qualifier	Equipment	Qualifier
Z None	0 Tinnitus Masker	5 Hearing Aid Selection/Fitting/Test Z None	Z None
Z None	1 Monaural Hearing Aid 2 Binaural Hearing Aid 5 Assistive Listening Device	1 Audiometer 2 Sound Field/Booth 5 Hearing Aid Selection/Fitting/Test K Audiovisual L Assistive Listening Z None	Z None
Z None	3 Augmentative/Alternative Communication System	M Augmentative/Alternative Communication	Z None
Z None	4 Voice Prosthetic	S Voice Analysis V Speech Prosthesis	Z None
Z None	6 Dynamic Orthosis 7 Static Orthosis 8 Prosthesis 9 Assistive, Adaptive, Supportive or Protective Devices	E Orthosis F Assistive, Adaptive, Supportive or Protective U Prosthesis Z None	Z None

◀ New ◀ Revised ~~deleted~~ Deleted ♀ Females Only ♂ Males Only
🅝 Noncovered 🅛 Limited Coverage 🅗 Hospital-Acquired Condition **Coding Clinic**

SECTION: F PHYSICAL REHABILITATION AND DIAGNOSTIC AUDIOLOGY

SECTION QUALIFIER: 0 REHABILITATION

TYPE: F CAREGIVER TRAINING: Training in activities to support patient's optimal level of function

Body System – Body Region	Type Qualifier	Equipment	Qualifier
Z None	0 Bathing/Showering Technique 1 Dressing 2 Feeding and Eating 3 Grooming/Personal Hygiene 4 Bed Mobility 5 Transfer 6 Wheelchair Mobility 7 Therapeutic Exercise 8 Airway Clearance Techniques 9 Wound Management B Vocational Activities and Functional Community or Work Reintegration Skills C Gait Training/Functional Ambulation D Application, Proper Use and Care Devices F Application, Proper Use and Care of Orthoses G Application, Proper Use and Care of Prosthesis H Home Management	E Orthosis F Assistive, Adaptive, Supportive or Protective U Prosthesis Z None	Z None
Z None	J Communication Skills	K Audiovisual L Assistive Listening M Augmentative/Alternative Communication P Computer Z None	Z None

SECTION: F PHYSICAL REHABILITATION AND DIAGNOSTIC AUDIOLOGY

SECTION QUALIFIER: 1 DIAGNOSTIC AUDIOLOGY

TYPE: 3 HEARING ASSESSMENT: Measurement of hearing and related functions

Body System – Body Region	Type Qualifier	Equipment	Qualifier
Z None	0 Hearing Screening	0 Occupational Hearing 1 Audiometer 2 Sound Field/Booth 3 Tympanometer 8 Vestibular/Balance 9 Cochlear Implant Z None	Z None
Z None	1 Pure Tone Audiometry, Air 2 Pure Tone Audiometry, Air and Bone	0 Occupational Hearing 1 Audiometer 2 Sound Field/Booth Z None	Z None
Z None	3 Bekesy Audiometry 6 Visual Reinforcement Audiometry 9 Short Increment Sensitivity Index B Stenger C Pure Tone Stenger	1 Audiometer 2 Sound Field/Booth Z None	Z None
Z None	4 Conditioned Play Audiometry 5 Select Picture Audiometry	1 Audiometer 2 Sound Field/Booth K Audiovisual Z None	Z None
Z None	7 Alternate Binaural or Monaural Loudness Balance	1 Audiometer K Audiovisual Z None	Z None
Z None	8 Tone Decay D Tympanometry F Eustachian Tube Function G Acoustic Reflex Patterns H Acoustic Reflex Threshold J Acoustic Reflex Decay	3 Tympanometer 4 Electroacoustic Immitance/ Acoustic Reflex Z None	Z None
Z None	K Electrocochleography L Auditory Evoked Potentials	7 Electrophysiologic Z None	Z None
Z None	M Evoked Otoacoustic Emissions, Screening N Evoked Otoacoustic Emissions, Diagnostic	6 Otoacoustic Emission (OAE) Z None	Z None
Z None	P Aural Rehabilitation Status	1 Audiometer 2 Sound Field/Booth 4 Electroacoustic Immitance/ Acoustic Reflex 9 Cochlear Implant K Audiovisual L Assistive Listening P Computer Z None	Z None
Z None	Q Auditory Processing	K Audiovisual P Computer Y Other Equipment Z None	Z None

◀ New ◀ Revised ~~deleted~~ Deleted ♀ Females Only ♂ Males Only
 Noncovered Limited Coverage Hospital-Acquired Condition **Coding Clinic**

SECTION: F PHYSICAL REHABILITATION AND DIAGNOSTIC AUDIOLOGY
SECTION QUALIFIER: 1 DIAGNOSTIC AUDIOLOGY
TYPE: 4 **HEARING AID ASSESSMENT:** Measurement of the appropriateness and/or effectiveness of a hearing device

Body System – Body Region	Type Qualifier	Equipment	Qualifier
Z None	0 Cochlear Implant	1 Audiometer 2 Sound Field/Booth 3 Tympanometer 4 Electroacoustic Immitance/ Acoustic Reflex 5 Hearing Aid Selection/ Fitting/Test 7 Electrophysiologic 9 Cochlear Implant K Audiovisual L Assistive Listening P Computer Y Other Equipment Z None	Z None
Z None	1 Ear Canal Probe Microphone 6 Binaural Electroacoustic Hearing Aid Check 8 Monaural Electroacoustic Hearing Aid Check	5 Hearing Aid Selection/ Fitting/Test Z None	Z None
Z None	2 Monaural Hearing Aid 3 Binaural Hearing Aid	1 Audiometer 2 Sound Field/Booth 3 Tympanometer 4 Electroacoustic Immitance/ Acoustic Reflex 5 Hearing Aid Selection/ Fitting/Test K Audiovisual L Assistive Listening P Computer Z None	Z None
Z None	4 Assistive Listening System/ Device Selection	1 Audiometer 2 Sound Field/Booth 3 Tympanometer 4 Electroacoustic Immitance/ Acoustic Reflex K Audiovisual L Assistive Listening Z None	Z None
Z None	5 Sensory Aids	1 Audiometer 2 Sound Field/Booth 3 Tympanometer 4 Electroacoustic Immitance/ Acoustic Reflex 5 Hearing Aid Selection/ Fitting/Test K Audiovisual L Assistive Listening Z None	Z None
Z None	7 Ear Protector Attentuation	0 Occupational Hearing Z None	Z None

◀ New ◀▦ Revised ~~deleted~~ Deleted ♀ Females Only ♂ Males Only
Ⓝⓒ Noncovered Ⓛⓒ Limited Coverage Ⓗⓐⓒ Hospital-Acquired Condition **Coding Clinic**

SECTION: F PHYSICAL REHABILITATION AND DIAGNOSTIC AUDIOLOGY

SECTION QUALIFIER: 1 DIAGNOSTIC AUDIOLOGY

TYPE: 5 VESTIBULAR ASSESSMENT: Measurement of the vestibular system and related functions

Body System – Body Region	Type Qualifier	Equipment	Qualifier
Z None	0 Bithermal, Binaural Caloric Irrigation 1 Bithermal, Monaural Caloric Irrigation 2 Unithermal Binaural Screen 3 Oscillating Tracking 4 Sinusoidal Vertical Axis Rotational 5 Dix-Hallpike Dynamic 6 Computerized Dynamic Posturography	8 Vestibular/Balance Z None	Z None
Z None	7 Tinnitus Masker	5 Hearing Aid Selection/ Fitting/Test Z None	Z None

◀ New   ◀ Revised   ~~deleted~~ Deleted   ♀ Females Only   ♂ Males Only
℞ Noncovered   ℞ Limited Coverage   ℞ Hospital-Acquired Condition   **Coding Clinic**

| ◀ New | ◀▮▮ Revised | ~~deleted~~ Deleted | ♀ Females Only | ♂ Males Only |
| 🅺 Noncovered | 🅻 Limited Coverage | 🅷 Hospital-Acquired Condition | **Coding Clinic** |

661

1; 2; 3; 5

Z: NONE

G: MENTAL HEALTH

SECTION: **G MENTAL HEALTH**

SECTION QUALIFIER: Z NONE

TYPE: 1 **PSYCHOLOGICAL TESTS:** The administration and interpretation of standardized psychological tests and measurement instruments for the assessment of psychological function

Qualifier	Qualifier	Qualifier	Qualifier
0 Developmental 1 Personality and Behavioral 2 Intellectual and Psychoeducational 3 Neuropsychological 4 Neurobehavioral and Cognitive Status	Z None	Z None	Z None

SECTION: **G MENTAL HEALTH**

SECTION QUALIFIER: Z NONE

TYPE: 2 **CRISIS INTERVENTION:** Treatment of a traumatized, acutely disturbed or distressed individual for the purpose of short-term stabilization

Qualifier	Qualifier	Qualifier	Qualifier
Z None	Z None	Z None	Z None

SECTION: **G MENTAL HEALTH**

SECTION QUALIFIER: Z NONE

TYPE: 3 **MEDICATION MANAGEMENT:** Monitoring and adjusting the use of medications for the treatment of a mental health disorder

Qualifier	Qualifier	Qualifier	Qualifier
Z None	Z None	Z None	Z None

SECTION: **G MENTAL HEALTH**

SECTION QUALIFIER: Z NONE

TYPE: 5 **INDIVIDUAL PSYCHOTHERAPY:** Treatment of an individual with a mental health disorder by behavioral, cognitive, psychoanalytic, psychodynamic or psychophysiological means to improve functioning or well-being

Qualifier	Qualifier	Qualifier	Qualifier
0 Interactive 1 Behavioral 2 Cognitive 3 Interpersonal 4 Psychoanalysis 5 Psychodynamic 6 Supportive 8 Cognitive-Behavioral 9 Psychophysiological	Z None	Z None	Z None

◀ New ◀ Revised ~~deleted~~ Deleted ♀ Females Only ♂ Males Only
℞ Noncovered ℞ Limited Coverage ℞ Hospital-Acquired Condition **Coding Clinic**

SECTION: G MENTAL HEALTH
SECTION QUALIFIER: Z NONE
TYPE: 6 **COUNSELING:** The application of psychological methods to treat an individual with normal developmental issues and psychological problems in order to increase function, improve well-being, alleviate distress, maladjustment or resolve crises

Qualifier	Qualifier	Qualifier	Qualifier
0 Educational 1 Vocational 3 Other Counseling	Z None	Z None	Z None

SECTION: G MENTAL HEALTH
SECTION QUALIFIER: Z NONE
TYPE: 7 **FAMILY PSYCHOTHERAPY:** Treatment that includes one or more family members of an individual with a mental health disorder by behavioral, cognitive, psychoanalytic, psychodynamic or psychophysiological means to improve functioning or well-being

Qualifier	Qualifier	Qualifier	Qualifier
2 Other Family Psychotherapy	Z None	Z None	Z None

SECTION: G MENTAL HEALTH
SECTION QUALIFIER: Z NONE
TYPE: B **ELECTROCONVULSIVE THERAPY:** The application of controlled electrical voltages to treat a mental health disorder

Qualifier	Qualifier	Qualifier	Qualifier
0 Unilateral-Single Seizure 1 Unilateral-Multiple Seizure 2 Bilateral-Single Seizure 3 Bilateral-Multiple Seizure 4 Other Electroconvulsive Therapy	Z None	Z None	Z None

SECTION: G MENTAL HEALTH
SECTION QUALIFIER: Z NONE
TYPE: C **BIOFEEDBACK:** Provision of information from the monitoring and regulating of physiological processes in conjunction with cognitive-behavioral techniques to improve patient functioning or well-being

Qualifier	Qualifier	Qualifier	Qualifier
9 Other Biofeedback	Z None	Z None	Z None

SECTION: **G MENTAL HEALTH**
SECTION QUALIFIER: Z   NONE
TYPE: **F HYPNOSIS:** Induction of a state of heightened suggestibility by auditory, visual, and tactile techniques to elicit an emotional or behavioral response

Qualifier	Qualifier	Qualifier	Qualifier
Z None	Z None	Z None	Z None

SECTION: **G MENTAL HEALTH**
SECTION QUALIFIER: Z   NONE
TYPE: **G NARCOSYNTHESIS:** Administration of intravenous barbiturates in order to release suppressed or repressed thoughts

Qualifier	Qualifier	Qualifier	Qualifier
Z None	Z None	Z None	Z None

SECTION: **G MENTAL HEALTH**
SECTION QUALIFIER: Z   NONE
TYPE: **H GROUP PSYCHOTHERAPY:** Treatment of two or more individuals with a mental health disorder by behavioral, cognitive, psychoanalytic, psychodynamic, or psychophysiological means to improve functioning or well-being

Qualifier	Qualifier	Qualifier	Qualifier
Z None	Z None	Z None	Z None

SECTION: **G MENTAL HEALTH**
SECTION QUALIFIER: Z   NONE
TYPE: **J LIGHT THERAPY:** Application of specialized light treatments to improve functioning or well-being

Qualifier	Qualifier	Qualifier	Qualifier
Z None	Z None	Z None	Z None

◀ New   ◀ Revised   ~~deleted~~ Deleted   ♀ Females Only   ♂ Males Only
Ⓝc Noncovered   Ⓛc Limited Coverage   Ⓗ Hospital-Acquired Condition   **Coding Clinic**

F; G; H; J

Z: NONE

G: MENTAL HEALTH

SECTION: H SUBSTANCE ABUSE TREATMENT
SECTION QUALIFIER: Z NONE
TYPE: 2 DETOXIFICATION SERVICES: Detoxification from alcohol and/or drugs

Qualifier	Qualifier	Qualifier	Qualifier
Z None	Z None	Z None	Z None

SECTION: H SUBSTANCE ABUSE TREATMENT
SECTION QUALIFIER: Z NONE
TYPE: 3 INDIVIDUAL COUNSELING: The application of psychological methods to treat an individual with addictive behavior

Qualifier	Qualifier	Qualifier	Qualifier
0 Cognitive 1 Behavioral 2 Cognitive-Behavioral 3 12-Step 4 Interpersonal 5 Vocational 6 Psychoeducation 7 Motivational Enhancement 8 Confrontational 9 Continuing Care B Spiritual C Pre/Post-Test Infectious Disease	Z None	Z None	Z None

SECTION: H SUBSTANCE ABUSE TREATMENT
SECTION QUALIFIER: Z NONE
TYPE: 4 GROUP COUNSELING: The application of psychological methods to treat two or more individuals with addictive behavior

Qualifier	Qualifier	Qualifier	Qualifier
0 Cognitive 1 Behavioral 2 Cognitive-Behavioral 3 12-Step 4 Interpersonal 5 Vocational 6 Psychoeducation 7 Motivational Enhancement 8 Confrontational 9 Continuing Care B Spiritual C Pre/Post-Test Infectious Disease	Z None	Z None	Z None

◀ New   ◀▥ Revised   ~~deleted~~ Deleted   ♀ Females Only   ♂ Males Only
Ⓠ Noncovered   Ⓠ Limited Coverage   Ⓠ Hospital-Acquired Condition   **Coding Clinic**

SECTION: H SUBSTANCE ABUSE TREATMENT
SECTION QUALIFIER: Z NONE
TYPE: 5 **INDIVIDUAL PSYCHOTHERAPY:** Treatment of an individual with addictive behavior by behavioral, cognitive, psychoanalytic, psychodynamic, or psychophysiological means

Qualifier	Qualifier	Qualifier	Qualifier
0 Cognitive 1 Behavioral 2 Cognitive-Behavioral 3 12-Step 4 Interpersonal 5 Interactive 6 Psychoeducation 7 Motivational Enhancement 8 Confrontational 9 Supportive B Psychoanalysis C Psychodynamic D Psychophysiological	Z None	Z None	Z None

SECTION: H SUBSTANCE ABUSE TREATMENT
SECTION QUALIFIER: Z NONE
TYPE: 6 **FAMILY COUNSELING:** The application of psychological methods that includes one or more family members to treat an individual with addictive behavior

Qualifier	Qualifier	Qualifier	Qualifier
3 Other Family Counseling	Z None	Z None	Z None

SECTION: H SUBSTANCE ABUSE TREATMENT
SECTION QUALIFIER: Z NONE
TYPE: 8 **MEDICATION MANAGEMENT:** Monitoring and adjusting the use of replacement medications for the treatment of addiction

Qualifier	Qualifier	Qualifier	Qualifier
0 Nicotine Replacement 1 Methadone Maintenance 2 Levo-alpha-acetyl-methadol (LAAM) 3 Antabuse 4 Naltrexone 5 Naloxone 6 Clonidine 7 Bupropion 8 Psychiatric Medication 9 Other Replacement Medication	Z None	Z None	Z None

H: SUBSTANCE ABUSE TREATMENT

Z: NONE

5; 6; 8

SECTION:　　　H SUBSTANCE ABUSE TREATMENT
SECTION QUALIFIER: Z　NONE
TYPE:　　　　　　9　**PHARMACOTHERAPY:** The use of replacement medications for the treatment of addiction

Qualifier	Qualifier	Qualifier	Qualifier
0　Nicotine Replacement 1　Methadone Maintenance 2　Levo-alpha-acetyl-methadol (LAAM) 3　Antabuse 4　Naltrexone 5　Naloxone 6　Clonidine 7　Bupropion 8　Psychiatric Medication 9　Other Replacement Medication	Z　None	Z　None	Z　None

9: PHARMACOTHERAPY

Z: NONE

H: SUBSTANCE ABUSE TREATMENT

◀ New　　◀▥ Revised　　~~deleted~~ Deleted　　♀ Females Only　　♂ Males Only
 Noncovered　　 Limited Coverage　　 Hospital-Acquired Condition　　**Coding Clinic**

INDEX

3

3f (Aortic) Bioprosthesis valve *use* Zooplastic Tissue in Heart and Great Vessels

A

Abdominal aortic plexus *use* Nerve, Abdominal Sympathetic
Abdominal esophagus *use* Esophagus, Lower
Abdominohysterectomy
  see Excision, Uterus 0UB9
  see Resection, Uterus 0UT9
Abdominoplasty
  see Alteration, Abdominal Wall, 0W0F
  see Repair, Abdominal Wall, 0WQF
  see Supplement, Abdominal Wall, 0WUF
Abductor hallucis muscle
  use Muscle, Foot, Right
  use Muscle, Foot, Left
AbioCor® Total Replacement Heart *use* Synthetic Substitute
Ablation *see* Destruction
Abortion
  Products of Conception 10A0
  Abortifacient 10A07ZX
  Laminaria 10A07ZW
  Vacuum 10A07Z6
Abrasion *see* Extraction
Absolute Pro Vascular (OTW) Self-Expanding Stent System *use* Intraluminal Device ◄
Accessory cephalic vein
  use Vein, Cephalic, Right
  use Vein, Cephalic, Left
Accessory obturator nerve *use* Nerve, Lumbar Plexus
Accessory phrenic nerve *use* Nerve, Phrenic
Accessory spleen *use* Spleen
Acculink (RX) Carotid Stent System *use* Intraluminal Device ◄
Acellular Hydrated Dermis *use* Nonautologous Tissue Substitute
Acetabulectomy
  see Excision, Lower Bones 0QB
  see Resection, Lower Bones 0QT
Acetabulofemoral joint
  use Joint, Hip, Right
  use Joint, Hip, Left
Acetabuloplasty
  see Repair, Lower Bones 0QQ
  see Replacement, Lower Bones 0QR
  see Supplement, Lower Bones 0QU
Achilles tendon
  use Tendon, Lower Leg, Left
  use Tendon, Lower Leg, Right
Achillorrhaphy *use* Repair, Tendons 0LQ
Achillotenotomy, achillotomy
  see Division, Tendons 0L8
  see Drainage, Tendons 0L9
Acromioclavicular ligament
  use Bursa and Ligament, Shoulder, Right
  use Bursa and Ligament, Shoulder, Left
Acromion (process)
  use Scapula, Left
  use Scapula, Right
Acromionectomy
  see Excision, Upper Joints 0RB
  see Resection, Upper Joints 0RT
Acromioplasty
  see Repair, Upper Joints 0RQ
  see Replacement, Upper Joints 0RR
  see Supplement, Upper Joints 0RU
Activa PC neurostimulator *use* Stimulator Generator, Multiple Array in 0JH
Activa RC neurostimulator *use* Stimulator Generator, Multiple Array Rechargeable in 0JH
Activa SC neurostimulator *use* Stimulator Generator, Single Array in 0JH
Activities of Daily Living Assessment F02

Activities of Daily Living Treatment F08
ACUITY™ Steerable Lead
  use Cardiac Lead, Defibrillator in 02H
  use Cardiac Lead, Pacemaker in 02H
Acupuncture
  Breast
    Anesthesia 8E0H300
    No Qualifier 8E0H30Z
  Integumentary System
    Anesthesia 8E0H300
    No Qualifier 8E0H30Z
Adductor brevis muscle
  use Muscle, Upper Leg, Left
  use Muscle, Upper Leg, Right
Adductor hallucis muscle
  use Muscle, Foot, Left
  use Muscle, Foot, Right
Adductor longus muscle
  use Muscle, Upper Leg, Right
  use Muscle, Upper Leg, Left
Adductor magnus muscle
  use Muscle, Upper Leg, Right
  use Muscle, Upper Leg, Left
Adenohypophysis *use* Gland, Pituitary
Adenoidectomy
  see Excision, Adenoids 0CBQ
  see Resection, Adenoids 0CTQ
Adenoidotomy *see* Drainage, Adenoids 0C9Q
Adhesiolysis *see* Release
Administration
  Blood products *see* Transfusion
  Other substance *see* Introduction of substance in or on
Adrenalectomy
  see Excision, Endocrine System 0GB
  see Resection, Endocrine System 0GT
Adrenalorrhaphy *see* Repair, Endocrine System 0GQ
Adrenalotomy *see* Drainage, Endocrine System 0G9
Advancement
  see Reposition
  see Transfer
Advisa (MRI) *use* Pacemaker, Dual Chamber in 0JH ◄
AIGISRx Antibacterial Envelope *use* Anti-Infective Envelope ◄
Alar ligament of axis *use* Bursa and Ligament, Head and Neck
Alimentation *see* Introduction of substance in or on
Alteration
  Abdominal Wall 0W0F
  Ankle Region
    Left 0Y0L
    Right 0Y0K
  Arm
    Lower
      Left 0X0F
      Right 0X0D
    Upper
      Left 0X09
      Right 0X08
  Axilla
    Left 0X05
    Right 0X04
  Back
    Lower 0W0L
    Upper 0W0K
  Breast
    Bilateral 0H0V
    Left 0H0U
    Right 0H0T
  Buttock
    Left 0Y01
    Right 0Y00
  Chest Wall 0W08
  Ear
    Bilateral 0902
    Left 0901
    Right 0900

Alteration *(Continued)*
  Elbow Region
    Left 0X0C
    Right 0X0B
  Extremity
    Lower
      Left 0Y0B
      Right 0Y09
    Upper
      Left 0X07
      Right 0X06
  Eyelid
    Lower
      Left 080R
      Right 080Q
    Upper
      Left 080P
      Right 080N
  Face 0W02
  Head 0W00
  Jaw
    Lower 0W05
    Upper 0W04
  Knee Region
    Left 0Y0G
    Right 0Y0F
  Leg
    Lower
      Left 0Y0J
      Right 0Y0H
    Upper
      Left 0Y0D
      Right 0Y0C
  Lip
    Lower 0C01X
    Upper 0C00X
  Neck 0W06
  Nose 090K
  Perineum
    Female 0W0N
    Male 0W0M
  Shoulder Region
    Left 0X03
    Right 0X02
  Subcutaneous Tissue and Fascia
    Abdomen 0J08
    Back 0J07
    Buttock 0J09
    Chest 0J06
    Face 0J01
    Lower Arm
      Left 0J0H
      Right 0J0G
    Lower Leg
      Left 0J0P
      Right 0J0N
    Neck
      Anterior 0J04
      Posterior 0J05
    Upper Arm
      Left 0J0F
      Right 0J0D
    Upper Leg
      Left 0J0M
      Right 0J0L
  Wrist Region
    Left 0X0H
    Right 0X0G
Alveolar process of mandible
  use Mandible, Left
  use Mandible, Right
Alveolar process of maxilla
  use Maxilla, Right
  use Maxilla, Left
Alveolectomy
  see Excision, Head and Facial Bones 0NB
  see Resection, Head and Facial Bones 0NT
Alveoloplasty
  see Repair, Head and Facial Bones 0NQ
  see Replacement, Head and Facial Bones 0NR
  see Supplement, Head and Facial Bones 0NU

Alveolotomy
  see Division, Head and Facial Bones 0N8
  see Drainage, Head and Facial Bones 0N9
Ambulatory cardiac monitoring 4A12X45
Amniocentesis *see* Drainage, Products of
  Conception 1090
Amnioinfusion *see* Introduction of substance in
  or on, Products of Conception 3E0E
Amnioscopy 10J08ZZ
Amniotomy *see* Drainage, Products of
  Conception 1090
AMPLATZER® Muscular VSD Occluder *use*
  Synthetic Substitute
Amputation *see* Detachment
AMS 800® Urinary Control System *use*
  Artificial Sphincter in Urinary System
Anal orifice *use* Anus
Analog radiography *see* Plain Radiography
Analog radiology *see* Plain Radiography
Anastomosis *see* Bypass
Anatomical snuffbox
  use Muscle, Lower Arm and Wrist, Left
  use Muscle, Lower Arm and Wrist, Right
AneuRx® AAA Advantage® *use* Intraluminal
  Device
Angiectomy
  see Excision, Heart and Great Vessels 02B
  see Excision, Upper Arteries 03B
  see Excision, Lower Arteries 04B
  see Excision, Upper Veins 05B
  see Excision, Lower Veins 06B
Angiocardiography
  Combined right and left heart *see*
    Fluoroscopy, Heart, Right and Left B216
  Left Heart *see* Fluoroscopy, Heart, Left B215
  Right Heart *see* Fluoroscopy, Heart, Right B214
  SPY *see* Fluoroscopy, Heart B21
Angiography
  see Plain Radiography, Heart B20
  see Fluoroscopy, Heart B21
Angioplasty
  see Dilation, Heart and Great Vessels 027
  see Repair, Heart and Great Vessels 02Q
  see Replacement, Heart and Great Vessels 02R
  see Dilation, Upper Arteries 037
  see Repair, Upper Arteries 03Q
  see Replacement, Upper Arteries 03R
  see Dilation, Lower Arteries 047
  see Repair, Lower Arteries 04Q
  see Replacement, Lower Arteries 04R
  see Supplement, Heart and Great Vessels 02U
  see Supplement, Upper Arteries 03U
  see Supplement, Lower Arteries 04U
Angiorrhaphy
  see Repair, Heart and Great Vessels 02Q
  see Repair, Upper Arteries 03Q
  see Repair, Lower Arteries 04Q
Angioscopy
  02JY4ZZ
  03JY4ZZ
  04JY4ZZ
Angiotripsy
  see Occlusion, Upper Arteries 03L
  see Occlusion, Lower Arteries 04L
Angular artery *use* Artery, Face
Angular vein
  use Vein, Face, Left
  use Vein, Face, Right
Annular ligament
  use Bursa and Ligament, Elbow, Left
  use Bursa and Ligament, Elbow, Right
Annuloplasty
  see Repair, Heart and Great Vessels 02Q
  see Supplement, Heart and Great Vessels 02U
Annuloplasty ring *use* Synthetic Substitute
Anoplasty
  see Repair, Anus 0DQQ
  see Supplement, Anus 0DUQ
Anorectal junction *use* Rectum
Anoscopy 0DJD8ZZ
Ansa cervicalis *use* Plexus, Cervical
Antabuse therapy HZ93ZZZ

Antebrachial fascia
  use Subcutaneous Tissue and Fascia, Lower
    Arm, Left
  use Subcutaneous Tissue and Fascia, Lower
    Arm, Right
Anterior (pectoral) lymph node
  use Lymphatic, Axillary, Right
  use Lymphatic, Axillary, Left
Anterior cerebral artery *use* Artery, Intracranial
Anterior cerebral vein *use* Vein, Intracranial
Anterior choroidal artery *use* Artery,
  Intracranial
Anterior circumflex humeral artery
  use Artery, Axillary, Left
  use Artery, Axillary, Right
Anterior communicating artery *use* Artery,
  Intracranial
Anterior cruciate ligament (ACL)
  use Bursa and Ligament, Knee, Left
  use Bursa and Ligament, Knee, Right
Anterior crural nerve *use* Nerve, Femoral
Anterior facial vein
  use Vein, Face, Left
  use Vein, Face, Right
Anterior intercostal artery
  use Artery, Internal Mammary, Right
  use Artery, Internal Mammary, Left
Anterior interosseous nerve *use* Nerve, Median
Anterior lateral malleolar artery
  use Artery, Anterior Tibial, Right
  use Artery, Anterior Tibial, Left
Anterior lingual gland *use* Gland, Minor
  Salivary
Anterior medial malleolar artery
  use Artery, Anterior Tibial, Right
  use Artery, Anterior Tibial, Left
Anterior spinal artery
  use Artery, Vertebral, Right
  use Artery, Vertebral, Left
Anterior tibial recurrent artery
  use Artery, Anterior Tibial, Right
  use Artery, Anterior Tibial, Left
Anterior ulnar recurrent artery
  use Artery, Ulnar, Right
  use Artery, Ulnar, Left
Anterior vagal trunk *use* Nerve, Vagus
Anterior vertebral muscle
  use Muscle, Neck, Left
  use Muscle, Neck, Right
Antihelix
  use Ear, External, Right
  use Ear, External, Left
  use Ear, External, Bilateral
Antimicrobial envelope *use* Anti-Infective
  Envelope ◄
Antitragus
  use Ear, External, Bilateral
  use Ear, External, Right
  use Ear, External, Left
Antrostomy *see* Drainage, Ear, Nose, Sinus 099
Antrotomy *see* Drainage, Ear, Nose, Sinus 099
Antrum of Highmore
  use Sinus, Maxillary, Left
  use Sinus, Maxillary, Right
Aortic annulus *use* Valve, Aortic
Aortic arch *use* Aorta, Thoracic
Aortic intercostal artery *use* Aorta, Thoracic
Aortography
  see Plain Radiography, Upper Arteries B30
  see Fluoroscopy, Upper Arteries B31
  see Plain Radiography, Lower Arteries B40
  see Fluoroscopy, Lower Arteries B41
Aortoplasty
  see Repair, Aorta, Thoracic 02QW
  see Replacement, Aorta, Thoracic 02RW
  see Supplement, Aorta, Thoracic 02UW
  see Repair, Aorta, Abdominal 04Q0
  see Replacement, Aorta, Abdominal 04R0
  see Supplement, Aorta, Abdominal 04U0
Apical (subclavicular) lymph node
  use Lymphatic, Axillary, Left
  use Lymphatic, Axillary, Right

Apneustic center *use* Pons
Appendectomy
  see Excision, Appendix 0DBJ
  see Resection, Appendix 0DTJ
Appendicolysis *see* Release, Appendix 0DNJ
Appendicotomy *see* Drainage, Appendix 0D9J
Application *see* Introduction of substance in
  or on
Aquapheresis 6A550Z3
Aqueduct of Sylvius *use* Cerebral Ventricle
Aqueous humour
  use Anterior Chamber, Right
  use Anterior Chamber, Left
Arachnoid mater
  use Spinal Meninges
  use Cerebral Meninges
Arcuate artery
  use Artery, Foot, Left
  use Artery, Foot, Right
Areola
  use Nipple, Left
  use Nipple, Right
AROM (artificial rupture of membranes)
  10907ZC
Arterial canal (duct) *use* Artery, Pulmonary, Left
Arterial pulse tracing *see* Measurement,
  Arterial 4A03
Arteriectomy
  see Excision, Heart and Great Vessels 02B
  see Excision, Upper Arteries 03B
  see Excision, Lower Arteries 04B
Arteriography
  see Plain Radiography, Heart B20
  see Fluoroscopy, Heart B21
  see Plain Radiography, Upper Arteries B30
  see Fluoroscopy, Upper Arteries B31
  see Plain Radiography, Lower Arteries B40
  see Fluoroscopy, Lower Arteries B41
Arterioplasty
  see Repair, Heart and Great Vessels 02Q
  see Replacement, Heart and Great Vessels 02R
  see Repair, Upper Arteries 03Q
  see Replacement, Upper Arteries 03R
  see Repair, Lower Arteries 04Q
  see Replacement, Lower Arteries 04R
  see Supplement, Upper Arteries 03U
  see Supplement, Lower Arteries 04U
  see Supplement, Heart and Great Vessels 02U
Arteriorrhaphy
  see Repair, Heart and Great Vessels 02Q
  see Repair, Upper Arteries 03Q
  see Repair, Lower Arteries 04Q
Arterioscopy
  02JY4ZZ
  03JY4ZZ
  04JY4ZZ
Arthrectomy
  see Excision, Upper Joints 0RB
  see Resection, Upper Joints 0RT
  see Excision, Lower Joints 0SB
  see Resection, Lower Joints 0ST
Arthrocentesis
  see Drainage, Upper Joints 0R9
  see Drainage, Lower Joints 0S9
Arthrodesis
  see Fusion, Upper Joints 0RG
  see Fusion, Lower Joints 0SG
Arthrography
  see Plain Radiography, Skull and Facial Bones
    BN0
  see Plain Radiography, Non-Axial Upper
    Bones BP0
  see Plain Radiography, Non-Axial Lower
    Bones BQ0
Arthrolysis
  see Release, Upper Joints 0RN
  see Release, Lower Joints 0SN
Arthropexy
  see Repair, Upper Joints 0RQ
  see Reposition, Upper Joints 0RS
  see Repair, Lower Joints 0SQ
  see Reposition, Lower Joints 0SS

A

Arthroplasty
  see Repair, Upper Joints 0RQ
  see Replacement, Upper Joints 0RR
  see Repair, Lower Joints 0SQ
  see Replacement, Lower Joints 0SR
  see Supplement, Lower Joints 0SU
  see Supplement, Upper Joints 0RU
Arthroscopy
  see Inspection, Upper Joints 0RJ
  see Inspection, Lower Joints 0SJ
Arthrotomy
  see Drainage, Upper Joints 0R9
  see Drainage, Lower Joints 0S9
Artificial anal sphincter (AAS) *use* Artificial
  Sphincter in Gastrointestinal System
Artificial bowel sphincter (neosphincter) *use*
  Artificial Sphincter in Gastrointestinal
  System
Artificial Sphincter
  Insertion of device in
    Anus 0DHQ
    Bladder 0THB
    Bladder Neck 0THC
    Urethra 0THD
  Removal of device from
    Anus 0DPQ
    Bladder 0TPB
    Urethra 0TPD
  Revision of device in
    Anus 0DWQ
    Bladder 0TWB
    Urethra 0TWD
Artificial urinary sphincter (AUS) *use* Artificial
  Sphincter in Urinary System
Aryepiglottic fold *use* Larynx
Arytenoid cartilage *use* Larynx
Arytenoid muscle
  use Muscle, Neck, Left
  use Muscle, Neck, Right
Arytenoidectomy *see* Excision, Larynx
  0CBS
Arytenoidopexy *see* Repair, Larynx
  0CQS
Ascenda Intrathecal Catheter *use* Infusion
  Device ◄
Ascending aorta *use* Aorta, Thoracic
Ascending palatine artery *use* Artery,
  Face
Ascending pharyngeal artery
  use Artery, External Carotid, Left
  use Artery, External Carotid, Right
Aspiration *see* Drainage
Assessment
  Activities of daily living *see* Activities of
    Daily Living Assessment, Rehabilitation
    F02
  Hearing *see* Hearing Assessment, Diagnostic
    Audiology F13
  Hearing aid *see* Hearing Aid Assessment,
    Diagnostic Audiology F14
  Motor function *see* Motor Function
    Assessment, Rehabilitation F01
  Nerve function *see* Motor Function
    Assessment, Rehabilitation F01
  Speech *see* Speech Assessment, Rehabilitation
    F00
  Vestibular *see* Vestibular Assessment,
    Diagnostic Audiology F15
  Vocational *see* Activities of Daily Living
    Treatment, Rehabilitation F08

Assistance
  Cardiac
    Continuous
      Balloon Pump 5A02210
      Impeller Pump 5A0221D
      Other Pump 5A02216
      Pulsatile Compression 5A02215
    Intermittent
      Balloon Pump 5A02110
      Impeller Pump 5A0211D
      Other Pump 5A02116
      Pulsatile Compression 5A02115
  Circulatory
    Continuous
      Hyperbaric 5A05221
      Supersaturated 5A0522C
    Intermittent
      Hyperbaric 5A05121
      Supersaturated 5A0512C
  Respiratory
    24-96 Consecutive Hours
      Continuous Negative Airway Pressure
        5A09459
      Continuous Positive Airway Pressure
        5A09457
      Intermittent Negative Airway Pressure
        5A0945B
      Intermittent Positive Airway Pressure
        5A09458
      No Qualifier 5A0945Z
    Greater than 96 Consecutive Hours
      Continuous Negative Airway Pressure
        5A09559
      Continuous Positive Airway Pressure
        5A09557
      Intermittent Negative Airway Pressure
        5A0955B
      Intermittent Positive Airway Pressure
        5A09558
      No Qualifier 5A0955Z
    Less than 24 Consecutive Hours
      Continuous Negative Airway Pressure
        5A09359
      Continuous Positive Airway Pressure
        5A09357
      Intermittent Negative Airway Pressure
        5A0935B
      Intermittent Positive Airway Pressure
        5A09358
      No Qualifier 5A0935Z
Assurant (Cobalt) stent *use* Intraluminal Device
Atherectomy
  see Extirpation, Heart and Great Vessels 02C
  see Extirpation, Upper Arteries 03C
  see Extirpation, Lower Arteries 04C
Atlantoaxial joint *use* Joint, Cervical Vertebral
Atmospheric Control 6A0Z
Atrioseptoplasty
  see Repair, Heart and Great Vessels 02Q
  see Replacement, Heart and Great Vessels 02R
  see Supplement, Heart and Great Vessels 02U
Atrioventricular node *use* Conduction
  Mechanism
Atrium dextrum cordis *use* Atrium, Right
Atrium pulmonale *use* Atrium, Left
Attain Ability® lead
  use Cardiac Lead, Pacemaker in 02H
  use Cardiac Lead, Defibrillator in 02H
Attain StarFix® (OTW) lead
  use Cardiac Lead, Defibrillator in O2H
  use Cardiac Lead, Pacemaker in 02H

Audiology, diagnostic
  see Hearing Assessment, Diagnostic
    Audiology F13
  see Hearing Aid Assessment, Diagnostic
    Audiology F14
  see Vestibular Assessment, Diagnostic
    Audiology F15
Audiometry *see* Hearing Assessment,
  Diagnostic Audiology F13
Auditory tube
  use Eustachian Tube, Right
  use Eustachian Tube, Left
Auerbach's (myenteric) plexus *use* Nerve,
  Abdominal Sympathetic
Auricle
  use Ear, External, Left
  use Ear, External, Bilateral
  use Ear, External, Right
Auricularis muscle *use* Muscle, Head
Autograft *use* Autologous Tissue Substitute
Autologous artery graft
  use Autologous Arterial Tissue in Lower
    Arteries
  use Autologous Arterial Tissue in Upper
    Veins
  use Autologous Arterial Tissue in Lower
    Veins
  use Autologous Arterial Tissue in Heart and
    Great Vessels
  use Autologous Arterial Tissue in Upper
    Arteries
Autologous vein graft
  use Autologous Venous Tissue in Lower
    Arteries
  use Autologous Venous Tissue in Upper
    Veins
  use Autologous Venous Tissue in Lower
    Veins
  use Autologous Venous Tissue in Heart and
    Great Vessels
  use Autologous Venous Tissue in Upper
    Arteries
Autotransfusion *see* Transfusion
Autotransplant
  Adrenal tissue *see* Reposition, Endocrine
    System 0GS
  Kidney
    see Reposition, Urinary System 0TS
  Pancreatic tissue *see* Reposition, Pancreas
    0FSG
  Parathyroid tissue *see* Reposition, Endocrine
    System 0GS
  Thyroid tissue *see* Reposition, Endocrine
    System 0GS
  Tooth *see* Reattachment, Mouth and Throat
    0CM
Avulsion *see* Extraction
Axial Lumbar Interbody Fusion System
  use Interbody Fusion Device in Lower
    Joints
AxiaLIF® System *use* Interbody Fusion Device
  in Lower Joints
Axillary fascia
  use Subcutaneous Tissue and Fascia, Upper
    Arm, Left
  use Subcutaneous Tissue and Fascia, Upper
    Arm, Right
Axillary nerve *use* Nerve, Brachial Plexus

B

BAK/C® Interbody Cervical Fusion System *use* Interbody Fusion Device in Upper Joints
BAL (bronchial alveolar lavage), diagnostic *see* Drainage, Respiratory System 0B9
Balanoplasty
   see Repair, Penis 0VQS
   see Supplement, Penis 0VUS
Balloon Pump
   Continuous, Output 5A02210
   Intermittent, Output 5A02110
Bandage, Elastic *see* Compression
Banding ◀▥
   see Restriction ◀
   see Occlusion ◀
Bard® Composix® (E/X) (LP) mesh *use* Synthetic Substitute
Bard® Composix® Kugel® patch *use* Synthetic Substitute
Bard® Dulex™ mesh *use* Synthetic Substitute
Bard® Ventralex™ hernia patch *use* Synthetic Substitute
Barium swallow *see* Fluoroscopy, Gastrointestinal System BD1
Baroreflex Activation Therapy® (BAT®)
   use Stimulator Generator in Subcutaneous Tissue and Fascia ◀
   use Stimulator Lead in Upper Arteries
   ~~use Cardiac Rhythm Related Device in Subcutaneous Tissue and Fascia~~
Bartholin's (greater vestibular) gland *use* Gland, Vestibular
Basal (internal) cerebral vein *use* Vein, Intracranial
Basal metabolic rate (BMR) *see* Measurement, Physiological Systems 4A0Z
Basal nuclei *use* Basal Ganglia
Basilar artery *use* Artery, Intracranial
Basis pontis *use* Pons
Beam Radiation
   Abdomen DW03
      Intraoperative DW033Z0
   Adrenal Gland DG02
      Intraoperative DG023Z0
   Bile Ducts DF02
      Intraoperative DF023Z0
   Bladder DT02
      Intraoperative DT023Z0
   Bone
      Other DP0C
         Intraoperative DP0C3Z0
   Bone Marrow D700
      Intraoperative D7003Z0
   Brain D000
      Intraoperative D0003Z0
   Brain Stem D001
      Intraoperative D0013Z0
   Breast
      Left DM00
         Intraoperative DM003Z0
      Right DM01
         Intraoperative DM013Z0
   Bronchus DB01
      Intraoperative DB013Z0
   Cervix DU01
      Intraoperative DU013Z0
   Chest DW02
      Intraoperative DW023Z0
   Chest Wall DB07
      Intraoperative DB073Z0
   Colon DD05
      Intraoperative DD053Z0
   Diaphragm DB08
      Intraoperative DB083Z0
   Duodenum DD02
      Intraoperative DD023Z0
   Ear D900
      Intraoperative D9003Z0
   Esophagus DD00
      Intraoperative DD003Z0

Beam Radiation *(Continued)*
   Eye D800
      Intraoperative D8003Z0
   Femur DP09
      Intraoperative DP093Z0
   Fibula DP0B
      Intraoperative DP0B3Z0
   Gallbladder DF01
      Intraoperative DF013Z0
   Gland
      Adrenal DG02
         Intraoperative DG023Z0
      Parathyroid DG04
         Intraoperative DG043Z0
      Pituitary DG00
         Intraoperative DG003Z0
      Thyroid DG05
         Intraoperative DG053Z0
   Glands
      Salivary D906
         Intraoperative D9063Z0
   Head and Neck DW01
      Intraoperative DW013Z0
   Hemibody DW04
      Intraoperative DW043Z0
   Humerus DP06
      Intraoperative DP063Z0
   Hypopharynx D903
      Intraoperative D9033Z0
   Ileum DD04
      Intraoperative DD043Z0
   Jejunum DD03
      Intraoperative DD033Z0
   Kidney DT00
      Intraoperative DT003Z0
   Larynx D90B
      Intraoperative D90B3Z0
   Liver DF00
      Intraoperative DF003Z0
   Lung DB02
      Intraoperative DB023Z0
   Lymphatics
      Abdomen D706
         Intraoperative D7063Z0
      Axillary D704
         Intraoperative D7043Z0
      Inguinal D708
         Intraoperative D7083Z0
      Neck D703
         Intraoperative D7033Z0
      Pelvis D707
         Intraoperative D7073Z0
      Thorax D705
         Intraoperative D7053Z0
   Mandible DP03
      Intraoperative DP033Z0
   Maxilla DP02
      Intraoperative DP023Z0
   Mediastinum DB06
      Intraoperative DB063Z0
   Mouth D904
      Intraoperative D9043Z0
   Nasopharynx D90D
      Intraoperative D90D3Z0
   Neck and Head DW01
      Intraoperative DW013Z0
   Nerve
      Peripheral D007
         Intraoperative D0073Z0
   Nose D901
      Intraoperative D9013Z0
   Oropharynx D90F
      Intraoperative D90F3Z0
   Ovary DU00
      Intraoperative DU003Z0
   Palate
      Hard D908
         Intraoperative D9083Z0
      Soft D909
         Intraoperative D9093Z0
   Pancreas DF03
      Intraoperative DF033Z0

Beam Radiation *(Continued)*
   Parathyroid Gland DG04
      Intraoperative DG043Z0
   Pelvic Bones DP08
      Intraoperative DP083Z0
   Pelvic Region DW06
      Intraoperative DW063Z0
   Pineal Body DG01
      Intraoperative DG013Z0
   Pituitary Gland DG00
      Intraoperative DG003Z0
   Pleura DB05
      Intraoperative DB053Z0
   Prostate DV00
      Intraoperative DV003Z0
   Radius DP07
      Intraoperative DP073Z0
   Rectum DD07
      Intraoperative DD073Z0
   Rib DP05
      Intraoperative DP053Z0
   Sinuses D907
      Intraoperative D9073Z0
   Skin
      Abdomen DH08
         Intraoperative DH083Z0
      Arm DH04
         Intraoperative DH043Z0
      Back DH07
         Intraoperative DH073Z0
      Buttock DH09
         Intraoperative DH093Z0
      Chest DH06
         Intraoperative DH063Z0
      Face DH02
         Intraoperative DH023Z0
      Leg DH0B
         Intraoperative DH0B3Z0
      Neck DH03
         Intraoperative DH033Z0
   Skull DP00
      Intraoperative DP003Z0
   Spinal Cord D006
      Intraoperative D0063Z0
   Spleen D702
      Intraoperative D7023Z0
   Sternum DP04
      Intraoperative DP043Z0
   Stomach DD01
      Intraoperative DD013Z0
   Testis DV01
      Intraoperative DV013Z0
   Thymus D701
      Intraoperative D7013Z0
   Thyroid Gland DG05
      Intraoperative DG053Z0
   Tibia DP0B
      Intraoperative DP0B3Z0
   Tongue D905
      Intraoperative D9053Z0
   Trachea DB00
      Intraoperative DB003Z0
   Ulna DP07
      Intraoperative DP073Z0
   Ureter DT01
      Intraoperative DT013Z0
   Urethra DT03
      Intraoperative DT033Z0
   Uterus DU02
      Intraoperative DU023Z0
   Whole Body DW05
      Intraoperative DW053Z0
Bedside swallow F00ZJWZ ◀
Berlin Heart Ventricular Assist Device *use* Implantable Heart Assist System in Heart and Great Vessels
Biceps brachii muscle
   use Muscle, Upper Arm, Right
   use Muscle, Upper Arm, Left
Biceps femoris muscle
   use Muscle, Upper Leg, Right
   use Muscle, Upper Leg, Left

Bicipital aponeurosis
  use Subcutaneous Tissue and Fascia, Lower
    Arm, Left
  use Subcutaneous Tissue and Fascia, Lower
    Arm, Right
Bicuspid valve *use* Valve, Mitral
Bililite therapy *see* Ultraviolet Light Therapy,
    Skin 6A80
Bioactive embolization coil(s) *use* Intraluminal
    Device, Bioactive in Upper Arteries
Biofeedback GZC9ZZZ
Biopsy
  see Drainage with qualifier Diagnostic
  see Excision with qualifier Diagnostic
  Bone Marrow *see* Extraction with qualifier
    Diagnostic
BiPAP *see* Assistance, Respiratory 5A09
Bisection *see* Division
Biventricular external heart assist system *use*
    External Heart Assist System in Heart and
    Great Vessels
Blepharectomy
  see Excision, Eye 08B
  see Resection, Eye 08T
Blepharoplasty
  see Repair, Eye 08Q
  see Replacement, Eye 08R
  see Supplement, Eye 08U
  see Reposition, Eye 08S
Blepharorrhaphy *see* Repair, Eye 08Q
Blepharotomy *see* Drainage, Eye 089
Block, Nerve, anesthetic injection 3E0T3CZ
Blood glucose monitoring system *use*
    Monitoring Device
Blood pressure *see* Measurement, Arterial 4A03
BMR (basal metabolic rate) *see* Measurement,
    Physiological Systems 4A0Z
Body of femur
  use Femoral Shaft, Right
  use Femoral Shaft, Left
Body of fibula
  use Fibula, Right
  use Fibula, Left
Bone anchored hearing device
  use Hearing Device, Bone Conduction in 09H
  use Hearing Device, in Head and Facial
    Bones
Bone bank bone graft *use* Nonautologous
    Tissue Substitute
Bone Growth Stimulator
  Insertion of device in
    Bone
      Facial 0NHW
      Lower 0QHY
      Nasal 0NHB
      Upper 0PHY
    Skull 0NH0
  Removal of device from
    Bone
      Facial 0NPW
      Lower 0QPY
      Nasal 0NPB
      Upper 0PPY
    Skull 0NP0
  Revision of device in
    Bone
      Facial 0NWW
      Lower 0QWY
      Nasal 0NWB
      Upper 0PWY
    Skull 0NW0
Bone marrow transplant *see* Transfusion
Bone morphogenetic protein 2 (BMP 2) *use*
    Recombinant Bone Morphogenetic
    Protein ◄
Bone screw (interlocking) (lag) (pedicle)
    (recessed)
  use Internal Fixation Device in Head and
    Facial Bones
  use Internal Fixation Device in Upper Bones
  use Internal Fixation Device in Lower Bones

Bony labyrinth
  use Ear, Inner, Left
  use Ear, Inner, Right
Bony orbit
  use Orbit, Right
  use Orbit, Left
Bony vestibule
  use Ear, Inner, Right
  use Ear, Inner, Left
Botallo's duct *use* Artery, Pulmonary, Left
Bovine pericardial valve *use* Zooplastic Tissue
    in Heart and Great Vessels
Bovine pericardium graft *use* Zooplastic Tissue
    in Heart and Great Vessels
BP (blood pressure) *see* Measurement, Arterial
    4A03
Brachial (lateral) lymph node
  use Lymphatic, Axillary, Left
  use Lymphatic, Axillary, Right
Brachialis muscle
  use Muscle, Upper Arm, Right
  use Muscle, Upper Arm, Left
Brachiocephalic artery *use* Artery, Innominate
Brachiocephalic trunk *use* Artery, Innominate
Brachiocephalic vein
  use Vein, Innominate, Right
  use Vein, Innominate, Left
Brachioradialis muscle
  use Muscle, Lower Arm and Wrist, Right
  use Muscle, Lower Arm and Wrist, Left
Brachytherapy
  Abdomen DW13
  Adrenal Gland DG12
  Bile Ducts DF12
  Bladder DT12
  Bone Marrow D710
  Brain D010
  Brain Stem D011
  Breast
    Left DM10
    Right DM11
  Bronchus DB11
  Cervix DU11
  Chest DW12
  Chest Wall DB17
  Colon DD15
  Diaphragm DB18
  Duodenum DD12
  Ear D910
  Esophagus DD10
  Eye D810
  Gallbladder DF11
  Gland
    Adrenal DG12
    Parathyroid DG14
    Pituitary DG10
    Thyroid DG15
  Glands, Salivary D916
  Head and Neck DW11
  Hypopharynx D913
  Ileum DD14
  Jejunum DD13
  Kidney DT10
  Larynx D91B
  Liver DF10
  Lung DB12
  Lymphatics
    Abdomen D716
    Axillary D714
    Inguinal D718
    Neck D713
    Pelvis D717
    Thorax D715
  Mediastinum DB16
  Mouth D914
  Nasopharynx D91D
  Neck and Head DW11
  Nerve, Peripheral D017
  Nose D911
  Oropharynx D91F
  Ovary DU10

Brachytherapy (*Continued*)
  Palate
    Hard D918
    Soft D919
  Pancreas DF13
  Parathyroid Gland DG14
  Pelvic Region DW16
  Pineal Body DG11
  Pituitary Gland DG10
  Pleura DB15
  Prostate DV10
  Rectum DD17
  Sinuses D917
  Spinal Cord D016
  Spleen D712
  Stomach DD11
  Testis DV11
  Thymus D711
  Thyroid Gland DG15
  Tongue D915
  Trachea DB10
  Ureter DT11
  Urethra DT13
  Uterus DU12
Brachytherapy seeds *use* Radioactive
    Element
Broad ligament *use* Uterine Supporting
    Structure
Bronchial artery *use* Aorta, Thoracic
Bronchography
  see Plain Radiography, Respiratory System
    BB0
  see Fluoroscopy, Respiratory System BB1
Bronchoplasty
  see Repair, Respiratory System 0BQ
  see Supplement, Respiratory System 0BU
Bronchorrhaphy *see* Repair, Respiratory System
    0BQ
Bronchoscopy 0BJ08ZZ
Bronchotomy *see* Drainage, Respiratory System
    0B9
BRYAN® Cervical Disc System *use* Synthetic
    Substitute
Buccal gland *use* Buccal Mucosa
Buccinator lymph node *use* Lymphatic,
    Head
Buccinator muscle *use* Muscle, Facial
Buckling, scleral with implant *see* Supplement,
    Eye 08U
Bulbospongiosus muscle *use* Muscle,
    Perineum
Bulbourethral (Cowper's) gland *use* Urethra
Bundle of His *use* Conduction Mechanism
Bundle of Kent *use* Conduction Mechanism
Bunionectomy *see* Excision, Lower Bones
    0QB
Bursectomy
  see Excision, Bursae and Ligaments 0MB
  see Resection, Bursae and Ligaments 0MT
Bursocentesis *see* Drainage, Bursae and
    Ligaments 0M9
Bursography
  see Plain Radiography, Non-Axial Upper
    Bones BP0
  see Plain Radiography, Non-Axial Lower
    Bones BQ0
Bursotomy
  see Division, Bursae and Ligaments
    0M8
  see Drainage, Bursae and Ligaments
    0M9
BVS 5000 Ventricular Assist Device *use*
    External Heart Assist System in Heart
    and Great Vessels
Bypass
  Anterior Chamber
    Left 08133
    Right 08123
  Aorta
    Abdominal 0410
    Thoracic 021W

Bypass (*Continued*)
  Artery
    Axillary
      Left 03160
      Right 03150
    Brachial
      Left 03180
      Right 03170
    Common Carotid
      Left 031J0
      Right 031H0
    Common Iliac
      Left 041D
      Right 041C
    Coronary
      Four or More Sites 0213
      One Site 0210
      Three Sites 0212
      Two Sites 0211
    External Carotid
      Left 031N0
      Right 031M0
    External Iliac
      Left 041J
      Right 041H
    Femoral
      Left 041L
      Right 041K
    Innominate 03120
    Internal Carotid
      Left 031L0
      Right 031K0
    Internal Iliac
      Left 041F
      Right 041E
    Intracranial 031G0
    Popliteal
      Left 041N
      Right 041M
    Radial
      Left 031C0
      Right 031B0
    Splenic 0414
    Subclavian
      Left 03140
      Right 03130
    Temporal
      Left 031T0
      Right 031S0
    Ulnar
      Left 031A0
      Right 03190
  Atrium
    Left 0217
    Right 0216
  Bladder 0T1B
  Cavity, Cranial 0W110J
  Cecum 0D1H
  Cerebral Ventricle 0016
  Colon
    Ascending 0D1K
    Descending 0D1M
    Sigmoid 0D1N
    Transverse 0D1L

Bypass (*Continued*)
  Duct
    Common Bile 0F19
    Cystic 0F18
    Hepatic
      Left 0F16
      Right 0F15
    Lacrimal
      Left 081Y
      Right 081X
    Pancreatic 0F1D
      Accessory 0F1F
  Duodenum 0D19
  Ear
    Left 091E0
    Right 091D0
  Esophagus 0D15
    Lower 0D13
    Middle 0D12
    Upper 0D11
  Fallopian Tube
    Left 0U16
    Right 0U15
  Gallbladder 0F14
  Ileum 0D1B
  Jejunum 0D1A
  Kidney Pelvis
    Left 0T14
    Right 0T13
  Pancreas 0F1G
  Pelvic Cavity 0W1J
  Peritoneal Cavity 0W1G
  Pleural Cavity
    Left 0W1B
    Right 0W19
  Spinal Canal 001U
  Stomach 0D16
  Trachea 0B11
  Ureter
    Left 0T17
    Right 0T16
  Ureters, Bilateral 0T18
  Vas Deferens
    Bilateral 0V1Q
    Left 0V1P
    Right 0V1N
  Vein
    Axillary
      Left 0518
      Right 0517
    Azygos 0510
    Basilic
      Left 051C
      Right 051B
    Brachial
      Left 051A
      Right 0519
    Cephalic
      Left 051F
      Right 051D
    Colic 0617
    Common Iliac
      Left 061D
      Right 061C

Bypass (*Continued*)
  Vein (*Continued*)
    Esophageal 0613
    External Iliac
      Left 061G
      Right 061F
    External Jugular
      Left 051Q
      Right 051P
    Face
      Left 051V
      Right 051T
    Femoral
      Left 061N
      Right 061M
    Foot
      Left 061V
      Right 061T
    Gastric 0612
    Greater Saphenous
      Left 061Q
      Right 061P
    Hand
      Left 051H
      Right 051G
    Hemiazygos 0511
    Hepatic 0614
    Hypogastric
      Left 061J
      Right 061H
    Inferior Mesenteric 0616
    Innominate
      Left 0514
      Right 0513
    Internal Jugular
      Left 051N
      Right 051M
    Intracranial 051L
    Lesser Saphenous
      Left 061S
      Right 061R
    Portal 0618
    Renal
      Left 061B
      Right 0619
    Splenic 0611
    Subclavian
      Left 0516
      Right 0515
    Superior Mesenteric 0615
    Vertebral
      Left 051S
      Right 051R
  Vena Cava
    Inferior 0610
    Superior 021V
  Ventricle
    Left 021L
    Right 021K
Bypass, cardiopulmonary 5A1221Z

C

Caesarean section see Extraction, Products of
Conception 10D0
Calcaneocuboid joint
use Joint, Tarsal, Left
use Joint, Tarsal, Right
Calcaneocuboid ligament
use Bursa and Ligament, Foot, Right
use Bursa and Ligament, Foot, Left
Calcaneofibular ligament
use Bursa and Ligament, Ankle, Left
use Bursa and Ligament, Ankle, Right
Calcaneus
use Tarsal, Right
use Tarsal, Left
Cannulation
see Bypass
see Dilation
see Drainage
see Irrigation
Canthorrhaphy see Repair, Eye 08Q
Canthotomy see Release, Eye 08N
Capitate bone
use Carpal, Left
use Carpal, Right
Capsulectomy, lens see Excision, Eye 08B
Capsulorrhaphy, joint
see Repair, Upper Joints 0RQ
see Repair, Lower Joints 0SQ
Cardia use Esophagogastric Junction
Cardiac contractility modulation lead use
Cardiac Lead in Heart and Great Vessels
Cardiac event recorder use Monitoring Device
Cardiac Lead
Defibrillator
Atrium
Left 02H7
Right 02H6
Pericardium 02HN
Vein, Coronary 02H4
Ventricle
Left 02HL
Right 02HK
Insertion of device in
Atrium
Left 02H7
Right 02H6
Pericardium 02HN
Vein, Coronary 02H4
Ventricle
Left 02HL
Right 02HK
Pacemaker
Atrium
Left 02H7
Right 02H6
Pericardium 02HN
Vein, Coronary 02H4
Ventricle
Left 02HL
Right 02HK
Removal of device from, Heart 02PA
Revision of device in, Heart 02WA
Cardiac plexus use Nerve, Thoracic
Sympathetic
Cardiac Resynchronization Defibrillator Pulse
Generator
Abdomen 0JH8
Chest 0JH6
Cardiac Resynchronization Pacemaker Pulse
Generator
Abdomen 0JH8
Chest 0JH6
Cardiac resynchronization therapy (CRT) lead
use Cardiac Lead, Pacemaker in 02H
use Cardiac Lead, Defibrillator in 02H
Cardiac Rhythm Related Device
Insertion of device in
Abdomen 0JH8
Chest 0JH6

Cardiac Rhythm Related Device (Continued)
Removal of device from, Subcutaneous Tissue
and Fascia, Trunk 0JPT
Revision of device in, Subcutaneous Tissue
and Fascia, Trunk 0JWT
Cardiocentesis see Drainage, Pericardial Cavity
0W9D
Cardioesophageal junction use
Esophagogastric Junction
Cardiolysis see Release, Heart and Great Vessels
02N
CardioMEMS® pressure sensor use Monitoring
Device, Pressure Sensor in 02H
Cardiomyotomy see Division, Esophagogastric
Junction 0D84
Cardioplegia see Introduction of substance in or
on, Heart 3E08
Cardiorrhaphy see Repair, Heart and Great
Vessels 02Q
Cardioversion 5A2204Z
Caregiver Training F0FZ
Caroticotympanic artery
use Artery, Internal Carotid, Right
use Artery, Internal Carotid, Left
Carotid (artery) sinus (baroreceptor) lead use
Stimulator Lead in Upper Arteries
Carotid glomus
use Carotid Bodies, Bilateral
use Carotid Body, Right
use Carotid Body, Left
Carotid sinus
use Artery, Internal Carotid, Left
use Artery, Internal Carotid, Right
Carotid sinus nerve use Nerve,
Glossopharyngeal
Carotid WALLSTENT® Monorail®
Endoprosthesis use Intraluminal
Device
Carpectomy
see Excision, Upper Bones 0PB
see Resection, Upper Bones 0PT
Carpometacarpal (CMC) joint
use Joint, Metacarpocarpal, Left
use Joint, Metacarpocarpal, Right
Carpometacarpal ligament
use Bursa and Ligament, Hand, Left
use Bursa and Ligament, Hand, Right
Casting see Immobilization
CAT scan see Computerized Tomography
(CT Scan)
Catheterization
see Dilation
see Drainage
see Irrigation
see Insertion of device in
Heart see Measurement, Cardiac 4A02
Umbilical vein, for infusion 06H033T
Cauda equina use Spinal Cord, Lumbar
Cauterization
see Destruction
see Repair
Cavernous plexus use Nerve, Head and Neck
Sympathetic
Cecectomy
see Excision, Cecum 0DBH
see Resection, Cecum 0DTH
Cecocolostomy
see Bypass, Gastrointestinal System 0D1
see Drainage, Gastrointestinal System
0D9
Cecopexy
see Repair, Cecum 0DQH
see Reposition, Cecum 0DSH
Cecoplication see Restriction, Cecum 0DVH
Cecorrhaphy see Repair, Cecum 0DQH
Cecostomy
see Bypass, Cecum 0D1H
see Drainage, Cecum 0D9H
Cecotomy see Drainage, Cecum 0D9H
Celiac (solar) plexus use Nerve, Abdominal
Sympathetic

Celiac ganglion use Nerve, Abdominal
Sympathetic
Celiac lymph node use Lymphatic, Aortic
Celiac trunk use Artery, Celiac
Central axillary lymph node
use Lymphatic, Axillary, Left
use Lymphatic, Axillary, Right
Central venous pressure see Measurement,
Venous 4A04
Centrimag® Blood Pump use External Heart
Assist System in Heart and Great Vessels ◄▥▥
Cephalogram BN00ZZZ
Cerclage see Restriction
Cerebral aqueduct (Sylvius) use Cerebral
Ventricle
Cerebrum use Brain
Cervical esophagus use Esophagus, Upper
Cervical facet joint
use Joint, Cervical Vertebral
use Joint, Cervical Vertebral, 2 or more
Cervical ganglion use Nerve, Head and Neck
Sympathetic
Cervical interspinous ligament use Bursa and
Ligament, Head and Neck
Cervical intertransverse ligament use Bursa
and Ligament, Head and Neck
Cervical ligamentum flavum use Bursa and
Ligament, Head and Neck
Cervical lymph node
use Lymphatic, Neck, Right
use Lymphatic, Neck, Left
Cervicectomy
see Excision, Cervix 0UBC
see Resection, Cervix 0UTC
Cervicothoracic facet joint use Joint,
Cervicothoracic Vertebral
Cesarean section see Extraction, Products of
Conception 10D0
Change device in
Abdominal Wall 0W2FX
Back
Lower 0W2LX
Upper 0W2KX
Bladder 0T2BX
Bone
Facial 0N2WX
Lower 0Q2YX
Nasal 0N2BX
Upper 0P2YX
Bone Marrow 072TX
Brain 0020X
Breast
Left 0H2UX
Right 0H2TX
Bursa and Ligament
Lower 0M2YX
Upper 0M2XX
Cavity, Cranial 0W21X
Chest Wall 0W28X
Cisterna Chyli 072LX
Diaphragm 0B2TX
Duct
Hepatobiliary 0F2BX
Pancreatic 0F2DX
Ear
Left 092JX
Right 092HX
Epididymis and Spermatic Cord 0V2MX
Extremity
Lower
Left 0Y2BX
Right 0Y29X
Upper
Left 0X27X
Right 0X26X
Eye
Left 0821X
Right 0820X
Face 0W22X
Fallopian Tube 0U28X
Gallbladder 0F24X

◄ New   ◄▥▥ Revised   ~~deleted~~ Deleted

Change device in *(Continued)*
  Gland
    Adrenal 0G25X
    Endocrine 0G2SX
    Pituitary 0G20X
    Salivary 0C2AX
  Head 0W20X
  Intestinal Tract
    Lower 0D2DXUZ
    Upper 0D20XUZ
  Jaw
    Lower 0W25X
    Upper 0W24X
  Joint
    Lower 0S2YX
    Upper 0R2YX
  Kidney 0T25X
  Larynx 0C2SX
  Liver 0F20X
  Lung
    Left 0B2LX
    Right 0B2KX
  Lymphatic 072NX
    Thoracic Duct 072KX
  Mediastinum 0W2CX
  Mesentery 0D2VX
  Mouth and Throat 0C2YX
  Muscle
    Lower 0K2YX
    Upper 0K2XX
  Neck 0W26X
  Nerve
    Cranial 002EX
    Peripheral 012YX
  Nose 092KX
  Omentum 0D2UX
  Ovary 0U23X
  Pancreas 0F2GX
  Parathyroid Gland 0G2RX
  Pelvic Cavity 0W2JX
  Penis 0V2SX
  Pericardial Cavity 0W2DX
  Perineum
    Female 0W2NX
    Male 0W2MX
  Peritoneal Cavity 0W2GX
  Peritoneum 0D2WX
  Pineal Body 0G21X
  Pleura 0B2QX
  Pleural Cavity
    Left 0W2BX
    Right 0W29X
  Products of Conception 10207
  Prostate and Seminal Vesicles 0V24X
  Retroperitoneum 0W2HX
  Scrotum and Tunica Vaginalis
    0V28X
  Sinus 092YX
  Skin 0H2PX
  Skull 0N20X
  Spinal Canal 002UX
  Spleen 072PX
  Subcutaneous Tissue and Fascia
    Head and Neck 0J2SX
    Lower Extremity 0J2WX
    Trunk 0J2TX
    Upper Extremity 0J2VX
  Tendon
    Lower 0L2YX
    Upper 0L2XX
  Testis 0V2DX
  Thymus 072MX
  Thyroid Gland 0G2KX
  Trachea 0B21
  Tracheobronchial Tree 0B20X
  Ureter 0T29X
  Urethra 0T2DX
  Uterus and Cervix 0U2DXHZ
  Vagina and Cul-de-sac 0U2HXGZ
  Vas Deferens 0V2RX
  Vulva 0U2MX

Change device in or on
  Abdominal Wall 2W03X
  Anorectal 2Y03X5Z
  Arm
    Lower
      Left 2W0DX
      Right 2W0CX
    Upper
      Left 2W0BX
      Right 2W0AX
  Back 2W05X
  Chest Wall 2W04X
  Ear 2Y02X5Z
  Extremity
    Lower
      Left 2W0MX
      Right 2W0LX
    Upper
      Left 2W09X
      Right 2W08X
  Face 2W01X
  Finger
    Left 2W0KX
    Right 2W0JX
  Foot
    Left 2W0TX
    Right 2W0SX
  Genital Tract, Female 2Y04X5Z
  Hand
    Left 2W0FX
    Right 2W0EX
  Head 2W00X
  Inguinal Region
    Left 2W07X
    Right 2W06X
  Leg
    Lower
      Left 2W0RX
      Right 2W0QX
    Upper
      Left 2W0PX
      Right 2W0NX
  Mouth and Pharynx 2Y00X5Z
  Nasal 2Y01X5Z
  Neck 2W02X
  Thumb
    Left 2W0HX
    Right 2W0GX
  Toe
    Left 2W0VX
    Right 2W0UX
  Urethra 2Y05X5Z
Chemoembolization *see* Introduction of
  substance in or on
Chemosurgery, Skin 3E00XTZ
Chemothalamectomy *see* Destruction,
  Thalamus 0059
Chemotherapy, Infusion for cancer *see*
  Introduction of substance in or on
Chest x-ray *see* Plain Radiography, Chest BW03
Chiropractic Manipulation
  Abdomen 9WB9X
  Cervical 9WB1X
  Extremities
    Lower 9WB6X
    Upper 9WB7X
  Head 9WB0X
  Lumbar 9WB3X
  Pelvis 9WB5X
  Rib Cage 9WB8X
  Sacrum 9WB4X
  Thoracic 9WB2X
Choana *use* Nasopharynx
Cholangiogram
  see Plain Radiography, Hepatobiliary System
    and Pancreas BF0
  see Fluoroscopy, Hepatobiliary System and
    Pancreas BF1
Cholecystectomy
  see Excision, Gallbladder 0FB4
  see Resection, Gallbladder 0FT4

Cholecystojejunostomy
  see Bypass, Hepatobiliary System and
    Pancreas 0F1
  see Drainage, Hepatobiliary System and
    Pancreas 0F9
Cholecystopexy
  see Repair, Gallbladder 0FQ4
  see Reposition, Gallbladder 0FS4
Cholecystoscopy 0FJ44ZZ
Cholecystostomy
  see Drainage, Gallbladder 0F94
  see Bypass, Gallbladder 0F14
Cholecystotomy *see* Drainage, Gallbladder 0F94
Choledochectomy
  see Excision, Hepatobiliary System and
    Pancreas 0FB
  see Resection, Hepatobiliary System and
    Pancreas 0FT
Choledocholithotomy *see* Extirpation, Duct,
  Common Bile 0FC9
Choledochoplasty
  see Repair, Hepatobiliary System and
    Pancreas 0FQ
  see Replacement, Hepatobiliary System and
    Pancreas 0FR
  see Supplement, Hepatobiliary System and
    Pancreas 0FU
Choledochoscopy 0FJB8ZZ
Choledochotomy *see* Drainage, Hepatobiliary
  System and Pancreas 0F9
Cholelithotomy *see* Extirpation, Hepatobiliary
  System and Pancreas 0FC
Chondrectomy
  see Excision, Upper Joints 0RB
  see Excision, Lower Joints 0SB
  Knee *see* Excision, Lower Joints 0SB
  Semilunar cartilage *see* Excision, Lower Joints
    0SB
Chondroglossus muscle *use* Muscle, Tongue,
  Palate, Pharynx
Chorda tympani *use* Nerve, Facial
Chordotomy *see* Division, Central Nervous
  System 008
Choroid plexus *use* Cerebral Ventricle
Choroidectomy
  see Excision, Eye 08B
  see Resection, Eye 08T
Ciliary body
  use Eye, Right
  use Eye, Left
Ciliary ganglion *use* Nerve, Head and Neck
  Sympathetic
Circle of Willis *use* Artery, Intracranial
Circumflex iliac artery
  use Artery, Femoral, Right
  use Artery, Femoral, Left
Clamp and rod internal fixation system (CRIF)
  use Internal Fixation Device in Upper Bones
  use Internal Fixation Device in Lower
    Bones
Clamping *see* Occlusion
Claustrum *use* Basal Ganglia
Claviculectomy
  see Excision, Upper Bones 0PB
  see Resection, Upper Bones 0PT
Claviculotomy
  see Division, Upper Bones 0P8
  see Drainage, Upper Bones 0P9
Clipping, aneurysm *see* Restriction using
  Extraluminal Device
Clitorectomy, clitoridectomy
  see Excision, Clitoris 0UBJ
  see Resection, Clitoris 0UTJ
Clolar *use* Clofarabine ◀
Closure
  see Occlusion
  see Repair
Clysis *see* Introduction of substance in or on
Coagulation *see* Destruction
CoAxia NeuroFlo catheter *use* Intraluminal
  Device

Cobalt/chromium head and polyethylene socket *use* Synthetic Substitute, Metal on Polyethylene in 0SR
Cobalt/chromium head and socket *use* Synthetic Substitute, Metal in 0SR
Coccygeal body *use* Coccygeal Glomus
Coccygeus muscle
  use Muscle, Trunk, Left
  use Muscle, Trunk, Right
Cochlea
  use Ear, Inner, Left
  use Ear, Inner, Right
Cochlear implant (CI), multiple channel (electrode) *use* Hearing Device, Multiple Channel Cochlear Prosthesis in 09H
Cochlear implant (CI), single channel (electrode) *use* Hearing Device, Single Channel Cochlear Prosthesis in 09H
Cochlear Implant Treatment F0BZ0
Cochlear nerve *use* Nerve, Acoustic
COGNIS® CRT-D *use* Cardiac Resynchronization Defibrillator Pulse Generator in 0JH
Colectomy
  see Excision, Gastrointestinal System 0DB
  see Resection, Gastrointestinal System 0DT
Collapse *see* Occlusion
Collection from
  Breast, Breast Milk 8E0HX62
  Indwelling Device
    Circulatory System
      Blood 8C02X6K
      Other Fluid 8C02X6L
    Nervous System
      Cerebrospinal Fluid 8C01X6J
      Other Fluid 8C01X6L
  Integumentary System, Breast Milk 8E0HX62
  Reproductive System, Male, Sperm 8E0VX63
Colocentesis *see* Drainage, Gastrointestinal System 0D9
Colofixation
  see Repair, Gastrointestinal System 0DQ
  see Reposition, Gastrointestinal System 0DS
Cololysis *see* Release, Gastrointestinal System 0DN
Colonic Z-Stent® *use* Intraluminal Device
Colonoscopy 0DJD8ZZ
Colopexy
  see Repair, Gastrointestinal System 0DQ
  see Reposition, Gastrointestinal System 0DS
Coloplication *see* Restriction, Gastrointestinal System 0DV
Coloproctectomy
  see Excision, Gastrointestinal System 0DB
  see Resection, Gastrointestinal System 0DT
Coloproctostomy
  see Bypass, Gastrointestinal System 0D1
  see Drainage, Gastrointestinal System 0D9
Colopuncture *see* Drainage, Gastrointestinal System 0D9
Colorrhaphy *see* Repair, Gastrointestinal System 0DQ
Colostomy
  see Bypass, Gastrointestinal System 0D1
  see Drainage, Gastrointestinal System 0D9
Colpectomy
  see Excision, Vagina 0UBG
  see Resection, Vagina 0UTG
Colpocentesis *see* Drainage, Vagina 0U9G
Colpopexy
  see Repair, Vagina 0UQG
  see Reposition, Vagina 0USG
Colpoplasty
  see Repair, Vagina 0UQG
  see Supplement, Vagina 0UUG
Colporrhaphy *see* Repair, Vagina 0UQG
Colposcopy 0UJH8ZZ
Columella *use* Nose
Common digital vein
  use Vein, Foot, Right
  use Vein, Foot, Left

Common facial vein
  use Vein, Face, Left
  use Vein, Face, Right
Common fibular nerve *use* Nerve, Peroneal
Common hepatic artery *use* Artery, Hepatic
Common iliac (subaortic) lymph node *use* Lymphatic, Pelvis
Common interosseous artery
  use Artery, Ulnar, Left
  use Artery, Ulnar, Right
Common peroneal nerve *use* Nerve, Peroneal
Complete (SE) stent *use* Intraluminal Device
Compression *see* Restriction
  Abdominal Wall 2W13X
  Arm
    Lower
      Left 2W1DX
      Right 2W1CX
    Upper
      Left 2W1BX
      Right 2W1AX
  Back 2W15X
  Chest Wall 2W14X
  Extremity
    Lower
      Left 2W1MX
      Right 2W1LX
    Upper
      Left 2W19X
      Right 2W18X
  Face 2W11X
  Finger
    Left 2W1KX
    Right 2W1JX
  Foot
    Left 2W1TX
    Right 2W1SX
  Hand
    Left 2W1FX
    Right 2W1EX
  Head 2W10X
  Inguinal Region
    Left 2W17X
    Right 2W16X
  Leg
    Lower
      Left 2W1RX
      Right 2W1QX
    Upper
      Left 2W1PX
      Right 2W1NX
  Neck 2W12X
  Thumb
    Left 2W1HX
    Right 2W1GX
  Toe
    Left 2W1VX
    Right 2W1UX
Computer Assisted Procedure
  Extremity
    Lower
      No Qualifier 8E0YXBZ
      With Computerized Tomography 8E0YXBG
      With Fluoroscopy 8E0YXBF
      With Magnetic Resonance Imaging 8E0YXBH
    Upper
      No Qualifier 8E0XXBZ
      With Computerized Tomography 8E0XXBG
      With Fluoroscopy 8E0XXBF
      With Magnetic Resonance Imaging 8E0XXBH
  Head and Neck Region
    No Qualifier 8E09XBZ
    With Computerized Tomography 8E09XBG
    With Fluoroscopy 8E09XBF
    With Magnetic Resonance Imaging 8E09XBH

Computer Assisted Procedure
  (Continued)
  Trunk Region
    No Qualifier 8E0WXBZ
    With Computerized Tomography 8E0WXBG
    With Fluoroscopy 8E0WXBF
    With Magnetic Resonance Imaging 8E0WXBH
Computerized Tomography (CT Scan)
  Abdomen BW20
    Chest and Pelvis BW25
  Abdomen and Chest BW24
  Abdomen and Pelvis BW21
  Airway, Trachea BB2F
  Ankle
    Left BQ2H
    Right BQ2G
  Aorta
    Abdominal B420
      Intravascular Optical Coherence B420Z2Z
    Thoracic B320
      Intravascular Optical Coherence B320Z2Z
  Arm
    Left BP2F
    Right BP2E
  Artery
    Celiac B421
      Intravascular Optical Coherence B421Z2Z
    Common Carotid
      Bilateral B325
      Intravascular Optical Coherence B325Z2Z
    Coronary
      Bypass Graft
        Multiple B223
        Intravascular Optical Coherence B223Z2Z
      Multiple B221
        Intravascular Optical Coherence B221Z2Z
    Internal Carotid
      Bilateral B328
      Intravascular Optical Coherence B328Z2Z
    Intracranial B32R
      Intravascular Optical Coherence B32RZ2Z
    Lower Extremity
      Bilateral B42H
      Intravascular Optical Coherence B42HZ2Z
      Left B42G
      Intravascular Optical Coherence B42GZ2Z
      Right B42F
      Intravascular Optical Coherence B42FZ2Z
    Pelvic B42C
      Intravascular Optical Coherence B42CZ2Z
    Pulmonary
      Left B32T
      Intravascular Optical Coherence B32TZ2Z
      Right B32S
      Intravascular Optical Coherence B32SZ2Z
    Renal
      Bilateral B428
      Intravascular Optical Coherence B428Z2Z
    Transplant B42M
      Intravascular Optical Coherence B42MZ2Z
    Superior Mesenteric B424
      Intravascular Optical Coherence B424Z2Z

◀ New   ◀ Revised   ~~deleted~~ Deleted

Computerized Tomography (*Continued*)
Artery (*Continued*)
  Vertebral
    Bilateral B32G
    Intravascular Optical Coherence
      B32GZ2Z
Bladder BT20
Bone
  Facial BN25
  Temporal BN2F
Brain B020
Calcaneus
  Left BQ2K
  Right BQ2J
Cerebral Ventricle B028
Chest, Abdomen and Pelvis BW25
Chest and Abdomen BW24
Cisterna B027
Clavicle
  Left BP25
  Right BP24
Coccyx BR2F
Colon BD24
Ear B920
Elbow
  Left BP2H
  Right BP2G
Extremity
  Lower
    Left BQ2S
    Right BQ2R
  Upper
    Bilateral BP2V
    Left BP2U
    Right BP2T
Eye
  Bilateral B827
  Left B826
  Right B825
Femur
  Left BQ24
  Right BQ23
Fibula
  Left BQ2C
  Right BQ2B
Finger
  Left BP2S
  Right BP2R
Foot
  Left BQ2M
  Right BQ2L
Forearm
  Left BP2K
  Right BP2J
Gland
  Adrenal, Bilateral BG22
  Parathyroid BG23
  Parotid, Bilateral B926
  Salivary, Bilateral B92D
  Submandibular, Bilateral B929
  Thyroid BG24
Hand
  Left BP2P
  Right BP2N
Hands and Wrists, Bilateral BP2Q
Head BW28
Head and Neck BW29
Heart
  Right and Left B226
  Intravascular Optical Coherence B226Z2Z
Hepatobiliary System, All BF2C
Hip
  Left BQ21
  Right BQ20
Humerus
  Left BP2B
  Right BP2A
Intracranial Sinus B522
  Intravascular Optical Coherence B522Z2Z
Joint
  Acromioclavicular, Bilateral BP23

Computerized Tomography (*Continued*)
Joint (*Continued*)
  Finger
    Left BP2DZZZ
    Right BP2CZZZ
  Foot
    Left BQ2Y
    Right BQ2X
  Hand
    Left BP2DZZZ
    Right BP2CZZZ
  Sacroiliac BR2D
  Sternoclavicular
    Bilateral BP22
    Left BP21
    Right BP20
  Temporomandibular, Bilateral BN29
  Toe
    Left BQ2Y
    Right BQ2X
Kidney
  Bilateral BT23
  Left BT22
  Right BT21
  Transplant BT29
Knee
  Left BQ28
  Right BQ27
Larynx B92J
Leg
  Left BQ2F
  Right BQ2D
Liver BF25
Liver and Spleen BF26
Lung, Bilateral BB24
Mandible BN26
Nasopharynx B92F
Neck BW2F
Neck and Head BW29
Orbit, Bilateral BN23
Oropharynx B92F
Pancreas BF27
Patella
  Left BQ2W
  Right BQ2V
Pelvic Region BW2G
Pelvis BR2C
  Chest and Abdomen BW25
Pelvis and Abdomen BW21
Pituitary Gland B029
Prostate BV23
Ribs
  Left BP2Y
  Right BP2X
Sacrum BR2F
Scapula
  Left BP27
  Right BP26
Sella Turcica B029
Shoulder
  Left BP29
  Right BP28
Sinus
  Intracranial B522
    Intravascular Optical Coherence B522Z2Z
  Paranasal B922
Skull BN20
Spinal Cord B02B
Spine
  Cervical BR20
  Lumbar BR29
  Thoracic BR27
Spleen and Liver BF26
Thorax BP2W
Tibia
  Left BQ2C
  Right BQ2B
Toe
  Left BQ2Q
  Right BQ2P
Trachea BB2F

Computerized Tomography (*Continued*)
Tracheobronchial Tree
  Bilateral BB29
  Left BB28
  Right BB27
Vein
  Pelvic (Iliac)
    Left B52G
      Intravascular Optical Coherence
        B52GZ2Z
    Right B52F
      Intravascular Optical Coherence
        B52FZ2Z
  Pelvic (Iliac) Bilateral B52H
    Intravascular Optical Coherence
      B52HZ2Z
  Portal B52T
    Intravascular Optical Coherence
      B52TZ2Z
  Pulmonary
    Bilateral B52S
      Intravascular Optical Coherence
        B52SZ2Z
    Left B52R
      Intravascular Optical Coherence
        B52RZ2Z
    Right B52Q
      Intravascular Optical Coherence
        B52QZ2Z
  Renal
    Bilateral B52L
      Intravascular Optical Coherence
        B52LZ2Z
    Left B52K
      Intravascular Optical Coherence
        B52KZ2Z
    Right B52J
      Intravascular Optical Coherence
        B52JZ2Z
  Spanchnic B52T
    Intravascular Optical Coherence
      B52TZ2Z
  Vena Cava
    Inferior B529
      Intravascular Optical Coherence
        B529Z2Z
    Superior B528
      Intravascular Optical Coherence
        B528Z2Z
Ventricle, Cerebral B028
Wrist
  Left BP2M
  Right BP2L
Concerto II CRT-D *use* Cardiac
  Resynchronization Defibrillator Pulse
  Generator in 0JH
Condylectomy
  see Excision, Head and Facial Bones 0NB
  see Excision, Upper Bones 0PB
  see Excision, Lower Bones 0QB
Condyloid process
  use Mandible, Left
  use Mandible, Right
Condylotomy
  see Division, Head and Facial Bones 0N8
  see Drainage, Head and Facial Bones 0N9
  see Division, Upper Bones 0P8
  see Drainage, Upper Bones 0P9
  see Division, Lower Bones 0Q8
  see Drainage, Lower Bones 0Q9
Condylysis
  see Release, Head and Facial Bones 0NN
  see Release, Upper Bones 0PN
  see Release, Lower Bones 0QN
Conization, cervix *see* Excision, Uterus 0UB9
Conjunctivoplasty
  see Repair, Eye 08Q
  see Replacement, Eye 08R
**CONSERVE® PLUS Total Resurfacing Hip
  System** *use* Resurfacing Device in Lower
  Joints

Construction
　Auricle, ear *see* Replacement, Ear, Nose, Sinus
　　09R
　Ileal conduit *see* Bypass, Urinary System 0T1
Consulta CRT-D *use* Cardiac Resynchronization
　Defibrillator Pulse Generator in 0JH
Consulta CRT-P *use* Cardiac Resynchronization
　Pacemaker Pulse Generator in 0JH
Contact Radiation
　Abdomen DWY37ZZ
　Adrenal Gland DGY27ZZ
　Bile Ducts DFY27ZZ
　Bladder DTY27ZZ
　Bone, Other DPYC7ZZ
　Brain D0Y07ZZ
　Brain Stem D0Y17ZZ
　Breast
　　Left DMY07ZZ
　　Right DMY17ZZ
　Bronchus DBY17ZZ
　Cervix DUY17ZZ
　Chest DWY27ZZ
　Chest Wall DBY77ZZ
　Colon DDY57ZZ
　Diaphragm DBY87ZZ
　Duodenum DDY27ZZ
　Ear D9Y07ZZ
　Esophagus DDY07ZZ
　Eye D8Y07ZZ
　Femur DPY97ZZ
　Fibula DPYB7ZZ
　Gallbladder DFY17ZZ
　Gland
　　Adrenal DGY27ZZ
　　Parathyroid DGY47ZZ
　　Pituitary DGY07ZZ
　　Thyroid DGY57ZZ
　Glands, Salivary D9Y67ZZ
　Head and Neck DWY17ZZ
　Hemibody DWY47ZZ
　Humerus DPY67ZZ
　Hypopharynx D9Y37ZZ
　Ileum DDY47ZZ
　Jejunum DDY37ZZ
　Kidney DTY07ZZ
　Larynx D9YB7ZZ
　Liver DFY07ZZ
　Lung DBY27ZZ
　Mandible DPY37ZZ
　Maxilla DPY27ZZ
　Mediastinum DBY67ZZ
　Mouth D9Y47ZZ
　Nasopharynx D9YD7ZZ
　Neck and Head DWY17ZZ
　Nerve, Peripheral D0Y77ZZ
　Nose D9Y17ZZ
　Oropharynx D9YF7ZZ
　Ovary DUY07ZZ
　Palate
　　Hard D9Y87ZZ
　　Soft D9Y97ZZ
　Pancreas DFY37ZZ
　Parathyroid Gland DGY47ZZ
　Pelvic Bones DPY87ZZ
　Pelvic Region DWY67ZZ
　Pineal Body DGY17ZZ
　Pituitary Gland DGY07ZZ
　Pleura DBY57ZZ
　Prostate DVY07ZZ
　Radius DPY77ZZ
　Rectum DDY77ZZ
　Rib DPY57ZZ
　Sinuses D9Y77ZZ
　Skin
　　Abdomen DHY87ZZ
　　Arm DHY47ZZ
　　Back DHY77ZZ
　　Buttock DHY97ZZ
　　Chest DHY67ZZ
　　Face DHY27ZZ
　　Leg DHYB7ZZ
　　Neck DHY37ZZ

Contact Radiation *(Continued)*
　Skull DPY07ZZ
　Spinal Cord D0Y67ZZ
　Sternum DPY47ZZ
　Stomach DDY17ZZ
　Testis DVY17ZZ
　Thyroid Gland DGY57ZZ
　Tibia DPYB7ZZ
　Tongue D9Y57ZZ
　Trachea DBY07ZZ
　Ulna DPY77ZZ
　Ureter DTY17ZZ
　Urethra DTY37ZZ
　Uterus DUY27ZZ
　Whole Body DWY57ZZ
CONTAK RENEWAL® 3 RF (HE) CRT-D *use*
　Cardiac Resynchronization Defibrillator
　Pulse Generator in
　0JH
Contegra Pulmonary Valved Conduit *use*
　Zooplastic Tissue in Heart and Great
　Vessels
Continuous Glucose Monitoring (CGM)
　device *use* Monitoring Device
Continuous Negative Airway Pressure
　24-96 Consecutive Hours, Ventilation
　　5A09459
　Greater than 96 Consecutive Hours,
　　Ventilation 5A09559
　Less than 24 Consecutive Hours, Ventilation
　　5A09359
Continuous Positive Airway Pressure
　24-96 Consecutive Hours, Ventilation 5A09457
　Greater than 96 Consecutive Hours,
　　Ventilation 5A09557
　Less than 24 Consecutive Hours, Ventilation
　　5A09357
Contraceptive Device
　Change device in, Uterus and Cervix
　　0U2DXHZ
　Insertion of device in
　　Cervix 0UHC
　　Subcutaneous Tissue and Fascia
　　　Abdomen 0JH8
　　　Chest 0JH6
　　　Lower Arm
　　　　Left 0JHH
　　　　Right 0JHG
　　　Lower Leg
　　　　Left 0JHP
　　　　Right 0JHN
　　　Upper Arm
　　　　Left 0JHF
　　　　Right 0JHD
　　　Upper Leg
　　　　Left 0JHM
　　　　Right 0JHL
　　Uterus 0UH9
　Removal of device from
　　Subcutaneous Tissue and Fascia
　　　Lower Extremity 0JPW
　　　Trunk 0JPT
　　　Upper Extremity 0JPV
　　Uterus and Cervix 0UPD
　Revision of device in
　　Subcutaneous Tissue and Fascia
　　　Lower Extremity 0JWW
　　　Trunk 0JWT
　　　Upper Extremity 0JWV
　　Uterus and Cervix 0UWD
Contractility Modulation Device
　Abdomen 0JH8
　Chest 0JH6
Control postprocedural bleeding in
　Abdominal Wall 0W3F
　Ankle Region
　　Left 0Y3L
　　Right 0Y3K
　Arm
　　Lower
　　　Left 0X3F
　　　Right 0X3D

Control postprocedural bleeding in *(Continued)*
　Arm *(Continued)*
　　Upper
　　　Left 0X39
　　　Right 0X38
　Axilla
　　Left 0X35
　　Right 0X34
　Back
　　Lower 0W3L
　　Upper 0W3K
　Buttock
　　Left 0Y31
　　Right 0Y30
　Cavity, Cranial 0W31
　Chest Wall 0W38
　Elbow Region
　　Left 0X3C
　　Right 0X3B
　Extremity
　　Lower
　　　Left 0Y3B
　　　Right 0Y39
　　Upper
　　　Left 0X37
　　　Right 0X36
　Face 0W32
　Femoral Region
　　Left 0Y38
　　Right 0Y37
　Foot
　　Left 0Y3N
　　Right 0Y3M
　Gastrointestinal Tract 0W3P
　Genitourinary Tract 0W3R
　Hand
　　Left 0X3K
　　Right 0X3J
　Head 0W30
　Inguinal Region
　　Left 0Y36
　　Right 0Y35
　Jaw
　　Lower 0W35
　　Upper 0W34
　Knee Region
　　Left 0Y3G
　　Right 0Y3F
　Leg
　　Lower
　　　Left 0Y3J
　　　Right 0Y3H
　　Upper
　　　Left 0Y3D
　　　Right 0Y3C
　Mediastinum 0W3C
　Neck 0W36
　Oral Cavity and Throat 0W33
　Pelvic Cavity 0W3J
　Pericardial Cavity 0W3D
　Perineum
　　Female 0W3N
　　Male 0W3M
　Peritoneal Cavity 0W3G
　Pleural Cavity
　　Left 0W3B
　　Right 0W39
　Respiratory Tract 0W3Q
　Retroperitoneum 0W3H
　Shoulder Region
　　Left 0X33
　　Right 0X32
　Wrist Region
　　Left 0X3H
　　Right 0X3G
Conus arteriosus *use* Ventricle, Right
Conus medullaris *use* Spinal Cord, Lumbar
Conversion
　Cardiac rhythm 5A2204Z
　Gastrostomy to jejunostomy feeding device
　　see Insertion of device in, Jejunum 0DHA

◀ New　◀▥ Revised　~~deleted~~ Deleted

Coracoacromial ligament
  use Bursa and Ligament, Shoulder, Right
  use Bursa and Ligament, Shoulder, Left
Coracobrachialis muscle
  use Muscle, Upper Arm, Left
  use Muscle, Upper Arm, Right
Coracoclavicular ligament
  use Bursa and Ligament, Shoulder, Left
  use Bursa and Ligament, Shoulder, Right
Coracohumeral ligament
  use Bursa and Ligament, Shoulder, Left
  use Bursa and Ligament, Shoulder, Right
Coracoid process
  use Scapula, Right
  use Scapula, Left
Cordotomy *see* Division, Central Nervous
  System 008
Core needle biopsy *see* Excision with qualifier
  Diagnostic
CoreValve transcatheter aortic valve *use*
  Zooplastic Tissue in Heart and Great Vessels
Cormet Hip Resurfacing System *use*
  Resurfacing Device in Lower Joints
Corniculate cartilage *use* Larynx
CoRoent® XL *use* Interbody Fusion Device in
  Lower Joints
Coronary arteriography
  see Plain Radiography, Heart B20
  see Fluoroscopy, Heart B21
Corox (OTW) Bipolar Lead
  use Cardiac Lead, Pacemaker in 02H
  use Cardiac Lead, Defibrillator in 02H
Corpus callosum *use* Brain
Corpus cavernosum *use* Penis
Corpus spongiosum *use* Penis
Corpus striatum *use* Basal Ganglia
Corrugator supercilii muscle *use* Muscle, Facial
Cortical strip neurostimulator lead *use*
  Neurostimulator Lead in Central Nervous
  System
Costatectomy
  see Excision, Upper Bones 0PB
  see Resection, Upper Bones 0PT
Costectomy
  see Excision, Upper Bones 0PB
  see Resection, Upper Bones 0PT
Costocervical trunk
  use Artery, Subclavian, Left
  use Artery, Subclavian, Right
Costochondrectomy
  see Excision, Upper Bones 0PB
  see Resection, Upper Bones 0PT
Costoclavicular ligament
  use Bursa and Ligament, Shoulder, Left
  use Bursa and Ligament, Shoulder, Right
Costosternoplasty
  see Repair, Upper Bones 0PQ
  see Replacement, Upper Bones 0PR
  see Supplement, Upper Bones 0PU
Costotomy
  see Division, Upper Bones 0P8
  see Drainage, Upper Bones 0P9
Costotransverse joint *use* Joint, Thoracic
  Vertebral ◀▥
  ~~use Joint, Thoracic Vertebral~~
  ~~use Joint, Thoracic Vertebral, 2 to 7~~
  ~~use Joint, Thoracic Vertebral, 8 or more~~
Costotransverse ligament
  use Bursa and Ligament, Thorax, Right
  use Bursa and Ligament, Thorax, Left
Costovertebral joint *use* Joint, Thoracic
  Vertebral ◀▥
  ~~use Joint, Thoracic Vertebral, 8 or more~~
  ~~use Joint, Thoracic Vertebral, 2 to 7~~
  ~~use Joint, Thoracic Vertebral~~
Costoxiphoid ligament
  use Bursa and Ligament, Thorax, Right
  use Bursa and Ligament, Thorax, Left
Counseling
  Family, for substance abuse, Other Family
    Counseling HZ63ZZZ

Counseling *(Continued)*
  Group
    12-Step HZ43ZZZ
    Behavioral HZ41ZZZ
    Cognitive HZ40ZZZ
    Cognitive-Behavioral HZ42ZZZ
    Confrontational HZ48ZZZ
    Continuing Care HZ49ZZZ
    Infectious Disease
      Post-Test HZ4CZZZ
      Pre-Test HZ4CZZZ
    Interpersonal HZ44ZZZ
    Motivational Enhancement HZ47ZZZ
    Psychoeducation HZ46ZZZ
    Spiritual HZ4BZZZ
    Vocational HZ45ZZZ
  Individual
    12-Step HZ33ZZZ
    Behavioral HZ31ZZZ
    Cognitive HZ30ZZZ
    Cognitive-Behavioral HZ32ZZZ
    Confrontational HZ38ZZZ
    Continuing Care HZ39ZZZ
    Infectious Disease
      Post-Test HZ3CZZZ
      Pre-Test HZ3CZZZ
    Interpersonal HZ34ZZZ
    Motivational Enhancement HZ37ZZZ
    Psychoeducation HZ36ZZZ
    Spiritual HZ3BZZZ
    Vocational HZ35ZZZ
  Mental Health Services
    Educational GZ60ZZZ
    Other Counseling GZ63ZZZ
    Vocational GZ61ZZZ
Countershock, cardiac 5A2204Z
Cowper's (bulbourethral) gland *use* Urethra
CPAP (continuous positive airway pressure)
  see Assistance, Respiratory 5A09
Cranial dura mater *use* Dura Mater
Cranial epidural space *use* Epidural Space
Cranial subarachnoid space *use* Subarachnoid
  Space
Cranial subdural space *use* Subdural Space
Craniectomy
  see Excision, Head and Facial Bones 0NB
  see Resection, Head and Facial Bones 0NT
Cranioplasty
  see Repair, Head and Facial Bones 0NQ
  see Replacement, Head and Facial Bones 0NR
  see Supplement, Head and Facial Bones 0NU
Craniotomy
  see Drainage, Central Nervous System 009
  see Division, Head and Facial Bones 0N8
  see Drainage, Head and Facial Bones 0N9
Creation
  Female 0W4N0
  Male 0W4M0
Cremaster muscle *use* Muscle, Perineum
Cribriform plate
  use Bone, Ethmoid, Left
  use Bone, Ethmoid, Right
Cricoid cartilage *use* Larynx
Cricoidectomy *see* Excision, Larynx 0CBS
Cricothyroid artery
  use Artery, Thyroid, Left
  use Artery, Thyroid, Right
Cricothyroid muscle
  use Muscle, Neck, Right
  use Muscle, Neck, Left
Crisis Intervention GZ2ZZZZ
Crural fascia
  use Subcutaneous Tissue and Fascia, Upper
    Leg, Right
  use Subcutaneous Tissue and Fascia, Upper
    Leg, Left
Crushing, nerve
  Cranial *see* Destruction, Central Nervous
    System 005
  Peripheral *see* Destruction, Peripheral
    Nervous System 015

Cryoablation *see* Destruction
Cryotherapy *see* Destruction
Cryptorchidectomy
  see Excision, Male Reproductive System 0VB
  see Resection, Male Reproductive System 0VT
Cryptorchiectomy
  see Excision, Male Reproductive System 0VB
  see Resection, Male Reproductive System 0VT
Cryptotomy
  see Division, Gastrointestinal System 0D8
  see Drainage, Gastrointestinal System 0D9
CT scan *see* Computerized Tomography (CT
  Scan)
CT sialogram *see* Computerized Tomography
  (CT Scan), Ear, Nose, Mouth and Throat
  B92
Cubital lymph node
  use Lymphatic, Upper Extremity, Left
  use Lymphatic, Upper Extremity, Right
Cubital nerve *use* Nerve, Ulnar
Cuboid bone
  use Tarsal, Left
  use Tarsal, Right
Cuboideonavicular joint
  use Joint, Tarsal, Right
  use Joint, Tarsal, Left
Culdocentesis *see* Drainage, Cul-de-sac 0U9F
Culdoplasty
  see Repair, Cul-de-sac 0UQF
  see Supplement, Cul-de-sac 0UUF
Culdoscopy 0UJH8ZZ
Culdotomy *see* Drainage, Cul-de-sac 0U9F
Culmen *use* Cerebellum
Cultured epidermal cell autograft *use*
  Autologous Tissue Substitute
Cuneiform cartilage *use* Larynx
Cuneonavicular joint
  use Joint, Tarsal, Left
  use Joint, Tarsal, Right
Cuneonavicular ligament
  use Bursa and Ligament, Foot, Left
  use Bursa and Ligament, Foot, Right
Curettage
  see Excision
  see Extraction
Cutaneous (transverse) cervical nerve *use*
  Nerve, Cervical Plexus
CVP (central venous pressure) *see*
  Measurement, Venous 4A04
Cyclodiathermy *see* Destruction, Eye 085
Cyclophotocoagulation *see* Destruction, Eye 085
CYPHER® Stent *use* Intraluminal Device, Drug-
  eluting in Heart and Great Vessels
Cystectomy
  see Excision, Bladder 0TBB
  see Resection, Bladder 0TTB
Cystocele repair *see* Repair, Subcutaneous
  Tissue and Fascia, Pelvic Region 0JQC
Cystography
  see Plain Radiography, Urinary System BT0
  see Fluoroscopy, Urinary System BT1
Cystolithotomy *see* Extirpation, Bladder 0TCB
Cystopexy
  see Repair, Bladder 0TQB
  see Reposition, Bladder 0TSB
Cystoplasty
  see Repair, Bladder 0TQB
  see Replacement, Bladder 0TRB
  see Supplement, Bladder 0TUB
Cystorrhaphy *see* Repair, Bladder 0TQB
Cystoscopy 0TJB8ZZ
Cystostomy *see* Bypass, Bladder 0T1B
Cystostomy tube *use* Drainage Device
Cystotomy *see* Drainage, Bladder 0T9B
Cystourethrography
  see Plain Radiography, Urinary System BT0
  see Fluoroscopy, Urinary System BT1
Cystourethroplasty
  see Repair, Urinary System 0TQ
  see Replacement, Urinary System 0TR
  see Supplement, Urinary System 0TU

D

DBS lead *use* Neurostimulator Lead in Central Nervous System
DeBakey Left Ventricular Assist Device *use* Implantable Heart Assist System in Heart and Great Vessels
Debridement
  Excisional *see* Excision
  Non-excisional *see* Extraction
Decompression, Circulatory 6A15
Decortication, lung *see* Excision, Respiratory System 0BD
Deep brain neurostimulator lead *use* Neurostimulator Lead in Central Nervous System
Deep cervical fascia *see* Subcutaneous Tissue and Fascia, Neck, Anterior
Deep cervical vein
  use Vein, Vertebral, Left
  use Vein, Vertebral, Right
Deep circumflex iliac artery
  use Artery, External Iliac, Left
  use Artery, External Iliac, Right
Deep facial vein
  use Vein, Face, Left
  use Vein, Face, Right
Deep femoral (profunda femoris) vein
  use Vein, Femoral, Left
  use Vein, Femoral, Right
Deep femoral artery
  use Artery, Femoral, Right
  use Artery, Femoral, Left
Deep Inferior Epigastric Artery Perforator Flap
  Bilateral 0HRV077
  Left 0HRU077
  Right 0HRT077
Deep palmar arch
  use Artery, Hand, Left
  use Artery, Hand, Right
Deep transverse perineal muscle *use* Muscle, Perineum
Deferential artery
  use Artery, Internal Iliac, Right
  use Artery, Internal Iliac, Left
Defibrillator Generator
  Abdomen 0JH8
  Chest 0JH6
Delivery
  Cesarean *see* Extraction, Products of Conception 10D0
  Forceps *see* Extraction, Products of Conception 10D0
  Manually assisted 10E0XZZ
  Products of Conception 10E0XZZ
  Vacuum assisted *see* Extraction, Products of Conception 10D0
Delta frame external fixator
  use External Fixation Device, Hybrid in 0PH
  use External Fixation Device, Hybrid in 0PS
  use External Fixation Device, Hybrid in 0QH
  use External Fixation Device, Hybrid in 0QS
Delta III Reverse shoulder prosthesis *use* Synthetic Substitute, Reverse Ball and Socket in 0RR
Deltoid fascia
  use Subcutaneous Tissue and Fascia, Upper Arm, Right
  use Subcutaneous Tissue and Fascia, Upper Arm, Left
Deltoid ligament
  use Bursa and Ligament, Ankle, Left
  use Bursa and Ligament, Ankle, Right
Deltoid muscle
  use Muscle, Shoulder, Left
  use Muscle, Shoulder, Right
Deltopectoral (infraclavicular) lymph node
  use Lymphatic, Upper Extremity, Right
  use Lymphatic, Upper Extremity, Left

Denervation
  Cranial nerve *see* Destruction, Central Nervous System 005
  Peripheral nerve *see* Destruction, Peripheral Nervous System 015
Densitometry
  Plain Radiography
    Femur
      Left BQ04ZZ1
      Right BQ03ZZ1
    Hip
      Left BQ01ZZ1
      Right BQ00ZZ1
    Spine
      Cervical BR00ZZ1
      Lumbar BR09ZZ1
      Thoracic BR07ZZ1
      Whole BR0GZZ1
  Ultrasonography
    Elbow
      Left BP4HZZ1
      Right BP4GZZ1
    Hand
      Left BP4PZZ1
      Right BP4NZZ1
    Shoulder
      Left BP49ZZ1
      Right BP48ZZ1
    Wrist
      Left BP4MZZ1
      Right BP4LZZ1
Dentate ligament *use* Dura Mater
Denticulate ligament *use* Spinal Meninges
Depressor anguli oris muscle *use* Muscle, Facial
Depressor labii inferioris muscle *use* Muscle, Facial
Depressor septi nasi muscle *use* Muscle, Facial
Depressor supercilii muscle *use* Muscle, Facial
Dermabrasion *see* Extraction, Skin and Breast 0HD
Dermis *see* Skin
Descending genicular artery
  use Artery, Femoral, Right
  use Artery, Femoral, Left
Destruction
  Acetabulum
    Left 0Q55
    Right 0Q54
  Adenoids 0C5Q
  Ampulla of Vater 0F5C
  Anal Sphincter 0D5R
  Anterior Chamber
    Left 08533ZZ
    Right 08523ZZ
  Anus 0D5Q
  Aorta
    Abdominal 0450
    Thoracic 025W
  Aortic Body 0G5D
  Appendix 0D5J
  Artery
    Anterior Tibial
      Left 045Q
      Right 045P
    Axillary
      Left 0356
      Right 0355
    Brachial
      Left 0358
      Right 0357
    Celiac 0451
    Colic
      Left 0457
      Middle 0458
      Right 0456
    Common Carotid
      Left 035J
      Right 035H

Destruction *(Continued)*
  Artery *(Continued)*
    Common Iliac
      Left 045D
      Right 045C
    External Carotid
      Left 035N
      Right 035M
    External Iliac
      Left 045J
      Right 045H
    Face 035R
    Femoral
      Left 045L
      Right 045K
    Foot
      Left 045W
      Right 045V
    Gastric 0452
    Hand
      Left 035F
      Right 035D
    Hepatic 0453
    Inferior Mesenteric 045B
    Innominate 0352
    Internal Carotid
      Left 035L
      Right 035K
    Internal Iliac
      Left 045F
      Right 045E
    Internal Mammary
      Left 0351
      Right 0350
    Intracranial 035G
    Lower 045Y
    Peroneal
      Left 045U
      Right 045T
    Popliteal
      Left 045N
      Right 045M
    Posterior Tibial
      Left 045S
      Right 045R
    Pulmonary
      Left 025R
      Right 025Q
    Pulmonary Trunk 025P
    Radial
      Left 035C
      Right 035B
    Renal
      Left 045A
      Right 0459
    Splenic 0454
    Subclavian
      Left 0354
      Right 0353
    Superior Mesenteric 0455
    Temporal
      Left 035T
      Right 035S
    Thyroid
      Left 035V
      Right 035U
    Ulnar
      Left 035A
      Right 0359
    Upper 035Y
    Vertebral
      Left 035Q
      Right 035P
  Atrium
    Left 0257
    Right 0256
  Auditory Ossicle
    Left 095A0ZZ
    Right 09590ZZ
  Basal Ganglia 0058
  Bladder 0T5B

◀ New   ◀▥▥ Revised   ~~deleted~~ Deleted

Destruction (*Continued*)
Bladder Neck 0T5C
Bone
  Ethmoid
    Left 0N5G
    Right 0N5F
  Frontal
    Left 0N52
    Right 0N51
  Hyoid 0N5X
  Lacrimal
    Left 0N5J
    Right 0N5H
  Nasal 0N5B
  Occipital
    Left 0N58
    Right 0N57
  Palatine
    Left 0N5L
    Right 0N5K
  Parietal
    Left 0N54
    Right 0N53
  Pelvic
    Left 0Q53
    Right 0Q52
  Sphenoid
    Left 0N5D
    Right 0N5C
  Temporal
    Left 0N56
    Right 0N55
  Zygomatic
    Left 0N5N
    Right 0N5M
Brain 0050
Breast
  Bilateral 0H5V
  Left 0H5U
  Right 0H5T
Bronchus
  Lingula 0B59
  Lower Lobe
    Left 0B5B
    Right 0B56
  Main
    Left 0B57
    Right 0B53
  Middle Lobe, Right 0B55
  Upper Lobe
    Left 0B58
    Right 0B54
Buccal Mucosa 0C54
Bursa and Ligament
  Abdomen
    Left 0M5J
    Right 0M5H
  Ankle
    Left 0M5R
    Right 0M5Q
  Elbow
    Left 0M54
    Right 0M53
  Foot
    Left 0M5T
    Right 0M5S
  Hand
    Left 0M58
    Right 0M57
  Head and Neck 0M50
  Hip
    Left 0M5M
    Right 0M5L
  Knee
    Left 0M5P
    Right 0M5N
  Lower Extremity
    Left 0M5W
    Right 0M5V
  Perineum 0M5K

Destruction (*Continued*)
Bursa and Ligament (*Continued*)
  Shoulder
    Left 0M52
    Right 0M51
  Thorax
    Left 0M5G
    Right 0M5F
  Trunk
    Left 0M5D
    Right 0M5C
  Upper Extremity
    Left 0M5B
    Right 0M59
  Wrist
    Left 0M56
    Right 0M55
Carina 0B52
Carotid Bodies, Bilateral 0G58
Carotid Body
  Left 0G56
  Right 0G57
Carpal
  Left 0P5N
  Right 0P5M
Cecum 0D5H
Cerebellum 005C
Cerebral Hemisphere 0057
Cerebral Meninges 0051
Cerebral Ventricle 0056
Cervix 0U5C
Chordae Tendineae 0259
Choroid
  Left 085B
  Right 085A
Cisterna Chyli 075L
Clavicle
  Left 0P5B
  Right 0P59
Clitoris 0U5J
Coccygeal Glomus 0G5B
Coccyx 0Q5S
Colon
  Ascending 0D5K
  Descending 0D5M
  Sigmoid 0D5N
  Transverse 0D5L
Conduction Mechanism 0258
Conjunctiva
  Left 085TXZZ
  Right 085SXZZ
Cord
  Bilateral 0V5H
  Left 0V5G
  Right 0V5F
Cornea
  Left 0859XZZ
  Right 0858XZZ
Cul-de-sac 0U5F
Diaphragm
  Left 0B5S
  Right 0B5R
Disc
  Cervical Vertebral 0R53
  Cervicothoracic Vertebral 0R55
  Lumbar Vertebral 0S52
  Lumbosacral 0S54
  Thoracic Vertebral 0R59
  Thoracolumbar Vertebral 0R5B
Duct
  Common Bile 0F59
  Cystic 0F58
  Hepatic
    Left 0F56
    Right 0F55
  Lacrimal
    Left 085Y
    Right 085X
  Pancreatic 0F5D
    Accessory 0F5F

Destruction (*Continued*)
Duct (*Continued*)
  Parotid
    Left 0C5C
    Right 0C5B
  Thoracic 075K
Duodenum 0D59
Dura Mater 0052
Ear
  External
    Left 0951
    Right 0950
  External Auditory Canal
    Left 0954
    Right 0953
  Inner
    Left 095E0ZZ
    Right 095D0ZZ
  Middle
    Left 09560ZZ
    Right 09550ZZ
Endometrium 0U5B
Epididymis
  Bilateral 0V5L
  Left 0V5K
  Right 0V5J
Epiglottis 0C5R
Esophagogastric Junction 0D54
Esophagus 0D55
  Lower 0D53
  Middle 0D52
  Upper 0D51
Eustachian Tube
  Left 095G
  Right 095F
Eye
  Left 0851XZZ
  Right 0850XZZ
Eyelid
  Lower
    Left 085R
    Right 085Q
  Upper
    Left 085P
    Right 085N
Fallopian Tube
  Left 0U56
  Right 0U55
Fallopian Tubes, Bilateral 0U57
Femoral Shaft
  Left 0Q59
  Right 0Q58
Femur
  Lower
    Left 0Q5C
    Right 0Q5B
  Upper
    Left 0Q57
    Right 0Q56
Fibula
  Left 0Q5K
  Right 0Q5J
Finger Nail 0H5QXZZ
Gallbladder 0F54
Gingiva
  Lower 0C56
  Upper 0C55
Gland
  Adrenal
    Bilateral 0G54
    Left 0G52
    Right 0G53
  Lacrimal
    Left 085W
    Right 085V
  Minor Salivary 0C5J
  Parotid
    Left 0C59
    Right 0C58
  Pituitary 0G50

Destruction (*Continued*)
Gland (*Continued*)
Sublingual
Left 0C5F
Right 0C5D
Submaxillary
Left 0C5H
Right 0C5G
Vestibular 0U5L
Glenoid Cavity
Left 0P58
Right 0P57
Glomus Jugulare 0G5C
Humeral Head
Left 0P5D
Right 0P5C
Humeral Shaft
Left 0P5G
Right 0P5F
Hymen 0U5K
Hypothalamus 005A
Ileocecal Valve 0D5C
Ileum 0D5B
Intestine
Large 0D5E
Left 0D5G
Right 0D5F
Small 0D58
Iris
Left 085D3ZZ
Right 085C3ZZ
Jejunum 0D5A
Joint
Acromioclavicular
Left 0R5H
Right 0R5G
Ankle
Left 0S5G
Right 0S5F
Carpal
Left 0R5R
Right 0R5Q
Cervical Vertebral 0R51
Cervicothoracic Vertebral 0R54
Coccygeal 0S56
Elbow
Left 0R5M
Right 0R5L
Finger Phalangeal
Left 0R5X
Right 0R5W
Hip
Left 0S5B
Right 0S59
Knee
Left 0S5D
Right 0S5C
Lumbar Vertebral 0S50
Lumbosacral 0S53
Metacarpocarpal
Left 0R5T
Right 0R5S
Metacarpophalangeal
Left 0R5V
Right 0R5U
Metatarsal-Phalangeal
Left 0S5N
Right 0S5M
Metatarsal-Tarsal
Left 0S5L
Right 0S5K
Occipital-cervical 0R50
Sacrococcygeal 0S55
Sacroiliac
Left 0S58
Right 0S57
Shoulder
Left 0R5K
Right 0R5J
Sternoclavicular
Left 0R5F
Right 0R5E

Destruction (*Continued*)
Joint (*Continued*)
Tarsal
Left 0S5J
Right 0S5H
Temporomandibular
Left 0R5D
Right 0R5C
Thoracic Vertebral 0R56
Thoracolumbar Vertebral 0R5A
Toe Phalangeal
Left 0S5Q
Right 0S5P
Wrist
Left 0R5P
Right 0R5N
Kidney
Left 0T51
Right 0T50
Kidney Pelvis
Left 0T54
Right 0T53
Larynx 0C5S
Lens
Left 085K3ZZ
Right 085J3ZZ
Lip
Lower 0C51
Upper 0C50
Liver 0F50
Left Lobe 0F52
Right Lobe 0F51
Lung
Bilateral 0B5M
Left 0B5L
Lower Lobe
Left 0B5J
Right 0B5F
Middle Lobe, Right 0B5D
Right 0B5K
Upper Lobe
Left 0B5G
Right 0B5C
Lung Lingula 0B5H
Lymphatic
Aortic 075D
Axillary
Left 0756
Right 0755
Head 0750
Inguinal
Left 075J
Right 075H
Internal Mammary
Left 0759
Right 0758
Lower Extremity
Left 075G
Right 075F
Mesenteric 075B
Neck
Left 0752
Right 0751
Pelvis 075C
Thorax 0757
Upper Extremity
Left 0754
Right 0753
Mandible
Left 0N5V
Right 0N5T
Maxilla
Left 0N5S
Right 0N5R
Medulla Oblongata 005D
Mesentery 0D5V
Metacarpal
Left 0P5Q
Right 0P5P
Metatarsal
Left 0Q5P
Right 0Q5N

Destruction (*Continued*)
Muscle
Abdomen
Left 0K5L
Right 0K5K
Extraocular
Left 085M
Right 085L
Facial 0K51
Foot
Left 0K5W
Right 0K5V
Hand
Left 0K5D
Right 0K5C
Head 0K50
Hip
Left 0K5P
Right 0K5N
Lower Arm and Wrist
Left 0K5B
Right 0K59
Lower Leg
Left 0K5T
Right 0K5S
Neck
Left 0K53
Right 0K52
Papillary 025D
Perineum 0K5M
Shoulder
Left 0K56
Right 0K55
Thorax
Left 0K5J
Right 0K5H
Tongue, Palate, Pharynx 0K54
Trunk
Left 0K5G
Right 0K5F
Upper Arm
Left 0K58
Right 0K57
Upper Leg
Left 0K5R
Right 0K5Q
Nasopharynx 095N
Nerve
Abdominal Sympathetic 015M
Abducens 005L
Accessory 005R
Acoustic 005N
Brachial Plexus 0153
Cervical 0151
Cervical Plexus 0153
Facial 005M
Femoral 015D
Glossopharyngeal 005P
Head and Neck Sympathetic 015K
Hypoglossal 005S
Lumbar 015B
Lumbar Plexus 0159
Lumbar Sympathetic 015N
Lumbosacral Plexus 015A
Median 0155
Oculomotor 005H
Olfactory 005F
Optic 005G
Peroneal 015H
Phrenic 0152
Pudendal 015C
Radial 0156
Sacral 015R
Sacral Plexus 015Q
Sacral Sympathetic 015P
Sciatic 015F
Thoracic 0158
Thoracic Sympathetic 015L
Tibial 015G
Trigeminal 005K
Trochlear 005J

◀ New ◀▥ Revised ~~deleted~~ Deleted

Destruction *(Continued)*
  Nerve *(Continued)*
    Ulnar 0154
    Vagus 005Q
  Nipple
    Left 0H5X
    Right 0H5W
  Nose 095K
  Omentum
    Greater 0D5S
    Lesser 0D5T
  Orbit
    Left 0N5Q
    Right 0N5P
  Ovary
    Bilateral 0U52
    Left 0U51
    Right 0U50
  Palate
    Hard 0C52
    Soft 0C53
  Pancreas 0F5G
  Para-aortic Body 0G59
  Paraganglion Extremity 0G5F
  Parathyroid Gland 0G5R
    Inferior
      Left 0G5P
      Right 0G5N
    Multiple 0G5Q
    Superior
      Left 0G5M
      Right 0G5L
  Patella
    Left 0Q5F
    Right 0Q5D
  Penis 0V5S
  Pericardium 025N
  Peritoneum 0D5W
  Phalanx
    Finger
      Left 0P5V
      Right 0P5T
    Thumb
      Left 0P5S
      Right 0P5R
    Toe
      Left 0Q5R
      Right 0Q5Q
  Pharynx 0C5M
  Pineal Body 0G51
  Pleura
    Left 0B5P
    Right 0B5N
  Pons 005B
  Prepuce 0V5T
  Prostate 0V50
  Radius
    Left 0P5J
    Right 0P5H
  Rectum 0D5P
  Retina
    Left 085F3ZZ
    Right 085E3ZZ
  Retinal Vessel
    Left 085H3ZZ
    Right 085G3ZZ
  Rib
    Left 0P52
    Right 0P51
  Sacrum 0Q51
  Scapula
    Left 0P56
    Right 0P55
  Sclera
    Left 0857XZZ
    Right 0856XZZ
  Scrotum 0V55
  Septum
    Atrial 0255
    Nasal 095M
    Ventricular 025M

Destruction *(Continued)*
  Sinus
    Accessory 095P
    Ethmoid
      Left 095V
      Right 095U
    Frontal
      Left 095T
      Right 095S
    Mastoid
      Left 095C
      Right 095B
    Maxillary
      Left 095R
      Right 095Q
    Sphenoid
      Left 095X
      Right 095W
  Skin
    Abdomen 0H57XZ
    Back 0H56XZ
    Buttock 0H58XZ
    Chest 0H55XZ
    Ear
      Left 0H53XZ
      Right 0H52XZ
    Face 0H51XZ
    Foot
      Left 0H5NXZ
      Right 0H5MXZ
    Genitalia 0H5AXZ
    Hand
      Left 0H5GXZ
      Right 0H5FXZ
    Lower Arm
      Left 0H5EXZ
      Right 0H5DXZ
    Lower Leg
      Left 0H5LXZ
      Right 0H5KXZ
    Neck 0H54XZ
    Perineum 0H59XZ
    Scalp 0H50XZ
    Upper Arm
      Left 0H5CXZ
      Right 0H5BXZ
    Upper Leg
      Left 0H5JXZ
      Right 0H5HXZ
  Skull 0N50
  Spinal Cord
    Cervical 005W
    Lumbar 005Y
    Thoracic 005X
  Spinal Meninges 005T
  Spleen 075P
  Sternum 0P50
  Stomach 0D56
    Pylorus 0D57
  Subcutaneous Tissue and Fascia
    Abdomen 0J58
    Back 0J57
    Buttock 0J59
    Chest 0J56
    Face 0J51
    Foot
      Left 0J5R
      Right 0J5Q
    Hand
      Left 0J5K
      Right 0J5J
    Lower Arm
      Left 0J5H
      Right 0J5G
    Lower Leg
      Left 0J5P
      Right 0J5N
    Neck
      Anterior 0J54
      Posterior 0J55
    Pelvic Region 0J5C

Destruction *(Continued)*
  Subcutaneous Tissue and Fascia *(Continued)*
    Perineum 0J5B
    Scalp 0J50
    Upper Arm
      Left 0J5F
      Right 0J5D
    Upper Leg
      Left 0J5M
      Right 0J5L
  Tarsal
    Left 0Q5M
    Right 0Q5L
  Tendon
    Abdomen
      Left 0L5G
      Right 0L5F
    Ankle
      Left 0L5T
      Right 0L5S
    Foot
      Left 0L5W
      Right 0L5V
    Hand
      Left 0L58
      Right 0L57
    Head and Neck 0L50
    Hip
      Left 0L5K
      Right 0L5J
    Knee
      Left 0L5R
      Right 0L5Q
    Lower Arm and Wrist
      Left 0L56
      Right 0L55
    Lower Leg
      Left 0L5P
      Right 0L5N
    Perineum 0L5H
    Shoulder
      Left 0L52
      Right 0L51
    Thorax
      Left 0L5D
      Right 0L5C
    Trunk
      Left 0L5B
      Right 0L59
    Upper Arm
      Left 0L54
      Right 0L53
    Upper Leg
      Left 0L5M
      Right 0L5L
  Testis
    Bilateral 0V5C
    Left 0V5B
    Right 0V59
  Thalamus 0059
  Thymus 075M
  Thyroid Gland
    Left Lobe 0G5G
    Right Lobe 0G5H
  Tibia
    Left 0Q5H
    Right 0Q5G
  Toe Nail 0H5RXZZ
  Tongue 0C57
  Tonsils 0C5P
  Tooth
    Lower 0C5X
    Upper 0C5W
  Trachea 0B51
  Tunica Vaginalis
    Left 0V57
    Right 0V56
  Turbinate, Nasal 095L
  Tympanic Membrane
    Left 0958
    Right 0959

Destruction (*Continued*)
Ulna
  Left 0P5L
  Right 0P5K
Ureter
  Left 0T57
  Right 0T56
Urethra 0T5D
Uterine Supporting Structure 0U54
Uterus 0U59
Uvula 0C5N
Vagina 0U5G
Valve
  Aortic 025F
  Mitral 025G
  Pulmonary 025H
  Tricuspid 025J
Vas Deferens
  Bilateral 0V5Q
  Left 0V5P
  Right 0V5N
Vein
  Axillary
    Left 0558
    Right 0557
  Azygos 0550
  Basilic
    Left 055C
    Right 055B
  Brachial
    Left 055A
    Right 0559
  Cephalic
    Left 055F
    Right 055D
  Colic 0657
  Common Iliac
    Left 065D
    Right 065C
  Coronary 0254
  Esophageal 0653
  External Iliac
    Left 065G
    Right 065F
  External Jugular
    Left 055Q
    Right 055P
  Face
    Left 055V
    Right 055T
  Femoral
    Left 065N
    Right 065M
  Foot
    Left 065V
    Right 065T
  Gastric 0652
  Greater Saphenous
    Left 065Q
    Right 065P
  Hand
    Left 055H
    Right 055G
  Hemiazygos 0551
  Hepatic 0654
  Hypogastric
    Left 065J
    Right 065H
  Inferior Mesenteric 0656
  Innominate
    Left 0554
    Right 0553
  Internal Jugular
    Left 055N
    Right 055M
  Intracranial 055L
  Lesser Saphenous
    Left 065S
    Right 065R
  Lower 065Y
  Portal 0658

Destruction (*Continued*)
Vein (*Continued*)
  Pulmonary
    Left 025T
    Right 025S
  Renal
    Left 065B
    Right 0659
  Splenic 0651
  Subclavian
    Left 0556
    Right 0555
  Superior Mesenteric 0655
  Upper 055Y
  Vertebral
    Left 055S
    Right 055R
Vena Cava
  Inferior 0650
  Superior 025V
Ventricle
  Left 025L
  Right 025K
Vertebra
  Cervical 0P53
  Lumbar 0Q50
  Thoracic 0P54
Vesicle
  Bilateral 0V53
  Left 0V52
  Right 0V51
Vitreous
  Left 08553ZZ
  Right 08543ZZ
Vocal Cord
  Left 0C5V
  Right 0C5T
Vulva 0U5M
Detachment
Arm
  Lower
    Left 0X6F0Z
    Right 0X6D0Z
  Upper
    Left 0X690Z
    Right 0X680Z
Elbow Region
  Left 0X6C0ZZ
  Right 0X6B0ZZ
Femoral Region
  Left 0Y680ZZ
  Right 0Y670ZZ
Finger
  Index
    Left 0X6P0Z
    Right 0X6N0Z
  Little
    Left 0X6W0Z
    Right 0X6V0Z
  Middle
    Left 0X6R0Z
    Right 0X6Q0Z
  Ring
    Left 0X6T0Z
    Right 0X6S0Z
Foot
  Left 0Y6N0Z
  Right 0Y6M0Z
Forequarter
  Left 0X610ZZ
  Right 0X600ZZ
Hand
  Left 0X6K0Z
  Right 0X6J0Z
Hindquarter
  Bilateral 0Y640ZZ
  Left 0Y630ZZ
  Right 0Y620ZZ
Knee Region
  Left 0Y6G0ZZ
  Right 0Y6F0ZZ

Detachment (*Continued*)
Leg
  Lower
    Left 0Y6J0Z
    Right 0Y6H0Z
  Upper
    Left 0Y6D0Z
    Right 0Y6C0Z
Shoulder Region
  Left 0X630ZZ
  Right 0X620ZZ
Thumb
  Left 0X6M0Z
  Right 0X6L0Z
Toe
  1st
    Left 0Y6Q0Z
    Right 0Y6P0Z
  2nd
    Left 0Y6S0Z
    Right 0Y6R0Z
  3rd
    Left 0Y6U0Z
    Right 0Y6T0Z
  4th
    Left 0Y6W0Z
    Right 0Y6V0Z
  5th
    Left 0Y6Y0Z
    Right 0Y6X0Z
Determination, Mental status GZ14ZZZ
Detorsion
  see Release
  see Reposition
Detoxification Services, for substance abuse
  HZ2ZZZZ
Device Fitting F0DZ
Diagnostic Audiology *see* Audiology,
  Diagnostic
Diagnostic imaging *see* Imaging, Diagnostic
Diagnostic radiology *see* Imaging, Diagnostic
Dialysis
  Hemodialysis 5A1D00Z
  Peritoneal 3E1M39Z
Diaphragma sellae *use* Dura Mater
Diaphragmatic pacemaker generator *use*
  Stimulator Generator in Subcutaneous
  Tissue and Fascia
Diaphragmatic Pacemaker Lead
  Insertion of device in
    Left 0BHS
    Right 0BHR
  Removal of device from, Diaphragm
    0BPT
  Revision of device in, Diaphragm 0BWT
Digital radiography, plain *see* Plain
  Radiography
Dilation
  Ampulla of Vater 0F7C
  Anus 0D7Q
  Aorta
    Abdominal 0470
    Thoracic 027W
  Artery
    Anterior Tibial
      Left 047Q
      Right 047P
    Axillary
      Left 0376
      Right 0375
    Brachial
      Left 0378
      Right 0377
    Celiac 0471
    Colic
      Left 0477
      Middle 0478
      Right 0476
    Common Carotid
      Left 037J
      Right 037H

◀ New   ⬅ Revised   ~~deleted~~ Deleted

Dilation *(Continued)*
  Artery *(Continued)*
    Common Iliac
      Left 047D
      Right 047C
    Coronary
      Four or More Sites 0273
      One Site 0270
      Three Sites 0272
      Two Sites 0271
    External Carotid
      Left 037N
      Right 037M
    External Iliac
      Left 047J
      Right 047H
    Face 037R
    Femoral
      Left 047L
      Right 047K
    Foot
      Left 047W
      Right 047V
    Gastric 0472
    Hand
      Left 037F
      Right 037D
    Hepatic 0473
    Inferior Mesenteric 047B
    Innominate 0372
    Internal Carotid
      Left 037L
      Right 037K
    Internal Iliac
      Left 047F
      Right 047E
    Internal Mammary
      Left 0371
      Right 0370
    Intracranial 037G
    Lower 047Y
    Peroneal
      Left 047U
      Right 047T
    Popliteal
      Left 047N
      Right 047M
    Posterior Tibial
      Left 047S
      Right 047R
    Pulmonary
      Left 027R
      Right 027Q
    Pulmonary Trunk 027P
    Radial
      Left 037C
      Right 037B
    Renal
      Left 047A
      Right 0479
    Splenic 0474
    Subclavian
      Left 0374
      Right 0373
    Superior Mesenteric 0475
    Temporal
      Left 037T
      Right 037S
    Thyroid
      Left 037V
      Right 037U
    Ulnar
      Left 037A
      Right 0379
    Upper 037Y
    Vertebral
      Left 037Q
      Right 037P
  Bladder 0T7B
  Bladder Neck 0T7C

Dilation *(Continued)*
  Bronchus
    Lingula 0B79
    Lower Lobe
      Left 0B7B
      Right 0B76
    Main
      Left 0B77
      Right 0B73
    Middle Lobe, Right 0B75
    Upper Lobe
      Left 0B78
      Right 0B74
  Carina 0B72
  Cecum 0D7H
  Cervix 0U7C
  Colon
    Ascending 0D7K
    Descending 0D7M
    Sigmoid 0D7N
    Transverse 0D7L
  Duct
    Common Bile 0F79
    Cystic 0F78
    Hepatic
      Left 0F76
      Right 0F75
    Lacrimal
      Left 087Y
      Right 087X
    Pancreatic 0F7D
      Accessory 0F7F
    Parotid
      Left 0C7C
      Right 0C7B
  Duodenum 0D79
  Esophagogastric Junction 0D74
  Esophagus 0D75
    Lower 0D73
    Middle 0D72
    Upper 0D71
  Eustachian Tube
    Left 097G
    Right 097F
  Fallopian Tube
    Left 0U76
    Right 0U75
  Fallopian Tubes, Bilateral 0U77
  Hymen 0U7K
  Ileocecal Valve 0D7C
  Ileum 0D7B
  Intestine
    Large 0D7E
      Left 0D7G
      Right 0D7F
    Small 0D78
  Jejunum 0D7A
  Kidney Pelvis
    Left 0T74
    Right 0T73
  Larynx 0C7S
  Pharynx 0C7M
  Rectum 0D7P
  Stomach 0D76
    Pylorus 0D77
  Trachea 0B71
  Ureter
    Left 0T77
    Right 0T76
  Ureters, Bilateral 0T78
  Urethra 0T7D
  Uterus 0U79
  Vagina 0U7G
  Valve
    Aortic 027F
    Ileocecal 0D7C
    Mitral 027G
    Pulmonary 027H
    Tricuspid 027J
  Vas Deferens
    Bilateral 0V7Q
    Left 0V7P
    Right 0V7N

Dilation *(Continued)*
  Vein
    Axillary
      Left 0578
      Right 0577
    Azygos 0570
    Basilic
      Left 057C
      Right 057B
    Brachial
      Left 057A
      Right 0579
    Cephalic
      Left 057F
      Right 057D
    Colic 0677
    Common Iliac
      Left 067D
      Right 067C
    Esophageal 0673
    External Iliac
      Left 067G
      Right 067F
    External Jugular
      Left 057Q
      Right 057P
    Face
      Left 057V
      Right 057T
    Femoral
      Left 067N
      Right 067M
    Foot
      Left 067V
      Right 067T
    Gastric 0672
    Greater Saphenous
      Left 067Q
      Right 067P
    Hand
      Left 057H
      Right 057G
    Hemiazygos 0571
    Hepatic 0674
    Hypogastric
      Left 067J
      Right 067H
    Inferior Mesenteric
      0676
    Innominate
      Left 0574
      Right 0573
    Internal Jugular
      Left 057N
      Right 057M
    Intracranial 057L
    Lesser Saphenous
      Left 067S
      Right 067R
    Lower 067Y
    Portal 0678
    Pulmonary
      Left 027T
      Right 027S
    Renal
      Left 067B
      Right 0679
    Splenic 0671
    Subclavian
      Left 0576
      Right 0575
    Superior Mesenteric
      0675
    Upper 057Y
    Vertebral
      Left 057S
      Right 057R
  Vena Cava
    Inferior 0670
    Superior 027V
  Ventricle, Right 027K

◀ New   ⬅ Revised   ~~deleted~~ Deleted

Direct Lateral Interbody Fusion (DLIF) device
  use Interbody Fusion Device in Lower
    Joints
Disarticulation *see* Detachment
Discectomy, diskectomy
  see Excision, Upper Joints 0RB
  see Resection, Upper Joints 0RT
  see Excision, Lower Joints 0SB
  see Resection, Lower Joints 0ST
Discography
  see Plain Radiography, Axial Skeleton,
    Except Skull and Facial Bones
    BR0
  see Fluoroscopy, Axial Skeleton, Except
    Skull and Facial Bones BR1
Distal humerus
  use Humeral Shaft, Right
  use Humeral Shaft, Left
Distal humerus, involving joint
  use Joint, Elbow, Right
  use Joint, Elbow, Left
Distal radioulnar joint
  use Joint, Wrist, Right
  use Joint, Wrist, Left
Diversion *see* Bypass
Diverticulectomy *see* Excision, Gastrointestinal
  System 0DB
Division
  Acetabulum
    Left 0Q85
    Right 0Q84
  Anal Sphincter 0D8R
  Basal Ganglia 0088
  Bladder Neck 0T8C
  Bone
    Ethmoid
      Left 0N8G
      Right 0N8F
    Frontal
      Left 0N82
      Right 0N81
    Hyoid 0N8X
    Lacrimal
      Left 0N8J
      Right 0N8H
    Nasal 0N8B
    Occipital
      Left 0N88
      Right 0N87
    Palatine
      Left 0N8L
      Right 0N8K
    Parietal
      Left 0N84
      Right 0N83
    Pelvic
      Left 0Q83
      Right 0Q82
    Sphenoid
      Left 0N8D
      Right 0N8C
    Temporal
      Left 0N86
      Right 0N85
    Zygomatic
      Left 0N8N
      Right 0N8M
  Brain 0080
  Bursa and Ligament
    Abdomen
      Left 0M8J
      Right 0M8H
    Ankle
      Left 0M8R
      Right 0M8Q
    Elbow
      Left 0M84
      Right 0M83
    Foot
      Left 0M8T
      Right 0M8S

Division *(Continued)*
  Bursa and Ligament *(Continued)*
    Hand
      Left 0M88
      Right 0M87
    Head and Neck 0M80
    Hip
      Left 0M8M
      Right 0M8L
    Knee
      Left 0M8P
      Right 0M8N
    Lower Extremity
      Left 0M8W
      Right 0M8V
    Perineum 0M8K
    Shoulder
      Left 0M82
      Right 0M81
    Thorax
      Left 0M8G
      Right 0M8F
    Trunk
      Left 0M8D
      Right 0M8C
    Upper Extremity
      Left 0M8B
      Right 0M89
    Wrist
      Left 0M86
      Right 0M85
  Carpal
    Left 0P8N
    Right 0P8M
  Cerebral Hemisphere 0087
  Chordae Tendineae 0289
  Clavicle
    Left 0P8B
    Right 0P89
  Coccyx 0Q8S
  Conduction Mechanism
    0288
  Esophagogastric Junction
    0D84
  Femoral Shaft
    Left 0Q89
    Right 0Q88
  Femur
    Lower
      Left 0Q8C
      Right 0Q8B
    Upper
      Left 0Q87
      Right 0Q86
  Fibula
    Left 0Q8K
    Right 0Q8J
  Gland, Pituitary 0G80
  Glenoid Cavity
    Left 0P88
    Right 0P87
  Humeral Head
    Left 0P8D
    Right 0P8C
  Humeral Shaft
    Left 0P8G
    Right 0P8F
  Hymen 0U8K
  Kidneys, Bilateral 0T82
  Mandible
    Left 0N8V
    Right 0N8T
  Maxilla
    Left 0N8S
    Right 0N8R
  Metacarpal
    Left 0P8Q
    Right 0P8P
  Metatarsal
    Left 0Q8P
    Right 0Q8N

Division *(Continued)*
  Muscle
    Abdomen
      Left 0K8L
      Right 0K8K
    Facial 0K81
    Foot
      Left 0K8W
      Right 0K8V
    Hand
      Left 0K8D
      Right 0K8C
    Head 0K80
    Hip
      Left 0K8P
      Right 0K8N
    Lower Arm and Wrist
      Left 0K8B
      Right 0K89
    Lower Leg
      Left 0K8T
      Right 0K8S
    Neck
      Left 0K83
      Right 0K82
    Papillary 028D
    Perineum 0K8M
    Shoulder
      Left 0K86
      Right 0K85
    Thorax
      Left 0K8J
      Right 0K8H
    Tongue, Palate, Pharynx 0K84
    Trunk
      Left 0K8G
      Right 0K8F
    Upper Arm
      Left 0K88
      Right 0K87
    Upper Leg
      Left 0K8R
      Right 0K8Q
  Nerve
    Abdominal Sympathetic
      018M
    Abducens 008L
    Accessory 008R
    Acoustic 008N
    Brachial Plexus 0183
    Cervical 0181
    Cervical Plexus 0180
    Facial 008M
    Femoral 018D
    Glossopharyngeal 008P
    Head and Neck Sympathetic
      018K
    Hypoglossal 008S
    Lumbar 018B
    Lumbar Plexus 0189
    Lumbar Sympathetic 018N
    Lumbosacral Plexus 018A
    Median 0185
    Oculomotor 008H
    Olfactory 008F
    Optic 008G
    Peroneal 018H
    Phrenic 0182
    Pudendal 018C
    Radial 0186
    Sacral 018R
    Sacral Plexus 018Q
    Sacral Sympathetic 018P
    Sciatic 018F
    Thoracic 0188
    Thoracic Sympathetic 018L
    Tibial 018G
    Trigeminal 008K
    Trochlear 008J
    Ulnar 0184
    Vagus 008Q

◀ New   ◀▥ Revised   ~~deleted~~ Deleted

◀ New   ◀▦ Revised   ~~deleted~~ Deleted

Drainage *(Continued)*
  Ear *(Continued)*
    External Auditory Canal
      Left 0994
      Right 0993
    Inner
      Left 099E
      Right 099D
    Middle
      Left 0996
      Right 0995
  Elbow Region
    Left 0X9C
    Right 0X9B
  Epididymis
    Bilateral 0V9L
    Left 0V9K
    Right 0V9J
  Epidural Space 0093
  Epiglottis 0C9R
  Esophagogastric Junction 0D94
  Esophagus 0D95
    Lower 0D93
    Middle 0D92
    Upper 0D91
  Eustachian Tube
    Left 099G
    Right 099F
  Extremity
    Lower
      Left 0Y9B
      Right 0Y99
    Upper
      Left 0X97
      Right 0X96
  Eye
    Left 0891
    Right 0890
  Eyelid
    Lower
      Left 089R
      Right 089Q
    Upper
      Left 089P
      Right 089N
  Face 0W92
  Fallopian Tube
    Left 0U96
    Right 0U95
  Fallopian Tubes, Bilateral 0U97
  Femoral Region
    Left 0Y98
    Right 0Y97
  Femoral Shaft
    Left 0Q99
    Right 0Q98
  Femur
    Lower
      Left 0Q9C
      Right 0Q9B
    Upper
      Left 0Q97
      Right 0Q96
  Fibula
    Left 0Q9K
    Right 0Q9J
  Finger Nail 0H9Q
  Foot
    Left 0Y9N
    Right 0Y9M
  Gallbladder 0F94
  Gingiva
    Lower 0C96
    Upper 0C95
  Gland
    Adrenal
      Bilateral 0G94
      Left 0G92
      Right 0G93
    Lacrimal
      Left 089W
      Right 089V

Drainage *(Continued)*
  Gland *(Continued)*
    Minor Salivary 0C9J
    Parotid
      Left 0C99
      Right 0C98
    Pituitary 0G90
    Sublingual
      Left 0C9F
      Right 0C9D
    Submaxillary
      Left 0C9H
      Right 0C9G
    Vestibular 0U9L
  Glenoid Cavity
    Left 0P98
    Right 0P97
  Glomus Jugulare 0G9C
  Hand
    Left 0X9K
    Right 0X9J
  Head 0W90
  Humeral Head
    Left 0P9D
    Right 0P9C
  Humeral Shaft
    Left 0P9G
    Right 0P9F
  Hymen 0U9K
  Hypothalamus 009A
  Ileocecal Valve 0D9C
  Ileum 0D9B
  Inguinal Region
    Left 0Y96
    Right 0Y95
  Intestine
    Large 0D9E
      Left 0D9G
      Right 0D9F
    Small 0D98
  Iris
    Left 089D
    Right 089C
  Jaw
    Lower 0W95
    Upper 0W94
  Jejunum 0D9A
  Joint
    Acromioclavicular
      Left 0R9H
      Right 0R9G
    Ankle
      Left 0S9G
      Right 0S9F
    Carpal
      Left 0R9R
      Right 0R9Q
    Cervical Vertebral 0R91
    Cervicothoracic Vertebral 0R94
    Coccygeal 0S96
    Elbow
      Left 0R9M
      Right 0R9L
    Finger Phalangeal
      Left 0R9X
      Right 0R9W
    Hip
      Left 0S9B
      Right 0S99
    Knee
      Left 0S9D
      Right 0S9C
    Lumbar Vertebral 0S90
    Lumbosacral 0S93
    Metacarpocarpal
      Left 0R9T
      Right 0R9S
    Metacarpophalangeal
      Left 0R9V
      Right 0R9U

Drainage *(Continued)*
  Joint *(Continued)*
    Metatarsal-Phalangeal
      Left 0S9N
      Right 0S9M
    Metatarsal-Tarsal
      Left 0S9L
      Right 0S9K
    Occipital-cervical 0R90
    Sacrococcygeal 0S95
    Sacroiliac
      Left 0S98
      Right 0S97
    Shoulder
      Left 0R9K
      Right 0R9J
    Sternoclavicular
      Left 0R9F
      Right 0R9E
    Tarsal
      Left 0S9J
      Right 0S9H
    Temporomandibular
      Left 0R9D
      Right 0R9C
    Thoracic Vertebral 0R96
    Thoracolumbar Vertebral 0R9A
    Toe Phalangeal
      Left 0S9Q
      Right 0S9P
    Wrist
      Left 0R9P
      Right 0R9N
  Kidney
    Left 0T91
    Right 0T90
  Kidney Pelvis
    Left 0T94
    Right 0T93
  Knee Region
    Left 0Y9G
    Right 0Y9F
  Larynx 0C9S
  Leg
    Lower
      Left 0Y9J
      Right 0Y9H
    Upper
      Left 0Y9D
      Right 0Y9C
  Lens
    Left 089K
    Right 089J
  Lip
    Lower 0C91
    Upper 0C90
  Liver 0F90
    Left Lobe 0F92
    Right Lobe 0F91
  Lung
    Bilateral 0B9M
    Left 0B9L
    Lower Lobe
      Left 0B9J
      Right 0B9F
    Middle Lobe, Right 0B9D
    Right 0B9K
    Upper Lobe
      Left 0B9G
      Right 0B9C
  Lung Lingula 0B9H
  Lymphatic
    Aortic 079D
    Axillary
      Left 0796
      Right 0795
    Head 0790
    Inguinal
      Left 079J
      Right 079H

Drainage *(Continued)*
  Lymphatic *(Continued)*
    Internal Mammary
      Left 0799
      Right 0798
    Lower Extremity
      Left 079G
      Right 079F
    Mesenteric 079B
    Neck
      Left 0792
      Right 0791
    Pelvis 079C
    Thoracic Duct 079K
    Thorax 0797
    Upper Extremity
      Left 0794
      Right 0793
  Mandible
    Left 0N9V
    Right 0N9T
  Maxilla
    Left 0N9S
    Right 0N9R
  Mediastinum 0W9C
  Medulla Oblongata 009D
  Mesentery 0D9V
  Metacarpal
    Left 0P9Q
    Right 0P9P
  Metatarsal
    Left 0Q9P
    Right 0Q9N
  Muscle
    Abdomen
      Left 0K9L
      Right 0K9K
    Extraocular
      Left 089M
      Right 089L
    Facial 0K91
    Foot
      Left 0K9W
      Right 0K9V
    Hand
      Left 0K9D
      Right 0K9C
    Head 0K90
    Hip
      Left 0K9P
      Right 0K9N
    Lower Arm and Wrist
      Left 0K9B
      Right 0K99
    Lower Leg
      Left 0K9T
      Right 0K9S
    Neck
      Left 0K93
      Right 0K92
    Perineum 0K9M
    Shoulder
      Left 0K96
      Right 0K95
    Thorax
      Left 0K9J
      Right 0K9H
    Tongue, Palate, Pharynx 0K94
    Trunk
      Left 0K9G
      Right 0K9F
    Upper Arm
      Left 0K98
      Right 0K97
    Upper Leg
      Left 0K9R
      Right 0K9Q
  Nasopharynx 099N
  Neck 0W96

Drainage *(Continued)*
  Nerve
    Abdominal Sympathetic 019M
    Abducens 009L
    Accessory 009R
    Acoustic 009N
    Brachial Plexus 0193
    Cervical 0191
    Cervical Plexus 0190
    Facial 009M
    Femoral 019D
    Glossopharyngeal 009P
    Head and Neck Sympathetic 019K
    Hypoglossal 009S
    Lumbar 019B
    Lumbar Plexus 0199
    Lumbar Sympathetic 019N
    Lumbosacral Plexus 019A
    Median 0195
    Oculomotor 009H
    Olfactory 009F
    Optic 009G
    Peroneal 019H
    Phrenic 0192
    Pudendal 019C
    Radial 0196
    Sacral 019R
    Sacral Sympathetic 019P
    Sciatic 019F
    Thoracic 0198
    Thoracic Sympathetic 019L
    Tibial 019G
    Trigeminal 009K
    Trochlear 009J
    Ulnar 0194
    Vagus 009Q
  Nipple
    Left 0H9X
    Right 0H9W
  Nose 099K
  Omentum
    Greater 0D9S
    Lesser 0D9T
  Oral Cavity and Throat 0W93
  Orbit
    Left 0N9Q
    Right 0N9P
  Ovary
    Bilateral 0U92
    Left 0U91
    Right 0U90
  Palate
    Hard 0C92
    Soft 0C93
  Pancreas 0F9G
  Para-aortic Body 0G99
  Paraganglion Extremity 0G9F
  Parathyroid Gland 0G9R
    Inferior
      Left 0G9P
      Right 0G9N
    Multiple 0G9Q
    Superior
      Left 0G9P
      Right 0G9L
  Patella
    Left 0Q9F
    Right 0Q9D
  Pelvic Cavity 0W9J
  Penis 0V9S
  Pericardial Cavity 0W9D
  Perineum
    Female 0W9N
    Male 0W9M
  Peritoneal Cavity 0W9G
  Peritoneum 0D9W
  Phalanx
    Finger
      Left 0P9V
      Right 0P9T

Drainage *(Continued)*
  Phalanx *(Continued)*
    Thumb
      Left 0P9S
      Right 0P9R
    Toe
      Left 0Q9R
      Right 0Q9Q
  Pharynx 0C9M
  Pineal Body 0G91
  Pleura
    Left 0B9P
    Right 0B9N
  Pleural Cavity
    Left 0W9B
    Right 0W99
  Pons 009B
  Prepuce 0V9T
  Products of Conception
    Amniotic Fluid
      Diagnostic 1090
      Therapeutic 1090
    Fetal Blood 1090
    Fetal Cerebrospinal Fluid 1090
    Fetal Fluid, Other 1090
    Fluid, Other 1090
  Prostate 0V90
  Radius
    Left 0P9J
    Right 0P9H
  Rectum 0D9P
  Retina
    Left 089F
    Right 089E
  Retinal Vessel
    Left 089H
    Right 089G
  Retroperitoneum 0W9H
  Rib
    Left 0P92
    Right 0P91
  Sacrum 0Q91
  Scapula
    Left 0P96
    Right 0P95
  Sclera
    Left 0897
    Right 0896
  Scrotum 0V95
  Septum, Nasal 099M
  Shoulder Region
    Left 0X93
    Right 0X92
  Sinus
    Accessory 099P
    Ethmoid
      Left 099V
      Right 099U
    Frontal
      Left 099T
      Right 099S
    Mastoid
      Left 099C
      Right 099B
    Maxillary
      Left 099R
      Right 099Q
    Sphenoid
      Left 099X
      Right 099W
  Skin
    Abdomen 0H97
    Back 0H96
    Buttock 0H98
    Chest 0H95
    Ear
      Left 0H93
      Right 0H92
    Face 0H91
    Foot
      Left 0H9N
      Right 0H9M

◀ New   ◀▥ Revised   ~~deleted~~ Deleted

Drainage *(Continued)*
  Skin *(Continued)*
    Genitalia 0H9A
    Hand
      Left 0H9G
      Right 0H9F
    Lower Arm
      Left 0H9E
      Right 0H9D
    Lower Leg
      Left 0H9L
      Right 0H9K
    Neck 0H94
    Perineum 0H99
    Scalp 0H90
    Upper Arm
      Left 0H9C
      Right 0H9B
    Upper Leg
      Left 0H9J
      Right 0H9H
  Skull 0N90
  Spinal Canal 009U
  Spinal Cord
    Cervical 009W
    Lumbar 009Y
    Thoracic 009X
  Spinal Meninges 009T
  Spleen 079P
  Sternum 0P90
  Stomach 0D96
    Pylorus 0D97
  Subarachnoid Space 0095
  Subcutaneous Tissue and
      Fascia
    Abdomen 0J98
    Back 0J97
    Buttock 0J99
    Chest 0J96
    Face 0J91
    Foot
      Left 0J9R
      Right 0J9Q
    Hand
      Left 0J9K
      Right 0J9J
    Lower Arm
      Left 0J9H
      Right 0J9G
    Lower Leg
      Left 0J9P
      Right 0J9N
    Neck
      Anterior 0J94
      Posterior 0J95
    Pelvic Region 0J9C
    Perineum 0J9B
    Scalp 0J90
    Upper Arm
      Left 0J9F
      Right 0J9D
    Upper Leg
      Left 0J9M
      Right 0J9L
  Subdural Space 0094
  Tarsal
    Left 0Q9M
    Right 0Q9L
  Tendon
    Abdomen
      Left 0L9G
      Right 0L9F
    Ankle
      Left 0L9T
      Right 0L9S
    Foot
      Left 0L9W
      Right 0L9V
    Hand
      Left 0L98
      Right 0L97

Drainage *(Continued)*
  Tendon *(Continued)*
    Head and Neck 0L90
    Hip
      Left 0L9K
      Right 0L9J
    Knee
      Left 0L9R
      Right 0L9Q
    Lower Arm and Wrist
      Left 0L96
      Right 0L95
    Lower Leg
      Left 0L9P
      Right 0L9N
    Perineum 0L9H
    Shoulder
      Left 0L92
      Right 0L91
    Thorax
      Left 0L9D
      Right 0L9C
    Trunk
      Left 0L9B
      Right 0L99
    Upper Arm
      Left 0L94
      Right 0L93
    Upper Leg
      Left 0L9M
      Right 0L9L
  Testis
    Bilateral 0V9C
    Left 0V9B
    Right 0V99
  Thalamus 0099
  Thymus 079M
  Thyroid Gland 0G9K
    Left Lobe 0G9G
    Right Lobe 0G9H
  Tibia
    Left 0Q9H
    Right 0Q9G
  Toe Nail 0H9R
  Tongue 0C97
  Tonsils 0C9P
  Tooth
    Lower 0C9X
    Upper 0C9W
  Trachea 0B91
  Tunica Vaginalis
    Left 0V97
    Right 0V96
  Turbinate, Nasal 099L
  Tympanic Membrane
    Left 0998
    Right 0997
  Ulna
    Left 0P9L
    Right 0P9K
  Ureter
    Left 0T97
    Right 0T96
  Ureters, Bilateral 0T98
  Urethra 0T9D
  Uterine Supporting Structure 0U94
  Uterus 0U99
  Uvula 0C9N
  Vagina 0U9G
  Vas Deferens
    Bilateral 0V9Q
    Left 0V9P
    Right 0V9N
  Vein
    Axillary
      Left 0598
      Right 0597
    Azygos 0590
    Basilic
      Left 059C
      Right 059B

Drainage *(Continued)*
  Vein *(Continued)*
    Brachial
      Left 059A
      Right 0599
    Cephalic
      Left 059F
      Right 059D
    Colic 0697
    Common Iliac
      Left 069D
      Right 069C
    Esophageal 0693
    External Iliac
      Left 069G
      Right 069F
    External Jugular
      Left 059Q
      Right 059P
    Face
      Left 059V
      Right 059T
    Femoral
      Left 069N
      Right 069M
    Foot
      Left 069V
      Right 069T
    Gastric 0692
    Greater Saphenous
      Left 069Q
      Right 069P
    Hand
      Left 059H
      Right 059G
    Hemiazygos 0591
    Hepatic 0694
    Hypogastric
      Left 069J
      Right 069H
    Inferior Mesenteric 0696
    Innominate
      Left 0594
      Right 0593
    Internal Jugular
      Left 059N
      Right 059M
    Intracranial 059L
    Lesser Saphenous
      Left 069S
      Right 069R
    Lower 069Y
    Portal 0698
    Renal
      Left 069B
      Right 0699
    Splenic 0691
    Subclavian
      Left 0596
      Right 0595
    Superior Mesenteric 0695
    Upper 059Y
    Vertebral
      Left 059S
      Right 059R
  Vena Cava, Inferior 0690
  Vertebra
    Cervical 0P93
    Lumbar 0Q90
    Thoracic 0P94
  Vesicle
    Bilateral 0V93
    Left 0V92
    Right 0V91
  Vitreous
    Left 0895
    Right 0894
  Vocal Cord
    Left 0C9V
    Right 0C9T
  Vulva 0U9M

Drainage *(Continued)*
  Wrist Region
    Left 0X9H
    Right 0X9G
Dressing
  Abdominal Wall 2W23X4Z
  Arm
    Lower
      Left 2W2DX4Z
      Right 2W2CX4Z
    Upper
      Left 2W2BX4Z
      Right 2W2AX4Z
  Back 2W25X4Z
  Chest Wall 2W24X4Z
  Extremity
    Lower
      Left 2W2MX4Z
      Right 2W2LX4Z
    Upper
      Left 2W29X4Z
      Right 2W28X4Z
  Face 2W21X4Z
  Finger
    Left 2W2KX4Z
    Right 2W2JX4Z
  Foot
    Left 2W2TX4Z
    Right 2W2SX4Z
  Hand
    Left 2W2FX4Z
    Right 2W2EX4Z
  Head 2W20X4Z

Dressing *(Continued)*
  Inguinal Region
    Left 2W27X4Z
    Right 2W26X4Z
  Leg
    Lower
      Left 2W2RX4Z
      Right 2W2QX4Z
    Upper
      Left 2W2PX4Z
      Right 2W2NX4Z
  Neck 2W22X4Z
  Thumb
    Left 2W2HX4Z
    Right 2W2GX4Z
  Toe
    Left 2W2VX4Z
    Right 2W2UX4Z
Driver stent (RX) (OTW) *use* Intraluminal Device
Drotrecogin alfa *see* Introduction of Recombinant Human-activated Protein C
Duct of Santorini *use* Duct, Pancreatic, Accessory
Duct of Wirsung *use* Duct, Pancreatic
Ductogram, mammary *see* Plain Radiography, Skin, Subcutaneous Tissue and Breast BH0
Ductography, mammary *see* Plain Radiography, Skin, Subcutaneous Tissue and Breast BH0
Ductus deferens
  use Vas Deferens, Left
  use Vas Deferens, Right

Ductus deferens *(Continued)*
  use Vas Deferens
  use Vas Deferens, Bilateral
Duodenal ampulla *use* Ampulla of Vater
Duodenectomy
  see Excision, Duodenum 0DB9
  see Resection, Duodenum 0DT9
Duodenocholedochotomy *see* Drainage, Gallbladder 0F94
Duodenocystostomy
  see Bypass, Gallbladder 0F14
  see Drainage, Gallbladder 0F94
Duodenoenterostomy
  see Bypass, Gastrointestinal System 0D1
  see Drainage, Gastrointestinal System 0D9
Duodenojejunal flexure *use* Jejunum
Duodenolysis *see* Release, Duodenum 0DN9
Duodenorrhaphy *see* Repair, Duodenum 0DQ9
Duodenostomy
  see Bypass, Duodenum 0D19
  see Drainage, Duodenum 0D99
Duodenotomy *see* Drainage, Duodenum 0D99
DuraHeart Left Ventricular Assist System *use* Implantable Heart Assist System in Heart and Great Vessels
Dural venous sinus *use* Vein, Intracranial
Durata® Defibrillation Lead *use* Cardiac Lead, Defibrillator in 02H
Dynesys® Dynamic Stabilization System
  use Spinal Stabilization Device, Pedicle-Based in 0RH
  use Spinal Stabilization Device, Pedicle-Based in 0SH

◀ New ◀▥ Revised ~~deleted~~ Deleted

E

E-Luminexx™ (Biliary) (Vascular) Stent *use* Intraluminal Device
Earlobe
   use Ear, External, Left
   use Ear, External, Bilateral
   use Ear, External, Right
Echocardiogram *see* Ultrasonography, Heart B24
Echography *see* Ultrasonography
ECMO *see* Performance, Circulatory 5A15
EEG (electroencephalogram) *see* Measurement, Central Nervous 4A00
EGD (esophagogastroduodenscopy) 0DJ08ZZ
Eighth cranial nerve *use* Nerve, Acoustic
Ejaculatory duct
   use Vas Deferens, Bilateral
   use Vas Deferens, Left
   use Vas Deferens, Right
   use Vas Deferens
EKG (electrocardiogram) *see* Measurement, Cardiac 4A02
Electrical bone growth stimulator (EBGS)
   use Bone Growth Stimulator in Head and Facial Bones
   use Bone Growth Stimulator in Upper Bones
   use Bone Growth Stimulator in Lower Bones
Electrical muscle stimulation (EMS) lead *use* Stimulator Lead in Muscles
Electrocautery
   Destruction *see* Destruction
   Repair *see* Repair
Electroconvulsive Therapy
   Bilateral-Multiple Seizure GZB3ZZZ
   Bilateral-Single Seizure GZB2ZZZ
   Electroconvulsive Therapy, Other GZB4ZZZ
   Unilateral-Multiple Seizure GZB1ZZZ
   Unilateral-Single Seizure GZB0ZZZ
Electroencephalogram (EEG) *see* Measurement, Central Nervous 4A00
Electromagnetic Therapy
   Central Nervous 6A22
   Urinary 6A21
Electronic muscle stimulator lead *use* Stimulator Lead in Muscles
Electrophysiologic stimulation (EPS) *see* Measurement, Cardiac 4A02
Electroshock therapy *see* Electroconvulsive Therapy
Elevation, bone fragments, skull *see* Reposition, Head and Facial Bones 0NS
Eleventh cranial nerve *use* Nerve, Accessory
Embolectomy *see* Extirpation
Embolization
   see Occlusion
   see Restriction
Embolization coil(s) *use* Intraluminal Device
EMG (electromyogram) *see* Measurement, Musculoskeletal 4A0F
Encephalon *use* Brain
Endarterectomy
   see Excision, Upper Arteries 03B
   see Excision, Lower Arteries 04B
Endeavor® (III) (IV) (Sprint) Zotarolimus-eluting Coronary Stent System *use* Intraluminal Device, Drug-eluting in Heart and Great Vessels
EndoSure® sensor *use* Monitoring Device, Pressure Sensor in 02H
ENDOTAK RELIANCE® (G) Defibrillation Lead *use* Cardiac Lead, Defibrillator in 02H
Endotracheal tube (cuffed) (double-lumen) *use* Intraluminal Device, Endotracheal Airway in Respiratory System
Endurant® Endovascular Stent Graft *use* Intraluminal Device
Enlargement
   see Dilation
   see Repair
EnRhythm *use* Pacemaker, Dual Chamber in 0JH

Enterorrhaphy *see* Repair, Gastrointestinal System 0DQ
Enterra gastric neurostimulator *use* Stimulator Generator, Multiple Array in 0JH
Enucleation
   Eyeball *see* Resection, Eye 08T
   Eyeball with prosthetic implant *see* Replacement, Eye 08R
Ependyma *use* Cerebral Ventricle
Epicel® cultured epidermal autograft *use* Autologous Tissue Substitute
Epic™ Stented Tissue Valve (aortic) *use* Zooplastic Tissue in Heart and Great Vessels
Epidermis *use* Skin
Epididymectomy
   see Excision, Male Reproductive System 0VB
   see Resection, Male Reproductive System 0VT
Epididymoplasty
   see Repair, Male Reproductive System 0VQ
   see Supplement, Male Reproductive System 0VU
Epididymorrhaphy *see* Repair, Male Reproductive System 0VQ
Epididymotomy *see* Drainage, Male Reproductive System 0V9
Epiphysiodesis
   see Fusion, Upper Joints 0RG
   see Fusion, Lower Joints 0SG
Epiploic foramen *use* Peritoneum
Epiretinal Visual Prosthesis
   use Epiretinal Visual Prosthesis in Eye
   Insertion of device in
      Left 08H105Z
      Right 08H005Z
Episiorrhaphy *see* Repair, Perineum, Female 0WQN
Episiotomy *see* Division, Perineum, Female 0W8N
Epithalamus *use* Thalamus
Epitroclear lymph node
   use Lymphatic, Upper Extremity, Left
   use Lymphatic, Upper Extremity, Right
EPS (electrophysiologic stimulation) *see* Measurement, Cardiac 4A02
Eptifibatide, infusion *see* Introduction of Platelet Inhibitor
ERCP (endoscopic retrograde cholangiopancreatography) *see* Fluoroscopy, Hepatobiliary System and Pancreas BF1
Erector spinae muscle
   use Muscle, Trunk, Left
   use Muscle, Trunk, Right
Esophageal artery *use* Aorta, Thoracic
Esophageal obturator airway (EOA)
   use Intraluminal Device, Airway in Gastrointestinal System
Esophageal plexus *use* Nerve, Thoracic Sympathetic
Esophagectomy
   see Excision, Gastrointestinal System 0DB
   see Resection, Gastrointestinal System 0DT
Esophagocoloplasty
   see Repair, Gastrointestinal System 0DQ
   see Supplement, Gastrointestinal System 0DU
Esophagoenterostomy
   see Bypass, Gastrointestinal System 0D1
   see Drainage, Gastrointestinal System 0D9
Esophagoesophagostomy
   see Bypass, Gastrointestinal System 0D1
   see Drainage, Gastrointestinal System 0D9
Esophagogastrectomy
   see Excision, Gastrointestinal System 0DB
   see Resection, Gastrointestinal System 0DT
Esophagogastroduodenscopy (EGD) 0DJ08ZZ
Esophagogastroplasty
   see Repair, Gastrointestinal System 0DQ
   see Supplement, Gastrointestinal System 0DU
Esophagogastroscopy 0DJ68ZZ
Esophagogastrostomy
   see Bypass, Gastrointestinal System 0D1
   see Drainage, Gastrointestinal System 0D9

Esophagojejunoplasty *see* Supplement, Gastrointestinal System 0DU
Esophagojejunostomy
   see Drainage, Gastrointestinal System 0D9
   see Bypass, Gastrointestinal System 0D1
Esophagomyotomy *see* Division, Esophagogastric Junction 0D84
Esophagoplasty
   see Repair, Gastrointestinal System 0DQ
   see Replacement, Esophagus 0DR5
   see Supplement, Gastrointestinal System 0DU
Esophagoplication *see* Restriction, Gastrointestinal System 0DV
Esophagorrhaphy *see* Repair, Gastrointestinal System 0DQ
Esophagoscopy 0DJ08ZZ
Esophagotomy *see* Drainage, Gastrointestinal System 0D9
Esteem® implantable hearing system *use* Hearing Device in Ear, Nose, Sinus
ESWL (extracorporeal shock wave lithotripsy) *see* Fragmentation
Ethmoidal air cell
   use Sinus, Ethmoid, Left
   use Sinus, Ethmoid, Right
Ethmoidectomy
   see Excision, Ear, Nose, Sinus 09B
   see Resection, Ear, Nose, Sinus 09T
   see Excision, Head and Facial Bones 0NB
   see Resection, Head and Facial Bones 0NT
Ethmoidotomy *see* Drainage, Ear, Nose, Sinus 099
Evacuation
   Hematoma *see* Extirpation
   Other Fluid *see* Drainage
Evera (XT)(S)(DR/VR) *use* Defibrillator Generator in 0JH ◀
Everolimus-eluting coronary stent *use* Intraluminal Device, Drug-eluting in Heart and Great Vessels
Evisceration
   Eyeball *see* Resection, Eye 08T
   Eyeball with prosthetic implant *see* Replacement, Eye 08R
Ex-PRESS™ mini glaucoma shunt *use* Synthetic Substitute
Examination *see* Inspection
Exchange *see* Change device in
Excision
   Abdominal Wall 0WBF
   Acetabulum
      Left 0QB5
      Right 0QB4
   Adenoids 0CBQ
   Ampulla of Vater 0FBC
   Anal Sphincter 0DBR
   Ankle Region
      Left 0YBL
      Right 0YBK
   Anus 0DBQ
   Aorta
      Abdominal 04B0
      Thoracic 02BW
   Aortic Body 0GBD
   Appendix 0DBJ
   Arm
      Lower
         Left 0XBF
         Right 0XBD
      Upper
         Left 0XB9
         Right 0XB8
   Artery
      Anterior Tibial
         Left 04BQ
         Right 04BP
      Axillary
         Left 03B6
         Right 03B5
      Brachial
         Left 03B8
         Right 03B7

Excision *(Continued)*
  Artery *(Continued)*
    Celiac 04B1
    Colic
      Left 04B7
      Middle 04B8
      Right 04B6
    Common Carotid
      Left 03BJ
      Right 03BH
    Common Iliac
      Left 04BD
      Right 04BC
    External Carotid
      Left 03BN
      Right 03BM
    External Iliac
      Left 04BJ
      Right 04BH
    Face 03BR
    Femoral
      Left 04BL
      Right 04BK
    Foot
      Left 04BW
      Right 04BV
    Gastric 04B2
    Hand
      Left 03BF
      Right 03BD
    Hepatic 04B3
    Inferior Mesenteric 04BB
    Innominate 03B2
    Internal Carotid
      Left 03BL
      Right 03BK
    Internal Iliac
      Left 04BF
      Right 04BE
    Internal Mammary
      Left 03B1
      Right 03B0
    Intracranial 03BG
    Lower 04BY
    Peroneal
      Left 04BU
      Right 04BT
    Popliteal
      Left 04BN
      Right 04BM
    Posterior Tibial
      Left 04BS
      Right 04BR
    Pulmonary
      Left 02BR
      Right 02BQ
    Pulmonary Trunk 02BP
    Radial
      Left 03BC
      Right 03BB
    Renal
      Left 04BA
      Right 04B9
    Splenic 04B4
    Subclavian
      Left 03B4
      Right 03B3
    Superior Mesenteric 04B5
    Temporal
      Left 03BT
      Right 03BS
    Thyroid
      Left 03BV
      Right 03BU
    Ulnar
      Left 03BA
      Right 03B9
    Upper 03BY
    Vertebral
      Left 03BQ
      Right 03BP

Excision *(Continued)*
  Atrium
    Left 02B7
    Right 02B6
  Auditory Ossicle
    Left 09BA0Z
    Right 09B90Z
  Axilla
    Left 0XB5
    Right 0XB4
  Back
    Lower 0WBL
    Upper 0WBK
  Basal Ganglia 00B8
  Bladder 0TBB
  Bladder Neck 0TBC
  Bone
    Ethmoid
      Left 0NBG
      Right 0NBF
    Frontal
      Left 0NB2
      Right 0NB1
    Hyoid 0NBX
    Lacrimal
      Left 0NBJ
      Right 0NBH
    Nasal 0NBB
    Occipital
      Left 0NB8
      Right 0NB7
    Palatine
      Left 0NBL
      Right 0NBK
    Parietal
      Left 0NB4
      Right 0NB3
    Pelvic
      Left 0QB3
      Right 0QB2
    Sphenoid
      Left 0NBD
      Right 0NBC
    Temporal
      Left 0NB6
      Right 0NB5
    Zygomatic
      Left 0NBN
      Right 0NBM
  Brain 00B0
  Breast
    Bilateral 0HBV
    Left 0HBU
    Right 0HBT
    Supernumerary 0HBY
  Bronchus
    Lingula 0BB9
    Lower Lobe
      Left 0BBB
      Right 0BB6
    Main
      Left 0BB7
      Right 0BB3
    Middle Lobe, Right 0BB5
    Upper Lobe
      Left 0BB8
      Right 0BB4
  Buccal Mucosa 0CB4
  Bursa and Ligament
    Abdomen
      Left 0MBJ
      Right 0MBH
    Ankle
      Left 0MBR
      Right 0MBQ
    Elbow
      Left 0MB4
      Right 0MB3
    Foot
      Left 0MBT
      Right 0MBS

Excision *(Continued)*
  Bursa and Ligament *(Continued)*
    Hand
      Left 0MB8
      Right 0MB7
    Head and Neck 0MB0
    Hip
      Left 0MBM
      Right 0MBL
    Knee
      Left 0MBP
      Right 0MBN
    Lower Extremity
      Left 0MBW
      Right 0MBV
    Perineum 0MBK
    Shoulder
      Left 0MB2
      Right 0MB1
    Thorax
      Left 0MBG
      Right 0MBF
    Trunk
      Left 0MBD
      Right 0MBC
    Upper Extremity
      Left 0MBB
      Right 0MB9
    Wrist
      Left 0MB6
      Right 0MB5
  Buttock
    Left 0YB1
    Right 0YB0
  Carina 0BB2
  Carotid Bodies, Bilateral 0GB8
  Carotid Body
    Left 0GB6
    Right 0GB7
  Carpal
    Left 0PBN
    Right 0PBM
  Cecum 0DBH
  Cerebellum 00BC
  Cerebral Hemisphere 00B7
  Cerebral Meninges 00B1
  Cerebral Ventricle 00B6
  Cervix 0UBC
  Chest Wall 0WB8
  Chordae Tendineae 02B9
  Choroid
    Left 08BB
    Right 08BA
  Cisterna Chyli 07BL
  Clavicle
    Left 0PBB
    Right 0PB9
  Clitoris 0UBJ
  Coccygeal Glomus 0GBB
  Coccyx 0QBS
  Colon
    Ascending 0DBK
    Descending 0DBM
    Sigmoid 0DBN
    Transverse 0DBL
  Conduction Mechanism 02B8
  Conjunctiva
    Left 08BTXZ
    Right 08BSXZ
  Cord
    Bilateral 0VBH
    Left 0VBG
    Right 0VBF
  Cornea
    Left 08B9XZ
    Right 08B8XZ
  Cul-de-sac 0UBF
  Diaphragm
    Left 0BBS
    Right 0BBR

◄ New   ◄||| Revised   ~~deleted~~ Deleted

Excision *(Continued)*
  Disc
    Cervical Vertebral 0RB3
    Cervicothoracic Vertebral 0RB5
    Lumbar Vertebral 0SB2
    Lumbosacral 0SB4
    Thoracic Vertebral 0RB9
    Thoracolumbar Vertebral 0RBB
  Duct
    Common Bile 0FB9
    Cystic 0FB8
    Hepatic
      Left 0FB6
      Right 0FB5
    Lacrimal
      Left 08BY
      Right 08BX
    Pancreatic 0FBD
      Accessory 0FBF
    Parotid
      Left 0CBC
      Right 0CBB
  Duodenum 0DB9
  Dura Mater 00B2
  Ear
    External
      Left 09B1
      Right 09B0
    External Auditory Canal
      Left 09B4
      Right 09B3
    Inner
      Left 09BE0Z
      Right 09BD0Z
    Middle
      Left 09B60Z
      Right 09B50Z
  Elbow Region
    Left 0XBC
    Right 0XBB
  Epididymis
    Bilateral 0VBL
    Left 0VBK
    Right 0VBJ
  Epiglottis 0CBR
  Esophagogastric Junction 0DB4
  Esophagus 0DB5
    Lower 0DB3
    Middle 0DB2
    Upper 0DB1
  Eustachian Tube
    Left 09BG
    Right 09BF
  Extremity
    Lower
      Left 0YBB
      Right 0YB9
    Upper
      Left 0XB7
      Right 0XB6
  Eye
    Left 08B1
    Right 08B0
  Eyelid
    Lower
      Left 08BR
      Right 08BQ
    Upper
      Left 08BP
      Right 08BN
  Face 0WB2
  Fallopian Tube
    Left 0UB6
    Right 0UB5
  Fallopian Tubes, Bilateral 0UB7
  Femoral Region
    Left 0YB8
    Right 0YB7
  Femoral Shaft
    Left 0QB9
    Right 0QB8

Excision *(Continued)*
  Femur
    Lower
      Left 0QBC
      Right 0QBB
    Upper
      Left 0QB7
      Right 0QB6
  Fibula
    Left 0QBK
    Right 0QBJ
  Finger Nail 0HBQXZ
  Foot
    Left 0YBN
    Right 0YBM
  Gallbladder 0FB4
  Gingiva
    Lower 0CB6
    Upper 0CB5
  Gland
    Adrenal
      Bilateral 0GB4
      Left 0GB2
      Right 0GB3
    Lacrimal
      Left 08BW
      Right 08BV
    Minor Salivary 0CBJ
    Parotid
      Left 0CB9
      Right 0CB8
    Pituitary 0GB0
    Sublingual
      Left 0CBF
      Right 0CBD
    Submaxillary
      Left 0CBH
      Right 0CBG
    Vestibular 0UBL
  Glenoid Cavity
    Left 0PB8
    Right 0PB7
  Glomus Jugulare 0GBC
  Hand
    Left 0XBK
    Right 0XBJ
  Head 0WB0
  Humeral Head
    Left 0PBD
    Right 0PBC
  Humeral Shaft
    Left 0PBG
    Right 0PBF
  Hymen 0UBK
  Hypothalamus 00BA
  Ileocecal Valve 0DBC
  Ileum 0DBB
  Inguinal Region
    Left 0YB6
    Right 0YB5
  Intestine
    Large 0DBE
      Left 0DBG
      Right 0DBF
    Small 0DB8
  Iris
    Left 08BD3Z
    Right 08BC3Z
  Jaw
    Lower 0WB5
    Upper 0WB4
  Jejunum 0DBA
  Joint
    Acromioclavicular
      Left 0RBH
      Right 0RBG
    Ankle
      Left 0SBG
      Right 0SBF
    Carpal
      Left 0RBR
      Right 0RBQ

Excision *(Continued)*
  Joint *(Continued)*
    Cervical Vertebral 0RB1
    Cervicothoracic Vertebral 0RB4
    Coccygeal 0SB6
    Elbow
      Left 0RBM
      Right 0RBL
    Finger Phalangeal
      Left 0RBX
      Right 0RBW
    Hip
      Left 0SBB
      Right 0SB9
    Knee
      Left 0SBD
      Right 0SBC
    Lumbar Vertebral 0SB0
    Lumbosacral 0SB3
    Metacarpocarpal
      Left 0RBT
      Right 0RBS
    Metacarpophalangeal
      Left 0RBV
      Right 0RBU
    Metatarsal-Phalangeal
      Left 0SBN
      Right 0SBM
    Metatarsal-Tarsal
      Left 0SBL
      Right 0SBK
    Occipital-cervical 0RB0
    Sacrococcygeal 0SB5
    Sacroiliac
      Left 0SB8
      Right 0SB7
    Shoulder
      Left 0RBK
      Right 0RBJ
    Sternoclavicular
      Left 0RBF
      Right 0RBE
    Tarsal
      Left 0SBJ
      Right 0SBH
    Temporomandibular
      Left 0RBD
      Right 0RBC
    Thoracic Vertebral 0RB6
    Thoracolumbar Vertebral 0RBA
    Toe Phalangeal
      Left 0SBQ
      Right 0SBP
    Wrist
      Left 0RBP
      Right 0RBN
  Kidney
    Left 0TB1
    Right 0TB0
  Kidney Pelvis
    Left 0TB4
    Right 0TB3
  Knee Region
    Left 0YBG
    Right 0YBF
  Larynx 0CBS
  Leg
    Lower
      Left 0YBJ
      Right 0YBH
    Upper
      Left 0YBD
      Right 0YBC
  Lens
    Left 08BK3Z
    Right 08BJ3Z
  Lip
    Lower 0CB1
    Upper 0CB0

Excision *(Continued)*
  Liver 0FB0
    Left Lobe 0FB2
    Right Lobe 0FB1
  Lung
    Bilateral 0BBM
    Left 0BBL
    Lower Lobe
      Left 0BBJ
      Right 0BBF
    Middle Lobe, Right 0BBD
    Right 0BBK
    Upper Lobe
      Left 0BBG
      Right 0BBC
  Lung Lingula 0BBH
  Lymphatic
    Aortic 07BD
    Axillary
      Left 07B6
      Right 07B5
    Head 07B0
    Inguinal
      Left 07BJ
      Right 07BH
    Internal Mammary
      Left 07B9
      Right 07B8
    Lower Extremity
      Left 07BG
      Right 07BF
    Mesenteric 07BB
    Neck
      Left 07B2
      Right 07B1
    Pelvis 07BC
    Thoracic Duct 07BK
    Thorax 07B7
    Upper Extremity
      Left 07B4
      Right 07B3
  Mandible
    Left 0NBV
    Right 0NBT
  Maxilla
    Left 0NBS
    Right 0NBR
  Mediastinum 0WBC
  Medulla Oblongata 00BD
  Mesentery 0DBV
  Metacarpal
    Left 0PBQ
    Right 0PBP
  Metatarsal
    Left 0QBP
    Right 0QBN
  Muscle
    Abdomen
      Left 0KBL
      Right 0KBK
    Extraocular
      Left 08BM
      Right 08BL
    Facial 0KB1
    Foot
      Left 0KBW
      Right 0KBV
    Hand
      Left 0KBD
      Right 0KBC
    Head 0KB0
    Hip
      Left 0KBP
      Right 0KBN
    Lower Arm and Wrist
      Left 0KBB
      Right 0KB9
    Lower Leg
      Left 0KBT
      Right 0KBS

Excision *(Continued)*
  Muscle *(Continued)*
    Neck
      Left 0KB3
      Right 0KB2
    Papillary 02BD
    Perineum 0KBM
    Shoulder
      Left 0KB6
      Right 0KB5
    Thorax
      Left 0KBJ
      Right 0KBH
    Tongue, Palate, Pharynx
      0KB4
    Trunk
      Left 0KBG
      Right 0KBF
    Upper Arm
      Left 0KB8
      Right 0KB7
    Upper Leg
      Left 0KBR
      Right 0KBQ
  Nasopharynx 09BN
  Neck 0WB6
  Nerve
    Abdominal Sympathetic 01BM
    Abducens 00BL
    Accessory 00BR
    Acoustic 00BN
    Brachial Plexus 01B3
    Cervical 01B1
    Cervical Plexus 01B0
    Facial 00BM
    Femoral 01BD
    Glossopharyngeal 00BP
    Head and Neck Sympathetic
      01BK
    Hypoglossal 00BS
    Lumbar 01BB
    Lumbar Plexus 01B9
    Lumbar Sympathetic 01BN
    Lumbosacral Plexus 01BA
    Median 01B5
    Oculomotor 00BH
    Olfactory 00BF
    Optic 00BG
    Peroneal 01BH
    Phrenic 01B2
    Pudendal 01BC
    Radial 01B6
    Sacral 01BR
    Sacral Plexus 01BQ
    Sacral Sympathetic 01BP
    Sciatic 01BF
    Thoracic 01B8
    Thoracic Sympathetic 01BL
    Tibial 01BG
    Trigeminal 00BK
    Trochlear 00BJ
    Ulnar 01B4
    Vagus 00BQ
  Nipple
    Left 0HBX
    Right 0HBW
  Nose 09BK
  Omentum
    Greater 0DBS
    Lesser 0DBT
  Orbit
    Left 0NBQ
    Right 0NBP
  Ovary
    Bilateral 0UB2
    Left 0UB1
    Right 0UB0
  Palate
    Hard 0CB2
    Soft 0CB3
  Pancreas 0FBG

Excision *(Continued)*
  Para-aortic Body 0GB9
  Paraganglion Extremity 0GBF
  Parathyroid Gland 0GBR
    Inferior
      Left 0GBP
      Right 0GBN
    Multiple 0GBQ
    Superior
      Left 0GBM
      Right 0GBL
  Patella
    Left 0QBF
    Right 0QBD
  Penis 0VBS
  Pericardium 02BN
  Perineum
    Female 0WBN
    Male 0WBM
  Peritoneum 0DBW
  Phalanx
    Finger
      Left 0PBV
      Right 0PBT
    Thumb
      Left 0PBS
      Right 0PBR
    Toe
      Left 0QBR
      Right 0QBQ
  Pharynx 0CBM
  Pineal Body 0GB1
  Pleura
    Left 0BBP
    Right 0BBN
  Pons 00BB
  Prepuce 0VBT
  Prostate 0VB0
  Radius
    Left 0PBJ
    Right 0PBH
  Rectum 0DBP
  Retina
    Left 08BF3Z
    Right 08BE3Z
  Retroperitoneum 0WBH
  Rib
    Left 0PB2
    Right 0PB1
  Sacrum 0QB1
  Scapula
    Left 0PB6
    Right 0PB5
  Sclera
    Left 08B7XZ
    Right 08B6XZ
  Scrotum 0VB5
  Septum
    Atrial 02B5
    Nasal 09BM
    Ventricular 02BM
  Shoulder Region
    Left 0XB3
    Right 0XB2
  Sinus
    Accessory 09BP
    Ethmoid
      Left 09BV
      Right 09BU
    Frontal
      Left 09BT
      Right 09BS
    Mastoid
      Left 09BC
      Right 09BB
    Maxillary
      Left 09BR
      Right 09BQ
    Sphenoid
      Left 09BX
      Right 09BW

◀ New ◀▥ Revised ~~deleted~~ Deleted

Excision *(Continued)*
　Skin
　　Abdomen 0HB7XZ
　　Back 0HB6XZ
　　Buttock 0HB8XZ
　　Chest 0HB5XZ
　　Ear
　　　Left 0HB3XZ
　　　Right 0HB2XZ
　　Face 0HB1XZ
　　Foot
　　　Left 0HBNXZ
　　　Right 0HBMXZ
　　Genitalia 0HBAXZ
　　Hand
　　　Left 0HBGXZ
　　　Right 0HBFXZ
　　Lower Arm
　　　Left 0HBEXZ
　　　Right 0HBDXZ
　　Lower Leg
　　　Left 0HBLXZ
　　　Right 0HBKXZ
　　Neck 0HB4XZ
　　Perineum 0HB9XZ
　　Scalp 0HB0XZ
　　Upper Arm
　　　Left 0HBCXZ
　　　Right 0HBBXZ
　　Upper Leg
　　　Left 0HBJXZ
　　　Right 0HBHXZ
　Skull 0NB0
　Spinal Cord
　　Cervical 00BW
　　Lumbar 00BY
　　Thoracic 00BX
　Spinal Meninges 00BT
　Spleen 07BP
　Sternum 0PB0
　Stomach 0DB6
　　Pylorus 0DB7
　Subcutaneous Tissue and Fascia
　　Abdomen 0JB8
　　Back 0JB7
　　Buttock 0JB9
　　Chest 0JB6
　　Face 0JB1
　　Foot
　　　Left 0JBR
　　　Right 0JBQ
　　Hand
　　　Left 0JBK
　　　Right 0JBJ
　　Lower Arm
　　　Left 0JBH
　　　Right 0JBG
　　Lower Leg
　　　Left 0JBP
　　　Right 0JBN
　　Neck
　　　Anterior 0JB4
　　　Posterior 0JB5
　　Pelvic Region 0JBC
　　Perineum 0JBB
　　Scalp 0JB0
　　Upper Arm
　　　Left 0JBF
　　　Right 0JBD
　　Upper Leg
　　　Left 0JBM
　　　Right 0JBL
　Tarsal
　　Left 0QBM
　　Right 0QBL
　Tendon
　　Abdomen
　　　Left 0LBG
　　　Right 0LBF
　　Ankle
　　　Left 0LBT
　　　Right 0LBS

Excision *(Continued)*
　Tendon *(Continued)*
　　Foot
　　　Left 0LBW
　　　Right 0LBV
　　Hand
　　　Left 0LB8
　　　Right 0LB7
　　Head and Neck 0LB0
　　Hip
　　　Left 0LBK
　　　Right 0LBJ
　　Knee
　　　Left 0LBR
　　　Right 0LBQ
　　Lower Arm and Wrist
　　　Left 0LB6
　　　Right 0LB5
　　Lower Leg
　　　Left 0LBP
　　　Right 0LBN
　　Perineum 0LBH
　　Shoulder
　　　Left 0LB2
　　　Right 0LB1
　　Thorax
　　　Left 0LBD
　　　Right 0LBC
　　Trunk
　　　Left 0LBB
　　　Right 0LB9
　　Upper Arm
　　　Left 0LB4
　　　Right 0LB3
　　Upper Leg
　　　Left 0LBM
　　　Right 0LBL
　Testis
　　Bilateral 0VBC
　　Left 0VBB
　　Right 0VB9
　Thalamus 00B9
　Thymus 07BM
　Thyroid Gland
　　Left Lobe 0GBG
　　Right Lobe 0GBH
　Tibia
　　Left 0QBH
　　Right 0QBG
　Toe Nail 0HBRXZ
　Tongue 0CB7
　Tonsils 0CBP
　Tooth
　　Lower 0CBX
　　Upper 0CBW
　Trachea 0BB1
　Tunica Vaginalis
　　Left 0VB7
　　Right 0VB6
　Turbinate, Nasal 09BL
　Tympanic Membrane
　　Left 09B8
　　Right 09B7
　Ulna
　　Left 0PBL
　　Right 0PBK
　Ureter
　　Left 0TB7
　　Right 0TB6
　Urethra 0TBD
　Uterine Supporting Structure
　　0UB4
　Uterus 0UB9
　Uvula 0CBN
　Vagina 0UBG
　Valve
　　Aortic 02BF
　　Mitral 02BG
　　Pulmonary 02BH
　　Tricuspid 02BJ

Excision *(Continued)*
　Vas Deferens
　　Bilateral 0VBQ
　　Left 0VBP
　　Right 0VBN
　Vein
　　Axillary
　　　Left 05B8
　　　Right 05B7
　　Azygos 05B0
　　Basilic
　　　Left 05BC
　　　Right 05BB
　　Brachial
　　　Left 05BA
　　　Right 05B9
　　Cephalic
　　　Left 05BF
　　　Right 05BD
　　Colic 06B7
　　Common Iliac
　　　Left 06BD
　　　Right 06BC
　　Coronary 02B4
　　Esophageal 06B3
　　External Iliac
　　　Left 06BG
　　　Right 06BF
　　External Jugular
　　　Left 05BQ
　　　Right 05BP
　　Face
　　　Left 05BV
　　　Right 05BT
　　Femoral
　　　Left 06BN
　　　Right 06BM
　　Foot
　　　Left 06BV
　　　Right 06BT
　　Gastric 06B2
　　Greater Saphenous
　　　Left 06BQ
　　　Right 06BP
　　Hand
　　　Left 05BH
　　　Right 05BG
　　Hemiazygos 05B1
　　Hepatic 06B4
　　Hypogastric
　　　Left 06BJ
　　　Right 06BH
　　Inferior Mesenteric 06B6
　　Innominate
　　　Left 05B4
　　　Right 05B3
　　Internal Jugular
　　　Left 05BN
　　　Right 05BM
　　Intracranial 05BL
　　Lesser Saphenous
　　　Left 06BS
　　　Right 06BR
　　Lower 06BY
　　Portal 06B8
　　Pulmonary
　　　Left 02BT
　　　Right 02BS
　　Renal
　　　Left 06BB
　　　Right 06B9
　　Splenic 06B1
　　Subclavian
　　　Left 05B6
　　　Right 05B5
　　Superior Mesenteric 06B5
　　Upper 05BY
　　Vertebral
　　　Left 05BS
　　　Right 05BR

◀ New　　◀▥ Revised　　~~deleted~~ Deleted

Excision (Continued)
  Vena Cava
    Inferior 06B0
    Superior 02BV
  Ventricle
    Left 02BL
    Right 02BK
  Vertebra
    Cervical 0PB3
    Lumbar 0QB0
    Thoracic 0PB4
  Vesicle
    Bilateral 0VB3
    Left 0VB2
    Right 0VB1
  Vitreous
    Left 08B53Z
    Right 08B43Z
  Vocal Cord
    Left 0CBV
    Right 0CBT
  Vulva 0UBM
  Wrist Region
    Left 0XBH
    Right 0XBG
Exclusion, Left atrial appendage (LAA) see
  Occlusion, Atrium, Left 02L7
Exercise, rehabilitation see Motor Treatment,
  Rehabilitation F07
Exploration see Inspection
Express® (LD) Premounted Stent System use
  Intraluminal Device
Express® Biliary SD Monorail® Premounted
  Stent System use Intraluminal Device
Express® SD Renal Monorail® Premounted
  Stent System use Intraluminal Device
Extensor carpi radialis muscle
  use Muscle, Lower Arm and Wrist, Left
  use Muscle, Lower Arm and Wrist, Right
Extensor carpi ulnaris muscle
  use Muscle, Lower Arm and Wrist, Left
  use Muscle, Lower Arm and Wrist, Right
Extensor digitorum brevis muscle
  use Muscle, Foot, Right
  use Muscle, Foot, Left
Extensor digitorum longus muscle
  use Muscle, Lower Leg, Left
  use Muscle, Lower Leg, Right
Extensor hallucis brevis muscle
  use Muscle, Foot, Right
  use Muscle, Foot, Left
Extensor hallucis longus muscle
  use Muscle, Lower Leg, Right
  use Muscle, Lower Leg, Left
External anal sphincter use Anal Sphincter
External auditory meatus
  use Ear, External Auditory Canal, Left
  use Ear, External Auditory Canal, Right
External fixator
  use External Fixation Device in Head and
    Facial Bones
  use External Fixation Device in Upper Bones
  use External Fixation Device in Lower Bones
  use External Fixation Device in Upper Joints
  use External Fixation Device in Lower Joints
External maxillary artery use Artery, Face
External naris use Nose
External oblique aponeurosis use
  Subcutaneous Tissue and Fascia, Trunk
External oblique muscle
  use Muscle, Abdomen, Left
  use Muscle, Abdomen, Right
External popliteal nerve use Nerve,
  Peroneal
External pudendal artery
  use Artery, Femoral, Right
  use Artery, Femoral, Left
External pudendal vein
  use Vein, Greater Saphenous, Right
  use Vein, Greater Saphenous, Left
External urethral sphincter use Urethra

Extirpation
  Acetabulum
    Left 0QC5
    Right 0QC4
  Adenoids 0CCQ
  Ampulla of Vater 0FCC
  Anal Sphincter 0DCR
  Anterior Chamber
    Left 08C3
    Right 08C2
  Anus 0DCQ
  Aorta
    Abdominal 04C0
    Thoracic 02CW
  Aortic Body 0GCD
  Appendix 0DCJ
  Artery
    Anterior Tibial
      Left 04CQ
      Right 04CP
    Axillary
      Left 03C6
      Right 03C5
    Brachial
      Left 03C8
      Right 03C7
    Celiac 04C1
    Colic
      Left 04C7
      Middle 04C8
      Right 04C6
    Common Carotid
      Left 03CJ
      Right 03CH
    Common Iliac
      Left 04CD
      Right 04CC
    Coronary
      Four or More Sites
        02C3
      One Site 02C0
      Three Sites 02C2
      Two Sites 02C1
    External Carotid
      Left 03CN
      Right 03CM
    External Iliac
      Left 04CJ
      Right 04CH
    Face 03CR
    Femoral
      Left 04CL
      Right 04CK
    Foot
      Left 04CW
      Right 04CV
    Gastric 04C2
    Hand
      Left 03CF
      Right 03CD
    Hepatic 04C3
    Inferior Mesenteric
      04CB
    Innominate 03C2
    Internal Carotid
      Left 03CL
      Right 03CK
    Internal Iliac
      Left 04CF
      Right 04CE
    Internal Mammary
      Left 03C1
      Right 03C0
    Intracranial 03CG
    Lower 04CY
    Peroneal
      Left 04CU
      Right 04CT
    Popliteal
      Left 04CN
      Right 04CM

Extirpation (Continued)
  Artery (Continued)
    Posterior Tibial
      Left 04CS
      Right 04CR
    Pulmonary
      Left 02CR
      Right 02CQ
    Pulmonary Trunk 02CP
    Radial
      Left 03CC
      Right 03CB
    Renal
      Left 04CA
      Right 04C9
    Splenic 04C4
    Subclavian
      Left 03C4
      Right 03C3
    Superior Mesenteric
      04C5
    Temporal
      Left 03CT
      Right 03CS
    Thyroid
      Left 03CV
      Right 03CU
    Ulnar
      Left 03CA
      Right 03C9
    Upper 03CY
    Vertebral
      Left 03CQ
      Right 03CP
  Atrium
    Left 02C7
    Right 02C6
  Auditory Ossicle
    Left 09CA0ZZ
    Right 09C90ZZ
  Basal Ganglia 00C8
  Bladder 0TCB
  Bladder Neck 0TCC
  Bone
    Ethmoid
      Left 0NCG
      Right 0NCF
    Frontal
      Left 0NC2
      Right 0NC1
    Hyoid 0NCX
    Lacrimal
      Left 0NCJ
      Right 0NCH
    Nasal 0NCB
    Occipital
      Left 0NC8
      Right 0NC7
    Palatine
      Left 0NCL
      Right 0NCK
    Parietal
      Left 0NC4
      Right 0NC3
    Pelvic
      Left 0QC3
      Right 0QC2
    Sphenoid
      Left 0NCD
      Right 0NCC
    Temporal
      Left 0NC6
      Right 0NC5
    Zygomatic
      Left 0NCN
      Right 0NCM
  Brain 00C0
  Breast
    Bilateral 0HCV
    Left 0HCU
    Right 0HCT

◄ New   ◄█ Revised   ~~deleted~~ Deleted

Extirpation (Continued)
  Bronchus
    Lingula 0BC9
    Lower Lobe
      Left 0BCB
      Right 0BC6
    Main
      Left 0BC7
      Right 0BC3
    Middle Lobe, Right 0BC5
    Upper Lobe
      Left 0BC8
      Right 0BC4
  Buccal Mucosa 0CC4
  Bursa and Ligament
    Abdomen
      Left 0MCJ
      Right 0MCH
    Ankle
      Left 0MCR
      Right 0MCQ
    Elbow
      Left 0MC4
      Right 0MC3
    Foot
      Left 0MCT
      Right 0MCS
    Hand
      Left 0MC8
      Right 0MC7
    Head and Neck 0MC0
    Hip
      Left 0MCM
      Right 0MCL
    Knee
      Left 0MCP
      Right 0MCN
    Lower Extremity
      Left 0MCW
      Right 0MCV
    Perineum 0MCK
    Shoulder
      Left 0MC2
      Right 0MC1
    Thorax
      Left 0MCG
      Right 0MCF
    Trunk
      Left 0MCD
      Right 0MCC
    Upper Extremity
      Left 0MCB
      Right 0MC9
    Wrist
      Left 0MC6
      Right 0MC5
  Carina 0BC2
  Carotid Bodies, Bilateral 0GC8
  Carotid Body
    Left 0GC6
    Right 0GC7
  Carpal
    Left 0PCN
    Right 0PCM
  Cavity, Cranial 0WC1
  Cecum 0DCH
  Cerebellum 00CC
  Cerebral Hemisphere 00C7
  Cerebral Meninges 00C1
  Cerebral Ventricle 00C6
  Cervix 0UCC
  Chordae Tendineae 02C9
  Choroid
    Left 08CB
    Right 08CA
  Cisterna Chyli 07CL
  Clavicle
    Left 0PCB
    Right 0PC9
  Clitoris 0UCJ
  Coccygeal Glomus 0GCB

Extirpation (Continued)
  Coccyx 0QCS
  Colon
    Ascending 0DCK
    Descending 0DCM
    Sigmoid 0DCN
    Transverse 0DCL
  Conduction Mechanism 02C8
  Conjunctiva
    Left 08CTXZZ
    Right 08CSXZZ
  Cord
    Bilateral 0VCH
    Left 0VCG
    Right 0VCF
  Cornea
    Left 08C9XZZ
    Right 08C8XZZ
  Cul-de-sac 0UCF
  Diaphragm
    Left 0BCS
    Right 0BCR
  Disc
    Cervical Vertebral 0RC3
    Cervicothoracic Vertebral 0RC5
    Lumbar Vertebral 0SC2
    Lumbosacral 0SC4
    Thoracic Vertebral 0RC9
    Thoracolumbar Vertebral 0RCB
  Duct
    Common Bile 0FC9
    Cystic 0FC8
    Hepatic
      Left 0FC6
      Right 0FC5
    Lacrimal
      Left 08CY
      Right 08CX
    Pancreatic 0FCD
      Accessory 0FCF
    Parotid
      Left 0CCC
      Right 0CCB
  Duodenum 0DC9
  Dura Mater 00C2
  Ear
    External
      Left 09C1
      Right 09C0
    External Auditory Canal
      Left 09C4
      Right 09C3
    Inner
      Left 09CE0ZZ
      Right 09CD0ZZ
    Middle
      Left 09C60ZZ
      Right 09C50ZZ
  Endometrium 0UCB
  Epididymis
    Bilateral 0VCL
    Left 0VCK
    Right 0VCJ
  Epidural Space 00C3
  Epiglottis 0CCR
  Esophagogastric Junction
    0DC4
  Esophagus 0DC5
    Lower 0DC3
    Middle 0DC2
    Upper 0DC1
  Eustachian Tube
    Left 09CG
    Right 09CF
  Eye
    Left 08C1XZZ
    Right 08C0XZZ
  Eyelid
    Lower
      Left 08CR
      Right 08CQ

Extirpation (Continued)
  Eyelid (Continued)
    Upper
      Left 08CP
      Right 08CN
  Fallopian Tube
    Left 0UC6
    Right 0UC5
  Fallopian Tubes, Bilateral 0UC7
  Femoral Shaft
    Left 0QC9
    Right 0QC8
  Femur
    Lower
      Left 0QCC
      Right 0QCB
    Upper
      Left 0QC7
      Right 0QC6
  Fibula
    Left 0QCK
    Right 0QCJ
  Finger Nail 0HCQXZZ
  Gallbladder 0FC4
  Gastrointestinal Tract 0WCP
  Genitourinary Tract 0WCR
  Gingiva
    Lower 0CC6
    Upper 0CC5
  Gland
    Adrenal
      Bilateral 0GC4
      Left 0GC2
      Right 0GC3
    Lacrimal
      Left 08CW
      Right 08CV
    Minor Salivary 0CCJ
    Parotid
      Left 0CC9
      Right 0CC8
    Pituitary 0GC0
    Sublingual
      Left 0CCF
      Right 0CCD
    Submaxillary
      Left 0CCH
      Right 0CCG
    Vestibular 0UCL
  Glenoid Cavity
    Left 0PC8
    Right 0PC7
  Glomus Jugulare 0GCC
  Humeral Head
    Left 0PCD
    Right 0PCC
  Humeral Shaft
    Left 0PCG
    Right 0PCF
  Hymen 0UCK
  Hypothalamus 00CA
  Ileocecal Valve 0DCC
  Ileum 0DCB
  Intestine
    Large 0DCE
      Left 0DCG
      Right 0DCF
    Small 0DC8
  Iris
    Left 08CD
    Right 08CC
  Jejunum 0DCA
  Joint
    Acromioclavicular
      Left 0RCH
      Right 0RCG
    Ankle
      Left 0SCG
      Right 0SCF
    Carpal
      Left 0RCR
      Right 0RCQ

◀ New   ◀▥ Revised   ~~deleted~~ Deleted

Extirpation (Continued)
  Joint (Continued)
    Cervical Vertebral 0RC1
    Cervicothoracic Vertebral
      0RC4
    Coccygeal 0SC6
    Elbow
      Left 0RCM
      Right 0RCL
    Finger Phalangeal
      Left 0RCX
      Right 0RCW
    Hip
      Left 0SCB
      Right 0SC9
    Knee
      Left 0SCD
      Right 0SCC
    Lumbar Vertebral 0SC0
    Lumbosacral 0SC3
    Metacarpocarpal
      Left 0RCT
      Right 0RCS
    Metacarpophalangeal
      Left 0RCV
      Right 0RCU
    Metatarsal-Phalangeal
      Left 0SCN
      Right 0SCM
    Metatarsal-Tarsal
      Left 0SCL
      Right 0SCK
    Occipital-cervical 0RC0
    Sacrococcygeal 0SC5
    Sacroiliac
      Left 0SC8
      Right 0SC7
    Shoulder
      Left 0RCK
      Right 0RCJ
    Sternoclavicular
      Left 0RCF
      Right 0RCE
    Tarsal
      Left 0SCJ
      Right 0SCH
    Temporomandibular
      Left 0RCD
      Right 0RCC
    Thoracic Vertebral 0RC6
    Thoracolumbar Vertebral 0RCA
    Toe Phalangeal
      Left 0SCQ
      Right 0SCP
    Wrist
      Left 0RCP
      Right 0RCN
  Kidney
    Left 0TC1
    Right 0TC0
  Kidney Pelvis
    Left 0TC4
    Right 0TC3
  Larynx 0CCS
  Lens
    Left 08CK
    Right 08CJ
  Lip
    Lower 0CC1
    Upper 0CC0
  Liver 0FC0
    Left Lobe 0FC2
    Right Lobe 0FC1
  Lung
    Bilateral 0BCM
    Left 0BCL
    Lower Lobe
      Left 0BCJ
      Right 0BCF
    Middle Lobe, Right 0BCD
    Right 0BCK

Extirpation (Continued)
  Lung (Continued)
    Upper Lobe
      Left 0BCG
      Right 0BCC
  Lung Lingula 0BCH
  Lymphatic
    Aortic 07CD
    Axillary
      Left 07C6
      Right 07C5
    Head 07C0
    Inguinal
      Left 07CJ
      Right 07CH
    Internal Mammary
      Left 07C9
      Right 07C8
    Lower Extremity
      Left 07CG
      Right 07CF
    Mesenteric 07CB
    Neck
      Left 07C2
      Right 07C1
    Pelvis 07CC
    Thoracic Duct 07CK
    Thorax 07C7
    Upper Extremity
      Left 07C4
      Right 07C3
  Mandible
    Left 0NCV
    Right 0NCT
  Maxilla
    Left 0NCS
    Right 0NCR
  Mediastinum 0WCC
  Medulla Oblongata 00CD
  Mesentery 0DCV
  Metacarpal
    Left 0PCQ
    Right 0PCP
  Metatarsal
    Left 0QCP
    Right 0QCN
  Muscle
    Abdomen
      Left 0KCL
      Right 0KCK
    Extraocular
      Left 08CM
      Right 08CL
    Facial 0KC1
    Foot
      Left 0KCW
      Right 0KCV
    Hand
      Left 0KCD
      Right 0KCC
    Head 0KC0
    Hip
      Left 0KCP
      Right 0KCN
    Lower Arm and Wrist
      Left 0KCB
      Right 0KC9
    Lower Leg
      Left 0KCT
      Right 0KCS
    Neck
      Left 0KC3
      Right 0KC2
    Papillary 02CD
    Perineum 0KCM
    Shoulder
      Left 0KC6
      Right 0KC5
    Thorax
      Left 0KCJ
      Right 0KCH

Extirpation (Continued)
  Muscle (Continued)
    Tongue, Palate, Pharynx 0KC4
    Trunk
      Left 0KCG
      Right 0KCF
    Upper Arm
      Left 0KC8
      Right 0KC7
    Upper Leg
      Left 0KCR
      Right 0KCQ
  Nasopharynx 09CN
  Nerve
    Abdominal Sympathetic 01CM
    Abducens 00CL
    Accessory 00CR
    Acoustic 00CN
    Brachial Plexus 01C3
    Cervical 01C1
    Cervical Plexus 01C0
    Facial 00CM
    Femoral 01CD
    Glossopharyngeal 00CP
    Head and Neck Sympathetic 01CK
    Hypoglossal 00CS
    Lumbar 01CB
    Lumbar Plexus 01C9
    Lumbar Sympathetic 01CN
    Lumbosacral Plexus 01CA
    Median 01C5
    Oculomotor 00CH
    Olfactory 00CF
    Optic 00CG
    Peroneal 01CH
    Phrenic 01C2
    Pudendal 01CC
    Radial 01C6
    Sacral 01CR
    Sacral Plexus 01CQ
    Sacral Sympathetic 01CP
    Sciatic 01CF
    Thoracic 01C8
    Thoracic Sympathetic 01CL
    Tibial 01CG
    Trigeminal 00CK
    Trochlear 00CJ
    Ulnar 01C4
    Vagus 00CQ
  Nipple
    Left 0HCX
    Right 0HCW
  Nose 09CK
  Omentum
    Greater 0DCS
    Lesser 0DCT
  Oral Cavity and Throat 0WC3
  Orbit
    Left 0NCQ
    Right 0NCP
  Ovary
    Bilateral 0UC2
    Left 0UC1
    Right 0UC0
  Palate
    Hard 0CC2
    Soft 0CC3
  Pancreas 0FCG
  Para-aortic Body 0GC9
  Paraganglion Extremity 0GCF
  Parathyroid Gland 0GCR
    Inferior
      Left 0GCP
      Right 0GCN
    Multiple 0GCQ
    Superior
      Left 0GCM
      Right 0GCL
  Patella
    Left 0QCF
    Right 0QCD

◀ New   ◀‖‖ Revised   ~~deleted~~ Deleted

Extirpation (Continued)
Pelvic Cavity 0WCJ
Penis 0VCS
Pericardial Cavity 0WCD
Pericardium 02CN
Peritoneal Cavity 0WCG
Peritoneum 0DCW
Phalanx
  Finger
    Left 0PCV
    Right 0PCT
  Thumb
    Left 0PCS
    Right 0PCR
  Toe
    Left 0QCR
    Right 0QCQ
Pharynx 0CCM
Pineal Body 0GC1
Pleura
  Left 0BCP
  Right 0BCN
Pleural Cavity
  Left 0WCB
  Right 0WC9
Pons 00CB
Prepuce 0VCT
Prostate 0VC0
Radius
  Left 0PCJ
  Right 0PCH
Rectum 0DCP
Respiratory Tract 0WCQ
Retina
  Left 08CF
  Right 08CE
Retinal Vessel
  Left 08CH
  Right 08CG
Rib
  Left 0PC2
  Right 0PC1
Sacrum 0QC1
Scapula
  Left 0PC6
  Right 0PC5
Sclera
  Left 08C7XZZ
  Right 08C6XZZ
Scrotum 0VC5
Septum
  Atrial 02C5
  Nasal 09CM
  Ventricular 02CM
Sinus
  Accessory 09CP
  Ethmoid
    Left 09CV
    Right 09CU
  Frontal
    Left 09CT
    Right 09CS
  Mastoid
    Left 09CC
    Right 09CB
  Maxillary
    Left 09CR
    Right 09CQ
  Sphenoid
    Left 09CX
    Right 09CW
Skin
  Abdomen 0HC7XZZ
  Back 0HC6XZZ
  Buttock 0HC8XZZ
  Chest 0HC5XZZ
  Ear
    Left 0HC3XZZ
    Right 0HC2XZZ
  Face 0HC1XZZ

Extirpation (Continued)
Skin (Continued)
  Foot
    Left 0HCNXZZ
    Right 0HCMXZZ
  Genitalia 0HCAXZZ
  Hand
    Left 0HCGXZZ
    Right 0HCFXZZ
  Lower Arm
    Left 0HCEXZZ
    Right 0HCDXZZ
  Lower Leg
    Left 0HCLXZZ
    Right 0HCKXZZ
  Neck 0HC4XZZ
  Perineum 0HC9XZZ
  Scalp 0HC0XZZ
  Upper Arm
    Left 0HCCXZZ
    Right 0HCBXZZ
  Upper Leg
    Left 0HCJXZZ
    Right 0HCHXZZ
Spinal Cord
  Cervical 00CW
  Lumbar 00CY
  Thoracic 00CX
Spinal Meninges 00CT
Spleen 07CP
Sternum 0PC0
Stomach 0DC6
  Pylorus 0DC7
Subarachnoid Space 00C5
Subcutaneous Tissue and Fascia
  Abdomen 0JC8
  Back 0JC7
  Buttock 0JC9
  Chest 0JC6
  Face 0JC1
  Foot
    Left 0JCR
    Right 0JCQ
  Hand
    Left 0JCK
    Right 0JCJ
  Lower Arm
    Left 0JCH
    Right 0JCG
  Lower Leg
    Left 0JCP
    Right 0JCN
  Neck
    Anterior 0JC4
    Posterior 0JC5
  Pelvic Region 0JCC
  Perineum 0JCB
  Scalp 0JC0
  Upper Arm
    Left 0JCF
    Right 0JCD
  Upper Leg
    Left 0JCM
    Right 0JCL
Subdural Space 00C4
Tarsal
  Left 0QCM
  Right 0QCL
Tendon
  Abdomen
    Left 0LCG
    Right 0LCF
  Ankle
    Left 0LCT
    Right 0LCS
  Foot
    Left 0LCW
    Right 0LCV
  Hand
    Left 0LC8
    Right 0LC7

Extirpation (Continued)
Tendon (Continued)
  Head and Neck 0LC0
  Hip
    Left 0LCK
    Right 0LCJ
  Knee
    Left 0LCR
    Right 0LCQ
  Lower Arm and Wrist
    Left 0LC6
    Right 0LC5
  Lower Leg
    Left 0LCP
    Right 0LCN
  Perineum 0LCH
  Shoulder
    Left 0LC2
    Right 0LC1
  Thorax
    Left 0LCD
    Right 0LCC
  Trunk
    Left 0LCB
    Right 0LC9
  Upper Arm
    Left 0LC4
    Right 0LC3
  Upper Leg
    Left 0LCM
    Right 0LCL
Testis
  Bilateral 0VCC
  Left 0VCB
  Right 0VC9
Thalamus 00C9
Thymus 07CM
Thyroid Gland 0GCK
  Left Lobe 0GCG
  Right Lobe 0GCH
Tibia
  Left 0QCH
  Right 0QCG
Toe Nail 0HCRXZZ
Tongue 0CC7
Tonsils 0CCP
Tooth
  Lower 0CCX
  Upper 0CCW
Trachea 0BC1
Tunica Vaginalis
  Left 0VC7
  Right 0VC6
Turbinate, Nasal 09CL
Tympanic Membrane
  Left 09C8
  Right 09C7
Ulna
  Left 0PCL
  Right 0PCK
Ureter
  Left 0TC7
  Right 0TC6
Urethra 0TCD
Uterine Supporting Structure 0UC4
Uterus 0UC9
Uvula 0CCN
Vagina 0UCG
Valve
  Aortic 02CF
  Mitral 02CG
  Pulmonary 02CH
  Tricuspid 02CJ
Vas Deferens
  Bilateral 0VCQ
  Left 0VCP
  Right 0VCN
Vein
  Axillary
    Left 05C8
    Right 05C7

◀ New   ◀▦ Revised   ~~deleted~~ Deleted

Extirpation (Continued)
  Vein (Continued)
    Azygos 05C0
    Basilic
      Left 05CC
      Right 05CB
    Brachial
      Left 05CA
      Right 05C9
    Cephalic
      Left 05CF
      Right 05CD
    Colic 06C7
    Common Iliac
      Left 06CD
      Right 06CC
    Coronary 02C4
    Esophageal 06C3
    External Iliac
      Left 06CG
      Right 06CF
    External Jugular
      Left 05CQ
      Right 05CP
    Face
      Left 05CV
      Right 05CT
    Femoral
      Left 06CN
      Right 06CM
    Foot
      Left 06CV
      Right 06CT
    Gastric 06C2
    Greater Saphenous
      Left 06CQ
      Right 06CP
    Hand
      Left 05CH
      Right 05CG
    Hemiazygos 05C1
    Hepatic 06C4
    Hypogastric
      Left 06CJ
      Right 06CH
    Inferior Mesenteric
      06C6
    Innominate
      Left 05C4
      Right 05C3
    Internal Jugular
      Left 05CN
      Right 05CM
    Intracranial 05CL
    Lesser Saphenous
      Left 06CS
      Right 06CR
    Lower 06CY
    Portal 06C8
    Pulmonary
      Left 02CT
      Right 02CS
    Renal
      Left 06CB
      Right 06C9
    Splenic 06C1
    Subclavian
      Left 05C6
      Right 05C5
    Superior Mesenteric
      06C5
    Upper 05CY
    Vertebral
      Left 05CS
      Right 05CR
  Vena Cava
    Inferior 06C0
    Superior 02CV
  Ventricle
    Left 02CL
    Right 02CK

Extirpation (Continued)
  Vertebra
    Cervical 0PC3
    Lumbar 0QC0
    Thoracic 0PC4
  Vesicle
    Bilateral 0VC3
    Left 0VC2
    Right 0VC1
  Vitreous
    Left 08C5
    Right 08C4
  Vocal Cord
    Left 0CCV
    Right 0CCT
  Vulva 0UCM
Extracorporeal shock wave lithotripsy see
  Fragmentation
Extracranial-intracranial bypass (EC-IC) see
  Bypass, Upper Arteries 031
Extraction
  Auditory Ossicle
    Left 09DA0ZZ
    Right 09D90ZZ
  Bone Marrow
    Iliac 07DR
    Sternum 07DQ
    Vertebral 07DS
  Bursa and Ligament
    Abdomen
      Left 0MDJ
      Right 0MDH
    Ankle
      Left 0MDR
      Right 0MDQ
    Elbow
      Left 0MD4
      Right 0MD3
    Foot
      Left 0MDT
      Right 0MDS
    Hand
      Left 0MD8
      Right 0MD7
    Head and Neck 0MD0
    Hip
      Left 0MDM
      Right 0MDL
    Knee
      Left 0MDP
      Right 0MDN
    Lower Extremity
      Left 0MDW
      Right 0MDV
    Perineum 0MDK
    Shoulder
      Left 0MD2
      Right 0MD1
    Thorax
      Left 0MDG
      Right 0MDF
    Trunk
      Left 0MDD
      Right 0MDC
    Upper Extremity
      Left 0MDB
      Right 0MD9
    Wrist
      Left 0MD6
      Right 0MD5
  Cerebral Meninges 00D1
  Cornea
    Left 08D9XZ
    Right 08D8XZ
  Dura Mater 00D2
  Endometrium 0UDB
  Finger Nail 0HDQXZZ
  Hair 0HDSXZZ
  Kidney
    Left 0TD1
    Right 0TD0

Extraction (Continued)
  Lens
    Left 08DK3ZZ
    Right 08DJ3ZZ
  Nerve
    Abdominal Sympathetic
      01DM
    Abducens 00DL
    Accessory 00DR
    Acoustic 00DN
    Brachial Plexus 01D3
    Cervical 01D1
    Cervical Plexus 01D0
    Facial 00DM
    Femoral 01DD
    Glossopharyngeal 00DP
    Head and Neck Sympathetic
      01DK
    Hypoglossal 00DS
    Lumbar 01DB
    Lumbar Plexus 01D9
    Lumbar Sympathetic 01DN
    Lumbosacral Plexus 01DA
    Median 01D5
    Oculomotor 00DH
    Olfactory 00DF
    Optic 00DG
    Peroneal 01DH
    Phrenic 01D2
    Pudendal 01DC
    Radial 01D6
    Sacral 01DR
    Sacral Plexus 01DQ
    Sacral Sympathetic 01DP
    Sciatic 01DF
    Thoracic 01D8
    Thoracic Sympathetic 01DL
    Tibial 01DG
    Trigeminal 00DK
    Trochlear 00DJ
    Ulnar 01D4
    Vagus 00DQ
  Ova 0UDN
  Pleura
    Left 0BDP
    Right 0BDN
  Products of Conception
    Classical 10D00Z0
    Ectopic 10D2
    Extraperitoneal 10D00Z2
    High Forceps 10D07Z5
    Internal Version 10D07Z7
    Low Cervical 10D00Z1
    Low Forceps 10D07Z3
    Mid Forceps 10D07Z4
    Other 10D07Z8
    Retained 10D1
    Vacuum 10D07Z6
  Septum, Nasal 09DM
  Sinus
    Accessory 09DP
    Ethmoid
      Left 09DV
      Right 09DU
    Frontal
      Left 09DT
      Right 09DS
    Mastoid
      Left 09DC
      Right 09DB
    Maxillary
      Left 09DR
      Right 09DQ
    Sphenoid
      Left 09DX
      Right 09DW
  Skin
    Abdomen 0HD7XZZ
    Back 0HD6XZZ
    Buttock 0HD8XZZ
    Chest 0HD5XZZ

Extraction *(Continued)*
  Skin *(Continued)*
    Ear
      Left 0HD3XZZ
      Right 0HD2XZZ
    Face 0HD1XZZ
    Foot
      Left 0HDNXZZ
      Right 0HDMXZZ
    Genitalia 0HDAXZZ
    Hand
      Left 0HDGXZZ
      Right 0HDFXZZ
    Lower Arm
      Left 0HDEXZZ
      Right 0HDDXZZ
    Lower Leg
      Left 0HDLXZZ
      Right 0HDKXZZ
    Neck 0HD4XZZ
    Perineum 0HD9XZZ
    Scalp 0HD0XZZ
    Upper Arm
      Left 0HDCXZZ
      Right 0HDBXZZ
    Upper Leg
      Left 0HDJXZZ
      Right 0HDHXZZ
  Spinal Meninges 00DT
  Subcutaneous Tissue and Fascia
    Abdomen 0JD8
    Back 0JD7
    Buttock 0JD9
    Chest 0JD6
    Face 0JD1

Extraction *(Continued)*
  Subcutaneous Tissue and Fascia *(Continued)*
    Foot
      Left 0JDR
      Right 0JDQ
    Hand
      Left 0JDK
      Right 0JDJ
    Lower Arm
      Left 0JDH
      Right 0JDG
    Lower Leg
      Left 0JDP
      Right 0JDN
    Neck
      Anterior 0JD4
      Posterior 0JD5
    Pelvic Region 0JDC
    Perineum 0JDB
    Scalp 0JD0
    Upper Arm
      Left 0JDF
      Right 0JDD
    Upper Leg
      Left 0JDM
      Right 0JDL
  Toe Nail 0HDRXZZ
  Tooth
    Lower 0CDXXZ
    Upper 0CDWXZ
  Turbinate, Nasal 09DL
  Tympanic Membrane
    Left 09D8
    Right 09D7

Extraction *(Continued)*
  Vein
    Basilic
      Left 05DC
      Right 05DB
    Brachial
      Left 05DA
      Right 05D9
    Cephalic
      Left 05DF
      Right 05DD
    Femoral
      Left 06DN
      Right 06DM
    Foot
      Left 06DV
      Right 06DT
    Greater Saphenous
      Left 06DQ
      Right 06DP
    Hand
      Left 05DH
      Right 05DG
    Lesser Saphenous
      Left 06DS
      Right 06DR
    Lower 06DY
    Upper 05DY
  Vocal Cord
    Left 0CDV
    Right 0CDT
Extradural space *use* Epidural Space
EXtreme Lateral Interbody Fusion (XLIF) device *use* Interbody Fusion Device in Lower Joints

F

Face lift *see* Alteration, Face 0W02
Facet replacement spinal stabilization device
  use Spinal Stabilization Device, Facet
    Replacement in 0RH
  use Spinal Stabilization Device, Facet
    Replacement in 0SH
Facial artery *use* Artery, Face
False vocal cord *use* Larynx
Falx cerebri *use* Dura Mater
Fascia lata
  use Subcutaneous Tissue and Fascia, Upper
    Leg, Left
  use Subcutaneous Tissue and Fascia, Upper
    Leg, Right
Fasciaplasty, fascioplasty
  see Repair, Subcutaneous Tissue and Fascia 0JQ
  see Replacement, Subcutaneous Tissue and
    Fascia 0JR
Fasciectomy
  see Excision, Subcutaneous Tissue and Fascia
    0JB
Fasciorrhaphy *see* Repair, Subcutaneous Tissue
  and Fascia 0JQ
Fasciotomy
  see Division, Subcutaneous Tissue and Fascia
    0J8
  see Drainage, Subcutaneous Tissue and Fascia
    0J9
Feeding Device
  Change device in
    Lower 0D2DXUZ
    Upper 0D20XUZ
  Insertion of device in
    Duodenum 0DH9
    Esophagus 0DH5
    Ileum 0DHB
    Intestine, Small 0DH8
    Jejunum 0DHA
    Stomach 0DH6
  Removal of device from
    Esophagus 0DP5
    Intestinal Tract
      Lower 0DPD
      Upper 0DP0
    Stomach 0DP6
  Revision of device in
    Intestinal Tract
      Lower 0DWD
      Upper 0DW0
    Stomach 0DW6
Femoral head
  use Femur, Upper, Right
  use Femur, Upper, Left
Femoral lymph node
  use Lymphatic, Lower Extremity, Left
  use Lymphatic, Lower Extremity, Right
Femoropatellar joint
  use Joint, Knee, Right
  use Joint, Knee, Right, Femoral Surface
  use Joint, Knee, Left
  use Joint, Knee, Left, Femoral Surface
Femorotibial joint
  use Joint, Knee, Right
  use Joint, Knee, Right, Tibial Surface
  use Joint, Knee, Left
  use Joint, Knee, Left, Tibial Surface
Fibular artery
  use Artery, Peroneal, Right
  use Artery, Peroneal, Left
Fibularis brevis muscle
  use Muscle, Lower Leg, Left
  use Muscle, Lower Leg, Right
Fibularis longus muscle
  use Muscle, Lower Leg, Left
  use Muscle, Lower Leg, Right
Fifth cranial nerve *use* Nerve, Trigeminal
Fimbriectomy
  see Excision, Female Reproductive System 0UB
  see Resection, Female Reproductive System
    0UT

First cranial nerve *use* Nerve, Olfactory
First intercostal nerve *use* Nerve, Brachial
  Plexus
Fistulization
  see Bypass
  see Drainage
  see Repair
Fitting
  Arch bars, for fracture reduction *see*
    Reposition, Mouth and Throat 0CS
  Arch bars, for immobilization *see*
    Immobilization, Face 2W31
  Artificial limb *see* Device Fitting,
    Rehabilitation F0D
  Hearing aid *see* Device Fitting, Rehabilitation
    F0D
  Ocular prosthesis F0DZ8UZ
  Prosthesis, limb *see* Device Fitting,
    Rehabilitation F0D
  Prosthesis, ocular F0DZ8UZ
Fixation, bone
  External, with fracture reduction *see* Reposition
  External, without fracture reduction *see*
    Insertion
  Internal, with fracture reduction *see*
    Reposition
  Internal, without fracture reduction *see*
    Insertion
FLAIR® Endovascular Stent Graft *use*
  Intraluminal Device
Flexible Composite Mesh *use* Synthetic
  Substitute
Flexor carpi radialis muscle
  use Muscle, Lower Arm and Wrist, Right
  use Muscle, Lower Arm and Wrist, Left
Flexor carpi ulnaris muscle
  use Muscle, Lower Arm and Wrist, Right
  use Muscle, Lower Arm and Wrist, Left
Flexor digitorum brevis muscle
  use Muscle, Foot, Left
  use Muscle, Foot, Right
Flexor digitorum longus muscle
  use Muscle, Lower Leg, Left
  use Muscle, Lower Leg, Right
Flexor hallucis brevis muscle
  use Muscle, Foot, Left
  use Muscle, Foot, Right
Flexor hallucis longus muscle
  use Muscle, Lower Leg, Right
  use Muscle, Lower Leg, Left
Flexor pollicis longus muscle
  use Muscle, Lower Arm and Wrist, Left
  use Muscle, Lower Arm and Wrist, Right
Fluoroscopy
  Abdomen and Pelvis BW11
  Airway, Upper BB1DZZZ
  Ankle
    Left BQ1H
    Right BQ1G
  Aorta
    Abdominal B410
      Laser, Intraoperative B410
    Thoracic B310
      Laser, Intraoperative B310
    Thoraco-Abdominal B31P
      Laser, Intraoperative B31P
  Aorta and Bilateral Lower Extremity Arteries
    B41D
    Laser, Intraoperative B41D
  Arm
    Left BP1FZZZ
    Right BP1EZZZ
  Artery
    Brachiocephalic-Subclavian
      Right B311
      Laser, Intraoperative B311
    Bronchial B31L
      Laser, Intraoperative B31L
    Bypass Graft, Other B21F
    Cervico-Cerebral Arch B31Q
      Laser, Intraoperative B31Q

Fluoroscopy *(Continued)*
  Artery *(Continued)*
    Common Carotid
      Bilateral B315
        Laser, Intraoperative B315
      Left B314
        Laser, Intraoperative B314
      Right B313
        Laser, Intraoperative B313
    Coronary
      Bypass Graft
        Multiple B213
          Laser, Intraoperative
            B213
        Single B212
          Laser, Intraoperative B212
      Multiple B211
        Laser, Intraoperative B211
      Single B210
        Laser, Intraoperative B210
    External Carotid
      Bilateral B31C
        Laser, Intraoperative B31C
      Left B31B
        Laser, Intraoperative B31B
      Right B319
        Laser, Intraoperative B319
    Hepatic B412
      Laser, Intraoperative B412
    Inferior Mesenteric B415
      Laser, Intraoperative B415
    Intercostal B31L
      Laser, Intraoperative B31L
    Internal Carotid
      Bilateral B318
        Laser, Intraoperative B318
      Left B317
        Laser, Intraoperative B317
      Right B316
        Laser, Intraoperative B316
    Internal Mammary Bypass Graft
      Left B218
      Right B217
    Intra-Abdominal
      Other B41B
      Laser, Intraoperative B41B
    Intracranial B31R
      Laser, Intraoperative B31R
    Lower
      Other B41J
      Laser, Intraoperative B41J
    Lower Extremity
      Bilateral and Aorta B41D
        Laser, Intraoperative B41D
      Left B41G
        Laser, Intraoperative B41G
      Right B41F
        Laser, Intraoperative B41F
    Lumbar B419
      Laser, Intraoperative B419
    Pelvic B41C
      Laser, Intraoperative B41C
    Pulmonary
      Left B31T
        Laser, Intraoperative B31T
      Right B31S
        Laser, Intraoperative B31S
    Renal
      Bilateral B418
        Laser, Intraoperative B418
      Left B417
        Laser, Intraoperative B417
      Right B416
        Laser, Intraoperative B416
    Spinal B31M
      Laser, Intraoperative B31M
    Splenic B413
      Laser, Intraoperative B413
    Subclavian, Left B312
      Left B312
      Laser, Intraoperative B312

◀ New   ◀ Revised   ~~deleted~~ Deleted

Fluoroscopy *(Continued)*
  Artery *(Continued)*
    Superior Mesenteric B414
      Laser, Intraoperative B414
    Upper
      Other B31N
      Laser, Intraoperative B31N
    Upper Extremity
      Bilateral B31K
        Laser, Intraoperative B31K
      Left B31J
        Laser, Intraoperative B31J
      Right B31H
        Laser, Intraoperative B31H
    Vertebral
      Bilateral B31G
        Laser, Intraoperative B31G
      Left B31F
        Laser, Intraoperative B31F
      Right B31D
        Laser, Intraoperative B31D
  Bile Duct BF10
    Pancreatic Duct and Gallbladder BF14
  Bile Duct and Gallbladder BF13
  Biliary Duct BF11
  Bladder BT10
    Kidney and Ureter BT14
      Left BT1F
      Right BT1D
  Bladder and Urethra BT1B
  Bowel, Small BD1
  Calcaneus
    Left BQ1KZZZ
    Right BQ1JZZZ
  Clavicle
    Left BP15ZZZ
    Right BP14ZZZ
  Coccyx BR1F
  Colon BD14
  Corpora Cavernosa BV10
  Dialysis Fistula B51W
  Dialysis Shunt B51W
  Diaphragm BB16ZZZ
  Disc
    Cervical BR11
    Lumbar BR13
    Thoracic BR12
  Duodenum BD19
  Elbow
    Left BP1H
    Right BP1G
  Epiglottis B91G
  Esophagus BD11
  Extremity
    Lower BW1C
    Upper BW1J
  Facet Joint
    Cervical BR14
    Lumbar BR16
    Thoracic BR15
  Fallopian Tube
    Bilateral BU12
    Left BU11
    Right BU10
  Fallopian Tube and Uterus BU18
  Femur
    Left BQ14ZZZ
    Right BQ13ZZZ
  Finger
    Left BP1SZZZ
    Right BP1RZZZ
  Foot
    Left BQ1MZZZ
    Right BQ1LZZZ
  Forearm
    Left BP1KZZZ
    Right BP1JZZZ
  Gallbladder BF12
    Bile Duct and Pancreatic Duct BF14
  Gallbladder and Bile Duct BF13
  Gastrointestinal, Upper BD1

Fluoroscopy *(Continued)*
  Hand
    Left BP1PZZZ
    Right BP1NZZZ
  Head and Neck BW19
  Heart
    Left B215
    Right B214
    Right and Left B216
  Hip
    Left BQ11
    Right BQ10
  Humerus
    Left BP1BZZZ
    Right BP1AZZZ
  Ileal Diversion Loop BT1C
  Ileal Loop, Ureters and Kidney BT1G
  Intracranial Sinus B512
  Joint
    Acromioclavicular, Bilateral BP13ZZZ
    Finger
      Left BP1D
      Right BP1C
    Foot
      Left BQ1Y
      Right BQ1X
    Hand
      Left BP1D
      Right BP1C
    Lumbosacral BR1B
    Sacroiliac BR1D
    Sternoclavicular
      Bilateral BP12ZZZ
      Left BP11ZZZ
      Right BP10ZZZ
    Temporomandibular
      Bilateral BN19
      Left BN18
      Right BN17
    Thoracolumbar BR18
    Toe
      Left BQ1Y
      Right BQ1X
  Kidney
    Bilateral BT13
    Ileal Loop and Ureter BT1G
    Left BT12
    Right BT11
    Ureter and Bladder BT14
      Left BT1F
      Right BT1D
  Knee
    Left BQ18
    Right BQ17
  Larynx B91J
  Leg
    Left BQ1FZZZ
    Right BQ1DZZZ
  Lung
    Bilateral BB14ZZZ
    Left BB13ZZZ
    Right BB12ZZZ
    Mediastinum BB1CZZZ
  Mouth BD1B
  Neck and Head BW19
  Oropharynx BD1B
  Pancreatic Duct BF1
    Gallbladder and Bile Buct BF14
  Patella
    Left BQ1WZZZ
    Right BQ1VZZZ
  Pelvis BR1C
  Pelvis and Abdomen BW11
  Pharynix B91G
  Ribs
    Left BP1YZZZ
    Right BP1XZZZ
  Sacrum BR1F
  Scapula
    Left BP17ZZZ
    Right BP16ZZZ

Fluoroscopy *(Continued)*
  Shoulder
    Left BP19
    Right BP18
  Sinus, Intracranial B512
  Spinal Cord B01B
  Spine
    Cervical BR10
    Lumbar BR19
    Thoracic BR17
    Whole BR1G
  Sternum BR1H
  Stomach BD12
  Toe
    Left BQ1QZZZ
    Right BQ1PZZZ
  Tracheobronchial Tree
    Bilateral BB19YZZ
    Left BB18YZZ
    Right BB17YZZ
  Ureter
    Ileal Loop and Kidney BT1G
    Kidney and Bladder BT14
      Left BT1F
      Right BT1D
    Left BT17
    Right BT16
  Urethra BT15
  Urethra and Bladder BT1B
  Uterus BU16
  Uterus and Fallopian Tube BU18
  Vagina BU19
  Vasa Vasorum BV18
  Vein
    Cerebellar B511
    Cerebral B511
    Epidural B510
    Jugular
      Bilateral B515
      Left B514
      Right B513
    Lower Extremity
      Bilateral B51D
      Left B51C
      Right B51B
    Other B51V
    Pelvic (Iliac)
      Left B51G
      Right B51F
    Pelvic (Iliac) Bilateral B51H
    Portal B51T
    Pulmonary
      Bilateral B51S
      Left B51R
      Right B51Q
    Renal
      Bilateral B51L
      Left B51K
      Right B51J
    Spanchnic B51T
    Subclavian
      Left B517
      Right B516
    Upper Extremity
      Bilateral B51P
      Left B51N
      Right B51M
  Vena Cava
    Inferior B519
    Superior B518
  Wrist
    Left BP1M
    Right BP1L
Flushing *see* Irrigation
Foley catheter *use* Drainage Device
Foramen magnum
  use Bone, Occipital, Right
  use Bone, Occipital, Left
Foramen of Monro (intraventricular) *use*
  Cerebral Ventricle
Foreskin *use* Prepuce

Formula™ Balloon-Expandable Renal Stent System *use* Intraluminal Device
Fossa of Rosenmuller *use* Nasopharynx
Fourth cranial nerve *use* Nerve, Trochlear
Fourth ventricle *use* Cerebral Ventricle
Fovea
  use Retina, Right
  use Retina, Left
Fragmentation
  Ampulla of Vater 0FFC
  Anus 0DFQ
  Appendix 0DFJ
  Bladder 0TFB
  Bladder Neck 0TFC
  Bronchus
    Lingula 0BF9
    Lower Lobe
      Left 0BFB
      Right 0BF6
    Main
      Left 0BF7
      Right 0BF3
    Middle Lobe, Right 0BF5
    Upper Lobe
      Left 0BF8
      Right 0BF4
  Carina 0BF2
  Cavity, Cranial 0WF1
  Cecum 0DFH
  Cerebral Ventricle 00F6
  Colon
    Ascending 0DFK
    Descending 0DFM
    Sigmoid 0DFN
    Transverse 0DFL
  Duct
    Common Bile 0FF9
    Cystic 0FF8
    Hepatic
      Left 0FF6
      Right 0FF5
    Pancreatic 0FFD
      Accessory 0FFF
    Parotid
      Left 0CFC
      Right 0CFB
  Duodenum 0DF9
  Epidural Space 00F3
  Esophagus 0DF5
  Fallopian Tube
    Left 0UF6
    Right 0UF5
  Fallopian Tubes, Bilateral 0UF7
  Gallbladder 0FF4
  Gastrointestinal Tract 0WFP
  Genitourinary Tract 0WFR
  Ileum 0DFB
  Intestine
    Large 0DFE
      Left 0DFG
      Right 0DFF
    Small 0DF8
  Jejunum 0DFA
  Kidney Pelvis
    Left 0TF4
    Right 0TF3

Fragmentation *(Continued)*
  Mediastinum 0WFC
  Oral Cavity and Throat 0WF3
  Pelvic Cavity 0WFJ
  Pericardial Cavity 0WFD
  Pericardium 02FN
  Peritoneal Cavity 0WFG
  Pleural Cavity
    Left 0WFB
    Right 0WF9
  Rectum 0DFP
  Respiratory Tract 0WFQ
  Spinal Canal 00FU
  Stomach 0DF6
  Subarachnoid Space 00F5
  Subdural Space 00F4
  Trachea 0BF1
  Ureter
    Left 0TF7
    Right 0TF6
  Urethra 0TFD
  Uterus 0UF9
  Vitreous
    Left 08F5
    Right 08F4
Freestyle (Stentless) Aortic Root Bioprosthesis *use* Zooplastic Tissue in Heart and Great Vessels
Frenectomy
  see Excision, Mouth and Throat 0CB
  see Resection, Mouth and Throat 0CT
Frenoplasty, frenuloplasty
  see Repair, Mouth and Throat 0CQ
  see Replacement, Mouth and Throat 0CR
  see Supplement, Mouth and Throat 0CU
Frenotomy
  see Drainage, Mouth and Throat 0C9
  see Release, Mouth and Throat 0CN
Frenulotomy
  see Drainage, Mouth and Throat 0C9
  see Release, Mouth and Throat 0CN
Frenulum labii inferioris *use* Lip, Lower
Frenulum labii superioris *use* Lip, Upper
Frenulum linguae *use* Tongue
Frenulumectomy
  see Excision, Mouth and Throat 0CB
  see Resection, Mouth and Throat 0CT
Frontal lobe *use* Cerebral Hemisphere
Frontal vein
  use Vein, Face, Right
  use Vein, Face, Left
Fulguration *see* Destruction
Fundoplication, gastroesophageal *see* Restriction, Esophagogastric Junction 0DV4
Fundus uteri *use* Uterus
Fusion
  Acromioclavicular
    Left 0RGH
    Right 0RGG
  Ankle
    Left 0SGG
    Right 0SGF

Fusion *(Continued)*
  Carpal
    Left 0RGR
    Right 0RGQ
  Cervical Vertebral 0RG1
    2 or more 0RG2
  Cervicothoracic Vertebral 0RG4
  Coccygeal 0SG6
  Elbow
    Left 0RGM
    Right 0RGL
  Finger Phalangeal
    Left 0RGX
    Right 0RGW
  Hip
    Left 0SGB
    Right 0SG9
  Knee
    Left 0SGD
    Right 0SGC
  Lumbar Vertebral 0SG0
    2 or more 0SG1
  Lumbosacral 0SG3
  Metacarpocarpal
    Left 0RGT
    Right 0RGS
  Metacarpophalangeal
    Left 0RGV
    Right 0RGU
  Metatarsal-Phalangeal
    Left 0SGN
    Right 0SGM
  Metatarsal-Tarsal
    Left 0SGL
    Right 0SGK
  Occipital-cervical 0RG0
  Sacrococcygeal 0SG5
  Sacroiliac
    Left 0SG8
    Right 0SG7
  Shoulder
    Left 0RGK
    Right 0RGJ
  Sternoclavicular
    Left 0RGF
    Right 0RGE
  Tarsal
    Left 0SGJ
    Right 0SGH
  Temporomandibular
    Left 0RGD
    Right 0RGC
  Thoracic Vertebral 0RG6
    2 to 7 0RG7
    8 or more 0RG8
  Thoracolumbar Vertebral 0RGA
  Toe Phalangeal
    Left 0SGQ
    Right 0SGP
  Wrist
    Left 0RGP
    Right 0RGN
Fusion screw (compression) (lag) (locking)
  use Internal Fixation Device in Upper Joints
  use Internal Fixation Device in Lower Joints

◀ New   ◀▥ Revised   ~~deleted~~ Deleted

G

Gait training *see* Motor Treatment, Rehabilitation F07

Galea aponeurotica *use* Subcutaneous Tissue and Fascia, Scalp

Ganglion impar (ganglion of Walther) *use* Nerve, Sacral Sympathetic

Ganglionectomy
Destruction of lesion *see* Destruction
Excision of lesion *see* Excision

Gasserian ganglion *use* Nerve, Trigeminal

Gastrectomy
Partial *see* Excision, Stomach 0DB6
Total *see* Resection, Stomach 0DT6
Vertical (sleeve) *see* Excision, Stomach 0DB6

Gastric electrical stimulation (GES) lead *use* Stimulator Lead in Gastrointestinal System

Gastric lymph node *use* Lymphatic, Aortic

Gastric pacemaker lead *use* Stimulator Lead in Gastrointestinal System

Gastric plexus *see* Nerve, Abdominal Sympathetic

Gastrocnemius muscle
use Muscle, Lower Leg, Left
use Muscle, Lower Leg, Right

Gastrocolic ligament *use* Omentum, Greater

Gastrocolic omentum *use* Omentum, Greater

Gastrocolostomy
see Bypass, Gastrointestinal System 0D1
see Drainage, Gastrointestinal System 0D9

Gastroduodenal artery *use* Artery, Hepatic

Gastroduodenectomy
see Excision, Gastrointestinal System 0DB
see Resection, Gastrointestinal System 0DT

Gastroduodenoscopy 0DJ08ZZ

Gastroenteroplasty
see Repair, Gastrointestinal System 0DQ
see Supplement, Gastrointestinal System 0DU

Gastroenterostomy
see Bypass, Gastrointestinal System 0D1
see Drainage, Gastrointestinal System 0D9

Gastroesophageal (GE) junction *use* Esophagogastric Junction

Gastrogastrostomy
see Bypass, Stomach 0D16
see Drainage, Stomach 0D96

Gastrohepatic omentum *use* Omentum, Lesser

Gastrojejunostomy
see Bypass, Stomach 0D16
see Drainage, Stomach 0D96

Gastrolysis *see* Release, Stomach 0DN6

Gastropexy
see Repair, Stomach 0DQ6
see Reposition, Stomach 0DS6

Gastrophrenic ligament *use* Omentum, Greater

Gastroplasty
see Repair, Stomach 0DQ6
see Supplement, Stomach 0DU6

Gastroplication *see* Restriction, Stomach 0DV6

Gastropylorectomy *see* Excision, Gastrointestinal System 0DB

Gastrorrhaphy *see* Repair, Stomach 0DQ6

Gastroscopy 0DJ68ZZ

Gastrosplenic ligament *use* Omentum, Greater

Gastrostomy
see Bypass, Stomach 0D16
see Drainage, Stomach 0D96

Gastrotomy *see* Drainage, Stomach 0D96

Gemellus muscle
use Muscle, Hip, Left
use Muscle, Hip, Right

Geniculate ganglion *use* Nerve, Facial

Geniculate nucleus *use* Thalamus

Genioglossus muscle *use* Muscle, Tongue, Palate, Pharynx

Genioplasty *see* Alteration, Jaw, Lower 0W05

Genitofemoral nerve *use* Nerve, Lumbar Plexus

Gingivectomy *see* Excision, Mouth and Throat 0CB

Gingivoplasty
see Repair, Mouth and Throat 0CQ
see Replacement, Mouth and Throat 0CR
see Supplement, Mouth and Throat 0CU

Glans penis *use* Prepuce

Glenohumeral joint
use Joint, Shoulder, Left
use Joint, Shoulder, Right

Glenohumeral ligament
use Bursa and Ligament, Shoulder, Right
use Bursa and Ligament, Shoulder, Left

Glenoid fossa (of scapula)
use Glenoid Cavity, Left
use Glenoid Cavity, Right

Glenoid ligament (labrum)
use Bursa and Ligament, Shoulder, Right
use Bursa and Ligament, Shoulder, Left

Globus pallidus *use* Basal Ganglia

Glomectomy
see Excision, Endocrine System 0GB
see Resection, Endocrine System 0GT

Glossectomy
see Excision, Tongue 0CB7
see Resection, Tongue 0CT7

Glossoepiglottic fold *use* Epiglottis

Glossopexy
see Repair, Tongue 0CQ7
see Reposition, Tongue 0CS7

Glossoplasty
see Repair, Tongue 0CQ7
see Replacement, Tongue 0CR7
see Supplement, Tongue 0CU7

Glossorrhaphy *see* Repair, Tongue 0CQ7

Glossotomy *see* Drainage, Tongue 0C97

Glottis *use* Larynx

Gluteal Artery Perforator Flap
Bilateral 0HRV079
Left 0HRU079
Right 0HRT079

Gluteal lymph node *use* Lymphatic, Pelvis

Gluteal vein
use Vein, Hypogastric, Right
use Vein, Hypogastric, Left

Gluteus maximus muscle
use Muscle, Hip, Right
use Muscle, Hip, Left

Gluteus medius muscle
use Muscle, Hip, Right
use Muscle, Hip, Left

Gluteus minimus muscle
use Muscle, Hip, Left
use Muscle, Hip, Right

GORE® DUALMESH® *use* Synthetic Substitute

Gracilis muscle
use Muscle, Upper Leg, Left
use Muscle, Upper Leg, Right

Graft
see Replacement
see Supplement

Great auricular nerve *use* Nerve, Lumbar Plexus

Great cerebral vein *use* Vein, Intracranial

Great saphenous vein
use Vein, Greater Saphenous, Left
use Vein, Greater Saphenous, Right

Greater alar cartilage *use* Nose

Greater occipital nerve *use* Nerve, Cervical

Greater splanchnic nerve *use* Nerve, Thoracic Sympathetic

Greater superficial petrosal nerve *use* Nerve, Facial

Greater trochanter
use Femur, Upper, Left
use Femur, Upper, Right

Greater tuberosity
use Humeral Head, Right
use Humeral Head, Left

Greater vestibular (Bartholin's) gland
use Gland, Vestibular

Greater wing
use Bone, Sphenoid, Left
use Bone, Sphenoid, Right

Guedel airway *use* Intraluminal Device, Airway in Mouth and Throat

Guidance, catheter placement
EKG *see* Measurement, Physiological Systems 4A0
Fluoroscopy *see* Fluoroscopy, Veins B51
Ultrasound *see* Ultrasonography, Veins B54

H

Hallux
  use Toe, 1st, Right
  use Toe, 1st, Left
Hamate bone
  use Carpal, Right
  use Carpal, Left
Hancock Bioprosthesis (aortic) (mitral) valve
  use Zooplastic Tissue in Heart and Great
  Vessels
Hancock Bioprosthetic Valved Conduit *use*
  Zooplastic Tissue in Heart and Great
  Vessels
Harvesting, stem cells *see* Pheresis, Circulatory
  6A55
Head of fibula
  use Fibula, Right
  use Fibula, Left
Hearing Aid Assessment F14Z
Hearing Assessment F13Z
Hearing Device
  Bone Conduction
    Left 09HE
    Right 09HD
  Insertion of device in
    Left 0NH6[034]SZ
    Right 0NH5[034]SZ
  Multiple Channel Cochlear Prosthesis
    Left 09HE
    Right 09HD
  Removal of device from, Skull 0NP0
  Revision of device in, Skull 0NW0
  Single Channel Cochlear Prosthesis
    Left 09HE
    Right 09HD
Hearing Treatment F09Z
Heart Assist System
  External
    Insertion of device in, Heart
      02HA
    Removal of device from, Heart
      02PA
    Revision of device in, Heart
      02WA
  Implantable
    Insertion of device in, Heart
      02HA
    Removal of device from, Heart
      02PA
    Revision of device in, Heart
      02WA
HeartMate II® Left Ventricular Assist
  Device (LVAD) *use* Implantable Heart
  Assist System in Heart and Great
  Vessels
HeartMate XVE® Left Ventricular Assist
  Device (LVAD) *use* Implantable Heart
  Assist System in Heart and Great
  Vessels
HeartMate® implantable heart assist system
  see Insertion of device in, Heart 02HA
Helix
  use Ear, External, Bilateral
  use Ear, External, Right
  use Ear, External, Left
Hemicolectomy *see* Resection, Gastrointestinal
  System 0DT
Hemicystectomy *see* Excision, Urinary System
  0TB
Hemigastrectomy *see* Excision, Gastrointestinal
  System 0DB
Hemiglossectomy *see* Excision, Mouth and
  Throat 0CB
Hemilaminectomy
  see Excision, Upper Bones 0PB
  see Excision, Lower Bones 0QB
  see Release, Central Nervous System 00N ◄
  see Release, Peripheral Nervous System
    01N ◄
  see Drainage, Upper Bones 0P9 ◄

Hemilaminectomy *(Continued)*
  see Release, Upper Bones 0PN ◄
  see Drainage, Lower Bones 0Q9 ◄
  see Release, Lower Bones 0QN ◄
Hemilaryngectomy *see* Excision, Larynx
  0CBS
Hemimandibulectomy *see* Excision, Head and
  Facial Bones 0NB
Hemimaxillectomy *see* Excision, Head and
  Facial Bones 0NB
Hemipylorectomy *see* Excision, Gastrointestinal
  System 0DB
Hemispherectomy
  see Excision, Central Nervous System
    00B
  see Resection, Central Nervous System
    00T
Hemithyroidectomy
  see Resection, Endocrine System 0GT
  see Excision, Endocrine System 0GB
Hemodialysis 5A1D00Z
Hepatectomy
  see Excision, Hepatobiliary System and
    Pancreas 0FB
  see Resection, Hepatobiliary System and
    Pancreas 0FT
Hepatic artery proper *use* Artery,
  Hepatic
Hepatic flexure *use* Colon, Ascending
Hepatic lymph node *use* Lymphatic,
  Aortic
Hepatic plexus *use* Nerve, Abdominal
  Sympathetic
Hepatic portal vein *use* Vein, Portal
Hepaticoduodenostomy
  see Bypass, Hepatobiliary System and
    Pancreas 0F1
  see Drainage, Hepatobiliary System and
    Pancreas 0F9
Hepaticotomy *see* Drainage, Hepatobiliary
  System and Pancreas 0F9
Hepatocholedochostomy *see* Drainage, Duct,
  Common Bile 0F99
Hepatogastric ligament *use* Omentum,
  Lesser
Hepatopancreatic ampulla *use* Ampulla of
  Vater
Hepatopexy
  see Repair, Hepatobiliary System and
    Pancreas 0FQ
  see Reposition, Hepatobiliary System and
    Pancreas 0FS
Hepatorrhaphy *see* Repair, Hepatobiliary
  System and Pancreas 0FQ
Hepatotomy *see* Drainage, Hepatobiliary
  System and Pancreas 0F9
Herculink (RX) Elite Renal Stent System *use*
  Intraluminal Device ◄
Herniorrhaphy
  see Repair, Anatomical Regions, General
    0WQ
  see Repair, Anatomical Regions, Lower
    Extremities 0YQ
  with synthetic substitute
    see Supplement, Anatomical Regions,
      General 0WU
    see Supplement, Anatomical Regions,
      Lower Extremities 0YU
Hip (joint) liner *use* Liner in Lower Joints
Holter monitoring 4A12X45
Holter valve ventricular shunt *use* Synthetic
  Substitute
Humeroradial joint
  use Joint, Elbow, Right
  use Joint, Elbow, Left
Humeroulnar joint
  use Joint, Elbow, Left
  use Joint, Elbow, Right
Humerus, distal
  use Humeral Shaft, Right
  use Humeral Shaft, Left

Hydrocelectomy *see* Excision, Male
  Reproductive System 0VB
Hydrotherapy
  Assisted exercise in pool *see* Motor Treatment,
    Rehabilitation F07
  Whirlpool *see* Activities of Daily Living
    Treatment, Rehabilitation F08
Hymenectomy
  see Excision, Hymen 0UBK
  see Resection, Hymen 0UTK
Hymenoplasty
  see Repair, Hymen 0UQK
  see Supplement, Hymen 0UUK
Hymenorrhaphy *see* Repair, Hymen 0UQK
Hymenotomy
  see Division, Hymen 0U8K
  see Drainage, Hymen 0U9K
Hyoglossus muscle *use* Muscle, Tongue, Palate,
  Pharynx
Hyoid artery
  use Artery, Thyroid, Right
  use Artery, Thyroid, Left
Hyperalimentation *see* Introduction of
  substance in or on
Hyperbaric oxygenation
  Decompression sickness treatment *see*
    Decompression, Circulatory 6A15
  Wound treatment *see* Assistance, Circulatory
    5A05
Hyperthermia
  Radiation Therapy
    Abdomen DWY38ZZ
    Adrenal Gland DGY28ZZ
    Bile Ducts DFY28ZZ
    Bladder DTY28ZZ
    Bone, Other DPYC8ZZ
    Bone Marrow D7Y08ZZ
    Brain D0Y08ZZ
    Brain Stem D0Y18ZZ
    Breast
      Left DMY08ZZ
      Right DMY18ZZ
    Bronchus DBY18ZZ
    Cervix DUY18ZZ
    Chest DWY28ZZ
    Chest Wall DBY78ZZ
    Colon DDY58ZZ
    Diaphragm DBY88ZZ
    Duodenum DDY28ZZ
    Ear D9Y08ZZ
    Esophagus DDY08ZZ
    Eye D8Y08ZZ
    Femur DPY98ZZ
    Fibula DPYB8ZZ
    Gallbladder DFY18ZZ
    Gland
      Adrenal DGY28ZZ
      Parathyroid DGY48ZZ
      Pituitary DGY08ZZ
      Thyroid DGY58ZZ
    Glands, Salivary D9Y68ZZ
    Head and Neck DWY18ZZ
    Hemibody DWY48ZZ
    Humerus DPY68ZZ
    Hypopharynx D9Y38ZZ
    Ileum DDY48ZZ
    Jejunum DDY38ZZ
    Kidney DTY08ZZ
    Larynx D9YB8ZZ
    Liver DFY08ZZ
    Lung DBY28ZZ
    Lymphatics
      Abdomen D7Y68ZZ
      Axillary D7Y48ZZ
      Inguinal D7Y88ZZ
      Neck D7Y38ZZ
      Pelvis D7Y78ZZ
      Thorax D7Y58ZZ
    Mandible DPY38ZZ
    Maxilla DPY28ZZ
    Mediastinum DBY68ZZ

◄ New   ◄▦ Revised   ~~deleted~~ Deleted

Hyperthermia *(Continued)*
  Radiation Therapy *(Continued)*
    Mouth D9Y48ZZ
    Nasopharynx D9YD8ZZ
    Neck and Head DWY18ZZ
    Nerve, Peripheral D0Y78ZZ
    Nose D9Y18ZZ
    Oropharynx D9YF8ZZ
    Ovary DUY08ZZ
    Palate
      Hard D9Y88ZZ
      Soft D9Y98ZZ
    Pancreas DFY38ZZ
    Parathyroid Gland DGY48ZZ
    Pelvic Bones DPY88ZZ
    Pelvic Region DWY68ZZ
    Pineal Body DGY18ZZ
    Pituitary Gland DGY08ZZ
    Pleura DBY58ZZ
    Prostate DVY08ZZ
    Radius DPY78ZZ
    Rectum DDY78ZZ
    Rib DPY58ZZ
    Sinuses D9Y78ZZ
    Skin
      Abdomen DHY88ZZ
      Arm DHY48ZZ
      Back DHY78ZZ
      Buttock DHY98ZZ

Hyperthermia *(Continued)*
  Radiation Therapy *(Continued)*
    Skin *(Continued)*
      Chest DHY68ZZ
      Face DHY28ZZ
      Leg DHYB8ZZ
      Neck DHY38ZZ
    Skull DPY08ZZ
    Spinal Cord D0Y68ZZ
    Spleen D7Y28ZZ
    Sternum DPY48ZZ
    Stomach DDY18ZZ
    Testis DVY18ZZ
    Thymus D7Y18ZZ
    Thyroid Gland DGY58ZZ
    Tibia DPYB8ZZ
    Tongue D9Y58ZZ
    Trachea DBY08ZZ
    Ulna DPY78ZZ
    Ureter DTY18ZZ
    Urethra DTY38ZZ
    Uterus DUY28ZZ
    Whole Body DWY58ZZ
    Whole Body 6A3Z
Hypnosis GZFZZZZ
Hypogastric artery
  use Artery, Internal Iliac, Right
  use Artery, Internal Iliac, Left
Hypopharynx *use* Pharynx

Hypophysectomy
  see Excision, Gland, Pituitary 0GB0
  see Resection, Gland, Pituitary 0GT0
Hypophysis *use* Gland, Pituitary
Hypothalamotomy *see* Destruction, Thalamus 0059
Hypothenar muscle
  use Muscle, Hand, Right
  use Muscle, Hand, Left
Hypothermia, Whole Body 6A4Z
Hysterectomy
  see Excision, Uterus 0UB9
  see Resection, Uterus 0UT9
Hysterolysis *see* Release, Uterus 0UN9
Hysteropexy
  see Repair, Uterus 0UQ9
  see Reposition, Uterus 0US9
Hysteroplasty
  see Repair, Uterus 0UQ9
Hysterorrhaphy *see* Repair, Uterus 0UQ9
Hysteroscopy 0UJD8ZZ
Hysterotomy
  see Drainage, Uterus 0U99
Hysterotrachelectomy *see* Resection, Uterus 0UT9
Hysterotracheloplasty
  see Repair, Uterus 0UQ9
Hysterotrachelorrhaphy *see* Repair, Uterus 0UQ9

I

IABP (Intra-aortic balloon pump) *see*
Assistance, Cardiac 5A02
**IAEMT (Intraoperative anesthetic effect
monitoring and titration)** *see* Monitoring,
Central Nervous 4A10
Ileal artery *use* Artery, Superior Mesenteric
Ileectomy
see Excision, Ileum 0DBB
see Resection, Ileum 0DTB
Ileocolic artery *use* Artery, Superior Mesenteric
Ileocolic vein *use* Vein, Colic
Ileopexy
see Repair, Ileum 0DQB
see Reposition, Ileum 0DSB
Ileorrhaphy *see* Repair, Ileum 0DQB
Ileoscopy 0DJD8ZZ
Ileostomy
see Bypass, Ileum 0D1B
see Drainage, Ileum 0D9B
Ileotomy *see* Drainage, Ileum 0D9B
Ileoureterostomy *see* Bypass, Bladder 0T1B
Iliac crest
use Bone, Pelvic, Left
use Bone, Pelvic, Right
Iliac fascia
use Subcutaneous Tissue and Fascia, Upper
Leg, Left
use Subcutaneous Tissue and Fascia, Upper
Leg, Right
Iliac lymph node *use* Lymphatic, Pelvis
Iliacus muscle
use Muscle, Hip, Right
use Muscle, Hip, Left
Iliofemoral ligament
use Bursa and Ligament, Hip, Left
use Bursa and Ligament, Hip, Right
Iliohypogastric nerve *use* Nerve, Lumbar
Plexus
Ilioinguinal nerve *use* Nerve, Lumbar Plexus
Iliolumbar artery
use Artery, Internal Iliac, Left
use Artery, Internal Iliac, Right
Iliolumbar ligament
use Bursa and Ligament, Trunk, Left
use Bursa and Ligament, Trunk, Right
Iliotibial tract (band)
use Subcutaneous Tissue and Fascia, Upper
Leg, Right
use Subcutaneous Tissue and Fascia, Upper
Leg, Left
Ilium
use Bone, Pelvic, Left
use Bone, Pelvic, Right
Ilizarov external fixator
use External Fixation Device, Ring in 0PH
use External Fixation Device, Ring in 0PS
use External Fixation Device, Ring in 0QH
use External Fixation Device, Ring in 0QS
Ilizarov-Vecklich device
use External Fixation Device, Limb
Lengthening in 0PH
use External Fixation Device, Limb
Lengthening in 0QH
Imaging, diagnostic
see Plain Radiography
see Fluoroscopy
see Computerized Tomography (CT Scan)
see Magnetic Resonance Imaging (MRI)
see Ultrasonography
Immobilization
Abdominal Wall 2W33X
Arm
Lower
Left 2W3DX
Right 2W3CX
Upper
Left 2W3BX
Right 2W3AX
Back 2W35X

Immobilization *(Continued)*
Chest Wall 2W34X
Extremity
Lower
Left 2W3MX
Right 2W3LX
Upper
Left 2W39X
Right 2W38X
Face 2W31X
Finger
Left 2W3KX
Right 2W3JX
Foot
Left 2W3TX
Right 2W3SX
Hand
Left 2W3FX
Right 2W3EX
Head 2W30X
Inguinal Region
Left 2W37X
Right 2W36X
Leg
Lower
Left 2W3RX
Right 2W3QX
Upper
Left 2W3PX
Right 2W3NX
Neck 2W32X
Thumb
Left 2W3HX
Right 2W3GX
Toe
Left 2W3VX
Right 2W3UX
Immunization *see* Introduction of Serum,
Toxoid, and Vaccine
Immunotherapy *see* Introduction of
Immunotherapeutic Substance
Immunotherapy, antineoplastic
Interferon *see* Introduction of Low-dose
Interleukin-2
Interleukin-2 of high-dose *see* Introduction,
High-dose Interleukin-2
Interleukin-2, low-dose *see* Introduction of
Low-dose Interleukin-2
Monoclonal antibody *see* Introduction of
Monoclonal Antibody
Proleukin, high-dose *see* Introduction of
High-dose Interleukin-2
Proleukin, low-dose *see* Introduction of Low-
dose Interleukin-2
~~Impella® (2.5)(5.0)(LD) cardiac assist device use
Intraluminal Device~~
Impeller Pump
Continuous, Output 5A0221D
Intermittent, Output 5A0211D
Implantable cardioverter-defibrillator (ICD)
use Defibrillator Generator in 0JH
**Implantable drug infusion pump (anti-
spasmodic) (chemotherapy) (pain)** *use*
Infusion Device, Pump in Subcutaneous
Tissue and Fascia
Implantable glucose monitoring device *use*
Monitoring Device
Implantable hemodynamic monitor (IHM) *use*
Monitoring Device, Hemodynamic in 0JH
**Implantable hemodynamic monitoring
system (IHMS)** *use* Monitoring Device,
Hemodynamic in 0JH
Implantable Miniature Telescope™ (IMT) use
Synthetic Substitute, Intraocular Telescope
in 08R
Implantation
see Insertion
see Replacement
Implanted (venous) (access) port *use* Vascular
Access Device, Reservoir in Subcutaneous
Tissue and Fascia
IMV (intermittent mandatory ventilation) *see*
Assistance, Respiratory 5A09

In Vitro Fertilization 8E0ZXY1
Incision, abscess *see* Drainage
Incudectomy
see Excision, Ear, Nose, Sinus 09B
see Resection, Ear, Nose, Sinus 09T
Incudopexy
see Reposition, Ear, Nose, Sinus 09S
see Repair, Ear, Nose, Sinus 09Q
Incus
use Ossicle, Auditory, Left
use Ossicle, Auditory, Right
Induction of labor
Artificial rupture of membranes *see* Drainage,
Pregnancy 109
Oxytocin *see* Introduction of Hormone
InDura, intrathecal catheter (1P) (spinal) *use*
Infusion Device
Inferior cardiac nerve *use* Nerve, Thoracic
Sympathetic
Inferior cerebellar vein *use* Vein, Intracranial
Inferior cerebral vein *use* Vein, Intracranial
Inferior epigastric artery
use Artery, External Iliac, Right
use Artery, External Iliac, Left
Inferior epigastric lymph node *use* Lymphatic,
Pelvis
Inferior genicular artery
use Artery, Popliteal, Left
use Artery, Popliteal, Right
Inferior gluteal artery
use Artery, Internal Iliac, Right
use Artery, Internal Iliac, Left
Inferior gluteal nerve *use* Nerve, Sacral Plexus
Inferior hypogastric plexus *use* Nerve,
Abdominal Sympathetic
Inferior labial artery *use* Artery, Face
Inferior longitudinal muscle *use* Muscle,
Tongue, Palate, Pharynx
Inferior mesenteric ganglion *use* Nerve,
Abdominal Sympathetic
Inferior mesenteric lymph node *use* Lymphatic,
Mesenteric
Inferior mesenteric plexus *use* Nerve,
Abdominal Sympathetic
Inferior oblique muscle
use Muscle, Extraocular, Right
use Muscle, Extraocular, Left
Inferior pancreaticoduodenal artery *use* Artery,
Superior Mesenteric
Inferior phrenic artery *use* Aorta, Abdominal
Inferior rectus muscle
use Muscle, Extraocular, Right
use Muscle, Extraocular, Left
Inferior suprarenal artery
use Artery, Renal, Left
use Artery, Renal, Right
Inferior tarsal plate
use Eyelid, Lower, Right
use Eyelid, Lower, Left
Inferior thyroid vein
use Vein, Innominate, Left
use Vein, Innominate, Right
Inferior tibiofibular joint
use Joint, Ankle, Right
use Joint, Ankle, Left
Inferior turbinate *use* Turbinate, Nasal
Inferior ulnar collateral artery
use Artery, Brachial, Right
use Artery, Brachial, Left
Inferior vesical artery
use Artery, Internal Iliac, Right
use Artery, Internal Iliac, Left
Infraauricular lymph node *use* Lymphatic,
Head
Infraclavicular (deltopectoral) lymph node
use Lymphatic, Upper Extremity, Left
use Lymphatic, Upper Extremity, Right
Infrahyoid muscle
use Muscle, Neck, Left
use Muscle, Neck, Right
Infraparotid lymph node *use* Lymphatic, Head

◀ New   ◀▥ Revised   ~~deleted~~ Deleted

Insertion of device in (Continued)

Bone (Continued)
  Temporal
    Left 0NH6
    Right 0NH5
  Upper 0PHY
  Zygomatic
    Left 0NHN
    Right 0NHM
Brain 00H0
Breast
  Bilateral 0HHV
  Left 0HHU
  Right 0HHT
Bronchus
  Lingula 0BH9
  Lower Lobe
    Left 0BHB
    Right 0BH6
  Main
    Left 0BH7
    Right 0BH3
  Middle Lobe, Right 0BH5
  Upper Lobe
    Left 0BH8
    Right 0BH4
Buttock
  Left 0YH1
  Right 0YH0
Carpal
  Left 0PHN
  Right 0PHM
Cavity, Cranial 0WH1
Cerebral Ventricle 00H6
Cervix 0UHC
Chest Wall 0WH8
Cisterna Chyli 07HL
Clavicle
  Left 0PHB
  Right 0PH9
Coccyx 0QHS
Cul-de-sac 0UHF
Diaphragm
  Left 0BHS
  Right 0BHR
Disc
  Cervical Vertebral 0RH3
  Cervicothoracic Vertebral 0RH5
  Lumbar Vertebral 0SH2
  Lumbosacral 0SH4
  Thoracic Vertebral 0RH9
  Thoracolumbar Vertebral 0RHB
Duct
  Hepatobiliary 0FHB
  Pancreatic 0FHD
Duodenum 0DH9
Ear
  Left 09HE
  Right 09HD
Elbow Region
  Left 0XHC
  Right 0XHB
Epididymis and Spermatic Cord 0VHM
Esophagus 0DH5
Extremity
  Lower
    Left 0YHB
    Right 0YH9
  Upper
    Left 0XH7
    Right 0XH6
Eye
  Left 08H1
  Right 08H0
Face 0WH2
Fallopian Tube 0UH8
Femoral Region
  Left 0YH8
  Right 0YH7
Femoral Shaft
  Left 0QH9
  Right 0QH8

Insertion of device in (Continued)

Femur
  Lower
    Left 0QHC
    Right 0QHB
  Upper
    Left 0QH7
    Right 0QH6
Fibula
  Left 0QHK
  Right 0QHJ
Foot
  Left 0YHN
  Right 0YHM
Gallbladder 0FH4
Gastrointestinal Tract 0WHP
Genitourinary Tract 0WHR
Gland, Endocrine 0GHS
Glenoid Cavity
  Left 0PH8
  Right 0PH7
Hand
  Left 0XHK
  Right 0XHJ
Head 0WH0
Heart 02HA
Humeral Head
  Left 0PHD
  Right 0PHC
Humeral Shaft
  Left 0PHG
  Right 0PHF
Ileum 0DHB
Inguinal Region
  Left 0YH6
  Right 0YH5
Intestine
  Large 0DHE
  Small 0DH8
Jaw
  Lower 0WH5
  Upper 0WH4
Jejunum 0DHA
Joint
  Acromioclavicular
    Left 0RHH
    Right 0RHG
  Ankle
    Left 0SHG
    Right 0SHF
  Carpal
    Left 0RHR
    Right 0RHQ
  Cervical Vertebral 0RH1
  Cervicothoracic Vertebral 0RH4
  Coccygeal 0SH6
  Elbow
    Left 0RHM
    Right 0RHL
  Finger Phalangeal
    Left 0RHX
    Right 0RHW
  Hip
    Left 0SHB
    Right 0SH9
  Knee
    Left 0SHD
    Right 0SHC
  Lumbar Vertebral 0SH0
  Lumbosacral 0SH3
  Metacarpocarpal
    Left 0RHT
    Right 0RHS
  Metacarpophalangeal
    Left 0RHV
    Right 0RHU
  Metatarsal-Phalangeal
    Left 0SHN
    Right 0SHM
  Metatarsal-Tarsal
    Left 0SHL
    Right 0SHK

Insertion of device in (Continued)

Joint (Continued)
  Occipital-cervical 0RH0
  Sacrococcygeal 0SH5
  Sacroiliac
    Left 0SH8
    Right 0SH7
  Shoulder
    Left 0RHK
    Right 0RHJ
  Sternoclavicular
    Left 0RHF
    Right 0RHE
  Tarsal
    Left 0SHJ
    Right 0SHH
  Temporomandibular
    Left 0RHD
    Right 0RHC
  Thoracic Vertebral 0RH6
  Thoracolumbar Vertebral 0RHA
  Toe Phalangeal
    Left 0SHQ
    Right 0SHP
  Wrist
    Left 0RHP
    Right 0RHN
Kidney 0TH5
Knee Region
  Left 0YHG
  Right 0YHF
Leg
  Lower
    Left 0YHJ
    Right 0YHH
  Upper
    Left 0YHD
    Right 0YHC
Liver 0FH0
  Left Lobe 0FH2
  Right Lobe 0FH1
Lung
  Left 0BHL
  Right 0BHK
Lymphatic 07HN
  Thoracic Duct 07HK
Mandible
  Left 0NHV
  Right 0NHT
Maxilla
  Left 0NHS
  Right 0NHR
Mediastinum 0WHC
Metacarpal
  Left 0PHQ
  Right 0PHP
Metatarsal
  Left 0QHP
  Right 0QHN
Mouth and Throat 0CHY
Muscle
  Lower 0KHY
  Upper 0KHX
Nasopharynx 09HN
Neck 0WH6
Nerve
  Cranial 00HE
  Peripheral 01HY
Nipple
  Left 0HHX
  Right 0HHW
Oral Cavity and Throat
  0WH3
Orbit
  Left 0NHQ
  Right 0NHP
Ovary 0UH3
Pancreas 0FHG
Patella
  Left 0QHF
  Right 0QHD

◀ New   ◀▥▥ Revised   ~~deleted~~ Deleted

Inspection (*Continued*)

Duct
  Hepatobiliary 0FJB
  Pancreatic 0FJD
Ear
  Inner
    Left 09JE
    Right 09JD
  Left 09JJ
  Right 09JH
Elbow Region
  Left 0XJC
  Right 0XJB
Epididymis and Spermatic Cord
    0VJM
Extremity
  Lower
    Left 0YJB
    Right 0YJ9
  Upper
    Left 0XJ7
    Right 0XJ6
Eye
  Left 08J1XZZ
  Right 08J0XZZ
Face 0WJ2
Fallopian Tube 0UJ8
Femoral Region
  Bilateral 0YJE
  Left 0YJ8
  Right 0YJ7
Finger Nail 0HJQXZZ
Foot
  Left 0YJN
  Right 0YJM
Gallbladder 0FJ4
Gastrointestinal Tract 0WJP
Genitourinary Tract 0WJR
Gland
  Adrenal 0GJ5
  Endocrine 0GJS
  Pituitary 0GJ0
  Salivary 0CJA
Great Vessel 02JY
Hand
  Left 0XJK
  Right 0XJJ
Head 0WJ0
Heart 02JA
Inguinal Region
  Bilateral 0YJA
  Left 0YJ6
  Right 0YJ5
Intestinal Tract
  Lower 0DJD
  Upper 0DJ0
Jaw
  Lower 0WJ5
  Upper 0WJ4
Joint
  Acromioclavicular
    Left 0RJH
    Right 0RJG
  Ankle
    Left 0SJG
    Right 0SJF
  Carpal
    Left 0RJR
    Right 0RJQ
  Cervical Vertebral 0RJ1
  Cervicothoracic Vertebral 0RJ4
  Coccygeal 0SJ6
  Elbow
    Left 0RJM
    Right 0RJL
  Finger Phalangeal
    Left 0RJX
    Right 0RJW
  Hip
    Left 0SJB
    Right 0SJ9

Inspection (*Continued*)

Joint (*Continued*)
  Knee
    Left 0SJD
    Right 0SJC
  Lumbar Vertebral 0SJ0
  Lumbosacral 0SJ3
  Metacarpocarpal
    Left 0RJT
    Right 0RJS
  Metacarpophalangeal
    Left 0RJV
    Right 0RJU
  Metatarsal-Phalangeal
    Left 0SJN
    Right 0SJM
  Metatarsal-Tarsal
    Left 0SJL
    Right 0SJK
  Occipital-cervical 0RJ0
  Sacrococcygeal 0SJ5
  Sacroiliac
    Left 0SJ8
    Right 0SJ7
  Shoulder
    Left 0RJK
    Right 0RJJ
  Sternoclavicular
    Left 0RJF
    Right 0RJE
  Tarsal
    Left 0SJJ
    Right 0SJH
  Temporomandibular
    Left 0RJD
    Right 0RJC
  Thoracic Vertebral 0RJ6
  Thoracolumbar Vertebral
    0RJA
  Toe Phalangeal
    Left 0SJQ
    Right 0SJP
  Wrist
    Left 0RJP
    Right 0RJN
Kidney 0TJ5
Knee Region
  Left 0YJG
  Right 0YJF
Larynx 0CJS
Leg
  Lower
    Left 0YJJ
    Right 0YJH
  Upper
    Left 0YJD
    Right 0YJC
Lens
  Left 08JKXZZ
  Right 08JJXZZ
Liver 0FJ0
Lung
  Left 0BJL
  Right 0BJK
Lymphatic 07JN
  Thoracic Duct 07JK
Mediastinum 0WJC
Mesentery 0DJV
Mouth and Throat 0CJY
Muscle
  Extraocular
    Left 08JM
    Right 08JL
  Lower 0KJY
  Upper 0KJX
Neck 0WJ6
Nerve
  Cranial 00JE
  Peripheral 01JY
Nose 09JK
Omentum 0DJU

Inspection (*Continued*)

Oral Cavity and Throat 0WJ3
Ovary 0UJ3
Pancreas 0FJG
Parathyroid Gland 0GJR
Pelvic Cavity 0WJD
Penis 0VJS
Pericardial Cavity 0WJD
Perineum
  Female 0WJN
  Male 0WJM
Peritoneal Cavity 0WJG
Peritoneum 0DJW
Pineal Body 0GJ1
Pleura 0BJQ
Pleural Cavity
  Left 0WJB
  Right 0WJ9
Products of Conception 10J0
  Ectopic 10J2
  Retained 10J1
Prostate and Seminal Vesicles 0VJ4
Respiratory Tract 0WJQ
Retroperitoneum 0WJH
Scrotum and Tunica Vaginalis 0VJ8
Shoulder Region
  Left 0XJ3
  Right 0XJ2
Sinus 09JY
Skin 0HJPXZZ
Skull 0NJ0
Spinal Canal 00JU
Spinal Cord 00JV
Spleen 07JP
Stomach 0DJ6
Subcutaneous Tissue and Fascia
  Head and Neck 0JJS
  Lower Extremity 0JJW
  Trunk 0JJT
  Upper Extremity 0JJV
Tendon
  Lower 0LJY
  Upper 0LJX
Testis 0VJD
Thymus 07JM
Thyroid Gland 0GJK
Toe Nail 0HJRXZZ
Trachea 0BJ1
Tracheobronchial Tree 0BJ0
Tympanic Membrane
  Left 09J8
  Right 09J7
Ureter 0TJ9
Urethra 0TJD
Uterus and Cervix 0UJD
Vagina and Cul-de-sac 0UJH
Vas Deferens 0VJR
Vein
  Lower 06JY
  Upper 05JY
Vulva 0UJM
Wall
  Abdominal 0WJF
  Chest 0WJ8
Wrist Region
  Left 0XJH
  Right 0XJG
Instillation *see* Introduction of substance in or
    on
Insufflation *see* Introduction of substance in
    or on
Interatrial septum *use* Septum, Atrial
Interbody fusion (spine) cage
    use Interbody Fusion Device in Upper Joints
    use Interbody Fusion Device in Lower Joints
Intercarpal joint
    use Joint, Carpal, Right
    use Joint, Carpal, Left
Intercarpal ligament
    use Bursa and Ligament, Hand, Right
    use Bursa and Ligament, Hand, Left

◀ New   ◀▥▥ Revised   ~~deleted~~ Deleted

Interclavicular ligament
use Bursa and Ligament, Shoulder, Right
use Bursa and Ligament, Shoulder, Left
Intercostal lymph node *use* Lymphatic, Thorax
Intercostal muscle
use Muscle, Thorax, Right
use Muscle, Thorax, Left
Intercostal nerve *use* Nerve, Thoracic
Intercostobrachial nerve *use* Nerve,
Thoracic
Intercuneiform joint
use Joint, Tarsal, Right
use Joint, Tarsal, Left
Intercuneiform ligament
use Bursa and Ligament, Foot, Left
use Bursa and Ligament, Foot, Right
Intermediate cuneiform bone
use Tarsal, Right
use Tarsal, Left
Intermittent mandatory ventilation *see*
Assistance, Respiratory 5A09
Intermittent Negative Airway Pressure
24-96 Consecutive Hours, Ventilation 5A0945B
Greater than 96 Consecutive Hours,
Ventilation 5A0955B
Less than 24 Consecutive Hours, Ventilation
5A0935B
Intermittent Positive Airway Pressure
24-96 Consecutive Hours, Ventilation 5A09458
Greater than 96 Consecutive Hours,
Ventilation 5A09558
Less than 24 Consecutive Hours, Ventilation
5A09358
Intermittent positive pressure breathing *see*
Assistance, Respiratory 5A09
Internal (basal) cerebral vein *use* Vein,
Intracranial
Internal anal sphincter *use* Anal Sphincter
Internal carotid plexus *use* Nerve, Head and
Neck Sympathetic
Internal iliac vein
use Vein, Hypogastric, Right
use Vein, Hypogastric, Left
Internal maxillary artery
use Artery, External Carotid, Left
use Artery, External Carotid, Right
Internal naris *use* Nose
Internal oblique muscle
use Muscle, Abdomen, Right
use Muscle, Abdomen, Left
Internal pudendal artery
use Artery, Internal Iliac, Right
use Artery, Internal Iliac, Left
Internal pudendal vein
use Vein, Hypogastric, Right
use Vein, Hypogastric, Left
Internal thoracic artery
use Artery, Subclavian, Right
use Artery, Subclavian, Left
use Artery, Internal Mammary, Left
use Artery, Internal Mammary, Right
Internal urethral sphincter *use* Urethra
Interphalangeal (IP) joint
use Joint, Finger Phalangeal, Left
use Joint, Toe Phalangeal, Right
use Joint, Toe Phalangeal, Left
use Joint, Finger Phalangeal, Right
Interphalangeal ligament
use Bursa and Ligament, Hand, Left
use Bursa and Ligament, Hand, Right
use Bursa and Ligament, Foot, Right
use Bursa and Ligament, Foot, Left
Interrogation, cardiac rhythm related device
Interrogation only *see* Measurement, Cardiac
4B02
With cardiac function testing *see*
Measurement, Cardiac 4A02
Interruption *see* Occlusion
Interspinalis muscle
use Muscle, Trunk, Right
use Muscle, Trunk, Left

Interspinous ligament
use Bursa and Ligament, Trunk, Right
use Bursa and Ligament, Trunk, Left
**Interspinous process spinal stabilization
device**
use Spinal Stabilization Device, Interspinous
Process in 0RH
use Spinal Stabilization Device, Interspinous
Process in 0SH
InterStim® Therapy lead *use* Neurostimulator
Lead in Peripheral Nervous System
InterStim® Therapy neurostimulator, *use*
Stimulator Generator, Single Array in
0JH
Intertransversarius muscle
use Muscle, Trunk, Left
use Muscle, Trunk, Right
Intertransverse ligament
use Bursa and Ligament, Trunk, Right
use Bursa and Ligament, Trunk, Left
Interventricular foramen (Monro) *use* Cerebral
Ventricle
Interventricular septum *use* Septum,
Ventricular
Intestinal lymphatic trunk *use* Cisterna
Chyli
Intraluminal Device
Airway
Esophagus 0DH5
Mouth and Throat 0CHY
Nasopharynx 09HN
Bioactive
Occlusion
Common Carotid
Left 03LJ
Right 03LH
External Carotid
Left 03LN
Right 03LM
Internal Carotid
Left 03LL
Right 03LK
Intracranial 03LG
Vertebral
Left 03LQ
Right 03LP
Restriction
Common Carotid
Left 03VJ
Right 03VH
External Carotid
Left 03VN
Right 03VM
Internal Carotid
Left 03VL
Right 03VK
Intracranial 03VG
Vertebral
Left 03VQ
Right 03VP
Endobronchial Valve
Lingula 0BH9
Lower Lobe
Left 0BHB
Right 0BH6
Main
Left 0BH7
Right 0BH3
Middle Lobe, Right 0BH5
Upper Lobe
Left 0BH8
Right 0BH4
Endotracheal Airway
Change device in, Trachea 0B21XEZ
Insertion of device in, Trachea 0BH1
Pessary
Change device in, Vagina and Cul-de-sac
0U2HXGZ
Insertion of device in
Cul-de-sac 0UHF
Vagina 0UHG

Intramedullary (IM) rod (nail)
use Internal Fixation Device, Intramedullary
in Upper Bones
use Internal Fixation Device, Intramedullary
in Lower Bones
**Intramedullary skeletal kinetic distractor
(ISKD)**
use Internal Fixation Device, Intramedullary
in Upper Bones
use Internal Fixation Device, Intramedullary
in Lower Bones
Intraocular Telescope
Left 08RK30Z
Right 08RJ30Z
Intraoperative Radiation Therapy (IORT)
Anus DDY8CZZ
Bile Ducts DFY2CZZ
Bladder DTY2CZZ
Cervix DUY1CZZ
Colon DDY5CZZ
Duodenum DDY2CZZ
Gallbladder DFY1CZZ
Ileum DDY4CZZ
Jejunum DDY3CZZ
Kidney DTY0CZZ
Larynx D9YBCZZ
Liver DFY0CZZ
Mouth D9Y4CZZ
Nasopharynx D9YDCZZ
Ovary DUY0CZZ
Pancreas DFY3CZZ
Pharynx D9YCCZZ
Prostate DVY0CZZ
Rectum DDY7CZZ
Stomach DDY1CZZ
Ureter DTY1CZZ
Urethra DTY3CZZ
Uterus DUY2CZZ
Intrauterine device (IUD) *use* Contraceptive
Device in Female Reproductive System
Introduction of substance in or on
Artery
Central 3E06
Analgesics 3E06
Anesthetic, Intracirculatory 3E06
Anti-infective 3E06
Anti-inflammatory 3E06
Antiarrhythmic 3E06
Antineoplastic 3E06
Destructive Agent 3E06
Diagnostic Substance, Other 3E06
Electrolytic Substance 3E06
Hormone 3E06
Hypnotics 3E06
Immunotherapeutic 3E06
Nutritional Substance 3E06
Platelet Inhibitor 3E06
Radioactive Substance 3E06
Sedatives 3E06
Serum 3E06
Thrombolytic 3E06
Toxoid 3E06
Vaccine 3E06
Vasopressor 3E06
Water Balance Substance 3E06
Coronary 3E07
Diagnostic Substance, Other
3E07
Platelet Inhibitor 3E07
Thrombolytic 3E07
Peripheral 3E05
Analgesics 3E05
Anesthetic, Intracirculatory
3E05
Anti-infective 3E05
Anti-inflammatory 3E05
Antiarrhythmic 3E05
Antineoplastic 3E05
Destructive Agent 3E05
Diagnostic Substance, Other
3E05

◀ New   ◀⫴ Revised   ~~deleted~~ Deleted

Introduction of substance in or on *(Continued)*
    Muscle 3E023GC
        Analgesics 3E023NZ
        Anesthetic, Local 3E023BZ
        Anti-infective 3E0232
        Anti-inflammatory 3E0233Z
        Antineoplastic 3E0230
        Destructive Agent 3E023TZ
        Diagnostic Substance, Other 3E023KZ
        Electrolytic Substance 3E0237Z
        Hypnotics 3E023NZ
        Nutritional Substance 3E0236Z
        Radioactive Substance 3E023HZ
        Sedatives 3E023NZ
        Serum 3E0234Z
        Toxoid 3E0234Z
        Vaccine 3E0234Z
        Water Balance Substance 3E0237Z
    Nerve
        Cranial 3E0X3GC
            Anesthetic
                Local 3E0X3BZ
                Regional 3E0X3CZ
            Anti-inflammatory 3E0X33Z
            Destructive Agent 3E0X3TZ
        Peripheral 3E0T3GC
            Anesthetic
                Local 3E0T3BZ
                Regional 3E0T3CZ
            Anti-inflammatory 3E0T33Z
            Destructive Agent 3E0T3TZ
        Plexus 3E0T3GC
            Anesthetic
                Local 3E0T3BZ
                Regional 3E0T3CZ
            Anti-inflammatory 3E0T33Z
            Destructive Agent 3E0T3TZ
    Nose 3E09
        Analgesics 3E09
        Anesthetic, Local 3E09
        Anti-infective 3E09
        Anti-inflammatory 3E09
        Antineoplastic 3E09
        Destructive Agent 3E09
        Diagnostic Substance, Other 3E09
        Hypnotics 3E09
        Radioactive Substance 3E09
        Sedatives 3E09
        Serum 3E09
        Toxoid 3E09
        Vaccine 3E09
    Pancreatic Tract 3E0J
        Analgesics 3E0J
        Anesthetic, Local 3E0J
        Anti-infective 3E0J
        Anti-inflammatory 3E0J
        Antineoplastic 3E0J
        Destructive Agent 3E0J
        Diagnostic Substance, Other 3E0J
        Electrolytic Substance 3E0J
        Gas 3E0J
        Hypnotics 3E0J
        Islet Cells, Pancreatic 3E0J
        Nutritional Substance 3E0J
        Radioactive Substance 3E0J
        Sedatives 3E0J
        Water Balance Substance 3E0J
    Pericardial Cavity 3E0Y3GC
        Analgesics 3E0Y3NZ
        Anesthetic, Local 3E0Y3BZ
        Anti-infective 3E0Y32
        Anti-inflammatory 3E0Y33Z
        Antineoplastic 3E0Y
        Destructive Agent 3E0Y3TZ
        Diagnostic Substance, Other 3E0Y3KZ
        Electrolytic Substance 3E0Y37Z
        Gas 3E0Y
        Hypnotics 3E0Y3NZ
        Nutritional Substance 3E0Y36Z
        Radioactive Substance 3E0Y3HZ
        Sedatives 3E0Y3NZ
        Water Balance Substance 3E0Y37Z

Introduction of substance in or on *(Continued)*
    Peritoneal Cavity 3E0M3GC
        Adhesion Barrier 3E0M05Z
        Analgesics 3E0M3NZ
        Anesthetic, Local 3E0M3BZ
        Anti-infective 3E0M32
        Anti-inflammatory 3E0M33Z
        Antineoplastic 3E0M
        Destructive Agent 3E0M3TZ
        Diagnostic Substance, Other 3E0M3KZ
        Electrolytic Substance 3E0M37Z
        Gas 3E0M
        Hypnotics 3E0M3NZ
        Nutritional Substance 3E0M36Z
        Radioactive Substance 3E0M3HZ
        Sedatives 3E0M3NZ
        Water Balance Substance 3E0M37Z
    Pharynx 3E0D
        Analgesics 3E0D
        Anesthetic, Local 3E0D
        Anti-infective 3E0D
        Anti-inflammatory 3E0D
        Antiarrhythmic 3E0D
        Antineoplastic 3E0D
        Destructive Agent 3E0D
        Diagnostic Substance, Other 3E0D
        Electrolytic Substance 3E0D
        Hypnotics 3E0D
        Nutritional Substance 3E0D
        Radioactive Substance 3E0D
        Sedatives 3E0D
        Serum 3E0D
        Toxoid 3E0D
        Vaccine 3E0D
        Water Balance Substance 3E0D
    Pleural Cavity 3E0L3GC
        Adhesion Barrier 3E0L05Z
        Analgesics 3E0L3NZ
        Anesthetic, Local 3E0L3BZ
        Anti-infective 3E0L32
        Anti-inflammatory 3E0L33Z
        Antineoplastic 3E0L
        Destructive Agent 3E0L3TZ
        Diagnostic Substance, Other 3E0L3KZ
        Electrolytic Substance 3E0L37Z
        Gas 3E0L
        Hypnotics 3E0L3NZ
        Nutritional Substance 3E0L36Z
        Radioactive Substance 3E0L3HZ
        Sedatives 3E0L3NZ
        Water Balance Substance 3E0L37Z
    Products of Conception 3E0E
        Analgesics 3E0E
        Anesthetic, Local 3E0E
        Anti-infective 3E0E
        Anti-inflammatory 3E0E
        Antineoplastic 3E0E
        Destructive Agent 3E0E
        Diagnostic Substance, Other 3E0E
        Electrolytic Substance 3E0E
        Gas 3E0E
        Hypnotics 3E0E
        Nutritional Substance 3E0E
        Radioactive Substance 3E0E
        Sedatives 3E0E
        Water Balance Substance 3E0E
    Reproductive
        Female 3E0P
            Adhesion Barrier 3E0P05Z
            Analgesics 3E0P
            Anesthetic, Local 3E0P
            Anti-infective 3E0P
            Anti-inflammatory 3E0P
            Antineoplastic 3E0P
            Destructive Agent 3E0P
            Diagnostic Substance, Other 3E0P
            Electrolytic Substance 3E0P
            Gas 3E0P
            Hypnotics 3E0P
            Nutritional Substance 3E0P
            Ovum, Fertilized 3E0P

Introduction of substance in or on *(Continued)*
    Reproductive *(Continued)*
        Female *(Continued)*
            Radioactive Substance 3E0P
            Sedatives 3E0P
            Sperm 3E0P
            Water Balance Substance 3E0P
        Male 3E0N
            Analgesics 3E0N
            Anesthetic, Local 3E0N
            Anti-infective 3E0N
            Anti-inflammatory 3E0N
            Antineoplastic 3E0N
            Destructive Agent 3E0N
            Diagnostic Substance, Other 3E0N
            Electrolytic Substance 3E0N
            Gas 3E0N
            Hypnotics 3E0N
            Nutritional Substance 3E0N
            Radioactive Substance 3E0N
            Sedatives 3E0N
            Water Balance Substance 3E0N
    Respiratory Tract 3E0F
        Analgesics 3E0F
        Anesthetic
            Inhalation 3E0F
            Local 3E0F
        Anti-infective 3E0F
        Anti-inflammatory 3E0F
        Antineoplastic 3E0F
        Destructive Agent 3E0F
        Diagnostic Substance, Other 3E0F
        Electrolytic Substance 3E0F
        Gas 3E0F
        Hypnotics 3E0F
        Nutritional Substance 3E0F
        Radioactive Substance 3E0F
        Sedatives 3E0F
        Water Balance Substance 3E0F
    Skin 3E00XGC
        Analgesics 3E00XNZ
        Anesthetic, Local 3E00XBZ
        Anti-infective 3E00X2
        Anti-inflammatory 3E00X3Z
        Antineoplastic 3E00X0
        Destructive Agent 3E00XTZ
        Diagnostic Substance, Other 3E00XKZ
        Hypnotics 3E00XNZ
        Pigment 3E00XMZ
        Sedatives 3E00XNZ
        Serum 3E00X4Z
        Toxoid 3E00X4Z
        Vaccine 3E00X4Z
    Spinal Canal 3E0R3GC
        Analgesics 3E0R3NZ
        Anesthetic
            Local 3E0R3BZ
            Regional 3E0R3CZ
        Anti-infective 3E0R32
        Anti-inflammatory 3E0R33Z
        Antineoplastic 3E0R30
        Destructive Agent 3E0R3TZ
        Diagnostic Substance, Other 3E0R3KZ
        Electrolytic Substance 3E0R37Z
        Gas 3E0R
        Hypnotics 3E0R3NZ
        Nutritional Substance 3E0R36Z
        Radioactive Substance 3E0R3HZ
        Sedatives 3E0R3NZ
        Stem Cells
            Embryonic 3E0R
            Somatic 3E0R
        Water Balance Substance 3E0R37Z
    Subcutaneous Tissue 3E013GC
        Analgesics 3E013NZ
        Anesthetic, Local 3E013BZ
        Anti-infective 3E01
        Anti-inflammatory 3E0133Z
        Antineoplastic 3E0130
        Destructive Agent 3E013TZ
        Diagnostic Substance, Other 3E013KZ

◀ New   ◀▦ Revised   ~~deleted~~ Deleted

Introduction of substance in or on *(Continued)*
  Subcutaneous Tissue *(Continued)*
    Electrolytic Substance 3E0137Z
    Hormone 3E013V
    Hypnotics 3E013NZ
    Nutritional Substance 3E0136Z
    Radioactive Substance 3E013HZ
    Sedatives 3E013NZ
    Serum 3E0134Z
    Toxoid 3E0134Z
    Vaccine 3E0134Z
    Water Balance Substance 3E0137Z
  Vein
    Central 3E04
      Analgesics 3E04
      Anesthetic, Intracirculatory 3E04
      Anti-infective 3E04
      Anti-inflammatory 3E04
      Antiarrhythmic 3E04
      Antineoplastic 3E04
      Destructive Agent 3E04
      Diagnostic Substance, Other 3E04
      Electrolytic Substance 3E04
      Hormone 3E04
      Hypnotics 3E04
      Immunotherapeutic 3E04
      Nutritional Substance 3E04
      Platelet Inhibitor 3E04
      Radioactive Substance 3E04
      Sedatives 3E04
      Serum 3E04
      Thrombolytic 3E04
      Toxoid 3E04
      Vaccine 3E04
      Vasopressor 3E04
      Water Balance Substance 3E04
    Peripheral 3E03
      Analgesics 3E03
      Anesthetic, Intracirculatory 3E03
      Anti-infective 3E03
      Anti-inflammatory 3E03
      Antiarrhythmic 3E03
      Antineoplastic 3E03
      Destructive Agent 3E03
      Diagnostic Substance, Other 3E03
      Electrolytic Substance 3E03
      Hormone 3E03
      Hypnotics 3E03
      Immunotherapeutic 3E03
      Islet Cells, Pancreatic 3E03
      Nutritional Substance 3E03
      Platelet Inhibitor 3E03
      Radioactive Substance 3E03
      Sedatives 3E03
      Serum 3E03
      Thrombolytic 3E03
      Toxoid 3E03
      Vaccine 3E03
      Vasopressor 3E03
      Water Balance Substance 3E03
Intubation
  Airway
    see Insertion of device in, Trachea 0BH1
    see Insertion of device in, Mouth and
      Throat 0CHY
    see Insertion of device in, Esophagus 0DH5

Intubation *(Continued)*
  Drainage device *see* Drainage
  Feeding Device *see* Insertion of device in,
    Gastrointestinal System 0DH
IPPB (intermittent positive pressure
  breathing) *see* Assistance, Respiratory
  5A09
Iridectomy
  see Excision, Eye 08B
  see Resection, Eye 08T
Iridoplasty
  see Repair, Eye 08Q
  see Replacement, Eye 08R
  see Supplement, Eye 08U
Iridotomy *see* Drainage, Eye 089
Irrigation
  Biliary Tract, Irrigating Substance 3E1J
  Brain, Irrigating Substance 3E1Q38Z
  Cranial Cavity, Irrigating Substance 3E1Q38Z
  Ear, Irrigating Substance 3E1B
  Epidural Space, Irrigating Substance 3E1S38Z
  Eye, Irrigating Substance 3E1C
  Gastrointestinal Tract
    Lower, Irrigating Substance 3E1H
    Upper, Irrigating Substance 3E1G
  Genitourinary Tract, Irrigating Substance
    3E1K
  Irrigating Substance 3C1ZX8Z
  Joint, Irrigating Substance 3E1U38Z
  Mucous Membrane, Irrigating Substance
    3E10
  Nose, Irrigating Substance 3E19
  Pancreatic Tract, Irrigating Substance 3E1J
  Pericardial Cavity, Irrigating Substance
    3E1Y38Z
  Peritoneal Cavity
    Dialysate 3E1M39Z
    Irrigating Substance 3E1M38Z
  Pleural Cavity, Irrigating Substance
    3E1L38Z
  Reproductive
    Female, Irrigating Substance 3E1P
    Male, Irrigating Substance 3E1N
  Respiratory Tract, Irrigating Substance 3E1F
  Skin, Irrigating Substance 3E10
  Spinal Canal, Irrigating Substance 3E1R38Z
Ischiatic nerve *use* Nerve, Sciatic
Ischiocavernosus muscle *use* Muscle,
  Perineum
Ischiofemoral ligament
  use Bursa and Ligament, Hip, Left
  use Bursa and Ligament, Hip, Right
Ischium
  use Bone, Pelvic, Right
  use Bone, Pelvic, Left
Isolation 8E0ZXY6
Isotope Administration, Whole Body DWY5G
Itrel (3) (4) neurostimulator *use* Stimulator
  Generator, Single Array in 0JH

J

Jejunal artery *use* Artery, Superior Mesenteric
Jejunectomy
  see Excision, Jejunum 0DBA
  see Resection, Jejunum 0DTA

Jejunocolostomy
  see Bypass, Gastrointestinal System 0D1
  see Drainage, Gastrointestinal System 0D9
Jejunopexy
  see Repair, Jejunum 0DQA
  see Reposition, Jejunum 0DSA
Jejunostomy
  see Bypass, Jejunum 0D1A
  see Drainage, Jejunum 0D9A
Jejunotomy *see* Drainage, Jejunum 0D9A
Joint fixation plate
  use Internal Fixation Device in Upper
    Joints
  use Internal Fixation Device in Lower
    Joints
Joint liner (insert) *use* Liner in Lower
  Joints
Joint spacer (antibiotic)
  use Spacer in Upper Joints
  use Spacer in Lower Joints
Jugular body *use* Glomus Jugulare
Jugular lymph node
  use Lymphatic, Neck, Left
  use Lymphatic, Neck, Right

K

Kappa *use* Pacemaker, Dual Chamber in
  0JH
Kcentra *use* 4-Factor Prothrombin Complex
  Concentrate ◀
Keratectomy, kerectomy
  see Excision, Eye 08B
  see Resection, Eye 08T
Keratocentesis *see* Drainage, Eye 089
Keratoplasty
  see Repair, Eye 08Q
  see Replacement, Eye 08R
  see Supplement, Eye 08U
Keratotomy
  see Drainage, Eye 089
  see Repair, Eye 08Q
~~Kinetra® neurostimulator use Stimulator~~
  ~~Generator, Multiple Array in 0JH~~
Kirschner wire (K-wire)
  use Internal Fixation Device in Head and
    Facial Bones
  use Internal Fixation Device in Upper
    Bones
  use Internal Fixation Device in Lower
    Bones
  use Internal Fixation Device in Upper
    Joints
  use Internal Fixation Device in Lower
    Joints
Knee (implant) insert *use* Liner in Lower
  Joints
KUB x-ray *see* Plain Radiography, Kidney,
  Ureter and Bladder BT04
Kuntscher nail
  use Internal Fixation Device, Intramedullary
    in Upper Bones
  use Internal Fixation Device, Intramedullary
    in Lower Bones

L

Labia majora *use* Vulva
Labia minora *use* Vulva
Labial gland
  use Lip, Upper
  use Lip, Lower
Labiectomy
  see Excision, Female Reproductive System 0UB
  see Resection, Female Reproductive System 0UT
Lacrimal canaliculus
  use Duct, Lacrimal, Left
  use Duct, Lacrimal, Right
Lacrimal punctum
  use Duct, Lacrimal, Right
  use Duct, Lacrimal, Left
Lacrimal sac
  use Duct, Lacrimal, Right
  use Duct, Lacrimal, Left
Laminectomy
  see Excision, Upper Bones 0PB
  see Excision, Lower Bones 0QB
Laminotomy
  see Drainage, Upper Bones 0P9 ◄
  ~~*see* Drainage, Upper Joints 0R9~~
  see Drainage, Lower Bones 0Q9 ◄
  ~~*see* Drainage, Lower Joints 0S9~~
  see Release, Upper Bones 0PN ◄
  ~~*see* Release, Upper Joints 0RN~~
  see Release, Lower Bones 0QN ◄
  ~~*see* Release, Lower Joints 0SN~~
  see Release, Central Nervous System 00N
  see Release, Peripheral Nervous System 01N
  see Excision, Upper Bones 0PB ◄
  see Excision, Lower Bones 0QB ◄
LAP-BAND® adjustable gastric banding system *use* Extraluminal Device
Laparoscopy *see* Inspection
Laparotomy
  Drainage *see* Drainage, Peritoneal Cavity 0W9G
  Exploratory *see* Inspection, Peritoneal *use* Nerve, Lumbar Plexus 0WJG
Laryngectomy
  see Excision, Larynx 0CBS
  see Resection, Larynx 0CTS
Laryngocentesis *see* Drainage, Larynx 0C9S
Laryngogram *see* Fluoroscopy, Larynx B91J
Laryngopexy
  see Repair, Larynx 0CQS
Laryngopharynx *use* Pharynx
Laryngoplasty
  see Repair, Larynx 0CQS
  see Replacement, Larynx 0CRS
  see Supplement, Larynx 0CUS
Laryngorrhaphy *see* Repair, Larynx 0CQS
Laryngoscopy 0CJS8ZZ
Laryngotomy *see* Drainage, Larynx 0C9S
Laser Interstitial Thermal Therapy
  Adrenal Gland DGY2KZZ
  Anus DDY8KZZ
  Bile Ducts DFY2KZZ
  Brain D0Y0KZZ
  Brain Stem D0Y1KZZ
  Breast
    Left DMY0KZZ
    Right DMY1KZZ
  Bronchus DBY1KZZ
  Chest Wall DBY7KZZ
  Colon DDY5KZZ
  Diaphragm DBY8KZZ
  Duodenum DDY2KZZ
  Esophagus DDY0KZZ
  Gallbladder DFY1KZZ
  Gland
    Adrenal DGY2KZZ
    Parathyroid DGY4KZZ
    Pituitary DGY0KZZ
    Thyroid DGY5KZZ
  Ileum DDY4KZZ
  Jejunum DDY3KZZ

Laser Interstitial Thermal Therapy
  (Continued)
  Liver DFY0KZZ
  Lung DBY2KZZ
  Mediastinum DBY6KZZ
  Nerve, Peripheral D0Y7KZZ
  Pancreas DFY3KZZ
  Parathyroid Gland DGY4KZZ
  Pineal Body DGY1KZZ
  Pituitary Gland DGY0KZZ
  Pleura DBY5KZZ
  Prostate DVY0KZZ
  Rectum DDY7KZZ
  Spinal Cord D0Y6KZZ
  Stomach DDY1KZZ
  Thyroid Gland DGY5KZZ
  Trachea DBY0KZZ
Lateral (brachial) lymph node
  use Lymphatic, Axillary, Left
  use Lymphatic, Axillary, Right
Lateral canthus
  use Eyelid, Upper, Right
  use Eyelid, Upper, Left
Lateral collateral ligament (LCL)
  use Bursa and Ligament, Knee, Right
  use Bursa and Ligament, Knee, Left
Lateral condyle of femur
  use Femur, Lower, Right
  use Femur, Lower, Left
Lateral condyle of tibia
  use Tibia, Left
  use Tibia, Right
Lateral cuneiform bone
  use Tarsal, Right
  use Tarsal, Left
Lateral epicondyle of femur
  use Femur, Lower, Left
  use Femur, Lower, Right
Lateral epicondyle of humerus
  use Humeral Shaft, Right
  use Humeral Shaft, Left
Lateral femoral cutaneous nerve *use* Nerve, Lumbar Plexus
Lateral malleolus
  use Fibula, Right
  use Fibula, Left
Lateral meniscus
  use Joint, Knee, Left
  use Joint, Knee, Right
Lateral nasal cartilage *use* Nose
Lateral plantar artery
  use Artery, Foot, Left
  use Artery, Foot, Right
Lateral plantar nerve *use* Nerve, Tibial
Lateral rectus muscle
  use Muscle, Extraocular, Left
  use Muscle, Extraocular, Right
Lateral sacral artery
  use Artery, Internal Iliac, Left
  use Artery, Internal Iliac, Right
Lateral sacral vein
  use Vein, Hypogastric, Left
  use Vein, Hypogastric, Right
Lateral sural cutaneous nerve *use* Nerve, Peroneal
Lateral tarsal artery
  use Artery, Foot, Right
  use Artery, Foot, Left
Lateral temporomandibular ligament
  use Bursa and Ligament, Head and Neck
Lateral thoracic artery
  use Artery, Axillary, Left
  use Artery, Axillary, Right
Latissimus dorsi muscle
  use Muscle, Trunk, Left
  use Muscle, Trunk, Right
Latissimus Dorsi Myocutaneous Flap
  Bilateral 0HRV075
  Left 0HRU075
  Right 0HRT075

Lavage
  see Irrigation
  bronchial alveolar, diagnostic *see* Drainage, Respiratory System 0B9
Least splanchnic nerve *use* Nerve, Thoracic Sympathetic
Left ascending lumbar vein *use* Vein, Hemiazygos
Left atrioventricular valve *use* Valve, Mitral
Left auricular appendix *use* Atrium, Left
Left colic vein *use* Vein, Colic
Left coronary sulcus *use* Heart, Left
Left gastric artery *use* Artery, Gastric
Left gastroepiploic artery *use* Artery, Splenic
Left gastroepiploic vein *use* Vein, Splenic
Left inferior phrenic vein *use* Vein, Renal, Left
Left inferior pulmonary vein *use* Vein, Pulmonary, Left
Left jugular trunk *use* Duct, Thoracic
Left lateral ventricle *use* Ventricle, Cerebral
Left ovarian vein *use* Vein, Renal, Left
Left second lumbar vein *use* Vein, Renal, Left
Left subclavian trunk *use* Lymphatic, Thoracic Duct
Left subcostal vein *use* Vein, Hemiazygos
Left superior pulmonary vein *use* Vein, Pulmonary, Left
Left suprarenal vein *use* Vein, Renal, Left
Left testicular vein *use* Vein, Renal, Left
Lengthening
  Bone, with device *see* Insertion of Limb Lengthening Device
  Muscle, by incision *see* Division, Muscles 0K8
  Tendon, by incision *see* Division, Tendons 0L8
Leptomeninges
  use Meninges, Cerebral
  use Meninges, Spinal
Lesser alar cartilage *use* Nose
Lesser occipital nerve *use* Nerve, Cervical Plexus
Lesser splanchnic nerve *use* Nerve, Thoracic Sympathetic
Lesser trochanter
  use Femur, Upper, Right
  use Femur, Upper, Left
Lesser tuberosity
  use Humeral Head, Left
  use Humeral Head, Right
Lesser wing
  use Bone, Sphenoid, Right
  use Bone, Sphenoid, Left
Leukopheresis, therapeutic *see* Pheresis, Circulatory 6A55
Levator anguli oris muscle *use* Muscle, Facial
Levator ani muscle
  use Muscle, Trunk, Left
  use Muscle, Trunk, Right
Levator labii superioris alaeque nasi muscle *use* Muscle, Facial
Levator labii superioris muscle *use* Muscle, Facial
Levator palpebrae superioris muscle
  use Eyelid, Upper, Left
  use Eyelid, Upper, Right
Levator scapulae muscle
  use Muscle, Neck, Left
  use Muscle, Neck, Right
Levator veli palatini muscle *use* Muscle, Tongue, Palate, Pharynx
Levatores costarum muscle
  use Muscle, Thorax, Left
  use Muscle, Thorax, Right
LifeStent® (Flexstar) (XL) Vascular Stent System *use* Intraluminal Device
Ligament of head of fibula
  use Bursa and Ligament, Knee, Right
  use Bursa and Ligament, Knee, Left
Ligament of the lateral malleolus
  use Bursa and Ligament, Ankle, Left
  use Bursa and Ligament, Ankle, Right

Ligamentum flavum
  use Bursa and Ligament, Trunk, Left
  use Bursa and Ligament, Trunk, Right
Ligation *see* Occlusion
Ligation, hemorrhoid *see* Occlusion, Lower
  Veins, Hemorrhoidal Plexus
Light Therapy GZJZZZZ
Liner
  Removal of device from
    Hip
      Left 0SPB09Z
      Right 0SP909Z
    Knee
      Left 0SPD09Z
      Right 0SPC09Z
  Revision of device in
    Hip
      Left 0SWB09Z
      Right 0SW909Z
    Knee
      Left 0SWD09Z
      Right 0SWC09Z
  Supplement
    Hip
      Left 0SUB09Z
        Acetabular Surface 0SUE09Z
        Femoral Surface 0SUS09Z
      Right 0SU909Z
        Acetabular Surface 0SUA09Z
        Femoral Surface 0SUR09Z
    Knee
      Left 0SUD09
        Femoral Surface 0SUU09Z
        Tibial Surface 0SUW09Z
      Right 0SUC09
        Femoral Surface 0SUT09Z
        Tibial Surface 0SUV09Z
Lingual artery
  use Artery, External Carotid, Right
  use Artery, External Carotid, Left

Lingual tonsil *use* Tongue
Lingulectomy, lung
  see Excision, Lung Lingula 0BBH
  see Resection, Lung Lingula 0BTH
Lithotripsy
  see Fragmentation
  with removal of fragments *see* Extirpation
LIVIAN™ CRT-D *use* Cardiac
  Resynchronization Defibrillator Pulse
  Generator in 0JH
Lobectomy
  see Excision, Central Nervous System
    00B
  see Excision, Respiratory System 0BB
  see Resection, Respiratory System 0BT
  see Excision, Hepatobiliary System and
    Pancreas 0FB
  see Resection, Hepatobiliary System and
    Pancreas 0FT
  see Excision, Endocrine System 0GB
  see Resection, Endocrine System 0GT
Lobotomy *see* Division, Brain 0080
Localization
  see Map
  see Imaging
Locus ceruleus *use* Pons
Long thoracic nerve *use* Nerve, Brachial
Plexus
Loop ileostomy *see* Bypass, Ileum 0D1B
Loop recorder, implantable *use* Monitoring
  Device
Lower GI series *see* Fluoroscopy, Colon
  BD14
Lumbar artery *use* Aorta, Abdominal
Lumbar facet joint *use* Joint, Lumbar
  Vertebral ◄▥
  ~~use Joint, Lumbar Vertebral, 2 or more~~
  ~~use Joint, Lumbar Vertebral~~
Lumbar ganglion *use* Nerve, Lumbar
  Sympathetic

Lumbar lymph node *use* Lymphatic, Aortic
Lumbar lymphatic trunk *use* Cisterna Chyli
Lumbar splanchnic nerve *use* Nerve, Lumbar
  Sympathetic
Lumbosacral facet joint *use* Joint, Lumbosacral
Lumbosacral trunk *use* Nerve, Lumbar
Lumpectomy
  see Excision
Lunate bone
  use Carpal, Left
  use Carpal, Right
Lunotriquetral ligament
  use Bursa and Ligament, Hand, Left
  use Bursa and Ligament, Hand, Right
Lymphadenectomy
  see Excision, Lymphatic and Hemic Systems
    07B
  see Resection, Lymphatic and Hemic Systems
    07T
Lymphadenotomy *see* Drainage, Lymphatic and
  Hemic Systems 079
Lymphangiectomy
  see Excision, Lymphatic and Hemic Systems
    07B
  see Resection, Lymphatic and Hemic Systems
    07T
Lymphangiogram *see* Plain Radiography,
  Lymphatic System B70
Lymphangioplasty
  see Repair, Lymphatic and Hemic Systems
    07Q
  see Supplement, Lymphatic and Hemic
    Systems 07U
Lymphangiorrhaphy *see* Repair, Lymphatic and
  Hemic Systems 07Q
Lymphangiotomy *see* Drainage, Lymphatic and
  Hemic Systems 079
Lysis *see* Release

◄ New   ◄▥ Revised   ~~deleted~~ Deleted

M

Macula
use Retina, Right
use Retina, Left
Magnet extraction, ocular foreign body *see*
Extirpation, Eye 08C
Magnetic Resonance Imaging (MRI)
Abdomen BW30
Ankle
Left BQ3H
Right BQ3G
Aorta
Abdominal B430
Thoracic B330
Arm
Left BP3F
Right BP3E
Artery
Celiac B431
Cervico-Cerebral Arch B33Q
Common Carotid, Bilateral B335
Coronary
Bypass Graft, Multiple B233
Multiple B231
Internal Carotid, Bilateral B338
Intracranial B33R
Lower Extremity
Bilateral B43H
Left B43G
Right B43F
Pelvic B43C
Renal, Bilateral B438
Spinal B33M
Superior Mesenteric B434
Upper Extremity
Bilateral B33K
Left B33J
Right B33H
Vertebral, Bilateral B33G
Bladder BT30
Brachial Plexus BW3P
Brain B030
Breast
Bilateral BH32
Left BH31
Right BH30
Calcaneus
Left BQ3K
Right BQ3J
Chest BW33Y
Coccyx BR3F
Connective Tissue
Lower Extremity BL31
Upper Extremity BL30
Corpora Cavernosa BV30
Disc
Cervical BR31
Lumbar BR33
Thoracic BR32
Ear B930
Elbow
Left BP3H
Right BP3G
Eye
Bilateral B837
Left B836
Right B835
Femur
Left BQ34
Right BQ33
Fetal Abdomen BY33
Fetal Extremity BY35
Fetal Head BY30
Fetal Heart BY31
Fetal Spine BY34
Fetal Thorax BY32
Fetus, Whole BY36
Foot
Left BQ3M
Right BQ3L

Magnetic Resonance Imaging (MRI)
(Continued)
Forearm
Left BP3K
Right BP3J
Gland
Adrenal, Bilateral BG32
Parathyroid BG33
Parotid, Bilateral B936
Salivary, Bilateral B93D
Submandibular, Bilateral B939
Thyroid BG34
Head BW38
Heart, Right and Left B236
Hip
Left BQ31
Right BQ30
Intracranial Sinus B532
Joint
Finger
Left BP3D
Right BP3C
Hand
Left BP3D
Right BP3C
Temporomandibular, Bilateral BN39
Kidney
Bilateral BT33
Left BT32
Right BT31
Transplant BT39
Knee
Left BQ38
Right BQ37
Larynx B93J
Leg
Left BQ3F
Right BQ3D
Liver BF35
Liver and Spleen BF36
Lung Apices BB3G
Nasopharynx B93F
Neck BW3F
Nerve
Acoustic B03C
Brachial Plexus BW3P
Oropharynx B93F
Ovary
Bilateral BU35
Left BU34
Right BU33
Ovary and Uterus BU3C
Pancreas BF37
Patella
Left BQ3W
Right BQ3V
Pelvic Region BW3G
Pelvis BR3C
Pituitary Gland B039
Plexus, Brachial BW3P
Prostate BV33
Retroperitoneum BW3H
Sacrum BR3F
Scrotum BV34
Sella Turcica B039
Shoulder
Left BP39
Right BP38
Sinus
Intracranial B532
Paranasal B932
Spinal Cord B03B
Spine
Cervical BR30
Lumbar BR39
Thoracic BR37
Spleen and Liver BF36
Subcutaneous Tissue
Abdomen BH3H
Extremity
Lower BH3J
Upper BH3F

Magnetic Resonance Imaging (MRI)
(Continued)
Subcutaneous Tissue *(Continued)*
Head BH3D
Neck BH3D
Pelvis BH3H
Thorax BH3G
Tendon
Lower Extremity BL33
Upper Extremity BL32
Testicle
Bilateral BV37
Left BV36
Right BV35
Toe
Left BQ3Q
Right BQ3P
Uterus BU36
Pregnant BU3B
Uterus and Ovary BU3C
Vagina BU39
Vein
Cerebellar B531
Cerebral B531
Jugular, Bilateral B535
Lower Extremity
Bilateral B53D
Left B53C
Right B53B
Other B53V
Pelvic (Iliac) Bilateral B53H
Portal B53T
Pulmonary, Bilateral B53S
Renal, Bilateral B53L
Spanchnic B53T
Upper Extremity
Bilateral B53P
Left B53N
Right B53M
Vena Cava
Inferior B539
Superior B538
Wrist
Left BP3M
Right BP3L
Malleotomy *see* Drainage, Ear, Nose, Sinus 099
Malleus
use Auditory Ossicle, Right
use Auditory Ossicle, Left
Mammaplasty, mammoplasty
see Alteration, Skin and Breast 0H0
see Repair, Skin and Breast 0HQ
see Replacement, Skin and Breast 0HR
see Supplement, Skin and Breast 0HU
Mammary duct
use Breast, Bilateral
use Breast, Right
use Breast, Left
Mammary gland
use Breast, Bilateral
use Breast, Right
use Breast, Left
Mammectomy
see Excision, Skin and Breast 0HB
see Resection, Skin and Breast 0HT
Mammillary body *use* Hypothalamus
Mammography *see* Plain Radiography, Skin, Subcutaneous Tissue and Breast BH0
Mammotomy *see* Drainage, Skin and Breast 0H9
Mandibular nerve *use* Nerve, Trigeminal
Mandibular notch
use Mandible, Right
use Mandible, Left
Mandibulectomy
see Excision, Head and Facial Bones 0NB
see Resection, Head and Facial Bones 0NT
Manipulation
Adhesions *see* Release
Chiropractic *see* Chiropractic Manipulation
Manubrium *use* Sternum

M

Map

Basal Ganglia 00K8
Brain 00K0
Cerebellum 00KC
Cerebral Hemisphere 00K7
Conduction Mechanism 02K8
Hypothalamus 00KA
Medulla Oblongata 00KD
Pons 00KB
Thalamus 00K9

Mapping
Doppler ultrasound *see* Ultrasonography
Electrocardiogram only *see* Measurement, Cardiac 4A02

Mark IV Breathing Pacemaker System *use* Stimulator Generator in Subcutaneous Tissue and Fascia

Marsupialization
see Drainage
see Excision

Massage, cardiac
External 5A12012
Open 02QA0ZZ

Masseter muscle *use* Muscle, Head
Masseteric fascia *use* Subcutaneous Tissue and Fascia, Face

Mastectomy
see Excision, Skin and Breast 0HB
see Resection, Skin and Breast 0HT

Mastoid (postauricular) lymph node
use Lymphatic, Neck, Left
use Lymphatic, Neck, Right

Mastoid air cells
use Sinus, Mastoid, Left
use Sinus, Mastoid, Right

Mastoid process
use Bone, Temporal, Right
use Bone, Temporal, Left

Mastoidectomy
see Excision, Ear, Nose, Sinus 09B
see Resection, Ear, Nose, Sinus 09T

Mastoidotomy *see* Drainage, Ear, Nose, Sinus 099

Mastopexy
see Reposition, Skin and Breast 0HS
see Repair, Skin and Breast 0HQ

Mastorrhaphy *see* Repair, Skin and Breast 0HQ

Mastotomy *see* Drainage, Skin and Breast 0H9

Maxillary artery
use Artery, External Carotid, Right
use Artery, External Carotid, Left

Maxillary nerve *use* Nerve, Trigeminal

Maximo II DR (VR) *use* Defibrillator Generator in 0JH

Maximo II DR CRT-D *use* Cardiac Resynchronization Defibrillator Pulse Generator in 0JH

Measurement
Arterial
  Flow
    Coronary 4A03
    Peripheral 4A03
    Pulmonary 4A03
  Pressure
    Coronary 4A03
    Peripheral 4A03
    Pulmonary 4A03
    Thoracic, Other 4A03
  Pulse
    Coronary 4A03
    Peripheral 4A03
    Pulmonary 4A03
  Saturation, Peripheral 4A03
  Sound, Peripheral 4A03
Biliary
  Flow 4A0C
  Pressure 4A0C
Cardiac
  Action Currents 4A02
  Defibrillator 4B02XTZ

Measurement *(Continued)*
Cardiac *(Continued)*
  Electrical Activity 4A02
    Guidance 4A02X4A
    No Qualifier 4A02X4Z
  Output 4A02
  Pacemaker 4B02XSZ
  Rate 4A02
  Rhythm 4A02
  Sampling and Pressure
    Bilateral 4A02
    Left Heart 4A02
    Right Heart 4A02
  Sound 4A02
  Total Activity, Stress 4A02XM4
Central Nervous
  Conductivity 4A00
  Electrical Activity 4A00
  Pressure 4A000BZ
    Intracranial 4A00
  Saturation, Intracranial 4A00
  Stimulator 4B00XVZ
  Temperature, Intracranial 4A00
Circulatory, Volume 4A05XLZ
Gastrointestinal
  Motility 4A0B
  Pressure 4A0B
  Secretion 4A0B
Lymphatic
  Flow 4A06
  Pressure 4A06
Metabolism 4A0Z
Musculoskeletal
  Contractility 4A0F
  Stimulator 4B0FXVZ
Olfactory, Acuity 4A08X0Z
Peripheral Nervous
  Conductivity
    Motor 4A01
    Sensory 4A01
  Electrical Activity 4A01
  Stimulator 4B01XVZ
Products of Conception
  Cardiac
    Electrical Activity 4A0H
    Rate 4A0H
    Rhythm 4A0H
    Sound 4A0H
  Nervous
    Conductivity 4A0J
    Electrical Activity 4A0J
    Pressure 4A0J
Respiratory
  Capacity 4A09
  Flow 4A09
  Pacemaker 4B09XSZ
  Rate 4A09
  Resistance 4A09
  Total Activity 4A09
  Volume 4A09
Sleep 4A0ZXQZ
Temperature 4A0Z
Urinary
  Contractility 4A0D73Z
  Flow 4A0D75Z
  Pressure 4A0D7BZ
  Resistance 4A0D7DZ
  Volume 4A0D7LZ
Venous
  Flow
    Central 4A04
    Peripheral 4A04
    Portal 4A04
    Pulmonary 4A04
  Pressure
    Central 4A04
    Peripheral 4A04
    Portal 4A04
    Pulmonary 4A04

Measurement *(Continued)*
Venous *(Continued)*
  Pulse
    Central 4A04
    Peripheral 4A04
    Portal 4A04
    Pulmonary 4A04
  Saturation, Peripheral 4A04
  Visual
    Acuity 4A07X0Z
    Mobility 4A07X7Z
    Pressure 4A07XBZ

Meatoplasty, urethra *see* Repair, Urethra 0TQD
Meatotomy *see* Drainage, Urinary System 0T9
Mechanical ventilation *see* Performance, Respiratory 5A19

Medial canthus
use Eyelid, Lower, Left
use Eyelid, Lower, Right

Medial collateral ligament (MCL)
use Bursa and Ligament, Knee, Left
use Bursa and Ligament, Knee, Right

Medial condyle of femur
use Femur, Lower, Right
use Femur, Lower, Left

Medial condyle of tibia
use Tibia, Left
use Tibia, Right

Medial cuneiform bone
use Tarsal, Right
use Tarsal, Left

Medial epicondyle of femur
use Femur, Lower, Right
use Femur, Lower, Left

Medial epicondyle of humerus
use Humeral Shaft, Left
use Humeral Shaft, Right

Medial malleolus
use Tibia, Right
use Tibia, Left

Medial meniscus
use Joint, Knee, Right
use Joint, Knee, Left

Medial plantar artery
use Artery, Foot, Right
use Artery, Foot, Left

Medial plantar nerve *use* Nerve, Tibial
Medial popliteal nerve *use* Nerve, Tibial

Medial rectus muscle
use Muscle, Extraocular, Right
use Muscle, Extraocular, Left

Medial sural cutaneous nerve *use* Nerve, Tibial

Median antebrachial vein
use Vein, Basilic, Left
use Vein, Basilic, Right

Median cubital vein
use Vein, Basilic, Left
use Vein, Basilic, Right

Median sacral artery *use* Aorta, Abdominal

Mediastinal lymph node *use* Lymphatic, Thorax

Mediastinoscopy 0WJC4ZZ

Medication Management GZ3ZZZZ
for substance abuse
  Antabuse HZ83ZZZ
  Bupropion HZ87ZZZ
  Clonidine HZ86ZZZ
  Levo-alpha-acetyl-methadol (LAAM) HZ82ZZZ
  Methadone Maintenance HZ81ZZZ
  Naloxone HZ85ZZZ
  Naltrexone HZ84ZZZ
  Nicotine Replacement HZ80ZZZ
  Other Replacement Medication HZ89ZZZ
  Psychiatric Medication HZ88ZZZ

Meditation 8E0ZXY5

Meissner's (submucous) plexus *use* Nerve, Abdominal Sympathetic

Melody® transcatheter pulmonary valve *use* Zooplastic Tissue in Heart and Great Vessels

◄ New   ◄⫴ Revised   ~~deleted~~ Deleted

Membranous urethra *use* Urethra
Meningeorrhaphy
  see Repair, Cerebral Meninges 00Q1
  see Repair, Spinal Meninges 00QT
Meniscectomy
  see Excision, Lower Joints 0SB
  see Resection, Lower Joints 0ST
Mental foramen
  use Mandible, Left
  use Mandible, Right
Mentalis muscle *use* Muscle, Facial
Mentoplasty *see* Alteration, Jaw, Lower 0W05
Mesenterectomy *see* Excision, Mesentery 0DBV
Mesenteriorrhaphy, mesenterorrhaphy *see*
  Repair, Mesentery 0DQV
Mesenteriplication *see* Repair, Mesentery
  0DQV
Mesoappendix *use* Mesentery
Mesocolon *use* Mesentery
Metacarpal ligament
  use Bursa and Ligament, Hand, Left
  use Bursa and Ligament, Hand, Right
Metacarpophalangeal ligament
  use Bursa and Ligament, Hand, Right
  use Bursa and Ligament, Hand, Left
Metatarsal ligament
  use Bursa and Ligament, Foot, Right
  use Bursa and Ligament, Foot, Left
Metatarsectomy
  see Excision, Lower Bones 0QB
  see Resection, Lower Bones 0QT
Metatarsophalangeal (MTP) joint
  use Joint, Metatarsal-Phalangeal, Left
  use Joint, Metatarsal-Phalangeal, Right
Metatarsophalangeal ligament
  use Bursa and Ligament, Foot, Right
  use Bursa and Ligament, Foot, Left
Metathalamus *use* Thalamus
Micro-Driver stent (RX) (OTW) *use*
  Intraluminal Device
MicroMed HeartAssist *use* Implantable Heart
  Assist System in Heart and Great Vessels
Micrus CERECYTE microcoil *use* Intraluminal
  Device, Bioactive in Upper Arteries
Midcarpal joint
  use Joint, Carpal, Right
  use Joint, Carpal, Left
Middle cardiac nerve *use* Nerve, Thoracic
  Sympathetic
Middle cerebral artery *use* Artery, Intracranial
Middle cerebral vein *use* Vein, Intracranial
Middle colic vein *use* Vein, Colic
Middle genicular artery
  use Artery, Popliteal, Left
  use Artery, Popliteal, Right
Middle hemorrhoidal vein
  use Vein, Hypogastric, Left
  use Vein, Hypogastric, Right
Middle rectal artery
  use Artery, Internal Iliac, Right
  use Artery, Internal Iliac, Left
Middle suprarenal artery *use* Aorta,
  Abdominal
Middle temporal artery
  use Artery, Temporal, Left
  use Artery, Temporal, Right
Middle turbinate *use* Turbinate, Nasal
MitraClip valve repair system *use* Synthetic
  Substitute
Mitral annulus *use* Valve, Mitral
Mitroflow® Aortic Pericardial Heart Valve
  use Zooplastic Tissue in Heart and Great
  Vessels
Mobilization, adhesions *see* Release
Molar gland *use* Buccal Mucosa
Monitoring
  Arterial
    Flow
      Coronary 4A13
      Peripheral 4A13
      Pulmonary 4A13

Monitoring *(Continued)*
  Arterial *(Continued)*
    Pressure
      Coronary 4A13
      Peripheral 4A13
      Pulmonary 4A13
    Pulse
      Coronary 4A13
      Peripheral 4A13
      Pulmonary 4A13
    Saturation, Peripheral 4A13
    Sound, Peripheral 4A13
  Cardiac
    Electrical Activity 4A12
      Ambulatory 4A12X45
      No Qualifier 4A12X4Z
    Output 4A12
    Rate 4A12
    Rhythm 4A12
    Sound 4A12
    Total Activity, Stress 4A12XM4
  Central Nervous
    Conductivity 4A10
    Electrical Activity
      Intraoperative 4A10
      No Qualifier 4A10
    Pressure 4A100BZ
      Intracranial 4A10
    Saturation, Intracranial 4A10
    Temperature, Intracranial 4A10
  Gastrointestinal
    Motility 4A1B
    Pressure 4A1B
    Secretion 4A1B
  Lymphatic
    Flow 4A16
    Pressure 4A16
  Peripheral Nervous
    Conductivity
      Motor 4A11
      Sensory 4A11
    Electrical Activity Intraoperative 4A11
    No Qualifier 4A11
  Products of Conception
    Cardiac
      Electrical Activity 4A1H
      Rate 4A1H
      Rhythm 4A1H
      Sound 4A1H
    Nervous
      Conductivity 4A1J
      Electrical Activity 4A1J
      Pressure 4A1J
  Respiratory
    Capacity 4A19
    Flow 4A19
    Rate 4A19
    Resistance 4A19
    Volume 4A19
  Sleep 4A1ZXQZ
  Temperature 4A1Z
  Urinary
    Contractility 4A1D73Z
    Flow 4A1D75Z
    Pressure 4A1D7BZ
    Resistance 4A1D7DZ
    Volume 4A1D7LZ
  Venous
    Flow
      Central 4A14
      Peripheral 4A14
      Portal 4A14
      Pulmonary 4A14
    Pressure
      Central 4A14
      Peripheral 4A14
      Portal 4A14
      Pulmonary 4A14
    Pulse
      Central 4A14
      Peripheral 4A14

Monitoring *(Continued)*
  Venous *(Continued)*
    Pulse *(Continued)*
      Portal 4A14
      Pulmonary 4A14
    Saturation
      Central 4A14
      Portal 4A14
      Pulmonary 4A14
~~**Monitoring Device**~~
  ~~Abdomen 0JH8~~
  ~~Chest 0JH6~~
Monitoring Device, Hemodynamic ◄
  Abdomen 0JH8 ◄
  Chest 0JH6 ◄
Mosaic Bioprosthesis (aortic) (mitral) valve *use*
  Zooplastic Tissue in Heart and Great
  Vessels ◄
Motor Function Assessment F01
Motor Treatment F07
MR Angiography
  see Magnetic Resonance Imaging (MRI),
    Heart B23
  see Magnetic Resonance Imaging (MRI),
    Upper Arteries B33
  see Magnetic Resonance Imaging (MRI),
    Lower Arteries B43
MULTI-LINK (VISION)(MINI-VISION)
  (ULTRA) Coronary Stent System *use*
  Intraluminal Device ◄
Multiple sleep latency test 4A0ZXQZ
Musculocutaneous nerve *use* Nerve, Brachial
  Plexus
Musculopexy
  see Repair, Muscles 0KQ
  see Reposition, Muscles 0KS
Musculophrenic artery
  use Artery, Internal Mammary, Left
  use Artery, Internal Mammary, Right
Musculoplasty
  see Repair, Muscles 0KQ
  see Supplement, Muscles 0KU
Musculorrhaphy *see* Repair, Muscles
  0KQ
Musculospiral nerve *use* Nerve, Radial
Myectomy
  see Excision, Muscles 0KB
  see Resection, Muscles 0KT
Myelencephalon *use* Medulla Oblongata
Myelogram
  CT *see* Computerized Tomography (CT Scan),
    Central Nervous System B02
  MRI *see* Magnetic Resonance Imaging (MRI),
    Central Nervous System B03
Myenteric (Auerbach's) plexus *use* Nerve,
  Abdominal Sympathetic
Myomectomy *see* Excision, Female
  Reproductive System 0UB
Myometrium *use* Uterus
Myopexy
  see Repair, Muscles 0KQ
  see Reposition, Muscles 0KS
Myoplasty
  see Repair, Muscles 0KQ
  see Supplement, Muscles 0KU
Myorrhaphy *see* Repair, Muscles 0KQ
Myoscopy *see* Inspection, Muscles 0KJ
Myotomy
  see Division, Muscles 0K8
  see Drainage, Muscles 0K9
Myringectomy
  see Excision, Ear, Nose, Sinus 09B
  see Resection, Ear, Nose, Sinus 09T
Myringoplasty
  see Repair, Ear, Nose, Sinus 09Q
  see Replacement, Ear, Nose, Sinus 09R
  see Supplement, Ear, Nose, Sinus 09U
Myringostomy *see* Drainage, Ear, Nose, Sinus
  099
Myringotomy *see* Drainage, Ear, Nose, Sinus
  099

◄ New   ◄▧ Revised   ~~deleted~~ Deleted

N

Nail bed
use Finger Nail
use Toe Nail
Nail plate
use Finger Nail
use Toe Nail
Narcosynthesis GZGZZZZ
Nasal cavity *use* Nose
Nasal concha *use* Turbinate, Nasal
Nasalis muscle *use* Muscle, Facial
Nasolacrimal duct
use Duct, Lacrimal, Right
use Duct, Lacrimal, Left
Nasopharyngeal airway (NPA) *use* Intraluminal
Device, Airway in Ear, Nose, Sinus
Navicular bone
use Tarsal, Left
use Tarsal, Right
Near Infrared Spectroscopy, Circulatory
System 8E023DZ
Neck of femur
use Femur, Upper, Right
use Femur, Upper, Left
Neck of humerus (anatomical)(surgical)
use Humeral Head, Right
use Humeral Head, Left
Nephrectomy
see Excision, Urinary System 0TB
see Resection, Urinary System 0TT
Nephrolithotomy *see* Extirpation, Urinary
System 0TC
Nephrolysis *see* Release, Urinary System 0TN
Nephropexy
see Repair, Urinary System 0TQ
see Reposition, Urinary System 0TS
Nephroplasty
see Repair, Urinary System 0TQ
see Supplement, Urinary System 0TU
Nephropyeloureterostomy
see Bypass, Urinary System 0T1
see Drainage, Urinary System 0T9
Nephrorrhaphy *see* Repair, Urinary System 0TQ
Nephroscopy, transurethral 0TJ58ZZ
Nephrostomy
see Bypass, Urinary System 0T1
see Drainage, Urinary System 0T9
Nephrotomography
see Plain Radiography, Urinary System BT0
see Fluoroscopy, Urinary System BT1
Nephrotomy
see Drainage, Urinary System 0T9
see Division, Urinary System 0T8
Nerve conduction study
see Measurement, Central Nervous 4A00
see Measurement, Peripheral Nervous 4A01
Nerve Function Assessment F01
Nerve to the stapedius *use* Nerve, Facial
Nesiritide *use* Human B-type Natriuretic
Peptide ◀
Neurectomy
see Excision, Central Nervous System 00B
see Excision, Peripheral Nervous System 01B
Neurexeresis
see Extraction, Central Nervous System 00D
see Extraction, Peripheral Nervous System
01D
Neurohypophysis *use* Gland, Pituitary
Neurolysis
see Release, Central Nervous System 00N
see Release, Peripheral Nervous System 01N

Neuromuscular electrical stimulation (NEMS)
lead *use* Stimulator Lead in Muscles
Neurophysiologic monitoring *see* Monitoring,
Central Nervous 4A10
Neuroplasty
see Repair, Central Nervous System 00Q
see Repair, Peripheral Nervous System 01Q
see Supplement, Central Nervous System 00U
see Supplement, Peripheral Nervous System
01U
Neurorrhaphy
see Repair, Central Nervous System 00Q
see Repair, Peripheral Nervous System 01Q
Neurostimulator Generator
Insertion of device in, Skull 0NH00NZ
Removal of device from, Skull 0NP00NZ
Revision of device in, Skull 0NW00NZ
Neurostimulator generator, multiple channel
use Stimulator Generator, Multiple Array
in 0JH
Neurostimulator generator, multiple channel
rechargeable *use* Stimulator Generator,
Multiple Array Rechargeable in 0JH
Neurostimulator generator, single channel *use*
Stimulator Generator, Single Array in 0JH
Neurostimulator generator, single channel
rechargeable *use* Stimulator Generator,
Single Array Rechargeable in 0JH
Neurostimulator Lead
Insertion of device in
Brain 00H0
Canal, Spinal 00HU
Cerebral Ventricle 00H6
Nerve
Cranial 00HE
Peripheral 01HY
Spinal Canal 00HU
Spinal Cord 00HV
Removal of device from
Brain 00P0
Cerebral Ventricle 00P6
Nerve
Cranial 00PE
Peripheral 01PY
Spinal Canal 00PU
Spinal Cord 00PV
Revision of device in
Brain 00W0
Cerebral Ventricle 00W6
Nerve
Cranial 00WE
Peripheral 01WY
Spinal Canal 00WU
Spinal Cord 00WV
Neurotomy
see Division, Central Nervous System 008
see Division, Peripheral Nervous System
018
Neurotripsy
see Destruction, Central Nervous System
005
see Destruction, Peripheral Nervous System
015
Neutralization plate
use Internal Fixation Device in Head and
Facial Bones
use Internal Fixation Device in Upper Bones
use Internal Fixation Device in Lower Bones
Ninth cranial nerve *use* Nerve,
Glossopharyngeal

Nitinol framed polymer mesh *use* Synthetic
Substitute
Non-tunneled central venous catheter *use*
Infusion Device
Nonimaging Nuclear Medicine Assay
Bladder, Kidneys and Ureters CT63
Blood C763
Kidneys, Ureters and Bladder CT63
Lymphatics and Hematologic System
C76YYZZ
Ureters, Kidneys and Bladder CT63
Urinary System CT6YYZZ
Nonimaging Nuclear Medicine Probe
CP5YYZZ
Abdomen CW50
Abdomen and Chest CW54
Abdomen and Pelvis CW51
Brain C050
Central Nervous System C05YYZZ
Chest CW53
Chest and Abdomen CW54
Chest and Neck CW56
Extremity
Lower CP5
Upper CP5
Head and Neck CW5B
Heart C25YYZZ
Right and Left C256
Lymphatics
Head C75J
Head and Neck C755
Lower Extremity C75P
Neck C75K
Pelvic C75D
Trunk C75M
Upper Chest C75L
Upper Extremity C75N
Lymphatics and Hematologic System
C75YYZZ
Neck and Chest CW56
Neck and Head CW5B
Pelvic Region CW5J
Pelvis and Abdomen CW51
Spine CP55ZZZ
Nonimaging Nuclear Medicine Uptake
Endocrine System CG4YYZZ
Gland, Thyroid CG42
Nostril *use* Nose
Novacor Left Ventricular Assist Device *use*
Implantable Heart Assist System in Heart
and Great Vessels
Novation® Ceramic AHS® (Articulation Hip
System) *use* Synthetic Substitute, Ceramic
in 0SR
Nuclear medicine
see Planar Nuclear Medicine Imaging
see Tomographic (Tomo) Nuclear Medicine
Imaging
see Positron Emission Tomographic (PET)
Imaging
see Nonimaging Nuclear Medicine Uptake
see Nonimaging Nuclear Medicine Probe
see Nonimaging Nuclear Medicine Assay
see Systemic Nuclear Medicine Therapy
Nuclear scintigraphy *see* Nuclear Medicine
Nutrition, concentrated substances
Enteral infusion 3E0G36Z
Parenteral (peripheral) infusion *see*
Introduction of Nutritional Substance

◀ New ◀▥ Revised ~~deleted~~ Deleted

O

Obliteration *see* Destruction
Obturator artery
  use Artery, Internal Iliac, Left
  use Artery, Internal Iliac, Right
Obturator lymph node *use* Lymphatic,
  Pelvis
Obturator muscle
  use Muscle, Hip, Left
  use Muscle, Hip, Right
Obturator nerve *use* Nerve, Lumbar
  Plexus
Obturator vein
  use Vein, Hypogastric, Right
  use Vein, Hypogastric, Left
Obtuse margin *use* Heart, Left
Occipital artery
  use Artery, External Carotid, Right
  use Artery, External Carotid, Left
Occipital lobe *use* Cerebral Hemisphere
Occipital lymph node
  use Lymphatic, Neck, Left
  use Lymphatic, Neck, Right
Occipitofrontalis muscle *use* Muscle,
  Facial
Occlusion
  Ampulla of Vater 0FLC
  Anus 0DLQ
  Aorta, Abdominal 04L0
  Artery
    Anterior Tibial
      Left 04LQ
      Right 04LP
    Axillary
      Left 03L6
      Right 03L5
    Brachial
      Left 03L8
      Right 03L7
    Celiac 04L1
    Colic
      Left 04L7
      Middle 04L8
      Right 04L6
    Common Carotid
      Left 03LJ
      Right 03LH
    Common Iliac
      Left 04LD
      Right 04LC
    External Carotid
      Left 03LN
      Right 03LM
    External Iliac
      Left 04LJ
      Right 04LH
    Face 03LR
    Femoral
      Left 04LL
      Right 04LK
    Foot
      Left 04LW
      Right 04LV
    Gastric 04L2
    Hand
      Left 03LF
      Right 03LD
    Hepatic 04L3
    Inferior Mesenteric 04LB
    Innominate 03L2
    Internal Carotid
      Left 03LL
      Right 03LK
    Internal Iliac
      Left, Uterine Artery, Left 04LF
      Right, Uterine Artery, Right 04LE
    Internal Mammary
      Left 03L1
      Right 03L0
    Intracranial 03LG

Occlusion *(Continued)*
  Artery *(Continued)*
    Lower 04LY
    Peroneal
      Left 04LU
      Right 04LT
    Popliteal
      Left 04LN
      Right 04LM
    Posterior Tibial
      Left 04LS
      Right 04LR
    Pulmonary, Left 02LR
    Radial
      Left 03LC
      Right 03LB
    Renal
      Left 04LA
      Right 04L9
    Splenic 04L4
    Subclavian
      Left 03L4
      Right 03L3
    Superior Mesenteric 04L5
    Temporal
      Left 03LT
      Right 03LS
    Thyroid
      Left 03LV
      Right 03LU
    Ulnar
      Left 03LA
      Right 03L9
    Upper 03LY
    Vertebral
      Left 03LQ
      Right 03LP
  Atrium, Left 02L7
  Bladder 0TLB
  Bladder Neck 0TLC
  Bronchus
    Lingula 0BL9
    Lower Lobe
      Left 0BLB
      Right 0BL6
    Main
      Left 0BL7
      Right 0BL3
    Middle Lobe, Right 0BL5
    Upper Lobe
      Left 0BL8
      Right 0BL4
  Carina 0BL2
  Cecum 0DLH
  Cisterna Chyli 07LL
  Colon
    Ascending 0DLK
    Descending 0DLM
    Sigmoid 0DLN
    Transverse 0DLL
  Cord
    Bilateral 0VLH
    Left 0VLG
    Right 0VLF
  Cul-de-sac 0ULF
  Duct
    Common Bile 0FL9
    Cystic 0FL8
    Hepatic
      Left 0FL6
      Right 0FL5
    Lacrimal
      Left 08LY
      Right 08LX
    Pancreatic 0FLD
      Accessory 0FLF
    Parotid
      Left 0CLC
      Right 0CLB
  Duodenum 0DL9
  Esophagogastric Junction 0DL4

Occlusion *(Continued)*
  Esophagus 0DL5
    Lower 0DL3
    Middle 0DL2
    Upper 0DL1
  Fallopian Tube
    Left 0UL6
    Right 0UL5
  Fallopian Tubes, Bilateral
    0UL7
  Ileocecal Valve 0DLC
  Ileum 0DLB
  Intestine
    Large 0DLE
      Left 0DLG
      Right 0DLF
    Small 0DL8
  Jejunum 0DLA
  Kidney Pelvis
    Left 0TL4
    Right 0TL3
  Left atrial appendage (LAA) *see*
    Occlusion, Atrium, Left
    02L7
  Lymphatic
    Aortic 07LD
    Axillary
      Left 07L6
      Right 07L5
    Head 07L0
    Inguinal
      Left 07LJ
      Right 07LH
    Internal Mammary
      Left 07L9
      Right 07L8
    Lower Extremity
      Left 07LG
      Right 07LF
    Mesenteric 07LB
    Neck
      Left 07L2
      Right 07L1
    Pelvis 07LC
    Thoracic Duct 07LK
    Thorax 07L7
    Upper Extremity
      Left 07L4
      Right 07L3
  Rectum 0DLP
  Stomach 0DL6
    Pylorus 0DL7
  Trachea 0BL1
  Ureter
    Left 0TL7
    Right 0TL6
  Urethra 0TLD
  Vagina 0ULG
  Vas Deferens
    Bilateral 0VLQ
    Left 0VLP
    Right 0VLN
  Vein
    Axillary
      Left 05L8
      Right 05L7
    Azygos 05L0
    Basilic
      Left 05LC
      Right 05LB
    Brachial
      Left 05LA
      Right 05L9
    Cephalic
      Left 05LF
      Right 05LD
    Colic 06L7
    Common Iliac
      Left 06LD
      Right 06LC
    Esophageal 06L3

Occlusion *(Continued)*
  Vein *(Continued)*
    External Iliac
      Left 06LG
      Right 06LF
    External Jugular
      Left 05LQ
      Right 05LP
    Face
      Left 05LV
      Right 05LT
    Femoral
      Left 06LN
      Right 06LM
    Foot
      Left 06LV
      Right 06LT
    Gastric 06L2
    Greater Saphenous
      Left 06LQ
      Right 06LP
    Hand
      Left 05LH
      Right 05LG
    Hemiazygos 05L1
    Hepatic 06L4
    Hypogastric
      Left 06LJ
      Right 06LH
    Inferior Mesenteric 06L6
    Innominate
      Left 05L4
      Right 05L3
    Internal Jugular
      Left 05LN
      Right 05LM
    Intracranial 05LL
    Lesser Saphenous
      Left 06LS
      Right 06LR
    Lower 06LY
    Portal 06L8
    Pulmonary
      Left 02LT
      Right 02LS
    Renal
      Left 06LB
      Right 06L9
    Splenic 06L1
    Subclavian
      Left 05L6
      Right 05L5
    Superior Mesenteric 06L5
    Upper 05LY
    Vertebral
      Left 05LS
      Right 05LR
  Vena Cava
    Inferior 06L0
    Superior 02LV
Occupational therapy *see* Activities of Daily Living Treatment, Rehabilitation F08
Odentectomy
  see Excision, Mouth and Throat 0CB
  see Resection, Mouth and Throat 0CT
Olecranon bursa
  use Bursa and Ligament, Elbow, Left
  use Bursa and Ligament, Elbow, Right
Olecranon process
  use Ulna, Left
  use Ulna, Right
Olfactory bulb *use* Nerve, Olfactory
Omentectomy, omentumectomy
  see Excision, Gastrointestinal System 0DB
  see Resection, Gastrointestinal System 0DT
Omentofixation *see* Repair, Gastrointestinal System 0DQ

Omentoplasty
  see Repair, Gastrointestinal System 0DQ
  see Replacement, Gastrointestinal System 0DR
  see Supplement, Gastrointestinal System 0DU
Omentorrhaphy *see* Repair, Gastrointestinal System 0DQ
Omentotomy *see* Drainage, Gastrointestinal System 0D9
Omnilink Elite Vascular Balloon Expandable Stent System *use* Intraluminal Device ◀
Onychectomy
  see Excision, Skin and Breast 0HB
  see Resection, Skin and Breast 0HT
Onychoplasty
  see Repair, Skin and Breast 0HQ
  see Replacement, Skin and Breast 0HR
Onychotomy *see* Drainage, Skin and Breast 0H9
Oophorectomy
  see Excision, Female Reproductive System 0UB
  see Resection, Female Reproductive System 0UT
Oophoropexy
  see Repair, Female Reproductive System 0UQ
  see Reposition, Female Reproductive System 0US
Oophoroplasty
  see Repair, Female Reproductive System 0UQ
  see Supplement, Female Reproductive System 0UU
Oophororrhaphy *see* Repair, Female Reproductive System 0UQ
Oophorostomy *see* Drainage, Female Reproductive System 0U9
Oophorotomy
  see Drainage, Female Reproductive System 0U9
  see Division, Female Reproductive System 0U8
Oophorrhaphy *see* Repair, Female Reproductive System 0UQ
Open Pivot (mechanical) valve *use* Synthetic Substitute ◀
Open Pivot Aortic Valve Graft (AVG) *use* Synthetic Substitute ◀
Ophthalmic artery
  use Artery, Internal Carotid, Right
  use Artery, Internal Carotid, Left
Ophthalmic nerve *use* Nerve, Trigeminal
Ophthalmic vein *use* Vein, Intracranial
Opponensplasty
  Tendon replacement *see* Replacement, Tendons 0LR
  Tendon transfer *see* Transfer, Tendons 0LX
Optic chiasma *use* Nerve, Optic
Optic disc
  use Retina, Left
  use Retina, Right
Optic foramen
  use Bone, Sphenoid, Right
  use Bone, Sphenoid, Left
Optical coherence tomography, intravascular *see* Computerized Tomography (CT Scan)
Optimizer™ III implantable pulse generator *use* Contractility Modulation Device in 0JH
Orbicularis oculi muscle
  use Eyelid, Upper, Left
  use Eyelid, Upper, Right
Orbicularis oris muscle *use* Muscle, Facial
Orbital fascia *use* Subcutaneous Tissue and Fascia, Face
Orbital portion of ethmoid bone
  use Orbit, Left
  use Orbit, Right
Orbital portion of frontal bone
  use Orbit, Right
  use Orbit, Left
Orbital portion of lacrimal bone
  use Orbit, Left
  use Orbit, Right

Orbital portion of maxilla
  use Orbit, Left
  use Orbit, Right
Orbital portion of palatine bone
  use Orbit, Right
  use Orbit, Left
Orbital portion of sphenoid bone
  use Orbit, Right
  use Orbit, Left
Orbital portion of zygomatic bone
  use Orbit, Left
  use Orbit, Right
Orchectomy, orchidectomy, orchiectomy
  see Excision, Male Reproductive System 0VB
  see Resection, Male Reproductive System 0VT
Orchidoplasty, orchioplasty
  see Repair, Male Reproductive System 0VQ
  see Replacement, Male Reproductive System 0VR
  see Supplement, Male Reproductive System 0VU
Orchidorrhaphy, orchiorrhaphy *see* Repair, Male Reproductive System 0VQ
Orchidotomy, orchiotomy, orchotomy *see* Drainage, Male Reproductive System 0V9
Orchiopexy
  see Repair, Male Reproductive System 0VQ
  see Reposition, Male Reproductive System 0VS
Oropharyngeal airway (OPA) *use* Intraluminal Device, Airway in Mouth and Throat
Oropharynx *use* Pharynx
Ossicular chain
  use Auditory Ossicle, Left
  use Auditory Ossicle, Right
Ossiculectomy
  see Excision, Ear, Nose, Sinus 09B
  see Resection, Ear, Nose, Sinus 09T
Ossiculotomy *see* Drainage, Ear, Nose, Sinus 099
Ostectomy
  see Excision, Head and Facial Bones 0NB
  see Resection, Head and Facial Bones 0NT
  see Excision, Upper Bones 0PB
  see Resection, Upper Bones 0PT
  see Excision, Lower Bones 0QB
  see Resection, Lower Bones 0QT
Osteoclasis
  see Division, Head and Facial Bones 0N8
  see Division, Upper Bones 0P8
  see Division, Lower Bones 0Q8
Osteolysis
  see Release, Head and Facial Bones 0NN
  see Release, Upper Bones 0PN
  see Release, Lower Bones 0QN
Osteopathic Treatment
  Abdomen 7W09X
  Cervical 7W01X
  Extremity
    Lower 7W06X
    Upper 7W07X
  Head 7W00X
  Lumbar 7W03X
  Pelvis 7W05X
  Rib Cage 7W08X
  Sacrum 7W04X
  Thoracic 7W02X
Osteopexy
  see Repair, Head and Facial Bones 0NQ
  see Reposition, Head and Facial Bones 0NS
  see Repair, Upper Bones 0PQ
  see Reposition, Upper Bones 0PS
  see Repair, Lower Bones 0QQ
  see Reposition, Lower Bones 0QS
Osteoplasty
  see Repair, Head and Facial Bones 0NQ
  see Replacement, Head and Facial Bones 0NR
  see Repair, Upper Bones 0PQ
  see Replacement, Upper Bones 0PR

◀ New   ◀▥ Revised   ~~deleted~~ Deleted

Osteoplasty *(Continued)*
  see Repair, Lower Bones 0QQ
  see Replacement, Lower Bones 0QR
  see Supplement, Lower Bones 0QU
  see Supplement, Head and Facial Bones
    0NU
  see Supplement, Upper Bones 0PU
Osteorrhaphy
  see Repair, Head and Facial Bones 0NQ
  see Repair, Upper Bones 0PQ
  see Repair, Lower Bones 0QQ
Osteotomy, ostotomy
  see Division, Head and Facial Bones 0N8
  see Drainage, Head and Facial Bones 0N9
  see Division, Upper Bones 0P8
  see Drainage, Upper Bones 0P9
  see Division, Lower Bones 0Q8
  see Drainage, Lower Bones 0Q9
Otic ganglion *use* Nerve, Head and Neck
    Sympathetic
Otoplasty
  see Repair, Ear, Nose, Sinus 09Q
  see Replacement, Ear, Nose, Sinus 09R
  see Supplement, Ear, Nose, Sinus 09U

Otoscopy *see* Inspection, Ear, Nose, Sinus 09J
Oval window
  use Ear, Middle, Left
  use Ear, Middle, Right
Ovarian artery *use* Aorta, Abdominal
Ovarian ligament *use* Uterine Supporting
    Structure
Ovariectomy
  see Excision, Female Reproductive System
    0UB
  see Resection, Female Reproductive System
    0UT
Ovariocentesis *see* Drainage, Female
    Reproductive System 0U9
Ovariopexy
  see Repair, Female Reproductive System
    0UQ
  see Reposition, Female Reproductive System
    0US
Ovariotomy
  see Drainage, Female Reproductive System
    0U9
  see Division, Female Reproductive System
    0U8

Ovatio™ CRT-D *use* Cardiac Resynchronization
    Defibrillator Pulse Generator in 0JH
Oversewing
  Gastrointestinal ulcer *see* Repair,
    Gastrointestinal System 0DQ
  Pleural bleb *see* Repair, Respiratory System
    0BQ
Oviduct
  use Fallopian Tube, Right
  use Fallopian Tube, Left
**Oxidized zirconium ceramic hip bearing
    surface** *use* Synthetic Substitute, Ceramic
    on Polyethylene in 0SR
Oximetry, Fetal pulse 10H073Z
Oxygenation
  Extracorporeal membrane (ECMO) *see*
    Performance, Circulatory 5A15 ◄▥▥
  Hyperbaric *see* Assistance, Circulatory 5A05
  Supersaturated *see* Assistance, Circulatory
    5A05

P

Pacemaker
  Dual Chamber
    Abdomen 0JH8
    Chest 0JH6
  Single Chamber
    Abdomen 0JH8
    Chest 0JH6
  Single Chamber Rate Responsive
    Abdomen 0JH8
    Chest 0JH6
Packing
  Abdominal Wall 2W43X5Z
  Anorectal 2Y43X5Z
  Arm
    Lower
      Left 2W4DX5Z
      Right 2W4CX5Z
    Upper
      Left 2W4BX5Z
      Right 2W4AX5Z
  Back 2W45X5Z
  Chest Wall 2W44X5Z
  Ear 2Y42X5Z
  Extremity
    Lower
      Left 2W4MX5Z
      Right 2W4LX5Z
    Upper
      Left 2W49X5Z
      Right 2W48X5Z
  Face 2W41X5Z
  Finger
    Left 2W4KX5Z
    Right 2W4JX5Z
  Foot
    Left 2W4TX5Z
    Right 2W4SX5Z
  Genital Tract, Female 2Y44X5Z
  Hand
    Left 2W4FX5Z
    Right 2W4EX5Z
  Head 2W40X5Z
  Inguinal Region
    Left 2W47X5Z
    Right 2W46X5Z
  Leg
    Lower
      Left 2W4RX5Z
      Right 2W4QX5Z
    Upper
      Left 2W4PX5Z
      Right 2W4NX5Z
  Mouth and Pharynx 2Y40X5Z
  Nasal 2Y41X5Z
  Neck 2W42X5Z
  Thumb
    Left 2W4HX5Z
    Right 2W4GX5Z
  Toe
    Left 2W4VX5Z
    Right 2W4UX5Z
  Urethra 2Y45X5Z
Paclitaxel-eluting coronary stent
  use Intraluminal Device,
    Drug-eluting in Heart and
    Great Vessels
Paclitaxel-eluting peripheral stent
  use Intraluminal Device, Drug-eluting in
    Upper Arteries
  use Intraluminal Device, Drug-eluting in
    Lower Arteries
Palatine gland *use* Buccal Mucosa
Palatine tonsil *use* Tonsils
Palatine uvula *use* Uvula
Palatoglossal muscle *use* Muscle, Tongue,
  Palate, Pharynx
Palatopharyngeal muscle *use* Muscle, Tongue,
  Palate, Pharynx

Palatoplasty
  see Repair, Mouth and Throat 0CQ
  see Replacement, Mouth and Throat 0CR
  see Supplement, Mouth and Throat 0CU
Palatorrhaphy *see* Repair, Mouth and Throat 0CQ
Palmar (volar) digital vein
  use Vein, Hand, Right
  use Vein, Hand, Left
Palmar (volar) metacarpal vein
  use Vein, Hand, Left
  use Vein, Hand, Right
Palmar cutaneous nerve
  use Nerve, Radial
  use Nerve, Median
Palmar fascia (aponeurosis)
  use Subcutaneous Tissue and Fascia, Hand,
    Left
  use Subcutaneous Tissue and Fascia, Hand,
    Right
Palmar interosseous muscle
  use Muscle, Hand, Left
  use Muscle, Hand, Right
Palmar ulnocarpal ligament
  use Bursa and Ligament, Wrist, Right
  use Bursa and Ligament, Wrist, Left
Palmaris longus muscle
  use Muscle, Lower Arm and Wrist, Left
  use Muscle, Lower Arm and Wrist, Right
Pancreatectomy
  see Excision, Pancreas 0FBG
  see Resection, Pancreas 0FTG
Pancreatic artery *use* Artery, Splenic
Pancreatic plexus *use* Nerve, Abdominal
  Sympathetic
Pancreatic vein *use* Vein, Splenic
Pancreaticoduodenostomy *see* Bypass,
  Hepatobiliary System and Pancreas 0F1
Pancreaticosplenic lymph node *use* Lymphatic,
  Aortic
Pancreatogram, endoscopic retrograde *see*
  Fluoroscopy, Pancreatic Duct BF18
Pancreatolithotomy *see* Extirpation, Pancreas
  0FCG
Pancreatotomy
  see Drainage, Pancreas 0F9G
  see Division, Pancreas 0F8G
Panniculectomy
  see Excision, Skin, Abdomen 0HB7
  see Excision, Abdominal Wall 0WBF
Paraaortic lymph node *use* Lymphatic, Aortic
Paracentesis
  Eye *see* Drainage, Eye 089
  Peritoneal Cavity *see* Drainage, Peritoneal
    Cavity 0W9G
  Tympanum *see* Drainage, Ear, Nose, Sinus 099
Pararectal lymph node *use* Lymphatic,
  Mesenteric
Parasternal lymph node *use* Lymphatic, Thorax
Parathyroidectomy
  see Excision, Endocrine System 0GB
  see Resection, Endocrine System 0GT
Paratracheal lymph node *use* Lymphatic, Thorax
Paraurethral (Skene's) gland *use* Gland,
  Vestibular
Parenteral nutrition, total *see* Introduction of
  Nutritional Substance
Parietal lobe *use* Cerebral Hemisphere
Parotid lymph node *use* Lymphatic, Head
Parotid plexus *use* Nerve, Facial
Parotidectomy
  see Excision, Mouth and Throat 0CB
  see Resection, Mouth and Throat 0CT
Pars flaccida
  use Membrane, Tympanic, Right
  use Membrane, Tympanic, Left
Partial joint replacement
  Hip *see* Replacement, Lower Joints 0SR
  Knee *see* Replacement, Lower Joints 0SR
  Shoulder *see* Replacement, Upper Joints 0RR
Partially absorbable mesh *use* Synthetic
  Substitute
Patch, blood, spinal 3E0S3GC

Patellapexy
  see Repair, Lower Bones 0QQ
  see Reposition, Lower Bones 0QS
Patellaplasty
  see Repair, Lower Bones 0QQ
  see Replacement, Lower Bones 0QR
  see Supplement, Lower Bones 0QU
Patellar ligament
  use Bursa and Ligament, Knee, Right
  use Bursa and Ligament, Knee, Left
Patellar tendon
  use Tendon, Knee, Left
  use Tendon, Knee, Right
Patellectomy
  see Excision, Lower Bones 0QB
  see Resection, Lower Bones 0QT
Patellofemoral joint
  use Joint, Knee, Right
  use Joint, Knee, Left
  use Joint, Knee, Right, Femoral Surface
  use Joint, Knee, Left, Femoral Surface
Pectineus muscle
  use Muscle, Upper Leg, Left
  use Muscle, Upper Leg, Right
Pectoral (anterior) lymph node
  use Lymphatic, Axillary, Right
  use Lymphatic, Axillary, Left
Pectoral fascia *use* Subcutaneous Tissue and
  Fascia, Chest
Pectoralis major muscle
  use Muscle, Thorax, Left
  use Muscle, Thorax, Right
Pectoralis minor muscle
  use Muscle, Thorax, Right
  use Muscle, Thorax, Left
Pedicle-based dynamic stabilization device
  use Spinal Stabilization Device, Pedicle-Based
    in 0RH
  use Spinal Stabilization Device, Pedicle-Based
    in 0SH
PEEP (positive end expiratory pressure) *see*
  Assistance, Respiratory 5A09
PEG (percutaneous endoscopic gastrostomy)
  0DH64UZ
PEJ (percutaneous endoscopic jejunostomy)
  0DHA4UZ
Pelvic splanchnic nerve
  use Nerve, Abdominal Sympathetic
  use Nerve, Sacral Sympathetic
Penectomy
  see Excision, Male Reproductive System 0VB
  see Resection, Male Reproductive System 0VT
Penile urethra *use* Urethra
**Percutaneous endoscopic gastrojejunostomy
  (PEG/J) tube** *use* Feeding Device in
  Gastrointestinal System
**Percutaneous endoscopic gastrostomy (PEG)
  tube** *use* Feeding Device in Gastrointestinal
  System
Percutaneous nephrostomy catheter *use*
  Drainage Device
**Percutaneous transluminal coronary
  angioplasty (PTCA)** *see* Dilation, Heart
  and Great Vessels 027
Performance
  Biliary
    Multiple, Filtration 5A1C60Z
    Single, Filtration 5A1C00Z
  Cardiac
    Continuous
      Output 5A1221Z
      Pacing 5A1223Z
    Intermittent, Pacing 5A1213Z
    Single, Output, Manual 5A12012
  Circulatory, Continuous, Oxygenation,
    Membrane 5A15223
  Respiratory
    24-96 Consecutive Hours, Ventilation
      5A1945Z
    Greater than 96 Consecutive Hours,
      Ventilation 5A1955Z
    Less than 24 Consecutive Hours,
      Ventilation 5A1935Z

◄ New   ◄┅ Revised   ~~deleted~~ Deleted

Performance (Continued)
  Respiratory (Continued)
    Single, Ventilation, Nonmechanical
      5A19054
  Urinary
    Multiple, Filtration 5A1D60Z
    Single, Filtration 5A1D00Z
Perfusion see Introduction of substance in or on
Pericardiectomy
  see Excision, Pericardium 02BN
  see Resection, Pericardium 02TN
Pericardiocentesis
  see Drainage, Cavity, Pericardial 0W9D
Pericardiolysis see Release, Pericardium 02NN
Pericardiophrenic artery
  use Artery, Internal Mammary, Left
  use Artery, Internal Mammary, Right
Pericardioplasty
  see Repair, Pericardium 02QN
  see Replacement, Pericardium 02RN
  see Supplement, Pericardium 02UN
Pericardiorrhaphy see Repair, Pericardium
  02QN
Pericardiostomy see Drainage, Cavity,
  Pericardial 0W9D
Pericardiotomy see Drainage, Cavity, Pericardial
  0W9D
Perimetrium use Uterus
Peripheral parenteral nutrition see Introduction
  of Nutritional Substance
Peripherally inserted central catheter (PICC)
  use Infusion Device
Peritoneal dialysis 3E1M39Z
Peritoneocentesis
  see Drainage, Peritoneum 0D9W
  see Drainage, Cavity, Peritoneal 0W9G
Peritoneoplasty
  see Repair, Peritoneum 0DQW
  see Replacement, Peritoneum 0DRW
  see Supplement, Peritoneum 0DUW
Peritoneoscopy 0DJW4ZZ
Peritoneotomy see Drainage, Peritoneum 0D9W
Peritoneumectomy
  see Excision, Peritoneum 0DBW
Peroneus brevis muscle
  use Muscle, Lower Leg, Left
  use Muscle, Lower Leg, Right
Peroneus longus muscle
  use Muscle, Lower Leg, Right
  use Muscle, Lower Leg, Left
Pessary ring use Intraluminal Device, Pessary in
  Female Reproductive System
PET scan see Positron Emission Tomographic
  (PET) Imaging
Petrous part of temporal bone
  use Bone, Temporal, Right
  use Bone, Temporal, Left
Phacoemulsification, lens
  With IOL implant see Replacement, Eye 08R
  Without IOL implant see Extraction, Eye 08D
Phalangectomy
  see Excision, Upper Bones 0PB
  see Resection, Upper Bones 0PT
  see Excision, Lower Bones 0QB
  see Resection, Lower Bones 0QT
Phallectomy
  see Excision, Penis 0VBS
  see Resection, Penis 0VTS
Phalloplasty
  see Repair, Penis 0VQS
  see Supplement, Penis 0VUS
Phallotomy see Drainage, Penis 0V9S
~~Pharmacotherapy~~
  ~~Antabuse HZ93ZZZ~~
  ~~Bupropion HZ97ZZZ~~
  ~~Clonidine HZ96ZZZ~~
  ~~Levo-alpha-acetyl-methadol (LAAM)~~
    ~~HZ92ZZZ~~
  ~~Methadone Maintenance HZ91ZZZ~~
  ~~Naloxone HZ95ZZZ~~
  ~~Naltrexone HZ94ZZZ~~

~~Pharmacotherapy (Continued)~~
  ~~Nicotine Replacement HZ90ZZZ~~
  ~~Psychiatric Medication HZ98ZZZ~~
  ~~Replacement Medication, Other HZ99ZZZ~~
Pharmacotherapy, for substance abuse ◄
  Antabuse HZ93ZZZ ◄
  Bupropion HZ97ZZZ ◄
  Clonidine HZ96ZZZ ◄
  Levo-alpha-acetyl-methadol (LAAM)
    HZ92ZZZ ◄
  Methadone Maintenance HZ91ZZZ ◄
  Naloxone HZ95ZZZ ◄
  Naltrexone HZ94ZZZ ◄
  Nicotine Replacement HZ90ZZZ ◄
  Psychiatric Medication HZ98ZZZ ◄
  Replacement Medication, Other
    HZ99ZZZ ◄
Pharyngeal constrictor muscle use Muscle,
  Tongue, Palate, Pharynx
Pharyngeal plexus use Nerve, Vagus
Pharyngeal recess use Nasopharynx
Pharyngeal tonsil use Adenoids
Pharyngogram see Fluoroscopy, Pharynx B91G
Pharyngoplasty
  see Repair, Mouth and Throat 0CQ
  see Replacement, Mouth and Throat 0CR
  see Supplement, Mouth and Throat 0CU
Pharyngorrhaphy see Repair, Mouth and Throat
  0CQ
Pharyngotomy see Drainage, Mouth and Throat
  0C9
Pharyngotympanic tube
  use Eustachian Tube, Right
  use Eustachian Tube, Left
Pheresis
  Erythrocytes 6A55
  Leukocytes 6A55
  Plasma 6A55
  Platelets 6A55
  Stem Cells
    Cord Blood 6A55
    Hematopoietic 6A55
Phlebectomy
  see Excision, Upper Veins 05B
  see Extraction, Upper Veins 05D
  see Excision, Lower Veins 06B
  see Extraction, Lower Veins 06D
Phlebography
  see Plain Radiography, Veins B50
  Impedance 4A04X51
Phleborrhaphy
  see Repair, Upper Veins 05Q
  see Repair, Lower Veins 06Q
Phlebotomy
  see Drainage, Upper Veins 059
  see Drainage, Lower Veins 069
Photocoagulation
  for Destruction see Destruction
  for Repair see Repair
Photopheresis, therapeutic see Phototherapy,
  Circulatory 6A65
Phototherapy
  Circulatory 6A65
  Skin 6A60
Phrenectomy, phrenoneurectomy see Excision,
  Nerve, Phrenic 01B2
Phrenemphraxis see Destruction, Nerve,
  Phrenic 0152
Phrenic nerve stimulator generator use
  Stimulator Generator in Subcutaneous
  Tissue and Fascia
Phrenic nerve stimulator lead use
  Diaphragmatic Pacemaker Lead in
  Respiratory System
Phreniclasis see Destruction, Nerve, Phrenic
  0152
Phrenicoexeresis see Extraction, Nerve, Phrenic
  01D2
Phrenicotomy see Division, Nerve, Phrenic 0182
Phrenicotripsy see Destruction, Nerve, Phrenic
  0152

Phrenoplasty
  see Repair, Respiratory System 0BQ
  see Supplement, Respiratory System 0BU
Phrenotomy see Drainage, Respiratory System
  0B9
Physiatry see Motor Treatment, Rehabilitation
  F07
Physical medicine see Motor Treatment,
  Rehabilitation F07
Physical therapy see Motor Treatment,
  Rehabilitation F07
PHYSIOMESH™ Flexible Composite Mesh use
  Synthetic Substitute
Pia mater
  use Spinal Meninges
  use Cerebral Meninges
Pinealectomy
  see Excision, Pineal Body 0GB1
  see Resection, Pineal Body 0GT1
Pinealoscopy 0GJ14ZZ
Pinealotomy see Drainage, Pineal Body
  0G91
Pinna
  use Ear, External, Left
  use Ear, External, Bilateral
  use Ear, External, Right
Pipeline™ Embolization device (PED) use
  Intraluminal Device
Piriform recess (sinus) use Pharynx
Piriformis muscle
  use Muscle, Hip, Left
  use Muscle, Hip, Right
Pisiform bone
  use Carpal, Left
  use Carpal, Right
Pisohamate ligament
  use Bursa and Ligament, Hand, Right
  use Bursa and Ligament, Hand, Left
Pisometacarpal ligament
  use Bursa and Ligament, Hand, Left
  use Bursa and Ligament, Hand, Right
Pituitectomy
  see Excision, Gland, Pituitary 0GB0
  see Resection, Gland, Pituitary 0GT0
Plain film radiology see Plain Radiography
Plain Radiography
  Abdomen BW00ZZZ
  Abdomen and Pelvis BW01ZZZ
  Abdominal Lymphatic
    Bilateral B701
    Unilateral B700
  Airway, Upper BB0DZZZ
  Ankle
    Left BQ0H
    Right BQ0G
  Aorta
    Abdominal B400
    Thoracic B300
    Thoraco-Abdominal B30P
  Aorta and Bilateral Lower Extremity Arteries
    B40D
  Arch
    Bilateral BN0DZZZ
    Left BN0CZZZ
    Right BN0BZZZ
  Arm
    Left BP0FZZZ
    Right BP0EZZZ
  Artery
    Brachiocephalic-Subclavian, Right B301
    Bronchial B30L
    Bypass Graft, Other B20F
    Cervico-Cerebral Arch B30Q
    Common Carotid
      Bilateral B305
      Left B304
      Right B303
    Coronary
      Bypass Graft
        Multiple B203
        Single B202

◀ New   ◀▭ Revised   ~~deleted~~ Deleted

Plain Radiography (*Continued*)
  Spine
    Cervical, Densitometry BR00ZZ1
    Lumbar, Densitometry BR09ZZ1
    Thoracic, Densitometry BR07ZZ1
    Whole, Densitometry BR0GZZ1
  Sternum BR0HZZZ
  Teeth
    All BN0JZZZ
    Multiple BN0HZZZ
  Testicle
    Left BV06
    Right BV05
  Toe
    Left BQ0QZZZ
    Right BQ0PZZZ
  Tooth, Single BN0GZZZ
  Tracheobronchial Tree
    Bilateral BB09YZZ
    Left BB08YZZ
    Right BB07YZZ
  Ureter
    Bilateral BT08
    Kidney and Bladder BT04
    Left BT07
    Right BT06
  Urethra BT05
  Urethra and Bladder BT0B
  Uterus BU06
  Uterus and Fallopian Tube BU08
  Vagina BU09
  Vasa Vasorum BV08
  Vein
    Cerebellar B501
    Cerebral B501
    Epidural B500
    Jugular
      Bilateral B505
      Left B504
      Right B503
    Lower Extremity
      Bilateral B50D
      Left B50C
      Right B50B
    Other B50V
    Pelvic (Iliac)
      Left B50G
      Right B50F
    Pelvic (Iliac) Bilateral B50H
    Portal B50T
    Pulmonary
      Bilateral B50S
      Left B50R
      Right B50Q
    Renal
      Bilateral B50L
      Left B50K
      Right B50J
    Spanchnic B50T
    Subclavian
      Left B507
      Right B506
    Upper Extremity
      Bilateral B50P
      Left B50N
      Right B50M
  Vena Cava
    Inferior B509
    Superior B508
  Whole Body BW0KZZZ
    Infant BW0MZZZ
  Whole Skeleton BW0LZZZ
  Wrist
    Left BP0M
    Right BP0L
Planar Nuclear Medicine Imaging CP1
  Abdomen CW10
  Abdomen and Chest CW14
  Abdomen and Pelvis CW11
  Anatomical Regions, Multiple CW1YYZZ
  Bladder, Kidneys and Ureters CT13

Planar Nuclear Medicine Imaging (*Continued*)
  Bladder and Ureters CT1H
  Blood C713
  Bone Marrow C710
  Brain C010
  Breast CH1YYZZ
    Bilateral CH12
    Left CH11
    Right CH10
  Bronchi and Lungs CB12
  Central Nervous System C01YYZZ
  Cerebrospinal Fluid C015
  Chest CW13
  Chest and Abdomen CW14
  Chest and Neck CW16
  Digestive System CD1YYZZ
  Ducts, Lacrimal, Bilateral C819
  Ear, Nose, Mouth and Throat C91YYZZ
  Endocrine System CG1YYZZ
  Extremity
    Lower CW1D
      Bilateral CP1F
      Left CP1D
      Right CP1C
    Upper CW1M
      Bilateral CP1B
      Left CP19
      Right CP18
  Eye C81YYZZ
  Gallbladder CF14
  Gastrointestinal Tract CD17
    Upper CD15
  Gland
    Adrenal, Bilateral CG14
    Parathyroid CG11
    Thyroid CG12
  Glands, Salivary, Bilateral C91B
  Head and Neck CW1B
  Heart C21YYZZ
    Right and Left C216
  Hepatobiliary System, All CF1C
  Hepatobiliary System and Pancreas
      CF1YYZZ
  Kidneys, Ureters and Bladder CT13
  Liver CF15
  Liver and Spleen CF16
  Lungs and Bronchi CB12
  Lymphatics
    Head C71J
    Head and Neck C715
    Lower Extremity C71P
    Neck C71K
    Pelvic C71D
    Trunk C71M
    Upper Chest C71L
    Upper Extremity C71N
  Lymphatics and Hematologic System
      C71YYZZ
  Musculoskeletal System, All CP1Z
  Myocardium C21G
  Neck and Chest CW16
  Neck and Head CW1B
  Pancreas and Hepatobiliary System
      CF1YYZZ
  Pelvic Region CW1J
  Pelvis CP16
  Pelvis and Abdomen CW11
  Pelvis and Spine CP17
  Reproductive System, Male CV1YYZZ
  Respiratory System CB1YYZZ
  Skin CH1YYZZ
  Skull CP11
  Spine CP15
  Spine and Pelvis CP17
  Spleen C712
  Spleen and Liver CF16
  Subcutaneous Tissue CH1YYZZ
  Testicles, Bilateral CV19
  Thorax CP14
  Ureters, Kidneys and Bladder
      CT13

Planar Nuclear Medicine Imaging (*Continued*)
  Ureters and Bladder CT1H
  Urinary System CT1YYZZ
  Veins C51YYZZ
    Central C51R
    Lower Extremity
      Bilateral C51D
      Left C51C
      Right C51B
    Upper Extremity
      Bilateral C51Q
      Left C51P
      Right C51N
  Whole Body CW1N
Plantar digital vein
  use Vein, Foot, Right
  use Vein, Foot, Left
Plantar fascia (aponeurosis)
  use Subcutaneous Tissue and Fascia, Foot,
      Right
  use Subcutaneous Tissue and Fascia, Foot,
      Left
Plantar metatarsal vein
  use Vein, Foot, Right
  use Vein, Foot, Left
Plantar venous arch
  use Vein, Foot, Right
  use Vein, Foot, Left
Plaque Radiation
  Abdomen DWY3FZZ
  Adrenal Gland DGY2FZZ
  Anus DDY8FZZ
  Bile Ducts DFY2FZZ
  Bladder DTY2FZZ
  Bone, Other DPYCFZZ
  Bone Marrow D7Y0FZZ
  Brain D0Y0FZZ
  Brain Stem D0Y1FZZ
  Breast
    Left DMY0FZZ
    Right DMY1FZZ
  Bronchus DBY1FZZ
  Cervix DUY1FZZ
  Chest DWY2FZZ
  Chest Wall DBY7FZZ
  Colon DDY5FZZ
  Diaphragm DBY8FZZ
  Duodenum DDY2FZZ
  Ear D9Y0FZZ
  Esophagus DDY0FZZ
  Eye D8Y0FZZ
  Femur DPY9FZZ
  Fibula DPYBFZZ
  Gallbladder DFY1FZZ
  Gland
    Adrenal DGY2FZZ
    Parathyroid DGY4FZZ
    Pituitary DGY0FZZ
    Thyroid DGY5FZZ
  Glands, Salivary D9Y6FZZ
  Head and Neck DWY1FZZ
  Hemibody DWY4FZZ
  Humerus DPY6FZZ
  Ileum DDY4FZZ
  Jejunum DDY3FZZ
  Kidney DTY0FZZ
  Larynx D9YBFZZ
  Liver DFY0FZZ
  Lung DBY2FZZ
  Lymphatics
    Abdomen D7Y6FZZ
    Axillary D7Y4FZZ
    Inguinal D7Y8FZZ
    Neck D7Y3FZZ
    Pelvis D7Y7FZZ
    Thorax D7Y5FZZ
  Mandible DPY3FZZ
  Maxilla DPY2FZZ
  Mediastinum DBY6FZZ
  Mouth D9Y4FZZ
  Nasopharynx D9YDFZZ

Plaque Radiation *(Continued)*
  Neck and Head DWY1FZZ
  Nerve, Peripheral D0Y7FZZ
  Nose D9Y1FZZ
  Ovary DUY0FZZ
  Palate
    Hard D9Y8FZZ
    Soft D9Y9FZZ
  Pancreas DFY3FZZ
  Parathyroid Gland DGY4FZZ
  Pelvic Bones DPY8FZZ
  Pelvic Region DWY6FZZ
  Pharynx D9YCFZZ
  Pineal Body DGY1FZZ
  Pituitary Gland DGY0FZZ
  Pleura DBY5FZZ
  Prostate DVY0FZZ
  Radius DPY7FZZ
  Rectum DDY7FZZ
  Rib DPY5FZZ
  Sinuses D9Y7FZZ
  Skin
    Abdomen DHY8FZZ
    Arm DHY4FZZ
    Back DHY7FZZ
    Buttock DHY9FZZ
    Chest DHY6FZZ
    Face DHY2FZZ
    Foot DHYCFZZ
    Hand DHY5FZZ
    Leg DHYBFZZ
    Neck DHY3FZZ
  Skull DPY0FZZ
  Spinal Cord D0Y6FZZ
  Spleen D7Y2FZZ
  Sternum DPY4FZZ
  Stomach DDY1FZZ
  Testis DVY1FZZ
  Thymus D7Y1FZZ
  Thyroid Gland DGY5FZZ
  Tibia DPYBFZZ
  Tongue D9Y5FZZ
  Trachea DBY0FZZ
  Ulna DPY7FZZ
  Ureter DTY1FZZ
  Urethra DTY3FZZ
  Uterus DUY2FZZ
  Whole Body DWY5FZZ
Plasmapheresis, therapeutic 6A550Z3
Plateletpheresis, therapeutic 6A550Z2
Platysma muscle
  use Muscle, Neck, Left
  use Muscle, Neck, Right
Pleurectomy
  see Excision, Respiratory System 0BB
  see Resection, Respiratory System 0BT
Pleurocentesis *see* Drainage, Anatomical
    Regions, General 0W9
Pleurodesis, pleurosclerosis
  Chemical Injection *see* Introduction of
      substance in or on, Pleural Cavity
      3E0L
  Surgical *see* Destruction, Respiratory System
      0B5
Pleurolysis *see* Release, Respiratory System
    0BN
Pleuroscopy 0BJQ4ZZ
Pleurotomy *see* Drainage, Respiratory System
    0B9
Plica semilunaris
  use Conjunctiva, Left
  use Conjunctiva, Right
Plication *see* Restriction
Pneumectomy
  see Excision, Respiratory System 0BB
  see Resection, Respiratory System 0BT
Pneumocentesis *see* Drainage, Respiratory
    System 0B9
Pneumogastric nerve *use* Nerve, Vagus
Pneumolysis *see* Release, Respiratory System
    0BN

Pneumonectomy *see* Resection, Respiratory
    System 0BT
Pneumonolysis *see* Release, Respiratory System
    0BN
Pneumonopexy
  see Repair, Respiratory System 0BQ
  see Reposition, Respiratory System 0BS
Pneumonorrhaphy *see* Repair, Respiratory
    System 0BQ
Pneumonotomy *see* Drainage, Respiratory
    System 0B9
Pneumotaxic center *use* Pons
Pneumotomy *see* Drainage, Respiratory System
    0B9
Pollicization *see* Transfer, Anatomical Regions,
    Upper Extremities 0XX
Polyethylene socket *use* Synthetic Substitute,
    Polyethylene in 0SR
Polymethylmethacrylate (PMMA) *use*
    Synthetic Substitute
Polypectomy, gastrointestinal *see* Excision,
    Gastrointestinal System 0DB
Polypropylene mesh *use* Synthetic Substitute
Polysomnogram 4A1ZXQZ
Pontine tegmentum *use* Pons
Popliteal ligament
  use Bursa and Ligament, Knee, Right
  use Bursa and Ligament, Knee, Left
Popliteal lymph node
  use Lymphatic, Lower Extremity, Right
  use Lymphatic, Lower Extremity, Left
Popliteal vein
  use Vein, Femoral, Right
  use Vein, Femoral, Left
Popliteus muscle
  use Muscle, Lower Leg, Right
  use Muscle, Lower Leg, Left
Porcine (bioprosthetic) valve *use* Zooplastic
    Tissue in Heart and Great Vessels
Positive end expiratory pressure *see*
    Performance, Respiratory 5A19
**Positron Emission Tomographic (PET)
    Imaging**
  Brain C030
  Bronchi and Lungs CB32
  Central Nervous System C03YYZZ
  Heart C23YYZZ
  Lungs and Bronchi CB32
  Myocardium C23G
  Respiratory System CB3YYZZ
  Whole Body CW3NYZZ
Positron emission tomography *see* Positron
    Emission Tomographic (PET) Imaging
Postauricular (mastoid) lymph node
  use Lymphatic, Neck, Right
  use Lymphatic, Neck, Left
Postcava *use* Vena Cava, Inferior
Posterior (subscapular) lymph node
  use Lymphatic, Axillary, Left
  use Lymphatic, Axillary, Right
Posterior auricular artery
  use Artery, External Carotid, Right
  use Artery, External Carotid, Left
Posterior auricular nerve *use* Nerve,
    Facial
Posterior auricular vein
  use Vein, External Jugular, Left
  use Vein, External Jugular, Right
Posterior cerebral artery *use* Artery,
    Intracranial
Posterior chamber
  use Eye, Right
  use Eye, Left
Posterior circumflex humeral artery
  use Artery, Axillary, Right
  use Artery, Axillary, Left
Posterior communicating artery *use* Artery,
    Intracranial
Posterior cruciate ligament (PCL)
  use Bursa and Ligament, Knee, Right
  use Bursa and Ligament, Knee, Left

Posterior facial (retromandibular) vein
  use Vein, Face, Right
  use Vein, Face, Left
Posterior femoral cutaneous nerve *use* Nerve,
    Sacral Plexus
Posterior inferior cerebellar artery (PICA) *use*
    Artery, Intracranial
Posterior interosseous nerve *use* Nerve, Radial
Posterior labial nerve *use* Nerve, Pudendal
Posterior scrotal nerve *use* Nerve, Pudendal
Posterior spinal artery
  use Artery, Vertebral, Left
  use Artery, Vertebral, Right
Posterior tibial recurrent artery
  use Artery, Anterior Tibial, Right
  use Artery, Anterior Tibial, Left
Posterior ulnar recurrent artery
  use Artery, Ulnar, Left
  use Artery, Ulnar, Right
Posterior vagal trunk *use* Nerve, Vagus
PPN (peripheral parenteral nutrition) *see*
    Introduction of Nutritional Substance
Preauricular lymph node *use* Lymphatic, Head
Precava *use* Vena Cava, Superior
Prepatellar bursa
  use Bursa and Ligament, Knee, Right
  use Bursa and Ligament, Knee, Left
Preputiotomy *see* Drainage, Male Reproductive
    System 0V9
Pressure support ventilation *see* Performance,
    Respiratory 5A19
PRESTIGE® Cervical Disc *use* Synthetic
    Substitute
Pretracheal fascia *use* Subcutaneous Tissue and
    Fascia, Neck, Anterior
Prevertebral fascia *use* Subcutaneous Tissue
    and Fascia, Neck, Posterior
~~PrimeAdvanced neurostimulator use Stimulator
    Generator, Multiple Array in 0JH~~
**PrimeAdvanced neurostimulator (SureScan)
    (MRI Safe)** *use* Stimulator Generator,
    Multiple Array in 0JH ◀
Princeps pollicis artery
  use Artery, Hand, Left
  use Artery, Hand, Right
Probing, duct
  Diagnostic *see* Inspection
  Dilation *see* Dilation
PROCEED™ Ventral Patch *use* Synthetic
    Substitute
Procerus muscle *use* Muscle, Facial
Proctectomy
  see Excision, Rectum 0DBP
  see Resection, Rectum 0DTP
Proctoclysis *see* Introduction of substance in or
    on, Gastrointestinal Tract, Lower 3E0H
Proctocolectomy
  see Excision, Gastrointestinal System 0DB
  see Resection, Gastrointestinal System 0DT
Proctocolpoplasty
  see Repair, Gastrointestinal System 0DQ
  see Supplement, Gastrointestinal System 0DU
Proctoperineoplasty
  see Repair, Gastrointestinal System 0DQ
  see Supplement, Gastrointestinal System 0DU
Proctoperineorrhaphy *see* Repair,
    Gastrointestinal System 0DQ
Proctopexy
  see Repair, Rectum 0DQP
  see Reposition, Rectum 0DSP
Proctoplasty
  see Repair, Rectum 0DQP
  see Supplement, Rectum 0DUP
Proctorrhaphy *see* Repair, Rectum 0DQP
Proctoscopy 0DJD8ZZ
Proctosigmoidectomy
  see Excision, Gastrointestinal System 0DB
  see Resection, Gastrointestinal System 0DT
Proctosigmoidoscopy 0DJD8ZZ
Proctostomy *see* Drainage, Rectum 0D9P
Proctotomy *see* Drainage, Rectum 0D9P

◀ New   ◀▥▥ Revised   ~~deleted~~ Deleted

Prodisc-C *use* Synthetic Substitute
Prodisc-L *use* Synthetic Substitute
Production, atrial septal defect *see* Excision, Septum, Atrial 02B5
Profunda brachii
  use Artery, Brachial, Right
  use Artery, Brachial, Left
Profunda femoris (deep femoral) vein
  use Vein, Femoral, Right
  use Vein, Femoral, Left
PROLENE Polypropylene Hernia System (PHS) *use* Synthetic Substitute
Pronator quadratus muscle
  use Muscle, Lower Arm and Wrist, Left
  use Muscle, Lower Arm and Wrist, Right
Pronator teres muscle
  use Muscle, Lower Arm and Wrist, Right
  use Muscle, Lower Arm and Wrist, Left
Prostatectomy
  see Excision, Prostate 0VB0
  see Resection, Prostate 0VT0
Prostatic urethra *use* Urethra
Prostatomy, prostatotomy *see* Drainage, Prostate 0V90
Protecta XT CRT-D *use* Cardiac Resynchronization Defibrillator Pulse Generator in 0JH
Protecta XT DR (XT VR) *use* Defibrillator Generator in 0JH
Protégé® RX Carotid Stent System *use* Intraluminal Device
Proximal radioulnar joint
  use Joint, Elbow, Left
  use Joint, Elbow, Right
Psoas muscle
  use Muscle, Hip, Right
  use Muscle, Hip, Left
PSV (pressure support ventilation) *see* Performance, Respiratory 5A19
Psychoanalysis GZ54ZZZ
Psychological Tests
  Cognitive Status GZ14ZZZ
  Developmental GZ10ZZZ
  Intellectual and Psychoeducational GZ12ZZZ
  Neurobehavioral Status GZ14ZZZ
  Neuropsychological GZ13ZZZ
  Personality and Behavioral GZ11ZZZ
Psychotherapy
  Family, Mental Health Services GZ72ZZZ
  Group
    GZHZZZZ
    Mental Health Services GZHZZZZ
  Individual
    see Psychotherapy, Individual, Mental Health Services
    for substance abuse
      12-Step HZ53ZZZ
      Behavioral HZ51ZZZ
      Cognitive HZ50ZZZ
      Cognitive-Behavioral HZ52ZZZ

Psychotherapy *(Continued)*
  Individual *(Continued)*
    for substance abuse *(Continued)*
      Confrontational HZ58ZZZ
      Interactive HZ55ZZZ
      Interpersonal HZ54ZZZ
      Motivational Enhancement HZ57ZZZ
      Psychoanalysis HZ5BZZZ
      Psychodynamic HZ5CZZZ
      Psychoeducation HZ56ZZZ
      Psychophysiological HZ5DZZZ
      Supportive HZ59ZZZ
    Mental Health Services
      Behavioral GZ51ZZZ
      Cognitive GZ52ZZZ
      Cognitive-Behavioral GZ58ZZZ
      Interactive GZ50ZZZ
      Interpersonal GZ53ZZZ
      Psychoanalysis GZ54ZZZ
      Psychodynamic GZ55ZZZ
      Psychophysiological GZ59ZZZ
      Supportive GZ56ZZZ
PTCA (percutaneous transluminal coronary angioplasty) *see* Dilation, Heart and Great Vessels 027
Pterygoid muscle *use* Muscle, Head
Pterygoid process
  use Bone, Sphenoid, Right
  use Bone, Sphenoid, Left
Pterygopalatine (sphenopalatine) ganglion *use* Nerve, Head and Neck Sympathetic
Pubic ligament
  use Bursa and Ligament, Trunk, Right
  use Bursa and Ligament, Trunk, Left
Pubis
  use Bone, Pelvic, Right
  use Bone, Pelvic, Left
Pubofemoral ligament
  use Bursa and Ligament, Hip, Left
  use Bursa and Ligament, Hip, Right
Pudendal nerve *use* Nerve, Sacral Plexus
Pull-through, rectal *see* Resection, Rectum 0DTP
Pulmoaortic canal *use* Artery, Pulmonary, Left
Pulmonary annulus *use* Valve, Pulmonary
Pulmonary artery wedge monitoring *see* Monitoring, Arterial 4A13
Pulmonary plexus
  use Nerve, Vagus
  use Nerve, Thoracic Sympathetic
Pulmonic valve *use* Valve, Pulmonary
Pulpectomy *see* Excision, Mouth and Throat 0CB
Pulverization *see* Fragmentation
Pulvinar *use* Thalamus
Pump reservoir *use* Infusion Device, Pump in Subcutaneous Tissue and Fascia
Punch biopsy *see* Excision with qualifier Diagnostic

Puncture *see* Drainage
Puncture, lumbar *see* Drainage, Spinal Canal 009U
Pyelography
  see Plain Radiography, Urinary System BT0
  see Fluoroscopy, Urinary System BT1
Pyeloileostomy, urinary diversion *see* Bypass, Urinary System 0T1
Pyeloplasty
  see Repair, Urinary System 0TQ
  see Replacement, Urinary System 0TR
  see Supplement, Urinary System 0TU
Pyelorrhaphy *see* Repair, Urinary System 0TQ
Pyeloscopy 0TJ58ZZ
Pyelostomy
  see Drainage, Urinary System 0T9
  see Bypass, Urinary System 0T1
Pyelotomy *see* Drainage, Urinary System 0T9
Pylorectomy
  see Excision, Stomach, Pylorus 0DB7
  see Resection, Stomach, Pylorus 0DT7
Pyloric antrum *use* Stomach, Pylorus
Pyloric canal *use* Stomach, Pylorus
Pyloric sphincter *use* Stomach, Pylorus
Pylorodiosis *see* Dilation, Stomach, Pylorus 0D77
Pylorogastrectomy
  see Excision, Gastrointestinal System 0DB
  see Resection, Gastrointestinal System 0DT
Pyloroplasty
  see Repair, Stomach, Pylorus 0DQ7
  see Supplement, Stomach, Pylorus 0DU7
Pyloroscopy 0DJ68ZZ
Pylorotomy *see* Drainage, Stomach, Pylorus 0D97
Pyramidalis muscle
  use Muscle, Abdomen, Left
  use Muscle, Abdomen, Right

Q

Quadrangular cartilage *use* Septum, Nasal
Quadrant resection of breast *see* Excision, Skin and Breast 0HB
Quadrate lobe *use* Liver
Quadratus femoris muscle
  use Muscle, Hip, Left
  use Muscle, Hip, Right
Quadratus lumborum muscle
  use Muscle, Trunk, Left
  use Muscle, Trunk, Right
Quadratus plantae muscle
  use Muscle, Foot, Left
  use Muscle, Foot, Right
Quadriceps (femoris)
  use Muscle, Upper Leg, Left
  use Muscle, Upper Leg, Right
Quarantine 8E0ZXY6

R

Radial collateral carpal ligament
  use Bursa and Ligament, Wrist, Right
  use Bursa and Ligament, Wrist, Left
Radial collateral ligament
  use Bursa and Ligament, Elbow, Left
  use Bursa and Ligament, Elbow, Right
Radial notch
  use Ulna, Left
  use Ulna, Right
Radial recurrent artery
  use Artery, Radial, Right
  use Artery, Radial, Left
Radial vein
  use Vein, Brachial, Right
  use Vein, Brachial, Left
Radialis indicis
  use Artery, Hand, Right
  use Artery, Hand, Left
Radiation Therapy
  see Beam Radiation
  see Brachytherapy
Radiation treatment *see* Radiation
    Oncology
Radiocarpal joint
  use Joint, Wrist, Left
  use Joint, Wrist, Right
Radiocarpal ligament
  use Bursa and Ligament, Wrist, Left
  use Bursa and Ligament, Wrist, Right
Radiography *see* Plain Radiography
Radiology, analog *see* Plain
    Radiography
Radiology, diagnostic *see* Imaging,
    Diagnostic
Radioulnar ligament
  use Bursa and Ligament, Wrist, Right
  use Bursa and Ligament, Wrist, Left
Range of motion testing *see* Motor
    Function Assessment, Rehabilitation
    F01
REALIZE® Adjustable Gastric Band *use*
    Extraluminal Device
Reattachment
  Abdominal Wall 0WMF0ZZ
  Ampulla of Vater 0FMC
  Ankle Region
    Left 0YML0ZZ
    Right 0YMK0ZZ
  Arm
    Lower
      Left 0XMF0ZZ
      Right 0XMD0ZZ
    Upper
      Left 0XM90ZZ
      Right 0XM80ZZ
  Axilla
    Left 0XM50ZZ
    Right 0XM40ZZ
  Back
    Lower 0WML0ZZ
    Upper 0WMK0ZZ
  Bladder 0TMB
  Bladder Neck 0TMC
  Breast
    Bilateral 0HMVXZZ
    Left 0HMUXZZ
    Right 0HMTXZZ
  Bronchus
    Lingula 0BM90ZZ
    Lower Lobe
      Left 0BMB0ZZ
      Right 0BM60ZZ
    Main
      Left 0BM70ZZ
      Right 0BM30ZZ
    Middle Lobe, Right 0BM50ZZ
    Upper Lobe
      Left 0BM80ZZ
      Right 0BM40ZZ

Reattachment *(Continued)*
  Bursa and Ligament
    Abdomen
      Left 0MMJ
      Right 0MMH
    Ankle
      Left 0MMR
      Right 0MMQ
    Elbow
      Left 0MM4
      Right 0MM3
    Foot
      Left 0MMT
      Right 0MMS
    Hand
      Left 0MM8
      Right 0MM7
    Head and Neck 0MM0
    Hip
      Left 0MMM
      Right 0MML
    Knee
      Left 0MMP
      Right 0MMN
    Lower Extremity
      Left 0MMW
      Right 0MMV
    Perineum 0MMK
    Shoulder
      Left 0MM2
      Right 0MM1
    Thorax
      Left 0MMG
      Right 0MMF
    Trunk
      Left 0MMD
      Right 0MMC
    Upper Extremity
      Left 0MMB
      Right 0MM9
    Wrist
      Left 0MM6
      Right 0MM5
  Buttock
    Left 0YM10ZZ
    Right 0YM00ZZ
  Carina 0BM20ZZ
  Cecum 0DMH
  Cervix 0UMC
  Chest Wall 0WM80ZZ
  Clitoris 0UMJXZZ
  Colon
    Ascending 0DMK
    Descending 0DMM
    Sigmoid 0DMN
    Transverse 0DML
  Cord
    Bilateral 0VMH
    Left 0VMG
    Right 0VMF
  Cul-de-sac 0UMF
  Diaphragm
    Left 0BMS0ZZ
    Right 0BMR0ZZ
  Duct
    Common Bile 0FM9
    Cystic 0FM8
    Hepatic
      Left 0FM6
      Right 0FM5
    Pancreatic 0FMD
      Accessory 0FMF
  Duodenum 0DM9
  Ear
    Left 09M1XZZ
    Right 09M0XZZ
  Elbow Region
    Left 0XMC0ZZ
    Right 0XMB0ZZ
  Esophagus 0DM5

Reattachment *(Continued)*
  Extremity
    Lower
      Left 0YMB0ZZ
      Right 0YM90ZZ
    Upper
      Left 0XM70ZZ
      Right 0XM60ZZ
  Eyelid
    Lower
      Left 08MRXZZ
      Right 08MQXZZ
    Upper
      Left 08MPXZZ
      Right 08MNXZZ
  Face 0WM20ZZ
  Fallopian Tube
    Left 0UM6
    Right 0UM5
  Fallopian Tubes, Bilateral
    0UM7
  Femoral Region
    Left 0YM80ZZ
    Right 0YM70ZZ
  Finger
    Index
      Left 0XMP0ZZ
      Right 0XMN0ZZ
    Little
      Left 0XMW0ZZ
      Right 0XMV0ZZ
    Middle
      Left 0XMR0ZZ
      Right 0XMQ0ZZ
    Ring
      Left 0XMT0ZZ
      Right 0XMS0ZZ
  Foot
    Left 0YMN0ZZ
    Right 0YMM0ZZ
  Forequarter
    Left 0XM10ZZ
    Right 0XM00ZZ
  Gallbladder 0FM4
  Gland
    Adrenal
      Left 0GM2
      Right 0GM3
  Hand
    Left 0XMK0ZZ
    Right 0XMJ0ZZ
  Hindquarter
    Bilateral 0YM40ZZ
    Left 0YM30ZZ
    Right 0YM20ZZ
  Hymen 0UMK
  Ileum 0DMB
  Inguinal Region
    Left 0YM60ZZ
    Right 0YM50ZZ
  Intestine
    Large 0DME
      Left 0DMG
      Right 0DMF
    Small 0DM8
  Jaw
    Lower 0WM50ZZ
    Upper 0WM40ZZ
  Jejunum 0DMA
  Kidney
    Left 0TM1
    Right 0TM0
  Kidney Pelvis
    Left 0TM4
    Right 0TM3
  Kidneys, Bilateral 0TM2
  Knee Region
    Left 0YMG0ZZ
    Right 0YMF0ZZ

Reattachment (*Continued*)
Leg
  Lower
    Left 0YMJ0ZZ
    Right 0YMH0ZZ
  Upper
    Left 0YMD0ZZ
    Right 0YMC0ZZ
Lip
  Lower 0CM10ZZ
  Upper 0CM00ZZ
Liver 0FM0
  Left Lobe 0FM2
  Right Lobe 0FM1
Lung
  Left 0BML0ZZ
  Lower Lobe
    Left 0BMJ0ZZ
    Right 0BMF0ZZ
  Middle Lobe, Right 0BMD0ZZ
  Right 0BMK0ZZ
  Upper Lobe
    Left 0BMG0ZZ
    Right 0BMC0ZZ
Lung Lingula 0BMH0ZZ
Muscle
  Abdomen
    Left 0KML
    Right 0KMK
  Facial 0KM1
  Foot
    Left 0KMW
    Right 0KMV
  Hand
    Left 0KMD
    Right 0KMC
  Head 0KM0
  Hip
    Left 0KMP
    Right 0KMN
  Lower Arm and Wrist
    Left 0KMB
    Right 0KM9
  Lower Leg
    Left 0KMT
    Right 0KMS
  Neck
    Left 0KM3
    Right 0KM2
  Perineum 0KMM
  Shoulder
    Left 0KM6
    Right 0KM5
  Thorax
    Left 0KMJ
    Right 0KMH
  Tongue, Palate, Pharynx 0KM4
  Trunk
    Left 0KMG
    Right 0KMF
  Upper Arm
    Left 0KM8
    Right 0KM7
  Upper Leg
    Left 0KMR
    Right 0KMQ
Neck 0WM60ZZ
Nipple
  Left 0HMXXZZ
  Right 0HMWXZZ
Nose 09MKXZZ
Ovary
  Bilateral 0UM2
  Left 0UM1
  Right 0UM0
Palate, Soft 0CM30ZZ
Pancreas 0FMG
Parathyroid Gland 0GMR
  Inferior
    Left 0GMP
    Right 0GMN

Reattachment (*Continued*)
Parathyroid Gland (*Continued*)
  Multiple 0GMQ
  Superior
    Left 0GMM
    Right 0GML
Penis 0VMSXZZ
Perineum
  Female 0WMN0ZZ
  Male 0WMM0ZZ
Rectum 0DMP
Scrotum 0VM5XZZ
Shoulder Region
  Left 0XM30ZZ
  Right 0XM20ZZ
Skin
  Abdomen 0HM7XZZ
  Back 0HM6XZZ
  Buttock 0HM8XZZ
  Chest 0HM5XZZ
  Ear
    Left 0HM3XZZ
    Right 0HM2XZZ
  Face 0HM1XZZ
  Foot
    Left 0HMNXZZ
    Right 0HMMXZZ
  Genitalia 0HMAXZZ
  Hand
    Left 0HMGXZZ
    Right 0HMFXZZ
  Lower Arm
    Left 0HMEXZZ
    Right 0HMDXZZ
  Lower Leg
    Left 0HMLXZZ
    Right 0HMKXZZ
  Neck 0HM4XZZ
  Perineum 0HM9XZZ
  Scalp 0HM0XZZ
  Upper Arm
    Left 0HMCXZZ
    Right 0HMBXZZ
  Upper Leg
    Left 0HMJXZZ
    Right 0HMHXZZ
Stomach 0DM6
Tendon
  Abdomen
    Left 0LMG
    Right 0LMF
  Ankle
    Left 0LMT
    Right 0LMS
  Foot
    Left 0LMW
    Right 0LMV
  Hand
    Left 0LM8
    Right 0LM7
  Head and Neck 0LM0
  Hip
    Left 0LMK
    Right 0LMJ
  Knee
    Left 0LMR
    Right 0LMQ
  Lower Arm and Wrist
    Left 0LM6
    Right 0LM5
  Lower Leg
    Left 0LMP
    Right 0LMN
  Perineum 0LMH
  Shoulder
    Left 0LM2
    Right 0LM1
  Thorax
    Left 0LMD
    Right 0LMC
  Trunk
    Left 0LMB
    Right 0LM9

Reattachment (*Continued*)
Tendon (*Continued*)
  Upper Arm
    Left 0LM4
    Right 0LM3
  Upper Leg
    Left 0LMM
    Right 0LML
Testis
  Bilateral 0VMC
  Left 0VMB
  Right 0VM9
Thumb
  Left 0XMM0ZZ
  Right 0XML0ZZ
Thyroid Gland
  Left Lobe 0GMG
  Right Lobe 0GMH
Toe
  1st
    Left 0YMQ0ZZ
    Right 0YMP0ZZ
  2nd
    Left 0YMS0ZZ
    Right 0YMR0ZZ
  3rd
    Left 0YMU0ZZ
    Right 0YMT0ZZ
  4th
    Left 0YMW0ZZ
    Right 0YMV0ZZ
  5th
    Left 0YMY0ZZ
    Right 0YMX0ZZ
Tongue 0CM70ZZ
Tooth
  Lower 0CMX
  Upper 0CMW
Trachea 0BM10ZZ
Tunica Vaginalis
  Left 0VM7
  Right 0VM6
Ureter
  Left 0TM7
  Right 0TM6
Ureters, Bilateral 0TM8
Urethra 0TMD
Uterine Supporting Structure 0UM4
Uterus 0UM9
Uvula 0CMN0ZZ
Vagina 0UMG
Vulva 0UMMXZZ
Wrist Region
  Left 0XMH0ZZ
  Right 0XMG0ZZ
Rebound HRD® (Hernia Repair Device) *use* Synthetic Substitute
Recession
  see Repair
  see Reposition
Reclosure, disrupted abdominal wall 0WQFXZZ
Reconstruction
  see Repair
  see Replacement
  see Supplement
Rectectomy
  see Excision, Rectum 0DBP
  see Resection, Rectum 0DTP
Rectocele repair
  see Repair, Subcutaneous Tissue and Fascia, Pelvic Region 0JQC
Rectopexy
  see Repair, Gastrointestinal System 0DQ
  see Reposition, Gastrointestinal System 0DS
Rectoplasty
  see Repair, Gastrointestinal System 0DQ
  see Supplement, Gastrointestinal System 0DU

Rectorrhaphy *see* Repair, Gastrointestinal
   System 0DQ
Rectoscopy 0DJD8ZZ
Rectosigmoid junction *use* Colon, Sigmoid
Rectosigmoidectomy
  see Excision, Gastrointestinal System 0DB
  see Resection, Gastrointestinal System 0DT
Rectostomy *see* Drainage, Rectum 0D9P
Rectotomy *see* Drainage, Rectum 0D9P
Rectus abdominis muscle
  use Muscle, Abdomen, Left
  use Muscle, Abdomen, Right
Rectus femoris muscle
  use Muscle, Upper Leg, Left
  use Muscle, Upper Leg, Right
Recurrent laryngeal nerve *use* Nerve,
  Vagus
Reduction
  Dislocation *see* Reposition
  Fracture *see* Reposition
  Intussusception, intestinal *see* Reposition,
    Gastrointestinal System 0DS
  Mammoplasty *see* Excision, Skin and Breast
    0HB
  Prolapse *see* Reposition
  Torsion *see* Reposition
  Volvulus, gastrointestinal *see* Reposition,
    Gastrointestinal System 0DS
Refusion *see* Fusion
Reimplantation
  see Reposition
  see Transfer
  see Reattachment
Reinforcement
  see Repair
  see Supplement
Relaxation, scar tissue *see* Release
Release
  Acetabulum
    Left 0QN5
    Right 0QN4
  Adenoids 0CNQ
  Ampulla of Vater 0FNC
  Anal Sphincter 0DNR
  Anterior Chamber
    Left 08N33ZZ
    Right 08N23ZZ
  Anus 0DNQ
  Aorta
    Abdominal 04N0
    Thoracic 02NW
  Aortic Body 0GND
  Appendix 0DNJ
  Artery
    Anterior Tibial
      Left 04NQ
      Right 04NP
    Axillary
      Left 03N6
      Right 03N5
    Brachial
      Left 03N8
      Right 03N7
    Celiac 04N1
    Colic
      Left 04N7
      Middle 04N8
      Right 04N6
    Common Carotid
      Left 03NJ
      Right 03NH
    Common Iliac
      Left 04ND
      Right 04NC
    External Carotid
      Left 03NN
      Right 03NM
    External Iliac
      Left 04NJ
      Right 04NH
    Face 03NR

Release *(Continued)*
  Artery *(Continued)*
    Femoral
      Left 04NL
      Right 04NK
    Foot
      Left 04NW
      Right 04NV
    Gastric 04N2
    Hand
      Left 03NF
      Right 03ND
    Hepatic 04N3
    Inferior Mesenteric 04NB
    Innominate 03N2
    Internal Carotid
      Left 03NL
      Right 03NK
    Internal Iliac
      Left 04NF
      Right 04NE
    Internal Mammary
      Left 03N1
      Right 03N0
    Intracranial 03NG
    Lower 04NY
    Peroneal
      Left 04NU
      Right 04NT
    Popliteal
      Left 04NN
      Right 04NM
    Posterior Tibial
      Left 04NS
      Right 04NR
    Pulmonary
      Left 02NR
      Right 02NQ
    Pulmonary Trunk 02NP
    Radial
      Left 03NC
      Right 03NB
    Renal
      Left 04NA
      Right 04N9
    Splenic 04N4
    Subclavian
      Left 03N4
      Right 03N3
    Superior Mesenteric
      04N5
    Temporal
      Left 03NT
      Right 03NS
    Thyroid
      Left 03NV
      Right 03NU
    Ulnar
      Left 03NA
      Right 03N9
    Upper 03NY
    Vertebral
      Left 03NQ
      Right 03NP
  Atrium
    Left 02N7
    Right 02N6
  Auditory Ossicle
    Left 09NA0ZZ
    Right 09N90ZZ
  Basal Ganglia 00N8
  Bladder 0TNB
  Bladder Neck 0TNC
  Bone
    Ethmoid
      Left 0NNG
      Right 0NNF
    Frontal
      Left 0NN2
      Right 0NN1
    Hyoid 0NNX

Release *(Continued)*
  Bone *(Continued)*
    Lacrimal
      Left 0NNJ
      Right 0NNH
    Nasal 0NNB
    Occipital
      Left 0NN8
      Right 0NN7
    Palatine
      Left 0NNL
      Right 0NNK
    Parietal
      Left 0NN4
      Right 0NN3
    Pelvic
      Left 0QN3
      Right 0QN2
    Sphenoid
      Left 0NND
      Right 0NNC
    Temporal
      Left 0NN6
      Right 0NN5
    Zygomatic
      Left 0NNN
      Right 0NNM
  Brain 00N0
  Breast
    Bilateral 0HNV
    Left 0HNU
    Right 0HNT
  Bronchus
    Lingula 0BN9
    Lower Lobe
      Left 0BNB
      Right 0BN6
    Main
      Left 0BN7
      Right 0BN3
    Middle Lobe, Right 0BN5
    Upper Lobe
      Left 0BN8
      Right 0BN4
  Buccal Mucosa 0CN4
  Bursa and Ligament
    Abdomen
      Left 0MNJ
      Right 0MNH
    Ankle
      Left 0MNR
      Right 0MNQ
    Elbow
      Left 0MN4
      Right 0MN3
    Foot
      Left 0MNT
      Right 0MNS
    Hand
      Left 0MN8
      Right 0MN7
    Head and Neck 0MN0
    Hip
      Left 0MNM
      Right 0MNL
    Knee
      Left 0MNP
      Right 0MNN
    Lower Extremity
      Left 0MNW
      Right 0MNV
    Perineum 0MNK
    Shoulder
      Left 0MN2
      Right 0MN1
    Thorax
      Left 0MNG
      Right 0MNF
    Trunk
      Left 0MND
      Right 0MNC

◀ New   ◀▦ Revised   ~~deleted~~ Deleted

Release *(Continued)*
Bursa and Ligament *(Continued)*
Upper Extremity
Left 0MNB
Right 0MN9
Wrist
Left 0MN6
Right 0MN5
Carina 0BN2
Carotid Bodies, Bilateral 0GN8
Carotid Body
Left 0GN6
Right 0GN7
Carpal
Left 0PNN
Right 0PNM
Cecum 0DNH
Cerebellum 00NC
Cerebral Hemisphere 00N7
Cerebral Meninges 00N1
Cerebral Ventricle 00N6
Cervix 0UNC
Chordae Tendineae 02N9
Choroid
Left 08NB
Right 08NA
Cisterna Chyli 07NL
Clavicle
Left 0PNB
Right 0PN9
Clitoris 0UNJ
Coccygeal Glomus 0GNB
Coccyx 0QNS
Colon
Ascending 0DNK
Descending 0DNM
Sigmoid 0DNN
Transverse 0DNL
Conduction Mechanism 02N8
Conjunctiva
Left 08NTXZZ
Right 08NSXZZ
Cord
Bilateral 0VNH
Left 0VNG
Right 0VNF
Cornea
Left 08N9XZZ
Right 08N8XZZ
Cul-de-sac 0UNF
Diaphragm
Left 0BNS
Right 0BNR
Disc
Cervical Vertebral 0RN3
Cervicothoracic Vertebral
0RN5
Lumbar Vertebral 0SN2
Lumbosacral 0SN4
Thoracic Vertebral 0RN9
Thoracolumbar Vertebral 0RNB
Duct
Common Bile 0FN9
Cystic 0FN8
Hepatic
Left 0FN6
Right 0FN5
Lacrimal
Left 08NY
Right 08NX
Pancreatic 0FND
Accessory 0FNF
Parotid
Left 0CNC
Right 0CNB
Duodenum 0DN9
Dura Mater 00N2
Ear
External
Left 09N1
Right 09N0

Release *(Continued)*
Ear *(Continued)*
External Auditory Canal
Left 09N4
Right 09N3
Inner
Left 09NE0ZZ
Right 09ND0ZZ
Middle
Left 09N60ZZ
Right 09N50ZZ
Epididymis
Bilateral 0VNL
Left 0VNK
Right 0VNJ
Epiglottis 0CNR
Esophagogastric Junction
0DN4
Esophagus 0DN5
Lower 0DN3
Middle 0DN2
Upper 0DN1
Eustachian Tube
Left 09NG
Right 09NF
Eye
Left 08N1XZZ
Right 08N0XZZ
Eyelid
Lower
Left 08NR
Right 08NQ
Upper
Left 08NP
Right 08NN
Fallopian Tube
Left 0UN6
Right 0UN5
Fallopian Tubes, Bilateral 0UN7
Femoral Shaft
Left 0QN9
Right 0QN8
Femur
Lower
Left 0QNC
Right 0QNB
Upper
Left 0QN7
Right 0QN6
Fibula
Left 0QNK
Right 0QNJ
Finger Nail 0HNQXZZ
Gallbladder 0FN4
Gingiva
Lower 0CN6
Upper 0CN5
Gland
Adrenal
Bilateral 0GN4
Left 0GN2
Right 0GN3
Lacrimal
Left 08NW
Right 08NV
Minor Salivary 0CNJ
Parotid
Left 0CN9
Right 0CN8
Pituitary 0GN0
Sublingual
Left 0CNF
Right 0CND
Submaxillary
Left 0CNH
Right 0CNG
Vestibular 0UNL
Glenoid Cavity
Left 0PN8
Right 0PN7
Glomus Jugulare 0GNC

Release *(Continued)*
Humeral Head
Left 0PND
Right 0PNC
Humeral Shaft
Left 0PNG
Right 0PNF
Hymen 0UNK
Hypothalamus 00NA
Ileocecal Valve 0DNC
Ileum 0DNB
Intestine
Large 0DNE
Left 0DNG
Right 0DNF
Small 0DN8
Iris
Left 08ND3ZZ
Right 08NC3ZZ
Jejunum 0DNA
Joint
Acromioclavicular
Left 0RNH
Right 0RNG
Ankle
Left 0SNG
Right 0SNF
Carpal
Left 0RNR
Right 0RNQ
Cervical Vertebral 0RN1
Cervicothoracic Vertebral 0RN4
Coccygeal 0SN6
Elbow
Left 0RNM
Right 0RNL
Finger Phalangeal
Left 0RNX
Right 0RNW
Hip
Left 0SNB
Right 0SN9
Knee
Left 0SND
Right 0SNC
Lumbar Vertebral 0SN0
Lumbosacral 0SN3
Metacarpocarpal
Left 0RNT
Right 0RNS
Metacarpophalangeal
Left 0RNV
Right 0RNU
Metatarsal-Phalangeal
Left 0SNN
Right 0SNM
Metatarsal-Tarsal
Left 0SNL
Right 0SNK
Occipital-cervical 0RN0
Sacrococcygeal 0SN5
Sacroiliac
Left 0SN8
Right 0SN7
Shoulder
Left 0RNK
Right 0RNJ
Sternoclavicular
Left 0RNF
Right 0RNE
Tarsal
Left 0SNJ
Right 0SNH
Temporomandibular
Left 0RND
Right 0RNC
Thoracic Vertebral 0RN6
Thoracolumbar Vertebral 0RNA
Toe Phalangeal
Left 0SNQ
Right 0SNP

Release (*Continued*)
  Joint (*Continued*)
    Wrist
      Left 0RNP
      Right 0RNN
  Kidney
    Left 0TN1
    Right 0TN0
  Kidney Pelvis
    Left 0TN4
    Right 0TN3
  Larynx 0CNS
  Lens
    Left 08NK3ZZ
    Right 08NJ3ZZ
  Lip
    Lower 0CN1
    Upper 0CN0
  Liver 0FN0
    Left Lobe 0FN2
    Right Lobe 0FN1
  Lung
    Bilateral 0BNM
    Left 0BNL
    Lower Lobe
      Left 0BNJ
      Right 0BNF
    Middle Lobe, Right
      0BND
    Right 0BNK
    Upper Lobe
      Left 0BNG
      Right 0BNC
  Lung Lingula 0BNH
  Lymphatic
    Aortic 07ND
    Axillary
      Left 07N6
      Right 07N5
    Head 07N0
    Inguinal
      Left 07NJ
      Right 07NH
    Internal Mammary
      Left 07N9
      Right 07N8
    Lower Extremity
      Left 07NG
      Right 07NF
    Mesenteric 07NB
    Neck
      Left 07N2
      Right 07N1
    Pelvis 07NC
    Thoracic Duct 07NK
    Thorax 07N7
    Upper Extremity
      Left 07N4
      Right 07N3
  Mandible
    Left 0NNV
    Right 0NNT
  Maxilla
    Left 0NNS
    Right 0NNR
  Medulla Oblongata 00ND
  Mesentery 0DNV
  Metacarpal
    Left 0PNQ
    Right 0PNP
  Metatarsal
    Left 0QNP
    Right 0QNN
  Muscle
    Abdomen
      Left 0KNL
      Right 0KNK
    Extraocular
      Left 08NM
      Right 08NL
    Facial 0KN1

Release (*Continued*)
  Muscle (*Continued*)
    Foot
      Left 0KNW
      Right 0KNV
    Hand
      Left 0KND
      Right 0KNC
    Head 0KN0
    Hip
      Left 0KNP
      Right 0KNN
    Lower Arm and Wrist
      Left 0KNB
      Right 0KN9
    Lower Leg
      Left 0KNT
      Right 0KNS
    Neck
      Left 0KN3
      Right 0KN2
    Papillary 02ND
    Perineum 0KNM
    Shoulder
      Left 0KN6
      Right 0KN5
    Thorax
      Left 0KNJ
      Right 0KNH
    Tongue, Palate, Pharynx 0KN4
    Trunk
      Left 0KNG
      Right 0KNF
    Upper Arm
      Left 0KN8
      Right 0KN7
    Upper Leg
      Left 0KNR
      Right 0KNQ
  Nasopharynx 09NN
  Nerve
    Abdominal Sympathetic 01NM
    Abducens 00NL
    Accessory 00NR
    Acoustic 00NN
    Brachial Plexus 01N3
    Cervical 01N1
    Cervical Plexus 01N0
    Facial 00NM
    Femoral 01ND
    Glossopharyngeal 00NP
    Head and Neck Sympathetic 01NK
    Hypoglossal 00NS
    Lumbar 01NB
    Lumbar Plexus 01N9
    Lumbar Sympathetic 01NN
    Lumbosacral Plexus 01NA
    Median 01N5
    Oculomotor 00NH
    Olfactory 00NF
    Optic 00NG
    Peroneal 01NH
    Phrenic 01N2
    Pudendal 01NC
    Radial 01N6
    Sacral 01NR
    Sacral Plexus 01NQ
    Sacral Sympathetic 01NP
    Sciatic 01NF
    Thoracic 01N8
    Thoracic Sympathetic 01NL
    Tibial 01NG
    Trigeminal 00NK
    Trochlear 00NJ
    Ulnar 01N4
    Vagus 00NQ
  Nipple
    Left 0HNX
    Right 0HNW
  Nose 09NK

Release (*Continued*)
  Omentum
    Greater 0DNS
    Lesser 0DNT
  Orbit
    Left 0NNQ
    Right 0NNP
  Ovary
    Bilateral 0UN2
    Left 0UN1
    Right 0UN0
  Palate
    Hard 0CN2
    Soft 0CN3
  Pancreas 0FNG
  Para-aortic Body 0GN9
  Paraganglion Extremity 0GNF
  Parathyroid Gland 0GNR
    Inferior
      Left 0GNP
      Right 0GNN
    Multiple 0GNQ
    Superior
      Left 0GNM
      Right 0GNL
  Patella
    Left 0QNF
    Right 0QND
  Penis 0VNS
  Pericardium 02NN
  Peritoneum 0DNW
  Phalanx
    Finger
      Left 0PNV
      Right 0PNT
    Thumb
      Left 0PNS
      Right 0PNR
    Toe
      Left 0QNR
      Right 0QNQ
  Pharynx 0CNM
  Pineal Body 0GN1
  Pleura
    Left 0BNP
    Right 0BNN
  Pons 00NB
  Prepuce 0VNT
  Prostate 0VN0
  Radius
    Left 0PNJ
    Right 0PNH
  Rectum 0DNP
  Retina
    Left 08NF3ZZ
    Right 08NE3ZZ
  Retinal Vessel
    Left 08NH3ZZ
    Right 08NG3ZZ
  Rib
    Left 0PN2
    Right 0PN1
  Sacrum 0QN1
  Scapula
    Left 0PN6
    Right 0PN5
  Sclera
    Left 08N7XZZ
    Right 08N6XZZ
  Scrotum 0VN5
  Septum
    Atrial 02N5
    Nasal 09NM
    Ventricular 02NM
  Sinus
    Accessory 09NP
    Ethmoid
      Left 09NV
      Right 09NU

◀ New   ◀▮▮▮ Revised   ~~deleted~~ Deleted

Release *(Continued)*
Sinus *(Continued)*
Frontal
Left 09NT
Right 09NS
Mastoid
Left 09NC
Right 09NB
Maxillary
Left 09NR
Right 09NQ
Sphenoid
Left 09NX
Right 09NW
Skin
Abdomen 0HN7XZZ
Back 0HN6XZZ
Buttock 0HN8XZZ
Chest 0HN5XZZ
Ear
Left 0HN3XZZ
Right 0HN2XZZ
Face 0HN1XZZ
Foot
Left 0HNNXZZ
Right 0HNMXZZ
Genitalia 0HNAXZZ
Hand
Left 0HNGXZZ
Right 0HNFXZZ
Lower Arm
Left 0HNEXZZ
Right 0HNDXZZ
Lower Leg
Left 0HNLXZZ
Right 0HNKXZZ
Neck 0HN4XZZ
Perineum 0HN9XZZ
Scalp 0HN0XZZ
Upper Arm
Left 0HNCXZZ
Right 0HNBXZZ
Upper Leg
Left 0HNJXZZ
Right 0HNHXZZ
Spinal Cord
Cervical 00NW
Lumbar 00NY
Thoracic 00NX
Spinal Meninges 00NT
Spleen 07NP
Sternum 0PN0
Stomach 0DN6
Pylorus 0DN7
Subcutaneous Tissue and Fascia
Abdomen 0JN8
Back 0JN7
Buttock 0JN9
Chest 0JN6
Face 0JN1
Foot
Left 0JNR
Right 0JNQ
Hand
Left 0JNK
Right 0JNJ
Lower Arm
Left 0JNH
Right 0JNG
Lower Leg
Left 0JNP
Right 0JNN
Neck
Anterior 0JN4
Posterior 0JN5
Pelvic Region 0JNC
Perineum 0JNB
Scalp 0JN0
Upper Arm
Left 0JNF
Right 0JND

Release *(Continued)*
Subcutaneous Tissue and Fascia
(Continued)
Upper Leg
Left 0JNM
Right 0JNL
Tarsal
Left 0QNM
Right 0QNL
Tendon
Abdomen
Left 0LNG
Right 0LNF
Ankle
Left 0LNT
Right 0LNS
Foot
Left 0LNW
Right 0LNV
Hand
Left 0LN8
Right 0LN7
Head and Neck 0LN0
Hip
Left 0LNK
Right 0LNJ
Knee
Left 0LNR
Right 0LNQ
Lower Arm and Wrist
Left 0LN6
Right 0LN5
Lower Leg
Left 0LNP
Right 0LNN
Perineum 0LNH
Shoulder
Left 0LN2
Right 0LN1
Thorax
Left 0LND
Right 0LNC
Trunk
Left 0LNB
Right 0LN9
Upper Arm
Left 0LN4
Right 0LN3
Upper Leg
Left 0LNM
Right 0LNL
Testis
Bilateral 0VNC
Left 0VNB
Right 0VN9
Thalamus 00N9
Thymus 07NM
Thyroid Gland 0GNK
Left Lobe 0GNG
Right Lobe 0GNH
Tibia
Left 0QNH
Right 0QNG
Toe Nail 0HNRXZZ
Tongue 0CN7
Tonsils 0CNP
Tooth
Lower 0CNX
Upper 0CNW
Trachea 0BN1
Tunica Vaginalis
Left 0VN7
Right 0VN6
Turbinate, Nasal 09NL
Tympanic Membrane
Left 09N8
Right 09N7
Ulna
Left 0PNL
Right 0PNK

Release *(Continued)*
Ureter
Left 0TN7
Right 0TN6
Urethra 0TND
Uterine Supporting Structure 0UN4
Uterus 0UN9
Uvula 0CNN
Vagina 0UNG
Valve
Aortic 02NF
Mitral 02NG
Pulmonary 02NH
Tricuspid 02NJ
Vas Deferens
Bilateral 0VNQ
Left 0VNP
Right 0VNN
Vein
Axillary
Left 05N8
Right 05N7
Azygos 05N0
Basilic
Left 05NC
Right 05NB
Brachial
Left 05NA
Right 05N9
Cephalic
Left 05NF
Right 05ND
Colic 06N7
Common Iliac
Left 06ND
Right 06NC
Coronary 02N4
Esophageal 06N3
External Iliac
Left 06NG
Right 06NF
External Jugular
Left 05NQ
Right 05NP
Face
Left 05NV
Right 05NT
Femoral
Left 06NN
Right 06NM
Foot
Left 06NV
Right 06NT
Gastric 06N2
Greater Saphenous
Left 06NQ
Right 06NP
Hand
Left 05NH
Right 05NG
Hemiazygos 05N1
Hepatic 06N4
Hypogastric
Left 06NJ
Right 06NH
Inferior Mesenteric 06N6
Innominate
Left 05N4
Right 05N3
Internal Jugular
Left 05NN
Right 05NM
Intracranial 05NL
Lesser Saphenous
Left 06NS
Right 06NR
Lower 06NY
Portal 06N8
Pulmonary
Left 02NT
Right 02NS

Release *(Continued)*
  Vein *(Continued)*
    Renal
      Left 06NB
      Right 06N9
    Splenic 06N1
    Subclavian
      Left 05N6
      Right 05N5
    Superior Mesenteric 06N5
    Upper 05NY
    Vertebral
      Left 05NS
      Right 05NR
  Vena Cava
    Inferior 06N0
    Superior 02NV
  Ventricle
    Left 02NL
    Right 02NK
  Vertebra
    Cervical 0PN3
    Lumbar 0QN0
    Thoracic 0PN4
  Vesicle
    Bilateral 0VN3
    Left 0VN2
    Right 0VN1
  Vitreous
    Left 08N53ZZ
    Right 08N43ZZ
  Vocal Cord
    Left 0CNV
    Right 0CNT
  Vulva 0UNM
Relocation *see* Reposition
Removal
  Abdominal Wall 2W53X
  Anorectal 2Y53X5Z
  Arm
    Lower
      Left 2W5DX
      Right 2W5CX
    Upper
      Left 2W5BX
      Right 2W5AX
  Back 2W55X
  Chest Wall 2W54X
  Ear 2Y52X5Z
  Extremity
    Lower
      Left 2W5MX
      Right 2W5LX
    Upper
      Left 2W59X
      Right 2W58X
  Face 2W51X
  Finger
    Left 2W5KX
    Right 2W5JX
  Foot
    Left 2W5TX
    Right 2W5SX
  Genital Tract, Female 2Y54X5Z
  Hand
    Left 2W5FX
    Right 2W5EX
  Head 2W50X
  Inguinal Region
    Left 2W57X
    Right 2W56X
  Leg
    Lower
      Left 2W5RX
      Right 2W5QX
    Upper
      Left 2W5PX
      Right 2W5NX
  Mouth and Pharynx 2Y50X5Z
  Nasal 2Y51X5Z
  Neck 2W52X

Removal *(Continued)*
  Thumb
    Left 2W5HX
    Right 2W5GX
  Toe
    Left 2W5VX
    Right 2W5UX
  Urethra 2Y55X5Z
Removal of device from
  Abdominal Wall 0WPF
  Acetabulum
    Left 0QP5
    Right 0QP4
  Anal Sphincter 0DPR
  Anus 0DPQ
  Artery
    Lower 04PY
    Upper 03PY
  Back
    Lower 0WPL
    Upper 0WPK
  Bladder 0TPB
  Bone
    Facial 0NPW
    Lower 0QPY
    Nasal 0NPB
    Pelvic
      Left 0QP3
      Right 0QP2
    Upper 0PPY
  Bone Marrow 07PT
  Brain 00P0
  Breast
    Left 0HPU
    Right 0HPT
  Bursa and Ligament
    Lower 0MPY
    Upper 0MPX
  Carpal
    Left 0PPN
    Right 0PPM
  Cavity, Cranial 0WP1
  Cerebral Ventricle 00P6
  Chest Wall 0WP8
  Cisterna Chyli 07PL
  Clavicle
    Left 0PPB
    Right 0PP9
  Coccyx 0QPS
  Diaphragm 0BPT
  Disc
    Cervical Vertebral 0RP3
    Cervicothoracic Vertebral 0RP5
    Lumbar Vertebral 0SP2
    Lumbosacral 0SP4
    Thoracic Vertebral 0RP9
    Thoracolumbar Vertebral 0RPB
  Duct
    Hepatobiliary 0FPB
    Pancreatic 0FPD
  Ear
    Inner
      Left 09PE
      Right 09PD
    Left 09PJ
    Right 09PH
  Epididymis and Spermatic Cord 0VPM
  Esophagus 0DP5
  Extremity
    Lower
      Left 0YPB
      Right 0YP9
    Upper
      Left 0XP7
      Right 0XP6
  Eye
    Left 08P1
    Right 08P0
  Face 0WP2
  Fallopian Tube 0UP8

Removal of device from *(Continued)*
  Femoral Shaft
    Left 0QP9
    Right 0QP8
  Femur
    Lower
      Left 0QPC
      Right 0QPB
    Upper
      Left 0QP7
      Right 0QP6
  Fibula
    Left 0QPK
    Right 0QPJ
  Finger Nail 0HPQX
  Gallbladder 0FP4
  Gastrointestinal Tract 0WPP
  Genitourinary Tract 0WPR
  Gland
    Adrenal 0GP5
    Endocrine 0GPS
    Pituitary 0GP0
    Salivary 0CPA
  Glenoid Cavity
    Left 0PP8
    Right 0PP7
  Great Vessel 02PY
  Hair 0HPSX
  Head 0WP0
  Heart 02PA
  Humeral Head
    Left 0PPD
    Right 0PPC
  Humeral Shaft
    Left 0PPG
    Right 0PPF
  Intestinal Tract
    Lower 0DPD
    Upper 0DP0
  Jaw
    Lower 0WP5
    Upper 0WP4
  Joint
    Acromioclavicular
      Left 0RPH
      Right 0RPG
    Ankle
      Left 0SPG
      Right 0SPF
    Carpal
      Left 0RPR
      Right 0RPQ
    Cervical Vertebral 0RP1
    Cervicothoracic Vertebral 0RP4
    Coccygeal 0SP6
    Elbow
      Left 0RPM
      Right 0RPL
    Finger Phalangeal
      Left 0RPX
      Right 0RPW
    Hip
      Left 0SPB
      Right 0SP9
    Knee
      Left 0SPD
      Right 0SPC
    Lumbar Vertebral 0SP0
    Lumbosacral 0SP3
    Metacarpocarpal
      Left 0RPT
      Right 0RPS
    Metacarpophalangeal
      Left 0RPV
      Right 0RPU
    Metatarsal-Phalangeal
      Left 0SPN
      Right 0SPM
    Metatarsal-Tarsal
      Left 0SPL
      Right 0SPK

◀ New   ◀ⅲ Revised   ~~deleted~~ Deleted

Removal of device from (*Continued*)
 Joint (*Continued*)
  Occipital-cervical 0RP0
  Sacrococcygeal 0SP5
  Sacroiliac
   Left 0SP8
   Right 0SP7
  Shoulder
   Left 0RPK
   Right 0RPJ
  Sternoclavicular
   Left 0RPF
   Right 0RPE
  Tarsal
   Left 0SPJ
   Right 0SPH
  Temporomandibular
   Left 0RPD
   Right 0RPC
  Thoracic Vertebral 0RP6
  Thoracolumbar Vertebral
    0RPA
  Toe Phalangeal
   Left 0SPQ
   Right 0SPP
  Wrist
   Left 0RPP
   Right 0RPN
 Kidney 0TP5
 Larynx 0CPS
 Lens
  Left 08PK3JZ
  Right 08PJ3JZ
 Liver 0FP0
 Lung
  Left 0BPL
  Right 0BPK
 Lymphatic 07PN
  Thoracic Duct 07PK
 Mediastinum 0WPC
 Mesentery 0DPV
 Metacarpal
  Left 0PPQ
  Right 0PPP
 Metatarsal
  Left 0QPP
  Right 0QPN
 Mouth and Throat 0CPY
 Muscle
  Extraocular
   Left 08PM
   Right 08PL
  Lower 0KPY
  Upper 0KPX
 Neck 0WP6
 Nerve
  Cranial 00PE
  Peripheral 01PY
 Nose 09PK
 Omentum 0DPU
 Ovary 0UP3
 Pancreas 0FPG
 Parathyroid Gland 0GPR
 Patella
  Left 0QPF
  Right 0QPD
 Pelvic Cavity 0WPJ
 Penis 0VPS
 Pericardial Cavity 0WPD
 Perineum
  Female 0WPN
  Male 0WPM
 Peritoneal Cavity 0WPG
 Peritoneum 0DPW
 Phalanx
  Finger
   Left 0PPV
   Right 0PPT
  Thumb
   Left 0PPS
   Right 0PPR

Removal of device from (*Continued*)
 Phalanx (*Continued*)
  Toe
   Left 0QPR
   Right 0QPQ
 Pineal Body 0GP1
 Pleura 0BPQ
 Pleural Cavity
  Left 0WPB
  Right 0WP9
 Products of Conception 10P0
 Prostate and Seminal Vesicles 0VP4
 Radius
  Left 0PPJ
  Right 0PPH
 Rectum 0DPP
 Respiratory Tract 0WPQ
 Retroperitoneum 0WPH
 Rib
  Left 0PP2
  Right 0PP1
 Sacrum 0QP1
 Scapula
  Left 0PP6
  Right 0PP5
 Scrotum and Tunica Vaginalis 0VP8
 Sinus 09PY
 Skin 0HPPX
 Skull 0NP0
 Spinal Canal 00PU
 Spinal Cord 00PV
 Spleen 07PP
 Sternum 0PP0
 Stomach 0DP6
 Subcutaneous Tissue and Fascia
  Head and Neck 0JPS
  Lower Extremity 0JPW
  Trunk 0JPT
  Upper Extremity 0JPV
 Tarsal
  Left 0QPM
  Right 0QPL
 Tendon
  Lower 0LPY
  Upper 0LPX
 Testis 0VPD
 Thymus 07PM
 Thyroid Gland 0GPK
 Tibia
  Left 0QPH
  Right 0QPG
 Toe Nail 0HPRX
 Trachea 0BP1
 Tracheobronchial Tree 0BP0
 Tympanic Membrane
  Left 09P8
  Right 09P7
 Ulna
  Left 0PPL
  Right 0PPK
 Ureter 0TP9
 Urethra 0TPD
 Uterus and Cervix 0UPD
 Vagina and Cul-de-sac 0UPH
 Vas Deferens 0VPR
 Vein
  Lower 06PY
  Upper 05PY
 Vertebra
  Cervical 0PP3
  Lumbar 0QP0
  Thoracic 0PP4
 Vulva 0UPM
Renal calyx
 use Kidney
 use Kidneys, Bilateral
 use Kidney, Left
 use Kidney, Right
Renal capsule
 use Kidney, Left
 use Kidney

Renal capsule (*Continued*)
 use Kidney, Right
 use Kidneys, Bilateral
Renal cortex
 use Kidneys, Bilateral
 use Kidney, Left
 use Kidney, Right
 use Kidney
Renal dialysis *see* Performance, Urinary
  5A1D
Renal plexus *use* Nerve, Abdominal
  Sympathetic
Renal segment
 use Kidney
 use Kidney, Left
 use Kidney, Right
 use Kidneys, Bilateral
Renal segmental artery
 use Artery, Renal, Left
 use Artery, Renal, Right
Reopening, operative site
 Control of bleeding *see* Control
   postprocedural bleeding in
 Inspection only *see* Inspection
Repair
 Abdominal Wall 0WQF
 Acetabulum
  Left 0QQ5
  Right 0QQ4
 Adenoids 0CQQ
 Ampulla of Vater 0FQC
 Anal Sphincter 0DQR
 Ankle Region
  Left 0YQL
  Right 0YQK
 Anterior Chamber
  Left 08Q33ZZ
  Right 08Q23ZZ
 Anus 0DQQ
 Aorta
  Abdominal 04Q0
  Thoracic 02QW
 Aortic Body 0GQD
 Appendix 0DQJ
 Arm
  Lower
   Left 0XQF
   Right 0XQD
  Upper
   Left 0XQ9
   Right 0XQ8
 Artery
  Anterior Tibial
   Left 04QQ
   Right 04QP
  Axillary
   Left 03Q6
   Right 03Q5
  Brachial
   Left 03Q8
   Right 03Q7
  Celiac 04Q1
  Colic
   Left 04Q7
   Middle 04Q8
   Right 04Q6
  Common Carotid
   Left 03QJ
   Right 03QH
  Common Iliac
   Left 04QD
   Right 04QC
  Coronary
   Four or More Sites 02Q3
   One Site 02Q0
   Three Sites 02Q2
   Two Sites 02Q1
  External Carotid
   Left 03QN
   Right 03QM

Repair *(Continued)*
  Artery *(Continued)*
    External Iliac
      Left 04QJ
      Right 04QH
    Face 03QR
    Femoral
      Left 04QL
      Right 04QK
    Foot
      Left 04QW
      Right 04QV
    Gastric 04Q2
    Hand
      Left 03QF
      Right 03QD
    Hepatic 04Q3
    Inferior Mesenteric 04QB
    Innominate 03Q2
    Internal Carotid
      Left 03QL
      Right 03QK
    Internal Iliac
      Left 04QF
      Right 04QE
    Internal Mammary
      Left 03Q1
      Right 03Q0
    Intracranial 03QG
    Lower 04QY
    Peroneal
      Left 04QU
      Right 04QT
    Popliteal
      Left 04QN
      Right 04QM
    Posterior Tibial
      Left 04QS
      Right 04QR
    Pulmonary
      Left 02QR
      Right 02QQ
    Pulmonary Trunk 02QP
    Radial
      Left 03QC
      Right 03QB
    Renal
      Left 04QA
      Right 04Q9
    Splenic 04Q4
    Subclavian
      Left 03Q4
      Right 03Q3
    Superior Mesenteric 04Q5
    Temporal
      Left 03QT
      Right 03QS
    Thyroid
      Left 03QV
      Right 03QU
    Ulnar
      Left 03QA
      Right 03Q9
    Upper 03QY
    Vertebral
      Left 03QQ
      Right 03QP
  Atrium
    Left 02Q7
    Right 02Q6
  Auditory Ossicle
    Left 09QA0ZZ
    Right 09Q90ZZ
  Axilla
    Left 0XQ5
    Right 0XQ4
  Back
    Lower 0WQL
    Upper 0WQK
  Basal Ganglia 00Q8
  Bladder 0TQB

Repair *(Continued)*
  Bladder Neck 0TQC
  Bone
    Ethmoid
      Left 0NQG
      Right 0NQF
    Frontal
      Left 0NQ2
      Right 0NQ1
    Hyoid 0NQX
    Lacrimal
      Left 0NQJ
      Right 0NQH
    Nasal 0NQB
    Occipital
      Left 0NQ8
      Right 0NQ7
    Palatine
      Left 0NQL
      Right 0NQK
    Parietal
      Left 0NQ4
      Right 0NQ3
    Pelvic
      Left 0QQ3
      Right 0QQ2
    Sphenoid
      Left 0NQD
      Right 0NQC
    Temporal
      Left 0NQ6
      Right 0NQ5
    Zygomatic
      Left 0NQN
      Right 0NQM
  Brain 00Q0
  Breast
    Bilateral 0HQV
    Left 0HQU
    Right 0HQT
    Supernumerary 0HQY
  Bronchus
    Lingula 0BQ9
    Lower Lobe
      Left 0BQB
      Right 0BQ6
    Main
      Left 0BQ7
      Right 0BQ3
    Middle Lobe, Right 0BQ5
    Upper Lobe
      Left 0BQ8
      Right 0BQ4
  Buccal Mucosa 0CQ4
  Bursa and Ligament
    Abdomen
      Left 0MQJ
      Right 0MQH
    Ankle
      Left 0MQR
      Right 0MQQ
    Elbow
      Left 0MQ4
      Right 0MQ3
    Foot
      Left 0MQT
      Right 0MQS
    Hand
      Left 0MQ8
      Right 0MQ7
    Head and Neck 0MQ0
    Hip
      Left 0MQM
      Right 0MQL
    Knee
      Left 0MQP
      Right 0MQN
    Lower Extremity
      Left 0MQW
      Right 0MQV
    Perineum 0MQK

Repair *(Continued)*
  Bursa and Ligament *(Continued)*
    Shoulder
      Left 0MQ2
      Right 0MQ1
    Thorax
      Left 0MQG
      Right 0MQF
    Trunk
      Left 0MQD
      Right 0MQC
    Upper Extremity
      Left 0MQB
      Right 0MQ9
    Wrist
      Left 0MQ6
      Right 0MQ5
  Buttock
    Left 0YQ1
    Right 0YQ0
  Carina 0BQ2
  Carotid Bodies, Bilateral 0GQ8
  Carotid Body
    Left 0GQ6
    Right 0GQ7
  Carpal
    Left 0PQN
    Right 0PQM
  Cecum 0DQH
  Cerebellum 00QC
  Cerebral Hemisphere 00Q7
  Cerebral Meninges 00Q1
  Cerebral Ventricle 00Q6
  Cervix 0UQC
  Chest Wall 0WQ8
  Chordae Tendineae 02Q9
  Choroid
    Left 08QB
    Right 08QA
  Cisterna Chyli 07QL
  Clavicle
    Left 0PQB
    Right 0PQ9
  Clitoris 0UQJ
  Coccygeal Glomus 0GQB
  Coccyx 0QQS
  Colon
    Ascending 0DQK
    Descending 0DQM
    Sigmoid 0DQN
    Transverse 0DQL
  Conduction Mechanism 02Q8
  Conjunctiva
    Left 08QTXZZ
    Right 08QSXZZ
  Cord
    Bilateral 0VQH
    Left 0VQG
    Right 0VQF
  Cornea
    Left 08Q9XZZ
    Right 08Q8XZZ
  Cul-de-sac 0UQF
  Diaphragm
    Left 0BQS
    Right 0BQR
  Disc
    Cervical Vertebral 0RQ3
    Cervicothoracic Vertebral 0RQ5
    Lumbar Vertebral 0SQ2
    Lumbosacral 0SQ4
    Thoracic Vertebral 0RQ9
    Thoracolumbar Vertebral 0RQB
  Duct
    Common Bile 0FQ9
    Cystic 0FQ8
    Hepatic
      Left 0FQ6
      Right 0FQ5

Repair (Continued)
  Duct (Continued)
    Lacrimal
      Left 08QY
      Right 08QX
    Pancreatic 0FQD
      Accessory 0FQF
    Parotid
      Left 0CQC
      Right 0CQB
  Duodenum 0DQ9
  Dura Mater 00Q2
  Ear
    External
      Bilateral 09Q2
      Left 09Q1
      Right 09Q0
    External Auditory Canal
      Left 09Q4
      Right 09Q3
    Inner
      Left 09QE0ZZ
      Right 09QD0ZZ
    Middle
      Left 09Q60ZZ
      Right 09Q50ZZ
  Elbow Region
    Left 0XQC
    Right 0XQB
  Epididymis
    Bilateral 0VQL
    Left 0VQK
    Right 0VQJ
  Epiglottis 0CQR
  Esophagogastric Junction
    0DQ4
  Esophagus 0DQ5
    Lower 0DQ3
    Middle 0DQ2
    Upper 0DQ1
  Eustachian Tube
    Left 09QG
    Right 09QF
  Extremity
    Lower
      Left 0YQB
      Right 0YQ9
    Upper
      Left 0XQ7
      Right 0XQ6
  Eye
    Left 08Q1XZZ
    Right 08Q0XZZ
  Eyelid
    Lower
      Left 08QR
      Right 08QQ
    Upper
      Left 08QP
      Right 08QN
  Face 0WQ2
  Fallopian Tube
    Left 0UQ6
    Right 0UQ5
  Fallopian Tubes, Bilateral
    0UQ7
  Femoral Region
    Bilateral 0YQE
    Left 0YQ8
    Right 0YQ7
  Femoral Shaft
    Left 0QQ9
    Right 0QQ8
  Femur
    Lower
      Left 0QQC
      Right 0QQB
    Upper
      Left 0QQ7
      Right 0QQ6

Repair (Continued)
  Fibula
    Left 0QQK
    Right 0QQJ
  Finger
    Index
      Left 0XQP
      Right 0XQN
    Little
      Left 0XQW
      Right 0XQV
    Middle
      Left 0XQR
      Right 0XQQ
    Ring
      Left 0XQT
      Right 0XQS
  Finger Nail 0HQQXZZ
  Foot
    Left 0YQN
    Right 0YQM
  Gallbladder 0FQ4
  Gingiva
    Lower 0CQ6
    Upper 0CQ5
  Gland
    Adrenal
      Bilateral 0GQ4
      Left 0GQ2
      Right 0GQ3
    Lacrimal
      Left 08QW
      Right 08QV
    Minor Salivary 0CQJ
    Parotid
      Left 0CQ9
      Right 0CQ8
    Pituitary 0GQ0
    Sublingual
      Left 0CQF
      Right 0CQD
    Submaxillary
      Left 0CQH
      Right 0CQG
    Vestibular 0UQL
  Glenoid Cavity
    Left 0PQ8
    Right 0PQ7
  Glomus Jugulare 0GQC
  Hand
    Left 0XQK
    Right 0XQJ
  Head 0WQ0
  Heart 02QA
    Left 02QC
    Right 02QB
  Humeral Head
    Left 0PQD
    Right 0PQC
  Humeral Shaft
    Left 0PQG
    Right 0PQF
  Hymen 0UQK
  Hypothalamus 00QA
  Ileocecal Valve 0DQC
  Ileum 0DQB
  Inguinal Region
    Bilateral 0YQA
    Left 0YQ6
    Right 0YQ5
  Intestine
    Large 0DQE
      Left 0DQG
      Right 0DQF
    Small 0DQ8
  Iris
    Left 08QD3ZZ
    Right 08QC3ZZ
  Jaw
    Lower 0WQ5
    Upper 0WQ4

Repair (Continued)
  Jejunum 0DQA
  Joint
    Acromioclavicular
      Left 0RQH
      Right 0RQG
    Ankle
      Left 0SQG
      Right 0SQF
    Carpal
      Left 0RQR
      Right 0RQQ
    Cervical Vertebral 0RQ1
    Cervicothoracic Vertebral 0RQ4
    Coccygeal 0SQ6
    Elbow
      Left 0RQM
      Right 0RQL
    Finger Phalangeal
      Left 0RQX
      Right 0RQW
    Hip
      Left 0SQB
      Right 0SQ9
    Knee
      Left 0SQD
      Right 0SQC
    Lumbar Vertebral 0SQ0
    Lumbosacral 0SQ3
    Metacarpocarpal
      Left 0RQT
      Right 0RQS
    Metacarpophalangeal
      Left 0RQV
      Right 0RQU
    Metatarsal-Phalangeal
      Left 0SQN
      Right 0SQM
    Metatarsal-Tarsal
      Left 0SQL
      Right 0SQK
    Occipital-cervical 0RQ0
    Sacrococcygeal 0SQ5
    Sacroiliac
      Left 0SQ8
      Right 0SQ7
    Shoulder
      Left 0RQK
      Right 0RQJ
    Sternoclavicular
      Left 0RQF
      Right 0RQE
    Tarsal
      Left 0SQJ
      Right 0SQH
    Temporomandibular
      Left 0RQD
      Right 0RQC
    Thoracic Vertebral 0RQ6
    Thoracolumbar Vertebral
      0RQA
    Toe Phalangeal
      Left 0SQQ
      Right 0SQP
    Wrist
      Left 0RQP
      Right 0RQN
  Kidney
    Left 0TQ1
    Right 0TQ0
  Kidney Pelvis
    Left 0TQ4
    Right 0TQ3
  Knee Region
    Left 0YQG
    Right 0YQF
  Larynx 0CQS
  Leg
    Lower
      Left 0YQJ
      Right 0YQH

◀ New   ◀▥ Revised   ~~deleted~~ Deleted

Repair *(Continued)*
  Leg *(Continued)*
    Upper
      Left 0YQD
      Right 0YQC
  Lens
    Left 08QK3ZZ
    Right 08QJ3ZZ
  Lip
    Lower 0CQ1
    Upper 0CQ0
  Liver 0FQ0
    Left Lobe 0FQ2
    Right Lobe 0FQ1
  Lung
    Bilateral 0BQM
    Left 0BQL
    Lower Lobe
      Left 0BQJ
      Right 0BQF
    Middle Lobe, Right 0BQD
    Right 0BQK
    Upper Lobe
      Left 0BQG
      Right 0BQC
  Lung Lingula 0BQH
  Lymphatic
    Aortic 07QD
    Axillary
      Left 07Q6
      Right 07Q5
    Head 07Q0
    Inguinal
      Left 07QJ
      Right 07QH
    Internal Mammary
      Left 07Q9
      Right 07Q8
    Lower Extremity
      Left 07QG
      Right 07QF
    Mesenteric 07QB
    Neck
      Left 07Q2
      Right 07Q1
    Pelvis 07QC
    Thoracic Duct 07QK
    Thorax 07Q7
    Upper Extremity
      Left 07Q4
      Right 07Q3
  Mandible
    Left 0NQV
    Right 0NQT
  Maxilla
    Left 0NQS
    Right 0NQR
  Mediastinum 0WQC
  Medulla Oblongata 00QD
  Mesentery 0DQV
  Metacarpal
    Left 0PQQ
    Right 0PQP
  Metatarsal
    Left 0QQP
    Right 0QQN
  Muscle
    Abdomen
      Left 0KQL
      Right 0KQK
    Extraocular
      Left 08QM
      Right 08QL
    Facial 0KQ1
    Foot
      Left 0KQW
      Right 0KQV
    Hand
      Left 0KQD
      Right 0KQC
    Head 0KQ0

Repair *(Continued)*
  Muscle *(Continued)*
    Hip
      Left 0KQP
      Right 0KQN
    Lower Arm and Wrist
      Left 0KQB
      Right 0KQ9
    Lower Leg
      Left 0KQT
      Right 0KQS
    Neck
      Left 0KQ3
      Right 0KQ2
    Papillary 02QD
    Perineum 0KQM
    Shoulder
      Left 0KQ6
      Right 0KQ5
    Thorax
      Left 0KQJ
      Right 0KQH
    Tongue, Palate, Pharynx 0KQ4
    Trunk
      Left 0KQG
      Right 0KQF
    Upper Arm
      Left 0KQ8
      Right 0KQ7
    Upper Leg
      Left 0KQR
      Right 0KQQ
  Nasopharynx 09QN
  Neck 0WQ6
  Nerve
    Abdominal Sympathetic 01QM
    Abducens 00QL
    Accessory 00QR
    Acoustic 00QN
    Brachial Plexus 01Q3
    Cervical 01Q1
    Cervical Plexus 01Q0
    Facial 00QM
    Femoral 01QD
    Glossopharyngeal 00QP
    Head and Neck Sympathetic
      01QK
    Hypoglossal 00QS
    Lumbar 01QB
    Lumbar Plexus 01Q9
    Lumbar Sympathetic 01QN
    Lumbosacral Plexus 01QA
    Median 01Q5
    Oculomotor 00QH
    Olfactory 00QF
    Optic 00QG
    Peroneal 01QH
    Phrenic 01Q2
    Pudendal 01QC
    Radial 01Q6
    Sacral 01QR
    Sacral Plexus 01QQ
    Sacral Sympathetic 01QP
    Sciatic 01QF
    Thoracic 01Q8
    Thoracic Sympathetic 01QL
    Tibial 01QG
    Trigeminal 00QK
    Trochlear 00QJ
    Ulnar 01Q4
    Vagus 00QQ
  Nipple
    Left 0HQX
    Right 0HQW
  Nose 09QK
  Omentum
    Greater 0DQS
    Lesser 0DQT
  Orbit
    Left 0NQQ
    Right 0NQP

Repair *(Continued)*
  Ovary
    Bilateral 0UQ2
    Left 0UQ1
    Right 0UQ0
  Palate
    Hard 0CQ2
    Soft 0CQ3
  Pancreas 0FQG
  Para-aortic Body 0GQ9
  Paraganglion Extremity 0GQF
  Parathyroid Gland 0GQR
    Inferior
      Left 0GQP
      Right 0GQN
    Multiple 0GQQ
    Superior
      Left 0GQM
      Right 0GQL
  Patella
    Left 0QQF
    Right 0QQD
  Penis 0VQS
  Pericardium 02QN
  Perineum
    Female 0WQN
    Male 0WQM
  Peritoneum 0DQW
  Phalanx
    Finger
      Left 0PQV
      Right 0PQT
    Thumb
      Left 0PQS
      Right 0PQR
    Toe
      Left 0QQR
      Right 0QQQ
  Pharynx 0CQM
  Pineal Body 0GQ1
  Pleura
    Left 0BQP
    Right 0BQN
  Pons 00QB
  Prepuce 0VQT
  Products of Conception
    10Q0
  Prostate 0VQ0
  Radius
    Left 0PQJ
    Right 0PQH
  Rectum 0DQP
  Retina
    Left 08QF3ZZ
    Right 08QE3ZZ
  Retinal Vessel
    Left 08QH3ZZ
    Right 08QG3ZZ
  Rib
    Left 0PQ2
    Right 0PQ1
  Sacrum 0QQ1
  Scapula
    Left 0PQ6
    Right 0PQ5
  Sclera
    Left 08Q7XZZ
    Right 08Q6XZZ
  Scrotum 0VQ5
  Septum
    Atrial 02Q5
    Nasal 09QM
    Ventricular 02QM
  Shoulder Region
    Left 0XQ3
    Right 0XQ2
  Sinus
    Accessory 09QP
    Ethmoid
      Left 09QV
      Right 09QU

◀ New   ◀▥ Revised   ~~deleted~~ Deleted

Repair *(Continued)*
  Vein *(Continued)*
    Hand
      Left 05QH
      Right 05QG
    Hemiazygos 05Q1
    Hepatic 06Q4
    Hypogastric
      Left 06QJ
      Right 06QH
    Inferior Mesenteric 06Q6
    Innominate
      Left 05Q4
      Right 05Q3
    Internal Jugular
      Left 05QN
      Right 05QM
    Intracranial 05QL
    Lesser Saphenous
      Left 06QS
      Right 06QR
    Lower 06QY
    Portal 06Q8
    Pulmonary
      Left 02QT
      Right 02QS
    Renal
      Left 06QB
      Right 06Q9
    Splenic 06Q1
    Subclavian
      Left 05Q6
      Right 05Q5
    Superior Mesenteric 06Q5
    Upper 05QY
    Vertebral
      Left 05QS
      Right 05QR
  Vena Cava
    Inferior 06Q0
    Superior 02QV
  Ventricle
    Left 02QL
    Right 02QK
  Vertebra
    Cervical 0PQ3
    Lumbar 0QQ0
    Thoracic 0PQ4
  Vesicle
    Bilateral 0VQ3
    Left 0VQ2
    Right 0VQ1
  Vitreous
    Left 08Q53ZZ
    Right 08Q43ZZ
  Vocal Cord
    Left 0CQV
    Right 0CQT
  Vulva 0UQM
  Wrist Region
    Left 0XQH
    Right 0XQG
Replacement
  Acetabulum
    Left 0QR5
    Right 0QR4
  Ampulla of Vater 0FRC
  Anal Sphincter 0DRR
  Aorta
    Abdominal 04R0
    Thoracic 02RW
  Artery
    Anterior Tibial
      Left 04RQ
      Right 04RP
    Axillary
      Left 03R6
      Right 03R5
    Brachial
      Left 03R8
      Right 03R7

Replacement *(Continued)*
  Artery *(Continued)*
    Celiac 04R1
    Colic
      Left 04R7
      Middle 04R8
      Right 04R6
    Common Carotid
      Left 03RJ
      Right 03RH
    Common Iliac
      Left 04RD
      Right 04RC
    External Carotid
      Left 03RN
      Right 03RM
    External Iliac
      Left 04RJ
      Right 04RH
    Face 03RR
    Femoral
      Left 04RL
      Right 04RK
    Foot
      Left 04RW
      Right 04RV
    Gastric 04R2
    Hand
      Left 03RF
      Right 03RD
    Hepatic 04R3
    Inferior Mesenteric 04RB
    Innominate 03R2
    Internal Carotid
      Left 03RL
      Right 03RK
    Internal Iliac
      Left 04RF
      Right 04RE
    Internal Mammary
      Left 03R1
      Right 03R0
    Intracranial 03RG
    Lower 04RY
    Peroneal
      Left 04RU
      Right 04RT
    Popliteal
      Left 04RN
      Right 04RM
    Posterior Tibial
      Left 04RS
      Right 04RR
    Pulmonary
      Left 02RR
      Right 02RQ
    Pulmonary Trunk 02RP
    Radial
      Left 03RC
      Right 03RB
    Renal
      Left 04RA
      Right 04R9
    Splenic 04R4
    Subclavian
      Left 03R4
      Right 03R3
    Superior Mesenteric 04R5
    Temporal
      Left 03RT
      Right 03RS
    Thyroid
      Left 03RV
      Right 03RU
    Ulnar
      Left 03RA
      Right 03R9
    Upper 03RY
    Vertebral
      Left 03RQ
      Right 03RP

Replacement *(Continued)*
  Atrium
    Left 02R7
    Right 02R6
  Auditory Ossicle
    Left 09RA0
    Right 09R90
  Bladder 0TRB
  Bladder Neck 0TRC
  Bone
    Ethmoid
      Left 0NRG
      Right 0NRF
    Frontal
      Left 0NR2
      Right 0NR1
    Hyoid 0NRX
    Lacrimal
      Left 0NRJ
      Right 0NRH
    Nasal 0NRB
    Occipital
      Left 0NR8
      Right 0NR7
    Palatine
      Left 0NRL
      Right 0NRK
    Parietal
      Left 0NR4
      Right 0NR3
    Pelvic
      Left 0QR3
      Right 0QR2
    Sphenoid
      Left 0NRD
      Right 0NRC
    Temporal
      Left 0NR6
      Right 0NR5
    Zygomatic
      Left 0NRN
      Right 0NRM
  Breast
    Bilateral 0HRV
    Left 0HRU
    Right 0HRT
  Buccal Mucosa 0CR4
  Carpal
    Left 0PRN
    Right 0PRM
  Chordae Tendineae 02R9
  Choroid
    Left 08RB
    Right 08RA
  Clavicle
    Left 0PRB
    Right 0PR9
  Coccyx 0QRS
  Conjunctiva
    Left 08RTX
    Right 08RSX
  Cornea
    Left 08R9
    Right 08R8
  Disc
    Cervical Vertebral 0RR30
    Cervicothoracic Vertebral 0RR50
    Lumbar Vertebral 0SR20
    Lumbosacral 0SR40
    Thoracic Vertebral 0RR90
    Thoracolumbar Vertebral 0RRB0
  Duct
    Common Bile 0FR9
    Cystic 0FR8
    Hepatic
      Left 0FR6
      Right 0FR5
    Lacrimal
      Left 08RY
      Right 08RX

◀ New   ⬅ Revised   ~~deleted~~ Deleted

Replacement *(Continued)*
  Duct *(Continued)*
    Pancreatic 0FRD
      Accessory 0FRF
    Parotid
      Left 0CRC
      Right 0CRB
  Ear
    External
      Bilateral 09R2
      Left 09R1
      Right 09R0
    Inner
      Left 09RE0
      Right 09RD0
    Middle
      Left 09R60
      Right 09R50
  Epiglottis 0CRR
  Esophagus 0DR5
  Eye
    Left 08R1
    Right 08R0
  Eyelid
    Lower
      Left 08RR
      Right 08RQ
    Upper
      Left 08RP
      Right 08RN
  Femoral Shaft
    Left 0QR9
    Right 0QR8
  Femur
    Lower
      Left 0QRC
      Right 0QRB
    Upper
      Left 0QR7
      Right 0QR6
  Fibula
    Left 0QRK
    Right 0QRJ
  Finger Nail 0HRQX
  Gingiva
    Lower 0CR6
    Upper 0CR5
  Glenoid Cavity
    Left 0PR8
    Right 0PR7
  Hair 0HRSX
  Humeral Head
    Left 0PRD
    Right 0PRC
  Humeral Shaft
    Left 0PRG
    Right 0PRF
  Iris
    Left 08RD3
    Right 08RC3
  Joint
    Acromioclavicular
      Left 0RRH0
      Right 0RRG0
    Ankle
      Left 0SRG
      Right 0SRF
    Carpal
      Left 0RRR0
      Right 0RRQ0
    Cervical Vertebral 0RR10
    Cervicothoracic Vertebral
      0RR40
    Coccygeal 0SR60
    Elbow
      Left 0RRM0
      Right 0RRL0
    Finger Phalangeal
      Left 0RRX0
      Right 0RRW0

Replacement *(Continued)*
  Joint *(Continued)*
    Hip
      Left 0SRB
        Acetabular Surface 0SRE
        Femoral Surface 0SRS
      Right 0SR9
        Acetabular Surface 0SRA
        Femoral Surface 0SRR
    Knee
      Left 0SRD
        Femoral Surface 0SRU
        Tibial Surface 0SRW
      Right 0SRC
        Femoral Surface 0SRT
        Tibial Surface 0SRV
    Lumbar Vertebral 0SR00
    Lumbosacral 0SR30
    Metacarpocarpal
      Left 0RRT0
      Right 0RRS0
    Metacarpophalangeal
      Left 0RRV0
      Right 0RRU0
    Metatarsal-Phalangeal
      Left 0SRN0
      Right 0SRM0
    Metatarsal-Tarsal
      Left 0SRL0
      Right 0SRK0
    Occipital-cervical 0RR00
    Sacrococcygeal 0SR50
    Sacroiliac
      Left 0SR80
      Right 0SR70
    Shoulder
      Left 0RRK
      Right 0RRJ
    Sternoclavicular
      Left 0RRF0
      Right 0RRE0
    Tarsal
      Left 0SRJ0
      Right 0SRH0
    Temporomandibular
      Left 0RRD0
      Right 0RRC0
    Thoracic Vertebral 0RR60
    Thoracolumbar Vertebral
      0RRA0
    Toe Phalangeal
      Left 0SRQ0
      Right 0SRP0
    Wrist
      Left 0RRP0
      Right 0RRN0
  Kidney Pelvis
    Left 0TR4
    Right 0TR3
  Larynx 0CRS
  Lens
    Left 08RK30Z
    Right 08RJ30Z
  Lip
    Lower 0CR1
    Upper 0CR0
  Mandible
    Left 0NRV
    Right 0NRT
  Maxilla
    Left 0NRS
    Right 0NRR
  Mesentery 0DRV
  Metacarpal
    Left 0PRQ
    Right 0PRP
  Metatarsal
    Left 0QRP
    Right 0QRN
  Muscle, Papillary 02RD
  Nasopharynx 09RN

Replacement *(Continued)*
  Nipple
    Left 0HRX
    Right 0HRW
  Nose 09RK
  Omentum
    Greater 0DRS
    Lesser 0DRT
  Orbit
    Left 0NRQ
    Right 0NRP
  Palate
    Hard 0CR2
    Soft 0CR3
  Patella
    Left 0QRF
    Right 0QRD
  Pericardium 02RN
  Peritoneum 0DRW
  Phalanx
    Finger
      Left 0PRV
      Right 0PRT
    Thumb
      Left 0PRS
      Right 0PRR
    Toe
      Left 0QRR
      Right 0QRQ
  Pharynx 0CRM
  Radius
    Left 0PRJ
    Right 0PRH
  Retinal Vessel
    Left 08RH3
    Right 08RG3
  Rib
    Left 0PR2
    Right 0PR1
  Sacrum 0QR1
  Scapula
    Left 0PR6
    Right 0PR5
  Sclera
    Left 08R7X
    Right 08R6X
  Septum
    Atrial 02R5
    Nasal 09RM
    Ventricular 02RM
  Skin
    Abdomen 0HR7
    Back 0HR6
    Buttock 0HR8
    Chest 0HR5
    Ear
      Left 0HR3
      Right 0HR2
    Face 0HR1
    Foot
      Left 0HRN
      Right 0HRM
    Genitalia 0HRA
    Hand
      Left 0HRG
      Right 0HRF
    Lower Arm
      Left 0HRE
      Right 0HRD
    Lower Leg
      Left 0HRL
      Right 0HRK
    Neck 0HR4
    Perineum 0HR9
    Scalp 0HR0
    Upper Arm
      Left 0HRC
      Right 0HRB
    Upper Leg
      Left 0HRJ
      Right 0HRH

◀ New   ◀▥ Revised   ~~deleted~~ Deleted

Replacement (Continued)

Skull 0NR0
Sternum 0PR0
Subcutaneous Tissue and Fascia
  Abdomen 0JR8
  Back 0JR7
  Buttock 0JR9
  Chest 0JR6
  Face 0JR1
  Foot
    Left 0JRR
    Right 0JRQ
  Hand
    Left 0JRK
    Right 0JRJ
  Lower Arm
    Left 0JRH
    Right 0JRG
  Lower Leg
    Left 0JRP
    Right 0JRN
  Neck
    Anterior 0JR4
    Posterior 0JR5
  Pelvic Region 0JRC
  Perineum 0JRB
  Scalp 0JR0
  Upper Arm
    Left 0JRF
    Right 0JRD
  Upper Leg
    Left 0JRM
    Right 0JRL
Tarsal
  Left 0QRM
  Right 0QRL
Tendon
  Abdomen
    Left 0LRG
    Right 0LRF
  Ankle
    Left 0LRT
    Right 0LRS
  Foot
    Left 0LRW
    Right 0LRV
  Hand
    Left 0LR8
    Right 0LR7
  Head and Neck 0LR0
  Hip
    Left 0LRK
    Right 0LRJ
  Knee
    Left 0LRR
    Right 0LRQ
  Lower Arm and Wrist
    Left 0LR6
    Right 0LR5
  Lower Leg
    Left 0LRP
    Right 0LRN
  Perineum 0LRH
  Shoulder
    Left 0LR2
    Right 0LR1
  Thorax
    Left 0LRD
    Right 0LRC
  Trunk
    Left 0LRB
    Right 0LR9
  Upper Arm
    Left 0LR4
    Right 0LR3
  Upper Leg
    Left 0LRM
    Right 0LRL
Testis
  Bilateral 0VRC0JZ
  Left 0VRB0JZ
  Right 0VR90JZ

Replacement (Continued)

Thumb
  Left 0XRM
  Right 0XRL
Tibia
  Left 0QRH
  Right 0QRG
Toe Nail 0HRRX
Tongue 0CR7
Tooth
  Lower 0CRX
  Upper 0CRW
Turbinate, Nasal 09RL
Tympanic Membrane
  Left 09R8
  Right 09R7
Ulna
  Left 0PRL
  Right 0PRK
Ureter
  Left 0TR7
  Right 0TR6
Urethra 0TRD
Uvula 0CRN
Valve
  Aortic 02RF
  Mitral 02RG
  Pulmonary 02RH
  Tricuspid 02RJ
Vein
  Axillary
    Left 05R8
    Right 05R7
  Azygos 05R0
  Basilic
    Left 05RC
    Right 05RB
  Brachial
    Left 05RA
    Right 05R9
  Cephalic
    Left 05RF
    Right 05RD
  Colic 06R7
  Common Iliac
    Left 06RD
    Right 06RC
  Esophageal 06R3
  External Iliac
    Left 06RG
    Right 06RF
  External Jugular
    Left 05RQ
    Right 05RP
  Face
    Left 05RV
    Right 05RT
  Femoral
    Left 06RN
    Right 06RM
  Foot
    Left 06RV
    Right 06RT
  Gastric 06R2
  Greater Saphenous
    Left 06RQ
    Right 06RP
  Hand
    Left 05RH
    Right 05RG
  Hemiazygos 05R1
  Hepatic 06R4
  Hypogastric
    Left 06RJ
    Right 06RH
  Inferior Mesenteric 06R6
  Innominate
    Left 05R4
    Right 05R3
  Internal Jugular
    Left 05RN
    Right 05RM

Replacement (Continued)

Vein (Continued)
  Intracranial 05RL
  Lesser Saphenous
    Left 06RS
    Right 06RR
  Lower 06RY
  Portal 06R8
  Pulmonary
    Left 02RT
    Right 02RS
  Renal
    Left 06RB
    Right 06R9
  Splenic 06R1
  Subclavian
    Left 05R6
    Right 05R5
  Superior Mesenteric 06R5
  Upper 05RY
  Vertebral
    Left 05RS
    Right 05RR
Vena Cava
  Inferior 06R0
  Superior 02RV
Ventricle
  Left 02RL
  Right 02RK
Vertebra
  Cervical 0PR3
  Lumbar 0QR0
  Thoracic 0PR4
Vitreous
  Left 08R53
  Right 08R43
Vocal Cord
  Left 0CRV
  Right 0CRT
Replantation see Reposition
Replantation, scalp see Reattachment, Skin,
  Scalp 0HM0
Reposition
Acetabulum
  Left 0QS5
  Right 0QS4
Ampulla of Vater 0FSC
Anus 0DSQ
Aorta
  Abdominal 04S0
  Thoracic 02SW0ZZ
Artery
  Anterior Tibial
    Left 04SQ
    Right 04SP
  Axillary
    Left 03S6
    Right 03S5
  Brachial
    Left 03S8
    Right 03S7
  Celiac 04S1
  Colic
    Left 04S7
    Middle 04S8
    Right 04S6
  Common Carotid
    Left 03SJ
    Right 03SH
  Common Iliac
    Left 04SD
    Right 04SC
  External Carotid
    Left 03SN
    Right 03SM
  External Iliac
    Left 04SJ
    Right 04SH
  Face 03SR
  Femoral
    Left 04SL
    Right 04SK

◀ New   ◀▥▥ Revised   ~~deleted~~ Deleted

Reposition *(Continued)*
  Artery *(Continued)*
    Foot
      Left 04SW
      Right 04SV
    Gastric 04S2
    Hand
      Left 03SF
      Right 03SD
    Hepatic 04S3
    Inferior Mesenteric
      04SB
    Innominate 03S2
    Internal Carotid
      Left 03SL
      Right 03SK
    Internal Iliac
      Left 04SF
      Right 04SE
    Internal Mammary
      Left 03S1
      Right 03S0
    Intracranial 03SG
    Lower 04SY
    Peroneal
      Left 04SU
      Right 04ST
    Popliteal
      Left 04SN
      Right 04SM
    Posterior Tibial
      Left 04SS
      Right 04SR
    Pulmonary
      Left 02SR0ZZ
      Right 02SQ0ZZ
    Pulmonary Trunk 02SP0ZZ
    Radial
      Left 03SC
      Right 03SB
    Renal
      Left 04SA
      Right 04S9
    Splenic 04S4
    Subclavian
      Left 03S4
      Right 03S3
    Superior Mesenteric 04S5
    Temporal
      Left 03ST
      Right 03SS
    Thyroid
      Left 03SV
      Right 03SU
    Ulnar
      Left 03SA
      Right 03S9
    Upper 03SY
    Vertebral
      Left 03SQ
      Right 03SP
  Auditory Ossicle
    Left 09SA
    Right 09S9
  Bladder 0TSB
  Bladder Neck 0TSC
  Bone
    Ethmoid
      Left 0NSG
      Right 0NSF
    Frontal
      Left 0NS2
      Right 0NS1
    Hyoid 0NSX
    Lacrimal
      Left 0NSJ
      Right 0NSH
    Nasal 0NSB
    Occipital
      Left 0NS8
      Right 0NS7

Reposition *(Continued)*
  Bone *(Continued)*
    Palatine
      Left 0NSL
      Right 0NSK
    Parietal
      Left 0NS4
      Right 0NS3
    Pelvic
      Left 0QS3
      Right 0QS2
    Sphenoid
      Left 0NSD
      Right 0NSC
    Temporal
      Left 0NS6
      Right 0NS5
    Zygomatic
      Left 0NSN
      Right 0NSM
  Breast
    Bilateral 0HSV0ZZ
    Left 0HSU0ZZ
    Right 0HST0ZZ
  Bronchus
    Lingula 0BS90ZZ
    Lower Lobe
      Left 0BSB0ZZ
      Right 0BS60ZZ
    Main
      Left 0BS70ZZ
      Right 0BS30ZZ
    Middle Lobe, Right
      0BS50ZZ
    Upper Lobe
      Left 0BS80ZZ
      Right 0BS40ZZ
  Bursa and Ligament
    Abdomen
      Left 0MSJ
      Right 0MSH
    Ankle
      Left 0MSR
      Right 0MSQ
    Elbow
      Left 0MS4
      Right 0MS3
    Foot
      Left 0MST
      Right 0MSS
    Hand
      Left 0MS8
      Right 0MS7
    Head and Neck
      0MS0
    Hip
      Left 0MSM
      Right 0MSL
    Knee
      Left 0MSP
      Right 0MSN
    Lower Extremity
      Left 0MSW
      Right 0MSV
    Perineum 0MSK
    Shoulder
      Left 0MS2
      Right 0MS1
    Thorax
      Left 0MSG
      Right 0MSF
    Trunk
      Left 0MSD
      Right 0MSC
    Upper Extremity
      Left 0MSB
      Right 0MS9
    Wrist
      Left 0MS6
      Right 0MS5
  Carina 0BS20ZZ

Reposition *(Continued)*
  Carpal
    Left 0PSN
    Right 0PSM
  Cecum 0DSH
  Cervix 0USC
  Clavicle
    Left 0PSB
    Right 0PS9
  Coccyx 0QSS
  Colon
    Ascending 0DSK
    Descending 0DSM
    Sigmoid 0DSN
    Transverse 0DSL
  Cord
    Bilateral 0VSH
    Left 0VSG
    Right 0VSF
  Cul-de-sac 0USF
  Diaphragm
    Left 0BSS0ZZ
    Right 0BSR0ZZ
  Duct
    Common Bile 0FS9
    Cystic 0FS8
    Hepatic
      Left 0FS6
      Right 0FS5
    Lacrimal
      Left 08SY
      Right 08SX
    Pancreatic 0FSD
      Accessory 0FSF
    Parotid
      Left 0CSC
      Right 0CSB
  Duodenum 0DS9
  Ear
    Bilateral 09S2
    Left 09S1
    Right 09S0
  Epiglottis 0CSR
  Esophagus 0DS5
  Eustachian Tube
    Left 09SG
    Right 09SF
  Eyelid
    Lower
      Left 08SR
      Right 08SQ
    Upper
      Left 08SP
      Right 08SN
  Fallopian Tube
    Left 0US6
    Right 0US5
  Fallopian Tubes, Bilateral
    0US7
  Femoral Shaft
    Left 0QS9
    Right 0QS8
  Femur
    Lower
      Left 0QSC
      Right 0QSB
    Upper
      Left 0QS7
      Right 0QS6
  Fibula
    Left 0QSK
    Right 0QSJ
  Gallbladder 0FS4
  Gland
    Adrenal
      Left 0GS2
      Right 0GS3
    Lacrimal
      Left 08SW
      Right 08SV

Reposition (Continued)

Glenoid Cavity
  Left 0PS8
  Right 0PS7
Hair 0HSSXZZ
Humeral Head
  Left 0PSD
  Right 0PSC
Humeral Shaft
  Left 0PSG
  Right 0PSF
Ileum 0DSB
Iris
  Left 08SD3ZZ
  Right 08SC3ZZ
Jejunum 0DSA
Joint
  Acromioclavicular
    Left 0RSH
    Right 0RSG
  Ankle
    Left 0SSG
    Right 0SSF
  Carpal
    Left 0RSR
    Right 0RSQ
  Cervical Vertebral 0RS1
  Cervicothoracic Vertebral
    0RS4
  Coccygeal 0SS6
  Elbow
    Left 0RSM
    Right 0RSL
  Finger Phalangeal
    Left 0RSX
    Right 0RSW
  Hip
    Left 0SSB
    Right 0SS9
  Knee
    Left 0SSD
    Right 0SSC
  Lumbar Vertebral 0SS0
  Lumbosacral 0SS3
  Metacarpocarpal
    Left 0RST
    Right 0RSS
  Metacarpophalangeal
    Left 0RSV
    Right 0RSU
  Metatarsal-Phalangeal
    Left 0SSN
    Right 0SSM
  Metatarsal-Tarsal
    Left 0SSL
    Right 0SSK
  Occipital-cervical 0RS0
  Sacrococcygeal 0SS5
  Sacroiliac
    Left 0SS8
    Right 0SS7
  Shoulder
    Left 0RSK
    Right 0RSJ
  Sternoclavicular
    Left 0RSF
    Right 0RSE
  Tarsal
    Left 0SSJ
    Right 0SSH
  Temporomandibular
    Left 0RSD
    Right 0RSC
  Thoracic Vertebral 0RS6
  Thoracolumbar Vertebral 0RSA
  Toe Phalangeal
    Left 0SSQ
    Right 0SSP
  Wrist
    Left 0RSP
    Right 0RSN

Reposition (Continued)

Kidney
  Left 0TS1
  Right 0TS0
Kidney Pelvis
  Left 0TS4
  Right 0TS3
Kidneys, Bilateral 0TS2
Lens
  Left 08SK3ZZ
  Right 08SJ3ZZ
Lip
  Lower 0CS1
  Upper 0CS0
Liver 0FS0
Lung
  Left 0BSL0ZZ
  Lower Lobe
    Left 0BSJ0ZZ
    Right 0BSF0ZZ
  Middle Lobe, Right
    0BSD0ZZ
  Right 0BSK0ZZ
  Upper Lobe
    Left 0BSG0ZZ
    Right 0BSC0ZZ
Lung Lingula 0BSH0ZZ
Mandible
  Left 0NSV
  Right 0NST
Maxilla
  Left 0NSS
  Right 0NSR
Metacarpal
  Left 0PSQ
  Right 0PSP
Metatarsal
  Left 0QSP
  Right 0QSN
Muscle
  Abdomen
    Left 0KSL
    Right 0KSK
  Extraocular
    Left 08SM
    Right 08SL
  Facial 0KS1
  Foot
    Left 0KSW
    Right 0KSV
  Hand
    Left 0KSD
    Right 0KSC
  Head 0KS0
  Hip
    Left 0KSP
    Right 0KSN
  Lower Arm and Wrist
    Left 0KSB
    Right 0KS9
  Lower Leg
    Left 0KST
    Right 0KSS
  Neck
    Left 0KS3
    Right 0KS2
  Perineum 0KSM
  Shoulder
    Left 0KS6
    Right 0KS5
  Thorax
    Left 0KSJ
    Right 0KSH
  Tongue, Palate, Pharynx
    0KS4
  Trunk
    Left 0KSG
    Right 0KSF
  Upper Arm
    Left 0KS8
    Right 0KS7

Reposition (Continued)

Muscle (Continued)
  Upper Leg
    Left 0KSR
    Right 0KSQ
Nerve
  Abducens 00SL
  Accessory 00SR
  Acoustic 00SN
  Brachial Plexus 01S3
  Cervical 01S1
  Cervical Plexus 01S0
  Facial 00SM
  Femoral 01SD
  Glossopharyngeal 00SP
  Hypoglossal 00SS
  Lumbar 01SB
  Lumbar Plexus 01S9
  Lumbosacral Plexus 01SA
  Median 01S5
  Oculomotor 00SH
  Olfactory 00SF
  Optic 00SG
  Peroneal 01SH
  Phrenic 01S2
  Pudendal 01SC
  Radial 01S6
  Sacral 01SR
  Sacral Plexus 01SQ
  Sciatic 01SF
  Thoracic 01S8
  Tibial 01SG
  Trigeminal 00SK
  Trochlear 00SJ
  Ulnar 01S4
  Vagus 00SQ
Nipple
  Left 0HSXXZZ
  Right 0HSWXZZ
Nose 09SK
Orbit
  Left 0NSQ
  Right 0NSP
Ovary
  Bilateral 0US2
  Left 0US1
  Right 0US0
Palate
  Hard 0CS2
  Soft 0CS3
Pancreas 0FSG
Parathyroid Gland 0GSR
  Inferior
    Left 0GSP
    Right 0GSN
  Multiple 0GSQ
  Superior
    Left 0GSM
    Right 0GSL
Patella
  Left 0QSF
  Right 0QSD
Phalanx
  Finger
    Left 0PSV
    Right 0PST
  Thumb
    Left 0PSS
    Right 0PSR
  Toe
    Left 0QSR
    Right 0QSQ
Products of Conception 10S0
  Ectopic 10S2
Radius
  Left 0PSJ
  Right 0PSH
Rectum 0DSP
Retinal Vessel
  Left 08SH3ZZ
  Right 08SG3ZZ

◀ New   ◀▦ Revised   ~~deleted~~ Deleted

Reposition *(Continued)*
- Rib
  - Left 0PS2
  - Right 0PS1
- Sacrum 0QS1
- Scapula
  - Left 0PS6
  - Right 0PS5
- Septum, Nasal 09SM
- Skull 0NS0
- Spinal Cord
  - Cervical 00SW
  - Lumbar 00SY
  - Thoracic 00SX
- Spleen 07SP0ZZ
- Sternum 0PS0
- Stomach 0DS6
- Tarsal
  - Left 0QSM
  - Right 0QSL
- Tendon
  - Abdomen
    - Left 0LSG
    - Right 0LSF
  - Ankle
    - Left 0LST
    - Right 0LSS
  - Foot
    - Left 0LSW
    - Right 0LSV
  - Hand
    - Left 0LS8
    - Right 0LS7
  - Head and Neck 0LS0
  - Hip
    - Left 0LSK
    - Right 0LSJ
  - Knee
    - Left 0LSR
    - Right 0LSQ
  - Lower Arm and Wrist
    - Left 0LS6
    - Right 0LS5
  - Lower Leg
    - Left 0LSP
    - Right 0LSN
  - Perineum 0LSH
  - Shoulder
    - Left 0LS2
    - Right 0LS1
  - Thorax
    - Left 0LSD
    - Right 0LSC
  - Trunk
    - Left 0LSB
    - Right 0LS9
  - Upper Arm
    - Left 0LS4
    - Right 0LS3
  - Upper Leg
    - Left 0LSM
    - Right 0LSL
- Testis
  - Bilateral 0VSC
  - Left 0VSB
  - Right 0VS9
- Thymus 07SM0ZZ
- Thyroid Gland
  - Left Lobe 0GSG
  - Right Lobe 0GSH
- Tibia
  - Left 0QSH
  - Right 0QSG
- Tongue 0CS7
- Tooth
  - Lower 0CSX
  - Upper 0CSW
- Trachea 0BS10ZZ
- Turbinate, Nasal 09SL
- Tympanic Membrane
  - Left 09S8
  - Right 09S7

Reposition *(Continued)*
- Ulna
  - Left 0PSL
  - Right 0PSK
- Ureter
  - Left 0TS7
  - Right 0TS6
- Ureters, Bilateral 0TS8
- Urethra 0TSD
- Uterine Supporting Structure 0US4
- Uterus 0US9
- Uvula 0CSN
- Vagina 0USG
- Vein
  - Axillary
    - Left 05S8
    - Right 05S7
  - Azygos 05S0
  - Basilic
    - Left 05SC
    - Right 05SB
  - Brachial
    - Left 05SA
    - Right 05S9
  - Cephalic
    - Left 05SF
    - Right 05SD
  - Colic 06S7
  - Common Iliac
    - Left 06SD
    - Right 06SC
  - Esophageal 06S3
  - External Iliac
    - Left 06SG
    - Right 06SF
  - External Jugular
    - Left 05SQ
    - Right 05SP
  - Face
    - Left 05SV
    - Right 05ST
  - Femoral
    - Left 06SN
    - Right 06SM
  - Foot
    - Left 06SV
    - Right 06ST
  - Gastric 06S2
  - Greater Saphenous
    - Left 06SQ
    - Right 06SP
  - Hand
    - Left 05SH
    - Right 05SG
  - Hemiazygos 05S1
  - Hepatic 06S4
  - Hypogastric
    - Left 06SJ
    - Right 06SH
  - Inferior Mesenteric 06S6
  - Innominate
    - Left 05S4
    - Right 05S3
  - Internal Jugular
    - Left 05SN
    - Right 05SM
  - Intracranial 05SL
  - Lesser Saphenous
    - Left 06SS
    - Right 06SR
  - Lower 06SY
  - Portal 06S8
  - Pulmonary
    - Left 02ST0ZZ
    - Right 02SS0ZZ
  - Renal
    - Left 06SB
    - Right 06S9
  - Splenic 06S1
  - Subclavian
    - Left 05S6
    - Right 05S5

Reposition *(Continued)*
- Vein *(Continued)*
  - Superior Mesenteric 06S5
  - Upper 05SY
  - Vertebral
    - Left 05SS
    - Right 05SR
- Vena Cava
  - Inferior 06S0
  - Superior 02SV0ZZ
- Vertebra
  - Cervical 0PS3
  - Lumbar 0QS0
  - Thoracic 0PS4
- Vocal Cord
  - Left 0CSV
  - Right 0CST

Resection
- Acetabulum
  - Left 0QT50ZZ
  - Right 0QT40ZZ
- Adenoids 0CTQ
- Ampulla of Vater 0FTC
- Anal Sphincter 0DTR
- Anus 0DTQ
- Aortic Body 0GTD
- Appendix 0DTJ
- Auditory Ossicle
  - Left 09TA0ZZ
  - Right 09T90ZZ
- Bladder 0TTB
- Bladder Neck 0TTC
- Bone
  - Ethmoid
    - Left 0NTG0ZZ
    - Right 0NTF0ZZ
  - Frontal
    - Left 0NT20ZZ
    - Right 0NT10ZZ
  - Hyoid 0NTX0ZZ
  - Lacrimal
    - Left 0NTJ0ZZ
    - Right 0NTH0ZZ
  - Nasal 0NTB0ZZ
  - Occipital
    - Left 0NT80ZZ
    - Right 0NT70ZZ
  - Palatine
    - Left 0NTL0ZZ
    - Right 0NTK0ZZ
  - Parietal
    - Left 0NT40ZZ
    - Right 0NT30ZZ
  - Pelvic
    - Left 0QT30ZZ
    - Right 0QT20ZZ
  - Sphenoid
    - Left 0NTD0ZZ
    - Right 0NTC0ZZ
  - Temporal
    - Left 0NT60ZZ
    - Right 0NT50ZZ
  - Zygomatic
    - Left 0NTN0ZZ
    - Right 0NTM0ZZ
- Breast
  - Bilateral 0HTV0ZZ
  - Left 0HTU0ZZ
  - Right 0HTT0ZZ
  - Supernumerary 0HTY0ZZ
- Bronchus
  - Lingula 0BT9
  - Lower Lobe
    - Left 0BTB
    - Right 0BT6
  - Main
    - Left 0BT7
    - Right 0BT3
  - Middle Lobe, Right 0BT5
  - Upper Lobe
    - Left 0BT8
    - Right 0BT4

◀ New ⬅ Revised ~~deleted~~ Deleted

Resection (*Continued*)
Bursa and Ligament
Abdomen
Left 0MTJ
Right 0MTH
Ankle
Left 0MTR
Right 0MTQ
Elbow
Left 0MT4
Right 0MT3
Foot
Left 0MTT
Right 0MTS
Hand
Left 0MT8
Right 0MT7
Head and Neck 0MT0
Hip
Left 0MTM
Right 0MTL
Knee
Left 0MTP
Right 0MTN
Lower Extremity
Left 0MTW
Right 0MTV
Perineum 0MTK
Shoulder
Left 0MT2
Right 0MT1
Thorax
Left 0MTG
Right 0MTF
Trunk
Left 0MTD
Right 0MTC
Upper Extremity
Left 0MTB
Right 0MT9
Wrist
Left 0MT6
Right 0MT5
Carina 0BT2
Carotid Bodies, Bilateral
0GT8
Carotid Body
Left 0GT6
Right 0GT7
Carpal
Left 0PTN0ZZ
Right 0PTM0ZZ
Cecum 0DTH
Cerebral Hemisphere 00T7
Cervix 0UTC
Chordae Tendineae 02T9
Cisterna Chyli 07TL
Clavicle
Left 0PTB0ZZ
Right 0PT90ZZ
Clitoris 0UTJ
Coccygeal Glomus 0GTB
Coccyx 0QTS0ZZ
Colon
Ascending 0DTK
Descending 0DTM
Sigmoid 0DTN
Transverse 0DTL
Conduction Mechanism
02T8
Cord
Bilateral 0VTH
Left 0VTG
Right 0VTF
Cornea
Left 08T9XZZ
Right 08T8XZZ
Cul-de-sac 0UTF
Diaphragm
Left 0BTS
Right 0BTR

Resection (*Continued*)
Disc
Cervical Vertebral 0RT30ZZ
Cervicothoracic Vertebral 0RT50ZZ
Lumbar Vertebral 0ST20ZZ
Lumbosacral 0ST40ZZ
Thoracic Vertebral 0RT90ZZ
Thoracolumbar Vertebral 0RTB0ZZ
Duct
Common Bile 0FT9
Cystic 0FT8
Hepatic
Left 0FT6
Right 0FT5
Lacrimal
Left 08TY
Right 08TX
Pancreatic 0FTD
Accessory 0FTF
Parotid
Left 0CTC0ZZ
Right 0CTB0ZZ
Duodenum 0DT9
Ear
External
Left 09T1
Right 09T0
Inner
Left 09TE0ZZ
Right 09TD0ZZ
Middle
Left 09T60ZZ
Right 09T50ZZ
Epididymis
Bilateral 0VTL
Left 0VTK
Right 0VTJ
Epiglottis 0CTR
Esophagogastric Junction 0DT4
Esophagus 0DT5
Lower 0DT3
Middle 0DT2
Upper 0DT1
Eustachian Tube
Left 09TG
Right 09TF
Eye
Left 08T1XZZ
Right 08T0XZZ
Eyelid
Lower
Left 08TR
Right 08TQ
Upper
Left 08TP
Right 08TN
Fallopian Tube
Left 0UT6
Right 0UT5
Fallopian Tubes, Bilateral
0UT7
Femoral Shaft
Left 0QT90ZZ
Right 0QT80ZZ
Femur
Lower
Left 0QTC0ZZ
Right 0QTB0ZZ
Upper
Left 0QT70ZZ
Right 0QT60ZZ
Fibula
Left 0QTK0ZZ
Right 0QTJ0ZZ
Finger Nail 0HTQXZZ
Gallbladder 0FT4
Gland
Adrenal
Bilateral 0GT4
Left 0GT2
Right 0GT3

Resection (*Continued*)
Gland (*Continued*)
Lacrimal
Left 08TW
Right 08TV
Minor Salivary 0CTJ0ZZ
Parotid
Left 0CT90ZZ
Right 0CT80ZZ
Pituitary 0GT0
Sublingual
Left 0CTF0ZZ
Right 0CTD0ZZ
Submaxillary
Left 0CTH0ZZ
Right 0CTG0ZZ
Vestibular 0UTL
Glenoid Cavity
Left 0PT80ZZ
Right 0PT70ZZ
Glomus Jugulare 0GTC
Humeral Head
Left 0PTD0ZZ
Right 0PTC0ZZ
Humeral Shaft
Left 0PTG0ZZ
Right 0PTF0ZZ
Hymen 0UTK
Ileocecal Valve 0DTC
Ileum 0DTB
Intestine
Large 0DTE
Left 0DTG
Right 0DTF
Small 0DT8
Iris
Left 08TD3ZZ
Right 08TC3ZZ
Jejunum 0DTA
Joint
Acromioclavicular
Left 0RTH0ZZ
Right 0RTG0ZZ
Ankle
Left 0STG0ZZ
Right 0STF0ZZ
Carpal
Left 0RTR0ZZ
Right 0RTQ0ZZ
Cervicothoracic Vertebral
0RT40ZZ
Coccygeal 0ST60ZZ
Elbow
Left 0RTM0ZZ
Right 0RTL0ZZ
Finger Phalangeal
Left 0RTX0ZZ
Right 0RTW0ZZ
Hip
Left 0STB0ZZ
Right 0ST90ZZ
Knee
Left 0STD0ZZ
Right 0STC0ZZ
Metacarpocarpal
Left 0RTT0ZZ
Right 0RTS0ZZ
Metacarpophalangeal
Left 0RTV0ZZ
Right 0RTU0ZZ
Metatarsal-Phalangeal
Left 0STN0ZZ
Right 0STM0ZZ
Metatarsal-Tarsal
Left 0STL0ZZ
Right 0STK0ZZ
Sacrococcygeal 0ST50ZZ
Sacroiliac
Left 0ST80ZZ
Right 0ST70ZZ

◀ New ◀▥▥ Revised ~~deleted~~ Deleted

Resection *(Continued)*
  Joint *(Continued)*
    Shoulder
      Left 0RTK0ZZ
      Right 0RTJ0ZZ
    Sternoclavicular
      Left 0RTF0ZZ
      Right 0RTE0ZZ
    Tarsal
      Left 0STJ0ZZ
      Right 0STH0ZZ
    Temporomandibular
      Left 0RTD0ZZ
      Right 0RTC0ZZ
    Toe Phalangeal
      Left 0STQ0ZZ
      Right 0STP0ZZ
    Wrist
      Left 0RTP0ZZ
      Right 0RTN0ZZ
  Kidney
    Left 0TT1
    Right 0TT0
  Kidney Pelvis
    Left 0TT4
    Right 0TT3
  Kidneys, Bilateral 0TT2
  Larynx 0CTS
  Lens
    Left 08TK3ZZ
    Right 08TJ3ZZ
  Lip
    Lower 0CT1
    Upper 0CT0
  Liver 0FT0
    Left Lobe 0FT2
    Right Lobe 0FT1
  Lung
    Bilateral 0BTM
    Left 0BTL
    Lower Lobe
      Left 0BTJ
      Right 0BTF
    Middle Lobe, Right
      0BTD
    Right 0BTK
    Upper Lobe
      Left 0BTG
      Right 0BTC
  Lung Lingula 0BTH
  Lymphatic
    Aortic 07TD
    Axillary
      Left 07T6
      Right 07T5
    Head 07T0
    Inguinal
      Left 07TJ
      Right 07TH
    Internal Mammary
      Left 07T9
      Right 07T8
    Lower Extremity
      Left 07TG
      Right 07TF
    Mesenteric 07TB
    Neck
      Left 07T2
      Right 07T1
    Pelvis 07TC
    Thoracic Duct 07TK
    Thorax 07T7
    Upper Extremity
      Left 07T4
      Right 07T3
  Mandible
    Left 0NTV0ZZ
    Right 0NTT0ZZ
  Maxilla
    Left 0NTS0ZZ
    Right 0NTR0ZZ

Resection *(Continued)*
  Metacarpal
    Left 0PTQ0ZZ
    Right 0PTP0ZZ
  Metatarsal
    Left 0QTP0ZZ
    Right 0QTN0ZZ
  Muscle
    Abdomen
      Left 0KTL
      Right 0KTK
    Extraocular
      Left 08TM
      Right 08TL
    Facial 0KT1
    Foot
      Left 0KTW
      Right 0KTV
    Hand
      Left 0KTD
      Right 0KTC
    Head 0KT0
    Hip
      Left 0KTP
      Right 0KTN
    Lower Arm and Wrist
      Left 0KTB
      Right 0KT9
    Lower Leg
      Left 0KTT
      Right 0KTS
    Neck
      Left 0KT3
      Right 0KT2
    Papillary 02TD
    Perineum 0KTM
    Shoulder
      Left 0KT6
      Right 0KT5
    Thorax
      Left 0KTJ
      Right 0KTH
    Tongue, Palate, Pharynx 0KT4
    Trunk
      Left 0KTG
      Right 0KTF
    Upper Arm
      Left 0KT8
      Right 0KT7
    Upper Leg
      Left 0KTR
      Right 0KTQ
  Nasopharynx 09TN
  Nipple
    Left 0HTXXZZ
    Right 0HTWXZZ
  Nose 09TK
  Omentum
    Greater 0DTS
    Lesser 0DTT
  Orbit
    Left 0NTQ0ZZ
    Right 0NTP0ZZ
  Ovary
    Bilateral 0UT2
    Left 0UT1
    Right 0UT0
  Palate
    Hard 0CT2
    Soft 0CT3
  Pancreas 0FTG
  Para-aortic Body 0GT9
  Paraganglion Extremity 0GTF
  Parathyroid Gland 0GTR
    Inferior
      Left 0GTP
      Right 0GTN
    Multiple 0GTQ
    Superior
      Left 0GTM
      Right 0GTL

Resection *(Continued)*
  Patella
    Left 0QTF0ZZ
    Right 0QTD0ZZ
  Penis 0VTS
  Pericardium 02TN
  Phalanx
    Finger
      Left 0PTV0ZZ
      Right 0PTT0ZZ
    Thumb
      Left 0PTS0ZZ
      Right 0PTR0ZZ
    Toe
      Left 0QTR0ZZ
      Right 0QTQ0ZZ
  Pharynx 0CTM
  Pineal Body 0GT1
  Prepuce 0VTT
  Products of Conception, Ectopic
    10T2
  Prostate 0VT0
  Radius
    Left 0PTJ0ZZ
    Right 0PTH0ZZ
  Rectum 0DTP
  Rib
    Left 0PT20ZZ
    Right 0PT10ZZ
  Scapula
    Left 0PT60ZZ
    Right 0PT50ZZ
  Scrotum 0VT5
  Septum
    Atrial 02T5
    Nasal 09TM
    Ventricular 02TM
  Sinus
    Accessory 09TP
    Ethmoid
      Left 09TV
      Right 09TU
    Frontal
      Left 09TT
      Right 09TS
    Mastoid
      Left 09TC
      Right 09TB
    Maxillary
      Left 09TR
      Right 09TQ
    Sphenoid
      Left 09TX
      Right 09TW
  Spleen 07TP
  Sternum 0PT00ZZ
  Stomach 0DT6
    Pylorus 0DT7
  Tarsal
    Left 0QTM0ZZ
    Right 0QTL0ZZ
  Tendon
    Abdomen
      Left 0LTG
      Right 0LTF
    Ankle
      Left 0LTT
      Right 0LTS
    Foot
      Left 0LTW
      Right 0LTV
    Hand
      Left 0LT8
      Right 0LT7
    Head and Neck 0LT0
    Hip
      Left 0LTK
      Right 0LTJ
    Knee
      Left 0LTR
      Right 0LTQ

◀ New   ◀ Revised   ~~deleted~~ Deleted

Resection (Continued)
  Tendon (Continued)
    Lower Arm and Wrist
      Left 0LT6
      Right 0LT5
    Lower Leg
      Left 0LTP
      Right 0LTN
    Perineum 0LTH
    Shoulder
      Left 0LT2
      Right 0LT1
    Thorax
      Left 0LTD
      Right 0LTC
    Trunk
      Left 0LTB
      Right 0LT9
    Upper Arm
      Left 0LT4
      Right 0LT3
    Upper Leg
      Left 0LTM
      Right 0LTL
  Testis
    Bilateral 0VTC
    Left 0VTB
    Right 0VT9
  Thymus 07TM
  Thyroid Gland 0GTK
    Left Lobe 0GTG
    Right Lobe 0GTH
  Tibia
    Left 0QTH0ZZ
    Right 0QTG0ZZ
  Toe Nail 0HTRXZZ
  Tongue 0CT7
  Tonsils 0CTP
  Tooth
    Lower 0CTX0Z
    Upper 0CTW0Z
  Trachea 0BT1
  Tunica Vaginalis
    Left 0VT7
    Right 0VT6
  Turbinate, Nasal 09TL
  Tympanic Membrane
    Left 09T8
    Right 09T7
  Ulna
    Left 0PTL0ZZ
    Right 0PTK0ZZ
  Ureter
    Left 0TT7
    Right 0TT6
  Urethra 0TTD
  Uterine Supporting Structure 0UT4
  Uterus 0UT9
  Uvula 0CTN
  Vagina 0UTG
  Valve, Pulmonary 02TH
  Vas Deferens
    Bilateral 0VTQ
    Left 0VTP
    Right 0VTN
  Vesicle
    Bilateral 0VT3
    Left 0VT2
    Right 0VT1
  Vitreous
    Left 08T53ZZ
    Right 08T43ZZ
  Vocal Cord
    Left 0CTV
    Right 0CTT
  Vulva 0UTM
Restoration, Cardiac, Single, Rhythm 5A2204Z
~~RestoreAdvanced neurostimulator use Stimulator Generator, Multiple Array Rechargeable in 0JH~~

RestoreAdvanced neurostimulator (SureScan) (MRI Safe) use Stimulator Generator, Multiple Array Rechargeable in 0JH ◀
~~RestoreSensor neurostimulator use Stimulator Generator, Multiple Array Rechargeable in 0JH~~

RestoreSensor neurostimulator (SureScan) (MRI Safe) use Stimulator Generator, Multiple Array Rechargeable in 0JH ◀
~~RestoreUltra neurostimulator use Stimulator Generator, Multiple Array Rechargeable in 0JH~~

RestoreUltra neurostimulator (SureScan)(MRI Safe) use Stimulator Generator, Multiple Array Rechargeable in 0JH ◀
Restriction
  Ampulla of Vater 0FVC
  Anus 0DVQ
  Aorta
    Abdominal 04V0
    Thoracic 02VW [034][CDZ]Z
  Artery
    Anterior Tibial
      Left 04VQ
      Right 04VP
    Axillary
      Left 03V6
      Right 03V5
    Brachial
      Left 03V8
      Right 03V7
    Celiac 04V1
    Colic
      Left 04V7
      Middle 04V8
      Right 04V6
    Common Carotid
      Left 03VJ
      Right 03VH
    Common Iliac
      Left 04VD
      Right 04VC
    External Carotid
      Left 03VN
      Right 03VM
    External Iliac
      Left 04VJ
      Right 04VH
    Face 03VR
    Femoral
      Left 04VL
      Right 04VK
    Foot
      Left 04VW
      Right 04VV
    Gastric 04V2
    Hand
      Left 03VF
      Right 03VD
    Hepatic 04V3
    Inferior Mesenteric 04VB
    Innominate 03V2
    Internal Carotid
      Left 03VL
      Right 03VK
    Internal Iliac
      Left 04VF
      Right 04VE
    Internal Mammary
      Left 03V1
      Right 03V0
    Intracranial 03VG
    Lower 04VY
    Peroneal
      Left 04VU
      Right 04VT
    Popliteal
      Left 04VN
      Right 04VM
    Posterior Tibial
      Left 04VS
      Right 04VR

Restriction (Continued)
  Artery (Continued)
    Pulmonary
      Left 02VR
      Right 02VQ
    Pulmonary Trunk 02VP
    Radial
      Left 03VC
      Right 03VB
    Renal
      Left 04VA
      Right 04V9
    Splenic 04V4
    Subclavian
      Left 03V4
      Right 03V3
    Superior Mesenteric 04V5
    Temporal
      Left 03VT
      Right 03VS
    Thyroid
      Left 03VV
      Right 03VU
    Ulnar
      Left 03VA
      Right 03V9
    Upper 03VY
    Vertebral
      Left 03VQ
      Right 03VP
  Bladder 0TVB
  Bladder Neck 0TVC
  Bronchus
    Lingula 0BV9
    Lower Lobe
      Left 0BVB
      Right 0BV6
    Main
      Left 0BV7
      Right 0BV3
    Middle Lobe, Right 0BV5
    Upper Lobe
      Left 0BV8
      Right 0BV4
  Carina 0BV2
  Cecum 0DVH
  Cervix 0UVC
  Cisterna Chyli 07VL
  Colon
    Ascending 0DVK
    Descending 0DVM
    Sigmoid 0DVN
    Transverse 0DVL
  Duct
    Common Bile 0FV9
    Cystic 0FV8
    Hepatic
      Left 0FV6
      Right 0FV5
    Lacrimal
      Left 08VY
      Right 08VX
    Pancreatic 0FVD
      Accessory 0FVF
    Parotid
      Left 0CVC
      Right 0CVB
  Duodenum 0DV9
  Esophagogastric Junction 0DV4
  Esophagus 0DV5
    Lower 0DV3
    Middle 0DV2
    Upper 0DV1
  Heart 02VA
  Ileocecal Valve 0DVC
  Ileum 0DVB
  Intestine
    Large 0DVE
      Left 0DVG
      Right 0DVF
    Small 0DV8

◀ New   ◀= Revised   ~~deleted~~ Deleted

Restriction *(Continued)*
Jejunum 0DVA
Kidney Pelvis
  Left 0TV4
  Right 0TV3
Lymphatic
  Aortic 07VD
  Axillary
    Left 07V6
    Right 07V5
  Head 07V0
  Inguinal
    Left 07VJ
    Right 07VH
  Internal Mammary
    Left 07V9
    Right 07V8
  Lower Extremity
    Left 07VG
    Right 07VF
  Mesenteric 07VB
  Neck
    Left 07V2
    Right 07V1
  Pelvis 07VC
  Thoracic Duct 07VK
  Thorax 07V7
  Upper Extremity
    Left 07V4
    Right 07V3
Rectum 0DVP
Stomach 0DV6
  Pylorus 0DV7
Trachea 0BV1
Ureter
  Left 0TV7
  Right 0TV6
Urethra 0TVD
Vein
  Axillary
    Left 05V8
    Right 05V7
  Azygos 05V0
  Basilic
    Left 05VC
    Right 05VB
  Brachial
    Left 05VA
    Right 05V9
  Cephalic
    Left 05VF
    Right 05VD
  Colic 06V7
  Common Iliac
    Left 06VD
    Right 06VC
  Esophageal 06V3
  External Iliac
    Left 06VG
    Right 06VF
  External Jugular
    Left 05VQ
    Right 05VP
  Face
    Left 05VV
    Right 05VT
  Femoral
    Left 06VN
    Right 06VM
  Foot
    Left 06VV
    Right 06VT
  Gastric 06V2
  Greater Saphenous
    Left 06VQ
    Right 06VP
  Hand
    Left 05VH
    Right 05VG
  Hemiazygos 05V1
  Hepatic 06V4

Restriction *(Continued)*
Vein *(Continued)*
  Hypogastric
    Left 06VJ
    Right 06VH
  Inferior Mesenteric 06V6
  Innominate
    Left 05V4
    Right 05V3
  Internal Jugular
    Left 05VN
    Right 05VM
  Intracranial 05VL
  Lesser Saphenous
    Left 06VS
    Right 06VR
  Lower 06VY
  Portal 06V8
  Pulmonary
    Left 02VT
    Right 02VS
  Renal
    Left 06VB
    Right 06V9
  Splenic 06V1
  Subclavian
    Left 05V6
    Right 05V5
  Superior Mesenteric 06V5
  Upper 05VY
  Vertebral
    Left 05VS
    Right 05VR
  Vena Cava
    Inferior 06V0
    Superior 02VV
Resurfacing Device
Removal of device from
  Left 0SPB0BZ
  Right 0SP90BZ
Revision of device in
  Left 0SWB0BZ
  Right 0SW90BZ
Supplement
  Left 0SUB0BZ
    Acetabular Surface 0SUE0BZ
    Femoral Surface 0SUS0BZ
  Right 0SU90BZ
    Acetabular Surface 0SUA0BZ
    Femoral Surface 0SUR0BZ
Resuscitation
Cardiopulmonary *see* Assistance, Cardiac 5A02
Cardioversion 5A2204Z
Defibrillation 5A2204Z
Endotracheal intubation *see* Insertion of device in, Trachea 0BH1
External chest compression 5A12012
Pulmonary 5A19054
Resuture, Heart valve prosthesis *see* Revision of device in, Heart and Great Vessels 02W
Retraining
Cardiac *see* Motor Treatment, Rehabilitation F07
Vocational *see* Activities of Daily Living Treatment, Rehabilitation F08
Retrogasserian rhizotomy *see* Division, Nerve, Trigeminal 008K
Retroperitoneal lymph node *use* Lymphatic, Aortic
Retroperitoneal space *use* Retroperitoneum
Retropharyngeal lymph node
  use Lymphatic, Neck, Left
  use Lymphatic, Neck, Right
Retropubic space *use* Pelvic Cavity
Reveal (DX) (XT) *use* Monitoring Device
Reverse total shoulder replacement *see* Replacement, Upper Joints 0RR
Reverse® Shoulder Prosthesis *use* Synthetic Substitute, Reverse Ball and Socket in 0RR

Revision of device in
Abdominal Wall 0WWF
Acetabulum
  Left 0QW5
  Right 0QW4
Anal Sphincter 0DWR
Anus 0DWQ
Artery
  Lower 04WY
  Upper 03WY
Auditory Ossicle
  Left 09WA
  Right 09W9
Back
  Lower 0WWL
  Upper 0WWK
Bladder 0TWB
Bone
  Facial 0NWW
  Lower 0QWY
  Nasal 0NWB
  Pelvic
    Left 0QW3
    Right 0QW2
  Upper 0PWY
Bone Marrow 07WT
Brain 00W0
Breast
  Left 0HWU
  Right 0HWT
Bursa and Ligament
  Lower 0MWY
  Upper 0MWX
Carpal
  Left 0PWN
  Right 0PWM
Cavity, Cranial 0WW1
Cerebral Ventricle 00W6
Chest Wall 0WW8
Cisterna Chyli 07WL
Clavicle
  Left 0PWB
  Right 0PW9
Coccyx 0QWS
Diaphragm 0BWT
Disc
  Cervical Vertebral 0RW3
  Cervicothoracic Vertebral 0RW5
  Lumbar Vertebral 0SW2
  Lumbosacral 0SW4
  Thoracic Vertebral 0RW9
  Thoracolumbar Vertebral 0RWB
Duct
  Hepatobiliary 0FWB
  Pancreatic 0FWD
  Thoracic 07WK
Ear
  Inner
    Left 09WE
    Right 09WD
  Left 09WJ
  Right 09WH
Epididymis and Spermatic Cord 0VWM
Esophagus 0DW5
Extremity
  Lower
    Left 0YWB
    Right 0YW9
  Upper
    Left 0XW7
    Right 0XW6
Eye
  Left 08W1
  Right 08W0
Face 0WW2
Fallopian Tube 0UW8
Femoral Shaft
  Left 0QW9
  Right 0QW8

◀ New   ◀‖ Revised   ~~deleted~~ Deleted

Revision of device in *(Continued)*
- Femur
  - Lower
    - Left 0QWC
    - Right 0QWB
  - Upper
    - Left 0QW7
    - Right 0QW6
- Fibula
  - Left 0QWK
  - Right 0QWJ
- Finger Nail 0HWQX
- Gallbladder 0FW4
- Gastrointestinal Tract 0WWP
- Genitourinary Tract 0WWR
- Gland
  - Adrenal 0GW5
  - Endocrine 0GWS
  - Pituitary 0GW0
  - Salivary 0CWA
- Glenoid Cavity
  - Left 0PW8
  - Right 0PW7
- Great Vessel 02WY
- Hair 0HWSX
- Head 0WW0
- Heart 02WA
- Humeral Head
  - Left 0PWD
  - Right 0PWC
- Humeral Shaft
  - Left 0PWG
  - Right 0PWF
- Intestinal Tract
  - Lower 0DWD
  - Upper 0DW0
- Intestine
  - Large 0DWE
  - Small 0DW8
- Jaw
  - Lower 0WW5
  - Upper 0WW4
- Joint
  - Acromioclavicular
    - Left 0RWH
    - Right 0RWG
  - Ankle
    - Left 0SWG
    - Right 0SWF
  - Carpal
    - Left 0RWR
    - Right 0RWQ
  - Cervical Vertebral 0RW1
  - Cervicothoracic Vertebral 0RW4
  - Coccygeal 0SW6
  - Elbow
    - Left 0RWM
    - Right 0RWL
  - Finger Phalangeal
    - Left 0RWX
    - Right 0RWW
  - Hip
    - Left 0SWB
    - Right 0SW9
  - Knee
    - Left 0SWD
    - Right 0SWC
  - Lumbar Vertebral 0SW0
  - Lumbosacral 0SW3
  - Metacarpocarpal
    - Left 0RWT
    - Right 0RWS
  - Metacarpophalangeal
    - Left 0RWV
    - Right 0RWU
  - Metatarsal-Phalangeal
    - Left 0SWN
    - Right 0SWM
  - Metatarsal-Tarsal
    - Left 0SWL
    - Right 0SWK
  - Occipital-cervical 0RW0

- Joint *(Continued)*
  - Sacrococcygeal 0SW5
  - Sacroiliac
    - Left 0SW8
    - Right 0SW7
  - Shoulder
    - Left 0RWK
    - Right 0RWJ
  - Sternoclavicular
    - Left 0RWF
    - Right 0RWE
  - Tarsal
    - Left 0SWJ
    - Right 0SWH
  - Temporomandibular
    - Left 0RWD
    - Right 0RWC
  - Thoracic Vertebral 0RW6
  - Thoracolumbar Vertebral 0RWA
  - Toe Phalangeal
    - Left 0SWQ
    - Right 0SWP
  - Wrist
    - Left 0RWP
    - Right 0RWN
- Kidney 0TW5
- Larynx 0CWS
- Lens
  - Left 08WK
  - Right 08WJ
- Liver 0FW0
- Lung
  - Left 0BWL
  - Right 0BWK
- Lymphatic 07WN
  - Thoracic Duct 07WK
- Mediastinum 0WWC
- Mesentery 0DWV
- Metacarpal
  - Left 0PWQ
  - Right 0PWP
- Metatarsal
  - Left 0QWP
  - Right 0QWN
- Mouth and Throat 0CWY
- Muscle
  - Extraocular
    - Left 08WM
    - Right 08WL
  - Lower 0KWY
  - Upper 0KWX
- Neck 0WW6
- Nerve
  - Cranial 00WE
  - Peripheral 01WY
- Nose 09WK
- Omentum 0DWU
- Ovary 0UW3
- Pancreas 0FWG
- Parathyroid Gland 0GWR
- Patella
  - Left 0QWF
  - Right 0QWD
- Pelvic Cavity 0WWJ
- Penis 0VWS
- Pericardial Cavity 0WWD
- Perineum
  - Female 0WWN
  - Male 0WWM
- Peritoneal Cavity 0WWG
- Peritoneum 0DWW
- Phalanx
  - Finger
    - Left 0PWV
    - Right 0PWT
  - Thumb
    - Left 0PWS
    - Right 0PWR
  - Toe
    - Left 0QWR
    - Right 0QWQ

- Pineal Body 0GW1
- Pleura 0BWQ
- Pleural Cavity
  - Left 0WWB
  - Right 0WW9
- Prostate and Seminal Vesicles 0VW4
- Radius
  - Left 0PWJ
  - Right 0PWH
- Respiratory Tract 0WWQ
- Retroperitoneum 0WWH
- Rib
  - Left 0PW2
  - Right 0PW1
- Sacrum 0QW1
- Scapula
  - Left 0PW6
  - Right 0PW5
- Scrotum and Tunica Vaginalis 0VW8
- Septum
  - Atrial 02W5
  - Ventricular 02WM
- Sinus 09WY
- Skin 0HWPX
- Skull 0NW0
- Spinal Canal 00WU
- Spinal Cord 00WV
- Spleen 07WP
- Sternum 0PW0
- Stomach 0DW6
- Subcutaneous Tissue and Fascia
  - Head and Neck 0JWS
  - Lower Extremity 0JWW
  - Trunk 0JWT
  - Upper Extremity 0JWV
- Tarsal
  - Left 0QWM
  - Right 0QWL
- Tendon
  - Lower 0LWY
  - Upper 0LWX
- Testis 0VWD
- Thymus 07WM
- Thyroid Gland 0GWK
- Tibia
  - Left 0QWH
  - Right 0QWG
- Toe Nail 0HWRX
- Trachea 0BW1
- Tracheobronchial Tree 0BW0
- Tympanic Membrane
  - Left 09W8
  - Right 09W7
- Ulna
  - Left 0PWL
  - Right 0PWK
- Ureter 0TW9
- Urethra 0TWD
- Uterus and Cervix 0UWD
- Vagina and Cul-de-sac 0UWH
- Valve
  - Aortic 02WF
  - Mitral 02WG
  - Pulmonary 02WH
  - Tricuspid 02WJ
- Vas Deferens 0VWR
- Vein
  - Lower 06WY
  - Upper 05WY
- Vertebra
  - Cervical 0PW3
  - Lumbar 0QW0
  - Thoracic 0PW4
- Vulva 0UWM

Revo MRI™ SureScan® pacemaker *use*
Pacemaker, Dual Chamber in 0JH
rhBMP-2 *use* Recombinant Bone Morphogenetic Protein ◄

◄ New   ◄ Revised   ~~deleted~~ Deleted

Rheos® System device *use* Stimulator Generator in Subcutaneous Tissue and Fascia ◄▥
Rheos® System lead *use* Stimulator Lead in Upper Arteries
Rhinopharynx *use* Nasopharynx
Rhinoplasty
  see Alteration, Nose 090K
  see Repair, Nose 09QK
  see Replacement, Nose 09RK
  see Supplement, Nose 09UK
Rhinorrhaphy *see* Repair, Nose 09QK
Rhinoscopy 09JKXZZ
Rhizotomy
  see Division, Central Nervous System 008
  see Division, Peripheral Nervous System 018
Rhomboid major muscle
  use Muscle, Trunk, Left
  use Muscle, Trunk, Right
Rhomboid minor muscle
  use Muscle, Trunk, Right
  use Muscle, Trunk, Left
Rhythm electrocardiogram *see* Measurement, Cardiac 4A02
Rhytidectomy *see* Face lift
Right ascending lumbar vein *use* Vein, Azygos
Right atrioventricular valve *use* Valve, Tricuspid

Right auricular appendix *use* Atrium, Right
Right colic vein *use* Vein, Colic
Right coronary sulcus *use* Heart, Right
Right gastric artery *use* Artery, Gastric
Right gastroepiploic vein *use* Vein, Superior Mesenteric
Right inferior phrenic vein *use* Vena Cava, Inferior
Right inferior pulmonary vein *use* Vein, Pulmonary, Right
Right jugular trunk *use* Lymphatic, Neck, Right
Right lateral ventricle *use* Cerebral Ventricle
Right lymphatic duct *use* Lymphatic, Neck, Right
Right ovarian vein *use* Vena Cava, Inferior
Right second lumbar vein *use* Vena Cava, Inferior
Right subclavian trunk *use* Lymphatic, Neck, Right
Right subcostal vein *use* Vein, Azygos
Right superior pulmonary vein *use* Vein, Pulmonary, Right
Right suprarenal vein *use* Vena Cava, Inferior
Right testicular vein *use* Vena Cava, Inferior
Rima glottidis *use* Larynx
Risorius muscle *use* Muscle, Facial

RNS System lead *use* Neurostimulator Lead in Central Nervous System
RNS system neurostimulator generator *use* Neurostimulator Generator in Head and Facial Bones
Robotic Assisted Procedure
  Extremity
    Lower 8E0Y
    Upper 8E0X
  Head and Neck Region 8E09
  Trunk Region 8E0W
Rotation of fetal head
  Forceps 10S07ZZ
  Manual 10S0XZZ
Round ligament of uterus *use* Uterine Supporting Structure
Round window
  use Ear, Inner, Right
  use Ear, Inner, Left
Roux-en-Y operation
  see Bypass, Gastrointestinal System 0D1
  see Bypass, Hepatobiliary System and Pancreas 0F1
Rupture
  Adhesions *see* Release
  Fluid collection *see* Drainage

S

◀ New ◀▬ Revised ~~deleted~~ Deleted

Spacer *(Continued)*
Insertion of device in *(Continued)*
Joint
Acromioclavicular
Left 0RHH
Right 0RHG
Ankle
Left 0SHG
Right 0SHF
Carpal
Left 0RHR
Right 0RHQ
Cervical Vertebral 0RH1
Cervicothoracic Vertebral 0RH4
Coccygeal 0SH6
Elbow
Left 0RHM
Right 0RHL
Finger Phalangeal
Left 0RHX
Right 0RHW
Hip
Left 0SHB
Right 0SH9
Knee
Left 0SHD
Right 0SHC
Lumbar Vertebral 0SH0
Lumbosacral 0SH3
Metacarpocarpal
Left 0RHT
Right 0RHS
Metacarpophalangeal
Left 0RHV
Right 0RHU
Metatarsal-Phalangeal
Left 0SHN
Right 0SHM
Metatarsal-Tarsal
Left 0SHL
Right 0SHK
Occipital-cervical 0RH0
Sacrococcygeal 0SH5
Sacroiliac
Left 0SH8
Right 0SH7
Shoulder
Left 0RHK
Right 0RHJ
Sternoclavicular
Left 0RHF
Right 0RHE
Tarsal
Left 0SHJ
Right 0SHH
Temporomandibular
Left 0RHD
Right 0RHC
Thoracic Vertebral 0RH6
Thoracolumbar Vertebral
0RHA
Toe Phalangeal
Left 0SHQ
Right 0SHP
Wrist
Left 0RHP
Right 0RHN
Removal of device from
Acromioclavicular
Left 0RPH
Right 0RPG
Ankle
Left 0SPG
Right 0SPF
Carpal
Left 0RPR
Right 0RPQ
Cervical Vertebral 0RP1
Cervicothoracic Vertebral
0RP4
Coccygeal 0SP6

Spacer *(Continued)*
Removal of device from *(Continued)*
Elbow
Left 0RPM
Right 0RPL
Finger Phalangeal
Left 0RPX
Right 0RPW
Hip
Left 0SPB
Right 0SP9
Knee
Left 0SPD
Right 0SPC
Lumbar Vertebral 0SP0
Lumbosacral 0SP3
Metacarpocarpal
Left 0RPT
Right 0RPS
Metacarpophalangeal
Left 0RPV
Right 0RPU
Metatarsal-Phalangeal
Left 0SPN
Right 0SPM
Metatarsal-Tarsal
Left 0SPL
Right 0SPK
Occipital-cervical 0RP0
Sacrococcygeal 0SP5
Sacroiliac
Left 0SP8
Right 0SP7
Shoulder
Left 0RPK
Right 0RPJ
Sternoclavicular
Left 0RPF
Right 0RPE
Tarsal
Left 0SPJ
Right 0SPH
Temporomandibular
Left 0RPD
Right 0RPC
Thoracic Vertebral 0RP6
Thoracolumbar Vertebral 0RPA
Toe Phalangeal
Left 0SPQ
Right 0SPP
Wrist
Left 0RPP
Right 0RPN
Revision of device in
Acromioclavicular
Left 0RWH
Right 0RWG
Ankle
Left 0SWG
Right 0SWF
Carpal
Left 0RWR
Right 0RWQ
Cervical Vertebral 0RW1
Cervicothoracic Vertebral
0RW4
Coccygeal 0SW6
Elbow
Left 0RWM
Right 0RWL
Finger Phalangeal
Left 0RWX
Right 0RWW
Hip
Left 0SWB
Right 0SW9
Knee
Left 0SWD
Right 0SWC
Lumbar Vertebral 0SW0
Lumbosacral 0SW3

Spacer *(Continued)*
Revision of device in *(Continued)*
Metacarpocarpal
Left 0RWT
Right 0RWS
Metacarpophalangeal
Left 0RWV
Right 0RWU
Metatarsal-Phalangeal
Left 0SWN
Right 0SWM
Metatarsal-Tarsal
Left 0SWL
Right 0SWK
Occipital-cervical 0RW0
Sacrococcygeal 0SW5
Sacroiliac
Left 0SW8
Right 0SW7
Shoulder
Left 0RWK
Right 0RWJ
Sternoclavicular
Left 0RWF
Right 0RWE
Tarsal
Left 0SWJ
Right 0SWH
Temporomandibular
Left 0RWD
Right 0RWC
Thoracic Vertebral 0RW6
Thoracolumbar Vertebral 0RWA
Toe Phalangeal
Left 0SWQ
Right 0SWP
Wrist
Left 0RWP
Right 0RWN
Spectroscopy
Intravascular 8E023DZ
Near infrared 8E023DZ
Speech Assessment F00
Speech therapy *see* Speech Treatment,
Rehabilitation F06
Speech Treatment F06
Sphenoidectomy
see Excision, Ear, Nose, Sinus 09B
see Resection, Ear, Nose, Sinus 09T
see Excision, Head and Facial Bones 0NB
see Resection, Head and Facial Bones 0NT
Sphenoidotomy *see* Drainage, Ear, Nose, Sinus
099
Sphenomandibular ligament *use* Bursa and
Ligament, Head and Neck
Sphenopalatine (pterygopalatine) ganglion *use*
Nerve, Head and Neck Sympathetic
Sphincterorrhaphy, anal *see* Repair, Sphincter,
Anal 0DQR
Sphincterotomy, anal
see Drainage, Sphincter, Anal 0D9R
see Division, Sphincter, Anal 0D8R
Spinal cord neurostimulator lead *use*
Neurostimulator Lead in Central Nervous
System
Spinal dura mater *use* Dura Mater
Spinal epidural space *use* Epidural Space
Spinal nerve, cervical *use* Nerve, Cervical
Spinal nerve, lumbar *use* Nerve, Lumbar
Spinal nerve, sacral *use* Nerve Sacral
Spinal nerve, thoracic *use* Nerve,
Thoracic
Spinal Stabilization Device
Facet Replacement
Cervical Vertebral 0RH1
Cervicothoracic Vertebral 0RH4
Lumbar Vertebral 0SH0
Lumbosacral 0SH3
Occipital-cervical 0RH0
Thoracic Vertebral 0RH6
Thoracolumbar Vertebral 0RHA

Spinal Stabilization Device *(Continued)*
  Interspinous Process
    Cervical Vertebral 0RH1
    Cervicothoracic Vertebral 0RH4
    Lumbar Vertebral 0SH0
    Lumbosacral 0SH3
    Occipital-cervical 0RH0
    Thoracic Vertebral 0RH6
    Thoracolumbar Vertebral 0RHA
  Pedicle-Based
    Cervical Vertebral 0RH1
    Cervicothoracic Vertebral 0RH4
    Lumbar Vertebral 0SH0
    Lumbosacral 0SH3
    Occipital-cervical 0RH0
    Thoracic Vertebral 0RH6
    Thoracolumbar Vertebral 0RHA
Spinal subarachnoid space *use* Subarachnoid
    Space
Spinal subdural space *use* Subdural Space
Spinous process
  use Vertebra, Thoracic
  use Vertebra, Lumbar
  use Vertebra, Cervical
Spiral ganglion *use* Nerve, Acoustic
Spiration IBV™ Valve System *use* Intraluminal
    Device, Endobronchial Valve in
    Respiratory System
Splenectomy
  see Excision, Lymphatic and Hemic Systems
    07B
  see Resection, Lymphatic and Hemic Systems
    07T
Splenic flexure *use* Colon, Transverse
Splenic plexus *use* Nerve, Abdominal
    Sympathetic
Splenius capitis muscle *use* Muscle, Head
Splenius cervicis muscle
  use Muscle, Neck, Left
  use Muscle, Neck, Right
Splenolysis *see* Release, Lymphatic and Hemic
    Systems 07N
Splenopexy
  see Repair, Lymphatic and Hemic Systems 07Q
  see Reposition, Lymphatic and Hemic
    Systems 07S
Splenoplasty *see* Repair, Lymphatic and Hemic
    Systems 07Q
Splenorrhaphy *see* Repair, Lymphatic and
    Hemic Systems 07Q
Splenotomy *see* Drainage, Lymphatic and
    Hemic Systems 079
Splinting, musculoskeletal *see* Immobilization,
    Anatomical Regions 2W3
Stapedectomy
  see Excision, Ear, Nose, Sinus 09B
  see Resection, Ear, Nose, Sinus 09T
Stapediolysis *see* Release, Ear, Nose, Sinus 09N
Stapedioplasty
  see Repair, Ear, Nose, Sinus 09Q
  see Replacement, Ear, Nose, Sinus 09R
  see Supplement, Ear, Nose, Sinus 09U
Stapedotomy *see* Drainage, Ear, Nose, Sinus 099
Stapes
  use Auditory Ossicle, Right
  use Auditory Ossicle, Left
Stellate ganglion *use* Nerve, Head and Neck
    Sympathetic
Stensen's duct
  use Duct, Parotid, Right
  use Duct, Parotid, Left
~~Stent (angioplasty) (embolization) use~~
    ~~Intraluminal Device~~
Stent, intraluminal (cardiovascular)
    (gastrointestinal)(hepatobiliary)(urinary)
    use Intraluminal Device ◀
Stented tissue valve *use* Zooplastic Tissue in
    Heart and Great Vessels
Stereotactic Radiosurgery
  Gamma Beam
    Abdomen DW23JZZ
    Adrenal Gland DG22JZZ

Stereotactic Radiosurgery *(Continued)*
  Gamma Beam *(Continued)*
    Bile Ducts DF22JZZ
    Bladder DT22JZZ
    Bone Marrow D720JZZ
    Brain D020JZZ
    Brain Stem D021JZZ
    Breast
      Left DM20JZZ
      Right DM21JZZ
    Bronchus DB21JZZ
    Cervix DU21JZZ
    Chest DW22JZZ
    Chest Wall DB27JZZ
    Colon DD25JZZ
    Diaphragm DB28JZZ
    Duodenum DD22JZZ
    Ear D920JZZ
    Esophagus DD20JZZ
    Eye D820JZZ
    Gallbladder DF21JZZ
    Gland
      Adrenal DG22JZZ
      Parathyroid DG24JZZ
      Pituitary DG20JZZ
      Thyroid DG25JZZ
    Glands, Salivary D926JZZ
    Head and Neck DW21JZZ
    Ileum DD24JZZ
    Jejunum DD23JZZ
    Kidney DT20JZZ
    Larynx D92BJZZ
    Liver DF20JZZ
    Lung DB22JZZ
    Lymphatics
      Abdomen D726JZZ
      Axillary D724JZZ
      Inguinal D728JZZ
      Neck D723JZZ
      Pelvis D727JZZ
      Thorax D725JZZ
    Mediastinum DB26JZZ
    Mouth D924JZZ
    Nasopharynx D92DJZZ
    Neck and Head DW21JZZ
    Nerve, Peripheral D027JZZ
    Nose D921JZZ
    Ovary DU20JZZ
    Palate
      Hard D928JZZ
      Soft D929JZZ
    Pancreas DF23JZZ
    Parathyroid Gland DG24JZZ
    Pelvic Region DW26JZZ
    Pharynx D92CJZZ
    Pineal Body DG21JZZ
    Pituitary Gland DG20JZZ
    Pleura DB25JZZ
    Prostate DV20JZZ
    Rectum DD27JZZ
    Sinuses D927JZZ
    Spinal Cord D026JZZ
    Spleen D722JZZ
    Stomach DD21JZZ
    Testis DV21JZZ
    Thymus D721JZZ
    Thyroid Gland DG25JZZ
    Tongue D925JZZ
    Trachea DB20JZZ
    Ureter DT21JZZ
    Urethra DT23JZZ
    Uterus DU22JZZ
  Other Photon
    Abdomen DW23DZZ
    Adrenal Gland DG22DZZ
    Bile Ducts DF22DZZ
    Bladder DT22DZZ
    Bone Marrow D720DZZ
    Brain D020DZZ
    Brain Stem D021DZZ
    Breast
      Left DM20DZZ
      Right DM21DZZ

Stereotactic Radiosurgery *(Continued)*
  Other Photon *(Continued)*
    Bronchus DB21DZZ
    Cervix DU21DZZ
    Chest DW22DZZ
    Chest Wall DB27DZZ
    Colon DD25DZZ
    Diaphragm DB28DZZ
    Duodenum DD22DZZ
    Ear D920DZZ
    Esophagus DD20DZZ
    Eye D820DZZ
    Gallbladder DF21DZZ
    Gland
      Adrenal DG22DZZ
      Parathyroid DG24DZZ
      Pituitary DG20DZZ
      Thyroid DG25DZZ
    Glands, Salivary D926DZZ
    Head and Neck DW21DZZ
    Ileum DD24DZZ
    Jejunum DD23DZZ
    Kidney DT20DZZ
    Larynx D92BDZZ
    Liver DF20DZZ
    Lung DB22DZZ
    Lymphatics
      Abdomen D726DZZ
      Axillary D724DZZ
      Inguinal D728DZZ
      Neck D723DZZ
      Pelvis D727DZZ
      Thorax D725DZZ
    Mediastinum DB26DZZ
    Mouth D924DZZ
    Nasopharynx D92DDZZ
    Neck and Head DW21DZZ
    Nerve, Peripheral D027DZZ
    Nose D921DZZ
    Ovary DU20DZZ
    Palate
      Hard D928DZZ
      Soft D929DZZ
    Pancreas DF23DZZ
    Parathyroid Gland DG24DZZ
    Pelvic Region DW26DZZ
    Pharynx D92CDZZ
    Pineal Body DG21DZZ
    Pituitary Gland DG20DZZ
    Pleura DB25DZZ
    Prostate DV20DZZ
    Rectum DD27DZZ
    Sinuses D927DZZ
    Spinal Cord D026DZZ
    Spleen D722DZZ
    Stomach DD21DZZ
    Testis DV21DZZ
    Thymus D721DZZ
    Thyroid Gland DG25DZZ
    Tongue D925DZZ
    Trachea DB20DZZ
    Ureter DT21DZZ
    Urethra DT23DZZ
    Uterus DU22DZZ
  Particulate
    Abdomen DW23HZZ
    Adrenal Gland DG22HZZ
    Bile Ducts DF22HZZ
    Bladder DT22HZZ
    Bone Marrow D720HZZ
    Brain D020HZZ
    Brain Stem D021HZZ
    Breast
      Left DM20HZZ
      Right DM21HZZ
    Bronchus DB21HZZ
    Cervix DU21HZZ
    Chest DW22HZZ
    Chest Wall DB27HZZ
    Colon DD25HZZ
    Diaphragm DB28HZZ
    Duodenum DD22HZZ

◀ New ◀▥ Revised ~~deleted~~ Deleted

Stereotactic Radiosurgery *(Continued)*
  Particulate *(Continued)*
    Ear D920HZZ
    Esophagus DD20HZZ
    Eye D820HZZ
    Gallbladder DF21HZZ
    Gland
      Adrenal DG22HZZ
      Parathyroid DG24HZZ
      Pituitary DG20HZZ
      Thyroid DG25HZZ
    Glands, Salivary D926HZZ
    Head and Neck DW21HZZ
    Ileum DD24HZZ
    Jejunum DD23HZZ
    Kidney DT20HZZ
    Larynx D92BHZZ
    Liver DF20HZZ
    Lung DB22HZZ
    Lymphatics
      Abdomen D726HZZ
      Axillary D724HZZ
      Inguinal D728HZZ
      Neck D723HZZ
      Pelvis D727HZZ
      Thorax D725HZZ
    Mediastinum DB26HZZ
    Mouth D924HZZ
    Nasopharynx D92DHZZ
    Neck and Head DW21HZZ
    Nerve, Peripheral D027HZZ
    Nose D921HZZ
    Ovary DU20HZZ
    Palate
      Hard D928HZZ
      Soft D929HZZ
    Pancreas DF23HZZ
    Parathyroid Gland DG24HZZ
    Pelvic Region DW26HZZ
    Pharynx D92CHZZ
    Pineal Body DG21HZZ
    Pituitary Gland DG20HZZ
    Pleura DB25HZZ
    Prostate DV20HZZ
    Rectum DD27HZZ
    Sinuses D927HZZ
    Spinal Cord D026HZZ
    Spleen D722HZZ
    Stomach DD21HZZ
    Testis DV21HZZ
    Thymus D721HZZ
    Thyroid Gland DG25HZZ
    Tongue D925HZZ
    Trachea DB20HZZ
    Ureter DT21HZZ
    Urethra DT23HZZ
    Uterus DU22HZZ
Sternoclavicular ligament
  use Bursa and Ligament, Shoulder, Left
  use Bursa and Ligament, Shoulder, Right
Sternocleidomastoid artery
  use Artery, Thyroid, Left
  use Artery, Thyroid, Right
Sternocleidomastoid muscle
  use Muscle, Neck, Left
  use Muscle, Neck, Right
Sternocostal ligament
  use Bursa and Ligament, Thorax, Right
  use Bursa and Ligament, Thorax, Left
Sternotomy
  see Division, Sternum 0P80
  see Drainage, Sternum 0P90
Stimulation, cardiac
  Cardioversion 5A2204Z
  Electrophysiologic testing *see* Measurement,
    Cardiac 4A02
Stimulator Generator
  Insertion of device in
    Abdomen 0JH8
    Back 0JH7
    Chest 0JH6

Stimulator Generator *(Continued)*
  Multiple Array
    Abdomen 0JH8
    Back 0JH7
    Chest 0JH6
  Multiple Array Rechargeable
    Abdomen 0JH8
    Back 0JH7
    Chest 0JH6
  Removal of device from, Subcutaneous Tissue
    and Fascia, Trunk 0JPT
  Revision of device in, Subcutaneous Tissue
    and Fascia, Trunk 0JWT
  Single Array
    Abdomen 0JH8
    Back 0JH7
    Chest 0JH6
  Single Array Rechargeable
    Abdomen 0JH8
    Back 0JH7
    Chest 0JH6
Stimulator Lead
  Insertion of device in
    Anal Sphincter 0DHR
    Artery
      Left 03HL
      Right 03HK
    Bladder 0THB
    Muscle
      Lower 0KHY
      Upper 0KHX
    Stomach 0DH6
    Ureter 0TH9
  Removal of device from
    Anal Sphincter 0DPR
    Artery, Upper 03PY
    Bladder 0TPB
    Muscle
      Lower 0KPY
      Upper 0KPX
    Stomach 0DP6
    Ureter 0TP9
  Revision of device in
    Anal Sphincter 0DWR
    Artery, Upper 03WY
    Bladder 0TWB
    Muscle
      Lower 0KWY
      Upper 0KWX
    Stomach 0DW6
    Ureter 0TW9
Stoma
  Excision
    Abdominal Wall 0WBFXZ2
    Neck 0WB6XZ2
  Repair
    Abdominal Wall 0WQFXZ2
    Neck 0WQ6XZ2
Stomatoplasty
  see Repair, Mouth and Throat 0CQ
  see Replacement, Mouth and Throat 0CR
  see Supplement, Mouth and Throat 0CU
Stomatorrhaphy *see* Repair, Mouth and Throat
  0CQ
Stratos LV *use* Cardiac Resynchronization
  Pacemaker Pulse Generator in 0JH
Stress test
  4A02XM4
  4A12XM4
Stripping *see* Extraction
Study
  Electrophysiologic stimulation, cardiac *see*
    Measurement, Cardiac 4A02
  Ocular motility 4A07X7Z
  Pulmonary airway flow measurement *see*
    Measurement, Respiratory 4A09
  Visual acuity 4A07X0Z
Styloglossus muscle *use* Muscle, Tongue,
  Palate, Pharynx
Stylomandibular ligament *use* Bursa and
  Ligament, Head and Neck

Stylopharyngeus muscle *use* Muscle, Tongue,
  Palate, Pharynx
Subacromial bursa
  use Bursa and Ligament, Shoulder, Left
  use Bursa and Ligament, Shoulder, Right
Subaortic (common iliac) lymph node *use*
  Lymphatic, Pelvis
Subclavicular (apical) lymph node
  use Lymphatic, Axillary, Left
  use Lymphatic, Axillary, Right
Subclavius muscle
  use Muscle, Thorax, Left
  use Muscle, Thorax, Right
Subclavius nerve *use* Nerve, Brachial Plexus
Subcostal artery *use* Aorta, Thoracic
Subcostal muscle
  use Muscle, Thorax, Left
  use Muscle, Thorax, Right
Subcostal nerve *use* Nerve, Thoracic
Subcutaneous injection reservoir, port *use*
  Vascular Access Device, Reservoir in
  Subcutaneous Tissue and Fascia
Subcutaneous injection reservoir, pump *use*
  Infusion Device, Pump in Subcutaneous
  Tissue and Fascia
Subdermal progesterone implant *use*
  Contraceptive Device in Subcutaneous
  Tissue and Fascia
Submandibular ganglion
  use Nerve, Head and Neck Sympathetic
  use Nerve, Facial
Submandibular gland
  use Gland, Submaxillary, Left
  use Gland, Submaxillary, Right
Submandibular lymph node *use* Lymphatic,
  Head
Submaxillary ganglion *use* Nerve, Head and
  Neck Sympathetic
Submaxillary lymph node *use* Lymphatic,
  Head
Submental artery *use* Artery, Face
Submental lymph node *use* Lymphatic,
  Head
Submucous (Meissner's) plexus *use* Nerve,
  Abdominal Sympathetic
Suboccipital nerve *use* Nerve, Cervical
Suboccipital venous plexus
  use Vein, Vertebral, Left
  use Vein, Vertebral, Right
Subparotid lymph node *use* Lymphatic,
  Head
Subscapular (posterior) lymph node
  use Lymphatic, Axillary, Left
  use Lymphatic, Axillary, Right
Subscapular aponeurosis
  use Subcutaneous Tissue and Fascia, Upper
    Arm, Right
  use Subcutaneous Tissue and Fascia, Upper
    Arm, Left
Subscapular artery
  use Artery, Axillary, Left
  use Artery, Axillary, Right
Subscapularis muscle
  use Muscle, Shoulder, Left
  use Muscle, Shoulder, Right
Substance Abuse Treatment
  Counseling
    Family, for substance abuse, Other Family
      Counseling HZ63ZZZ
    Group
      12-Step HZ43ZZZ
      Behavioral HZ41ZZZ
      Cognitive HZ40ZZZ
      Cognitive-Behavioral HZ42ZZZ
      Confrontational HZ48ZZZ
      Continuing Care HZ49ZZZ
      Infectious Disease
        Post-Test HZ4CZZZ
        Pre-Test HZ4CZZZ
      Interpersonal HZ44ZZZ
      Motivational Enhancement HZ47ZZZ

◄ New   ◄▓ Revised   ~~deleted~~ Deleted

Substance Abuse Treatment *(Continued)*
  Counseling *(Continued)*
    Group *(Continued)*
      Psychoeducation HZ46ZZZ
      Spiritual HZ4BZZZ
      Vocational HZ45ZZZ
    Individual
      12-Step HZ33ZZZ
      Behavioral HZ31ZZZ
      Cognitive HZ30ZZZ
      Cognitive-Behavioral HZ32ZZZ
      Confrontational HZ38ZZZ
      Continuing Care HZ39ZZZ
      Infectious Disease
        Post-Test HZ3CZZZ
        Pre-Test HZ3CZZZ
      Interpersonal HZ34ZZZ
      Motivational Enhancement HZ37ZZZ
      Psychoeducation HZ36ZZZ
      Spiritual HZ3BZZZ
      Vocational HZ35ZZZ
  Detoxification Services, for substance abuse HZ2ZZZZ
  Medication Management
    Antabuse HZ83ZZZ
    Bupropion HZ87ZZZ
    Clonidine HZ86ZZZ
    Levo-alpha-acetyl-methadol (LAAM) HZ82ZZZ
    Methadone Maintenance HZ81ZZZ
    Naloxone HZ85ZZZ
    Naltrexone HZ84ZZZ
    Nicotine Replacement HZ80ZZZ
    Other Replacement Medication HZ89ZZZ
    Psychiatric Medication HZ88ZZZ
  Pharmacotherapy
    Antabuse HZ93ZZZ
    Bupropion HZ97ZZZ
    Clonidine HZ96ZZZ
    Levo-alpha-acetyl-methadol (LAAM) HZ92ZZZ
    Methadone Maintenance HZ91ZZZ
    Naloxone HZ95ZZZ
    Naltrexone HZ94ZZZ
    Nicotine Replacement HZ90ZZZ
    Psychiatric Medication HZ98ZZZ
    Replacement Medication, Other HZ99ZZZ
  Psychotherapy
    12-Step HZ53ZZZ
    Behavioral HZ51ZZZ
    Cognitive HZ50ZZZ
    Cognitive-Behavioral HZ52ZZZ
    Confrontational HZ58ZZZ
    Interactive HZ55ZZZ
    Interpersonal HZ54ZZZ
    Motivational Enhancement HZ57ZZZ
    Psychoanalysis HZ5BZZZ
    Psychodynamic HZ5CZZZ
    Psychoeducation HZ56ZZZ
    Psychophysiological HZ5DZZZ
    Supportive HZ59ZZZ
Substantia nigra *use* Basal Ganglia
Subtalar (talocalcaneal) joint
  use Joint, Tarsal, Right
  use Joint, Tarsal, Left
Subtalar ligament
  use Bursa and Ligament, Foot, Left
  use Bursa and Ligament, Foot, Right
Subthalamic nucleus *use* Basal Ganglia
Suction *see* Drainage
Suction curettage (D&C), nonobstetric *see* Extraction, Endometrium 0UDB
Suction curettage, obstetric post-delivery *see* Extraction, Products of Conception, Retained 10D1
Superficial circumflex iliac vein
  use Vein, Greater Saphenous, Right
  use Vein, Greater Saphenous, Left

Superficial epigastric artery
  use Artery, Femoral, Left
  use Artery, Femoral, Right
Superficial epigastric vein
  use Vein, Greater Saphenous, Right
  use Vein, Greater Saphenous, Left
Superficial Inferior Epigastric Artery Flap
  Bilateral 0HRV078
  Left 0HRU078
  Right 0HRT078
Superficial palmar arch
  use Artery, Hand, Left
  use Artery, Hand, Right
Superficial palmar venous arch
  use Vein, Hand, Left
  use Vein, Hand, Right
Superficial temporal artery
  use Artery, Temporal, Right
  use Artery, Temporal, Left
Superficial transverse perineal muscle *use* Muscle, Perineum
Superior cardiac nerve *use* Nerve, Thoracic Sympathetic
Superior cerebellar vein *use* Vein, Intracranial
Superior cerebral vein *use* Vein, Intracranial
Superior clunic (cluneal) nerve *use* Nerve, Lumbar
Superior epigastric artery
  use Artery, Internal Mammary, Right
  use Artery, Internal Mammary, Left
Superior genicular artery
  use Artery, Popliteal, Left
  use Artery, Popliteal, Right
Superior gluteal artery
  use Artery, Internal Iliac, Left
  use Artery, Internal Iliac, Right
Superior gluteal nerve *use* Nerve, Lumbar Plexus
Superior hypogastric plexus *use* Nerve, Abdominal Sympathetic
Superior labial artery *use* Artery, Face
Superior laryngeal artery
  use Artery, Thyroid, Left
  use Artery, Thyroid, Right
Superior laryngeal nerve *use* Nerve, Vagus
Superior longitudinal muscle *use* Muscle, Tongue, Palate, Pharynx
Superior mesenteric ganglion *use* Nerve, Abdominal Sympathetic
Superior mesenteric lymph node *use* Lymphatic, Mesenteric
Superior mesenteric plexus *use* Nerve, Abdominal Sympathetic
Superior oblique muscle
  use Muscle, Extraocular, Left
  use Muscle, Extraocular, Right
Superior olivary nucleus *use* Pons
Superior rectal artery *use* Artery, Inferior Mesenteric
Superior rectal vein *use* Vein, Inferior Mesenteric
Superior rectus muscle
  use Muscle, Extraocular, Left
  use Muscle, Extraocular, Right
Superior tarsal plate
  use Eyelid, Upper, Right
  use Eyelid, Upper, Left
Superior thoracic artery
  use Artery, Axillary, Left
  use Artery, Axillary, Right
Superior thyroid artery
  use Artery, Thyroid, Right
  use Artery, External Carotid, Right
  use Artery, Thyroid, Left
  use Artery, External Carotid, Left
Superior turbinate *use* Turbinate, Nasal
Superior ulnar collateral artery
  use Artery, Brachial, Right
  use Artery, Brachial, Left

Supplement
  Abdominal Wall 0WUF
  Acetabulum
    Left 0QU5
    Right 0QU4
  Ampulla of Vater 0FUC
  Anal Sphincter 0DUR
  Ankle Region
    Left 0YUL
    Right 0YUK
  Anus 0DUQ
  Aorta
    Abdominal 04U0
    Thoracic 02UW
  Arm
    Lower
      Left 0XUF
      Right 0XUD
    Upper
      Left 0XU9
      Right 0XU8
  Artery
    Anterior Tibial
      Left 04UQ
      Right 04UP
    Axillary
      Left 03U6
      Right 03U5
    Brachial
      Left 03U8
      Right 03U7
    Celiac 04U1
    Colic
      Left 04U7
      Middle 04U8
      Right 04U6
    Common Carotid
      Left 03UJ
      Right 03UH
    Common Iliac
      Left 04UD
      Right 04UC
    External Carotid
      Left 03UN
      Right 03UM
    External Iliac
      Left 04UJ
      Right 04UH
    Face 03UR
    Femoral
      Left 04UL
      Right 04UK
    Foot
      Left 04UW
      Right 04UV
    Gastric 04U2
    Hand
      Left 03UF
      Right 03UD
    Hepatic 04U3
    Inferior Mesenteric 04UB
    Innominate 03U2
    Internal Carotid
      Left 03UL
      Right 03UK
    Internal Iliac
      Left 04UF
      Right 04UE
    Internal Mammary
      Left 03U1
      Right 03U0
    Intracranial 03UG
    Lower 04UY
    Peroneal
      Left 04UU
      Right 04UT
    Popliteal
      Left 04UN
      Right 04UM
    Posterior Tibial
      Left 04US
      Right 04UR

◀ New   ⬅ Revised   ~~deleted~~ Deleted

Supplement *(Continued)*
Artery *(Continued)*
Pulmonary
Left 02UR
Right 02UQ
Pulmonary Trunk 02UP
Radial
Left 03UC
Right 03UB
Renal
Left 04UA
Right 04U9
Splenic 04U4
Subclavian
Left 03U4
Right 03U3
Superior Mesenteric 04U5
Temporal
Left 03UT
Right 03US
Thyroid
Left 03UV
Right 03UU
Ulnar
Left 03UA
Right 03U9
Upper 03UY
Vertebral
Left 03UQ
Right 03UP
Atrium
Left 02U7
Right 02U6
Auditory Ossicle
Left 09UA0
Right 09U90
Axilla
Left 0XU5
Right 0XU4
Back
Lower 0WUL
Upper 0WUK
Bladder 0TUB
Bladder Neck 0TUC
Bone
Ethmoid
Left 0NUG
Right 0NUF
Frontal
Left 0NU2
Right 0NU1
Hyoid 0NUX
Lacrimal
Left 0NUJ
Right 0NUH
Nasal 0NUB
Occipital
Left 0NU8
Right 0NU7
Palatine
Left 0NUL
Right 0NUK
Parietal
Left 0NU4
Right 0NU3
Pelvic
Left 0QU3
Right 0QU2
Sphenoid
Left 0NUD
Right 0NUC
Temporal
Left 0NU6
Right 0NU5
Zygomatic
Left 0NUN
Right 0NUM
Breast
Bilateral 0HUV
Left 0HUU
Right 0HUT

Supplement *(Continued)*
Bronchus
Lingula 0BU9
Lower Lobe
Left 0BUB
Right 0BU6
Main
Left 0BU7
Right 0BU3
Middle Lobe, Right
0BU5
Upper Lobe
Left 0BU8
Right 0BU4
Buccal Mucosa 0CU4
Bursa and Ligament
Abdomen
Left 0MUJ
Right 0MUH
Ankle
Left 0MUR
Right 0MUQ
Elbow
Left 0MU4
Right 0MU3
Foot
Left 0MUT
Right 0MUS
Hand
Left 0MU8
Right 0MU7
Head and Neck 0MU0
Hip
Left 0MUM
Right 0MUL
Knee
Left 0MUP
Right 0MUN
Lower Extremity
Left 0MUW
Right 0MUV
Perineum 0MUK
Shoulder
Left 0MU2
Right 0MU1
Thorax
Left 0MUG
Right 0MUF
Trunk
Left 0MUD
Right 0MUC
Upper Extremity
Left 0MUB
Right 0MU9
Wrist
Left 0MU6
Right 0MU5
Buttock
Left 0YU1
Right 0YU0
Carina 0BU2
Carpal
Left 0PUN
Right 0PUM
Cecum 0DUH
Cerebral Meninges
00U1
Chest Wall 0WU8
Chordae Tendineae
02U9
Cisterna Chyli 07UL
Clavicle
Left 0PUB
Right 0PU9
Clitoris 0UUJ
Coccyx 0QUS
Colon
Ascending 0DUK
Descending 0DUM
Sigmoid 0DUN
Transverse 0DUL

Supplement *(Continued)*
Cord
Bilateral 0VUH
Left 0VUG
Right 0VUF
Cornea
Left 08U9
Right 08U8
Cul-de-sac 0UUF
Diaphragm
Left 0BUS
Right 0BUR
Disc
Cervical Vertebral 0RU3
Cervicothoracic Vertebral
0RU5
Lumbar Vertebral 0SU2
Lumbosacral 0SU4
Thoracic Vertebral 0RU9
Thoracolumbar Vertebral
0RUB
Duct
Common Bile 0FU9
Cystic 0FU8
Hepatic
Left 0FU6
Right 0FU5
Lacrimal
Left 08UY
Right 08UX
Pancreatic 0FUD
Accessory 0FUF
Duodenum 0DU9
Dura Mater 00U2
Ear
External
Bilateral 09U2
Left 09U1
Right 09U0
Inner
Left 09UE0
Right 09UD0
Middle
Left 09U60
Right 09U50
Elbow Region
Left 0XUC
Right 0XUB
Epididymis
Bilateral 0VUL
Left 0VUK
Right 0VUJ
Epiglottis 0CUR
Esophagogastric Junction
0DU4
Esophagus 0DU5
Lower 0DU3
Middle 0DU2
Upper 0DU1
Extremity
Lower
Left 0YUB
Right 0YU9
Upper
Left 0XU7
Right 0XU6
Eye
Left 08U1
Right 08U0
Eyelid
Lower
Left 08UR
Right 08UQ
Upper
Left 08UP
Right 08UN
Face 0WU2
Fallopian Tube
Left 0UU6
Right 0UU5
Fallopian Tubes, Bilateral 0UU7

Supplement (*Continued*)
Femoral Region
  Bilateral 0YUE
  Left 0YU8
  Right 0YU7
Femoral Shaft
  Left 0QU9
  Right 0QU8
Femur
  Lower
    Left 0QUC
    Right 0QUB
  Upper
    Left 0QU7
    Right 0QU6
Fibula
  Left 0QUK
  Right 0QUJ
Finger
  Index
    Left 0XUP
    Right 0XUN
  Little
    Left 0XUW
    Right 0XUV
  Middle
    Left 0XUR
    Right 0XUQ
  Ring
    Left 0XUT
    Right 0XUS
Foot
  Left 0YUN
  Right 0YUM
Gingiva
  Lower 0CU6
  Upper 0CU5
Glenoid Cavity
  Left 0PU8
  Right 0PU7
Hand
  Left 0XUK
  Right 0XUJ
Head 0WU0
Heart 02UA
Humeral Head
  Left 0PUD
  Right 0PUC
Humeral Shaft
  Left 0PUG
  Right 0PUF
Hymen 0UUK
Ileocecal Valve 0DUC
Ileum 0DUB
Inguinal Region
  Bilateral 0YUA
  Left 0YU6
  Right 0YU5
Intestine
  Large 0DUE
    Left 0DUG
    Right 0DUF
  Small 0DU8
Iris
  Left 08UD
  Right 08UC
Jaw
  Lower 0WU5
  Upper 0WU4
Jejunum 0DUA
Joint
  Acromioclavicular
    Left 0RUH
    Right 0RUG
  Ankle
    Left 0SUG
    Right 0SUF
  Carpal
    Left 0RUR
    Right 0RUQ
  Cervical Vertebral 0RU1

Supplement (*Continued*)
Joint (*Continued*)
  Cervicothoracic Vertebral 0RU4
  Coccygeal 0SU6
  Elbow
    Left 0RUM
    Right 0RUL
  Finger Phalangeal
    Left 0RUX
    Right 0RUW
  Hip
    Left 0SUB
      Acetabular Surface 0SUE
      Femoral Surface 0SUS
    Right 0SU9
      Acetabular Surface 0SUA
      Femoral Surface 0SUR
  Knee
    Left 0SUD
      Femoral Surface 0SUU09Z
      Tibial Surface 0SUW09Z
    Right 0SUC
      Femoral Surface 0SUT09Z
      Tibial Surface 0SUV09Z
  Lumbar Vertebral 0SU0
  Lumbosacral 0SU3
  Metacarpocarpal
    Left 0RUT
    Right 0RUS
  Metacarpophalangeal
    Left 0RUV
    Right 0RUU
  Metatarsal-Phalangeal
    Left 0SUN
    Right 0SUM
  Metatarsal-Tarsal
    Left 0SUL
    Right 0SUK
  Occipital-cervical 0RU0
  Sacrococcygeal 0SU5
  Sacroiliac
    Left 0SU8
    Right 0SU7
  Shoulder
    Left 0RUK
    Right 0RUJ
  Sternoclavicular
    Left 0RUF
    Right 0RUE
  Tarsal
    Left 0SUJ
    Right 0SUH
  Temporomandibular
    Left 0RUD
    Right 0RUC
  Thoracic Vertebral 0RU6
  Thoracolumbar Vertebral
    0RUA
  Toe Phalangeal
    Left 0SUQ
    Right 0SUP
  Wrist
    Left 0RUP
    Right 0RUN
Kidney Pelvis
  Left 0TU4
  Right 0TU3
Knee Region
  Left 0YUG
  Right 0YUF
Larynx 0CUS
Leg
  Lower
    Left 0YUJ
    Right 0YUH
  Upper
    Left 0YUD
    Right 0YUC
Lip
  Lower 0CU1
  Upper 0CU0

Supplement (*Continued*)
Lymphatic
  Aortic 07UD
  Axillary
    Left 07U6
    Right 07U5
  Head 07U0
  Inguinal
    Left 07UJ
    Right 07UH
  Internal Mammary
    Left 07U9
    Right 07U8
  Lower Extremity
    Left 07UG
    Right 07UF
  Mesenteric 07UB
  Neck
    Left 07U2
    Right 07U1
  Pelvis 07UC
  Thoracic Duct 07UK
  Thorax 07U7
  Upper Extremity
    Left 07U4
    Right 07U3
Mandible
  Left 0NUV
  Right 0NUT
Maxilla
  Left 0NUS
  Right 0NUR
Mediastinum 0WUC
Mesentery 0DUV
Metacarpal
  Left 0PUQ
  Right 0PUP
Metatarsal
  Left 0QUP
  Right 0QUN
Muscle
  Abdomen
    Left 0KUL
    Right 0KUK
  Extraocular
    Left 08UM
    Right 08UL
  Facial 0KU1
  Foot
    Left 0KUW
    Right 0KUV
  Hand
    Left 0KUD
    Right 0KUC
  Head 0KU0
  Hip
    Left 0KUP
    Right 0KUN
  Lower Arm and Wrist
    Left 0KUB
    Right 0KU9
  Lower Leg
    Left 0KUT
    Right 0KUS
  Neck
    Left 0KU3
    Right 0KU2
  Papillary 02UD
  Perineum 0KUM
  Shoulder
    Left 0KU6
    Right 0KU5
  Thorax
    Left 0KUJ
    Right 0KUH
  Tongue, Palate, Pharynx
    0KU4
  Trunk
    Left 0KUG
    Right 0KUF

◀ New   ◀▦ Revised   ~~deleted~~ Deleted

Supplement (*Continued*)
  Muscle (*Continued*)
    Upper Arm
      Left 0KU8
      Right 0KU7
    Upper Leg
      Left 0KUR
      Right 0KUQ
  Nasopharynx 09UN
  Neck 0WU6
  Nerve
    Abducens 00UL
    Accessory 00UR
    Acoustic 00UN
    Cervical 01U1
    Facial 00UM
    Femoral 01UD
    Glossopharyngeal
      00UP
    Hypoglossal 00US
    Lumbar 01UB
    Median 01U5
    Oculomotor 00UH
    Olfactory 00UF
    Optic 00UG
    Peroneal 01UH
    Phrenic 01U2
    Pudendal 01UC
    Radial 01U6
    Sacral 01UR
    Sciatic 01UF
    Thoracic 01U8
    Tibial 01UG
    Trigeminal 00UK
    Trochlear 00UJ
    Ulnar 01U4
    Vagus 00UQ
  Nipple
    Left 0HUX
    Right 0HUW
  Nose 09UK
  Omentum
    Greater 0DUS
    Lesser 0DUT
  Orbit
    Left 0NUQ
    Right 0NUP
  Palate
    Hard 0CU2
    Soft 0CU3
  Patella
    Left 0QUF
    Right 0QUD
  Penis 0VUS
  Pericardium 02UN
  Perineum
    Female 0WUN
    Male 0WUM
  Peritoneum 0DUW
  Phalanx
    Finger
      Left 0PUV
      Right 0PUT
    Thumb
      Left 0PUS
      Right 0PUR
    Toe
      Left 0QUR
      Right 0QUQ
  Pharynx 0CUM
  Prepuce 0VUT
  Radius
    Left 0PUJ
    Right 0PUH
  Rectum 0DUP
  Retina
    Left 08UF
    Right 08UE
  Retinal Vessel
    Left 08UH
    Right 08UG

Supplement (*Continued*)
  Rib
    Left 0PU2
    Right 0PU1
  Sacrum 0QU1
  Scapula
    Left 0PU6
    Right 0PU5
  Scrotum 0VU5
  Septum
    Atrial 02U5
    Nasal 09UM
    Ventricular 02UM
  Shoulder Region
    Left 0XU3
    Right 0XU2
  Skull 0NU0
  Spinal Meninges 00UT
  Sternum 0PU0
  Stomach 0DU6
    Pylorus 0DU7
  Subcutaneous Tissue and Fascia
    Abdomen 0JU8
    Back 0JU7
    Buttock 0JU9
    Chest 0JU6
    Face 0JU1
    Foot
      Left 0JUR
      Right 0JUQ
    Hand
      Left 0JUK
      Right 0JUJ
    Lower Arm
      Left 0JUH
      Right 0JUG
    Lower Leg
      Left 0JUP
      Right 0JUN
    Neck
      Anterior 0JU4
      Posterior 0JU5
    Pelvic Region 0JUC
    Perineum 0JUB
    Scalp 0JU0
    Upper Arm
      Left 0JUF
      Right 0JUD
    Upper Leg
      Left 0JUM
      Right 0JUL
  Tarsal
    Left 0QUM
    Right 0QUL
  Tendon
    Abdomen
      Left 0LUG
      Right 0LUF
    Ankle
      Left 0LUT
      Right 0LUS
    Foot
      Left 0LUW
      Right 0LUV
    Hand
      Left 0LU8
      Right 0LU7
    Head and Neck 0LU0
    Hip
      Left 0LUK
      Right 0LUJ
    Knee
      Left 0LUR
      Right 0LUQ
    Lower Arm and Wrist
      Left 0LU6
      Right 0LU5
    Lower Leg
      Left 0LUP
      Right 0LUN
    Perineum 0LUH

Supplement (*Continued*)
  Tendon (*Continued*)
    Shoulder
      Left 0LU2
      Right 0LU1
    Thorax
      Left 0LUD
      Right 0LUC
    Trunk
      Left 0LUB
      Right 0LU9
    Upper Arm
      Left 0LU4
      Right 0LU3
    Upper Leg
      Left 0LUM
      Right 0LUL
  Testis
    Bilateral 0VUC0
    Left 0VUB0
    Right 0VU90
  Thumb
    Left 0XUM
    Right 0XUL
  Tibia
    Left 0QUH
    Right 0QUG
  Toe
    1st
      Left 0YUQ
      Right 0YUP
    2nd
      Left 0YUS
      Right 0YUR
    3rd
      Left 0YUU
      Right 0YUT
    4th
      Left 0YUW
      Right 0YUV
    5th
      Left 0YUY
      Right 0YUX
  Tongue 0CU7
  Trachea 0BU1
  Tunica Vaginalis
    Left 0VU7
    Right 0VU6
  Turbinate, Nasal 09UL
  Tympanic Membrane
    Left 09U8
    Right 09U7
  Ulna
    Left 0PUL
    Right 0PUK
  Ureter
    Left 0TU7
    Right 0TU6
  Urethra 0TUD
  Uterine Supporting Structure
    0UU4
  Uvula 0CUN
  Vagina 0UUG
  Valve
    Aortic 02UF
    Mitral 02UG
    Pulmonary 02UH
    Tricuspid 02UJ
  Vas Deferens
    Bilateral 0VUQ
    Left 0VUP
    Right 0VUN
  Vein
    Axillary
      Left 05U8
      Right 05U7
    Azygos 05U0
    Basilic
      Left 05UC
      Right 05UB

◀ New   ◀▦ Revised   ~~deleted~~ Deleted

Supplement (*Continued*)
  Vein (*Continued*)
    Brachial
      Left 05UA
      Right 05U9
    Cephalic
      Left 05UF
      Right 05UD
    Colic 06U7
    Common Iliac
      Left 06UD
      Right 06UC
    Esophageal 06U3
    External Iliac
      Left 06UG
      Right 06UF
    External Jugular
      Left 05UQ
      Right 05UP
    Face
      Left 05UV
      Right 05UT
    Femoral
      Left 06UN
      Right 06UM
    Foot
      Left 06UV
      Right 06UT
    Gastric 06U2
    Greater Saphenous
      Left 06UQ
      Right 06UP
    Hand
      Left 05UH
      Right 05UG
    Hemiazygos 05U1
    Hepatic 06U4
    Hypogastric
      Left 06UJ
      Right 06UH
    Inferior Mesenteric 06U6
    Innominate
      Left 05U4
      Right 05U3
    Internal Jugular
      Left 05UN
      Right 05UM
    Intracranial 05UL
    Lesser Saphenous
      Left 06US
      Right 06UR
    Lower 06UY
    Portal 06U8
    Pulmonary
      Left 02UT
      Right 02US

Supplement (*Continued*)
  Vein (*Continued*)
    Renal
      Left 06UB
      Right 06U9
    Splenic 06U1
    Subclavian
      Left 05U6
      Right 05U5
    Superior Mesenteric 06U5
    Upper 05UY
    Vertebral
      Left 05US
      Right 05UR
    Vena Cava
      Inferior 06U0
      Superior 02UV
    Ventricle
      Left 02UL
      Right 02UK
    Vertebra
      Cervical 0PU3
      Lumbar 0QU0
      Thoracic 0PU4
    Vesicle
      Bilateral 0VU3
      Left 0VU2
      Right 0VU1
    Vocal Cord
      Left 0CUV
      Right 0CUT
    Vulva 0UUM
    Wrist Region
      Left 0XUH
      Right 0XUG
Supraclavicular (Virchow's) lymph node
  use Lymphatic, Neck, Left
  use Lymphatic, Neck, Right
Supraclavicular nerve *use* Nerve, Cervical
  Plexus
Suprahyoid lymph node *use* Lymphatic, Head
Suprahyoid muscle
  use Muscle, Neck, Right
  use Muscle, Neck, Left
Suprainguinal lymph node *use* Lymphatic,
  Pelvis
Supraorbital vein
  use Vein, Face, Left
  use Vein, Face, Right
Suprarenal gland
  use Gland, Adrenal, Left
  use Gland, Adrenal, Right
  use Gland, Adrenal, Bilateral
  use Gland, Adrenal
Suprarenal plexus *use* Nerve, Abdominal
  Sympathetic

Suprascapular nerve *use* Nerve, Brachial Plexus
Supraspinatus fascia
  use Subcutaneous Tissue and Fascia, Upper
    Arm, Right
  use Subcutaneous Tissue and Fascia, Upper
    Arm, Left
Supraspinatus muscle
  use Muscle, Shoulder, Right
  use Muscle, Shoulder, Left
Supraspinous ligament
  use Bursa and Ligament, Trunk, Right
  use Bursa and Ligament, Trunk, Left
Suprasternal notch *use* Sternum
Supratrochlear lymph node
  use Lymphatic, Upper Extremity, Right
  use Lymphatic, Upper Extremity, Left
Sural artery
  use Artery, Popliteal, Right
  use Artery, Popliteal, Left
Suspension
  Bladder Neck *see* Reposition, Bladder Neck
    0TSC
  Kidney *see* Reposition, Urinary System 0TS
  Urethra *see* Reposition, Urinary System 0TS
  Urethrovesical *see* Reposition, Bladder Neck
    0TSC
  Uterus *see* Reposition, Uterus 0US9
  Vagina *see* Reposition, Vagina 0USG
Suture
  Laceration repair *see* Repair
  Ligation *see* Occlusion
Suture Removal
  Extremity
    Lower 8E0YXY8
    Upper 8E0XXY8
  Head and Neck Region 8E09XY8
  Trunk Region 8E0WXY8
Sweat gland *use* Skin
Sympathectomy
  see Excision, Peripheral Nervous System 01B
SynCardia Total Artificial Heart *use* Synthetic
  Substitute
Synchra CRT-P *use* Cardiac Resynchronization
  Pacemaker Pulse Generator in 0JH
SynchroMed pump *use* Infusion Device, Pump
  in Subcutaneous Tissue and Fascia ◀
Synechiotomy, iris *see* Release, Eye 08N
Synovectomy
  Lower joint *see* Excision, Lower Joints 0SB
  Upper joint *see* Excision, Upper Joints 0RB
Systemic Nuclear Medicine Therapy
  Abdomen CW70
  Anatomical Regions, Multiple CW7YYZZ
  Chest CW73
  Thyroid CW7G
  Whole Body CW7N

T

Takedown
  Arteriovenous shunt *see* Removal of device from, Upper Arteries 03P
  Arteriovenous shunt, with creation of new shunt *see* Bypass, Upper Arteries 031
  Stoma *see* Repair
Talent® Converter *use* Intraluminal Device
Talent® Occluder *use* Intraluminal Device
Talent® Stent Graft (abdominal) (thoracic) *use* Intraluminal Device
Talocalcaneal (subtalar) joint
  use Joint, Tarsal, Left
  use Joint, Tarsal, Right
Talocalcaneal ligament
  use Bursa and Ligament, Foot, Left
  use Bursa and Ligament, Foot, Right
Talocalcaneonavicular joint
  use Joint, Tarsal, Right
  use Joint, Tarsal, Left
Talocalcaneonavicular ligament
  use Bursa and Ligament, Foot, Left
  use Bursa and Ligament, Foot, Right
Talocrural joint
  use Joint, Ankle, Right
  use Joint, Ankle, Left
Talofibular ligament
  use Bursa and Ligament, Ankle, Right
  use Bursa and Ligament, Ankle, Left
Talus bone
  use Tarsal, Right
  use Tarsal, Left
TandemHeart® System *use* External Heart Assist System in Heart and Great Vessels
Tarsectomy
  see Excision, Lower Bones 0QB
  see Resection, Lower Bones 0QT
Tarsometatarsal joint
  use Joint, Metatarsal-Tarsal, Right
  use Joint, Metatarsal-Tarsal, Left
Tarsometatarsal ligament
  use Bursa and Ligament, Foot, Right
  use Bursa and Ligament, Foot, Left
Tarsorrhaphy *see* Repair, Eye 08Q
Tattooing
  Cornea 3E0CXMZ
  Skin *see* Introduction of substance in or on Skin 3E00
TAXUS® Liberté® Paclitaxel-eluting Coronary Stent System *use* Intraluminal Device, Drug-eluting in Heart and Great Vessels
TBNA (transbronchial needle aspiration) *see* Drainage, Respiratory System 0B9
Telemetry
  4A12X4Z
  Ambulatory 4A12X45
Temperature gradient study 4A0ZXKZ
Temporal lobe *use* Cerebral Hemisphere
Temporalis muscle *use* Muscle, Head
Temporoparietalis muscle *use* Muscle, Head
Tendolysis *see* Release, Tendons 0LN
Tendonectomy
  see Excision, Tendons 0LB
  see Resection, Tendons 0LT
Tendonoplasty, tenoplasty
  see Repair, Tendons 0LQ
  see Replacement, Tendons 0LR
  see Supplement, Tendons 0LU
Tendorrhaphy *see* Repair, Tendons 0LQ
Tendototomy
  see Division, Tendons 0L8
  see Drainage, Tendons 0L9
Tenectomy, tenonectomy
  see Excision, Tendons 0LB
  see Resection, Tendons 0LT
Tenolysis *see* Release, Tendons 0LN
Tenontorrhaphy *see* Repair, Tendons 0LQ
Tenontotomy
  see Division, Tendons 0L8
  see Drainage, Tendons 0L9
Tenorrhaphy *see* Repair, Tendons 0LQ

Tenosynovectomy
  see Excision, Tendons 0LB
  see Resection, Tendons 0LT
Tenotomy
  see Division, Tendons 0L8
  see Drainage, Tendons 0L9
Tensor fasciae latae muscle
  use Muscle, Hip, Left
  use Muscle, Hip, Right
Tensor veli palatini muscle *use* Muscle, Tongue, Palate, Pharynx
Tenth cranial nerve *use* Nerve, Vagus
Tentorium cerebelli *use* Dura Mater
Teres major muscle
  use Muscle, Shoulder, Left
  use Muscle, Shoulder, Right
Teres minor muscle
  use Muscle, Shoulder, Right
  use Muscle, Shoulder, Left
Termination of pregnancy
  Aspiration curettage 10A07ZZ
  Dilation and curettage 10A07ZZ
  Hysterotomy 10A00ZZ
  Intra-amniotic injection 10A03ZZ
  Laminaria 10A07ZW
  Vacuum 10A07Z6
Testectomy
  see Excision, Male Reproductive System 0VB
  see Resection, Male Reproductive System 0VT
Testicular artery *use* Aorta, Abdominal
Testing
  Glaucoma 4A07XBZ
  Hearing *see* Hearing Assessment, Diagnostic Audiology F13
  Mental health *see* Psychological Tests
  Muscle function, electromyography (EMG) *see* Measurement, Musculoskeletal 4A0F
  Muscle function, manual *see* Motor Function Assessment, Rehabilitation F01
  Neurophysiologic monitoring, intra-operative *see* Monitoring, Physiological Systems 4A1
  Range of motion *see* Motor Function Assessment, Rehabilitation F01
  Vestibular function *see* Vestibular Assessment, Diagnostic Audiology F15
Thalamectomy *see* Excision, Thalamus 00B9
Thalamotomy
  see Drainage, Thalamus 0099
Thenar muscle
  use Muscle, Hand, Right
  use Muscle, Hand, Left
Therapeutic Massage
  Musculoskeletal System 8E0KX1Z
  Reproductive System
    Prostate 8E0VX1C
    Rectum 8E0VX1D
Therapeutic occlusion coil(s) *use* Intraluminal Device
Thermography 4A0ZXKZ
Thermotherapy, prostate *see* Destruction, Prostate 0V50
Third cranial nerve *use* Nerve, Oculomotor
Third occipital nerve *use* Nerve, Cervical
Third ventricle *use* Cerebral Ventricle
Thoracectomy *see* Excision, Anatomical Regions, General 0WB
Thoracentesis *see* Drainage, Anatomical Regions, General 0W9
Thoracic aortic plexus *use* Nerve, Thoracic Sympathetic
Thoracic esophagus *use* Esophagus, Middle
Thoracic facet joint *use* Joint, Thoracic Vertebral ◀▥
  ~~use Joint, Thoracic Vertebral, 2 to 7~~
  ~~use Joint, Thoracic Vertebral, 8 or more~~
  ~~use Joint, Thoracic Vertebral~~
Thoracic ganglion *use* Nerve, Thoracic Sympathetic
Thoracoacromial artery
  use Artery, Axillary, Right
  use Artery, Axillary, Left

Thoracocentesis *see* Drainage, Anatomical Regions, General 0W9
Thoracolumbar facet joint *use* Joint, Thoracolumbar Vertebral
Thoracoplasty
  see Repair, Anatomical Regions, General 0WQ
  see Supplement, Anatomical Regions, General 0WU
Thoracostomy tube *use* Drainage Device
Thoracostomy, for lung collapse *see* Drainage, Respiratory System 0B9
Thoracotomy *see* Drainage, Anatomical Regions, General 0W9
Thoratec IVAD (Implantable Ventricular Assist Device) *use* Implantable Heart Assist System in Heart and Great Vessels
Thoratec Paracorporeal Ventricular Assist Device *use* External Heart Assist System in Heart and Great Vessels
Thrombectomy *see* Extirpation
Thymectomy
  see Excision, Lymphatic and Hemic Systems 07B
  see Resection, Lymphatic and Hemic Systems 07T
Thymopexy
  see Repair, Lymphatic and Hemic Systems 07Q
  see Reposition, Lymphatic and Hemic Systems 07S
Thymus gland *use* Thymus
Thyroarytenoid muscle
  use Muscle, Neck, Right
  use Muscle, Neck, Left
Thyrocervical trunk
  use Artery, Thyroid, Right
  use Artery, Thyroid, Left
Thyroid cartilage *use* Larynx
Thyroidectomy
  see Excision, Endocrine System 0GB
  see Resection, Endocrine System 0GT
Thyroidorrhaphy *see* Repair, Endocrine System 0GQ
Thyroidoscopy 0GJK4ZZ
Thyroidotomy *see* Drainage, Endocrine System 0G9
Tibialis anterior muscle
  use Muscle, Lower Leg, Right
  use Muscle, Lower Leg, Left
Tibialis posterior muscle
  use Muscle, Lower Leg, Right
  use Muscle, Lower Leg, Left
Tibiofemoral joint
  use Joint, Knee, Right, Tibial Surface
  use Joint, Knee, Left, Tibial Surface
  use Joint, Knee, Right
  use Joint, Knee, Left
TigerPaw® system for closure of left atrial appendage *use* Extraluminal Device
Tissue bank graft *use* Nonautologous Tissue Substitute
Tissue Expander
  Insertion of device in
    Breast
      Bilateral 0HHV
      Left 0HHU
      Right 0HHT
    Nipple
      Left 0HHX
      Right 0HHW
    Subcutaneous Tissue and Fascia
      Abdomen 0JH8
      Back 0JH7
      Buttock 0JH9
      Chest 0JH6
      Face 0JH1
      Foot
        Left 0JHR
        Right 0JHQ
      Hand
        Left 0JHK
        Right 0JHJ

◄ New ◄▦ Revised ~~deleted~~ Deleted

Transfer (Continued)
  Bursa and Ligament (Continued)
    Knee
      Left 0MXP
      Right 0MXN
    Lower Extremity
      Left 0MXW
      Right 0MXV
    Perineum 0MXK
    Shoulder
      Left 0MX2
      Right 0MX1
    Thorax
      Left 0MXG
      Right 0MXF
    Trunk
      Left 0MXD
      Right 0MXC
    Upper Extremity
      Left 0MXB
      Right 0MX9
    Wrist
      Left 0MX6
      Right 0MX5
  Finger
    Left 0XXP0ZM
    Right 0XXN0ZL
  Gingiva
    Lower 0CX6
    Upper 0CX5
  Intestine
    Large 0DXE
    Small 0DX8
  Lip
    Lower 0CX1
    Upper 0CX0
  Muscle
    Abdomen
      Left 0KXL
      Right 0KXK
    Extraocular
      Left 08XM
      Right 08XL
    Facial 0KX1
    Foot
      Left 0KXW
      Right 0KXV
    Hand
      Left 0KXD
      Right 0KXC
    Head 0KX0
    Hip
      Left 0KXP
      Right 0KXN
    Lower Arm and Wrist
      Left 0KXB
      Right 0KX9
    Lower Leg
      Left 0KXT
      Right 0KXS
    Neck
      Left 0KX3
      Right 0KX2
    Perineum 0KXM
    Shoulder
      Left 0KX6
      Right 0KX5
    Thorax
      Left 0KXJ
      Right 0KXH
    Tongue, Palate, Pharynx
      0KX4
    Trunk
      Left 0KXG
      Right 0KXF
    Upper Arm
      Left 0KX8
      Right 0KX7
    Upper Leg
      Left 0KXR
      Right 0KXQ

Transfer (Continued)
  Nerve
    Abducens 00XL
    Accessory 00XR
    Acoustic 00XN
    Cervical 01X1
    Facial 00XM
    Femoral 01XD
    Glossopharyngeal 00XP
    Hypoglossal 00XS
    Lumbar 01XB
    Median 01X5
    Oculomotor 00XH
    Olfactory 00XF
    Optic 00XG
    Peroneal 01XH
    Phrenic 01X2
    Pudendal 01XC
    Radial 01X6
    Sciatic 01XF
    Thoracic 01X8
    Tibial 01XG
    Trigeminal 00XK
    Trochlear 00XJ
    Ulnar 01X4
    Vagus 00XQ
  Palate, Soft 0CX3
  Skin
    Abdomen 0HX7XZZ
    Back 0HX6XZZ
    Buttock 0HX8XZZ
    Chest 0HX5XZZ
    Ear
      Left 0HX3XZZ
      Right 0HX2XZZ
    Face 0HX1XZZ
    Foot
      Left 0HXNXZZ
      Right 0HXMXZZ
    Genitalia 0HXAXZZ
    Hand
      Left 0HXGXZZ
      Right 0HXFXZZ
    Lower Arm
      Left 0HXEXZZ
      Right 0HXDXZZ
    Lower Leg
      Left 0HXLXZZ
      Right 0HXKXZZ
    Neck 0HX4XZZ
    Perineum 0HX9XZZ
    Scalp 0HX0XZZ
    Upper Arm
      Left 0HXCXZZ
      Right 0HXBXZZ
    Upper Leg
      Left 0HXJXZZ
      Right 0HXHXZZ
  Stomach 0DX6
  Subcutaneous Tissue and Fascia
    Abdomen 0JX8
    Back 0JX7
    Buttock 0JX9
    Chest 0JX6
    Face 0JX1
    Foot
      Left 0JXR
      Right 0JXQ
    Hand
      Left 0JXK
      Right 0JXJ
    Lower Arm
      Left 0JXH
      Right 0JXG
    Lower Leg
      Left 0JXP
      Right 0JXN
    Neck
      Anterior 0JX4
      Posterior 0JX5
    Pelvic Region 0JXC

Transfer (Continued)
  Subcutaneous Tissue and Fascia (Continued)
    Perineum 0JXB
    Scalp 0JX0
    Upper Arm
      Left 0JXF
      Right 0JXD
    Upper Leg
      Left 0JXM
      Right 0JXL
  Tendon
    Abdomen
      Left 0LXG
      Right 0LXF
    Ankle
      Left 0LXT
      Right 0LXS
    Foot
      Left 0LXW
      Right 0LXV
    Hand
      Left 0LX8
      Right 0LX7
    Head and Neck 0LX0
    Hip
      Left 0LXK
      Right 0LXJ
    Knee
      Left 0LXR
      Right 0LXQ
    Lower Arm and Wrist
      Left 0LX6
      Right 0LX5
    Lower Leg
      Left 0LXP
      Right 0LXN
    Perineum 0LXH
    Shoulder
      Left 0LX2
      Right 0LX1
    Thorax
      Left 0LXD
      Right 0LXC
    Trunk
      Left 0LXB
      Right 0LX9
    Upper Arm
      Left 0LX4
      Right 0LX3
    Upper Leg
      Left 0LXM
      Right 0LXL
  Tongue 0CX7
Transfusion
  Artery
    Central
      Antihemophilic Factors 3026
      Blood
        Platelets 3026
        Red Cells 3026
          Frozen 3026
        White Cells 3026
        Whole 3026
      Bone Marrow 3026
      Factor IX 3026
      Fibrinogen 3026
      Globulin 3026
      Plasma
        Fresh 3026
        Frozen 3026
      Plasma Cryoprecipitate 3026
      Serum Albumin 3026
      Stem Cells
        Cord Blood 3026
        Hematopoietic 3026
    Peripheral
      Antihemophilic Factors 3025
      Blood
        Platelets 3025
        Red Cells 3025
          Frozen 3025

Transfusion *(Continued)*
  Artery *(Continued)*
    Peripheral *(Continued)*
      Blood *(Continued)*
        White Cells 3025
        Whole 3025
      Bone Marrow 3025
      Factor IX 3025
      Fibrinogen 3025
      Globulin 3025
      Plasma
        Fresh 3025
        Frozen 3025
      Plasma Cryoprecipitate 3025
      Serum Albumin 3025
      Stem Cells
        Cord Blood 3025
        Hematopoietic 3025
  Products of Conception
    Antihemophilic Factors 3027
    Blood
      Platelets 3027
      Red Cells 3027
        Frozen 3027
      White Cells 3027
      Whole 3027
    Factor IX 3027
    Fibrinogen 3027
    Globulin 3027
    Plasma
      Fresh 3027
      Frozen 3027
    Plasma Cryoprecipitate 3027
    Serum Albumin 3027
  Vein
    4-Factor Prothrombin Complex
      Concentrate 3028[03]B1
    Central
      Antihemophilic Factors 3024
      Blood
        Platelets 3024
        Red Cells 3024
          Frozen 3024
        White Cells 3024
        Whole 3024
      Bone Marrow 3024
      Factor IX 3024
      Fibrinogen 3024
      Globulin 3024
      Plasma
        Fresh 3024
        Frozen 3024
      Plasma Cryoprecipitate 3024
      Serum Albumin 3024
      Stem Cells
        Cord Blood 3024
        Embryonic 3024
        Hematopoietic 3024
    Peripheral
      Antihemophilic Factors 3023
      Blood
        Platelets 3023
        Red Cells 3023
          Frozen 3023
        White Cells 3023
        Whole 3023
      Bone Marrow 3023
      Factor IX 3023
      Fibrinogen 3023
      Globulin 3023
      Plasma
        Fresh 3023
        Frozen 3023
      Plasma Cryoprecipitate 3023

Transfusion *(Continued)*
  Vein *(Continued)*
    Peripheral *(Continued)*
      Serum Albumin 3023
      Stem Cells
        Cord Blood 3023
        Embryonic 3023
        Hematopoietic 3023
Transplantation
  Esophagus 0DY50Z
  Heart 02YA0Z
  Intestine
    Large 0DYE0Z
    Small 0DY80Z
  Kidney
    Left 0TY10Z
    Right 0TY00Z
  Liver 0FY00Z
  Lung
    Bilateral 0BYM0Z
    Left 0BYL0Z
    Lower Lobe
      Left 0BYJ0Z
      Right 0BYF0Z
    Middle Lobe, Right 0BYD0Z
    Right 0BYK0Z
    Upper Lobe
      Left 0BYG0Z
      Right 0BYC0Z
  Lung Lingula 0BYH0Z
  Ovary
    Left 0UY10Z
    Right 0UY00Z
  Pancreas 0FYG0Z
  Products of Conception 10Y0
  Spleen 07YP0Z
  Stomach 0DY60Z
  Thymus 07YM0Z
Transposition
  see Reposition
  see Transfer
Transversalis fascia *use* Subcutaneous Tissue
  and Fascia, Trunk
Transverse (cutaneous) cervical nerve *use*
  Nerve, Cervical Plexus
Transverse acetabular ligament
  use Bursa and Ligament, Hip, Left
  use Bursa and Ligament, Hip, Right
Transverse facial artery
  use Artery, Temporal, Left
  use Artery, Temporal, Right
Transverse humeral ligament
  use Bursa and Ligament, Shoulder, Left
  use Bursa and Ligament, Shoulder,
    Right
Transverse ligament of atlas *use* Bursa and
  Ligament, Head and Neck
Transverse Rectus Abdominis Myocutaneous
  Flap
  Replacement
    Bilateral 0HRV076
    Left 0HRU076
    Right 0HRT076
  Transfer
    Left 0KXL
    Right 0KXK
Transverse scapular ligament
  use Bursa and Ligament, Shoulder,
    Left
  use Bursa and Ligament, Shoulder,
    Right
Transverse thoracis muscle
  use Muscle, Thorax, Right
  use Muscle, Thorax, Left

Transversospinalis muscle
  use Muscle, Trunk, Right
  use Muscle, Trunk, Left
Transversus abdominis muscle
  use Muscle, Abdomen, Left
  use Muscle, Abdomen, Right
Trapezium bone
  use Carpal, Right
  use Carpal, Left
Trapezius muscle
  use Muscle, Trunk, Right
  use Muscle, Trunk, Left
Trapezoid bone
  use Carpal, Right
  use Carpal, Left
Triceps brachii muscle
  use Muscle, Upper Arm, Right
  use Muscle, Upper Arm, Left
Tricuspid annulus *use* Valve, Tricuspid
Trifacial nerve *use* Nerve, Trigeminal
Trifecta™ Valve (aortic) *use* Zooplastic Tissue in
  Heart and Great Vessels
Trigone of bladder *use* Bladder
Trimming, excisional *see* Excision
Triquetral bone
  use Carpal, Right
  use Carpal, Left
Trochanteric bursa
  use Bursa and Ligament, Hip, Right
  use Bursa and Ligament, Hip, Left
TUMT (Transurethral microwave
  thermotherapy of prostate) 0V507ZZ
TUNA (transurethral needle ablation of
  prostate) 0V507ZZ
Tunneled central venous catheter *use* Vascular
  Access Device in Subcutaneous Tissue and
  Fascia
Tunneled spinal (intrathecal) catheter *use*
  Infusion Device
Turbinectomy
  see Excision, Ear, Nose, Sinus 09B
  see Resection, Ear, Nose, Sinus 09T
Turbinoplasty
  see Repair, Ear, Nose, Sinus 09Q
  see Replacement, Ear, Nose, Sinus 09R
  see Supplement, Ear, Nose, Sinus 09U
Turbinotomy
  see Drainage, Ear, Nose, Sinus 099
  see Division, Ear, Nose, Sinus 098
TURP (transurethral resection of prostate) ◀▥
  see Excision, Prostate 0VB0 ◀
  see Resection, Prostate 0VT0 ◀
Twelfth cranial nerve *use* Nerve, Hypoglossal
Two lead pacemaker *use* Pacemaker, Dual
  Chamber in 0JH
Tympanic cavity
  use Ear, Middle, Left
  use Ear, Middle, Right
Tympanic nerve *use* Nerve, Glossopharyngeal
Tympanic part of temoporal bone
  use Bone, Temporal, Right
  use Bone, Temporal, Left
Tympanogram *see* Hearing Assessment,
  Diagnostic Audiology F13
Tympanoplasty
  see Repair, Ear, Nose, Sinus 09Q
  see Replacement, Ear, Nose, Sinus 09R
  see Supplement, Ear, Nosc, Sinus 09U
Tympanosympathectomy *see* Excision,
  Nerve, Head and Neck Sympathetic
  01BK
Tympanotomy *see* Drainage, Ear, Nose, Sinus
  099

◀ New   ◀▥ Revised   ~~deleted~~ Deleted

U

Ulnar collateral carpal ligament
use Bursa and Ligament, Wrist, Left
use Bursa and Ligament, Wrist, Right
Ulnar collateral ligament
use Bursa and Ligament, Elbow, Right
use Bursa and Ligament, Elbow, Left
Ulnar notch
use Radius, Left
use Radius, Right
Ulnar vein
use Vein, Brachial, Left
use Vein, Brachial, Right
Ultrafiltration
Hemodialysis *see* Performance, Urinary 5A1D
Therapeutic plasmapheresis *see* Pheresis,
Circulatory 6A55
Ultraflex™ Precision Colonic Stent System *use*
Intraluminal Device
ULTRAPRO Hernia System (UHS) *use*
Synthetic Substitute
**ULTRAPRO Partially Absorbable Lightweight
Mesh** *use* Synthetic Substitute
ULTRAPRO Plug *use* Synthetic Substitute
Ultrasonic osteogenic stimulator
use Bone Growth Stimulator in Upper Bones
use Bone Growth Stimulator in Head and
Facial Bones
use Bone Growth Stimulator in Lower Bones
Ultrasonography
Abdomen BW40ZZZ
Abdomen and Pelvis BW41ZZZ
Abdominal Wall BH49ZZZ
Aorta
Abdominal, Intravascular B440ZZ3
Thoracic, Intravascular B340ZZ3
Appendix BD48ZZZ
Artery
Brachiocephalic-Subclavian, Right,
Intravascular B341ZZ3
Celiac and Mesenteric, Intravascular
B44KZZ3
Common Carotid
Bilateral, Intravascular B345ZZ3
Left, Intravascular B344ZZ3
Right, Intravascular B343ZZ3
Coronary
Multiple B241YZZ
Intravascular B241ZZ3
Transesophageal B241ZZ4
Single B240YZZ
Intravascular B240ZZ3
Transesophageal B240ZZ4
Femoral, Intravascular B44LZZ3
Inferior Mesenteric, Intravascular B445ZZ3
Internal Carotid
Bilateral, Intravascular B348ZZ3
Left, Intravascular B347ZZ3
Right, Intravascular B346ZZ3
Intra-Abdominal, Other, Intravascular
B44BZZ3
Intracranial, Intravascular B34RZZ3
Lower Extremity
Bilateral, Intravascular B44HZZ3
Left, Intravascular B44GZZ3
Right, Intravascular B44FZZ3
Mesenteric and Celiac, Intravascular
B44KZZ3
Ophthalmic, Intravascular B34VZZ3
Penile, Intravascular B44NZZ3
Pulmonary
Left, Intravascular B34TZZ3
Right, Intravascular B34SZZ3
Renal
Bilateral, Intravascular B448ZZ3
Left, Intravascular B447ZZ3
Right, Intravascular B446ZZ3
Subclavian, Left, Intravascular B342ZZ3
Superior Mesenteric, Intravascular
B444ZZ3

Ultrasonography *(Continued)*
Artery *(Continued)*
Upper Extremity
Bilateral, Intravascular
B34KZZ3
Left, Intravascular B34JZZ3
Right, Intravascular B34HZZ3
Bile Duct BF40ZZZ
Bile Duct and Gallbladder BF43ZZZ
Bladder BT40ZZZ
and Kidney BT4JZZZ
Brain B040ZZZ
Breast
Bilateral BH42ZZZ
Left BH41ZZZ
Right BH40ZZZ
Chest Wall BH4BZZZ
Coccyx BR4FZZZ
Connective Tissue
Lower Extremity BL41ZZZ
Upper Extremity BL40ZZZ
Duodenum BD49ZZZ
Elbow
Left, Densitometry BP4HZZ1
Right, Densitometry BP4GZZ1
Esophagus BD41ZZZ
Extremity
Lower BH48ZZZ
Upper BH47ZZZ
Eye
Bilateral B847ZZZ
Left B846ZZZ
Right B845ZZZ
Fallopian Tube
Bilateral BU42
Left BU41
Right BU40
Fetal Umbilical Cord BY47ZZZ
Fetus
First Trimester, Multiple Gestation
BY4BZZZ
Second Trimester, Multiple Gestation
BY4DZZZ
Single
First Trimester BY49ZZZ
Second Trimester BY4CZZZ
Third Trimester BY4FZZZ
Third Trimester, Multiple Gestation
BY4GZZZ
Gallbladder BF42ZZZ
Gallbladder and Bile Duct BF43ZZZ
Gastrointestinal Tract BD47ZZZ
Gland
Adrenal
Bilateral BG42ZZZ
Left BG41ZZZ
Right BG40ZZZ
Parathyroid BG43ZZZ
Thyroid BG44ZZZ
Hand
Left, Densitometry BP4PZZ1
Right, Densitometry BP4NZZ1
Head and Neck BH4CZZZ
Heart
Left B245YZZ
Intravascular B245ZZ3
Transesophageal B245ZZ4
Pediatric B24DYZZ
Intravascular B24DZZ3
Transesophageal B24DZZ4
Right B244YZZ
Intravascular B244ZZ3
Transesophageal B244ZZ4
Right and Left B246YZZ
Intravascular B246ZZ3
Transesophageal B246ZZ4
Heart with Aorta B24BYZZ
Intravascular B24BZZ3
Transesophageal B24BZZ4
Hepatobiliary System, All
BF4CZZZ

Ultrasonography *(Continued)*
Hip
Bilateral BQ42ZZZ
Left BQ41ZZZ
Right BQ40ZZZ
Kidney
and Bladder BT4JZZZ
Bilateral BT43ZZZ
Left BT42ZZZ
Right BT41ZZZ
Transplant BT49ZZZ
Knee
Bilateral BQ49ZZZ
Left BQ48ZZZ
Right BQ47ZZZ
Liver BF45ZZZ
Liver and Spleen BF46ZZZ
Mediastinum BB4CZZZ
Neck BW4FZZZ
Ovary
Bilateral BU45
Left BU44
Right BU43
Ovary and Uterus BU4C
Pancreas BF47ZZZ
Pelvic Region BW4GZZZ
Pelvis and Abdomen BW41ZZZ
Penis BV4BZZZ
Pericardium B24CYZZ
Intravascular B24CZZ3
Transesophageal B24CZZ4
Placenta BY48ZZZ
Pleura BB4BZZZ
Prostate and Seminal Vesicle
BV49ZZZ
Rectum BD4CZZZ
Sacrum BR4FZZZ
Scrotum BV44ZZZ
Seminal Vesicle and Prostate
BV49ZZZ
Shoulder
Left, Densitometry BP49ZZ1
Right, Densitometry BP48ZZ1
Spinal Cord B04BZZZ
Spine
Cervical BR40ZZZ
Lumbar BR49ZZZ
Thoracic BR47ZZZ
Spleen and Liver BF46ZZZ
Stomach BD42ZZZ
Tendon
Lower Extremity BL43ZZZ
Upper Extremity BL42ZZZ
Ureter
Bilateral BT48ZZZ
Left BT47ZZZ
Right BT46ZZZ
Urethra BT45ZZZ
Uterus BU46
Uterus and Ovary BU4C
Vein
Jugular
Left, Intravascular B544ZZ3
Right, Intravascular B543ZZ3
Lower Extremity
Bilateral, Intravascular B54DZZ3
Left, Intravascular B54CZZ3
Right, Intravascular B54BZZ3
Portal, Intravascular B54TZZ3
Renal
Bilateral, Intravascular B54LZZ3
Left, Intravascular B54KZZ3
Right, Intravascular B54JZZ3
Spanchnic, Intravascular B54TZZ3
Subclavian
Left, Intravascular B547ZZ3
Right, Intravascular B546ZZ3
Upper Extremity
Bilateral, Intravascular B54PZZ3
Left, Intravascular B54NZZ3
Right, Intravascular B54MZZ3

Ultrasonography (Continued)
  Vena Cava
    Inferior, Intravascular B549ZZ3
    Superior, Intravascular B548ZZ3
  Wrist
    Left, Densitometry BP4MZZ1
    Right, Densitometry BP4LZZ1
Ultrasound bone healing system
  use Bone Growth Stimulator in Upper Bones
  use Bone Growth Stimulator in Head and
    Facial Bones
  use Bone Growth Stimulator in Lower Bones
Ultrasound Therapy
  Heart 6A75
  No Qualifier 6A75
  Vessels
    Head and Neck 6A75
    Other 6A75
    Peripheral 6A75
Ultraviolet Light Therapy, Skin 6A80
Umbilical artery
  use Artery, Internal Iliac, Left
  use Artery, Internal Iliac, Right
Uniplanar external fixator
  use External Fixation Device, Monoplanar in
    0PH
  use External Fixation Device, Monoplanar
    in 0PS
  use External Fixation Device, Monoplanar in
    0QH
  use External Fixation Device, Monoplanar
    in 0QS
Upper GI series *see* Fluoroscopy,
  Gastrointestinal, Upper BD15
Ureteral orifice
  use Ureter, Left
  use Ureter
  use Ureter, Right
  use Ureters, Bilateral
Ureterectomy
  see Excision, Urinary System 0TB
  see Resection, Urinary System 0TT
Ureterocolostomy *see* Bypass, Urinary System
  0T1
Ureterocystostomy *see* Bypass, Urinary System
  0T1
Ureteroenterostomy *see* Bypass, Urinary System
  0T1
Ureteroileostomy *see* Bypass, Urinary System
  0T1
Ureterolithotomy *see* Extirpation, Urinary
  System 0TC
Ureterolysis *see* Release, Urinary System 0TN
Ureteroneocystostomy
  see Bypass, Urinary System 0T1
  see Reposition, Urinary System 0TS
Ureteropelvic junction (UPJ)
  use Kidney Pelvis, Right
  use Kidney Pelvis, Left
Ureteropexy
  see Repair, Urinary System 0TQ
  see Reposition, Urinary System 0TS
Ureteroplasty
  see Repair, Urinary System 0TQ
  see Replacement, Urinary System 0TR
  see Supplement, Urinary System 0TU
Ureteroplication *see* Restriction, Urinary
  System 0TV
Ureteropyelography *see* Fluoroscopy, Urinary
  System BT1
Ureterorrhaphy *see* Repair, Urinary System 0TQ
Ureteroscopy 0TJ98ZZ
Ureterostomy
  see Bypass, Urinary System 0T1
  see Drainage, Urinary System 0T9
Ureterotomy *see* Drainage, Urinary System 0T9
Ureteroureterostomy *see* Bypass, Urinary
  System 0T1
Ureterovesical orifice
  use Ureter, Right
  use Ureter, Left

Ureterovesical orifice (Continued)
  use Ureters, Bilateral
  use Ureter
Urethral catheterization, indwelling
  0T9B70Z
Urethrectomy
  see Excision, Urethra 0TBD
  see Resection, Urethra 0TTD
Urethrolithotomy *see* Extirpation, Urethra
  0TCD
Urethrolysis *see* Release, Urethra 0TND
Urethropexy
  see Repair, Urethra 0TQD
  see Reposition, Urethra 0TSD
Urethroplasty
  see Repair, Urethra 0TQD
  see Replacement, Urethra 0TRD
  see Supplement, Urethra 0TUD
Urethrorrhaphy *see* Repair, Urethra 0TQD
Urethroscopy 0TJD8ZZ
Urethrotomy *see* Drainage, Urethra 0T9D
Urinary incontinence stimulator lead *use*
  Stimulator Lead in Urinary System
Urography *see* Fluoroscopy, Urinary System
  BT1
Uterine Artery
  use Artery, Internal Iliac, Left
  use Artery, Internal Iliac, Right
  Left, Occlusion, Artery, Internal Iliac, Left
    04LF
  Right, Occlusion, Artery, Internal Iliac, Right
    04LE
Uterine artery embolization (UAE) *see*
  Occlusion, Lower Arteries 04L
Uterine cornu *use* Uterus
Uterine tube
  use Fallopian Tube, Left
  use Fallopian Tube, Right
Uterine vein
  use Vein, Hypogastric, Left
  use Vein, Hypogastric, Right
Uvulectomy
  see Excision, Uvula 0CBN
  see Resection, Uvula 0CTN
Uvulorrhaphy *see* Repair, Uvula 0CQN
Uvulotomy *see* Drainage, Uvula 0C9N

V

Vaccination *see* Introduction of Serum, Toxoid,
  and Vaccine
Vacuum extraction, obstetric 10D07Z6
Vaginal artery
  use Artery, Internal Iliac, Right
  use Artery, Internal Iliac, Left
Vaginal pessary *use* Intraluminal Device,
  Pessary in Female Reproductive System
Vaginal vein
  use Vein, Hypogastric, Right
  use Vein, Hypogastric, Left
Vaginectomy
  see Excision, Vagina 0UBG
  see Resection, Vagina 0UTG
Vaginofixation
  see Repair, Vagina 0UQG
  see Reposition, Vagina 0USG
Vaginoplasty
  see Repair, Vagina 0UQG
  see Supplement, Vagina 0UUG
Vaginorrhaphy *see* Repair, Vagina 0UQG
Vaginoscopy 0UJH8ZZ
Vaginotomy *see* Drainage, Female Reproductive
  System 0U9
Vagotomy *see* Division, Nerve, Vagus 008Q
Valiant Thoracic Stent Graft *use* Intraluminal
  Device
Valvotomy, valvulotomy
  see Division, Heart and Great Vessels
    028
  see Release, Heart and Great Vessels
    02N

Valvuloplasty
  see Repair, Heart and Great Vessels 02Q
  see Replacement, Heart and Great Vessels 02R
  see Supplement, Heart and Great Vessels 02U
Vascular Access Device
  Insertion of device in
    Abdomen 0JH8
    Chest 0JH6
    Lower Arm
      Left 0JHH
      Right 0JHG
    Lower Leg
      Left 0JHP
      Right 0JHN
    Upper Arm
      Left 0JHF
      Right 0JHD
    Upper Leg
      Left 0JHM
      Right 0JHL
  Removal of device from
    Lower Extremity 0JPW
    Trunk 0JPT
    Upper Extremity 0JPV
  Reservoir
    Insertion of device in
      Abdomen 0JH8
      Chest 0JH6
      Lower Arm
        Left 0JHH
        Right 0JHG
      Lower Leg
        Left 0JHP
        Right 0JHN
      Upper Arm
        Left 0JHF
        Right 0JHD
      Upper Leg
        Left 0JHM
        Right 0JHL
    Removal of device from
      Lower Extremity 0JPW
      Trunk 0JPT
      Upper Extremity 0JPV
    Revision of device in
      Lower Extremity 0JWW
      Trunk 0JWT
      Upper Extremity 0JWV
  Revision of device in
    Lower Extremity 0JWW
    Trunk 0JWT
    Upper Extremity 0JWV
Vasectomy *see* Excision, Male Reproductive
  System 0VB
Vasography
  see Plain Radiography, Male Reproductive
    System BV0
  see Fluoroscopy, Male Reproductive System
    BV1
Vasoligation *see* Occlusion, Male Reproductive
  System 0VL
Vasorrhaphy *see* Repair, Male Reproductive
  System 0VQ
Vasostomy *see* Bypass, Male Reproductive
  System 0V1
Vasotomy
  Drainage *see* Drainage, Male Reproductive
    System 0V9
  With ligation *see* Occlusion, Male
    Reproductive System 0VL
Vasovasostomy *see* Repair, Male Reproductive
  System 0VQ
Vastus intermedius muscle
  use Muscle, Upper Leg, Right
  use Muscle, Upper Leg, Left
Vastus lateralis muscle
  use Muscle, Upper Leg, Left
  use Muscle, Upper Leg, Right
Vastus medialis muscle
  use Muscle, Upper Leg, Right
  use Muscle, Upper Leg, Left

◀ New ◀ Revised ~~deleted~~ Deleted

VCG (vectorcardiogram) *see* Measurement, Cardiac 4A02
Vectra® Vascular Access Graft *use* Vascular Access Device in Subcutaneous Tissue and Fascia
Venectomy
   see Excision, Upper Veins 05B
   see Excision, Lower Veins 06B
Venography
   see Plain Radiography, Veins B50
   see Fluoroscopy, Veins B51
Venorrhaphy
   see Repair, Upper Veins 05Q
   see Repair, Lower Veins 06Q
Venotripsy
   see Occlusion, Upper Veins 05L
   see Occlusion, Lower Veins 06L
Ventricular fold *use* Larynx
Ventriculoatriostomy *see* Bypass, Central Nervous System 001
Ventriculocisternostomy *see* Bypass, Central Nervous System 001
Ventriculogram, cardiac
   Combined left and right heart *see* Fluoroscopy, Heart, Right and Left B216
   Left ventricle *see* Fluoroscopy, Heart, Left B215
   Right ventricle *see* Fluoroscopy, Heart, Right B214
Ventriculopuncture, through previously implanted catheter 8C01X6J
Ventriculoscopy 00J04ZZ
Ventriculostomy
   External drainage *see* Drainage, Cerebral Ventricle 0096
   Internal shunt *see* Bypass, Cerebral Ventricle 0016
Ventriculovenostomy *see* Bypass, Cerebral Ventricle 0016
Ventrio™ Hernia Patch *use* Synthetic Substitute
VEP (visual evoked potential) 4A07X0Z
Vermiform appendix *use* Appendix
Vermilion border
   use Lip, Lower
   use Lip, Upper
Versa *use* Pacemaker, Dual Chamber in 0JH
Version, obstetric
   External 10S0XZZ
   Internal 10S07ZZ
Vertebral arch
   use Vertebra, Thoracic
   use Vertebra, Lumbar
   use Vertebra, Cervical
Vertebral canal *use* Spinal Canal
Vertebral foramen
   use Vertebra, Thoracic
   use Vertebra, Lumbar
   use Vertebra, Cervical
Vertebral lamina
   use Vertebra, Thoracic
   use Vertebra, Cervical
   use Vertebra, Lumbar
Vertebral pedicle
   use Vertebra, Lumbar
   use Vertebra, Thoracic
   use Vertebra, Cervical

Vesical vein
   use Vein, Hypogastric, Left
   use Vein, Hypogastric, Right
Vesicotomy *see* Drainage, Urinary System 0T9
Vesiculectomy
   see Excision, Male Reproductive System 0VB
   see Resection, Male Reproductive System 0VT
Vesiculogram, seminal *see* Plain Radiography, Male Reproductive System BV0
Vesiculotomy *see* Drainage, Male Reproductive System 0V9
Vestibular (Scarpa's) ganglion *use* Nerve, Acoustic
Vestibular Assessment F15Z
Vestibular nerve *use* Nerve, Acoustic
Vestibular Treatment F0C
Vestibulocochlear nerve *use* Nerve, Acoustic
Virchow's (supraclavicular) lymph node
   use Lymphatic, Neck, Left
   use Lymphatic, Neck, Right
Virtuoso (II) (DR) (VR) *use* Defibrillator Generator in 0JH
Vitrectomy
   see Excision, Eye 08B
   see Resection, Eye 08T
Vitreous body
   use Vitreous, Left
   use Vitreous, Right
Viva (XT)(S) *use* Cardiac Resynchronization Defibrillator Pulse Generator in 0JH ◀
Vocal fold
   use Vocal Cord, Left
   use Vocal Cord, Right
Vocational
   Assessment *see* Activities of Daily Living Assessment, Rehabilitation F02
   Retraining *see* Activities of Daily Living Treatment, Rehabilitation F08
Volar (palmar) digital vein
   use Vein, Hand, Left
   use Vein, Hand, Right
Volar (palmar) metacarpal vein
   use Vein, Hand, Right
   use Vein, Hand, Left
Vomer
   use Bone, Nasal
   use Septum, Nasal
Voraxaze *use* Glucarpidase ◀
Vulvectomy
   see Excision, Female Reproductive System 0UB
   see Resection, Female Reproductive System 0UT

W

WALLSTENT® Endoprosthesis *use* Intraluminal Device
Washing *see* Irrigation
Wedge resection, pulmonary *see* Excision, Respiratory System 0BB
Window *see* Drainage
Wiring, dental 2W31X9Z

X

Xact Carotid Stent System *use* Intraluminal Device ◀
X-ray *see* Plain Radiography
X-STOP® Spacer
   use Spinal Stabilization Device, Interspinous Process in 0RH
   use Spinal Stabilization Device, Interspinous Process in 0SH
Xenograft *use* Zooplastic Tissue in Heart and Great Vessels
~~XIENCE V Everolimus Eluting Coronary Stent System use Intraluminal Device, Drug-eluting in Heart and Great Vessels~~
XIENCE Everolimus Eluting Coronary Stent System *use* Intraluminal Device, Drug-eluting in Heart and Great Vessels ◀
Xiphoid process *use* Sternum
XLIF® System *use* Interbody Fusion Device in Lower Joints

Y

Yoga Therapy 8E0ZXY4

Z

Z-plasty, skin for scar contracture *see* Release, Skin and Breast 0HN
Zenith Flex® AAA Endovascular Graft *use* Intraluminal Device
Zenith TX2® TAA Endovascular Graft *use* Intraluminal Device
Zenith® Renu™ AAA Ancillary Graft *use* Intraluminal Device
Zilver® PTX® (paclitaxel) Drug-Eluting Peripheral Stent
   use Intraluminal Device, Drug-eluting in Upper Arteries
   use Intraluminal Device, Drug-eluting in Lower Arteries
Zimmer® NexGen® LPS Mobile Bearing Knee *use* Synthetic Substitute
Zimmer® NexGen® LPS-Flex Mobile Knee *use* Synthetic Substitute
Zonule of Zinn
   use Lens, Left
   use Lens, Right
Zotarolimus-eluting coronary stent *use* Intraluminal Device, Drug-eluting in Heart and Great Vessels
Zygomatic process of frontal bone
   use Bone, Frontal, Left
   use Bone, Frontal, Right
Zygomatic process of temporal bone
   use Bone, Temporal, Right
   use Bone, Temporal, Left
Zygomaticus muscle *use* Muscle, Facial
Zyvox *use* Oxazolidinones ◀

Appendices

DEFINITIONS
SECTION-CHARACTER

◀ New   ◀▥ Revised   ~~deleted~~ Deleted

SECTION 0 - MEDICAL AND SURGICAL
CHARACTER 3 - OPERATION

Alteration	**Definition:** Modifying the anatomic structure of a body part without affecting the function of the body part **Explanation:** Principal purpose is to improve appearance **Includes/Examples:** Face lift, breast augmentation
Bypass	**Definition:** Altering the route of passage of the contents of a tubular body part **Explanation:** Rerouting contents of a body part to a downstream area of the normal route, to a similar route and body part, or to an abnormal route and dissimilar body part. Includes one or more anastomoses, with or without the use of a device **Includes/Examples:** Coronary artery bypass, colostomy formation
Change	**Definition:** Taking out or off a device from a body part and putting back an identical or similar device in or on the same body part without cutting or puncturing the skin or a mucous membrane **Explanation:** All CHANGE procedures are coded using the approach EXTERNAL **Includes/Examples:** Urinary catheter change, gastrostomy tube change
Control	**Definition:** Stopping, or attempting to stop, postprocedural bleeding **Explanation:** The site of the bleeding is coded as an anatomical region and not to a specific body part **Includes/Examples:** Control of post-prostatectomy hemorrhage, control of post-tonsillectomy hemorrhage
Creation	**Definition:** Making a new genital structure that does not take over the function of a body part **Explanation:** Used only for sex change operations **Includes/Examples:** Creation of vagina in a male, creation of penis in a female
Destruction	**Definition:** Physical eradication of all or a portion of a body part by the direct use of energy, force, or a destructive agent **Explanation:** None of the body part is physically taken out **Includes/Examples:** Fulguration of rectal polyp, cautery of skin lesion

Detachment	**Definition:** Cutting off all or a portion of the upper or lower extremities **Explanation:** The body part value is the site of the detachment, with a qualifier if applicable to further specify the level where the extremity was detached **Includes/Examples:** Below knee amputation, disarticulation of shoulder
Dilation	**Definition:** Expanding an orifice or the lumen of a tubular body part **Explanation:** The orifice can be a natural orifice or an artificially created orifice. Accomplished by stretching a tubular body part using intraluminal pressure or by cutting part of the orifice or wall of the tubular body part **Includes/Examples:** Percutaneous transluminal angioplasty, pyloromyotomy
Division	**Definition:** Cutting into a body part, without draining fluids and/or gases from the body part, in order to separate or transect a body part **Explanation:** All or a portion of the body part is separated into two or more portions **Includes/Examples:** Spinal cordotomy, osteotomy
Drainage	**Definition:** Taking or letting out fluids and/or gases from a body part **Explanation:** The qualifier DIAGNOSTIC is used to identify drainage procedures that are biopsies **Includes/Examples:** Thoracentesis, incision and drainage
Excision	**Definition:** Cutting out or off, without replacement, a portion of a body part **Explanation:** The qualifier DIAGNOSTIC is used to identify excision procedures that are biopsies **Includes/Examples:** Partial nephrectomy, liver biopsy
Extirpation	**Definition:** Taking or cutting out solid matter from a body part **Explanation:** The solid matter may be an abnormal byproduct of a biological function or a foreign body; it may be imbedded in a body part or in the lumen of a tubular body part. The solid matter may or may not have been previously broken into pieces **Includes/Examples:** Thrombectomy, choledocholithotomy
Extraction	**Definition:** Pulling or stripping out or off all or a portion of a body part by the use of force **Explanation:** The qualifier DIAGNOSTIC is used to identify extraction procedures that are biopsies **Includes/Examples:** Dilation and curettage, vein stripping

◀ New ◀ Revised ~~deleted~~ Deleted

SECTION 0 - MEDICAL AND SURGICAL
CHARACTER 3 - OPERATION

Fragmentation	**Definition:** Breaking solid matter in a body part into pieces **Explanation:** Physical force (e.g., manual, ultrasonic) applied directly or indirectly is used to break the solid matter into pieces. The solid matter may be an abnormal byproduct of a biological function or a foreign body. The pieces of solid matter are not taken out **Includes/Examples:** Extracorporeal shockwave lithotripsy, transurethral lithotripsy
Fusion	**Definition:** Joining together portions of an articular body part rendering the articular body part immobile **Explanation:** The body part is joined together by fixation device, bone graft, or other means **Includes/Examples:** Spinal fusion, ankle arthrodesis
Insertion	**Definition:** Putting in a nonbiological appliance that monitors, assists, performs, or prevents a physiological function but does not physically take the place of a body part **Includes/Examples:** Insertion of radioactive implant, insertion of central venous catheter
Inspection	**Definition:** Visually and/or manually exploring a body part **Explanation:** Visual exploration may be performed with or without optical instrumentation. Manual exploration may be performed directly or through intervening body layers **Includes/Examples:** Diagnostic arthroscopy, exploratory laparotomy
Map	**Definition:** Locating the route of passage of electrical impulses and/or locating functional areas in a body part **Explanation:** Applicable only to the cardiac conduction mechanism and the central nervous system **Includes/Examples:** Cardiac mapping, cortical mapping
Occlusion	**Definition:** Completely closing an orifice or the lumen of a tubular body part **Explanation:** The orifice can be a natural orifice or an artificially created orifice **Includes/Examples:** Fallopian tube ligation, ligation of inferior vena cava
Reattachment	**Definition:** Putting back in or on all or a portion of a separated body part to its normal location or other suitable location **Explanation:** Vascular circulation and nervous pathways may or may not be reestablished **Includes/Examples:** Reattachment of hand, reattachment of avulsed kidney

Release	**Definition:** Freeing a body part from an abnormal physical constraint by cutting or by the use of force **Explanation:** Some of the restraining tissue may be taken out but none of the body part is taken out **Includes/Examples:** Adhesiolysis, carpal tunnel release
Removal	**Definition:** Taking out or off a device from a body part **Explanation:** If a device is taken out and a similar device put in without cutting or puncturing the skin or mucous membrane, the procedure is coded to the root operation CHANGE. Otherwise, the procedure for taking out a device is coded to the root operation REMOVAL **Includes/Examples:** Drainage tube removal, cardiac pacemaker removal
Repair	**Definition:** Restoring, to the extent possible, a body part to its normal anatomic structure and function **Explanation:** Used only when the method to accomplish the repair is not one of the other root operations **Includes/Examples:** Colostomy takedown, suture of laceration
Replacement	**Definition:** Putting in or on biological or synthetic material that physically takes the place and/or function of all or a portion of a body part **Explanation:** The body part may have been taken out or replaced, or may be taken out, physically eradicated, or rendered nonfunctional during the Replacement procedure. A Removal procedure is coded for taking out the device used in a previous replacement procedure **Includes/Examples:** Total hip replacement, bone graft, free skin graft
Reposition	**Definition:** Moving to its normal location, or other suitable location, all or a portion of a body part **Explanation:** The body part is moved to a new location from an abnormal location, or from a normal location where it is not functioning correctly. The body part may or may not be cut out or off to be moved to the new location **Includes/Examples:** Reposition of undescended testicle, fracture reduction
Resection	**Definition:** Cutting out or off, without replacement, all of a body part **Includes/Examples:** Total nephrectomy, total lobectomy of lung

SECTION 0 - MEDICAL AND SURGICAL
CHARACTER 3 - OPERATION

Restriction	**Definition:** Partially closing an orifice or the lumen of a tubular body part **Explanation:** The orifice can be a natural orifice or an artificially created orifice **Includes/Examples:** Esophagogastric fundoplication, cervical cerclage
Revision	**Definition:** Correcting, to the extent possible, a portion of a malfunctioning device or the position of a displaced device **Explanation:** Revision can include correcting a malfunctioning or displaced device by taking out or putting in components of the device such as a screw or pin **Includes/Examples:** Adjustment of position of pacemaker lead, recementing of hip prosthesis
Supplement	**Definition:** Putting in or on biological or synthetic material that physically reinforces and/or augments the function of a portion of a body part **Explanation:** The biological material is non-living, or is living and from the same individual. The body part may have been previously replaced, and the Supplement procedure is performed to physically reinforce and/or augment the function of the replaced body part **Includes/Examples:** Herniorrhaphy using mesh, free nerve graft, mitral valve ring annuloplasty, put a new acetabular liner in a previous hip replacement
Transfer	**Definition:** Moving, without taking out, all or a portion of a body part to another location to take over the function of all or a portion of a body part **Explanation:** The body part transferred remains connected to its vascular and nervous supply **Includes/Examples:** Tendon transfer, skin pedicle flap transfer
Transplantation	**Definition:** Putting in or on all or a portion of a living body part taken from another individual or animal to physically take the place and/or function of all or a portion of a similar body part **Explanation:** The native body part may or may not be taken out, and the transplanted body part may take over all or a portion of its function **Includes/Examples:** Kidney transplant, heart transplant

SECTION 0 - MEDICAL AND SURGICAL
CHARACTER 4 - BODY PART

1st Toe, Left 1st Toe, Right	**Includes:** Hallux
Abdomen Muscle, Left Abdomen Muscle, Right	**Includes:** External oblique muscle Internal oblique muscle Pyramidalis muscle Rectus abdominis muscle Transversus abdominis muscle
Abdominal Aorta	**Includes:** Inferior phrenic artery Lumbar artery Median sacral artery Middle suprarenal artery Ovarian artery Testicular artery
Abdominal Sympathetic Nerve	**Includes:** Abdominal aortic plexus Auerbach's (myenteric) plexus Celiac (solar) plexus Celiac ganglion Gastric plexus Hepatic plexus Inferior hypogastric plexus Inferior mesenteric ganglion Inferior mesenteric plexus Meissner's (submucous) plexus Myenteric (Auerbach's) plexus Pancreatic plexus Pelvic splanchnic nerve Renal plexus Solar (celiac) plexus Splenic plexus Submucous (Meissner's) plexus Superior hypogastric plexus Superior mesenteric ganglion Superior mesenteric plexus Suprarenal plexus

◀ New ◀▬ Revised ~~deleted~~ Deleted

SECTION 0, CHARACTER 3; 4

SECTION 0 - MEDICAL AND SURGICAL
CHARACTER 4 - BODY PART

Abducens Nerve	**Includes:** Sixth cranial nerve
Accessory Nerve	**Includes:** Eleventh cranial nerve
Acoustic Nerve	**Includes:** Cochlear nerve Eighth cranial nerve Scarpa's (vestibular) ganglion Spiral ganglion Vestibular (Scarpa's) ganglion Vestibular nerve Vestibulocochlear nerve
Adenoids	**Includes:** Pharyngeal tonsil
Adrenal Gland Adrenal Gland, Left Adrenal Gland, Right Adrenal Glands, Bilateral	**Includes:** Suprarenal gland
Ampulla of Vater	**Includes:** Duodenal ampulla Hepatopancreatic ampulla
Anal Sphincter	**Includes:** External anal sphincter Internal anal sphincter
Ankle Bursa and Ligament, Left Ankle Bursa and Ligament, Right	**Includes:** Calcaneofibular ligament Deltoid ligament Ligament of the lateral malleolus Talofibular ligament
Ankle Joint, Left Ankle Joint, Right	**Includes:** Inferior tibiofibular joint Talocrural joint
Anterior Chamber, Left Anterior Chamber, Right	**Includes:** Aqueous humour
Anterior Tibial Artery, Left Anterior Tibial Artery, Right	**Includes:** Anterior lateral malleolar artery Anterior medial malleolar artery Anterior tibial recurrent artery Dorsalis pedis artery Posterior tibial recurrent artery
Anus	**Includes:** Anal orifice
Aortic Valve	**Includes:** Aortic annulus

Appendix	**Includes:** Vermiform appendix
Ascending Colon	**Includes:** Hepatic flexure
Atrial Septum	**Includes:** Interatrial septum
Atrium, Left	**Includes:** Atrium pulmonale Left auricular appendix
Atrium, Right	**Includes:** Atrium dextrum cordis Right auricular appendix Sinus venosus
Auditory Ossicle, Left Auditory Ossicle, Right	**Includes:** Incus Malleus Ossicular chain Stapes
Axillary Artery, Left Axillary Artery, Right	**Includes:** Anterior circumflex humeral artery Lateral thoracic artery Posterior circumflex humeral artery Subscapular artery Superior thoracic artery Thoracoacromial artery
Azygos Vein	**Includes:** Right ascending lumbar vein Right subcostal vein
Basal Ganglia	**Includes:** Basal nuclei Claustrum Corpus striatum Globus pallidus Substantia nigra Subthalamic nucleus
Basilic Vein, Left Basilic Vein, Right	**Includes:** Median antebrachial vein Median cubital vein
Bladder	**Includes:** Trigone of bladder
Brachial Artery, Left Brachial Artery, Right	**Includes:** Inferior ulnar collateral artery Profunda brachii Superior ulnar collateral artery

◄ New   ◄ Revised   ~~deleted~~ Deleted

SECTION 0 - MEDICAL AND SURGICAL
CHARACTER 4 - BODY PART

Brachial Plexus	**Includes:** Axillary nerve Dorsal scapular nerve First intercostal nerve Long thoracic nerve Musculocutaneous nerve Subclavius nerve Suprascapular nerve
Brachial Vein, Left Brachial Vein, Right	**Includes:** Radial vein Ulnar vein
Brain	**Includes:** Cerebrum Corpus callosum Encephalon
Breast, Bilateral Breast, Left Breast, Right	**Includes:** Mammary duct Mammary gland
Buccal Mucosa	**Includes:** Buccal gland Molar gland Palatine gland
Carotid Bodies, Bilateral Carotid Body, Left Carotid Body, Right	**Includes:** Carotid glomus
Carpal Joint, Left Carpal Joint, Right	**Includes:** Intercarpal joint Midcarpal joint
Carpal, Left Carpal, Right	**Includes:** Capitate bone Hamate bone Lunate bone Pisiform bone Scaphoid bone Trapezium bone Trapezoid bone Triquetral bone
Celiac Artery	**Includes:** Celiac trunk
Cephalic Vein, Left Cephalic Vein, Right	**Includes:** Accessory cephalic vein
Cerebellum	**Includes:** Culmen
Cerebral Hemisphere	**Includes:** Frontal lobe Occipital lobe Parietal lobe Temporal lobe

Cerebral Meninges	**Includes:** Arachnoid mater Leptomeninges Pia mater
Cerebral Ventricle	**Includes:** Aqueduct of Sylvius Cerebral aqueduct (Sylvius) Choroid plexus Ependyma Foramen of Monro (intraventricular) Fourth ventricle Interventricular foramen (Monro) Left lateral ventricle Right lateral ventricle Third ventricle
Cervical Nerve	**Includes:** Greater occipital nerve Spinal nerve, cervical Suboccipital nerve Third occipital nerve
Cervical Plexus	**Includes:** Ansa cervicalis Cutaneous (transverse) cervical nerve Great auricular nerve Lesser occipital nerve Supraclavicular nerve Transverse (cutaneous) cervical nerve
Cervical Vertebra	**Includes:** Spinous process Vertebral arch Vertebral foramen Vertebral lamina Vertebral pedicle
Cervical Vertebral Joint	**Includes:** Atlantoaxial joint Cervical facet joint
Cervical Vertebral Joints, 2 or more	**Includes:** Cervical facet joint
Cervicothoracic Vertebral Joint	**Includes:** Cervicothoracic facet joint
Cisterna Chyli	**Includes:** Intestinal lymphatic trunk Lumbar lymphatic trunk
Coccygeal Glomus	**Includes:** Coccygeal body
Colic Vein	**Includes:** Ileocolic vein Left colic vein Middle colic vein Right colic vein

◀ New   ◀▬ Revised   ~~deleted~~ Deleted

SECTION 0 - MEDICAL AND SURGICAL
CHARACTER 4 - BODY PART

Conduction Mechanism	**Includes:** Atrioventricular node Bundle of His Bundle of Kent Sinoatrial node
Conjunctiva, Left Conjunctiva, Right	**Includes:** Plica semilunaris
Dura Mater	**Includes:** Cranial dura mater Dentate ligament Diaphragma sellae Falx cerebri Spinal dura mater Tentorium cerebelli
Elbow Bursa and Ligament, Left Elbow Bursa and Ligament, Right	**Includes:** Annular ligament Olecranon bursa Radial collateral ligament Ulnar collateral ligament
Elbow Joint, Left Elbow Joint, Right	**Includes:** Distal humerus, involving joint Humeroradial joint Humeroulnar joint Proximal radioulnar joint
Epidural Space	**Includes:** Cranial epidural space Extradural space Spinal epidural space
Epiglottis	**Includes:** Glossoepiglottic fold
Esophagogastric Junction	**Includes:** Cardia Cardioesophageal junction Gastroesophageal (GE) junction
Esophagus, Lower	**Includes:** Abdominal esophagus
Esophagus, Middle	**Includes:** Thoracic esophagus
Esophagus, Upper	**Includes:** Cervical esophagus
Ethmoid Bone, Left Ethmoid Bone, Right	**Includes:** Cribriform plate
Ethmoid Sinus, Left Ethmoid Sinus, Right	**Includes:** Ethmoidal air cell

Eustachian Tube, Left Eustachian Tube, Right	**Includes:** Auditory tube Pharyngotympanic tube
External Auditory Canal, Left External Auditory Canal, Right	**Includes:** External auditory meatus
External Carotid Artery, Left External Carotid Artery, Right	**Includes:** Ascending pharyngeal artery Internal maxillary artery Lingual artery Maxillary artery Occipital artery Posterior auricular artery Superior thyroid artery
External Ear, Bilateral External Ear, Left External Ear, Right	**Includes:** Antihelix Antitragus Auricle Earlobe Helix Pinna Tragus
External Iliac Artery, Left External Iliac Artery, Right	**Includes:** Deep circumflex iliac artery Inferior epigastric artery
External Jugular Vein, Left External Jugular Vein, Right	**Includes:** Posterior auricular vein
Extraocular Muscle, Left Extraocular Muscle, Right	**Includes:** Inferior oblique muscle Inferior rectus muscle Lateral rectus muscle Medial rectus muscle Superior oblique muscle Superior rectus muscle
Eye, Left Eye, Right	**Includes:** Ciliary body Posterior chamber
Face Artery	**Includes:** Angular artery Ascending palatine artery External maxillary artery Facial artery Inferior labial artery Submental artery Superior labial artery

SECTION 0 - MEDICAL AND SURGICAL
CHARACTER 4 - BODY PART

SECTION 0 - MEDICAL AND
CHARACTER 4 - BODY PART

Face Vein, Left Face Vein, Right	**Includes:** Angular vein Anterior facial vein Common facial vein Deep facial vein Frontal vein Posterior facial (retromandibular) vein Supraorbital vein
Facial Muscle	**Includes:** Buccinator muscle Corrugator supercilii muscle Depressor anguli oris muscle Depressor labii inferioris muscle Depressor septi nasi muscle Depressor supercilii muscle Levator anguli oris muscle Levator labii superioris alaeque nasi muscle Levator labii superioris muscle Mentalis muscle Nasalis muscle Occipitofrontalis muscle Orbicularis oris muscle Procerus muscle Risorius muscle Zygomaticus muscle
Facial Nerve	**Includes:** Chorda tympani Geniculate ganglion Greater superficial petrosal nerve Nerve to the stapedius Parotid plexus Posterior auricular nerve Seventh cranial nerve Submandibular ganglion
Fallopian Tube, Left Fallopian Tube, Right	**Includes:** Oviduct Salpinx Uterine tube
Femoral Artery, Left Femoral Artery, Right	**Includes:** Circumflex iliac artery Deep femoral artery Descending genicular artery External pudendal artery Superficial epigastric artery
Femoral Nerve	**Includes:** Anterior crural nerve Saphenous nerve
Femoral Shaft, Left Femoral Shaft, Right	**Includes:** Body of femur

Femoral Vein, Left Femoral Vein, Right	**Includes:** Deep femoral (profunda femoris) vein Popliteal vein Profunda femoris (deep femoral) vein
Fibula, Left Fibula, Right	**Includes:** Body of fibula Head of fibula Lateral malleolus
Finger Nail	**Includes:** Nail bed Nail plate
Finger Phalangeal Joint, Left Finger Phalangeal Joint, Right	**Includes:** Interphalangeal (IP) joint
Foot Artery, Left Foot Artery, Right	**Includes:** Arcuate artery Dorsal metatarsal artery Lateral plantar artery Lateral tarsal artery Medial plantar artery
Foot Bursa and Ligament, Left Foot Bursa and Ligament, Right	**Includes:** Calcaneocuboid ligament Cuneonavicular ligament Intercuneiform ligament Interphalangeal ligament Metatarsal ligament Metatarsophalangeal ligament Subtalar ligament Talocalcaneal ligament Talocalcaneonavicular ligament Tarsometatarsal ligament
Foot Muscle, Left Foot Muscle, Right	**Includes:** Abductor hallucis muscle Adductor hallucis muscle Extensor digitorum brevis muscle Extensor hallucis brevis muscle Flexor digitorum brevis muscle Flexor hallucis brevis muscle Quadratus plantae muscle
Foot Vein, Left Foot Vein, Right	**Includes:** Common digital vein Dorsal metatarsal vein Dorsal venous arch Plantar digital vein Plantar metatarsal vein Plantar venous arch
Frontal Bone, Left Frontal Bone, Right	**Includes:** Zygomatic process of frontal bone

◄ New   ◄ Revised   ~~deleted~~ Deleted

SECTION 0 - MEDICAL AND SURGICAL
CHARACTER 4 - BODY PART

Gastric Artery	**Includes:** Left gastric artery Right gastric artery
Glenoid Cavity, Left Glenoid Cavity, Right	**Includes:** Glenoid fossa (of scapula)
Glomus Jugulare	**Includes:** Jugular body
Glossopharyngeal Nerve	**Includes:** Carotid sinus nerve Ninth cranial nerve Tympanic nerve
Greater Omentum	**Includes:** Gastrocolic ligament Gastrocolic omentum Gastrophrenic ligament Gastrosplenic ligament
Greater Saphenous Vein, Left Greater Saphenous Vein, Right	**Includes:** External pudendal vein Great saphenous vein Superficial circumflex iliac vein Superficial epigastric vein
Hand Artery, Left Hand Artery, Right	**Includes:** Deep palmar arch Princeps pollicis artery Radialis indicis Superficial palmar arch
Hand Bursa and Ligament, Left Hand Bursa and Ligament, Right	**Includes:** Carpometacarpal ligament Intercarpal ligament Interphalangeal ligament Lunotriquetral ligament Metacarpal ligament Metacarpophalangeal ligament Pisohamate ligament Pisometacarpal ligament Scapholunate ligament Scaphotrapezium ligament
Hand Muscle, Left Hand Muscle, Right	**Includes:** Hypothenar muscle Palmar interosseous muscle Thenar muscle
Hand Vein, Left Hand Vein, Right	**Includes:** Dorsal metacarpal vein Palmar (volar) digital vein Palmar (volar) metacarpal vein Superficial palmar venous arch Volar (palmar) digital vein Volar (palmar) metacarpal vein
Head and Neck Bursa and Ligament	**Includes:** Alar ligament of axis Cervical interspinous ligament Cervical intertransverse ligament Cervical ligamentum flavum Lateral temporomandibular ligament Sphenomandibular ligament Stylomandibular ligament Transverse ligament of atlas
Head and Neck Sympathetic Nerve	**Includes:** Cavernous plexus Cervical ganglion Ciliary ganglion Internal carotid plexus Otic ganglion Pterygopalatine (sphenopalatine) ganglion Sphenopalatine (pterygopalatine) ganglion Stellate ganglion Submandibular ganglion Submaxillary ganglion
Head Muscle	**Includes:** Auricularis muscle Masseter muscle Pterygoid muscle Splenius capitis muscle Temporalis muscle Temporoparietalis muscle
Heart, Left	**Includes:** Left coronary sulcus Obtuse margin
Heart, Right	**Includes:** Right coronary sulcus
Hemiazygos Vein	**Includes** Left ascending lumbar vein Left subcostal vein
Hepatic Artery	**Includes:** Common hepatic artery Gastroduodenal artery Hepatic artery proper
Hip Bursa and Ligament, Left Hip Bursa and Ligament, Right	**Includes:** Iliofemoral ligament Ischiofemoral ligament Pubofemoral ligament Transverse acetabular ligament Trochanteric bursa
Hip Joint, Left Hip Joint, Right	**Includes:** Acetabulofemoral joint

SECTION 0 - MEDICAL AND SURGICAL
CHARACTER 4 - BODY PART

Hip Muscle, Left Hip Muscle, Right	**Includes:** Gemellus muscle Gluteus maximus muscle Gluteus medius muscle Gluteus minimus muscle Iliacus muscle Obturator muscle Piriformis muscle Psoas muscle Quadratus femoris muscle Tensor fasciae latae muscle
Humeral Head, Left Humeral Head, Right	**Includes:** Greater tuberosity Lesser tuberosity Neck of humerus (anatomical) (surgical)
Humeral Shaft, Left Humeral Shaft, Right	**Includes:** Distal humerus Humerus, distal Lateral epicondyle of humerus Medial epicondyle of humerus
Hypogastric Vein, Left Hypogastric Vein, Right	**Includes:** Gluteal vein Internal iliac vein Internal pudendal vein Lateral sacral vein Middle hemorrhoidal vein Obturator vein Uterine vein Vaginal vein Vesical vein
Hypoglossal Nerve	**Includes:** Twelfth cranial nerve
Hypothalamus	**Includes:** Mammillary body
Inferior Mesenteric Artery	**Includes:** Sigmoid artery Superior rectal artery
Inferior Mesenteric Vein	**Includes:** Sigmoid vein Superior rectal vein
Inferior Vena Cava	**Includes:** Postcava Right inferior phrenic vein Right ovarian vein Right second lumbar vein Right suprarenal vein Right testicular vein

Inguinal Region, Bilateral Inguinal Region, Left Inguinal Region, Right	**Includes:** Inguinal canal Inguinal triangle
Inner Ear, Left Inner Ear, Right	**Includes:** Bony labyrinth Bony vestibule Cochlea Round window Semicircular canal
Innominate Artery	**Includes:** Brachiocephalic artery Brachiocephalic trunk
Innominate Vein, Left Innominate Vein, Right	**Includes:** Brachiocephalic vein Inferior thyroid vein
Internal Carotid Artery, Left Internal Carotid Artery, Right	**Includes:** Caroticotympanic artery Carotid sinus Ophthalmic artery
Internal Iliac Artery, Left Internal Iliac Artery, Right	**Includes:** Deferential artery Hypogastric artery Iliolumbar artery Inferior gluteal artery Inferior vesical artery Internal pudendal artery Lateral sacral artery Middle rectal artery Obturator artery Superior gluteal artery Umbilical artery Uterine artery Vaginal artery
Internal Mammary Artery, Left Internal Mammary Artery, Right	**Includes:** Anterior intercostal artery Internal thoracic artery Musculophrenic artery Pericardiophrenic artery Superior epigastric artery
Intracranial Artery	**Includes:** Anterior cerebral artery Anterior choroidal artery Anterior communicating artery Basilar artery Circle of Willis Middle cerebral artery Posterior cerebral artery Posterior communicating artery Posterior inferior cerebellar artery (PICA)

◀ New   ◀||| Revised   ~~deleted~~ Deleted

SECTION 0 - MEDICAL AND SURGICAL
CHARACTER 4 - BODY PART

Intracranial Vein	**Includes:** Anterior cerebral vein Basal (internal) cerebral vein Dural venous sinus Great cerebral vein Inferior cerebellar vein Inferior cerebral vein Internal (basal) cerebral vein Middle cerebral vein Ophthalmic vein Superior cerebellar vein Superior cerebral vein
Jejunum	**Includes:** Duodenojejunal flexure
Kidney	**Includes:** Renal calyx Renal capsule Renal cortex Renal segment
Kidney Pelvis, Left Kidney Pelvis, Right	**Includes:** Ureteropelvic junction (UPJ)
Kidney, Left Kidney, Right Kidneys, Bilateral	**Includes:** Renal calyx Renal capsule Renal cortex Renal segment
Knee Bursa and Ligament, Left Knee Bursa and Ligament, Right	**Includes:** Anterior cruciate ligament (ACL) Lateral collateral ligament (LCL) Ligament of head of fibula Medial collateral ligament (MCL) Patellar ligament Popliteal ligament Posterior cruciate ligament (PCL) Prepatellar bursa
Knee Joint, Femoral Surface, Left Knee Joint, Femoral Surface, Right	**Includes:** Femoropatellar joint Patellofemoral joint
Knee Joint, Left Knee Joint, Right	**Includes:** Femoropatellar joint Femorotibial joint Lateral meniscus Medial meniscus Patellofemoral joint Tibiofemoral joint
Knee Joint, Tibial Surface, Left Knee Joint, Tibial Surface, Right	**Includes:** Femorotibial joint Tibiofemoral joint

Knee Tendon, Left Knee Tendon, Right	**Includes:** Patellar tendon
Lacrimal Duct, Left Lacrimal Duct, Right	**Includes:** Lacrimal canaliculus Lacrimal punctum Lacrimal sac Nasolacrimal duct
Larynx	**Includes:** Aryepiglottic fold Arytenoid cartilage Corniculate cartilage Cricoid cartilage Cuneiform cartilage False vocal cord Glottis Rima glottidis Thyroid cartilage Ventricular fold
Lens, Left Lens, Right	**Includes:** Zonule of Zinn
Lesser Omentum	**Includes:** Gastrohepatic omentum Hepatogastric ligament
Lesser Saphenous Vein, Left Lesser Saphenous Vein, Right	**Includes:** Small saphenous vein
Liver	**Includes:** Quadrate lobe
Lower Arm and Wrist Muscle, Left Lower Arm and Wrist Muscle, Right	**Includes:** Anatomical snuffbox Brachioradialis muscle Extensor carpi radialis muscle Extensor carpi ulnaris muscle Flexor carpi radialis muscle Flexor carpi ulnaris muscle Flexor pollicis longus muscle Palmaris longus muscle Pronator quadratus muscle Pronator teres muscle
Lower Eyelid, Left Lower Eyelid, Right	**Includes:** Inferior tarsal plate Medial canthus
Lower Femur, Left Lower Femur, Right	**Includes:** Lateral condyle of femur Lateral epicondyle of femur Medial condyle of femur Medial epicondyle of femur

SECTION 0 - MEDICAL AND SURGICAL
CHARACTER 4 - BODY PART

Body Part	Includes
Lower Leg Muscle, Left Lower Leg Muscle, Right	**Includes:** Extensor digitorum longus muscle Extensor hallucis longus muscle Fibularis brevis muscle Fibularis longus muscle Flexor digitorum longus muscle Flexor hallucis longus muscle Gastrocnemius muscle Peroneus brevis muscle Peroneus longus muscle Popliteus muscle Soleus muscle Tibialis anterior muscle Tibialis posterior muscle
Lower Leg Tendon, Left Lower Leg Tendon, Right	**Includes:** Achilles tendon
Lower Lip	**Includes:** Frenulum labii inferioris Labial gland Vermilion border
Lumbar Nerve	**Includes:** Lumbosacral trunk Spinal nerve, lumbar Superior clunic (cluneal) nerve
Lumbar Plexus	**Includes:** Accessory obturator nerve Genitofemoral nerve Iliohypogastric nerve Ilioinguinal nerve Lateral femoral cutaneous nerve Obturator nerve Superior gluteal nerve
Lumbar Spinal Cord	**Includes:** Cauda equina Conus medullaris
Lumbar Sympathetic Nerve	**Includes:** Lumbar ganglion Lumbar splanchnic nerve
Lumbar Vertebra	**Includes:** Spinous process Vertebral arch Vertebral foramen Vertebral lamina Vertebral pedicle
~~Lumbar Vertebral Joint~~ ~~Lumbar Vertebral Joints, 2 or more~~	~~Includes:~~ ~~Lumbar facet joint~~
Lumbar Vertebral Joint ◄	**Includes:** Lumbar facet joint ◄

Body Part	Includes
Lumbosacral Joint	**Includes:** Lumbosacral facet joint
Lymphatic, Aortic	**Includes:** Celiac lymph node Gastric lymph node Hepatic lymph node Lumbar lymph node Pancreaticosplenic lymph node Paraaortic lymph node Retroperitoneal lymph node
Lymphatic, Head	**Includes:** Buccinator lymph node Infraauricular lymph node Infraparotid lymph node Parotid lymph node Preauricular lymph node Submandibular lymph node Submaxillary lymph node Submental lymph node Subparotid lymph node Suprahyoid lymph node
Lymphatic, Left Axillary	**Includes:** Anterior (pectoral) lymph node Apical (subclavicular) lymph node Brachial (lateral) lymph node Central axillary lymph node Lateral (brachial) lymph node Pectoral (anterior) lymph node Posterior (subscapular) lymph node Subclavicular (apical) lymph node Subscapular (posterior) lymph node
Lymphatic, Left Lower Extremity	**Includes:** Femoral lymph node Popliteal lymph node
Lymphatic, Left Neck	**Includes:** Cervical lymph node Jugular lymph node Mastoid (postauricular) lymph node Occipital lymph node Postauricular (mastoid) lymph node Retropharyngeal lymph node Supraclavicular (Virchow's) lymph node Virchow's (supraclavicular) lymph node
Lymphatic, Left Upper Extremity	**Includes:** Cubital lymph node Deltopectoral (infraclavicular) lymph node Epitrochlear lymph node Infraclavicular (deltopectoral) lymph node Supratrochlear lymph node
Lymphatic, Mesenteric	**Includes:** Inferior mesenteric lymph node Pararectal lymph node Superior mesenteric lymph node

◄ New   ⇐ Revised   ~~deleted~~ Deleted

SECTION 0 - MEDICAL AND SURGICAL
CHARACTER 4 - BODY PART

Lymphatic, Pelvis	**Includes:** Common iliac (subaortic) lymph node Gluteal lymph node Iliac lymph node Inferior epigastric lymph node Obturator lymph node Sacral lymph node Subaortic (common iliac) lymph node Suprainguinal lymph node
Lymphatic, Right Axillary	**Includes:** Anterior (pectoral) lymph node Apical (subclavicular) lymph node Brachial (lateral) lymph node Central axillary lymph node Lateral (brachial) lymph node Pectoral (anterior) lymph node Posterior (subscapular) lymph node Subclavicular (apical) lymph node Subscapular (posterior) lymph node
Lymphatic, Right Lower Extremity	**Includes:** Femoral lymph node Popliteal lymph node
Lymphatic, Right Neck	**Includes:** Cervical lymph node Jugular lymph node Mastoid (postauricular) lymph node Occipital lymph node Postauricular (mastoid) lymph node Retropharyngeal lymph node Right jugular trunk Right lymphatic duct Right subclavian trunk Supraclavicular (Virchow's) lymph node Virchow's (supraclavicular) lymph node
Lymphatic, Right Upper Extremity	**Includes:** Cubital lymph node Deltopectoral (infraclavicular) lymph node Epitrochlear lymph node Infraclavicular (deltopectoral) lymph node Supratrochlear lymph node
Lymphatic, Thorax	**Includes:** Intercostal lymph node Mediastinal lymph node Parasternal lymph node Paratracheal lymph node Tracheobronchial lymph node
Mandible, Left Mandible, Right	**Includes:** Alveolar process of mandible Condyloid process Mandibular notch Mental foramen
Mastoid Sinus, Left Mastoid Sinus, Right	**Includes:** Mastoid air cells
Maxilla, Left Maxilla, Right	**Includes:** Alveolar process of maxilla
Maxillary Sinus, Left Maxillary Sinus, Right	**Includes:** Antrum of Highmore
Median Nerve	**Includes:** Anterior interosseous nerve Palmar cutaneous nerve
Medulla Oblongata	**Includes:** Myelencephalon
Mesentery	**Includes:** Mesoappendix Mesocolon
Metacarpocarpal Joint, Left Metacarpocarpal Joint, Right	**Includes:** Carpometacarpal (CMC) joint
Metatarsal-Phalangeal Joint, Left Metatarsal-Phalangeal Joint, Right	**Includes:** Metatarsophalangeal (MTP) joint
Metatarsal-Tarsal Joint, Left Metatarsal-Tarsal Joint, Right	**Includes:** Tarsometatarsal joint
Middle Ear, Left Middle Ear, Right	**Includes:** Oval window Tympanic cavity
Minor Salivary Gland	**Includes:** Anterior lingual gland
Mitral Valve	**Includes:** Bicuspid valve Left atrioventricular valve Mitral annulus
Nasal Bone	**Includes:** Vomer of nasal septum
Nasal Septum	**Includes:** Quadrangular cartilage Septal cartilage Vomer bone

SECTION 0 - MEDICAL AND SURGICAL
CHARACTER 4 - BODY PART

Nasal Turbinate	**Includes:** Inferior turbinate Middle turbinate Nasal concha Superior turbinate	**Pancreatic Duct**	**Includes:** Duct of Wirsung
Nasopharynx	**Includes:** Choana Fossa of Rosenmuller Pharyngeal recess Rhinopharynx	**Pancreatic Duct, Accessory**	**Includes:** Duct of Santorini
Neck Muscle, Left **Neck Muscle, Right**	**Includes:** Anterior vertebral muscle Arytenoid muscle Cricothyroid muscle Infrahyoid muscle Levator scapulae muscle Platysma muscle Scalene muscle Splenius cervicis muscle Sternocleidomastoid muscle Suprahyoid muscle Thyroarytenoid muscle	**Parotid Duct, Left** **Parotid Duct, Right**	**Includes:** Stensen's duct
		Pelvic Bone, Left **Pelvic Bone, Right**	**Includes:** Iliac crest Ilium Ischium Pubis
		Pelvic Cavity	**Includes:** Retropubic space
		Penis	**Includes:** Corpus cavernosum Corpus spongiosum
Nipple, Left **Nipple, Right**	**Includes:** Areola	**Perineum Muscle**	**Includes:** Bulbospongiosus muscle Cremaster muscle Deep transverse perineal muscle Ischiocavernosus muscle Superficial transverse perineal muscle
Nose	**Includes:** Columella External naris Greater alar cartilage Internal naris Lateral nasal cartilage Lesser alar cartilage Nasal cavity Nostril		
		Peritoneum	**Includes:** Epiploic foramen
		Peroneal Artery, Left **Peroneal Artery, Right**	**Includes:** Fibular artery
Occipital Bone, Left **Occipital Bone, Right**	**Includes:** Foramen magnum		
Oculomotor Nerve	**Includes:** Third cranial nerve	**Peroneal Nerve**	**Includes:** Common fibular nerve Common peroneal nerve External popliteal nerve Lateral sural cutaneous nerve
Olfactory Nerve	**Includes:** First cranial nerve Olfactory bulb		
		Pharynx	**Includes:** Hypopharynx Laryngopharynx Oropharynx Piriform recess (sinus)
Optic Nerve	**Includes:** Optic chiasma Second cranial nerve		
		Phrenic Nerve	**Includes:** Accessory phrenic nerve
Orbit, Left **Orbit, Right**	**Includes:** Bony orbit Orbital portion of ethmoid bone Orbital portion of frontal bone Orbital portion of lacrimal bone Orbital portion of maxilla Orbital portion of palatine bone Orbital portion of sphenoid bone Orbital portion of zygomatic bone	**Pituitary Gland**	**Includes:** Adenohypophysis Hypophysis Neurohypophysis

◀ New   ◀III Revised   ~~deleted~~ Deleted

SECTION 0 - MEDICAL AND SURGICAL
CHARACTER 4 - BODY PART

Pons	**Includes:** Apneustic center Basis pontis Locus ceruleus Pneumotaxic center Pontine tegmentum Superior olivary nucleus
Popliteal Artery, Left Popliteal Artery, Right	**Includes:** Inferior genicular artery Middle genicular artery Superior genicular artery Sural artery
Portal Vein	**Includes:** Hepatic portal vein
Prepuce	**Includes:** Foreskin Glans penis
Pudendal Nerve	**Includes:** Posterior labial nerve Posterior scrotal nerve
Pulmonary Artery, Left	**Includes:** Arterial canal (duct) Botallo's duct Pulmoaortic canal
Pulmonary Valve	**Includes:** Pulmonary annulus Pulmonic valve
Pulmonary Vein, Left	**Includes:** Left inferior pulmonary vein Left superior pulmonary vein
Pulmonary Vein, Right	**Includes:** Right inferior pulmonary vein Right superior pulmonary vein
Radial Artery, Left Radial Artery, Right	**Includes:** Radial recurrent artery
Radial Nerve	**Includes:** Dorsal digital nerve Musculospiral nerve Palmar cutaneous nerve Posterior interosseous nerve
Radius, Left Radius, Right	**Includes:** Ulnar notch
Rectum	**Includes:** Anorectal junction
Renal Artery, Left Renal Artery, Right	**Includes:** Inferior suprarenal artery Renal segmental artery

Renal Vein, Left	**Includes:** Left inferior phrenic vein Left ovarian vein Left second lumbar vein Left suprarenal vein Left testicular vein
Retina, Left Retina, Right	**Includes:** Fovea Macula Optic disc
Retroperitoneum	**Includes:** Retroperitoneal space
Sacral Nerve	**Includes:** Spinal nerve, sacral
Sacral Plexus	**Includes:** Inferior gluteal nerve Posterior femoral cutaneous nerve Pudendal nerve
Sacral Sympathetic Nerve	**Includes:** Ganglion impar (ganglion of Walther) Pelvic splanchnic nerve Sacral ganglion Sacral splanchnic nerve
Sacrococcygeal Joint	**Includes:** Sacrococcygeal symphysis
Scapula, Left Scapula, Right	**Includes:** Acromion (process) Coracoid process
Sciatic Nerve	**Includes:** Ischiatic nerve
Shoulder Bursa and Ligament, Left Shoulder Bursa and Ligament, Right	**Includes:** Acromioclavicular ligament Coracoacromial ligament Coracoclavicular ligament Coracohumeral ligament Costoclavicular ligament Glenohumeral ligament Glenoid ligament (labrum) Interclavicular ligament Sternoclavicular ligament Subacromial bursa Transverse humeral ligament Transverse scapular ligament
Shoulder Joint, Left Shoulder Joint, Right	**Includes:** Glenohumeral joint

SECTION 0 - MEDICAL AND SURGICAL
CHARACTER 4 - BODY PART

Shoulder Muscle, Left **Shoulder Muscle, Right**	**Includes:** Deltoid muscle Infraspinatus muscle Subscapularis muscle Supraspinatus muscle Teres major muscle Teres minor muscle
Sigmoid Colon	**Includes:** Rectosigmoid junction Sigmoid flexure
Skin	**Includes:** Dermis Epidermis Sebaceous gland Sweat gland
Sphenoid Bone, Left **Sphenoid Bone, Right**	**Includes:** Greater wing Lesser wing Optic foramen Pterygoid process Sella turcica
Spinal Canal	**Includes:** Vertebral canal
Spinal Meninges	**Includes:** Arachnoid mater Denticulate ligament Leptomeninges Pia mater
Spleen	**Includes:** Accessory spleen
Splenic Artery	**Includes:** Left gastroepiploic artery Pancreatic artery Short gastric artery
Splenic Vein	**Includes:** Left gastroepiploic vein Pancreatic vein
Sternum	**Includes:** Manubrium Suprasternal notch Xiphoid process
Stomach, Pylorus	**Includes:** Pyloric antrum Pyloric canal Pyloric sphincter
Subarachnoid Space	**Includes:** Cranial subarachnoid space Spinal subarachnoid space

Subclavian Artery, Left **Subclavian Artery, Right**	**Includes:** Costocervical trunk Dorsal scapular artery Internal thoracic artery
Subcutaneous Tissue and Fascia, Anterior Neck	**Includes:** Deep cervical fascia Pretracheal fascia
Subcutaneous Tissue and Fascia, Chest	**Includes:** Pectoral fascia
Subcutaneous Tissue and Fascia, Face	**Includes:** Masseteric fascia Orbital fascia
Subcutaneous Tissue and Fascia, Left Foot	**Includes:** Plantar fascia (aponeurosis)
Subcutaneous Tissue and Fascia, Left Hand	**Includes:** Palmar fascia (aponeurosis)
Subcutaneous Tissue and Fascia, Left Lower Arm	**Includes:** Antebrachial fascia Bicipital aponeurosis
Subcutaneous Tissue and Fascia, Left Upper Arm	**Includes:** Axillary fascia Deltoid fascia Infraspinatus fascia Subscapular aponeurosis Supraspinatus fascia
Subcutaneous Tissue and Fascia, Left Upper Leg	**Includes:** Crural fascia Fascia lata Iliac fascia Iliotibial tract (band)
Subcutaneous Tissue and Fascia, Posterior Neck	**Includes:** Prevertebral fascia
Subcutaneous Tissue and Fascia, Right Foot	**Includes:** Plantar fascia (aponeurosis)
Subcutaneous Tissue and Fascia, Right Hand	**Includes:** Palmar fascia (aponeurosis)
Subcutaneous Tissue and Fascia, Right Lower Arm	**Includes:** Antebrachial fascia Bicipital aponeurosis

◀ New   ◀▪▪ Revised   ~~deleted~~ Deleted

SECTION 0 - MEDICAL AND SURGICAL
CHARACTER 4 - BODY PART

Subcutaneous Tissue and Fascia, Right Upper Arm	**Includes:** Axillary fascia Deltoid fascia Infraspinatus fascia Subscapular aponeurosis Supraspinatus fascia
Subcutaneous Tissue and Fascia, Right Upper Leg	**Includes:** Crural fascia Fascia lata Iliac fascia Iliotibial tract (band)
Subcutaneous Tissue and Fascia, Scalp	**Includes:** Galea aponeurotica
Subcutaneous Tissue and Fascia, Trunk	**Includes:** External oblique aponeurosis Transversalis fascia
Subdural Space	**Includes:** Cranial subdural space Spinal subdural space
Submaxillary Gland, Left Submaxillary Gland, Right	**Includes:** Submandibular gland
Superior Mesenteric Artery	**Includes:** Ileal artery Ileocolic artery Inferior pancreaticoduodenal artery Jejunal artery
Superior Mesenteric Vein	**Includes:** Right gastroepiploic vein
Superior Vena Cava	**Includes:** Precava
Tarsal Joint, Left Tarsal Joint, Right	**Includes:** Calcaneocuboid joint Cuboideonavicular joint Cuneonavicular joint Intercuneiform joint Subtalar (talocalcaneal) joint Talocalcaneal (subtalar) joint Talocalcaneonavicular joint
Tarsal, Left Tarsal, Right	**Includes:** Calcaneus Cuboid bone Intermediate cuneiform bone Lateral cuneiform bone Medial cuneiform bone Navicular bone Talus bone

Temporal Artery, Left Temporal Artery, Right	**Includes:** Middle temporal artery Superficial temporal artery Transverse facial artery
Temporal Bone, Left Temporal Bone, Right	**Includes:** Mastoid process Petrous part of temporal bone Tympanic part of temporal bone Zygomatic process of temporal bone
Thalamus	**Includes:** Epithalamus Geniculate nucleus Metathalamus Pulvinar
Thoracic Aorta	**Includes:** Aortic arch Aortic intercostal artery Ascending aorta Bronchial artery Esophageal artery Subcostal artery
Thoracic Duct	**Includes:** Left jugular trunk Left subclavian trunk
Thoracic Nerve	**Includes:** Intercostal nerve Intercostobrachial nerve Spinal nerve, thoracic Subcostal nerve
Thoracic Sympathetic Nerve	**Includes:** Cardiac plexus Esophageal plexus Greater splanchnic nerve Inferior cardiac nerve Least splanchnic nerve Lesser splanchnic nerve Middle cardiac nerve Pulmonary plexus Superior cardiac nerve Thoracic aortic plexus Thoracic ganglion
Thoracic Vertebra	**Includes:** Spinous process Vertebral arch Vertebral foramen Vertebral lamina Vertebral pedicle

◀ New   ◀|||| Revised   ~~deleted~~ Deleted

SECTION 0 - MEDICAL AND SURGICAL
CHARACTER 4 - BODY PART

~~Thoracic Vertebral Joint~~ ~~Thoracic Vertebral Joints, 2 to 7~~ ~~Thoracic Vertebral Joints, 8 or more~~	~~Includes:~~ ~~Costotransverse joint~~ ~~Costovertebral joint~~ ~~Thoracic facet joint~~
Thoracic Vertebral Joint ◄	**Includes:** Costotransverse joint ◄ Costovertebral joint ◄ Thoracic facet joint ◄
Thoracolumbar Vertebral Joint	**Includes:** Thoracolumbar facet joint
Thorax Bursa and Ligament, Left Thorax Bursa and Ligament, Right	**Includes:** Costotransverse ligament Costoxiphoid ligament Sternocostal ligament
Thorax Muscle, Left Thorax Muscle, Right	**Includes:** Intercostal muscle Levatores costarum muscle Pectoralis major muscle Pectoralis minor muscle Serratus anterior muscle Subclavius muscle Subcostal muscle Transverse thoracis muscle
Thymus	**Includes:** Thymus gland
Thyroid Artery, Left Thyroid Artery, Right	**Includes:** Cricothyroid artery Hyoid artery Sternocleidomastoid artery Superior laryngeal artery Superior thyroid artery Thyrocervical trunk
Tibia, Left Tibia, Right	**Includes:** Lateral condyle of tibia Medial condyle of tibia Medial malleolus
Tibial Nerve	**Includes:** Lateral plantar nerve Medial plantar nerve Medial popliteal nerve Medial sural cutaneous nerve
Toe Nail	**Includes:** Nail bed Nail plate

Toe Phalangeal Joint, Left Toe Phalangeal Joint, Right	**Includes:** Interphalangeal (IP) joint
Tongue	**Includes:** Frenulum linguae Lingual tonsil
Tongue, Palate, Pharynx Muscle	**Includes:** Chrondroglossus muscle Genioglossus muscle Hyoglossus muscle Inferior longitudinal muscle Levator veli palatini muscle Palatoglossal muscle Palatopharyngeal muscle Pharyngeal constrictor muscle Salpingopharyngeus muscle Styloglossus muscle Stylopharyngeus muscle Superior longitudinal muscle Tensor veli palatini muscle
Tonsils	**Includes:** Palatine tonsil
Transverse Colon	**Includes:** Splenic flexure
Tricuspid Valve	**Includes:** Right atrioventricular valve Tricuspid annulus
Trigeminal Nerve	**Includes:** Fifth cranial nerve Gasserian ganglion Mandibular nerve Maxillary nerve Ophthalmic nerve Trifacial nerve
Trochlear Nerve	**Includes:** Fourth cranial nerve
Trunk Bursa and Ligament, Left Trunk Bursa and Ligament, Right	**Includes:** Iliolumbar ligament Interspinous ligament Intertransverse ligament Ligamentum flavum Pubic ligament Sacrococcygeal ligament Sacroiliac ligament Sacrospinous ligament Sacrotuberous ligament Supraspinous ligament

◄ New   ◄▥ Revised   ~~deleted~~ Deleted

SECTION 0 - MEDICAL AND SURGICAL
CHARACTER 4 - BODY PART

Trunk Muscle, Left Trunk Muscle, Right	**Includes:** Coccygeus muscle Erector spinae muscle Interspinalis muscle Intertransversarius muscle Latissimus dorsi muscle Levator ani muscle Quadratus lumborum muscle Rhomboid major muscle Rhomboid minor muscle Serratus posterior muscle Transversospinalis muscle Trapezius muscle
Tympanic Membrane, Left Tympanic Membrane, Right	**Includes:** Pars flaccida
Ulna, Left Ulna, Right	**Includes:** Olecranon process Radial notch
Ulnar Artery, Left Ulnar Artery, Right	**Includes:** Anterior ulnar recurrent artery Common interosseous artery Posterior ulnar recurrent artery
Ulnar Nerve	**Includes:** Cubital nerve
Upper Arm Muscle, Left Upper Arm Muscle, Right	**Includes:** Biceps brachii muscle Brachialis muscle Coracobrachialis muscle Triceps brachii muscle
Upper Eyelid, Left Upper Eyelid, Right	**Includes:** Lateral canthus Levator palpebrae superioris muscle Orbicularis oculi muscle Superior tarsal plate
Upper Femur, Left Upper Femur, Right	**Includes:** Femoral head Greater trochanter Lesser trochanter Neck of femur

Upper Leg Muscle, Left Upper Leg Muscle, Right	**Includes:** Adductor brevis muscle Adductor longus muscle Adductor magnus muscle Biceps femoris muscle Gracilis muscle Pectineus muscle Quadriceps (femoris) Rectus femoris muscle Sartorius muscle Semimembranosus muscle Semitendinosus muscle Vastus intermedius muscle Vastus lateralis muscle Vastus medialis muscle
Upper Lip	**Includes:** Frenulum labii superioris Labial gland Vermilion border
Ureter Ureter, Left Ureter, Right Ureters, Bilateral	**Includes:** Ureteral orifice Ureterovesical orifice
Urethra	**Includes:** Bulbourethral (Cowper's) gland Cowper's (bulbourethral) gland External urethral sphincter Internal urethral sphincter Membranous urethra Penile urethra Prostatic urethra
Uterine Supporting Structure	**Includes:** Broad ligament Infundibulopelvic ligament Ovarian ligament Round ligament of uterus
Uterus	**Includes:** Fundus uteri Myometrium Perimetrium Uterine cornu
Uvula	**Includes:** Palatine uvula
Vagus Nerve	**Includes:** Anterior vagal trunk Pharyngeal plexus Pneumogastric nerve Posterior vagal trunk Pulmonary plexus Recurrent laryngeal nerve Superior laryngeal nerve Tenth cranial nerve

◀ New   ◀▥ Revised   ~~deleted~~ Deleted

SECTION 0 - MEDICAL AND SURGICAL
CHARACTER 4 - BODY PART

Vas Deferens Vas Deferens, Bilateral Vas Deferens, Left Vas Deferens, Right	**Includes:** Ductus deferens Ejaculatory duct
Ventricle, Right	**Includes:** Conus arteriosus
Ventricular Septum	**Includes:** Interventricular septum
Vertebral Artery, Left Vertebral Artery, Right	**Includes:** Anterior spinal artery Posterior spinal artery
Vertebral Vein, Left Vertebral Vein, Right	**Includes:** Deep cervical vein Suboccipital venous plexus
Vestibular Gland	**Includes:** Bartholin's (greater vestibular) gland Greater vestibular (Bartholin's) gland Paraurethral (Skene's) gland Skene's (paraurethral) gland

Vitreous, Left Vitreous, Right	**Includes:** Vitreous body
Vocal Cord, Left Vocal Cord, Right	**Includes:** Vocal fold
Vulva	**Includes:** Labia majora Labia minora
Wrist Bursa and Ligament, Left Wrist Bursa and Ligament, Right	**Includes:** Palmar ulnocarpal ligament Radial collateral carpal ligament Radiocarpal ligament Radioulnar ligament Ulnar collateral carpal ligament
Wrist Joint, Left Wrist Joint, Right	**Includes:** Distal radioulnar joint Radiocarpal joint

SECTION 0 - MEDICAL AND SURGICAL
CHARACTER 5 - APPROACH

External	**Definition:** Procedures performed directly on the skin or mucous membrane and procedures performed indirectly by the application of external force through the skin or mucous membrane
Open	**Definition:** Cutting through the skin or mucous membrane and any other body layers necessary to expose the site of the procedure
Percutaneous	**Definition:** Entry, by puncture or minor incision, of instrumentation through the skin or mucous membrane and any other body layers necessary to reach the site of the procedure
Percutaneous Endoscopic	**Definition:** Entry, by puncture or minor incision, of instrumentation through the skin or mucous membrane and any other body layers necessary to reach and visualize the site of the procedure

Via Natural or Artificial Opening	**Definition:** Entry of instrumentation through a natural or artificial external opening to reach the site of the procedure
Via Natural or Artificial Opening Endoscopic	**Definition:** Entry of instrumentation through a natural or artificial external opening to reach and visualize the site of the procedure
Via Natural or Artificial Opening With Percutaneous Endoscopic Assistance	**Definition:** Entry of instrumentation through a natural or artificial external opening and entry, by puncture or minor incision, of instrumentation through the skin or mucous membrane and any other body layers necessary to aid in the performance of the procedure

◀ New ◀▥ Revised ~~deleted~~ Deleted

SECTION 0, CHARACTER 4; 5

SECTION 0 - MEDICAL AND SURGICAL
CHARACTER 6 - DEVICE

Artificial Sphincter in Gastrointestinal System	**Includes:** Artificial anal sphincter (AAS) Artificial bowel sphincter (neosphincter)
Artificial Sphincter in Urinary System	**Includes:** AMS 800® Urinary Control System Artificial urinary sphincter (AUS)
Autologous Arterial Tissue in Heart and Great Vessels	**Includes:** Autologous artery graft
Autologous Arterial Tissue in Lower Arteries	**Includes:** Autologous artery graft
Autologous Arterial Tissue in Lower Veins	**Includes:** Autologous artery graft
Autologous Arterial Tissue in Upper Arteries	**Includes:** Autologous artery graft
Autologous Arterial Tissue in Upper Veins	**Includes:** Autologous artery graft
Autologous Tissue Substitute	**Includes:** Autograft Cultured epidermal cell autograft Epicel® cultured epidermal autograft
Autologous Venous Tissue in Heart and Great Vessels	**Includes:** Autologous vein graft
Autologous Venous Tissue in Lower Arteries	**Includes:** Autologous vein graft
Autologous Venous Tissue in Lower Veins	**Includes:** Autologous vein graft
Autologous Venous Tissue in Upper Arteries	**Includes:** Autologous vein graft
Autologous Venous Tissue in Upper Veins	**Includes:** Autologous vein graft
Bone Growth Stimulator in Head and Facial Bones	**Includes:** Electrical bone growth stimulator (EBGS) Ultrasonic osteogenic stimulator Ultrasound bone healing system

Bone Growth Stimulator in Lower Bones	**Includes:** Electrical bone growth stimulator (EBGS) Ultrasonic osteogenic stimulator Ultrasound bone healing system
Bone Growth Stimulator in Upper Bones	**Includes:** Electrical bone growth stimulator (EBGS) Ultrasonic osteogenic stimulator Ultrasound bone healing system
Cardiac Lead in Heart and Great Vessels	**Includes:** Cardiac contractility modulation lead
Cardiac Lead, Defibrillator for Insertion in Heart and Great Vessels	**Includes:** ACUITY™ Steerable Lead Attain Ability® lead Attain StarFix® (OTW) lead Cardiac resynchronization therapy (CRT) lead Corox (OTW) Bipolar Lead Durata® Defibrillation Lead ENDOTAK RELIANCE® (G) Defibrillation Lead
Cardiac Lead, Pacemaker for Insertion in Heart and Great Vessels	**Includes:** ACUITY™ Steerable Lead Attain Ability® Lead Attain StarFix® (OTW) lead Cardiac resynchronization therapy (CRT) lead Corox (OTW) Bipolar Lead
Cardiac Resynchronization Defibrillator Pulse Generator for Insertion in Subcutaneous Tissue and Fascia	**Includes:** COGNIS® CRT-D Concerto II CRT-D Consulta CRT-D CONTAK RENEWAL® 3 RF (HE) CRT-D LIVIAN™ CRT-D Maximo II DR CRT-D Ovatio™ CRT-D Protecta XT CRT-D Viva (XT)(S) ◄
Cardiac Resynchronization Pacemaker Pulse Generator for Insertion in Subcutaneous Tissue and Fascia	**Includes:** Consulta CRT-P Stratos LV Synchra CRT-P
~~Cardiac Rhythm Related Device in Subcutaneous Tissue and Fascia~~	~~Includes:~~ ~~Baroreflex Activation Therapy® (BAT®)~~ ~~Rheos® System device~~
Contraceptive Device in Female Reproductive System	**Includes:** Intrauterine device (IUD)

APPENDIX A

◄ New   ◄▥ Revised   ~~deleted~~ Deleted

SECTION 0 - MEDICAL AND SURGICAL
CHARACTER 6 - DEVICE

Contraceptive Device in Subcutaneous Tissue and Fascia	**Includes:** Subdermal progesterone implant
Contractility Modulation Device for Insertion in Subcutaneous Tissue and Fascia	**Includes:** Optimizer™ III implantable pulse generator
Defibrillator Generator for Insertion in Subcutaneous Tissue and Fascia	**Includes:** Implantable cardioverter-defibrillator (ICD) Maximo II DR (VR) Protecta XT DR (XT VR) S ecura (DR) (VR) Evera (XT)(S)(DR/VR) ◄ Virtuoso (II) (DR) (VR)
Diaphragmatic Pacemaker Lead in Respiratory System	**Includes:** Phrenic nerve stimulator lead
Drainage Device	**Includes:** Cystostomy tube Foley catheter Percutaneous nephrostomy catheter Thoracostomy tube
Epiretinal Visual Prosthesis in Eye	**Includes:** Epiretinal visual prosthesis
External Fixation Device in Head and Facial Bones	**Includes:** External fixator
External Fixation Device in Lower Bones	**Includes:** External fixator
External Fixation Device in Lower Joints	**Includes:** External fixator
External Fixation Device in Upper Bones	**Includes:** External fixator
External Fixation Device in Upper Joints	**Includes:** External fixator
External Fixation Device, Hybrid for Insertion in Upper Bones	**Includes:** Delta frame external fixator Sheffield hybrid external fixator
External Fixation Device, Hybrid for Insertion in Lower Bones	**Includes:** Delta frame external fixator Sheffield hybrid external fixator

External Fixation Device, Hybrid for Reposition in Upper Bones	**Includes:** Delta frame external fixator Sheffield hybrid external fixator
External Fixation Device, Hybrid for Reposition in Lower Bones	**Includes:** Delta frame external fixator Sheffield hybrid external fixator
External Fixation Device, Limb Lengthening for Insertion in Upper Bones	**Includes:** Ilizarov-Vecklich device
External Fixation Device, Limb Lengthening for Insertion in Lower Bones	**Includes:** Ilizarov-Vecklich device
External Fixation Device, Monoplanar for Insertion in Upper Bones	**Includes:** Uniplanar external fixator
External Fixation Device, Monoplanar for Insertion in Lower Bones	**Includes:** Uniplanar external fixator
External Fixation Device, Monoplanar for Reposition in Upper Bones	**Includes:** Uniplanar external fixator
External Fixation Device, Monoplanar for Reposition in Lower Bones	**Includes:** Uniplanar external fixator
External Fixation Device, Ring for Insertion in Upper Bones	**Includes:** Ilizarov external fixator Sheffield ring external fixator
External Fixation Device, Ring for Insertion in Lower Bones	**Includes:** Ilizarov external fixator Sheffield ring external fixator
External Fixation Device, Ring for Reposition in Upper Bones	**Includes:** Ilizarov external fixator Sheffield ring external fixator
External Fixation Device, Ring for Reposition in Lower Bones	**Includes:** Ilizarov external fixator Sheffield ring external fixator

◄ New　◄▥ Revised　~~deleted~~ Deleted

SECTION 0 - MEDICAL AND SURGICAL
CHARACTER 6 - DEVICE

External Heart Assist System in Heart and Great Vessels	**Includes:** Biventricular external heart assist system BVS 5000 Ventricular Assist Device Centrimag® Blood Pump ◀ TandemHeart® System Thoratec Paracorporeal Ventricular Assist Device
Extraluminal Device	**Includes:** LAP-BAND® adjustable gastric banding system REALIZE® Adjustable Gastric Band TigerPaw® system for closure of left atrial appendage
Feeding Device in Gastrointestinal System	**Includes:** Percutaneous endoscopic gastrojejunostomy (PEG/J) tube Percutaneous endoscopic gastrostomy (PEG) tube
Hearing Device in Ear, Nose, Sinus	**Includes:** Esteem® implantable hearing system
Hearing Device in Head and Facial Bones	**Includes:** Bone anchored hearing device
Hearing Device, Bone Conduction for Insertion in Ear, Nose, Sinus	**Includes:** Bone anchored hearing device
Hearing Device, Multiple Channel Cochlear Prosthesis for Insertion in Ear, Nose, Sinus	**Includes:** Cochlear implant (CI), multiple channel (electrode)
Hearing Device, Single Channel Cochlear Prosthesis for Insertion in Ear, Nose, Sinus	**Includes:** Cochlear implant (CI), single channel (electrode)
Implantable Heart Assist System in Heart and Great Vessels	**Includes:** Berlin Heart Ventricular Assist Device DeBakey Left Ventricular Assist Device DuraHeart Left Ventricular Assist System HeartMate II® Left Ventricular Assist Device (LVAD) HeartMate XVE® Left Ventricular Assist Device (LVAD) MicroMed HeartAssist Novacor Left Ventricular Assist Device Thoratec IVAD (Implantable Ventricular Assist Device)
Infusion Device	**Includes:** Ascenda Intrathecal Catheter ◀ InDura, intrathecal catheter (1P) (spinal) Non-tunneled central venous catheter Peripherally inserted central catheter (PICC) Tunneled spinal (intrathecal) catheter

Infusion Device, Pump in Subcutaneous Tissue and Fascia	**Includes:** Implantable drug infusion pump (anti-spasmodic) (chemotherapy) (pain) Injection reservoir, pump Pump reservoir Subcutaneous injection reservoir, pump SynchroMed pump ◀
Interbody Fusion Device in Lower Joints	**Includes:** Axial Lumbar Interbody Fusion System AxiaLIF® System CoRoent® XL Direct Lateral Interbody Fusion (DLIF) device EXtreme Lateral Interbody Fusion (XLIF) device Interbody fusion (spine) cage XLIF® System
Interbody Fusion Device in Upper Joints	**Includes:** BAK/C® Interbody Cervical Fusion System Interbody fusion (spine) cage
Internal Fixation Device in Head and Facial Bones	**Includes:** Bone screw (interlocking) (lag) (pedicle) (recessed) Kirschner wire (K-wire) Neutralization plate
Internal Fixation Device in Lower Bones	**Includes:** Bone screw (interlocking) (lag) (pedicle) (recessed) Clamp and rod internal fixation system (CRIF) Kirschner wire (K-wire) Neutralization plate
Internal Fixation Device in Lower Joints	**Includes:** Fusion screw (compression) (lag) (locking) Joint fixation plate Kirschner wire (K-wire)
Internal Fixation Device in Upper Bones	**Includes:** Bone screw (interlocking) (lag) (pedicle) (recessed) Clamp and rod internal fixation system (CRIF) Kirschner wire (K-wire) Neutralization plate
Internal Fixation Device in Upper Joints	**Includes:** Fusion screw (compression) (lag) (locking) Joint fixation plate Kirschner wire (K-wire)
Internal Fixation Device, Intramedullary in Lower Bones	**Includes:** Intramedullary (IM) rod (nail) Intramedullary skeletal kinetic distractor (ISKD) Kuntscher nail
Internal Fixation Device, Intramedullary in Upper Bones	**Includes:** Intramedullary (IM) rod (nail) Intramedullary skeletal kinetic distractor (ISKD) Kuntscher nail

◀ New   ◀▥ Revised   ~~deleted~~ Deleted

APPENDIX A

SECTION 0 - MEDICAL AND SURGICAL
CHARACTER 6 - DEVICE

Internal Fixation Device, Rigid Plate for Insertion in Upper Bones	**Includes:** Titanium Sternal Fixation System (TSFS)
Internal Fixation Device, Rigid Plate for Reposition in Upper Bones	**Includes:** Titanium Sternal Fixation System (TSFS)
Intraluminal Device	**Includes:** Absolute Pro Vascular (OTW) Self-Expanding Stent System ◄ Acculink (RX) Carotid Stent System ◄ AneuRx® AAA Advantage® Assurant (Cobalt) stent Carotid WALLSTENT® Monorail® Endoprosthesis Centrimag® Blood Pump CoAxia NeuroFlo catheter Colonic Z-Stent® Complete (SE) stent Driver stent (RX) (OTW) E-Luminexx™ (Biliary) (Vascular) Stent Embolization coil(s) Endurant® Endovascular Stent Graft Express® (LD) Premounted Stent System Express® Biliary SD Monorail® Premounted Stent System Express® SD Renal Monorail® Premounted Stent System FLAIR® Endovascular Stent Graft Formula™ Balloon-Expandable Renal Stent System Herculink (RX) Elite Renal Stent System ◄ Impella® (2.5)(5.0)(LD) cardiac assist device LifeStent® (Flexstar) (XL) Vascular Stent System Micro-Driver stent (RX) (OTW) MULTI-LINK (VISION)(MINI-VISION)(ULTRA) Coronary Stent System ◄ Omnilink Elite Vascular Balloon Expandable Stent System ◄ Pipeline™ Embolization device (PED) Protégé® RX Carotid Stent System Stent (angioplasty) (embolization) Stent, intraluminal (cardiovascular) (gastrointestinal)(hepatobiliary)(urinary) ◄ Talent® Converter Talent® Occluder Talent® Stent Graft (abdominal) (thoracic) Therapeutic occlusion coil(s) Ultraflex™ Precision Colonic Stent System Valiant Thoracic Stent Graft WALLSTENT® Endoprosthesis Xact Carotid Stent System ◄ Zenith Flex® AAA Endovascular Graft Zenith® Renu™ AAA Ancillary Graft Zenith TX2® TAA Endovascular Graft
Intraluminal Device, Pessary in Female Reproductive System	**Includes:** Pessary ring Vaginal pessary
Intraluminal Device, Airway in Ear, Nose, Sinus	**Includes:** Nasopharyngeal airway (NPA)
Intraluminal Device, Airway in Gastrointestinal System	**Includes:** Esophageal obturator airway (EOA)
Intraluminal Device, Airway in Mouth and Throat	**Includes:** Guedel airway Oropharyngeal airway (OPA)
Intraluminal Device, Bioactive in Upper Arteries	**Includes:** Bioactive embolization coil(s) Micrus CERECYTE microcoil
Intraluminal Device, Drug-eluting in Heart and Great Vessels	**Includes:** CYPHER® Stent Endeavor® (III) (IV) (Sprint) Zotarolimus-eluting Coronary Stent System Everolimus-eluting coronary stent Paclitaxel-eluting coronary stent Sirolimus-eluting coronary stent TAXUS® Liberté® Paclitaxel-eluting Coronary Stent System XIENCE V Everolimus Eluting Coronary Stent System XIENCE Everolimus Eluting Coronary Stent System ◄ Zotarolimus-eluting coronary stent
Intraluminal Device, Drug-eluting in Lower Arteries	**Includes:** Paclitaxel-eluting peripheral stent Zilver® PTX® (paclitaxel) Drug-Eluting Peripheral Stent
Intraluminal Device, Drug-eluting in Upper Arteries	**Includes:** Paclitaxel-eluting peripheral stent Zilver® PTX® (paclitaxel) Drug-Eluting Peripheral Stent
Intraluminal Device, Endobronchial Valve in Respiratory System	**Includes:** Spiration IBV™ Valve System
Intraluminal Device, Endotracheal Airway in Respiratory System	**Includes:** Endotracheal tube (cuffed) (double-lumen)

◄ New ⇐ Revised ~~deleted~~ Deleted

SECTION 0 - MEDICAL AND SURGICAL
CHARACTER 6 - DEVICE

Liner in Lower Joints	**Includes:** Hip (joint) liner Joint liner (insert) Knee (implant) insert	Pacemaker, Single Chamber Rate Responsive for Insertion in Subcutaneous Tissue and Fascia	**Includes:** Single lead rate responsive pacemaker (atrium) (ventricle)
Monitoring Device	**Includes:** Blood glucose monitoring system Cardiac event recorder Continuous Glucose Monitoring (CGM) device Implantable glucose monitoring device Loop recorder, implantable Reveal (DX) (XT)	Radioactive Element	**Includes:** Brachytherapy seeds
		Resurfacing Device in Lower Joints	**Includes:** CONSERVE® PLUS Total Resurfacing Hip System Cormet Hip Resurfacing System
Monitoring Device, Hemodynamic for Insertion in Subcutaneous Tissue and Fascia	**Includes:** Implantable hemodynamic monitor (IHM) Implantable hemodynamic monitoring system (IHMS)	Spacer in Lower Joints	**Includes:** Joint spacer (antibiotic)
		Spacer in Upper Joints	**Includes:** Joint spacer (antibiotic)
Monitoring Device, Pressure Sensor for Insertion in Heart and Great Vessels	**Includes:** CardioMEMS® pressure sensor EndoSure® sensor	Spinal Stabilization Device, Facet Replacement for Insertion in Upper Joints	**Includes:** Facet replacement spinal stabilization device
Neurostimulator Lead in Central Nervous System	**Includes:** Cortical strip neurostimulator lead DBS lead Deep brain neurostimulator lead RNS System lead Spinal cord neurostimulator lead	Spinal Stabilization Device, Facet Replacement for Insertion in Lower Joints	**Includes:** Facet replacement spinal stabilization device
Neurostimulator Lead in Peripheral Nervous System	**Includes:** InterStim® Therapy lead	Spinal Stabilization Device, Interspinous Process for Insertion in Upper Joints	**Includes:** Interspinous process spinal stabilization device X-STOP® Spacer
Neurostimulator Generator in Head and Facial Bones	**Includes:** RNS system neurostimulator generator	Spinal Stabilization Device, Interspinous Process for Insertion in Lower Joints	**Includes:** Interspinous process spinal stabilization device X-STOP® Spacer
Nonautologous Tissue Substitute	**Includes:** Acellular Hydrated Dermis Bone bank bone graft Tissue bank graft	Spinal Stabilization Device, Pedicle-Based for Insertion in Upper Joints	**Includes:** Dynesys® Dynamic Stabilization System Pedicle-based dynamic stabilization device
Pacemaker, Dual Chamber for Insertion in Subcutaneous Tissue and Fascia	**Includes:** Advisa (MRI) ◀ EnRhythm Kappa Revo MRI™ SureScan® pacemaker Two lead pacemaker Versa	Spinal Stabilization Device, Pedicle-Based for Insertion in Lower Joints	**Includes:** Dynesys® Dynamic Stabilization System Pedicle-based dynamic stabilization device
Pacemaker, Single Chamber for Insertion in Subcutaneous Tissue and Fascia	**Includes:** Single lead pacemaker (atrium) (ventricle)	Stimulator Generator in Subcutaneous Tissue and Fascia	**Includes:** Baroreflex Activation Therapy® (BAT®) ◀ Diaphragmatic pacemaker generator Mark IV Breathing Pacemaker System Phrenic nerve stimulator generator Rheos® System device ◀

APPENDIX A

SECTION 0 - MEDICAL AND SURGICAL
CHARACTER 6 - DEVICE

Stimulator Generator, Multiple Array for Insertion in Subcutaneous Tissue and Fascia	**Includes:** Activa PC neurostimulator Enterra gastric neurostimulator ~~Kinetra® neurostimulator~~ Neurostimulator generator, multiple channel ~~PrimeAdvanced neurostimulator~~ PrimeAdvanced neurostimulator (SureScan) (MRI Safe) ◄
Stimulator Generator, Multiple Array Rechargeable for Insertion in Subcutaneous Tissue and Fascia	**Includes:** Activa RC neurostimulator Neurostimulator generator, multiple channel rechargeable ~~RestoreAdvanced neurostimulator~~ RestoreAdvanced neurostimulator (SureScan) (MRI Safe) ◄ ~~RestoreSensor neurostimulator~~ RestoreSensor neurostimulator (SureScan) (MRI Safe) ◄ ~~RestoreUltra neurostimulator~~ RestoreUltra neurostimulator (SureScan) (MRI Safe) ◄
Stimulator Generator, Single Array for Insertion in Subcutaneous Tissue and Fascia	**Includes:** Activa SC neurostimulator InterStim® Therapy neurostimulator Itrel (3) (4) neurostimulator Neurostimulator generator, single channel ~~Soletra® neurostimulator~~
Stimulator Generator, Single Array Rechargeable for Insertion in Subcutaneous Tissue and Fascia	**Includes:** Neurostimulator generator, single channel rechargeable
Stimulator Lead in Gastrointestinal System	**Includes:** Gastric electrical stimulation (GES) lead Gastric pacemaker lead
Stimulator Lead in Muscles	**Includes:** Electrical muscle stimulation (EMS) lead Electronic muscle stimulator lead Neuromuscular electrical stimulation (NEMS) lead
Stimulator Lead in Upper Arteries	**Includes:** Baroreflex Activation Therapy® (BAT®) Carotid (artery) sinus (baroreceptor) lead Rheos® System lead
Stimulator Lead in Urinary System	**Includes:** Sacral nerve modulation (SNM) lead Sacral neuromodulation lead Urinary incontinence stimulator lead

Synthetic Substitute	**Includes:** AbioCor® Total Replacement Heart AMPLATZER® Muscular VSD Occluder Annuloplasty ring Bard® Composix® (E/X) (LP) mesh Bard® Composix® Kugel® patch Bard® Dulex™ mesh Bard® Ventralex™ hernia patch BRYAN® Cervical Disc System Ex-PRESS™ mini glaucoma shunt Flexible Composite Mesh GORE® DUALMESH® Holter valve ventricular shunt MitraClip valve repair system Nitinol framed polymer mesh Open Pivot (mechanical) valve ◄ Open Pivot Aortic Valve Graft (AVG) ◄ Partially absorbable mesh PHYSIOMESH™ Flexible Composite Mesh Polymethylmethacrylate (PMMA) Polypropylene mesh PRESTIGE® Cervical Disc PROCEED™ Ventral Patch Prodisc-C Prodisc-L PROLENE Polypropylene Hernia System (PHS) Rebound HRD® (Hernia Repair Device) SynCardia Total Artificial Heart Total artificial (replacement) heart ULTRAPRO Hernia System (UHS) ULTRAPRO Partially Absorbable Lightweight Mesh ULTRAPRO Plug Ventrio™ Hernia Patch Zimmer® NexGen® LPS Mobile Bearing Knee Zimmer® NexGen® LPS-Flex Mobile Knee
Synthetic Substitute, Ceramic for Replacement in Lower Joints	**Includes:** Novation® Ceramic AHS® (Articulation Hip System)
Synthetic Substitute, Ceramic on Polyethylene for Replacement in Lower Joints	**Includes:** Oxidized zirconium ceramic hip bearing surface
Synthetic Substitute, Intraocular Telescope for Replacement in Eye	**Includes:** Implantable Miniature Telescope™ (IMT)

◄ New   ◄▬ Revised   ~~deleted~~ Deleted

SECTION 0 - MEDICAL AND SURGICAL
CHARACTER 6 - DEVICE

Synthetic Substitute, Metal for Replacement in Lower Joints	**Includes:** Cobalt/chromium head and socket
Synthetic Substitute, Metal on Polyethylene for Replacement in Lower Joints	**Includes:** Cobalt/chromium head and polyethylene socket
Synthetic Substitute, Polyethylene for Replacement in Lower Joints	**Includes:** Polyethylene socket
Synthetic Substitute, Reverse Ball and Socket for Replacement in Upper Joints	**Includes:** Delta III Reverse shoulder prosthesis Reverse® Shoulder Prosthesis
Tissue Expander in Skin and Breast	**Includes:** Tissue expander (inflatable) (injectable)
Tissue Expander in Subcutaneous Tissue and Fascia	**Includes:** Tissue expander (inflatable) (injectable)
Tracheostomy Device in Respiratory System	**Includes:** Tracheostomy tube

Vascular Access Device in Subcutaneous Tissue and Fascia	**Includes:** Tunneled central venous catheter Vectra® Vascular Access Graft
Vascular Access Device, Reservoir in Subcutaneous Tissue and Fascia	**Includes:** Implanted (venous) (access) port Injection reservoir, port Subcutaneous injection reservoir, port
Zooplastic Tissue in Heart and Great Vessels	**Includes:** 3f (Aortic) Bioprosthesis valve Bovine pericardial valve Bovine pericardium graft Contegra Pulmonary Valved Conduit CoreValve transcatheter aortic valve Epic™ Stented Tissue Valve (aortic) Freestyle (Stentless) Aortic Root Bioprosthesis Hancock Bioprosthesis (aortic) (mitral) valve Hancock Bioprosthetic Valved Conduit Melody® transcatheter pulmonary valve Mitroflow® Aortic Pericardial Heart Valve Mosaic Bioprosthesis (aortic) (mitral) valve ◄ Porcine (bioprosthetic) valve SAPIEN transcatheter aortic valve SJM Biocor® Stented Valve System Stented tissue valve Trifecta™ Valve (aortic) Xenograft

SECTION 1 - OBSTETRICS
CHARACTER 3 - OPERATION

Abortion	**Definition:** Artificially terminating a pregnancy
Change	**Definition:** Taking out or off a device from a body part and putting back an identical or similar device in or on the same body part without cutting or puncturing the skin or a mucous membrane **Explanation:** All CHANGE procedures are coded using the approach EXTERNAL
Delivery	**Definition:** Assisting the passage of the products of conception from the genital canal
Drainage	**Definition:** Taking or letting out fluids and/or gases from a body part by the use of force **Explanation:** The qualifier DIAGNOSTIC is used to identify drainage procedures that are biopsies

Extraction	**Definition:** Pulling or stripping out or off all or a portion of a body part **Explanation:** The qualifier DIAGNOSTIC is used to identify extraction procedures that are biopsies
Insertion	**Definition:** Putting in a nonbiological appliance that monitors, assists, performs, or prevents a physiological function but does not physically take the place of a body part
Inspection	**Definition:** Visually and/or manually exploring a body part **Explanation:** Visual exploration may be performed with or without optical instrumentation. Manual exploration may be performed directly or through intervening body layers

◄ New   ◄▦ Revised   ~~deleted~~ Deleted

SECTION 1 - OBSTETRICS
CHARACTER 3 - OPERATION

Removal	**Definition:** Taking out or off a device from a body part, region or orifice **Explanation:** If a device is taken out and a similar device put in without cutting or puncturing the skin or mucous membrane, the procedure is coded to the root operation CHANGE. Otherwise, the procedure for taking out a device is coded to the root operation REMOVAL
Repair	**Definition:** Restoring, to the extent possible, a body part to its normal anatomic structure and function **Explanation:** Used only when the method to accomplish the repair is not one of the other root operations

Reposition	**Definition:** Moving to its normal location or other suitable location all or a portion of a body part **Explanation:** The body part is moved to a new location from an abnormal location, or from a normal location where it is not functioning correctly. The body part may or may not be cut out or off to be moved to the new location
Resection	**Definition:** Cutting out or off, without replacement, all of a body part
Transplantation	**Definition:** Putting in or on all or a portion of a living body part taken from another individual or animal to physically take the place and/or function of all or a portion of a similar body part **Explanation:** The native body part may or may not be taken out, and the transplanted body part may take over all or a portion of its function

SECTION 1 - OBSTETRICS
CHARACTER 5 - APPROACH

External	**Definition:** Procedures performed directly on the skin or mucous membrane and procedures performed indirectly by the application of external force through the skin or mucous membrane
Open	**Definition:** Cutting through the skin or mucous membrane and any other body layers necessary to expose the site of the procedure
Percutaneous	**Definition:** Entry, by puncture or minor incision, of instrumentation through the skin or mucous membrane and any other body layers necessary to reach the site of the procedure

Percutaneous Endoscopic	**Definition:** Entry, by puncture or minor incision, of instrumentation through the skin or mucous membrane and any other body layers necessary to reach and visualize the site of the procedure
Via Natural or Artificial Opening	**Definition:** Entry of instrumentation through a natural or artificial external opening to reach the site of the procedure
Via Natural or Artificial Opening Endoscopic	**Definition:** Entry of instrumentation through a natural or artificial external opening to reach and visualize the site of the procedure

SECTION 2 - PLACEMENT
CHARACTER 3 - OPERATION

Change	**Definition:** Taking out or off a device from a body part and putting back an identical or similar device in or on the same body part without cutting or puncturing the skin or a mucous membrane
Compression	**Definition:** Putting pressure on a body region
Dressing	**Definition:** Putting material on a body region for protection

Immobilization	**Definition:** Limiting or preventing motion of a body region
Packing	**Definition:** Putting material in a body region or orifice
Removal	**Definition:** Taking out or off a device from a body part
Traction	**Definition:** Exerting a pulling force on a body region in a distal direction

◄ New   ⬅ Revised   ~~deleted~~ Deleted

SECTION 2 - PLACEMENT
CHARACTER 5 - APPROACH

External	**Definition:** Procedures performed directly on the skin or mucous membrane and procedures performed indirectly by the application of external force through the skin or mucous membrane

SECTION 3 - ADMINISTRATION
CHARACTER 3 - OPERATION

Introduction	**Definition:** Putting in or on a therapeutic, diagnostic, nutritional, physiological, or prophylactic substance except blood or blood products

Irrigation	**Definition:** Putting in or on a cleansing substance
Transfusion	**Definition:** Putting in blood or blood products

SECTION 3 - ADMINISTRATION
CHARACTER 5 - APPROACH

External	**Definition:** Procedures performed directly on the skin or mucous membrane and procedures performed indirectly by the application of external force through the skin or mucous membrane
Open	**Definition:** Cutting through the skin or mucous membrane and any other body layers necessary to expose the site of the procedure
Percutaneous	**Definition:** Entry, by puncture or minor incision, of instrumentation through the skin or mucous membrane and any other body layers necessary to reach the site of the procedure

Via Natural or Artificial Opening	**Definition:** Entry of instrumentation through a natural or artificial external opening to reach the site of the procedure
Via Natural or Artificial Opening Endoscopic	**Definition:** Entry of instrumentation through a natural or artificial external opening to reach and visualize the site of the procedure

SECTION 3 - ADMINISTRATION ◀
CHARACTER 6 - SUBSTANCE ◀

4-Factor Prothrombin Complex Concentrate ◀	**Includes:** Kcentra ◀
Adhesion Barrier ◀	**Includes:** Seprafilm ◀
Anti-Infective Envelope ◀	**Includes:** AIGISRx Antibacterial Envelope ◀ Antimicrobial envelope ◀
Clofarabine ◀	**Includes:** Clolar ◀
Glucarpidase ◀	**Includes:** Voraxaze ◀

Human B-type Natriuretic Peptide ◀	**Includes:** Nesiritide ◀
Other Thrombolytic ◀	**Includes:** Tissue Plasminogen Activator (tPA)(r-tPA) ◀
Oxazolidinones ◀	**Includes:** Zyvox ◀
Recombinant Bone Morphogenetic Protein ◀	**Includes:** Bone morphogenetic protein 2 (BMP 2) ◀ rhBMP-2 ◀

◀ New ◀◀ Revised ~~deleted~~ Deleted

SECTION 4 - MEASUREMENT AND MONITORING
CHARACTER 3 - OPERATION

Measurement	**Definition:** Determining the level of a physiological or physical function at a point in time	Monitoring	**Definition:** Determining the level of a physiological or physical function repetitively over a period of time

SECTION 4 - MEASUREMENT AND MONITORING
CHARACTER 5 - APPROACH

External	**Definition:** Procedures performed directly on the skin or mucous membrane and procedures performed indirectly by the application of external force through the skin or mucous membrane	Percutaneous Endoscopic	**Definition:** Entry, by puncture or minor incision, of instrumentation through the skin or mucous membrane and any other body layers necessary to reach and visualize the site of the procedure
Open	**Definition:** Cutting through the skin or mucous membrane and any other body layers necessary to expose the site of the procedure	Via Natural or Artificial Opening	**Definition:** Entry of instrumentation through a natural or artificial external opening to reach the site of the procedure
Percutaneous	**Definition:** Entry, by puncture or minor incision, of instrumentation through the skin or mucous membrane and any other body layers necessary to reach the site of the procedure	Via Natural or Artificial Opening Endoscopic	**Definition:** Entry of instrumentation through a natural or artificial external opening to reach and visualize the site of the procedure

SECTION 5 - EXTRACORPOREAL ASSISTANCE AND PERFORMANCE
CHARACTER 3 - OPERATION

Assistance	**Definition:** Taking over a portion of a physiological function by extracorporeal means	Restoration	**Definition:** Returning, or attempting to return, a physiological function to its original state by extracorporeal means.
Performance	**Definition:** Completely taking over a physiological function by extracorporeal means		

◀ New ◀▥ Revised ~~deleted~~ Deleted

SECTION 6 - EXTRACORPOREAL THERAPIES
CHARACTER 3 - OPERATION

Atmospheric Control	**Definition:** Extracorporeal control of atmospheric pressure and composition
Decompression	**Definition:** Extracorporeal elimination of undissolved gas from body fluids
Electromagnetic Therapy	**Definition:** Extracorporeal treatment by electromagnetic rays
Hyperthermia	**Definition:** Extracorporeal raising of body temperature
Hypothermia	**Definition:** Extracorporeal lowering of body temperature

Pheresis	**Definition:** Extracorporeal separation of blood products
Phototherapy	**Definition:** Extracorporeal treatment by light rays
Shock Wave Therapy	**Definition:** Extracorporeal treatment by shock waves
Ultrasound Therapy	**Definition:** Extracorporeal treatment by ultrasound
Ultraviolet Light Therapy	**Definition:** Extracorporeal treatment by ultraviolet light

SECTION 7 - OSTEOPATHIC
CHARACTER 3 - OPERATION

Treatment	**Definition:** Manual treatment to eliminate or alleviate somatic dysfunction and related disorders

SECTION 7 - OSTEOPATHIC
CHARACTER 5 - APPROACH

External	**Definition:** Procedures performed directly on the skin or mucous membrane and procedures performed indirectly by the application of external force through the skin or mucous membrane

SECTION 8 - OTHER PROCEDURES
CHARACTER 3 - OPERATION

Other Procedures	**Definition:** Methodologies which attempt to remediate or cure a disorder or disease

SECTION 8 - OTHER PROCEDURES
CHARACTER 5 - APPROACH

External	**Definition:** Procedures performed directly on the skin or mucous membrane and procedures performed indirectly by the application of external force through the skin or mucous membrane
Percutaneous	**Definition:** Entry, by puncture or minor incision, of instrumentation through the skin or mucous membrane and any other body layers necessary to reach the site of the procedure
Percutaneous Endoscopic	**Definition:** Entry, by puncture or minor incision, of instrumentation through the skin or mucous membrane and any other body layers necessary to reach and visualize the site of the procedure

Via Natural or Artificial Opening	**Definition:** Entry of instrumentation through a natural or artificial external opening to reach the site of the procedure
Via Natural or Artificial Opening Endoscopic	**Definition:** Entry of instrumentation through a natural or artificial external opening to reach and visualize the site of the procedure

SECTION 9 - CHIROPRACTIC
CHARACTER 3 - OPERATION

Manipulation	**Definition:** Manual procedure that involves a directed thrust to move a joint past the physiological range of motion, without exceeding the anatomical limit

SECTION 9 - CHIROPRACTIC
CHARACTER 5 - APPROACH

External	**Definition:** Procedures performed directly on the skin or mucous membrane and procedures performed indirectly by the application of external force through the skin or mucous membrane

◀ New ◀◀ Revised ~~deleted~~ Deleted

SECTION 8; 9, CHARACTER 3; 5; 3; 5

SECTION B - IMAGING
CHARACTER 3 - TYPE

Computerized Tomography (CT Scan)	**Definition:** Computer reformatted digital display of multiplanar images developed from the capture of multiple exposures of external ionizing radiation
Fluoroscopy	**Definition:** Single plane or bi-plane real time display of an image developed from the capture of external ionizing radiation on a fluorescent screen. The image may also be stored by either digital or analog means
Magnetic Resonance Imaging (MRI)	**Definition:** Computer reformatted digital display of multiplanar images developed from the capture of radiofrequency signals emitted by nuclei in a body site excited within a magnetic field

Plain Radiography	**Definition:** Planar display of an image developed from the capture of external ionizing radiation on photographic or photoconductive plate
Ultrasonography	**Definition:** Real time display of images of anatomy or flow information developed from the capture of reflected and attenuated high frequency sound waves

SECTION C - NUCLEAR MEDICINE
CHARACTER 3 - TYPE

Nonimaging Nuclear Medicine Assay	**Definition:** Introduction of radioactive materials into the body for the study of body fluids and blood elements, by the detection of radioactive emissions
Nonimaging Nuclear Medicine Probe	**Definition:** Introduction of radioactive materials into the body for the study of distribution and fate of certain substances by the detection of radioactive emissions; or, alternatively, measurement of absorption of radioactive emissions from an external source
Nonimaging Nuclear Medicine Uptake	**Definition:** Introduction of radioactive materials into the body for measurements of organ function, from the detection of radioactive emissions

Planar Nuclear Medicine Imaging	**Definition:** Introduction of radioactive materials into the body for single plane display of images developed from the capture of radioactive emissions
Positron Emission Tomographic (PET) Imaging	**Definition:** Introduction of radioactive materials into the body for three dimensional display of images developed from the simultaneous capture, 180 degrees apart, of radioactive emissions
Systemic Nuclear Medicine Therapy	**Definition:** Introduction of unsealed radioactive materials into the body for treatment
Tomographic (Tomo) Nuclear Medicine Imaging	**Definition:** Introduction of radioactive materials into the body for three dimensional display of images developed from the capture of radioactive emissions

APPENDIX A

SECTION F - PHYSICAL REHABILITATION AND DIAGNOSTIC AUDIOLOGY

CHARACTER 3 - TYPE

Activities of Daily Living Assessment	**Definition:** Measurement of functional level for activities of daily living
Activities of Daily Living Treatment	**Definition:** Exercise or activities to facilitate functional competence for activities of daily living
Caregiver Training	**Definition:** Training in activities to support patient's optimal level of function
Cochlear Implant Treatment	**Definition:** Application of techniques to improve the communication abilities of individuals with cochlear implant
Device Fitting	**Definition:** Fitting of a device designed to facilitate or support achievement of a higher level of function
Hearing Aid Assessment	**Definition:** Measurement of the appropriateness and/or effectiveness of a hearing device
Hearing Assessment	**Definition:** Measurement of hearing and related functions

Hearing Treatment	**Definition:** Application of techniques to improve, augment, or compensate for hearing and related functional impairment
Motor and/or Nerve Function Assessment	**Definition:** Measurement of motor, nerve, and related functions
Motor Treatment	**Definition:** Exercise or activities to increase or facilitate motor function
Speech Assessment	**Definition:** Measurement of speech and related functions
Speech Treatment	**Definition:** Application of techniques to improve, augment, or compensate for speech and related functional impairment
Vestibular Assessment	**Definition:** Measurement of the vestibular system and related functions
Vestibular Treatment	**Definition:** Application of techniques to improve, augment, or compensate for vestibular and related functional impairment

SECTION F - PHYSICAL REHABILITATION AND DIAGNOSTIC AUDIOLOGY

CHARACTER 5 - TYPE QUALIFIER

Acoustic Reflex Decay	**Definition:** Measures reduction in size/strength of acoustic reflex over time **Includes/Examples:** Includes site of lesion test
Acoustic Reflex Patterns	**Definition:** Defines site of lesion based upon presence/absence of acoustic reflexes with ipsilateral vs. contralateral stimulation
Acoustic Reflex Threshold	**Definition:** Determines minimal intensity that acoustic reflex occurs with ipsilateral and/or contralateral stimulation
Aerobic Capacity and Endurance	**Definition:** Measures autonomic responses to positional changes; perceived exertion, dyspnea or angina during activity; performance during exercise protocols; standard vital signs; and blood gas analysis or oxygen consumption

Alternate Binaural or Monaural Loudness Balance	**Definition:** Determines auditory stimulus parameter that yields the same objective sensation **Includes/Examples:** Sound intensities that yield same loudness perception
Anthropometric Characteristics	**Definition:** Measures edema, body fat composition, height, weight, length and girth
Aphasia (Assessment)	**Definition:** Measures expressive and receptive speech and language function including reading and writing
Aphasia (Treatment)	**Definition:** Applying techniques to improve, augment, or compensate for receptive/expressive language impairments
Articulation/Phonology (Assessment)	**Definition:** Measures speech production

◀ New ⬅ Revised ~~deleted~~ Deleted

SECTION F - PHYSICAL REHABILITATION AND DIAGNOSTIC AUDIOLOGY
CHARACTER 5 - TYPE QUALIFIER

Articulation/Phonology (Treatment)	**Definition:** Applying techniques to correct, improve, or compensate for speech productive impairment
Assistive Listening Device	**Definition:** Assists in use of effective and appropriate assistive listening device/system
Assistive Listening System/Device Selection	**Definition:** Measures the effectiveness and appropriateness of assistive listening systems/devices
Assistive, Adaptive, Supportive or Protective Devices	**Explanation:** Devices to facilitate or support achievement of a higher level of function in wheelchair mobility; bed mobility; transfer or ambulation ability; bath and showering ability; dressing; grooming; personal hygiene; play or leisure
Auditory Evoked Potentials	**Definition:** Measures electric responses produced by the VIIIth cranial nerve and brainstem following auditory stimulation
Auditory Processing (Assessment)	**Definition:** Evaluates ability to receive and process auditory information and comprehension of spoken language
Auditory Processing (Treatment)	**Definition:** Applying techniques to improve the receiving and processing of auditory information and comprehension of spoken language
Augmentative/ Alternative Communication System (Assessment)	**Definition:** Determines the appropriateness of aids, techniques, symbols, and/or strategies to augment or replace speech and enhance communication **Includes/Examples:** Includes the use of telephones, writing equipment, emergency equipment, and TDD
Augmentative/ Alternative Communication System (Treatment)	**Includes/Examples:** Includes augmentative communication devices and aids
Aural Rehabilitation	**Definition:** Applying techniques to improve the communication abilities associated with hearing loss
Aural Rehabilitation Status	**Definition:** Measures impact of a hearing loss including evaluation of receptive and expressive communication skills

Bathing/Showering	**Includes/Examples:** Includes obtaining and using supplies; soaping, rinsing, and drying body parts; maintaining bathing position; and transferring to and from bathing positions
Bathing/Showering Techniques	**Definition:** Activities to facilitate obtaining and using supplies, soaping, rinsing and drying body parts, maintaining bathing position, and transferring to and from bathing positions
Bed Mobility (Assessment)	**Definition:** Transitional movement within bed
Bed Mobility (Treatment)	**Definition:** Exercise or activities to facilitate transitional movements within bed
Bedside Swallowing and Oral Function	**Includes/Examples:** Bedside swallowing includes assessment of sucking, masticating, coughing, and swallowing. Oral function includes assessment of musculature for controlled movements, structures and functions to determine coordination and phonation
Bekesy Audiometry	**Definition:** Uses an instrument that provides a choice of discrete or continuously varying pure tones; choice of pulsed or continuous signal
Binaural Electroacoustic Hearing Aid Check	**Definition:** Determines mechanical and electroacoustic function of bilateral hearing aids using hearing aid test box
Binaural Hearing Aid (Assessment)	**Definition:** Measures the candidacy, effectiveness, and appropriateness of a hearing aids **Explanation:** Measures bilateral fit
Binaural Hearing Aid (Treatment)	**Explanation:** Assists in achieving maximum understanding and performance
Bithermal, Binaural Caloric Irrigation	**Definition:** Measures the rhythmic eye movements stimulated by changing the temperature of the vestibular system
Bithermal, Monaural Caloric Irrigation	**Definition:** Measures the rhythmic eye movements stimulated by changing the temperature of the vestibular system in one ear

SECTION F - PHYSICAL REHABILITATION AND DIAGNOSTIC AUDIOLOGY

CHARACTER 5 - TYPE QUALIFIER

Brief Tone Stimuli	**Definition:** Measures specific central auditory process
Cerumen Management	**Definition:** Includes examination of external auditory canal and tympanic membrane and removal of cerumen from external ear canal
Cochlear Implant	**Definition:** Measures candidacy for cochlear implant
Cochlear Implant Rehabilitation	**Definition:** Applying techniques to improve the communication abilities of individuals with cochlear implant; includes programming the device, providing patients/families with information
Communicative/ Cognitive Integration Skills (Assessment)	**Definition:** Measures ability to use higher cortical functions **Includes/Examples:** Includes orientation, recognition, attention span, initiation and termination of activity, memory, sequencing, categorizing, concept formation, spatial operations, judgment, problem solving, generalization and pragmatic communication
Communicative/ Cognitive Integration Skills (Treatment)	**Definition:** Activities to facilitate the use of higher cortical functions **Includes/Examples:** Includes level of arousal, orientation, recognition, attention span, initiation and termination of activity, memory sequencing, judgment and problem solving, learning and generalization, and pragmatic communication
Computerized Dynamic Posturography	**Definition:** Measures the status of the peripheral and central vestibular system and the sensory/motor component of balance; evaluates the efficacy of vestibular rehabilitation
Conditioned Play Audiometry	**Definition:** Behavioral measures using nonspeech and speech stimuli to obtain frequency-specific and ear-specific information on auditory status from the patient **Explanation:** Obtains speech reception threshold by having patient point to pictures of spondaic words

Coordination/Dexterity (Assessment)	**Definition:** Measures large and small muscle groups for controlled goal-directed movements **Explanation:** Dexterity includes object manipulation
Coordination/Dexterity (Treatment)	**Definition:** Exercise or activities to facilitate gross coordination and fine coordination
Cranial Nerve Integrity	**Definition:** Measures cranial nerve sensory and motor functions, including tastes, smell and facial expression
Dichotic Stimuli	**Definition:** Measures specific central auditory process
Distorted Speech	**Definition:** Measures specific central auditory process
Dix-Hallpike Dynamic	**Definition:** Measures nystagmus following Dix-Hallpike maneuver
Dressing	**Includes/Examples:** Includes selecting clothing and accessories, obtaining clothing from storage, dressing and, fastening and adjusting clothing and shoes, and applying and removing personal devices, prosthesis or orthosis
Dressing Techniques	**Definition:** Activities to facilitate selecting clothing and accessories, dressing and undressing, adjusting clothing and shoes, applying and removing devices, prostheses or orthoses
Dynamic Orthosis	**Includes/Examples:** Includes customized and prefabricated splints, inhibitory casts, spinal and other braces, and protective devices; allows motion through transfer of movement from other body parts or by use of outside forces
Ear Canal Probe Microphone	**Definition:** Real ear measures
Ear Protector Attentuation	**Definition:** Measures ear protector fit and effectiveness
Electrocochleography	**Definition:** Measures the VIIIth cranial nerve action potential
Environmental, Home and Work Barriers	**Definition:** Measures current and potential barriers to optimal function, including safety hazards, access problems and home or office design

◀ New　◀⫶⫶ Revised　~~deleted~~ Deleted

SECTION F - PHYSICAL REHABILITATION AND DIAGNOSTIC AUDIOLOGY
CHARACTER 5 - TYPE QUALIFIER

Ergonomics and Body Mechanics	**Definition:** Ergonomic measurement of job tasks, work hardening or work conditioning needs; functional capacity; and body mechanics
Eustachian Tube Function	**Definition:** Measures eustachian tube function and patency of eustachian tube
Evoked Otoacoustic Emissions, Diagnostic	**Definition:** Measures auditory evoked potentials in a diagnostic format
Evoked Otoacoustic Emissions, Screening	**Definition:** Measures auditory evoked potentials in a screening format
Facial Nerve Function	**Definition:** Measures electrical activity of the VIIth cranial nerve (facial nerve)
Feeding/Eating (Assessment)	**Includes/Examples:** Includes setting up food, selecting and using utensils and tableware, bringing food or drink to mouth, cleaning face, hands, and clothing, and management of alternative methods of nourishment
Feeding/Eating (Treatment)	**Definition:** Exercise or activities to facilitate setting up food, selecting and using utensils and tableware, bringing food or drink to mouth, cleaning face, hands, and clothing, and management of alternative methods of nourishment
Filtered Speech	**Definition:** Uses high or low pass filtered speech stimuli to assess central auditory processing disorders, site of lesion testing
Fluency (Assessment)	**Definition:** Measures speech fluency or stuttering
Fluency (Treatment)	**Definition:** Applying techniques to improve and augment fluent speech
Gait and/or Balance	**Definition:** Measures biomechanical, arthrokinematic and other spatial and temporal characteristics of gait and balance
Gait Training/ Functional Ambulation	**Definition:** Exercise or activities to facilitate ambulation on a variety of surfaces and in a variety of environments
Grooming/Personal Hygiene (Assessment)	**Includes/Examples:** Includes ability to obtain and use supplies in a sequential fashion, general grooming, oral hygiene, toilet hygiene, personal care devices, including care for artificial airways
Grooming/Personal Hygiene (Treatment)	**Definition:** Activities to facilitate obtaining and using supplies in a sequential fashion: general grooming, oral hygiene, toilet hygiene, cleaning body, and personal care devices, including artificial airways
Hearing and Related Disorders Counseling	**Definition:** Provides patients/families/caregivers with information, support, referrals to facilitate recovery from a communication disorder **Includes/Examples:** Includes strategies for psychosocial adjustment to hearing loss for clients and families/caregivers
Hearing and Related Disorders Prevention	**Definition:** Provides patients/families/caregivers with information and support to prevent communication disorders
Hearing Screening	**Definition:** Pass/refer measures designed to identify need for further audiologic assessment
Home Management (Assessment)	**Definition:** Obtaining and maintaining personal and household possessions and environment **Includes/Examples:** Includes clothing care, cleaning, meal preparation and cleanup, shopping, money management, household maintenance, safety procedures, and childcare/parenting
Home Management (Treatment)	**Definition:** Activities to facilitate obtaining and maintaining personal household possessions and environment **Includes/Examples:** Includes clothing care, cleaning, meal preparation and clean-up, shopping, money management, household maintenance, safety procedures, childcare/parenting
Instrumental Swallowing and Oral Function	**Definition:** Measures swallowing function using instrumental diagnostic procedures **Explanation:** Methods include videofluoroscopy, ultrasound, manometry, endoscopy
Integumentary Integrity	**Includes/Examples:** Includes burns, skin conditions, ecchymosis, bleeding, blisters, scar tissue, wounds and other traumas, tissue mobility, turgor and texture

APPENDIX A

SECTION F - PHYSICAL REHABILITATION AND DIAGNOSTIC AUDIOLOGY
CHARACTER 5 - TYPE QUALIFIER

Term	Description
Manual Therapy Techniques	**Definition:** Techniques in which the therapist uses his/her hands to administer skilled movements **Includes/Examples:** Includes connective tissue massage, joint mobilization and manipulation, manual lymph drainage, manual traction, soft tissue mobilization and manipulation
Masking Patterns	**Definition:** Measures central auditory processing status
Monaural Electroacoustic Hearing Aid Check	**Definition:** Determines mechanical and electroacoustic function of one hearing aid using hearing aid test box
Monaural Hearing Aid (Assessment)	**Definition:** Measures the candidacy, effectiveness, and appropriateness of a hearing aid **Explanation:** Measures unilateral fit
Monaural Hearing Aid (Treatment)	**Explanation:** Assists in achieving maximum understanding and performance
Motor Function (Assessment)	**Definition:** Measures the body's functional and versatile movement patterns **Includes/Examples:** Includes motor assessment scales, analysis of head, trunk and limb movement, and assessment of motor learning
Motor Function (Treatment)	**Definition:** Exercise or activities to facilitate crossing midline, laterality, bilateral integration, praxis, neuromuscular relaxation, inhibition, facilitation, motor function and motor learning
Motor Speech (Assessment)	**Definition:** Measures neurological motor aspects of speech production
Motor Speech (Treatment)	**Definition:** Applying techniques to improve and augment the impaired neurological motor aspects of speech production
Muscle Performance (Assessment)	**Definition:** Measures muscle strength, power and endurance using manual testing, dynamometry or computer-assisted electromechanical muscle test; functional muscle strength, power and endurance; muscle pain, tone, or soreness; or pelvic-floor musculature **Explanation:** Muscle endurance refers to the ability to contract a muscle repeatedly over time
Muscle Performance (Treatment)	**Definition:** Exercise or activities to increase the capacity of a muscle to do work in terms of strength, power, and/or endurance **Explanation:** Muscle strength is the force exerted to overcome resistance in one maximal effort. Muscle power is work produced per unit of time, or the product of strength and speed. Muscle endurance is the ability to contract a muscle repeatedly over time
Neuromotor Development	**Definition:** Measures motor development, righting and equilibrium reactions, and reflex and equilibrium reactions
Neurophysiologic Intraoperative	**Definition:** Monitors neural status during surgery
Non-invasive Instrumental Status	**Definition:** Instrumental measures of oral, nasal, vocal, and velopharyngeal functions as they pertain to speech production
Nonspoken Language (Assessment)	**Definition:** Measures nonspoken language (print, sign, symbols) for communication
Nonspoken Language (Treatment)	**Definition:** Applying techniques that improve, augment, or compensate spoken communication
Oral Peripheral Mechanism	**Definition:** Structural measures of face, jaw, lips, tongue, teeth, hard and soft palate, pharynx as related to speech production
Orofacial Myofunctional (Assessment)	**Definition:** Measures orofacial myofunctional patterns for speech and related functions
Orofacial Myofunctional (Treatment)	**Definition:** Applying techniques to improve, alter, or augment impaired orofacial myofunctional patterns and related speech production errors
Oscillating Tracking	**Definition:** Measures ability to visually track
Pain	**Definition:** Measures muscle soreness, pain and soreness with joint movement, and pain perception **Includes/Examples:** Includes questionnaires, graphs, symptom magnification scales or visual analog scales

◀ New   ⬅ Revised   ~~deleted~~ Deleted

SECTION F - PHYSICAL REHABILITATION AND DIAGNOSTIC AUDIOLOGY
CHARACTER 5 - TYPE QUALIFIER

Perceptual Processing (Assessment)	**Definition:** Measures stereognosis, kinesthesia, body schema, right-left discrimination, form constancy, position in space, visual closure, figure-ground, depth perception, spatial relations and topographical orientation
Perceptual Processing (Treatment)	**Definition:** Exercise and activities to facilitate perceptual processing **Explanation:** Includes stereognosis, kinesthesia, body schema, right-left discrimination, form constancy, position in space, visual closure, figure-ground, depth perception, spatial relations, and topographical orientation **Includes/Examples:** Includes stereognosis, kinesthesia, body schema, right-left discrimination, form constancy, position in space, visual closure, figure-ground, depth perception, spatial relations, and topographical orientation
Performance Intensity Phonetically Balanced Speech Discrimination	**Definition:** Measures word recognition over varying intensity levels
Postural Control	**Definition:** Exercise or activities to increase postural alignment and control
Prosthesis	**Explanation:** Artificial substitutes for missing body parts that augment performance or function
Psychosocial Skills (Assessment)	**Definition:** The ability to interact in society and to process emotions **Includes/Examples:** Includes psychological (values, interests, self-concept); social (role performance, social conduct, interpersonal skills, self expression); self-management (coping skills, time management, self-control)
Psychosocial Skills (Treatment)	**Definition:** The ability to interact in society and to process emotions **Includes/Examples:** Includes psychological (values, interests, self-concept); social (role performance, social conduct, interpersonal skills, self expression); self-management (coping skills, time management, self-control)

Pure Tone Audiometry, Air	**Definition:** Air-conduction pure tone threshold measures with appropriate masking
Pure Tone Audiometry, Air and Bone	**Definition:** Air-conduction and bone-conduction pure tone threshold measures with appropriate masking
Pure Tone Stenger	**Definition:** Measures unilateral nonorganic hearing loss based on simultaneous presentation of pure tones of differing volume
Range of Motion and Joint Integrity	**Definition:** Measures quantity, quality, grade, and classification of joint movement and/or mobility **Explanation:** Range of Motion is the space, distance or angle through which movement occurs at a joint or series of joints. Joint integrity is the conformance of joints to expected anatomic, biomechanical and kinematic norms
Range of Motion and Joint Mobility	**Definition:** Exercise or activities to increase muscle length and joint mobility
Receptive/Expressive Language (Assessment)	**Definition:** Measures receptive and expressive language
Receptive/Expressive Language (Treatment)	**Definition:** Applying techniques tot improve and augment receptive/expressive language
Reflex Integrity	**Definition:** Measures the presence, absence, or exaggeration of developmentally appropriate, pathologic or normal reflexes
Select Picture Audiometry	**Definition:** Establishes hearing threshold levels for speech using pictures
Sensorineural Acuity Level	**Definition:** Measures sensorineural acuity masking presented via bone conduction
Sensory Aids	**Definition:** Determines the appropriateness of a sensory prosthetic device, other than a hearing aid or assistive listening system/device
Sensory Awareness/ Processing/Integrity	**Includes/Examples:** Includes light touch, pressure, temperature, pain, sharp/dull, proprioception, vestibular, visual, auditory, gustatory, and olfactory

APPENDIX A

SECTION F - PHYSICAL REHABILITATION AND DIAGNOSTIC AUDIOLOGY
CHARACTER 5 - TYPE QUALIFIER

Short Increment Sensitivity Index	**Definition:** Measures the ear's ability to detect small intensity changes; site of lesion test requiring a behavioral response	Synthetic Sentence Identification	**Definition:** Measures central auditory dysfunction using identification of third order approximations of sentences and competing messages
Sinusoidal Vertical Axis Rotational	**Definition:** Measures nystagmus following rotation	Temporal Ordering of Stimuli	**Definition:** Measures specific central auditory process
Somatosensory Evoked Potentials	**Definition:** Measures neural activity from sites throughout the body	Therapeutic Exercise	**Definition:** Exercise or activities to facilitate sensory awareness, sensory processing, sensory integration, balance training, conditioning, reconditioning **Includes/Examples:** Includes developmental activities, breathing exercises, aerobic endurance activities, aquatic exercises, stretching and ventilatory muscle training
Speech and/or Language Screening	**Definition:** Identifies need for further speech and/or language evaluation		
Speech Threshold	**Definition:** Measures minimal intensity needed to repeat spondaic words		
Speech-Language Pathology and Related Disorders Counseling	**Definition:** Provides patients/families with information, support, referrals to facilitate recovery from a communication disorder	Tinnitus Masker (Assessment)	**Definition:** Determines candidacy for tinnitus masker
Speech-Language Pathology and Related Disorders Prevention	**Definition:** Applying techniques to avoid or minimize onset and/or development of a communication disorder	Tinnitus Masker (Treatment)	**Explanation:** Used to verify physical fit, acoustic appropriateness, and benefit; assists in achieving maximum benefit
Speech/Word Recognition	**Definition:** Measures ability to repeat/identify single syllable words; scores given as a percentage; includes word recognition/speech discrimination	Tone Decay	**Definition:** Measures decrease in hearing sensitivity to a tone; site of lesion test requiring a behavioral response
Staggered Spondaic Word	**Definition:** Measures central auditory processing site of lesion based upon dichotic presentation of spondaic words	Transfer	**Definition:** Transitional movement from one surface to another
		Transfer Training	**Definition:** Exercise or activities to facilitate movement from one surface to another
Static Orthosis	**Includes/Examples:** Includes customized and prefabricated splints, inhibitory casts, spinal and other braces, and protective devices; has no moving parts, maintains joint(s) in desired position	Tympanometry	**Definition:** Measures the integrity of the middle ear; measures ease at which sound flows through the tympanic membrane while air pressure against the membrane is varied
Stenger	**Definition:** Measures unilateral nonorganic hearing loss based on simultaneous presentation of signals of differing volume	Unithermal Binaural Screen	**Definition:** Measures the rhythmic eye movements stimulated by changing the temperature of the vestibular system in both ears using warm water, screening format
Swallowing Dysfunction	**Definition:** Activities to improve swallowing function in coordination with respiratory function **Includes/Examples:** Includes function and coordination of sucking, mastication, coughing, swallowing		

◀ New   ◀||| Revised   ~~deleted~~ Deleted

SECTION F - PHYSICAL REHABILITATION AND DIAGNOSTIC AUDIOLOGY
CHARACTER 5 - TYPE QUALIFIER

Ventilation, Respiration and Circulation	**Definition:** Measures ventilatory muscle strength, power and endurance, pulmonary function and ventilatory mechanics **Includes/Examples:** Includes ability to clear airway, activities that aggravate or relieve edema, pain, dyspnea or other symptoms, chest wall mobility, cardiopulmonary response to performance of ADL and IAD, cough and sputum, standard vital signs
Vestibular	**Definition:** Applying techniques to compensate for balance disorders; includes habituation, exercise therapy, and balance retraining
Visual Motor Integration (Assessment)	**Definition:** Coordinating the interaction of information from the eyes with body movement during activity
Visual Motor Integration (Treatment)	**Definition:** Exercise or activities to facilitate coordinating the interaction of information from eyes with body movement during activity
Visual Reinforcement Audiometry	**Definition:** Behavioral measures using nonspeech and speech stimuli to obtain frequency/ear-specific information on auditory status **Includes/Examples:** Includes a conditioned response of looking toward a visual reinforcer (e.g., lights, animated toy) every time auditory stimuli are heard
Vocational Activities and Functional Community or Work Reintegration Skills (Assessment)	**Definition:** Measures environmental, home, work (job/school/play) barriers that keep patients from functioning optimally in their environment **Includes/Examples:** Includes assessment of vocational skill and interests, environment of work (job/school/play), injury potential and injury prevention or reduction, ergonomic stressors, transportation skills, and ability to access and use community resources

Vocational Activities and Functional Community or Work Reintegration Skills (Treatment)	**Definition:** Activities to facilitate vocational exploration, body mechanics training, job acquisition, and environmental or work (job/school/play) task adaptation **Includes/Examples:** Includes injury prevention and reduction, ergonomic stressor reduction, job coaching and simulation, work hardening and conditioning, driving training, transportation skills, and use of community resources
Voice (Assessment)	**Definition:** Measures vocal structure, function and production
Voice (Treatment)	**Definition:** Applying techniques to improve voice and vocal function
Voice Prosthetic (Assessment)	**Definition:** Determines the appropriateness of voice prosthetic/adaptive device to enhance or facilitate communication
Voice Prosthetic (Treatment)	**Includes/Examples:** Includes electrolarynx, and other assistive, adaptive, supportive devices
Wheelchair Mobility (Assessment)	**Definition:** Measures fit and functional abilities within wheelchair in a variety of environments
Wheelchair Mobility (Treatment)	**Definition:** Management, maintenance and controlled operation of a wheelchair, scooter or other device, in and on a variety of surfaces and environments
Wound Management	**Includes/Examples:** Includes non-selective and selective debridement (enzymes, autolysis, sharp debridement), dressings (wound coverings, hydrogel, vacuum-assisted closure), topical agents, etc.

APPENDIX A

SECTION G - MENTAL HEALTH
CHARACTER 3 - TYPE

Biofeedback	**Definition:** Provision of information from the monitoring and regulating of physiological processes in conjunction with cognitive-behavioral techniques to improve patient functioning or well-being **Includes/Examples:** Includes EEG, blood pressure, skin temperature or peripheral blood flow, ECG, electrooculogram, EMG, respirometry or capnometry, GSR/EDR, perineometry to monitor/regulate bowel/bladder activity, electrogastrogram to monitor/regulate gastric motility
Counseling	**Definition:** The application of psychological methods to treat an individual with normal developmental issues and psychological problems in order to increase function, improve well-being, alleviate distress, maladjustment or resolve crises
Crisis Intervention	**Definition:** Treatment of a traumatized, acutely disturbed or distressed individual for the purpose of short-term stabilization **Includes/Examples:** Includes defusing, debriefing, counseling, psychotherapy and/or coordination of care with other providers or agencies
Electroconvulsive Therapy	**Definition:** The application of controlled electrical voltages to treat a mental health disorder **Includes/Examples:** Includes appropriate sedation and other preparation of the individual
Family Psychotherapy	**Definition:** Treatment that includes one or more family members of an individual with a mental health disorder by behavioral, cognitive, psychoanalytic, psychodynamic or psychophysiological means to improve functioning or well-being **Explanation:** Remediation of emotional or behavioral problems presented by one or more family members in cases where psychotherapy with more than one family member is indicated

Group Psychotherapy	**Definition:** Treatment of two or more individuals with a mental health disorder by behavioral, cognitive, psychoanalytic, psychodynamic or psychophysiological means to improve functioning or well-being
Hypnosis	**Definition:** Induction of a state of heightened suggestibility by auditory, visual and tactile techniques to elicit an emotional or behavioral response
Individual Psychotherapy	**Definition:** Treatment of an individual with a mental health disorder by behavioral, cognitive, psychoanalytic, psychodynamic or psychophysiological means to improve functioning or well-being
Light Therapy	**Definition:** Application of specialized light treatments to improve functioning or well-being
Medication Management	**Definition:** Monitoring and adjusting the use of medications for the treatment of a mental health disorder
Narcosynthesis	**Definition:** Administration of intravenous barbiturates in order to release suppressed or repressed thoughts
Psychological Tests	**Definition:** The administration and interpretation of standardized psychological tests and measurement instruments for the assessment of psychological function

◀ New   ⬅ Revised   ~~deleted~~ Deleted

SECTION G - MENTAL HEALTH
CHARACTER 4 - QUALIFIER

Behavioral	**Definition:** Primarily to modify behavior **Includes/Examples:** Includes modeling and role playing, positive reinforcement of target behaviors, response cost, and training of self-management skills	Neuropsychological	**Definition:** Thinking, reasoning and judgment, acquired knowledge, attention, memory, visual spatial abilities, language functions, planning
Cognitive	**Definition:** Primarily to correct cognitive distortions and errors	Personality and Behavioral	**Definition:** Mood, emotion, behavior, social functioning, psychopathological conditions, personality traits and characteristics
Cognitive-Behavioral	**Definition:** Combining cognitive and behavioral treatment strategies to improve functioning **Explanation:** Maladaptive responses are examined to determine how cognitions relate to behavior patterns in response to an event. Uses learning principles and information-processing models	Psychoanalysis	**Definition:** Methods of obtaining a detailed account of past and present mental and emotional experiences to determine the source and eliminate or diminish the undesirable effects of unconscious conflicts **Explanation:** Accomplished by making the individual aware of their existence, origin, and inappropriate expression in emotions and behavior
Developmental	**Definition:** Age-normed developmental status of cognitive, social and adaptive behavior skills	Psychodynamic	**Definition:** Exploration of past and present emotional experiences to understand motives and drives using insight-oriented techniques to reduce the undesirable effects of internal conflicts on emotions and behavior **Explanation:** Techniques include empathetic listening, clarifying self-defeating behavior patterns, and exploring adaptive alternatives
Intellectual and Psychoeducational	**Definition:** Intellectual abilities, academic achievement and learning capabilities (including behaviors and emotional factors affecting learning		
Interactive	**Definition:** Uses primarily physical aids and other forms of non-oral interaction with a patient who is physically, psychologically or developmentally unable to use ordinary language for communication **Includes/Examples:** Includes the use of toys in symbolic play	Psychophysiological	**Definition:** Monitoring and alteration of physiological processes to help the individual associate physiological reactions combined with cognitive and behavioral strategies to gain improved control of these processes to help the individual cope more effectively
Interpersonal	**Definition:** Helps an individual make changes in interpersonal behaviors to reduce psychological dysfunction **Includes/Examples:** Includes exploratory techniques, encouragement of affective expression, clarification of patient statements, analysis of communication patterns, use of therapy relationship and behavior change techniques	Supportive	**Definition:** Formation of therapeutic relationship primarily for providing emotional support to prevent further deterioration in functioning during periods of particular stress **Explanation:** Often used in conjunction with other therapeutic approaches
Neurobehavioral and Cognitive Status	**Definition:** Includes neurobehavioral status exam, interview(s), and observation for the clinical assessment of thinking, reasoning and judgment, acquired knowledge, attention, memory, visual spatial abilities, language functions, and planning	Vocational	**Definition:** Exploration of vocational interests, aptitudes and required adaptive behavior skills to develop and carry out a plan for achieving a successful vocational placement **Includes/Examples:** Includes enhancing work related adjustment and/or pursuing viable options in training education or preparation

APPENDIX A

◀ New   ◀▥ Revised   ~~deleted~~ Deleted

SECTION H - SUBSTANCE ABUSE TREATMENT
CHARACTER 3 - TYPE

Detoxification Services	**Definition:** Detoxification from alcohol and/ or drugs **Explanation:** Not a treatment modality, but helps the patient stabilize physically and psychologically until the body becomes free of drugs and the effects of alcohol
Family Counseling	**Definition:** The application of psychological methods that includes one or more family members to treat an individual with addictive behavior **Explanation:** Provides support and education for family members of addicted individuals. Family member participation is seen as a critical area of substance abuse treatment
Group Counseling	**Definition:** The application of psychological methods to treat two or more individuals with addictive behavior **Explanation:** Provides structured group counseling sessions and healing power through the connection with others

Individual Counseling	**Definition:** The application of psychological methods to treat an individual with addictive behavior **Explanation:** Comprised of several different techniques, which apply various strategies to address drug addiction
Individual Psychotherapy	**Definition:** Treatment of an individual with addictive behavior by behavioral, cognitive, psychoanalytic, psychodynamic or psychophysiological means
Medication Management	**Definition:** Monitoring and adjusting the use of replacement medications for the treatment of addiction
Pharmacotherapy	**Definition:** The use of replacement medications for the treatment of addiction

◀ New   ◀⁣⁣⁣▮ Revised   ~~deleted~~ Deleted

BODY PART KEY

Abdominal aortic plexus	**Use:** Abdominal Sympathetic Nerve
Abdominal esophagus	**Use:** Esophagus, Lower
Abductor hallucis muscle	**Use:** Foot Muscle, Right Foot Muscle, Left
Accessory cephalic vein	**Use:** Cephalic Vein, Right Cephalic Vein, Left
Accessory obturator nerve	**Use:** Lumbar Plexus
Accessory phrenic nerve	**Use:** Phrenic Nerve
Accessory spleen	**Use:** Spleen
Acetabulofemoral joint	**Use:** Hip Joint, Right Hip Joint, Left
Achilles tendon	**Use:** Lower Leg Tendon, Right Lower Leg Tendon, Left
Acromioclavicular ligament	**Use:** Shoulder Bursa and Ligament, Right Shoulder Bursa and Ligament, Left
Acromion (process)	**Use:** Scapula, Right Scapula, Left
Adductor brevis muscle	**Use:** Upper Leg Muscle, Right Upper Leg Muscle, Left
Adductor hallucis muscle	**Use:** Foot Muscle, Right Foot Muscle, Left
Adductor longus muscle Adductor magnus muscle	**Use:** Upper Leg Muscle, Right Upper Leg Muscle, Left
Adenohypophysis	**Use:** Pituitary Gland
Alar ligament of axis	**Use:** Head and Neck Bursa and Ligament
Alveolar process of mandible	**Use:** Mandible, Right Mandible, Left

Alveolar process of maxilla	**Use:** Maxilla, Right Maxilla, Left
Anal orifice	**Use:** Anus
Anatomical snuffbox	**Use:** Lower Arm and Wrist Muscle, Right Lower Arm and Wrist Muscle, Left
Angular artery	**Use:** Face Artery
Angular vein	**Use:** Face Vein, Right Face Vein, Left
Annular ligament	**Use:** Elbow Bursa and Ligament, Right Elbow Bursa and Ligament, Left
Anorectal junction	**Use:** Rectum
Ansa cervicalis	**Use:** Cervical Plexus
Antebrachial fascia	**Use:** Subcutaneous Tissue and Fascia, Right Lower Arm Subcutaneous Tissue and Fascia, Left Lower Arm
Anterior (pectoral) lymph node	**Use:** Lymphatic, Right Axillary Lymphatic, Left Axillary
Anterior cerebral artery	**Use:** Intracranial Artery
Anterior cerebral vein	**Use:** Intracranial Vein
Anterior choroidal artery	**Use:** Intracranial Artery
Anterior circumflex humeral artery	**Use:** Axillary Artery, Right Axillary Artery, Left
Anterior communicating artery	**Use:** Intracranial Artery
Anterior cruciate ligament (ACL)	**Use:** Knee Bursa and Ligament, Right Knee Bursa and Ligament, Left
Anterior crural nerve	**Use:** Femoral Nerve

Appendix B, Body Part Key

BODY PART KEY

Anterior facial vein	**Use:** Face Vein, Right Face Vein, Left
Anterior intercostal artery	**Use:** Internal Mammary Artery, Right Internal Mammary Artery, Left
Anterior interosseous nerve	**Use:** Median Nerve
Anterior lateral malleolar artery	**Use:** Anterior Tibial Artery, Right Anterior Tibial Artery, Left
Anterior lingual gland	**Use:** Minor Salivary Gland
Anterior medial malleolar artery	**Use:** Anterior Tibial Artery, Right Anterior Tibial Artery, Left
Anterior spinal artery	**Use:** Vertebral Artery, Right Vertebral Artery, Left
Anterior tibial recurrent artery	**Use:** Anterior Tibial Artery, Right Anterior Tibial Artery, Left
Anterior ulnar recurrent artery	**Use:** Ulnar Artery, Right Ulnar Artery, Left
Anterior vagal trunk	**Use:** Vagus Nerve
Anterior vertebral muscle	**Use:** Neck Muscle, Right Neck Muscle, Left
Antihelix Antitragus	**Use:** External Ear, Right External Ear, Left External Ear, Bilateral
Antrum of Highmore	**Use:** Maxillary Sinus, Right Maxillary Sinus, Left
Aortic annulus	**Use:** Aortic Valve
Aortic arch Aortic intercostal artery	**Use:** Thoracic Aorta
Apical (subclavicular) lymph node	**Use:** Lymphatic, Right Axillary Lymphatic, Left Axillary
Apneustic center	**Use:** Pons
Aqueduct of Sylvius	**Use:** Cerebral Ventricle
Aqueous humour	**Use:** Anterior Chamber, Right Anterior Chamber, Left
Arachnoid mater	**Use:** Cerebral Meninges Spinal Meninges
Arcuate artery	**Use:** Foot Artery, Right Foot Artery, Left
Areola	**Use:** Nipple, Right Nipple, Left
Arterial canal (duct)	**Use:** Pulmonary Artery, Left
Aryepiglottic fold Arytenoid cartilage	**Use:** Larynx
Arytenoid muscle	**Use:** Neck Muscle, Right Neck Muscle, Left
Ascending aorta	**Use:** Thoracic Aorta
Ascending palatine artery	**Use:** Face Artery
Ascending pharyngeal artery	**Use:** External Carotid Artery, Right External Carotid Artery, Left
Atlantoaxial joint	**Use:** Cervical Vertebral Joint
Atrioventricular node	**Use:** Conduction Mechanism
Atrium dextrum cordis	**Use:** Atrium, Right
Atrium pulmonale	**Use:** Atrium, Left
Auditory tube	**Use:** Eustachian Tube, Right Eustachian Tube, Left
Auerbach's (myenteric) plexus	**Use:** Abdominal Sympathetic Nerve

New　　Revised　　deleted Deleted

BODY PART KEY

Auricle	**Use:** External Ear, Right External Ear, Left External Ear, Bilateral
Auricularis muscle	**Use:** Head Muscle
Axillary fascia	**Use:** Subcutaneous Tissue and Fascia, Right Upper Arm Subcutaneous Tissue and Fascia, Left Upper Arm
Axillary nerve	**Use:** Brachial Plexus
Bartholin's (greater vestibular) gland	**Use:** Vestibular Gland
Basal (internal) cerebral vein	**Use:** Intracranial Vein
Basal nuclei	**Use:** Basal Ganglia
Basilar artery	**Use:** Intracranial Artery
Basis pontis	**Use:** Pons
Biceps brachii muscle	**Use:** Upper Arm Muscle, Right Upper Arm Muscle, Left
Biceps femoris muscle	**Use:** Upper Leg Muscle, Right Upper Leg Muscle, Left
Bicipital aponeurosis	**Use:** Subcutaneous Tissue and Fascia, Right Lower Arm Subcutaneous Tissue and Fascia, Left Lower Arm
Bicuspid valve	**Use:** Mitral Valve
Body of femur	**Use:** Femoral Shaft, Right Femoral Shaft, Left
Body of fibula	**Use:** Fibula, Right Fibula, Left
Bony labyrinth	**Use:** Inner Ear, Right Inner Ear, Left

Bony orbit	**Use:** Orbit, Right Orbit, Left
Bony vestibule	**Use:** Inner Ear, Right Inner Ear, Left
Botallo's duct	**Use:** Pulmonary Artery, Left
Brachial (lateral) lymph node	**Use:** Lymphatic, Right Axillary Lymphatic, Left Axillary
Brachialis muscle	**Use:** Upper Arm Muscle, Right Upper Arm Muscle, Left
Brachiocephalic artery Brachiocephalic trunk	**Use:** Innominate Artery
Brachiocephalic vein	**Use:** Innominate Vein, Right Innominate Vein, Left
Brachioradialis muscle	**Use:** Lower Arm and Wrist Muscle, Right Lower Arm and Wrist Muscle, Left
Broad ligament	**Use:** Uterine Supporting Structure
Bronchial artery	**Use:** Thoracic Aorta
Buccal gland	**Use:** Buccal Mucosa
Buccinator lymph node	**Use:** Lymphatic, Head
Buccinator muscle	**Use:** Facial Muscle
Bulbospongiosus muscle	**Use:** Perineum Muscle
Bulbourethral (Cowper's) gland	**Use:** Urethra
Bundle of His Bundle of Kent	**Use:** Conduction Mechanism
Calcaneocuboid joint	**Use:** Tarsal Joint, Right Tarsal Joint, Left
Calcaneocuboid ligament	**Use:** Foot Bursa and Ligament, Right Foot Bursa and Ligament, Left

◀ New   ◀◀◀ Revised   ~~deleted~~ Deleted

BODY PART KEY

Calcaneofibular ligament	**Use:** Ankle Bursa and Ligament, Right Ankle Bursa and Ligament, Left
Calcaneus	**Use:** Tarsal, Right Tarsal, Left
Capitate bone	**Use:** Carpal, Right Carpal, Left
Cardia	**Use:** Esophagogastric Junction
Cardiac plexus	**Use:** Thoracic Sympathetic Nerve
Cardioesophageal junction	**Use:** Esophagogastric Junction
Caroticotympanic artery	**Use:** Internal Carotid Artery, Right Internal Carotid Artery, Left
Carotid glomus	**Use:** Carotid Body, Left Carotid Body, Right Carotid Bodies, Bilateral
Carotid sinus	**Use:** Internal Carotid Artery, Right Internal Carotid Artery, Left
Carotid sinus nerve	**Use:** Glossopharyngeal Nerve
Carpometacarpal (CMC) joint	**Use:** Metacarpocarpal Joint, Right Metacarpocarpal Joint, Left
Carpometacarpal ligament	**Use:** Hand Bursa and Ligament, Right Hand Bursa and Ligament, Left
Cauda equina	**Use:** Lumbar Spinal Cord
Cavernous plexus	**Use:** Head and Neck Sympathetic Nerve
Celiac (solar) plexus Celiac ganglion	**Use:** Abdominal Sympathetic Nerve
Celiac lymph node	**Use:** Lymphatic, Aortic
Celiac trunk	**Use:** Celiac Artery
Central axillary lymph node	**Use:** Lymphatic, Right Axillary Lymphatic, Left Axillary
Cerebral aqueduct (Sylvius)	**Use:** Cerebral Ventricle
Cerebrum	**Use:** Brain
Cervical esophagus	**Use:** Esophagus, Upper
Cervical facet joint	**Use:** Cervical Vertebral Joint Cervical Vertebral Joints, 2 or more
Cervical ganglion	**Use:** Head and Neck Sympathetic Nerve
Cervical interspinous ligament Cervical intertransverse ligament Cervical ligamentum flavum	**Use:** Head and Neck Bursa and Ligament
Cervical lymph node	**Use:** Lymphatic, Right Neck Lymphatic, Left Neck
Cervicothoracic facet joint	**Use:** Cervicothoracic Vertebral Joint
Choana	**Use:** Nasopharynx
Chondroglossus muscle	**Use:** Tongue, Palate, Pharynx Muscle
Chorda tympani	**Use:** Facial Nerve
Choroid plexus	**Use:** Cerebral Ventricle
Ciliary body	**Use:** Eye, Right Eye, Left
Ciliary ganglion	**Use:** Head and Neck Sympathetic Nerve
Circle of Willis	**Use:** Intracranial Artery
Circumflex iliac artery	**Use:** Femoral Artery, Right Femoral Artery, Left
Claustrum	**Use:** Basal Ganglia
Coccygeal body	**Use:** Coccygeal Glomus
Coccygeus muscle	**Use:** Trunk Muscle, Right Trunk Muscle, Left

◀ New ◀▥ Revised ~~deleted~~ Deleted

BODY PART KEY

Cochlea	**Use:** Inner Ear, Right Inner Ear, Left
Cochlear nerve	**Use:** Acoustic Nerve
Columella	**Use:** Nose
Common digital vein	**Use:** Foot Vein, Right Foot Vein, Left
Common facial vein	**Use:** Face Vein, Right Face Vein, Left
Common fibular nerve	**Use:** Peroneal Nerve
Common hepatic artery	**Use:** Hepatic Artery
Common iliac (subaortic) lymph node	**Use:** Lymphatic, Pelvis
Common interosseous artery	**Use:** Ulnar Artery, Right Ulnar Artery, Left
Common peroneal nerve	**Use:** Peroneal Nerve
Condyloid process	**Use:** Mandible, Right Mandible, Left
Conus arteriosus	**Use:** Ventricle, Right
Conus medullaris	**Use:** Lumbar Spinal Cord
Coracoacromial ligament	**Use:** Shoulder Bursa and Ligament, Right Shoulder Bursa and Ligament, Left
Coracobrachialis muscle	**Use:** Upper Arm Muscle, Right Upper Arm Muscle, Left
Coracoclavicular ligament Coracohumeral ligament	**Use:** Shoulder Bursa and Ligament, Right Shoulder Bursa and Ligament, Left
Coracoid process	**Use:** Scapula, Right Scapula, Left
Corniculate cartilage	**Use:** Larynx
Corpus callosum	**Use:** Brain
Corpus cavernosum Corpus spongiosum	**Use:** Penis
Corpus striatum	**Use:** Basal Ganglia
Corrugator supercilii muscle	**Use:** Facial Muscle
Costocervical trunk	**Use:** Subclavian Artery, Right Subclavian Artery, Left
Costoclavicular ligament	**Use:** Shoulder Bursa and Ligament, Right Shoulder Bursa and Ligament, Left
Costotransverse joint	**Use:** Thoracic Vertebral Joint Thoracic Vertebral Joints, 2 to 7 Thoracic Vertebral Joints, 8 or more
Costotransverse ligament	**Use:** Thorax Bursa and Ligament, Right Thorax Bursa and Ligament, Left
Costovertebral joint	**Use:** Thoracic Vertebral Joint Thoracic Vertebral Joints, 2 to 7 Thoracic Vertebral Joints, 8 or more
Costoxiphoid ligament	**Use:** Thorax Bursa and Ligament, Right Thorax Bursa and Ligament, Left
Cowper's (bulbourethral) gland	**Use:** Urethra
Cranial dura mater	**Use:** Dura Mater
Cranial epidural space	**Use:** Epidural Space
Cranial subarachnoid space	**Use:** Subarachnoid Space
Cranial subdural space	**Use:** Subdural Space
Cremaster muscle	**Use:** Perineum Muscle

APPENDIX B

BODY PART KEY

BODY PART KEY

BODY PART KEY

Cribriform plate	**Use:** Ethmoid Bone, Right Ethmoid Bone, Left
Cricoid cartilage	**Use:** Larynx
Cricothyroid artery	**Use:** Thyroid Artery, Right Thyroid Artery, Left
Cricothyroid muscle	**Use:** Neck Muscle, Right Neck Muscle, Left
Crural fascia	**Use:** Subcutaneous Tissue and Fascia, Right Upper Leg Subcutaneous Tissue and Fascia, Left Upper Leg
Cubital lymph node	**Use:** Lymphatic, Right Upper Extremity Lymphatic, Left Upper Extremity
Cubital nerve	**Use:** Ulnar Nerve
Cuboid bone	**Use:** Tarsal, Right Tarsal, Left
Cuboideonavicular joint	**Use:** Tarsal Joint, Right Tarsal Joint, Left
Culmen	**Use:** Cerebellum
Cuneiform cartilage	**Use:** Larynx
Cuneonavicular joint	**Use:** Tarsal Joint, Right Tarsal Joint, Left
Cuneonavicular ligament	**Use:** Foot Bursa and Ligament, Right Foot Bursa and Ligament, Left
Cutaneous (transverse) cervical nerve	**Use:** Cervical Plexus
Deep cervical fascia	**Use:** Subcutaneous Tissue and Fascia, Anterior Neck
Deep cervical vein	**Use:** Vertebral Vein, Right Vertebral Vein, Left
Deep circumflex iliac artery	**Use:** External Iliac Artery, Right External Iliac Artery, Left

Deep facial vein	**Use:** Face Vein, Right Face Vein, Left
Deep femoral (profunda femoris) vein	**Use:** Femoral Vein, Right Femoral Vein, Left
Deep femoral artery	**Use:** Femoral Artery, Right Femoral Artery, Left
Deep palmar arch	**Use:** Hand Artery, Right Hand Artery, Left
Deep transverse perineal muscle	**Use:** Perineum Muscle
Deferential artery	**Use:** Internal Iliac Artery, Right Internal Iliac Artery, Left
Deltoid fascia	**Use:** Subcutaneous Tissue and Fascia, Right Upper Arm Subcutaneous Tissue and Fascia, Left Upper Arm
Deltoid ligament	**Use:** Ankle Bursa and Ligament, Right Ankle Bursa and Ligament, Left
Deltoid muscle	**Use:** Shoulder Muscle, Right Shoulder Muscle, Left
Deltopectoral (infraclavicular) lymph node	**Use:** Lymphatic, Right Upper Extremity Lymphatic, Left Upper Extremity
Dentate ligament	**Use:** Dura Mater
Denticulate ligament	**Use:** Spinal Cord
Depressor anguli oris muscle Depressor labii inferioris muscle Depressor septi nasi muscle Depressor supercilii muscle	**Use:** Facial Muscle
Dermis	**Use:** Skin
Descending genicular artery	**Use:** Femoral Artery, Right Femoral Artery, Left
Diaphragma sellae	**Use:** Dura Mater
Distal humerus	**Use:** Humeral Shaft, Right Humeral Shaft, Left

◀ New   ◀▥ Revised   ~~deleted~~ Deleted

BODY PART KEY

Distal humerus, involving joint	**Use:** Elbow Joint, Right Elbow Joint, Left
Distal radioulnar joint	**Use:** Wrist Joint, Right Wrist Joint, Left
Dorsal digital nerve	**Use:** Radial Nerve
Dorsal metacarpal vein	**Use:** Hand Vein, Right Hand Vein, Left
Dorsal metatarsal artery	**Use:** Foot Artery, Right Foot Artery, Left
Dorsal metatarsal vein	**Use:** Foot Vein, Right Foot Vein, Left
Dorsal scapular artery	**Use:** Subclavian Artery, Right Subclavian Artery, Left
Dorsal scapular nerve	**Use:** Brachial Plexus
Dorsal venous arch	**Use:** Foot Vein, Right Foot Vein, Left
Dorsalis pedis artery	**Use:** Anterior Tibial Artery, Right Anterior Tibial Artery, Left
Duct of Santorini	**Use:** Pancreatic Duct, Accessory
Duct of Wirsung	**Use:** Pancreatic Duct
Ductus deferens	**Use:** Vas Deferens, Right Vas Deferens, Left Vas Deferens, Bilateral Vas Deferens
Duodenal ampulla	**Use:** Ampulla of Vater
Duodenojejunal flexure	**Use:** Jejunum
Dural venous sinus	**Use:** Intracranial Vein
Earlobe	**Use:** External Ear, Right External Ear, Left External Ear, Bilateral

Eighth cranial nerve	**Use:** Acoustic Nerve
Ejaculatory duct	**Use:** Vas Deferens, Right Vas Deferens, Left Vas Deferens, Bilateral Vas Deferens
Eleventh cranial nerve	**Use:** Accessory Nerve
Encephalon	**Use:** Brain
Ependyma	**Use:** Cerebral Ventricle
Epidermis	**Use:** Skin
Epiploic foramen	**Use:** Peritoneum
Epithalamus	**Use:** Thalamus
Epitrochlear lymph node	**Use:** Lymphatic, Right Upper Extremity Lymphatic, Left Upper Extremity
Erector spinae muscle	**Use:** Trunk Muscle, Right Trunk Muscle, Left
Esophageal artery	**Use:** Thoracic Aorta
Esophageal plexus	**Use:** Thoracic Sympathetic Nerve
Ethmoidal air cell	**Use:** Ethmoid Sinus, Right Ethmoid Sinus, Left
Extensor carpi radialis muscle Extensor carpi ulnaris muscle	**Use:** Lower Arm and Wrist Muscle, Right Lower Arm and Wrist Muscle, Left
Extensor digitorum brevis muscle	**Use:** Foot Muscle, Right Foot Muscle, Left
Extensor digitorum longus muscle	**Use:** Lower Leg Muscle, Right Lower Leg Muscle, Left
Extensor hallucis brevis muscle	**Use:** Foot Muscle, Right Foot Muscle, Left
Extensor hallucis longus muscle	**Use:** Lower Leg Muscle, Right Lower Leg Muscle, Left

◀ New   ◀▥ Revised   ~~deleted~~ Deleted

BODY PART KEY

External anal sphincter	**Use:** Anal Sphincter
External auditory meatus	**Use:** External Auditory Canal, Right External Auditory Canal, Left
External maxillary artery	**Use:** Face Artery
External naris	**Use:** Nose
External oblique aponeurosis	**Use:** Subcutaneous Tissue and Fascia, Trunk
External oblique muscle	**Use:** Abdomen Muscle, Right Abdomen Muscle, Left
External popliteal nerve	**Use:** Peroneal Nerve
External pudendal artery	**Use:** Femoral Artery, Right Femoral Artery, Left
External pudendal vein	**Use:** Greater Saphenous Vein, Right Greater Saphenous Vein, Left
External urethral sphincter	**Use:** Urethra
Extradural space	**Use:** Epidural Space
Facial artery	**Use:** Face Artery
False vocal cord	**Use:** Larynx
Falx cerebri	**Use:** Dura Mater
Fascia lata	**Use:** Subcutaneous Tissue and Fascia, Right Upper Leg Subcutaneous Tissue and Fascia, Left Upper Leg
Femoral head	**Use:** Upper Femur, Right Upper Femur, Left
Femoral lymph node	**Use:** Lymphatic, Right Lower Extremity Lymphatic, Left Lower Extremity

Femoropatellar joint Femorotibial joint	**Use:** Knee Joint, Right Knee Joint, Left
Fibular artery	**Use:** Peroneal Artery, Right Peroneal Artery, Left
Fibularis brevis muscle Fibularis longus muscle	**Use:** Lower Leg Muscle, Right Lower Leg Muscle, Left
Fifth cranial nerve	**Use:** Trigeminal Nerve
First cranial nerve	**Use:** Olfactory Nerve
First intercostal nerve	**Use:** Brachial Plexus
Flexor carpi radialis muscle Flexor carpi ulnaris muscle	**Use:** Lower Arm and Wrist Muscle, Right Lower Arm and Wrist Muscle, Left
Flexor digitorum brevis muscle	**Use:** Foot Muscle, Right Foot Muscle, Left
Flexor digitorum longus muscle	**Use:** Lower Leg Muscle, Right Lower Leg Muscle, Left
Flexor hallucis brevis muscle	**Use:** Foot Muscle, Right Foot Muscle, Left
Flexor hallucis longus muscle	**Use:** Lower Leg Muscle, Right Lower Leg Muscle, Left
Flexor pollicis longus muscle	**Use:** Lower Arm and Wrist Muscle, Right Lower Arm and Wrist Muscle, Left
Foramen magnum	**Use:** Occipital Bone, Right Occipital Bone, Left
Foramen of Monro (intraventricular)	**Use:** Cerebral Ventricle
Foreskin	**Use:** Prepuce
Fossa of Rosenmuller	**Use:** Nasopharynx
Fourth cranial nerve	**Use:** Trochlear Nerve

◀ New　◀|||| Revised　~~deleted~~ Deleted

BODY PART KEY

Fourth ventricle	**Use:** Cerebral Ventricle
Fovea	**Use:** Retina, Right Retina, Left
Frenulum labii inferioris	**Use:** Lower Lip
Frenulum labii superioris	**Use:** Upper Lip
Frenulum linguae	**Use:** Tongue
Frontal lobe	**Use:** Cerebral Hemisphere
Frontal vein	**Use:** Face Vein, Right Face Vein, Left
Fundus uteri	**Use:** Uterus
Galea aponeurotica	**Use:** Subcutaneous Tissue and Fascia, Scalp
Ganglion impar (ganglion of Walther)	**Use:** Sacral Sympathetic Nerve
Gasserian ganglion	**Use:** Trigeminal Nerve
Gastric lymph node	**Use:** Lymphatic, Aortic
Gastric plexus	**Use:** Abdominal Sympathetic Nerve
Gastrocnemius muscle	**Use:** Lower Leg Muscle, Right Lower Leg Muscle, Left
Gastrocolic ligament Gastrocolic omentum	**Use:** Greater Omentum
Gastroduodenal artery	**Use:** Hepatic Artery
Gastroesophageal (GE) junction	**Use:** Esophagogastric Junction
Gastrohepatic omentum	**Use:** Lesser Omentum
Gastrophrenic ligament Gastrosplenic ligament	**Use:** Greater Omentum

Gemellus muscle	**Use:** Hip Muscle, Right Hip Muscle, Left
Geniculate ganglion	**Use:** Facial Nerve
Geniculate nucleus	**Use:** Thalamus
Genioglossus muscle	**Use:** Tongue, Palate, Pharynx Muscle
Genitofemoral nerve	**Use:** Lumbar Plexus
Glans penis	**Use:** Prepuce
Glenohumeral joint	**Use:** Shoulder Joint, Right Shoulder Joint, Left
Glenohumeral ligament	**Use:** Shoulder Bursa and Ligament, Right Shoulder Bursa and Ligament, Left
Glenoid fossa (of scapula)	**Use:** Glenoid Cavity, Right Glenoid Cavity, Left
Glenoid ligament (labrum)	**Use:** Shoulder Bursa and Ligament, Right Shoulder Bursa and Ligament, Left
Globus pallidus	**Use:** Basal Ganglia
Glossoepiglottic fold	**Use:** Epiglottis
Glottis	**Use:** Larynx
Gluteal lymph node	**Use:** Lymphatic, Pelvis
Gluteal vein	**Use:** Hypogastric Vein, Right Hypogastric Vein, Left
Gluteus maximus muscle Gluteus medius muscle Gluteus minimus muscle	**Use:** Hip Muscle, Right Hip Muscle, Left
Gracilis muscle	**Use:** Upper Leg Muscle, Right Upper Leg Muscle, Left

BODY PART KEY

Great auricular nerve	**Use:** Cervical Plexus
Great cerebral vein	**Use:** Intracranial Vein
Great saphenous vein	**Use:** Greater Saphenous Vein, Right Greater Saphenous Vein, Left
Greater alar cartilage	**Use:** Nose
Greater occipital nerve	**Use:** Cervical Nerve
Greater splanchnic nerve	**Use:** Thoracic Sympathetic Nerve
Greater superficial petrosal nerve	**Use:** Facial Nerve
Greater trochanter	**Use:** Upper Femur, Right Upper Femur, Left
Greater tuberosity	**Use:** Humeral Head, Right Humeral Head, Left
Greater vestibular (Bartholin's) gland	**Use:** Vestibular Gland
Greater wing	**Use:** Sphenoid Bone, Right Sphenoid Bone, Left
Hallux	**Use:** 1st Toe, Right 1st Toe, Left
Hamate bone	**Use:** Carpal, Right Carpal, Left
Head of fibula	**Use:** Fibula, Right Fibula, Left
Helix	**Use:** External Ear, Right External Ear, Left External Ear, Bilateral
Hepatic artery proper	**Use:** Hepatic Artery
Hepatic flexure	**Use:** Ascending Colon

Hepatic lymph node	**Use:** Lymphatic, Aortic
Hepatic plexus	**Use:** Abdominal Sympathetic Nerve
Hepatic portal vein	**Use:** Portal Vein
Hepatogastric ligament	**Use:** Lesser Omentum
Hepatopancreatic ampulla	**Use:** Ampulla of Vater
Humeroradial joint Humeroulnar joint	**Use:** Elbow Joint, Right Elbow Joint, Left
Humerus, distal	**Use:** Humeral Shaft, Right Humeral Shaft, Left
Hyoglossus muscle	**Use:** Tongue, Palate, Pharynx Muscle
Hyoid artery	**Use:** Thyroid Artery, Right Thyroid Artery, Left
Hypogastric artery	**Use:** Internal Iliac Artery, Right Internal Iliac Artery, Left
Hypopharynx	**Use:** Pharynx
Hypophysis	**Use:** Pituitary Gland
Hypothenar muscle	**Use:** Hand Muscle, Right Hand Muscle, Left
Ileal artery Ileocolic artery	**Use:** Superior Mesenteric Artery
Ileocolic vein	**Use:** Colic Vein
Iliac crest	**Use:** Pelvic Bone, Right Pelvic Bone, Left
Iliac fascia	**Use:** Subcutaneous Tissue and Fascia, Right Upper Leg Subcutaneous Tissue and Fascia, Left Upper Leg

◀ New   ◀▥ Revised   ~~deleted~~ Deleted

BODY PART KEY

Iliac lymph node	**Use:** Lymphatic, Pelvis
Iliacus muscle	**Use:** Hip Muscle, Right Hip Muscle, Left
Iliofemoral ligament	**Use:** Hip Bursa and Ligament, Right Hip Bursa and Ligament, Left
Iliohypogastric nerve Ilioinguinal nerve	**Use:** Lumbar Plexus
Iliolumbar artery	**Use:** Internal Iliac Artery, Right Internal Iliac Artery, Left
Iliolumbar ligament	**Use:** Trunk Bursa and Ligament, Right Trunk Bursa and Ligament, Left

Iliotibial tract (band)	**Use:**
	Subcutaneous Tissue and Fascia,
	  Right Upper Leg
	Subcutaneous Tissue and Fascia,
	  Left Upper Leg

Ilium	**Use:** Pelvic Bone, Right Pelvic Bone, Left
Incus	**Use:** Auditory Ossicle, Right Auditory Ossicle, Left
Inferior cardiac nerve	**Use:** Thoracic Sympathetic Nerve
Inferior cerebellar vein Inferior cerebral vein	**Use:** Intracranial Vein
Inferior epigastric artery	**Use:** External Iliac Artery, Right External Iliac Artery, Left
Inferior epigastric lymph node	**Use:** Lymphatic, Pelvis
Inferior genicular artery	**Use:** Popliteal Artery, Right Popliteal Artery, Left
Inferior gluteal artery	**Use:** Internal Iliac Artery, Right Internal Iliac Artery, Left
Inferior gluteal nerve	**Use:** Sacral Plexus
Inferior hypogastric plexus	**Use:** Abdominal Sympathetic Nerve
Inferior labial artery	**Use:** Face Artery
Inferior longitudinal muscle	**Use:** Tongue, Palate, Pharynx Muscle
Inferior mesenteric ganglion	**Use:** Abdominal Sympathetic Nerve
Inferior mesenteric lymph node	**Use:** Lymphatic, Mesenteric
Inferior mesenteric plexus	**Use:** Abdominal Sympathetic Nerve
Inferior oblique muscle	**Use:** Extraocular Muscle, Right Extraocular Muscle, Left
Inferior pancreaticoduodenal artery	**Use:** Superior Mesenteric Artery
Inferior phrenic artery	**Use:** Abdominal Aorta
Inferior rectus muscle	**Use:** Extraocular Muscle, Right Extraocular Muscle, Left
Inferior suprarenal artery	**Use:** Renal Artery, Right Renal Artery, Left
Inferior tarsal plate	**Use:** Lower Eyelid, Right Lower Eyelid, Left
Inferior thyroid vein	**Use:** Innominate Vein, Right Innominate Vein, Left
Inferior tibiofibular joint	**Use:** Ankle Joint, Right Ankle Joint, Left
Inferior turbinate	**Use:** Nasal Turbinate
Inferior ulnar collateral artery	**Use:** Brachial Artery, Right Brachial Artery, Left
Inferior vesical artery	**Use:** Internal Iliac Artery, Right Internal Iliac Artery, Left

◀ New   ◀▥ Revised   ~~deleted~~ Deleted

BODY PART KEY

Infraauricular lymph node	**Use:** Lymphatic, Head
Infraclavicular (deltopectoral) lymph node	**Use:** Lymphatic, Right Upper Extremity Lymphatic, Left Upper Extremity
Infrahyoid muscle	**Use:** Neck Muscle, Right Neck Muscle, Left
Infraparotid lymph node	**Use:** Lymphatic, Head
Infraspinatus fascia	**Use:** Subcutaneous Tissue and Fascia, Right Upper Arm Subcutaneous Tissue and Fascia, Left Upper Arm
Infraspinatus muscle	**Use:** Shoulder Muscle, Right Shoulder Muscle, Left
Infundibulopelvic ligament	**Use:** Uterine Supporting Structure
Inguinal canal Inguinal triangle	**Use:** Inguinal Region, Right Inguinal Region, Left Inguinal Region, Bilateral
Interatrial septum	**Use:** Atrial Septum
Intercarpal joint	**Use:** Carpal Joint, Right Carpal Joint, Left
Intercarpal ligament	**Use:** Hand Bursa and Ligament, Right Hand Bursa and Ligament, Left
Interclavicular ligament	**Use:** Shoulder Bursa and Ligament, Right Shoulder Bursa and Ligament, Left
Intercostal lymph node	**Use:** Lymphatic, Thorax
Intercostal muscle	**Use:** Thorax Muscle, Right Thorax Muscle, Left
Intercostal nerve Intercostobrachial nerve	**Use:** Thoracic Nerve

Intercuneiform joint	**Use:** Tarsal Joint, Right Tarsal Joint, Left
Intercuneiform ligament	**Use:** Foot Bursa and Ligament, Right Foot Bursa and Ligament, Left
Intermediate cuneiform bone	**Use:** Tarsal, Right Tarsal, Left
Internal (basal) cerebral vein	**Use:** Intracranial Vein
Internal anal sphincter	**Use:** Anal Sphincter
Internal carotid plexus	**Use:** Head and Neck Sympathetic Nerve
Internal iliac vein	**Use:** Hypogastric Vein, Right Hypogastric Vein, Left
Internal maxillary artery	**Use:** External Carotid Artery, Right External Carotid Artery, Left
Internal naris	**Use:** Nose
Internal oblique muscle	**Use:** Abdomen Muscle, Right Abdomen Muscle, Left
Internal pudendal artery	**Use:** Internal Iliac Artery, Right Internal Iliac Artery, Left
Internal pudendal vein	**Use:** Hypogastric Vein, Right Hypogastric Vein, Left
Internal thoracic artery	**Use:** Internal Mammary Artery, Right Internal Mammary Artery, Left Subclavian Artery, Right Subclavian Artery, Left
Internal urethral sphincter	**Use:** Urethra
Interphalangeal (IP) joint	**Use:** Finger Phalangeal Joint, Right Finger Phalangeal Joint, Left Toe Phalangeal Joint, Right Toe Phalangeal Joint, Left

◀ New   ◀▬ Revised   ~~deleted~~ Deleted

BODY PART KEY

Interphalangeal ligament	**Use:** Hand Bursa and Ligament, Right Hand Bursa and Ligament, Left Foot Bursa and Ligament, Right Foot Bursa and Ligament, Left
Interspinalis muscle	**Use:** Trunk Muscle, Right Trunk Muscle, Left
Interspinous ligament	**Use:** Trunk Bursa and Ligament, Right Trunk Bursa and Ligament, Left
Intertransversarius muscle	**Use:** Trunk Muscle, Right Trunk Muscle, Left
Intertransverse ligament	**Use:** Trunk Bursa and Ligament, Right Trunk Bursa and Ligament, Left
Interventricular foramen (Monro)	**Use:** Cerebral Ventricle
Interventricular septum	**Use:** Ventricular Septum
Intestinal lymphatic trunk	**Use:** Cisterna Chyli
Ischiatic nerve	**Use:** Sciatic Nerve
Ischiocavernosus muscle	**Use:** Perineum Muscle
Ischiofemoral ligament	**Use:** Hip Bursa and Ligament, Right Hip Bursa and Ligament, Left
Ischium	**Use:** Pelvic Bone, Right Pelvic Bone, Left
Jejunal artery	**Use:** Superior Mesenteric Artery
Jugular body	**Use:** Glomus Jugulare
Jugular lymph node	**Use:** Lymphatic, Right Neck Lymphatic, Left Neck
Labia majora Labia minora	**Use:** Vulva
Labial gland	**Use:** Upper Lip Lower Lip

Lacrimal canaliculus Lacrimal punctum Lacrimal sac	**Use:** Lacrimal Duct, Right Lacrimal Duct, Left
Laryngopharynx	**Use:** Pharynx
Lateral (brachial) lymph node	**Use:** Lymphatic, Right Axillary Lymphatic, Left Axillary
Lateral canthus	**Use:** Upper Eyelid, Right Upper Eyelid, Left
Lateral collateral ligament (LCL)	**Use:** Knee Bursa and Ligament, Right Knee Bursa and Ligament, Left
Lateral condyle of femur	**Use:** Lower Femur, Right Lower Femur, Left
Lateral condyle of tibia	**Use:** Tibia, Right Tibia, Left
Lateral cuneiform bone	**Use:** Tarsal, Right Tarsal, Left
Lateral epicondyle of femur	**Use:** Lower Femur, Right Lower Femur, Left
Lateral epicondyle of humerus	**Use:** Humeral Shaft, Right Humeral Shaft, Left
Lateral femoral cutaneous nerve	**Use:** Lumbar Plexus
Lateral malleolus	**Use:** Fibula, Right Fibula, Left
Lateral meniscus	**Use:** Knee Joint, Right Knee Joint, Left
Lateral nasal cartilage	**Use:** Nose
Lateral plantar artery	**Use:** Foot Artery, Right Foot Artery, Left
Lateral plantar nerve	**Use:** Tibial Nerve

APPENDIX B

BODY PART KEY

Lateral rectus muscle	**Use:** Extraocular Muscle, Right Extraocular Muscle, Left
Lateral sacral artery	**Use:** Internal Iliac Artery, Right Internal Iliac Artery, Left
Lateral sacral vein	**Use:** Hypogastric Vein, Right Hypogastric Vein, Left
Lateral sural cutaneous nerve	**Use:** Peroneal Nerve
Lateral tarsal artery	**Use:** Foot Artery, Right Foot Artery, Left
Lateral temporomandibular ligament	**Use:** Head and Neck Bursa and Ligament
Lateral thoracic artery	**Use:** Axillary Artery, Right Axillary Artery, Left
Latissimus dorsi muscle	**Use:** Trunk Muscle, Right Trunk Muscle, Left
Least splanchnic nerve	**Use:** Thoracic Sympathetic Nerve
Left ascending lumbar vein	**Use:** Hemiazygos Vein
Left atrioventricular valve	**Use:** Mitral Valve
Left auricular appendix	**Use:** Atrium, Left
Left colic vein	**Use:** Colic Vein
Left coronary sulcus	**Use:** Heart, Left
Left gastric artery	**Use:** Gastric Artery
Left gastroepiploic artery	**Use:** Splenic Artery
Left gastroepiploic vein	**Use:** Splenic Vein
Left inferior phrenic vein	**Use:** Renal Vein, Left
Left inferior pulmonary vein	**Use:** Pulmonary Vein, Left

Left jugular trunk	**Use:** Thoracic Duct
Left lateral ventricle	**Use:** Cerebral Ventricle
Left ovarian vein Left second lumbar vein	**Use:** Renal Vein, Left
Left subclavian trunk	**Use:** Thoracic Duct
Left subcostal vein	**Use:** Hemiazygos Vein
Left superior pulmonary vein	**Use:** Pulmonary Vein, Left
Left suprarenal vein Left testicular vein	**Use:** Renal Vein, Left
Leptomeninges	**Use:** Cerebral Meninges Spinal Meninges
Lesser alar cartilage	**Use:** Nose
Lesser occipital nerve	**Use:** Cervical Plexus
Lesser splanchnic nerve	**Use:** Thoracic Sympathetic Nerve
Lesser trochanter	**Use:** Upper Femur, Right Upper Femur, Left
Lesser tuberosity	**Use:** Humeral Head, Right Humeral Head, Left
Lesser wing	**Use:** Sphenoid Bone, Right Sphenoid Bone, Left
Levator anguli oris muscle	**Use:** Facial Muscle
Levator ani muscle	**Use:** Trunk Muscle, Right Trunk Muscle, Left
Levator labii superioris alaeque nasi muscle Levator labii superioris muscle	**Use:** Facial Muscle
Levator palpebrae superioris muscle	**Use:** Upper Eyelid, Right Upper Eyelid, Left
Levator scapulae muscle	**Use:** Neck Muscle, Right Neck Muscle, Left

◀ New ◀▥ Revised ~~deleted~~ Deleted

BODY PART KEY

Levator veli palatini muscle	**Use:** Tongue, Palate, Pharynx Muscle
Levatores costarum muscle	**Use:** Thorax Muscle, Right Thorax Muscle, Left
Ligament of head of fibula	**Use:** Knee Bursa and Ligament, Right Knee Bursa and Ligament, Left
Ligament of the lateral malleolus	**Use:** Ankle Bursa and Ligament, Right Ankle Bursa and Ligament, Left
Ligamentum flavum	**Use:** Trunk Bursa and Ligament, Right Trunk Bursa and Ligament, Left
Lingual artery	**Use:** External Carotid Artery, Right External Carotid Artery, Left
Lingual tonsil	**Use:** Tongue
Locus ceruleus	**Use:** Pons
Long thoracic nerve	**Use:** Brachial Plexus
Lumbar artery	**Use:** Abdominal Aorta
Lumbar facet joint	**Use:** Lumbar Vertebral Joint Lumbar Vertebral Joints, 2 or more
Lumbar ganglion	**Use:** Lumbar Sympathetic Nerve
Lumbar lymph node	**Use:** Lymphatic, Aortic
Lumbar lymphatic trunk	**Use:** Cisterna Chyli
Lumbar splanchnic nerve	**Use:** Lumbar Sympathetic Nerve
Lumbosacral facet joint	**Use:** Lumbosacral Joint
Lumbosacral trunk	**Use:** Lumbar Nerve
Lunate bone	**Use:** Carpal, Right Carpal, Left
Lunotriquetral ligament	**Use:** Hand Bursa and Ligament, Right Hand Bursa and Ligament, Left

Macula	**Use:** Retina, Right Retina, Left
Malleus	**Use:** Auditory Ossicle, Right Auditory Ossicle, Left
Mammary duct Mammary gland	**Use:** Breast, Right Breast, Left Breast, Bilateral
Mammillary body	**Use:** Hypothalamus
Mandibular nerve	**Use:** Trigeminal Nerve
Mandibular notch	**Use:** Mandible, Right Mandible, Left
Manubrium	**Use:** Sternum
Masseter muscle	**Use:** Head Muscle
Masseteric fascia	**Use:** Subcutaneous Tissue and Fascia, Face
Mastoid (postauricular) lymph node	**Use:** Lymphatic, Right Neck Lymphatic, Left Neck
Mastoid air cells	**Use:** Mastoid Sinus, Right Mastoid Sinus, Left
Mastoid process	**Use:** Temporal Bone, Right Temporal Bone, Left
Maxillary artery	**Use:** External Carotid Artery, Right External Carotid Artery, Left
Maxillary nerve	**Use:** Trigeminal Nerve
Medial canthus	**Use:** Lower Eyelid, Right Lower Eyelid, Left
Medial collateral ligament (MCL)	**Use:** Knee Bursa and Ligament, Right Knee Bursa and Ligament, Left
Medial condyle of femur	**Use:** Lower Femur, Right Lower Femur, Left

◀ New   ◀▥ Revised   ~~deleted~~ Deleted

APPENDIX B

BODY PART KEY

BODY PART KEY

Medial condyle of tibia	**Use:** Tibia, Right Tibia, Left
Medial cuneiform bone	**Use:** Tarsal, Right Tarsal, Left
Medial epicondyle of femur	**Use:** Lower Femur, Right Lower Femur, Left
Medial epicondyle of humerus	**Use:** Humeral Shaft, Right Humeral Shaft, Left
Medial malleolus	**Use:** Tibia, Right Tibia, Left
Medial meniscus	**Use:** Knee Joint, Right Knee Joint, Left
Medial plantar artery	**Use:** Foot Artery, Right Foot Artery, Left
Medial plantar nerve Medial popliteal nerve	**Use:** Tibial Nerve
Medial rectus muscle	**Use:** Extraocular Muscle, Right Extraocular Muscle, Left
Medial sural cutaneous nerve	**Use:** Tibial Nerve
Median antebrachial vein Median cubital vein	**Use:** Basilic Vein, Right Basilic Vein, Left
Median sacral artery	**Use:** Abdominal Aorta
Mediastinal lymph node	**Use:** Lymphatic, Thorax
Meissner's (submucous) plexus	**Use:** Abdominal Sympathetic Nerve
Membranous urethra	**Use:** Urethra
Mental foramen	**Use:** Mandible, Right Mandible, Left
Mentalis muscle	**Use:** Facial Muscle
Mesoappendix Mesocolon	**Use:** Mesentery

Metacarpal ligament Metacarpophalangeal ligament	**Use:** Hand Bursa and Ligament, Right Hand Bursa and Ligament, Left
Metatarsal ligament	**Use:** Foot Bursa and Ligament, Right Foot Bursa and Ligament, Left
Metatarsophalangeal (MTP) joint	**Use:** Metatarsal-Phalangeal Joint, Right Metatarsal-Phalangeal Joint, Left
Metatarsophalangeal ligament	**Use:** Foot Bursa and Ligament, Right Foot Bursa and Ligament, Left
Metathalamus	**Use:** Thalamus
Midcarpal joint	**Use:** Carpal Joint, Right Carpal Joint, Left
Middle cardiac nerve	**Use:** Thoracic Sympathetic Nerve
Middle cerebral artery	**Use:** Intracranial Artery
Middle cerebral vein	**Use:** Intracranial Vein
Middle colic vein	**Use:** Colic Vein
Middle genicular artery	**Use:** Popliteal Artery, Right Popliteal Artery, Left
Middle hemorrhoidal vein	**Use:** Hypogastric Vein, Right Hypogastric Vein, Left
Middle rectal artery	**Use:** Internal Iliac Artery, Right Internal Iliac Artery, Left
Middle suprarenal artery	**Use:** Abdominal Aorta
Middle temporal artery	**Use:** Temporal Artery, Right Temporal Artery, Left
Middle turbinate	**Use:** Nasal Turbinate
Mitral annulus	**Use:** Mitral Valve
Molar gland	**Use:** Buccal Mucosa
Musculocutaneous nerve	**Use:** Brachial Plexus

◀ New   ◀◀ Revised   ~~deleted~~ Deleted

BODY PART KEY

Musculophrenic artery	**Use:** Internal Mammary Artery, Right Internal Mammary Artery, Left
Musculospiral nerve	**Use:** Radial Nerve
Myelencephalon	**Use:** Medulla Oblongata
Myenteric (Auerbach's) plexus	**Use:** Abdominal Sympathetic Nerve
Myometrium	**Use:** Uterus
Nail bed Nail plate	**Use:** Finger Nail Toe Nail
Nasal cavity	**Use:** Nose
Nasal concha	**Use:** Nasal Turbinate
Nasalis muscle	**Use:** Facial Muscle
Nasolacrimal duct	**Use:** Lacrimal Duct, Right Lacrimal Duct, Left
Navicular bone	**Use:** Tarsal, Right Tarsal, Left
Neck of femur	**Use:** Upper Femur, Right Upper Femur, Left
Neck of humerus (anatomical) (surgical)	**Use:** Humeral Head, Right Humeral Head, Left
Nerve to the stapedius	**Use:** Facial Nerve
Neurohypophysis	**Use:** Pituitary Gland
Ninth cranial nerve	**Use:** Glossopharyngeal Nerve
Nostril	**Use:** Nose
Obturator artery	**Use:** Internal Iliac Artery, Right Internal Iliac Artery, Left
Obturator lymph node	**Use:** Lymphatic, Pelvis

Obturator muscle	**Use:** Hip Muscle, Right Hip Muscle, Left
Obturator nerve	**Use:** Lumbar Plexus
Obturator vein	**Use:** Hypogastric Vein, Right Hypogastric Vein, Left
Obtuse margin	**Use:** Heart, Left
Occipital artery	**Use:** External Carotid Artery, Right External Carotid Artery, Left
Occipital lobe	**Use:** Cerebral Hemisphere
Occipital lymph node	**Use:** Lymphatic, Right Neck Lymphatic, Left Neck
Occipitofrontalis muscle	**Use:** Facial Muscle
Olecranon bursa	**Use:** Elbow Bursa and Ligament, Right Elbow Bursa and Ligament, Left
Olecranon process	**Use:** Ulna, Right Ulna, Left
Olfactory bulb	**Use:** Olfactory Nerve
Ophthalmic artery	**Use:** Internal Carotid Artery, Right Internal Carotid Artery, Left
Ophthalmic nerve	**Use:** Trigeminal Nerve
Ophthalmic vein	**Use:** Intracranial Vein
Optic chiasma	**Use:** Optic Nerve
Optic disc	**Use:** Retina, Right Retina, Left
Optic foramen	**Use:** Sphenoid Bone, Right Sphenoid Bone, Left
Orbicularis oculi muscle	**Use:** Upper Eyelid, Right Upper Eyelid, Left

APPENDIX B

BODY PART KEY

Orbicularis oris muscle	**Use:** Facial Muscle
Orbital fascia	**Use:** Subcutaneous Tissue and Fascia, Face
Orbital portion of ethmoid bone Orbital portion of frontal bone Orbital portion of lacrimal bone Orbital portion of maxilla Orbital portion of palatine bone Orbital portion of sphenoid bone Orbital portion of zygomatic bone	**Use:** Orbit, Right Orbit, Left
Oropharynx	**Use:** Pharynx
Ossicular chain	**Use:** Auditory Ossicle, Right Auditory Ossicle, Left
Otic ganglion	**Use:** Head and Neck Sympathetic Nerve
Oval window	**Use:** Middle Ear, Right Middle Ear, Left
Ovarian artery	**Use:** Abdominal Aorta
Ovarian ligament	**Use:** Uterine Supporting Structure
Oviduct	**Use:** Fallopian Tube, Right Fallopian Tube, Left
Palatine gland	**Use:** Buccal Mucosa
Palatine tonsil	**Use:** Tonsils
Palatine uvula	**Use:** Uvula
Palatoglossal muscle Palatopharyngeal muscle	**Use:** Tongue, Palate, Pharynx Muscle
Palmar (volar) digital vein Palmar (volar) metacarpal vein	**Use:** Hand Vein, Right Hand Vein, Left
Palmar cutaneous nerve	**Use:** Median Nerve Radial Nerve
Palmar fascia (aponeurosis)	**Use:** Subcutaneous Tissue and Fascia, Right Hand Subcutaneous Tissue and Fascia, Left Hand
Palmar interosseous muscle	**Use:** Hand Muscle, Right Hand Muscle, Left
Palmar ulnocarpal ligament	**Use:** Wrist Bursa and Ligament, Right Wrist Bursa and Ligament, Left
Palmaris longus muscle	**Use:** Lower Arm and Wrist Muscle, Right Lower Arm and Wrist Muscle, Left
Pancreatic artery	**Use:** Splenic Artery
Pancreatic plexus	**Use:** Abdominal Sympathetic Nerve
Pancreatic vein	**Use:** Splenic Vein
Pancreaticosplenic lymph node Paraaortic lymph node	**Use:** Lymphatic, Aortic
Pararectal lymph node	**Use:** Lymphatic, Mesenteric
Parasternal lymph node Paratracheal lymph node	**Use:** Lymphatic, Thorax
Paraurethral (Skene's) gland	**Use:** Vestibular Gland
Parietal lobe	**Use:** Cerebral Hemisphere
Parotid lymph node	**Use:** Lymphatic, Head
Parotid plexus	**Use:** Facial Nerve
Pars flaccida	**Use:** Tympanic Membrane, Right Tympanic Membrane, Left
Patellar ligament	**Use:** Knee Bursa and Ligament, Right Knee Bursa and Ligament, Left
Patellar tendon	**Use:** Knee Tendon, Right Knee Tendon, Left
Pectineus muscle	**Use:** Upper Leg Muscle, Right Upper Leg Muscle, Left
Pectoral (anterior) lymph node	**Use:** Lymphatic, Right Axillary Lymphatic, Left Axillary
Pectoral fascia	**Use:** Subcutaneous Tissue and Fascia, Chest

◄ New ◄∥∥ Revised ~~deleted~~ Deleted

BODY PART KEY

Pectoralis major muscle Pectoralis minor muscle	**Use:** Thorax Muscle, Right Thorax Muscle, Left
Pelvic splanchnic nerve	**Use:** Abdominal Sympathetic Nerve Sacral Sympathetic Nerve
Penile urethra	**Use:** Urethra
Pericardiophrenic artery	**Use:** Internal Mammary Artery, Right Internal Mammary Artery, Left
Perimetrium	**Use:** Uterus
Peroneus brevis muscle Peroneus longus muscle	**Use:** Lower Leg Muscle, Right Lower Leg Muscle, Left
Petrous part of temporal bone	**Use:** Temporal Bone, Right Temporal Bone, Left
Pharyngeal constrictor muscle	**Use:** Tongue, Palate, Pharynx Muscle
Pharyngeal plexus	**Use:** Vagus Nerve
Pharyngeal recess	**Use:** Nasopharynx
Pharyngeal tonsil	**Use:** Adenoids
Pharyngotympanic tube	**Use:** Eustachian Tube, Right Eustachian Tube, Left
Pia mater	**Use:** Cerebral Meninges Spinal Meninges
Pinna	**Use:** External Ear, Right External Ear, Left External Ear, Bilateral
Piriform recess (sinus)	**Use:** Pharynx
Piriformis muscle	**Use:** Hip Muscle, Right Hip Muscle, Left
Pisiform bone	**Use:** Carpal, Right Carpal, Left
Pisohamate ligament Pisometacarpal ligament	**Use:** Hand Bursa and Ligament, Right Hand Bursa and Ligament, Left
Plantar digital vein	**Use:** Foot Vein, Right Foot Vein, Left
Plantar fascia (aponeurosis)	**Use:** Subcutaneous Tissue and Fascia, Right Foot Subcutaneous Tissue and Fascia, Left Foot
Plantar metatarsal vein Plantar venous arch	**Use:** Foot Vein, Right Foot Vein, Left
Platysma muscle	**Use:** Neck Muscle, Right Neck Muscle, Left
Plica semilunaris	**Use:** Conjunctiva, Right Conjunctiva, Left
Pneumogastric nerve	**Use:** Vagus Nerve
Pneumotaxic center Pontine tegmentum	**Use:** Pons
Popliteal ligament	**Use:** Knee Bursa and Ligament, Right Knee Bursa and Ligament, Left
Popliteal lymph node	**Use:** Lymphatic, Right Lower Extremity Lymphatic, Left Lower Extremity
Popliteal vein	**Use:** Femoral Vein, Right Femoral Vein, Left
Popliteus muscle	**Use:** Lower Leg Muscle, Right Lower Leg Muscle, Left
Postauricular (mastoid) lymph node	**Use:** Lymphatic, Right Neck Lymphatic, Left Neck
Postcava	**Use:** Inferior Vena Cava
Posterior (subscapular) lymph node	**Use:** Lymphatic, Right Axillary Lymphatic, Left Axillary
Posterior auricular artery	**Use:** External Carotid Artery, Right External Carotid Artery, Left
Posterior auricular nerve	**Use:** Facial Nerve

APPENDIX B

BODY PART KEY

Posterior auricular vein	**Use:** External Jugular Vein, Right External Jugular Vein, Left
Posterior cerebral artery	**Use:** Intracranial Artery
Posterior chamber	**Use:** Eye, Right Eye, Left
Posterior circumflex humeral artery	**Use:** Axillary Artery, Right Axillary Artery, Left
Posterior communicating artery	**Use:** Intracranial Artery
Posterior cruciate ligament (PCL)	**Use:** Knee Bursa and Ligament, Right Knee Bursa and Ligament, Left
Posterior facial (retromandibular) vein	**Use:** Face Vein, Right Face Vein, Left
Posterior femoral cutaneous nerve	**Use:** Sacral Plexus
Posterior inferior cerebellar artery (PICA)	**Use:** Intracranial Artery
Posterior interosseous nerve	**Use:** Radial Nerve
Posterior labial nerve Posterior scrotal nerve	**Use:** Pudendal Nerve
Posterior spinal artery	**Use:** Vertebral Artery, Right Vertebral Artery, Left
Posterior tibial recurrent artery	**Use:** Anterior Tibial Artery, Right Anterior Tibial Artery, Left
Posterior ulnar recurrent artery	**Use:** Ulnar Artery, Right Ulnar Artery, Left
Posterior vagal trunk	**Use:** Vagus Nerve
Preauricular lymph node	**Use:** Lymphatic, Head
Precava	**Use:** Superior Vena Cava
Prepatellar bursa	**Use:** Knee Bursa and Ligament, Right Knee Bursa and Ligament, Left
Pretracheal fascia	**Use:** Subcutaneous Tissue and Fascia, Anterior Neck
Prevertebral fascia	**Use:** Subcutaneous Tissue and Fascia, Posterior Neck
Princeps pollicis artery	**Use:** Hand Artery, Right Hand Artery, Left
Procerus muscle	**Use:** Facial Muscle
Profunda brachii	**Use:** Brachial Artery, Right Brachial Artery, Left
Profunda femoris (deep femoral) vein	**Use:** Femoral Vein, Right Femoral Vein, Left
Pronator quadratus muscle Pronator teres muscle	**Use:** Lower Arm and Wrist Muscle, Right Lower Arm and Wrist Muscle, Left
Prostatic urethra	**Use:** Urethra
Proximal radioulnar joint	**Use:** Elbow Joint, Right Elbow Joint, Left
Psoas muscle	**Use:** Hip Muscle, Right Hip Muscle, Left
Pterygoid muscle	**Use:** Head Muscle
Pterygoid process	**Use:** Sphenoid Bone, Right Sphenoid Bone, Left
Pterygopalatine (sphenopalatine) ganglion	**Use:** Head and Neck Sympathetic Nerve
Pubic ligament	**Use:** Trunk Bursa and Ligament, Right Trunk Bursa and Ligament, Left
Pubis	**Use:** Pelvic Bone, Right Pelvic Bone, Left
Pubofemoral ligament	**Use:** Hip Bursa and Ligament, Right Hip Bursa and Ligament, Left
Pudendal nerve	**Use:** Sacral Plexus

◀ New ◀▥ Revised ~~deleted~~ Deleted

BODY PART KEY

Pulmoaortic canal	**Use:** Pulmonary Artery, Left
Pulmonary annulus	**Use:** Pulmonary Valve
Pulmonary plexus	**Use:** Vagus Nerve Thoracic Sympathetic Nerve
Pulmonic valve	**Use:** Pulmonary Valve
Pulvinar	**Use:** Thalamus
Pyloric antrum Pyloric canal Pyloric sphincter	**Use:** Stomach, Pylorus
Pyramidalis muscle	**Use:** Abdomen Muscle, Right Abdomen Muscle, Left
Quadrangular cartilage	**Use:** Nasal Septum
Quadrate lobe	**Use:** Liver
Quadratus femoris muscle	**Use:** Hip Muscle, Right Hip Muscle, Left
Quadratus lumborum muscle	**Use:** Trunk Muscle, Right Trunk Muscle, Left
Quadratus plantae muscle	**Use:** Foot Muscle, Right Foot Muscle, Left
Quadriceps (femoris)	**Use:** Upper Leg Muscle, Right Upper Leg Muscle, Left
Radial collateral carpal ligament	**Use:** Wrist Bursa and Ligament, Right Wrist Bursa and Ligament, Left
Radial collateral ligament	**Use:** Elbow Bursa and Ligament, Right Elbow Bursa and Ligament, Left
Radial notch	**Use:** Ulna, Right Ulna, Left
Radial recurrent artery	**Use:** Radial Artery, Right Radial Artery, Left

Radial vein	**Use:** Brachial Vein, Right Brachial Vein, Left
Radialis indicis	**Use:** Hand Artery, Right Hand Artery, Left
Radiocarpal joint	**Use:** Wrist Joint, Right Wrist Joint, Left
Radiocarpal ligament Radioulnar ligament	**Use:** Wrist Bursa and Ligament, Right Wrist Bursa and Ligament, Left
Rectosigmoid junction	**Use:** Sigmoid Colon
Rectus abdominis muscle	**Use:** Abdomen Muscle, Right Abdomen Muscle, Left
Rectus femoris muscle	**Use:** Upper Leg Muscle, Right Upper Leg Muscle, Left
Recurrent laryngeal nerve	**Use:** Vagus Nerve
Renal calyx Renal capsule Renal cortex	**Use:** Kidney, Right Kidney, Left Kidneys, Bilateral Kidney
Renal plexus	**Use:** Abdominal Sympathetic Nerve
Renal segment	**Use:** Kidney, Right Kidney, Left Kidneys, Bilateral Kidney
Renal segmental artery	**Use:** Renal Artery, Right Renal Artery, Left
Retroperitoneal lymph node	**Use:** Lymphatic, Aortic
Retroperitoneal space	**Use:** Retroperitoneum
Retropharyngeal lymph node	**Use:** Lymphatic, Right Neck Lymphatic, Left Neck
Retropubic space	**Use:** Pelvic Cavity
Rhinopharynx	**Use:** Nasopharynx

APPENDIX B

◀ New   ⬅ Revised   ~~deleted~~ Deleted

BODY PART KEY

Rhomboid major muscle Rhomboid minor muscle	**Use:** Trunk Muscle, Right Trunk Muscle, Left
Right ascending lumbar vein	**Use:** Azygos Vein
Right atrioventricular valve	**Use:** Tricuspid Valve
Right auricular appendix	**Use:** Atrium, Right
Right colic vein	**Use:** Colic Vein
Right coronary sulcus	**Use:** Heart, Right
Right gastric artery	**Use:** Gastric Artery
Right gastroepiploic vein	**Use:** Superior Mesenteric Vein
Right inferior phrenic vein	**Use:** Inferior Vena Cava
Right inferior pulmonary vein	**Use:** Pulmonary Vein, Right
Right jugular trunk	**Use:** Lymphatic, Right Neck
Right lateral ventricle	**Use:** Cerebral Ventricle
Right lymphatic duct	**Use:** Lymphatic, Right Neck
Right ovarian vein Right second lumbar vein	**Use:** Inferior Vena Cava
Right subclavian trunk	**Use:** Lymphatic, Right Neck
Right subcostal vein	**Use:** Azygos Vein
Right superior pulmonary vein	**Use:** Pulmonary Vein, Right
Right suprarenal vein Right testicular vein	**Use:** Inferior Vena Cava
Rima glottidis	**Use:** Larynx
Risorius muscle	**Use:** Facial Muscle
Round ligament of uterus	**Use:** Uterine Supporting Structure

Round window	**Use:** Inner Ear, Right Inner Ear, Left
Sacral ganglion	**Use:** Sacral Sympathetic Nerve
Sacral lymph node	**Use:** Lymphatic, Pelvis
Sacral splanchnic nerve	**Use:** Sacral Sympathetic Nerve
Sacrococcygeal ligament	**Use:** Trunk Bursa and Ligament, Right Trunk Bursa and Ligament, Left
Sacrococcygeal symphysis	**Use:** Sacrococcygeal Joint
Sacroiliac ligament Sacrospinous ligament Sacrotuberous ligament	**Use:** Trunk Bursa and Ligament, Right Trunk Bursa and Ligament, Left
Salpingopharyngeus muscle	**Use:** Tongue, Palate, Pharynx Muscle
Salpinx	**Use:** Fallopian Tube, Right Fallopian Tube, Left
Saphenous nerve	**Use:** Femoral Nerve
Sartorius muscle	**Use:** Upper Leg Muscle, Right Upper Leg Muscle, Left
Scalene muscle	**Use:** Neck Muscle, Right Neck Muscle, Left
Scaphoid bone	**Use:** Carpal, Right Carpal, Left
Scapholunate ligament Scaphotrapezium ligament	**Use:** Hand Bursa and Ligament, Right Hand Bursa and Ligament, Left
Scarpa's (vestibular) ganglion	**Use:** Acoustic Nerve
Sebaceous gland	**Use:** Skin
Second cranial nerve	**Use:** Optic Nerve
Sella turcica	**Use:** Sphenoid Bone, Right Sphenoid Bone, Left

◀ New   ◀▬ Revised   ~~deleted~~ Deleted

BODY PART KEY

Semicircular canal	**Use:** Inner Ear, Right Inner Ear, Left
Semimembranosus muscle Semitendinosus muscle	**Use:** Upper Leg Muscle, Right Upper Leg Muscle, Left
Septal cartilage	**Use:** Nasal Septum
Serratus anterior muscle	**Use:** Thorax Muscle, Right Thorax Muscle, Left
Serratus posterior muscle	**Use:** Trunk Muscle, Right Trunk Muscle, Left
Seventh cranial nerve	**Use:** Facial Nerve
Short gastric artery	**Use:** Splenic Artery
Sigmoid artery	**Use:** Inferior Mesenteric Artery
Sigmoid flexure	**Use:** Sigmoid Colon
Sigmoid vein	**Use:** Inferior Mesenteric Vein
Sinoatrial node	**Use:** Conduction Mechanism
Sinus venosus	**Use:** Atrium, Right
Sixth cranial nerve	**Use:** Abducens Nerve
Skene's (paraurethral) gland	**Use:** Vestibular Gland
Small saphenous vein	**Use:** Lesser Saphenous Vein, Right Lesser Saphenous Vein, Left
Solar (celiac) plexus	**Use:** Abdominal Sympathetic Nerve
Soleus muscle	**Use:** Lower Leg Muscle, Right Lower Leg Muscle, Left
Sphenomandibular ligament	**Use:** Head and Neck Bursa and Ligament
Sphenopalatine (pterygopalatine) ganglion	**Use:** Head and Neck Sympathetic Nerve

Spinal dura mater	**Use:** Dura Mater
Spinal epidural space	**Use:** Epidural Space
Spinal subarachnoid space	**Use:** Subarachnoid Space
Spinal subdural space	**Use:** Subdural Space
Spinous process	**Use:** Cervical Vertebra Thoracic Vertebra Lumbar Vertebra
Spiral ganglion	**Use:** Acoustic Nerve
Splenic flexure	**Use:** Transverse Colon
Splenic plexus	**Use:** Abdominal Sympathetic Nerve
Splenius capitis muscle	**Use:** Head Muscle
Splenius cervicis muscle	**Use:** Neck Muscle, Right Neck Muscle, Left
Stapes	**Use:** Auditory Ossicle, Right Auditory Ossicle, Left
Stellate ganglion	**Use:** Head and Neck Sympathetic Nerve
Stensen's duct	**Use:** Parotid Duct, Right Parotid Duct, Left
Sternoclavicular ligament	**Use:** Shoulder Bursa and Ligament, Right Shoulder Bursa and Ligament, Left
Sternocleidomastoid artery	**Use:** Thyroid Artery, Right Thyroid Artery, Left
Sternocleidomastoid muscle	**Use:** Neck Muscle, Right Neck Muscle, Left
Sternocostal ligament	**Use:** Thorax Bursa and Ligament, Right Thorax Bursa and Ligament, Left
Styloglossus muscle	**Use:** Tongue, Palate, Pharynx Muscle

APPENDIX B

BODY PART KEY

BODY PART KEY

Stylomandibular ligament	**Use:** Head and Neck Bursa and Ligament
Stylopharyngeus muscle	**Use:** Tongue, Palate, Pharynx Muscle
Subacromial bursa	**Use:** Shoulder Bursa and Ligament, Right Shoulder Bursa and Ligament, Left
Subaortic (common iliac) lymph node	**Use:** Lymphatic, Pelvis
Subclavicular (apical) lymph node	**Use:** Lymphatic, Right Axillary Lymphatic, Left Axillary
Subclavius muscle	**Use:** Thorax Muscle, Right Thorax Muscle, Left
Subclavius nerve	**Use:** Brachial Plexus
Subcostal artery	**Use:** Thoracic Aorta
Subcostal muscle	**Use:** Thorax Muscle, Right Thorax Muscle, Left
Subcostal nerve	**Use:** Thoracic Nerve
Submandibular ganglion	**Use:** Facial Nerve Head and Neck Sympathetic Nerve
Submandibular gland	**Use:** Submaxillary Gland, Right Submaxillary Gland, Left
Submandibular lymph node	**Use:** Lymphatic, Head
Submaxillary ganglion	**Use:** Head and Neck Sympathetic Nerve
Submaxillary lymph node	**Use:** Lymphatic, Head
Submental artery	**Use:** Face Artery
Submental lymph node	**Use:** Lymphatic, Head
Submucous (Meissner's) plexus	**Use:** Abdominal Sympathetic Nerve
Suboccipital nerve	**Use:** Cervical Nerve

Suboccipital venous plexus	**Use:** Vertebral Vein, Right Vertebral Vein, Left
Subparotid lymph node	**Use:** Lymphatic, Head
Subscapular (posterior) lymph node	**Use:** Lymphatic, Right Axillary Lymphatic, Left Axillary
Subscapular aponeurosis	**Use:** Subcutaneous Tissue and Fascia, Right Upper Arm Subcutaneous Tissue and Fascia, Left Upper Arm
Subscapular artery	**Use:** Axillary Artery, Right Axillary Artery, Left
Subscapularis muscle	**Use:** Shoulder Muscle, Right Shoulder Muscle, Left
Substantia nigra	**Use:** Basal Ganglia
Subtalar (talocalcaneal) joint	**Use:** Tarsal Joint, Right Tarsal Joint, Left
Subtalar ligament	**Use:** Foot Bursa and Ligament, Right Foot Bursa and Ligament, Left
Subthalamic nucleus	**Use:** Basal Ganglia
Superficial circumflex iliac vein	**Use:** Greater Saphenous Vein, Right Greater Saphenous Vein, Left
Superficial epigastric artery	**Use:** Femoral Artery, Right Femoral Artery, Left
Superficial epigastric vein	**Use:** Greater Saphenous Vein, Right Greater Saphenous Vein, Left
Superficial palmar arch	**Use:** Hand Artery, Right Hand Artery, Left
Superficial palmar venous arch	**Use:** Hand Vein, Right Hand Vein, Left
Superficial temporal artery	**Use:** Temporal Artery, Right Temporal Artery, Left

◀ New   ◀▦ Revised   ~~deleted~~ Deleted

BODY PART KEY

Superficial transverse perineal muscle	**Use:** Perineum Muscle
Superior cardiac nerve	**Use:** Thoracic Sympathetic Nerve
Superior cerebellar vein Superior cerebral vein	**Use:** Intracranial Vein
Superior clunic (cluneal) nerve	**Use:** Lumbar Nerve
Superior epigastric artery	**Use:** Internal Mammary Artery, Right Internal Mammary Artery, Left
Superior genicular artery	**Use:** Popliteal Artery, Right Popliteal Artery, Left
Superior gluteal artery	**Use:** Internal Iliac Artery, Right Internal Iliac Artery, Left
Superior gluteal nerve	**Use:** Lumbar Plexus
Superior hypogastric plexus	**Use:** Abdominal Sympathetic Nerve
Superior labial artery	**Use:** Face Artery
Superior laryngeal artery	**Use:** Thyroid Artery, Right Thyroid Artery, Left
Superior laryngeal nerve	**Use:** Vagus Nerve
Superior longitudinal muscle	**Use:** Tongue, Palate, Pharynx Muscle
Superior mesenteric ganglion	**Use:** Abdominal Sympathetic Nerve
Superior mesenteric lymph node	**Use:** Lymphatic, Mesenteric
Superior mesenteric plexus	**Use:** Abdominal Sympathetic Nerve
Superior oblique muscle	**Use:** Extraocular Muscle, Right Extraocular Muscle, Left
Superior olivary nucleus	**Use:** Pons
Superior rectal artery	**Use:** Inferior Mesenteric Artery
Superior rectal vein	**Use:** Inferior Mesenteric Vein
Superior rectus muscle	**Use:** Extraocular Muscle, Right Extraocular Muscle, Left
Superior tarsal plate	**Use:** Upper Eyelid, Right Upper Eyelid, Left
Superior thoracic artery	**Use:** Axillary Artery, Right Axillary Artery, Left
Superior thyroid artery	**Use:** External Carotid Artery, Right External Carotid Artery, Left Thyroid Artery, Right Thyroid Artery, Left
Superior turbinate	**Use:** Nasal Turbinate
Superior ulnar collateral artery	**Use:** Brachial Artery, Right Brachial Artery, Left
Supraclavicular (Virchow's) lymph node	**Use:** Lymphatic, Right Neck Lymphatic, Left Neck
Supraclavicular nerve	**Use:** Cervical Plexus
Suprahyoid lymph node	**Use:** Lymphatic, Head
Suprahyoid muscle	**Use:** Neck Muscle, Right Neck Muscle, Left
Suprainguinal lymph node	**Use:** Lymphatic, Pelvis
Supraorbital vein	**Use:** Face Vein, Right Face Vein, Left
Suprarenal gland	**Use:** Adrenal Gland, Left Adrenal Gland, Right Adrenal Glands, Bilateral Adrenal Gland
Suprarenal plexus	**Use:** Abdominal Sympathetic Nerve
Suprascapular nerve	**Use:** Brachial Plexus
Supraspinatus fascia	**Use:** Subcutaneous Tissue and Fascia, Right Upper Arm Subcutaneous Tissue and Fascia, Left Upper Arm

◀ New   ◀▥ Revised   ~~deleted~~ Deleted

BODY PART KEY

Supraspinatus muscle	**Use:** Shoulder Muscle, Right Shoulder Muscle, Left
Supraspinous ligament	**Use:** Trunk Bursa and Ligament, Right Trunk Bursa and Ligament, Left
Suprasternal notch	**Use:** Sternum
Supratrochlear lymph node	**Use:** Lymphatic, Right Upper Extremity Lymphatic, Left Upper Extremity
Sural artery	**Use:** Popliteal Artery, Right Popliteal Artery, Left
Sweat gland	**Use:** Skin
Talocalcaneal (subtalar) joint	**Use:** Tarsal Joint, Right Tarsal Joint, Left
Talocalcaneal ligament	**Use:** Foot Bursa and Ligament, Right Foot Bursa and Ligament, Left
Talocalcaneonavicular joint	**Use:** Tarsal Joint, Right Tarsal Joint, Left
Talocalcaneonavicular ligament	**Use:** Foot Bursa and Ligament, Right Foot Bursa and Ligament, Left
Talocrural joint	**Use:** Ankle Joint, Right Ankle Joint, Left
Talofibular ligament	**Use:** Ankle Bursa and Ligament, Right Ankle Bursa and Ligament, Left
Talus bone	**Use:** Tarsal, Right Tarsal, Left
Tarsometatarsal joint	**Use:** Metatarsal-Tarsal Joint, Right Metatarsal-Tarsal Joint, Left
Tarsometatarsal ligament	**Use:** Foot Bursa and Ligament, Right Foot Bursa and Ligament, Left
Temporal lobe	**Use:** Cerebral Hemisphere
Temporalis muscle Temporoparietalis muscle	**Use:** Head Muscle

Tensor fasciae latae muscle	**Use:** Hip Muscle, Right Hip Muscle, Left
Tensor veli palatini muscle	**Use:** Tongue, Palate, Pharynx Muscle
Tenth cranial nerve	**Use:** Vagus Nerve
Tentorium cerebelli	**Use:** Dura Mater
Teres major muscle Teres minor muscle	**Use:** Shoulder Muscle, Right Shoulder Muscle, Left
Testicular artery	**Use:** Abdominal Aorta
Thenar muscle	**Use:** Hand Muscle, Right Hand Muscle, Left
Third cranial nerve	**Use:** Oculomotor Nerve
Third occipital nerve	**Use:** Cervical Nerve
Third ventricle	**Use:** Cerebral Ventricle
Thoracic aortic plexus	**Use:** Thoracic Sympathetic Nerve
Thoracic esophagus	**Use:** Esophagus, Middle
Thoracic facet joint	**Use:** Thoracic Vertebral Joint Thoracic Vertebral Joints, 2 to 7 Thoracic Vertebral Joints, 8 or more
Thoracic ganglion	**Use:** Thoracic Sympathetic Nerve
Thoracoacromial artery	**Use:** Axillary Artery, Right Axillary Artery, Left
Thoracolumbar facet joint	**Use:** Thoracolumbar Vertebral Joint
Thymus gland	**Use:** Thymus
Thyroarytenoid muscle	**Use:** Neck Muscle, Right Neck Muscle, Left

◄ New ◄▥ Revised ~~deleted~~ Deleted

BODY PART KEY

Thyrocervical trunk	**Use:** Thyroid Artery, Right Thyroid Artery, Left
Thyroid cartilage	**Use:** Larynx
Tibialis anterior muscle Tibialis posterior muscle	**Use:** Lower Leg Muscle, Right Lower Leg Muscle, Left
Tracheobronchial lymph node	**Use:** Lymphatic, Thorax
Tragus	**Use:** External Ear, Right External Ear, Left External Ear, Bilateral
Transversalis fascia	**Use:** Subcutaneous Tissue and Fascia, Trunk
Transverse (cutaneous) cervical nerve	**Use:** Cervical Plexus
Transverse acetabular ligament	**Use:** Hip Bursa and Ligament, Right Hip Bursa and Ligament, Left
Transverse facial artery	**Use:** Temporal Artery, Right Temporal Artery, Left
Transverse humeral ligament	**Use:** Shoulder Bursa and Ligament, Right Shoulder Bursa and Ligament, Left
Transverse ligament of atlas	**Use:** Head and Neck Bursa and Ligament
Transverse scapular ligament	**Use:** Shoulder Bursa and Ligament, Right Shoulder Bursa and Ligament, Left
Transverse thoracis muscle	**Use:** Thorax Muscle, Right Thorax Muscle, Left
Transversospinalis muscle	**Use:** Trunk Muscle, Right Trunk Muscle, Left
Transversus abdominis muscle	**Use:** Abdomen Muscle, Right Abdomen Muscle, Left
Trapezium bone	**Use:** Carpal, Right Carpal, Left

Trapezius muscle	**Use:** Trunk Muscle, Right Trunk Muscle, Left
Trapezoid bone	**Use:** Carpal, Right Carpal, Left
Triceps brachii muscle	**Use:** Upper Arm Muscle, Right Upper Arm Muscle, Left
Tricuspid annulus	**Use:** Tricuspid Valve
Trifacial nerve	**Use:** Trigeminal Nerve
Trigone of bladder	**Use:** Bladder
Triquetral bone	**Use:** Carpal, Right Carpal, Left
Trochanteric bursa	**Use:** Hip Bursa and Ligament, Right Hip Bursa and Ligament, Left
Twelfth cranial nerve	**Use:** Hypoglossal Nerve
Tympanic cavity	**Use:** Middle Ear, Right Middle Ear, Left
Tympanic nerve	**Use:** Glossopharyngeal Nerve
Tympanic part of temporal bone	**Use:** Temporal Bone, Right Temporal Bone, Left
Ulnar collateral carpal ligament	**Use:** Wrist Bursa and Ligament, Right Wrist Bursa and Ligament, Left
Ulnar collateral ligament	**Use:** Elbow Bursa and Ligament, Right Elbow Bursa and Ligament, Left
Ulnar notch	**Use:** Radius, Right Radius, Left
Ulnar vein	**Use:** Brachial Vein, Right Brachial Vein, Left
Umbilical artery	**Use:** Internal Iliac Artery, Right Internal Iliac Artery, Left

APPENDIX B

◀ New ◀▥ Revised ~~deleted~~ Deleted

BODY PART KEY

Ureteral orifice	**Use:** Ureter, Right Ureter, Left Ureters, Bilateral Ureter
Ureteropelvic junction (UPJ)	**Use:** Kidney Pelvis, Right Kidney Pelvis, Left
Ureterovesical orifice	**Use:** Ureter, Right Ureter, Left Ureters, Bilateral Ureter
Uterine artery	**Use:** Internal Iliac Artery, Right Internal Iliac Artery, Left
Uterine cornu	**Use:** Uterus
Uterine tube	**Use:** Fallopian Tube, Right Fallopian Tube, Left
Uterine vein	**Use:** Hypogastric Vein, Right Hypogastric Vein, Left
Vaginal artery	**Use:** Internal Iliac Artery, Right Internal Iliac Artery, Left
Vaginal vein	**Use:** Hypogastric Vein, Right Hypogastric Vein, Left
Vastus intermedius muscle Vastus lateralis muscle Vastus medialis muscle	**Use:** Upper Leg Muscle, Right Upper Leg Muscle, Left
Ventricular fold	**Use:** Larynx
Vermiform appendix	**Use:** Appendix
Vermilion border	**Use:** Upper Lip Lower Lip
Vertebral arch	**Use:** Cervical Vertebra Thoracic Vertebra Lumbar Vertebra
Vertebral canal	**Use:** Spinal Canal
Vertebral foramen Vertebral lamina Vertebral pedicle	**Use:** Cervical Vertebra Thoracic Vertebra Lumbar Vertebra
Vesical vein	**Use:** Hypogastric Vein, Right Hypogastric Vein, Left
Vestibular (Scarpa's) ganglion Vestibular nerve Vestibulocochlear nerve	**Use:** Acoustic Nerve
Virchow's (supraclavicular) lymph node	**Use:** Lymphatic, Right Neck Lymphatic, Left Neck
Vitreous body	**Use:** Vitreous, Right Vitreous, Left
Vocal fold	**Use:** Vocal Cord, Right Vocal Cord, Left
Volar (palmar) digital vein Volar (palmar) metacarpal vein	**Use:** Hand Vein, Right Hand Vein, Left
Vomer bone	**Use:** Nasal Septum
Vomer of nasal septum	**Use:** Nasal Bone
Xiphoid process	**Use:** Sternum
Zonule of Zinn	**Use:** Lens, Right Lens, Left
Zygomatic process of frontal bone	**Use:** Frontal Bone, Right Frontal Bone, Left
Zygomatic process of temporal bone	**Use:** Temporal Bone, Right Temporal Bone, Left
Zygomaticus muscle	**Use:** Facial Muscle

BODY PART KEY

◀ New ◀▥ Revised ~~deleted~~ Deleted

DEVICE KEY

3f (Aortic) Bioprosthesis valve	**Use:** Zooplastic Tissue in Heart and Great Vessels
AbioCor® Total Replacement Heart	**Use:** Synthetic Substitute
Acellular Hydrated Dermis	**Use:** Nonautologous Tissue Substitute
Activa PC neurostimulator	**Use:** Stimulator Generator, Multiple Array for Insertion in Subcutaneous Tissue and Fascia
Activa RC neurostimulator	**Use:** Stimulator Generator, Multiple Array Rechargeable for Insertion in Subcutaneous Tissue and Fascia
Activa SC neurostimulator	**Use:** Stimulator Generator, Single Array for Insertion in Subcutaneous Tissue and Fascia
ACUITY™ Steerable Lead	**Use:** Cardiac Lead, Pacemaker for Insertion in Heart and Great Vessels Cardiac Lead, Defibrillator for Insertion in Heart and Great Vessels
AMPLATZER® Muscular VSD Occluder	**Use:** Synthetic Substitute
AMS 800® Urinary Control System	**Use:** Artificial Sphincter in Urinary System
AneuRx® AAA Advantage®	**Use:** Intraluminal Device
Annuloplasty ring	**Use:** Synthetic Substitute
Artificial anal sphincter (AAS)	**Use:** Artificial Sphincter in Gastrointestinal System
Artificial bowel sphincter (neosphincter)	**Use:** Artificial Sphincter in Gastrointestinal System
Artificial urinary sphincter (AUS)	**Use:** Artificial Sphincter in Urinary System
Assurant (Cobalt) stent	**Use:** Intraluminal Device
Attain Ability® lead	**Use:** Cardiac Lead, Pacemaker for Insertion in Heart and Great Vessels Cardiac Lead, Defibrillator for Insertion in Heart and Great Vessels
Attain StarFix® (OTW) lead	**Use:** Cardiac Lead, Pacemaker for Insertion in Heart and Great Vessels Cardiac Lead, Defibrillator for Insertion in Heart and Great Vessels
Autograft	**Use:** Autologous Tissue Substitute
Autologous artery graft	**Use:** Autologous Arterial Tissue in Heart and Great Vessels Autologous Arterial Tissue in Upper Arteries Autologous Arterial Tissue in Lower Arteries Autologous Arterial Tissue in Upper Veins Autologous Arterial Tissue in Lower Veins
Autologous vein graft	**Use:** Autologous Venous Tissue in Heart and Great Vessels Autologous Venous Tissue in Upper Arteries Autologous Venous Tissue in Lower Arteries Autologous Venous Tissue in Upper Veins Autologous Venous Tissue in Lower Veins
Axial Lumbar Interbody Fusion System	**Use:** Interbody Fusion Device in Lower Joints
AxiaLIF® System	**Use:** Interbody Fusion Device in Lower Joints
BAK/C® Interbody Cervical Fusion System	**Use:** Interbody Fusion Device in Upper Joints

DEVICE KEY

DEVICE KEY

Device	Use
Bard® Composix® (E/X) (LP) mesh	**Use:** Synthetic Substitute
Bard® Composix® Kugel® patch	**Use:** Synthetic Substitute
Bard® Dulex™ mesh	**Use:** Synthetic Substitute
Bard® Ventralex™ hernia patch	**Use:** Synthetic Substitute
Baroreflex Activation Therapy® (BAT®)	**Use:** Stimulator Lead in Upper Arteries Cardiac Rhythm Related Device in Subcutaneous Tissue and Fascia
Berlin Heart Ventricular Assist Device	**Use:** Implantable Heart Assist System in Heart and Great Vessels
Bioactive embolization coil(s)	**Use:** Intraluminal Device, Bioactive in Upper Arteries
Biventricular external heart assist system	**Use:** External Heart Assist System in Heart and Great Vessels
Blood glucose monitoring system	**Use:** Monitoring Device
Bone anchored hearing device	**Use:** Hearing Device, Bone Conduction for Insertion in Ear, Nose, Sinus Hearing Device in Head and Facial Bones
Bone bank bone graft	**Use:** Nonautologous Tissue Substitute
Bone screw (interlocking) (lag) (pedicle) (recessed)	**Use:** Internal Fixation Device in Head and Facial Bones Internal Fixation Device in Upper Bones Internal Fixation Device in Lower Bones
Bovine pericardial valve	**Use:** Zooplastic Tissue in Heart and Great Vessels
Bovine pericardium graft	**Use:** Zooplastic Tissue in Heart and Great Vessels
Brachytherapy seeds	**Use:** Radioactive Element

Device	Use
BRYAN® Cervical Disc System	**Use:** Synthetic Substitute
BVS 5000 Ventricular Assist Device	**Use:** External Heart Assist System in Heart and Great Vessels
Cardiac contractility modulation lead	**Use:** Cardiac Lead in Heart and Great Vessels
Cardiac event recorder	**Use:** Monitoring Device
Cardiac resynchronization therapy (CRT) lead	**Use:** Cardiac Lead, Pacemaker for Insertion in Heart and Great Vessels Cardiac Lead, Defibrillator for Insertion in Heart and Great Vessels
CardioMEMS® pressure sensor	**Use:** Monitoring Device, Pressure Sensor for Insertion in Heart and Great Vessels
Carotid (artery) sinus (baroreceptor) lead	**Use:** Stimulator Lead in Upper Arteries
Carotid WALLSTENT® Monorail® Endoprosthesis	**Use:** Intraluminal Device
Centrimag® Blood Pump	**Use:** Intraluminal Device
Clamp and rod internal fixation system (CRIF)	**Use:** Internal Fixation Device in Upper Bones Internal Fixation Device in Lower Bones
CoAxia NeuroFlo catheter	**Use:** Intraluminal Device
Cobalt/chromium head and polyethylene socket	**Use:** Synthetic Substitute, Metal on Polyethylene for Replacement in Lower Joints
Cobalt/chromium head and socket	**Use:** Synthetic Substitute, Metal for Replacement in Lower Joints
Cochlear implant (CI), multiple channel (electrode)	**Use:** Hearing Device, Multiple Channel Cochlear Prosthesis for Insertion in Ear, Nose, Sinus

◀ New   ◀▥ Revised   ~~deleted~~ Deleted

DEVICE KEY

Cochlear implant (CI), single channel (electrode)	**Use:** Hearing Device, Single Channel Cochlear Prosthesis for Insertion in Ear, Nose, Sinus
COGNIS® CRT-D	**Use:** Cardiac Resynchronization Defibrillator Pulse Generator for Insertion in Subcutaneous Tissue and Fascia
Colonic Z-Stent®	**Use:** Intraluminal Device
Complete (SE) stent	**Use:** Intraluminal Device
Concerto II CRT-D	**Use:** Cardiac Resynchronization Defibrillator Pulse Generator for Insertion in Subcutaneous Tissue and Fascia
CONSERVE® PLUS Total Resurfacing Hip System	**Use:** Resurfacing Device in Lower Joints
Consulta CRT-D	**Use:** Cardiac Resynchronization Defibrillator Pulse Generator for Insertion in Subcutaneous Tissue and Fascia
Consulta CRT-P	**Use:** Cardiac Resynchronization Pacemaker Pulse Generator for Insertion in Subcutaneous Tissue and Fascia
CONTAK RENEWAL® 3 RF (HE) CRT-D	**Use:** Cardiac Resynchronization Defibrillator Pulse Generator for Insertion in Subcutaneous Tissue and Fascia
Contegra Pulmonary Valved Conduit	**Use:** Zooplastic Tissue in Heart and Great Vessels
Continuous Glucose Monitoring (CGM) device	**Use:** Monitoring Device
CoreValve transcatheter aortic valve	**Use:** Zooplastic Tissue in Heart and Great Vessels
Cormet Hip Resurfacing System	**Use:** Resurfacing Device in Lower Joints

CoRoent® XL	**Use:** Interbody Fusion Device in Lower Joints
Corox (OTW) Bipolar Lead	**Use:** Cardiac Lead, Pacemaker for Insertion in Heart and Great Vessels Cardiac Lead, Defibrillator for Insertion in Heart and Great Vessels
Cortical strip neurostimulator lead	**Use:** Neurostimulator Lead in Central Nervous System
Cultured epidermal cell autograft	**Use:** Autologous Tissue Substitute
CYPHER® Stent	**Use:** Intraluminal Device, Drug-eluting in Heart and Great Vessels
Cystostomy tube	**Use:** Drainage Device
DBS lead	**Use:** Neurostimulator Lead in Central Nervous System
DeBakey Left Ventricular Assist Device	**Use:** Implantable Heart Assist System in Heart and Great Vessels
Deep brain neurostimulator lead	**Use:** Neurostimulator Lead in Central Nervous System
Delta frame external fixator	**Use:** External Fixation Device, Hybrid for Insertion in Upper Bones External Fixation Device, Hybrid for Reposition in Upper Bones External Fixation Device, Hybrid for Insertion in Lower Bones External Fixation Device, Hybrid for Reposition in Lower Bones
Delta III Reverse shoulder prosthesis	**Use:** Synthetic Substitute, Reverse Ball and Socket for Replacement in Upper Joints
Diaphragmatic pacemaker generator	**Use:** Stimulator Generator in Subcutaneous Tissue and Fascia

◀ New ◀▥ Revised ~~deleted~~ Deleted

DEVICE KEY

DEVICE KEY

Direct Lateral Interbody Fusion (DLIF) device	**Use:** Interbody Fusion Device in Lower Joints
Driver stent (RX) (OTW)	**Use:** Intraluminal Device
DuraHeart Left Ventricular Assist System	**Use:** Implantable Heart Assist System in Heart and Great Vessels
Durata® Defibrillation Lead	**Use:** Cardiac Lead, Defibrillator for Insertion in Heart and Great Vessels
Dynesys® Dynamic Stabilization System	**Use:** Spinal Stabilization Device, Pedicle-Based for Insertion in Upper Joints Spinal Stabilization Device, Pedicle-Based for Insertion in Lower Joints
E-Luminexx™ (Biliary) (Vascular) Stent	**Use:** Intraluminal Device
Electrical bone growth stimulator (EBGS)	**Use:** Bone Growth Stimulator in Head and Facial Bones Bone Growth Stimulator in Upper Bones Bone Growth Stimulator in Lower Bones
Electrical muscle stimulation (EMS) lead	**Use:** Stimulator Lead in Muscles
Electronic muscle stimulator lead	**Use:** Stimulator Lead in Muscles
Embolization coil(s)	**Use:** Intraluminal Device
Endeavor® (III) (IV) (Sprint) Zotarolimus-eluting Coronary Stent System	**Use:** Intraluminal Device, Drug-eluting in Heart and Great Vessels
EndoSure® sensor	**Use:** Monitoring Device, Pressure Sensor for Insertion in Heart and Great Vessels
ENDOTAK RELIANCE® (G) Defibrillation Lead	**Use:** Cardiac Lead, Defibrillator for Insertion in Heart and Great Vessels
Endotracheal tube (cuffed) (double-lumen)	**Use:** Intraluminal Device, Endotracheal Airway in Respiratory System

Endurant® Endovascular Stent Graft	**Use:** Intraluminal Device
EnRhythm	**Use:** Pacemaker, Dual Chamber for Insertion in Subcutaneous Tissue and Fascia
Enterra gastric neurostimulator	**Use:** Stimulator Generator, Multiple Array for Insertion in Subcutaneous Tissue and Fascia
Epicel® cultured epidermal autograft	**Use:** Autologous Tissue Substitute
Epic™ Stented Tissue Valve (aortic)	**Use:** Zooplastic Tissue in Heart and Great Vessels
Esophageal obturator airway (EOA)	**Use:** Intraluminal Device, Airway in Gastrointestinal System
Esteem® implantable hearing system	**Use:** Hearing Device in Ear, Nose, Sinus
Everolimus-eluting coronary stent	**Use:** Intraluminal Device, Drug-eluting in Heart and Great Vessels
Ex-PRESS™ mini glaucoma shunt	**Use:** Synthetic Substitute
Express® (LD) Premounted Stent System	**Use:** Intraluminal Device
Express® Biliary SD Monorail® Premounted Stent System	**Use:** Intraluminal Device
Express® SD Renal Monorail® Premounted Stent System	**Use:** Intraluminal Device
External fixator	**Use:** External Fixation Device in Head and Facial Bones External Fixation Device in Upper Bones External Fixation Device in Lower Bones External Fixation Device in Upper Joints External Fixation Device in Lower Joints
EXtreme Lateral Interbody Fusion (XLIF) device	**Use:** Interbody Fusion Device in Lower Joints

◀ New ◀≡ Revised ~~deleted~~ Deleted

DEVICE KEY

Facet replacement spinal stabilization device	**Use:** Spinal Stabilization Device, Facet Replacement for Insertion in Upper Joints Spinal Stabilization Device, Facet Replacement for Insertion in Lower Joints
FLAIR® Endovascular Stent Graft	**Use:** Intraluminal Device
Flexible Composite Mesh	**Use:** Synthetic Substitute
Foley catheter	**Use:** Drainage Device
Formula™ Balloon-Expandable Renal Stent System	**Use:** Intraluminal Device
Freestyle (Stentless) Aortic Root Bioprosthesis	**Use:** Zooplastic Tissue in Heart and Great Vessels
Fusion screw (compression) (lag) (locking)	**Use:** Internal Fixation Device in Upper Joints Internal Fixation Device in Lower Joints
Gastric electrical stimulation (GES) lead	**Use:** Stimulator Lead in Gastrointestinal System
Gastric pacemaker lead	**Use:** Stimulator Lead in Gastrointestinal System
GORE® DUALMESH®	**Use:** Synthetic Substitute
Guedel airway	**Use:** Intraluminal Device, Airway in Mouth and Throat
Hancock Bioprosthesis (aortic) (mitral) valve	**Use:** Zooplastic Tissue in Heart and Great Vessels
Hancock Bioprosthetic Valved Conduit	**Use:** Zooplastic Tissue in Heart and Great Vessels
HeartMate II® Left Ventricular Assist Device (LVAD)	**Use:** Implantable Heart Assist System in Heart and Great Vessels
HeartMate XVE® Left Ventricular Assist Device (LVAD)	**Use:** Implantable Heart Assist System in Heart and Great Vessels

Hip (joint) liner	**Use:** Liner in Lower Joints
Holter valve ventricular shunt	**Use:** Synthetic Substitute
Ilizarov external fixator	**Use:** External Fixation Device, Ring for Insertion in Upper Bones External Fixation Device, Ring for Reposition in Upper Bones External Fixation Device, Ring for Insertion in Lower Bones External Fixation Device, Ring for Reposition in Lower Bones
Ilizarov-Vecklich device	**Use:** External Fixation Device, Limb Lengthening for Insertion in Upper Bones External Fixation Device, Limb Lengthening for Insertion in Lower Bones
Implantable cardioverter-defibrillator (ICD)	**Use:** Defibrillator Generator for Insertion in Subcutaneous Tissue and Fascia
Implantable drug infusion pump (anti-spasmodic) (chemotherapy) (pain)	**Use:** Infusion Device, Pump in Subcutaneous Tissue and Fascia
Implantable glucose monitoring device	**Use:** Monitoring Device
Implantable hemodynamic monitor (IHM)	**Use:** Monitoring Device, Hemodynamic for Insertion in Subcutaneous Tissue and Fascia
Implantable hemodynamic monitoring system (IHMS)	**Use:** Monitoring Device, Hemodynamic for Insertion in Subcutaneous Tissue and Fascia
Implantable Miniature Telescope™ (IMT)	**Use:** Synthetic Substitute, Intraocular Telescope for Replacement in Eye
Implanted (venous) (access) port	**Use:** Vascular Access Device, Reservoir in Subcutaneous Tissue and Fascia
InDura, intrathecal catheter (1P) (spinal)	**Use:** Infusion Device

APPENDIX C

◀ New   ◀▥ Revised   ~~deleted~~ Deleted

DEVICE KEY

Injection reservoir, port	**Use:** Vascular Access Device, Reservoir in Subcutaneous Tissue and Fascia
Injection reservoir, pump	**Use:** Infusion Device, Pump in Subcutaneous Tissue and Fascia
Interbody fusion (spine) cage	**Use:** Interbody Fusion Device in Upper Joints Interbody Fusion Device in Lower Joints
Interspinous process spinal stabilization device	**Use:** Spinal Stabilization Device, Interspinous Process for Insertion in Upper Joints Spinal Stabilization Device, Interspinous Process for Insertion in Lower Joints
InterStim® Therapy lead	**Use:** Neurostimulator Lead in Peripheral Nervous System
InterStim® Therapy neurostimulator	**Use:** Stimulator Generator, Single Array for Insertion in Subcutaneous Tissue and Fascia
Intramedullary (IM) rod (nail)	**Use:** Internal Fixation Device, Intramedullary in Upper Bones Internal Fixation Device, Intramedullary in Lower Bones
Intramedullary skeletal kinetic distractor (ISKD)	**Use:** Internal Fixation Device, Intramedullary in Upper Bones Internal Fixation Device, Intramedullary in Lower Bones
Intrauterine device (IUD)	**Use:** Contraceptive Device in Female Reproductive System
Itrel (3) (4) neurostimulator	**Use:** Stimulator Generator, Single Array for Insertion in Subcutaneous Tissue and Fascia
Joint fixation plate	**Use:** Internal Fixation Device in Upper Joints Internal Fixation Device in Lower Joints
Joint liner (insert)	**Use:** Liner in Lower Joints
Joint spacer (antibiotic)	**Use:** Spacer in Upper Joints Spacer in Lower Joints
Kappa	**Use:** Pacemaker, Dual Chamber for Insertion in Subcutaneous Tissue and Fascia
Kinetra® neurostimulator	**Use:** Stimulator Generator, Multiple Array for Insertion in Subcutaneous Tissue and Fascia
Kirschner wire (K-wire)	**Use:** Internal Fixation Device in Head and Facial Bones Internal Fixation Device in Upper Bones Internal Fixation Device in Lower Bones Internal Fixation Device in Upper Joints Internal Fixation Device in Lower Joints
Knee (implant) insert	**Use:** Liner in Lower Joints
Kuntscher nail	**Use:** Internal Fixation Device, Intramedullary in Upper Bones Internal Fixation Device, Intramedullary in Lower Bones
LAP-BAND® adjustable gastric banding system	**Use:** Extraluminal Device
LifeStent® (Flexstar) (XL) Vascular Stent System	**Use:** Intraluminal Device
LIVIAN™ CRT-D	**Use:** Cardiac Resynchronization Defibrillator Pulse Generator for Insertion in Subcutaneous Tissue and Fascia
Loop recorder, implantable	**Use:** Monitoring Device
Mark IV Breathing Pacemaker System	Stimulator Generator in Subcutaneous Tissue and Fascia
Maximo II DR (VR)	**Use:** Defibrillator Generator for Insertion in Subcutaneous Tissue and Fascia

◀ New   ◀▥ Revised   ~~deleted~~ Deleted

DEVICE KEY

Maximo II DR CRT-D	**Use:** Cardiac Resynchronization Defibrillator Pulse Generator for Insertion in Subcutaneous Tissue and Fascia
Melody® transcatheter pulmonary valve	**Use:** Zooplastic Tissue in Heart and Great Vessels
Micro-Driver stent (RX) (OTW)	**Use:** Intraluminal Device
Micrus CERECYTE microcoil	**Use:** Intraluminal Device, Bioactive in Upper Arteries
MitraClip valve repair system	**Use:** Synthetic Substitute
Mitroflow Aortic Pericardial Heart Valve	**Use:** Zooplastic Tissue in Heart and Great Vessels
Nasopharyngeal airway (NPA)	**Use:** Intraluminal Device, Airway in Ear, Nose, Sinus
Neuromuscular electrical stimulation (NEMS) lead	**Use:** Stimulator Lead in Muscles
Neurostimulator generator, multiple channel	**Use:** Stimulator Generator, Multiple Array for Insertion in Subcutaneous Tissue and Fascia
Neurostimulator generator, single channel	**Use:** Stimulator Generator, Single Array for Insertion in Subcutaneous Tissue and Fascia
Neurostimulator generator, multiple channel rechargeable	**Use:** Stimulator Generator, Multiple Array Rechargeable for Insertion in Subcutaneous Tissue and Fascia
Neurostimulator generator, single channel rechargeable	**Use:** Stimulator Generator, Single Array Rechargeable for Insertion in Subcutaneous Tissue and Fascia
Neutralization plate	**Use:** Internal Fixation Device in Head and Facial Bones Internal Fixation Device in Upper Bones Internal Fixation Device in Lower Bones
Nitinol framed polymer mesh	**Use:** Synthetic Substitute

Non-tunneled central venous catheter	**Use:** Infusion Device
Novacor Left Ventricular Assist Device	**Use:** Implantable Heart Assist System in Heart and Great Vessels
Novation® Ceramic AHS® (Articulation Hip System)	**Use:** Synthetic Substitute, Ceramic for Replacement in Lower Joints
Optimizer™ III implantable pulse generator	**Use:** Contractility Modulation Device for Insertion in Subcutaneous Tissue and Fascia
Oropharyngeal airway (OPA)	**Use:** Intraluminal Device, Airway in Mouth and Throat
Ovatio™ CRT-D	**Use:** Cardiac Resynchronization Defibrillator Pulse Generator for Insertion in Subcutaneous Tissue and Fascia
Oxidized zirconium ceramic hip bearing surface	**Use:** Synthetic Substitute, Ceramic on Polyethylene for Replacement in Lower Joints
Paclitaxel-eluting coronary stent	**Use:** Intraluminal Device, Drug-eluting in Heart and Great Vessels
Paclitaxel-eluting peripheral stent	**Use:** Intraluminal Device, Drug-eluting in Upper Arteries Intraluminal Device, Drug-eluting in Lower Arteries
Partially absorbable mesh	**Use:** Synthetic Substitute
Pedicle-based dynamic stabilization device	**Use:** Spinal Stabilization Device, Pedicle-Based for Insertion in Upper Joints Spinal Stabilization Device, Pedicle-Based for Insertion in Lower Joints
Percutaneous endoscopic gastrojejunostomy (PEG/J) tube	**Use:** Feeding Device in Gastrointestinal System
Percutaneous endoscopic gastrostomy (PEG) tube	**Use:** Feeding Device in Gastrointestinal System
Percutaneous nephrostomy catheter	**Use:** Drainage Device

◀ New　◀ Revised　~~deleted~~ Deleted

DEVICE KEY

DEVICE KEY

Peripherally inserted central catheter (PICC)	**Use:** Infusion Device
Pessary ring	**Use:** Intraluminal Device, Pessary in Female Reproductive System
Phrenic nerve stimulator generator	**Use:** Stimulator Generator in Subcutaneous Tissue and Fascia
Phrenic nerve stimulator lead	**Use:** Diaphragmatic Pacemaker Lead in Respiratory System
PHYSIOMESH™ Flexible Composite Mesh	**Use:** Synthetic Substitute
Pipeline™ Embolization device (PED)	**Use:** Intraluminal Device
Polyethylene socket	**Use:** Synthetic Substitute, Polyethylene for Replacement in Lower Joints
Polymethylmethacrylate (PMMA)	**Use:** Synthetic Substitute
Polypropylene mesh	**Use:** Synthetic Substitute
Porcine (bioprosthetic) valve	**Use:** Zooplastic Tissue in Heart and Great Vessels
PRESTIGE® Cervical Disc	**Use:** Synthetic Substitute
PrimeAdvanced neurostimulator	**Use:** Stimulator Generator, Multiple Array for Insertion in Subcutaneous Tissue and Fascia
PROCEED™ Ventral Patch	**Use:** Synthetic Substitute
Prodisc-C	**Use:** Synthetic Substitute
Prodisc-L	**Use:** Synthetic Substitute
PROLENE Polypropylene Hernia System (PHS)	**Use:** Synthetic Substitute
Protecta XT CRT-D	**Use:** Cardiac Resynchronization Defibrillator Pulse Generator for Insertion in Subcutaneous Tissue and Fascia
Protecta XT DR (XT VR)	**Use:** Defibrillator Generator for Insertion in Subcutaneous Tissue and Fascia
Protégé® RX Carotid Stent System	**Use:** Intraluminal Device
Pump reservoir	**Use:** Infusion Device, Pump in Subcutaneous Tissue and Fascia
PVAD™ Ventricular Assist Device	**Use:** External Heart Assist System in Heart and Great Vessels
REALIZE® Adjustable Gastric Band	**Use:** Extraluminal Device
Rebound HRD® (Hernia Repair Device)	**Use:** Synthetic Substitute
RestoreAdvanced neurostimulator	**Use:** Stimulator Generator, Multiple Array Rechargeable for Insertion in Subcutaneous Tissue and Fascia
RestoreSensor neurostimulator	**Use:** Stimulator Generator, Multiple Array Rechargeable for Insertion in Subcutaneous Tissue and Fascia
RestoreUltra neurostimulator	**Use:** Stimulator Generator, Multiple Array Rechargeable for Insertion in Subcutaneous Tissue and Fascia
Reveal (DX) (XT)	**Use:** Monitoring Device
Reverse® Shoulder Prosthesis	**Use:** Synthetic Substitute, Reverse Ball and Socket for Replacement in Upper Joints
Revo MRI™ SureScan® pacemaker	**Use:** Pacemaker, Dual Chamber for Insertion in Subcutaneous Tissue and Fascia
Rheos® System device	**Use:** Cardiac Rhythm Related Device in Subcutaneous Tissue and Fascia
Rheos® System lead	**Use:** Stimulator Lead in Upper Arteries

◀ New ◀‖‖ Revised ~~deleted~~ Deleted

DEVICE KEY

RNS System lead	**Use:** Neurostimulator Lead in Central Nervous System
RNS system neurostimulator generator	**Use:** Neurostimulator Generator in Head and Facial Bones
Sacral nerve modulation (SNM) lead	**Use:** Stimulator Lead in Urinary System
Sacral neuromodulation lead	**Use:** Stimulator Lead in Urinary System
SAPIEN transcatheter aortic valve	**Use:** Zooplastic Tissue in Heart and Great Vessels
Secura (DR) (VR)	**Use:** Defibrillator Generator for Insertion in Subcutaneous Tissue and Fascia
Sheffield hybrid external fixator	**Use:** External Fixation Device, Hybrid for Insertion in Upper Bones External Fixation Device, Hybrid for Reposition in Upper Bones External Fixation Device, Hybrid for Insertion in Lower Bones External Fixation Device, Hybrid for Reposition in Lower Bones
Sheffield ring external fixator	**Use:** External Fixation Device, Ring for Insertion in Upper Bones External Fixation Device, Ring for Reposition in Upper Bones External Fixation Device, Ring for Insertion in Lower Bones External Fixation Device, Ring for Reposition in Lower Bones
Single lead pacemaker (atrium) (ventricle)	**Use:** Pacemaker, Single Chamber for Insertion in Subcutaneous Tissue and Fascia
Single lead rate responsive pacemaker (atrium) (ventricle)	**Use:** Pacemaker, Single Chamber Rate Responsive for Insertion in Subcutaneous Tissue and Fascia
Sirolimus-eluting coronary stent	**Use:** Intraluminal Device, Drug-eluting in Heart and Great Vessels
SJM Biocor® Stented Valve System	**Use:** Zooplastic Tissue in Heart and Great Vessels

Soletra® neurostimulator	**Use:** Stimulator Generator, Single Array for Insertion in Subcutaneous Tissue and Fascia
Spinal cord neurostimulator lead	**Use:** Neurostimulator Lead in Central Nervous System
Spiration IBV™ Valve System	**Use:** Intraluminal Device, Endobronchial Valve in Respiratory System
Stent (angioplasty) (embolization)	**Use:** Intraluminal Device
Stented tissue valve	**Use:** Zooplastic Tissue in Heart and Great Vessels
Stratos LV	**Use:** Cardiac Resynchronization Pacemaker Pulse Generator for Insertion in Subcutaneous Tissue and Fascia
Subcutaneous injection reservoir, port	**Use:** Vascular Access Device, Reservoir in Subcutaneous Tissue and Fascia
Subcutaneous injection reservoir, pump	**Use:** Infusion Device, Pump in Subcutaneous Tissue and Fascia
Subdermal progesterone implant	**Use:** Contraceptive Device in Subcutaneous Tissue and Fascia
SynCardia Total Artificial Heart	**Use:** Synthetic Substitute
Synchra CRT-P	**Use:** Cardiac Resynchronization Pacemaker Pulse Generator for Insertion in Subcutaneous Tissue and Fascia
Talent® Converter	**Use:** Intraluminal Device
Talent® Occluder	**Use:** Intraluminal Device
Talent® Stent Graft (abdominal) (thoracic)	**Use:** Intraluminal Device
TandemHeart® System	**Use:** Intraluminal Device
TAXUS® Liberté® Paclitaxel-eluting Coronary Stent System	**Use:** Intraluminal Device, Drug-eluting in Heart and Great Vessels

◀ New ◀═ Revised ~~deleted~~ Deleted

APPENDIX C

DEVICE KEY

Therapeutic occlusion coil(s)	**Use:** Intraluminal Device
Thoracostomy tube	**Use:** Drainage Device
Thoratec IVAD (Implantable Ventricular Assist Device)	**Use:** Implantable Heart Assist System in Heart and Great Vessels
TigerPaw® system for closure of left atrial appendage	**Use:** Extraluminal Device
Tissue bank graft	**Use:** Nonautologous Tissue Substitute
Tissue expander (inflatable) (injectable)	**Use:** Tissue Expander in Skin and Breast Tissue Expander in Subcutaneous Tissue and Fascia
Titanium Sternal Fixation System (TSFS)	**Use:** Internal Fixation Device, Rigid Plate for Insertion in Upper Bones Internal Fixation Device, Rigid Plate for Reposition in Upper Bones
Total artificial (replacement) heart	**Use:** Synthetic Substitute
Tracheostomy tube	**Use:** Tracheostomy Device in Respiratory System
Trifecta™ Valve (aortic)	**Use:** Zooplastic Tissue in Heart and Great Vessels
Tunneled central venous catheter	**Use:** Vascular Access Device in Subcutaneous Tissue and Fascia
Tunneled spinal (intrathecal) catheter	**Use:** Infusion Device
Two lead pacemaker	**Use:** Pacemaker, Dual Chamber for Insertion in Subcutaneous Tissue and Fascia
Ultraflex™ Precision Colonic Stent System	**Use:** Intraluminal Device
ULTRAPRO Hernia System (UHS)	**Use:** Synthetic Substitute
ULTRAPRO Partially Absorbable Lightweight Mesh	**Use:** Synthetic Substitute
ULTRAPRO Plug	**Use:** Synthetic Substitute

Ultrasonic osteogenic stimulator	**Use:** Bone Growth Stimulator in Head and Facial Bones Bone Growth Stimulator in Upper Bones Bone Growth Stimulator in Lower Bones
Ultrasound bone healing system	**Use:** Bone Growth Stimulator in Head and Facial Bones Bone Growth Stimulator in Upper Bones Bone Growth Stimulator in Lower Bones
Uniplanar external fixator	**Use:** External Fixation Device, Monoplanar for Insertion in Upper Bones External Fixation Device, Monoplanar for Reposition in Upper Bones External Fixation Device, Monoplanar for Insertion in Lower Bones External Fixation Device, Monoplanar for Reposition in Lower Bones
Urinary incontinence stimulator lead	**Use:** Stimulator Lead in Urinary System
Vaginal pessary	**Use:** Intraluminal Device, Pessary in Female Reproductive System
Valiant Thoracic Stent Graft	**Use:** Intraluminal Device
Vectra® Vascular Access Graft	**Use:** Vascular Access Device in Subcutaneous Tissue and Fascia
Ventrio™ Hernia Patch	**Use:** Synthetic Substitute
Versa	**Use:** Pacemaker, Dual Chamber for Insertion in Subcutaneous Tissue and Fascia
Virtuoso (II) (DR) (VR)	**Use:** Defibrillator Generator for Insertion in Subcutaneous Tissue and Fascia
WALLSTENT® Endoprosthesis	**Use:** Intraluminal Device

◀ New   ◀▥ Revised   ~~deleted~~ Deleted

DEVICE KEY

X-STOP® Spacer	**Use:** Spinal Stabilization Device, Interspinous Process for Insertion in Upper Joints Spinal Stabilization Device, Interspinous Process for Insertion in Lower Joints
Xenograft	**Use:** Zooplastic Tissue in Heart and Great Vessels
XIENCE V Everolimus Eluting Coronary Stent System	**Use:** Intraluminal Device, Drug-eluting in Heart and Great Vessels
XLIF® System	**Use:** Interbody Fusion Device in Lower Joints
Zenith Flex® AAA Endovascular Graft	**Use:** Intraluminal Device

Zenith TX2® TAA Endovascular Graft	**Use:** Intraluminal Device
Zenith® Renu™ AAA Ancillary Graft	**Use:** Intraluminal Device
Zilver® PTX® (paclitaxel) Drug-Eluting Peripheral Stent	**Use:** Intraluminal Device, Drug-eluting in Upper Arteries Intraluminal Device, Drug-eluting in Lower Arteries
Zimmer® NexGen® LPS Mobile Bearing Knee	**Use:** Synthetic Substitute
Zimmer® NexGen® LPS-Flex Mobile Knee	**Use:** Synthetic Substitute
Zotarolimus-eluting coronary stent	**Use:** Intraluminal Device, Drug-eluting in Heart and Great Vessels

APPENDIX C

◄ New   ◄▥ Revised   deleted Deleted

DEVICE AGGREGATION TABLE

Specific Device	for Operation	in Body System	General Device
Autologous Arterial Tissue	All applicable	Heart and Great Vessels Lower Arteries Lower Veins Upper Arteries Upper Veins	**7** Autologous Tissue Substitute
Autologous Venous Tissue	All applicable	Heart and Great Vessels Lower Arteries Lower Veins Upper Arteries Upper Veins	**7** Autologous Tissue Substitute
Cardiac Lead, Defibrillator	Insertion	Heart and Great Vessels	**M** Cardiac Lead
Cardiac Lead, Pacemaker	Insertion	Heart and Great Vessels	**M** Cardiac Lead
Cardiac Resynchronization Defibrillator Pulse Generator	Insertion	Subcutaneous Tissue and Fascia	**P** Cardiac Rhythm Related Device
Cardiac Resynchronization Pacemaker Pulse Generator	Insertion	Subcutaneous Tissue and Fascia	**P** Cardiac Rhythm Related Device
Contractility Modulation Device	Insertion	Subcutaneous Tissue and Fascia	**P** Cardiac Rhythm Related Device
Defibrillator Generator	Insertion	Subcutaneous Tissue and Fascia	**P** Cardiac Rhythm Related Device
Epiretinal Visual Prosthesis	All applicable	Eye	**J** Synthetic Substitute
External Fixation Device, Hybrid	Insertion	Lower Bones Upper Bones	**5** External Fixation Device
External Fixation Device, Hybrid	Reposition	Lower Bones Upper Bones	**5** External Fixation Device
External Fixation Device, Limb Lengthening	Insertion	Lower Bones Upper Bones	**5** External Fixation Device
External Fixation Device, Monoplanar	Insertion	Lower Bones Upper Bones	**5** External Fixation Device
External Fixation Device, Monoplanar	Reposition	Lower Bones Upper Bones	**5** External Fixation Device
External Fixation Device, Ring	Insertion	Lower Bones Upper Bones	**5** External Fixation Device
External Fixation Device, Ring	Reposition	Lower Bones Upper Bones	**5** External Fixation Device
Hearing Device, Bone Conduction	Insertion	Ear, Nose, Sinus	**S** Hearing Device
Hearing Device, Multiple Channel Cochlear Prosthesis	Insertion	Ear, Nose, Sinus	**S** Hearing Device
Hearing Device, Single Channel Cochlear Prosthesis	Insertion	Ear, Nose, Sinus	**S** Hearing Device
Internal Fixation Device, Intramedullary	All applicable	Lower Bones Upper Bones	**4** Internal Fixation Device
Internal Fixation Device, Rigid Plate	Insertion	Upper Bones	**4** Internal Fixation Device
Internal Fixation Device, Rigid Plate	Reposition	Upper Bones	**4** Internal Fixation Device

◀ New   ◀▥ Revised   ~~deleted~~ Deleted

DEVICE AGGREGATION TABLE

Specific Device	for Operation	in Body System	General Device
Intraluminal Device, Pessary	All applicable	Female Reproductive System	**D** Intraluminal Device
Intraluminal Device, Airway	All applicable	Ear, Nose, Sinus Gastrointestinal System Mouth and Throat	**D** Intraluminal Device
Intraluminal Device, Bioactive	All applicable	Upper Arteries	**D** Intraluminal Device
Intraluminal Device, Drug-eluting	All applicable	Heart and Great Vessels Lower Arteries Upper Arteries	**D** Intraluminal Device
Intraluminal Device, Endobronchial Valve	All applicable	Respiratory System	**D** Intraluminal Device
Intraluminal Device, Endotracheal Airway	All applicable	Respiratory System	**D** Intraluminal Device
Intraluminal Device, Radioactive	All applicable	Heart and Great Vessels	**D** Intraluminal Device
Monitoring Device, Hemodynamic	Insertion	Subcutaneous Tissue and Fascia	**2** Monitoring Device
Monitoring Device, Pressure Sensor	Insertion	Heart and Great Vessels	**2** Monitoring Device
Pacemaker, Dual Chamber	Insertion	Subcutaneous Tissue and Fascia	**P** Cardiac Rhythm Related Device
Pacemaker, Single Chamber	Insertion	Subcutaneous Tissue and Fascia	**P** Cardiac Rhythm Related Device
Pacemaker, Single Chamber Rate Responsive	Insertion	Subcutaneous Tissue and Fascia	**P** Cardiac Rhythm Related Device
Spinal Stabilization Device, Facet Replacement	Insertion	Lower Joints Upper Joints	**4** Internal Fixation Device
Spinal Stabilization Device, Interspinous Process	Insertion	Lower Joints Upper Joints	**4** Internal Fixation Device
Spinal Stabilization Device, Pedicle-Based	Insertion	Lower Joints Upper Joints	**4** Internal Fixation Device
Stimulator Generator, Multiple Array	Insertion	Subcutaneous Tissue and Fascia	**M** Stimulator Generator
Stimulator Generator, Multiple Array Rechargeable	Insertion	Subcutaneous Tissue and Fascia	**M** Stimulator Generator
Stimulator Generator, Single Array	Insertion	Subcutaneous Tissue and Fascia	**M** Stimulator Generator
Stimulator Generator, Single Array Rechargeable	Insertion	Subcutaneous Tissue and Fascia	**M** Stimulator Generator
Synthetic Substitute, Ceramic	Replacement	Lower Joints	**J** Synthetic Substitute
Synthetic Substitute, Ceramic on Polyethylene	Replacement	Lower Joints	**J** Synthetic Substitute
Synthetic Substitute, Intraocular Telescope	Replacement	Eye	**J** Synthetic Substitute
Synthetic Substitute, Metal	Replacement	Lower Joints	**J** Synthetic Substitute
Synthetic Substitute, Metal on Polyethylene	Replacement	Lower Joints	**J** Synthetic Substitute
Synthetic Substitute, Polyethylene	Replacement	Lower Joints	**J** Synthetic Substitute
Synthetic Substitute, Reverse Ball and Socket	Replacement	Upper Joints	**J** Synthetic Substitute

APPENDIX D

◀ New ◀ Revised ~~deleted~~ Deleted

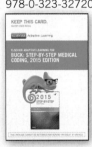
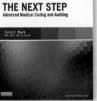
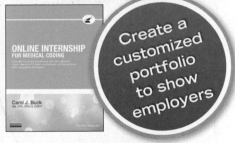
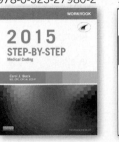
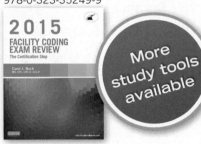
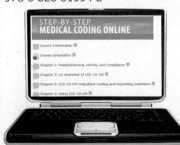
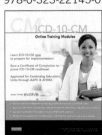
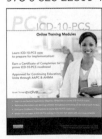